Pathology of the Hard Dental Tissues

Dedicated to my beloved wife Beatrice

Pathology of the Hard Dental Tissues

Albert Schuurs

ACTA (Academic Center for Dentistry Amsterdam)

Amsterdam

The Netherlands

With contributions from
Tommy Matos

WILEY-BLACKWELL

A John Wiley & Sons, Ltd., Publication

This edition first published 2013
© 2013 by Albert Schuurs

Wiley-Blackwell is an imprint of John Wiley & Sons, formed by the merger of Wiley's global Scientific, Technical and Medical
business with Blackwell Publishing.

Registered office: John Wiley & Sons, Ltd, The Atrium, Southern Gate, Chichester, West Sussex, PO19 8SQ, UK
Editorial offices: 9600 Garsington Road, Oxford, OX4 2DQ, UK
The Atrium, Southern Gate, Chichester, West Sussex, PO19 8SQ, UK
2121 State Avenue, Ames, Iowa 50014-8300, USA

For details of our global editorial offices, for customer services and for information about how to apply for permission
to reuse the copyright material in this book please see our website at www.wiley.com/wiley-blackwell.

Library of Congress Cataloging-in-Publication Data
Schuurs, A. H. B.
Pathology of the hard dental tissues / Albert Schuurs.
p. ; cm.
Includes bibliographical references and index.
ISBN 978-1-4051-5365-2 (hardback : alk. paper)
I. Title.
[DNLM: 1. Tooth Diseases–pathology. 2. Tooth Diseases–prevention & control. 3. Tooth Diseases–therapy. WU 140]
617.6'3–dc23
2012007476

A catalogue record for this book is available from the British Library.

Wiley also publishes its books in a variety of electronic formats. Some content that appears in print
may not be available in electronic books.

Cover images: courtesy of Albert Schuurs
Cover design by Steve Thompson

Set in 9.5/12 pt Sabon by Toppan Best-set Premedia Limited, Hong Kong
Printed and bound in Singapore by Markono Print Media Pte Ltd

1   2013

Contents

Introduction

Anomalies of the dental hard tissues are classified according to the time at which they develop:

- Prior to and during the development of the teeth within the jaws
- During the eruption of the teeth
- After the eruption of the teeth.

Prior to and during the development of the teeth within the jaws

Disturbances in odontogenesis *prior to* (that is, a failure of a tooth germ to develop) or *during tooth development* are commonly due to endogenous causes, i.e. causes within the body. The disturbances include deviations in the *number* of teeth, *morphological* anomalies and *structural* abnormalities of enamel and dentine, which are dealt with in Chapters 1, 2 and 3, respectively. The separate discussion of each group of anomalies may suggest that they occur independent of each other, but that is not the case. Anomalies in the size of some teeth, for instance, are probably associated with absence of other teeth,[33 37 79 198 199 455 497] implying a relation between tooth number and size. *Agenesis* of a (wisdom) tooth may be accompanied by delayed development of the premolars in the same or in another quadrant.[200 613] This may be because the number, size and morphology of the teeth are determined by interacting genes.

Traits, which are inherited poly-genetically, are distributed normally in the population (that is, statistically their distribution follows the normal bell curve).[33]

During the eruption of teeth

Anomalies of *eruption* may be due to disturbances in eruption times or the path and site of eruption. These anomalies may have either endogenous or exogenous (cause outside the body) causes and are described in Chapter 4.

After the eruption of the teeth

Post-developmental diseases and disturbances of the dental hard tissues, that is those developing after the eruption of the teeth are described in Chapters 5, 6, 7, 8 and 9. These are mostly caused by exogenous factors, but endogenous causes may also contribute. These disorders include *caries*, which despite a vast decline in incidence, is still likely the most frequently occurring of all diseases. The extensive knowledge that exists about caries warrants a separate book, but the disease cannot be neglected in a general book on dental hard tissue pathology.

Some other post-developmental dental diseases are: *erosion*, which is caused by the action of external acids on the dental hard tissues; *resorption*, which is caused by cells that commonly resorb (break down) the bony tissues; tooth *wear*; and *traumatic* conditions. *Discoloration* of the teeth (Chapter 10) may start in either the developmental or post-developmental phase.

Chapter 11 deals with the *syndromes* in which teeth are involved. For the purposes of this volume, a syndrome is defined as an inherited and causally related complex of somatic abnormalities and, occasionally, mental health and behavioural conditions. Because of the large number of such syndromes, only most commonly occurring ones are discussed in this book. The appendix provides an overview of the *chronology* of the individual teeth.

Additional information, for example, evolutionary aspects of the development of the dentition, about which reader is presumed to possess previous knowledge is presented in a smaller font to distinguish it from the main text.

Genetics

Since odontogenesis is under genetic (and environmental) control, an overview of the basics of genetics is necessary before considering the developmental anomalies.

Each human somatic cell nucleus contains DNA that is packaged into 22 pairs of autosomal chromosomes and one pair of sex chromosomes. The sex chromosome pair may consist of either X and X (female) or X and Y (male) chromosomes. The chromosomes are composed of the DNA polynucleotide chain, which resembles a spiral staircase (double helix). The DNA together with the mitochondrial chromosomes is called the genome. All hereditary information is transmitted by the genome. From the initial assumed number of 80 000–100 000 genes on the 46 chromosomes, a mere 30 000–35 000 were then estimated to exist,[544] but number of the protein-encoding genes that have been sequenced and mapped appears to be as low as 20 000–25 000.

A gene, which is a cluster of nucleotides within a chromosome, is a biological unit that carries hereditary information. All genes have roughly the same form, but they differ in the order and numbers of their four nucleotide building blocks, i.e. the four bases: adenosine, which is consistently paired with cytosine; and guanine, which is paired with thymine. Altogether, the current genome sequence contains 2.85 billion nucleotides, covering more than 99% of the genome with a very low error rate.[285]

Genes have two parts: the exon is the coding part, but the expression of the gene depends on the non-coding part (intron), the so-called junk-DNA. The introns splice the double helix, which allows the genes to be "read", and thus determine where the reading begins. Part of the function of this junk-DNA is still unknown. Transcription of the chromosomes (genes) by way of enzymatic synthesis of a complementary sequence of RNA nucleotides provides, outside the nucleus, the information necessary to synthesise the large number of different proteins. These proteins make up the trillion human cells, giving rise to the nearly 4000 anatomical structures constituting the body.[509]

Interpretation of family trees

The laws of heredity were first formulated by Mendel in 1865. Mendel had discovered that two "factors" (much later called "genes"), one from the mother and another from the father, determined the traits of their offspring. Genes have a regulatory developmental function, and are transmitted in the same way from generation to generation, the *genotype*. The way in which the genotype becomes manifest, the *phenotype*, varies however, because of the influence of environmental factors and mutations that occur not only between generations, but also between family members and within each individual. Knowledge about the chromosome and mutations responsible for hereditary anomalies is rapidly advancing and increasing.

A gene must be exactly copied: if not, a change in form occurs. Since genes encode protein(s), mutated genes will result in synthesis of abnormal proteins. Among the major kinds of gene mutations are:

- Point mutations – in which one base is substituted for another, for example adenosine for cytosine
- Frameshift mutations – in which one of the bases is deleted or inserted
- Deletions – in which a large segment of DNA is deleted and consequently the protein that the gene encodes for often is missing. Instead of being deleted, an extra (part of) a chromosome may be present.

Let us consider an example. The hereditary trait "hypocalcified enamel" may be designated as "**A**" (capital letter indicating dominant) and normally calcified enamel as "**a**" (lower case letter indicating recessive). All individuals receiving from their parents the combinations **AA** (i.e. both chromosomes of the autosomal pair of chromosomes contain the identical genes **A** and **A** = *homozygote*) or **Aa** (the chromosomes of an autosomal pair contain two different genes **A** and **a** = *heterozygote*) will have hypocalcified enamel (for the effect of "**A**" dominates over the effect of "**a**"). Individuals with both recessive homozygotes **aa** will possess normally calcified enamel.

According to Mendel's laws, the offspring of a father with **Aa** (and thus having sperm cells with either "**A**" or "**a**") and a mother with **aa** (each egg contains "**a**") will possess, in a statistical sense, the combinations of genes as shown in Table 0.1. The probability of a heterozygotic child developing hypocalcified enamel is 50%, due to the union of gametes of unlike genetic constitution. Likewise, the probability of homozygosity and therefore normal calcified enamel is also 50%.

If the X-chromosome of the father has the gene that determines the development of hypocalcified enamel, designated X^A, the possibility of the offsprings' enamel being hypocalcified is shown in Table 0.2. A father (X^AY) with poor-quality enamel cannot have a son with poorly calcified enamel because the son gets his X-chromosome from the mother. But all the daughters will have hypocalcified

Table 0.1 Autosomal inherited hypocalcified enamel (A)

| | | Father | |
		A	a
Mother	a	Aa	aa
	a	Aa	aa

"A" = hypocalcified enamel; "a" = normal enamel.

Table 0.2 Sex-chromosome (X-bound) inherited hypocalcified enamel

| | | Father | |
		X^A	Y
Mother	X	XX^A (daughter)	XY (son)
	X	XX^A (daughter)	XY (son)

X^A = hypocalcified enamel.

enamel (Table 0.2). This latter example clearly shows that the mother with $X^A X$ chromosomes will pass on the trait to her sons and daughters in equal proportions, assuming the father does not have X^A. In other words, the probability that a child, either male or female, receives X^A (= hypocalcified enamel) from the mother is 50%.

Based on the foregoing discussion, the following criteria may be used to interpret family trees:

1. Autosomal recessive traits:
   - Equal numbers of sons and daughters inherit the trait.
   - 25% of the second generation will show the trait.
2. Autosomal dominant traits:
   - Equal numbers of sons and daughters inherit the trait.
   - 50% of the offspring will show the trait when one of the parents is affected.
3. Sex-chromosome (X-linked) recessive traits:
   - Sons show the trait more frequently than daughters. In order to become manifest, women have to inherit the recessive gene from both the father and the mother; the daughters are "carriers" when either the father or the mother possesses the mutated gene.
   - The father transmits the defective gene to only his daughters.
4. Sex-chromosome (X-linked) dominant traits:
   - Daughters show the trait twice as often as the sons.
   - The father with the trait transmits it to all his daughters, but not to his sons.
   - The mother transmits the trait to her sons and daughters in equal proportions.
5. Sex-chromosome (X-linked) dominant father and mother:
   - 100% of the daughters will show the trait.
   - 50% of the sons are affected, unless both X-chromosomes of the mother contain the mutant gene, in which case all sons show the trait.
6. When the trait is linked to the Y-chromosome, all the sons will be affected but none of the daughters.

Studies of small groups (e.g. families) will favour the detection of a dominant rather than a recessive gene. Other important points to note are listed below:

- Expressivity – is the way in which an anomaly manifests itself, for instance a reduction in the size of a tooth may be more or less pronounced.
- Penetrance – denotes the proportion of the genotype that is phenotypically manifested. The penetrance is 50% when half of the descendants with the mutated gene show the trait.

Note: expressivity may be regarded as the individual measure and penetrance as the statistical measure.

- Lyon hypothesis – in each cell of a female, only one of the two X-chromosomes functions randomly. Her cells therefore essentially show a "mosaic pattern": in a cell either the X-chromosome of the father or that of the mother will be active;[367] a hereditary effect on the enamel may be represented as vertically alternating rows of normal and abnormal enamel.
- Allele – one of a pair (or series) of genes that may be present on a certain location in the chromosome. For instance, the allele for blue eyes or the allele for brown eyes is located in the same place.
- Polygenetic heredity – a dental trait is determined by more than one gene, for example "A" and "B" (if recessive, then "a" and "b").

In such cases, larger numbers of genotypes and phenotypes have to be distinguished. Suppose that two genes determine the tooth size (Table 0.3). After conception, the fertilised egg contains the two responsible genes from the father and the mother. The following combinations, in principle, are possible from the mother: AB, Ab, aB and ab. The same holds true for the two genes from the father. Table 0.3 shows all the possible combinations of genes that may occur in the offspring.[448] Five combinations with 4, 3, 2, 1 or 0 (capital A or B) are possible, thus five phenotypes exist (see the identical numbers in brackets). Table 0.3 also makes clear that the number of genotypes is larger, namely nine. For example, phenotype (4) includes the combinations with three capital letters and one small case letter. Phenotype (4) is present four times in Table 0.3. Altogether, the 16 combinations shown in the table represent nine genotypes.

Seven phenotypes are possible when three genes determine a trait. The number of phenotypes is given by the formula $2k + 1$, where k is the number of genes. Ludwig (1957) studied seven morphological traits of the mandibular second premolars in different races and in monozygotic and heterozygotic twins. Many combinations of the traits were evident.[365] The number of genes involved in the initiation, cell proliferation and morphogenesis of the teeth, is however much larger.

Table 0.3 Polygenetic heredity

Mother	Father			
	AB	**Ab**	**aB**	**ab**
AB	AB (5) AB	Ab (4) AB	aB (4) AB	ab (3) AB
Ab	AB (4) Ab	Ab (3) Ab	aB (3) Ab	ab (2) Ab
aB	AB (4) aB	Ab (3) aB	aB (3) aB	ab (2) aB
ab	AB (3) ab	Ab (2) ab	aB (2) ab	ab (1) ab

The numbers in parentheses are the numbers of phenotypes.

It is noteworthy that the regulatory genes sequentially exert their effects during the numerous developmental processes in an individual, depending on the time when and the tissue where they are expressed, that is to say, under the influence of the microenvironment of the cells. Information outside the cells is relayed through secretion and attachment of signalling molecules (for instance the fibroblast growth factors) to cell surface receptors and this determines the switching on and off of the expression of the genes within the cells. Thus, due to inductive interactions between cells originating from the embryonic epithelium and from the neural tube-derived mesenchymal tissues, genes turn on and off, depending on the stage of tooth development. In mice with a specific blocked-off gene (*MSX1* expressed in the dental mesenchyme), the expression of certain signals to the epithelium was inhibited, and not all the teeth developed. The importance of other genes has been established in the same way.[591] Up to a hundred genes and more are involved in the different stages of tooth development.[416] All these genes have a role in the mediation of cell communication, which occurs via small molecules to receptors and target genes.

To complicate matters, the external environment may modify the outcome of genetic regulation. The interaction between multiple genes and environmental factors results in complex diseases, such as type 1 diabetes mellitus. In this disease a familial clustering is assumed to involve at least 10 different genes, of which none is dominant.[544] References for this Introduction are included in the references for Chapter 1, beginning on page 293.

Section I
Developmental Anomalies

1

Anomalies of Number

1.1   Introduction

The human dentition may consist of fewer or more than the normal number of 20 deciduous or 32 permanent teeth. Fusion of two teeth may also give the impression of hypodontia (Section 1.2).

1.2   Hypodontia

Hypodontia is the term used for dentitions with fewer than the regular number of teeth due to *agenesis*, i.e. either absence of a tooth germ or failure of a tooth germ to develop. *Anodontia* is the congenital absence of all the teeth while the absence of many teeth is known as *oligodontia* or partial anodontia. *Isolated hypodontia* is the congenital absence of one or a few teeth. Incomplete dentitions not classified as having hypodontia by definition are those where teeth are absent due to failure of eruption, extraction due to caries or orthodontic treatment,[295] or where teeth have been lost due to trauma and other reasons.

Hypodontia is the most frequent of all congenital aberrations in humans, and also occurs in animals such as dogs.[245] The incidence of agenetic teeth in Caucasian populations seems to have increased during the twentieth century, but the available data are too limited to suggest a trend.[384]

The aetiology of hypodontia is not entirely clear, but genetic factors are most certainly involved. Because mutated genes associated with agenesis have developmental regulatory functions elsewhere in the embryo, associated defects in other tissues and organs are also possible.[591]

The skin develops from the ectoderm, one of the three primary germ layers, which is involved in the formation of the teeth. Patients with isolated dental agenesis may show unusual dermatoglyphic patterns of the palms of the hands and soles of the feet, suggesting a shared origin.[28]

The combination of freckles, thin eyebrows and hypodontia[609] suggests the same. Therefore, isolated dental agenesis might be a minor manifestation of a systemic disorder.

1.2.1   Isolated dental agenesis

As mentioned above, isolated dental agenesis is the result of the absence of one or a few tooth germ(s). Missing teeth can lead to diastema (interdental spaces) in the dental arches. Displacement and tilting of the neighbouring teeth may close these spaces.

Epidemiology
Primary dentition
Less than 1% of children exhibit hypodontia in the deciduous dentition. The teeth most often involved are the maxillary incisors, followed by the mandibular central or lateral incisors,[112 134 220 372 394 445 469] and also the first molars.[112] When the deciduous canines are agenetic,[205 608] a syndrome (see Chapter 11) such as cleft lip is usually present.[464] Around 50% of children with hypodontia are missing one tooth, usually the maxillary lateral incisor; in the rest usually two or more teeth are missing.[134] Japanese children show agenesis more frequently (5%), which may represent an ethnic trait.[112 158]

Permanent dentition
Surveys, often retrospective, of some 160 000 children and adolescents from different countries and populations indicate that 2% to 10% of the permanent dentitions show isolated dental agenesis, third molars excepted.[1 10 31 47 55 89 94 112 129 131 159 169 170 208 210 219 231 268 279 294 352 362 371 374 388 410 414 421 423 441 469 485 488 508 541 594 595 629 638 648] One study found that 13% of orthodontic patients had hypodontia,[476] however, this sample is not representative of the population and the finding may be considered as an outlier.

The main body of data has been collected from European and American Caucasian populations, although

Pathology of the Hard Dental Tissues, First Edition. Albert Schuurs.
© 2013 Albert Schuurs. Published 2013 by Blackwell Publishing Ltd.

some studies have included different ethnic and mixed populations. European and Australian children in general lack more teeth than North American Caucasians.[446] On average two teeth, frequently homologous teeth,[31] per individual are agenetic.[160]

Girls are significantly more susceptible to agenesis than boys,[1 31 47 169 200 219 279 476 485 488 452 566 664] but not all surveys have found a difference between the sexes.[159 374 497 501 574 665] Isolated dental agenesis may, however, occur about 1.4 times more often in girls than boys,[384 446] and agenesis of several teeth is also more common in girls.[210 585 595] In one study, the prevalence of hypodontia in Jewish children did not differ by sex, but girls lacked the maxillary lateral incisors more frequently and the boys the mandibular incisors.[170]

The overall prevalence of agenesis in the maxilla is comparable with that in the mandible, but there is a marked difference in the pattern of absence of tooth type between the jaws.[446] The five teeth most prone to agenesis in order of most to least prevalent, are: third molars > mandibular second premolars > maxillary lateral incisors > maxillary second premolars > mandibular lateral incisors.

However, other rank orders of agenesis of teeth, including teeth other than the ones mentioned above, have also been reported. Specific populations and inclusion of oligodont patients may account for the differences.[446]

Third molars Wisdom teeth are most often implicated in isolated dental agenesis, but the prevalence data vary. In 10–35% of adolescent and young adult dentitions, one to four third molars are absent.[5 33 34 73 129 200 231 234 250 260 255 276 308 412 441 455 511 535 554 594 596] In studies of third molar agenesis, subjects may not be very young since the teeth develop quite late in some individuals,[61 474] and older people may not recollect whether the teeth were extracted.

Third molar agenesis seems race-related.[33 132 260 524 554] For instance, 27% of the white population in the USA versus 2% of East Africans have missing wisdom teeth,[33] and more Chinese lack all four third molars than Caucasians.[132] Women lack wisdom teeth less often than men,[444] but some researchers did not find a sex difference.[346 354]

More so than other teeth, the third molars tends to show bilateral absence.[129 354 554] Almost 10% of subjects also lack other teeth when one or more third molars are agenetic.[73]

Mandibular second premolar Of the four frequently agenetic teeth (excluding third molars), 45% or more[47 466] are second mandibular premolars; they are bilaterally missing in almost half of the population missing these teeth.[574] The reported percentages for lower second premolar agenesis vary considerably, but may be as low as 3.5%. In some studies, the maxillary lateral incisors were the most frequently agenetic,[55 170 410 501 580 638] and in one study

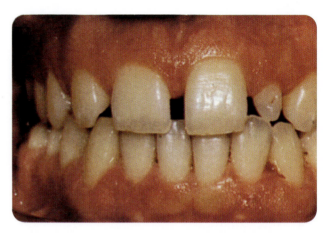

Figure 1.1 Agenetic right permanent maxillary lateral incisor; the contralateral tooth is underdeveloped.

it was the mandibular lateral incisors.[131] Such variations in findings might be due to ethnic differences.[444 524] Studies in Caucasians are more likely to show absence of the mandibular second premolar (and maxillary lateral incisor), and Asian studies of the mandibular incisors. A difference between the sexes has not been established.[574]

Maxillary lateral incisor A quarter of the four most frequently agenetic teeth (excluding third molars) are the maxillary lateral incisors. In some studies these teeth are reported to be missing even more often than the second mandibular premolars. A meta-analysis showed almost equal rates of agenesis of the maxillary lateral incisors and the maxillary second premolars.[384] In about 2.2% of Caucasians and Israelis the maxillary lateral incisor is absent.[170 580] Bilateral agenesis is common,[446] and the anomaly may be more common in women.[566]

Figure 1.1 shows a congenitally missing right maxillary lateral incisor and an underdeveloped contralateral incisor, which is rarer than bilateral agenesis.[566] The reduced, often conical, morphology may represent an incomplete expression of agenesis.[444]

Maxillary second premolar This tooth accounts for some 20% of the four frequently agenetic teeth, excluding the third molars. The variations in figures may be ascribed to small sample sizes, but the large differences in reported prevalences is substantial and remains unexplained. Bilateral agenesis occurs thrice as often as unilateral agenesis.[444]

Mandibular central incisor In order of frequency of agenesis in the permanent teeth, the mandibular central incisors usually come last, but not in Chinese children in Hong Kong.[131] Occasionally, the lateral incisor has been found to be missing more often than the central. Figures 1.2 and 1.3 show two and four retained deciduous mandibular incisors, respectively, due to absence of their successors.

Other teeth Any other tooth may be agenetic, and this is termed "aplasia of atypical elements".[524] For instance, absence of the maxillary first premolar,[159] second molar[47] [166 279 410] and the mandibular first premolar has been reported.[47 210] When the first permanent molar does not develop, other teeth tend to be missing too (oligodontia).[230 289 344] The maxillary central incisors are almost always present,[541] the canines being more often agenetic.[524] The condition in which there is presence of just one central incisor is described in Section 1.4.

Aetiology
Agenesis of teeth has been attributed to infectious diseases such as rubella, birth trauma, endocrine disorders, evolution and heredity.[268 572] For instance, one mother and her three daughters all had congenitally missing mandibular incisors, albeit different ones.[415]

Evolution
The relationship between agenesis and evolutionary processes is not clear.

Human teeth are diphyodont (two generation), except the permanent molars, which are monophyodont.[140] The last element of each tooth class (the third molars, second premolars and lateral incisors) is often agenetic or reduced in size. Bolk (1866–1930) therefore proposed the "terminal reduction theory": that is, during evolution, the *distal* element in each tooth class tends to disappear. However, of the four archetypal premolars per quadrant, the third and fourth premolars are present in the dentition of modern humans. The third molars would also have disappeared, but the primary fourth molar became the permanent first molar, accounting for the presence of three molars in modern humans.[524 628] Bolk's theory was eventually rejected but is summarised in Table 1.1, which also illustrates the current point of view.

Bolk also postulated that the teeth lost through evolution occasionally re-emerge in *Homo sapiens*. For instance, the lost lateral incisor reappears as an "additional tooth" between the central incisors (see Section 1.3).

Heredity
Hypodontia is usually a manifestation of an inherited trait (Figure 1.4) although it can occur sporadically, when it represents an acquired anomaly.[619] It is conceivable that certain mutated genes cause hypodontia.[591] Hypodontia

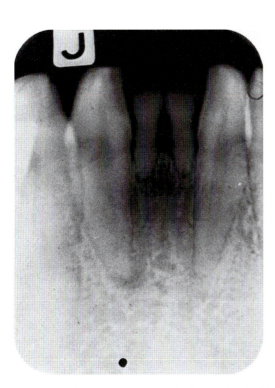

Figure 1.2 Agenetic permanent central incisors – the deciduous teeth are retained.

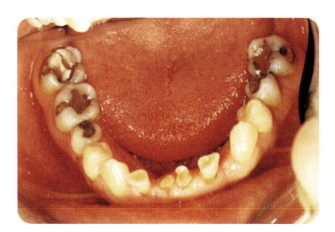

Figure 1.3 Four retained deciduous incisors in the mandible; the permanent successors are agenetic.

Table 1.1 Teeth per quadrant of the archetypal permanent dentition, the teeth remaining in modern humans according to Bolk, and present point of view[628]

Dentition	Incisors			Canines	Premolars and molars						
Archetypal	I_1	I_2	I_3	C	P_1	P_2	P_3	P_4	M_1	M_2	M_3
Human (Bolk)	–	I_2	I_3	C	P_1	P_2	–	m_4 (became M_1)	M_1	M_2	–
Human (the actual condition)	I_1	I_2	–	C	–	–	P_3	P_4	M_1	M_2	M_3

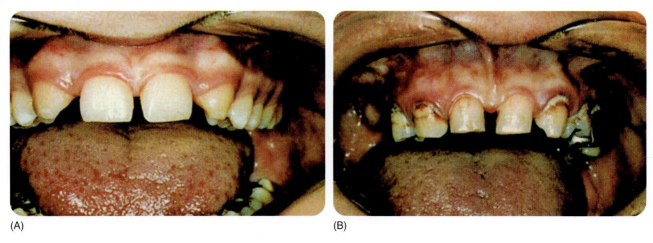

(A)   (B)

Figure 1.4 Mother (A) and daughter (B) with agenetic maxillary permanent lateral incisors.

follows an autosomal dominant mode of inheritance, but incomplete penetrance suggests interference of suppressor genes with the phenotypic expression.[92] Research has focused in particular on the maxillary lateral incisors, and, to a lesser degree, the premolars.

- Agenesis of maxillary lateral incisors is an autosomal dominant trait,[19 219 376] but other modes of inheritance have also been reported.[19 284 413]
- Agenesis of premolars is an autosomal dominant trait, with a complete penetrance, but varying expression.[577]
- Agenesis in particular affects the second premolars together with the lateral maxillary incisors, called the "incisor-premolar trait", with a penetrance of 86%.[284]

One study found that mutations in the genes for growth factors, which have a regulatory role during odontogenesis, were not responsible for dental agenesis.[25] Mutations in more than one gene and possibly multiple alleles are needed to explain the variations in dental agenesis.[37 480 488] One proposition is that to become manifest, agenesis must cross a "biological threshold"[110] and penetrance would require altered expression of more than one gene. A statistical analysis[575] in 171 families[185] concluded that hypodontia must be polygenetic.

- The *homeobox genes* regulate migration of the neural crest cells and tooth morphology. Mutations of the muscle-specific homeobox gene, *MSX1*, are linked to autosomal dominant agenesis of specific teeth.[357] Inactivation of *MSX1* has a highly selective effect on the dentition, but other genes must be involved for hypodontia to occur.[516] *MSX1* encodes transcription factors expressed in several tissues including the dental mesenchyme. *MSX1* mutations might be related to agenesis of premolars and molars.[357 626] *MSX1* is located on chromosome 4; the locus of *Notch2* for third molar

agenesis has been mapped to chromosome 3 in mice.[422] Multiple genes appear to contribute to interfamilial clinical variations in tooth agenesis.[619] Data on hypodontia fitted a polygenic model better than a single major gene model.[546] Several independent, defective genes acting alone or in combination, and eventually becoming antagonistic, may lead to a specific pattern of phenotypic agenesis.[625]

- Environmental factors are also implicated. Exposure in childhood to dioxin after an accident in a chemical factory (Seveso, Italy) resulted in increased incidence of hypodontia.[9] The association between different cleft types and hypodontia in twins was found to have a weak genetic component,[339] possibly because of the small sample size and the presence of environmental factors.
- Confounding factors also exist. Monozygotic twins, born from one fertilised egg, are in principle, genetically identical, but showed differential expression of hypodontia,[222 315 403] as mirrored agenesis of mandibular second premolars.[345] Regardless of tooth group concordance, mono- and dizygotic twins (born from two fertilised eggs) have similar prevalence rates of bilateral agenetic teeth.[64]

Dizygotic twins are no more similar than siblings. In the past, matched tooth anomalies were used as determinants of di- and monozygosity,[604] but cleavage of the egg can take place in the two-cell stage or later.[521] Monozygotic twins may have an abnormal number of (parts of) chromosomes.[560] Differing chromosomal compositions may exist through gene mutation or post-zygotic (partial) loss of a chromosome in one twin DNA (copy errors), while the other maintains the karyotype of the zygote. It has been established that monozygotic twins show mirror-image tooth anomalies but discordant hypodontia[222 244 312 339 345 403 604] and other dental features.[41 52 99 603 604] Moreover, lyonisation is a possibility in monozygotic female twins.

When multiple teeth are agenetic, associated deviant skeleto-dental patterns, such as a retruded maxilla,[45] have been hypothesised to be due to environmental effects. Horizontal and vertical pressure on the dental lamina during growth supposedly suppresses or distorts the tooth buds, likely affecting the last tooth in each tooth class.[397] One study concluded that in orthodontic patients, the frequency of maxillary and mandibular third molar agenesis is related to a decreased anterior–posterior dimension of solely the maxilla.[299]

Relationships between teeth

In isolated dental agenesis, the teeth that are present show smaller crowns, a "tendency" to agenesis.[308 524] A peg maxillary lateral incisor is also associated with non-eruption and a palatally erupted canine.[439 440]

- Agenesis of the maxillary lateral incisors increases the probability of other teeth being agenetic.[349] The same applies to an increasing number of agenetic wisdom teeth.[5 201 439 511 554 574] Such relationships are not always present,[319] and the reverse has also been reported.[491 532]
- When the wisdom teeth are agenetic, the anterior teeth in particular may be relatively small, but such findings are not consistent.[38 199 497 648]
- Agenesis of the maxillary lateral incisor seems to be compensated by a larger adjacent central incisor. When the lateral incisor is undersized, this compensation is not seen; in fact the adjacent central incisor also tends to be relatively small.[550]
- Agenetic wisdom teeth (in the Inuit) were not found to be associated with a reduced occlusal pattern of the other molars.[249]
- In at least 50% of patients with a missing deciduous lateral incisor, the successor is agenetic,[72 220 290 372 469] and if bilaterally absent, more permanent teeth may be agenetic, such as the rarely involved first and second molars.[133]

A division of mandibular tooth agenesis into three groups has been suggested, based on the radiological evidence of the mandibular canal. In the anterior part of maxillary jaw, a pronounced lack of teeth was found to be associated with absence or marked reduction in the size of the incisive foramen and nasopalatine canal.[320 532]

Tooth germ-related causes

For dental agenesis, a tooth germ must be affected during its earliest developmental stages. Likely causes are failure of mesenchyme condensation during the initiation of the tooth bud stage, absence of induction of the subsequent ectodermal reactions and an inability of the ameloblasts to produce enamel following reciprocal induction by the odontoblasts. On combining these tissues *in vitro*, there was development of tooth-like structures.[543] In experimental studies, the formation of the dental papilla was induced in the mandibular epithelial lamina through its contact with non-odontogenic mesenchyme.[401]

Odontogenesis is initiated in the epithelium and is guided by interactions with the neural crest cells.[529 593] Regulation of normal tooth development requires proteins produced by a number of genes for the series of reciprocal interactions between the dental epithelium and mesenchymal condensations, which are accumulations of proliferating cells originating from the neural tube. Some of these cells are pluripotent;[77] their absence is related to non-initiation of the tooth germ.[390 542]

The specific morphology of the teeth is also influenced by the cell condenstations.[390] Butler's "field theory" states that all tooth primordia are initially equivalent and that the morphology of the teeth is determined by morphogens in the antero–posterior axis.[93] Molecular investigations have identified single genes (such as the homeobox genes) with site-specific antero–posterior activity. A defective specific gene has been found to be associated with agenesis of specific posterior teeth, but not the anterior teeth. The developing maxillary dentition is not continuous: the upper incisors develop in the medial nasal processes of the first arch,[114] in the premaxilla.

The hypothesis that tooth agenesis is associated with prenatal brainstem anomalies has not been confirmed: the frequency of agenesis in such patients and the population was similar.[358]

Early disruption of the developmental processes is most probably a result of lack of (reciprocal) signals at the right time,[618] due to mutations in genes or an inability of the cells to respond appropriately.

Other causes

Dental development may be interrupted by diseases such as leprosy or the presence of congenital anomalies involving atrophy or disordered development of the anterior part of the maxilla. Figure 1.5 shows absence of a mandibular second premolar and arrested development of the contralateral tooth.

Ionising radiation (radiotherapy) can cause agenesis (and morphologic changes)[161] in humans[240 217 387 505] and animals[84 85] Just one treatment with 15 Gy leads to a temporary interruption in odontogenesis.[240 565] After *chemotherapy*, children showed marked tooth agenesis.[16]

Segmental odontomaxillary dysplasia is another condition with agenesis of one or both premolars in the affected jaw segment. The disorder consists of a unilateral maxillary enlargement from the canine region to the tuberosity, accompanied by gingival hyperplasia. Superiorly the enlargement occurs at the cost of the maxillary sinus. The spaced deciduous molars may be malformed, with splayed roots and pulp stones in enlarged pulp chambers. If the skin on the affected side contains more sweat glands than normal, the anomaly is called *hemimaxillofacial dysplasia*. The cause of the disorder is not known.[42 123 162 433 459 622 637]

Cutaneous abnormalities, such as "hairy nevus" of the skin and hypopigmentation of the lip border, are less frequently observed.[459 637] The anomalies originate *in utero* or in early childhood. Less common features are enlarged crowns and roots.[42 433] The condition seems to remain stable without significant progression.[123]

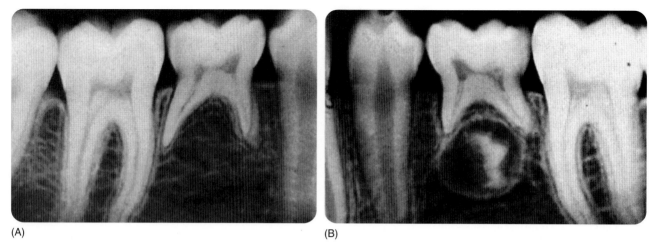

(A)   (B)

Figure 1.5 (A) Agenetic lower second premolar with retained deciduous second molar. (B) The development of the contralateral premolar is arrested.

Consequences

Consequences of isolated dental agenesis depend on the permanent tooth that is missing.

- When a permanent maxillary lateral incisor is agenetic, the predecessor will exfoliate, because the broad crown of the erupting permanent central incisor initiates and maintains the resorption of the roots of both the deciduous central and lateral incisors (Figure 1.4). The permanent canine frequently erupts partly mesially, and occasionally at the site of the lateral incisor, while the deciduous canines remain *in situ*.[138]
- If the mandibular central incisors are absent, the predecessors persist and may be functional for a long time.
- When the mandibular premolars are missing, the deciduous second molars are usually retained (Figure 1.5)[488] as root resorption is not initiated. In the maxilla, the deciduous second molar may exfoliate (due to resorption influenced by the first molar), but not as a rule.

A retained deciduous molar may function for many years, but undergoes wear and physiological changes, such as a reduction in the size of the pulp chamber and hypercementosis (Chapter 8).[506] Excessive wear or caries may lead to extraction. Another complication is infra-occlusion (Chapter 4), in which the occlusal surface of the retained tooth stays below the level of the occlusal plane, as the adjacent teeth continue to erupt. In 19–20-year-olds, more than half of the retained deciduous second molars showed 0.5–4.5 mm infra-occlusion.[53] The mesio-distal width of the retained tooth exceeds that of the missing mandibular second premolar, which causes a slight malocclusion.[53] After late extraction, there is tilting and migration of the neighbouring teeth and overeruption of the antagonist tooth, but this is minimal if the occlusion was stable to begin with.

An early diagnosis of premolar agenesis may be incorrect because these teeth may have delayed development.[12 117 393 648] In 6-year-olds, it is possible not to detect any trace of second mandibular premolar development[120] because initiation of calcification of mandibular second premolars may not start before the age of 9 years.[127]

Agenesis of wisdom teeth is often welcome, because a lack of space within the jaws may inhibit their eruption, causing secondary pathology (Chapter 4). A normal molar relationship (Class I) is observed in these cases.[151] Permanent teeth may erupt prematurely when the deciduous predecessors are agenetic.[464] Isolated dental agenesis may lead to malocclusion, but dentofacial deviations are mostly minor.[656] The alveolar process may be underdeveloped locally. In one study, patients lacking four or more teeth were found to have a smaller cranial base, a shorter maxillary length, a slightly prognathic mandible with anticlockwise rotation, and retroclination of the maxillary incisors.[172]

Prevention and treatment

Isolated agenesis in the deciduous dentition does not require treatment, but it is prudent to consider taking radiographs of the patient and their siblings, for counselling and timely treatment of agenetic permanent teeth.

Deciduous molars without successors must be extracted[214] at a young age,[395] taking into account the relationships between the maxillary and mandibular teeth. Early extraction allows the permanent first molar to move mesially spontaneously without excessive tilting, filling most of the extraction site. Spontaneous space closure occurs if the deciduous mandibular molar is extracted before the root of the mandibular first molar is completed and before the second molar erupts.[359] Deciduous second molar extraction at 10–13 years in dentitions with a normal occlusion was found to result in a diastema, which half closed within 1 year by the tilting and migration of the adjacent premolars and canines, and, in particular, mesial tilting of the first mandibular molars. The closure was enhanced by the displacement of the maxillary first molar due to growth in a downward direction.[375] [431] Two years later, 10% of maxillary and 20% of mandibular diastemata remained. In contrast with the mandible, a maxillary unilateral extraction did not result in a shift of midline.[375] The local width of the maxillary and mandibular alveolar arches decreases considerably after extraction.[431]

An unstable situation requires orthodontic closure of a diastema. Care must be taken that the anterior teeth do not tip lingually.[631] If the contralateral premolar is present, its extraction must be considered. An alternative approach is space maintenance, followed by the placement of an implant or a bridge. Long-term implant survival is around 90%, independent of its location.[167] Timing of implant placement depends on vertical alveolar growth, which continues beyond puberty: an implant-supported prosthesis inserted in adolescence will eventually become infra-occluded. Sometimes it is possible to transplant a tooth (Chapter 7) that must be extracted for orthodontic reasons into the site of an agenetic tooth.[340]

Extraction of retained deciduous molars in adulthood necessitates insertion of implants or bridges for function and aesthetics. However, deciduous second molars that are lacking successors and are retained into adulthood remain functional for a long time.[545] In one study, only a few retained second deciduous mandibular molars were lost because of caries or periodontal breakdown at the age of 48 years;[545] in a minority of cases root resorption of the deciduous molar will be a problem.[364] [666]

- A patient with agenesis of the permanent maxillary lateral incisors requires orthodontic space closure. In contrast with replacement with partial dentures, moving the permanent canines into contact with the central incisors (Figures 1.6 and 1.7) resulted in a healthier periodontium 7–10 years later[424] and greater patient satisfaction.[482] Restorative reshaping of such canines with composite creates a cosmetically acceptable emergent incisor profile on the canine.[490] If not treated orthodontically, a rather wide diastema will remain. Space maintenance is required to close the diastema with an adequate implant[546] or bridge after cessation of the (rapid) alveolar growth. The use of osseointegrated implants in children is problematic for reasons of jaw growth, but is presently under consideration.[643]
- When the permanent central mandibular incisors are absent, extraction of the predecessors is not indicated. An acceptable prosthetic solution after natural loss of the long-persisting deciduous teeth will require maintenance of the diastema.[180]

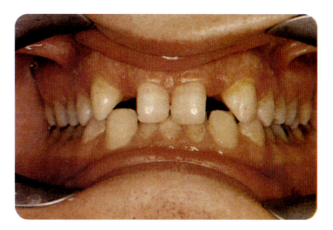

Figure 1.6 Patient with missing maxillary lateral incisors.

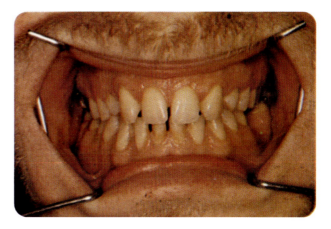

Figure 1.7 The canines of the patient in Figure 1.6 have been moved orthodontically into the locations of the agenetic maxillary lateral incisors. The morphology of the canines may be improved by grinding the cusps and building the lateral margins with composite so that the teeth resemble lateral incisors. Note the presence of only three lower incisors.

1.2.2 Oligodontia

The term *oligodontia* has been defined by various authors as the absence of either four or six and more or eight and more teeth, excluding agenesis of third molars.[263] [468] [648] [664] Oligodontia has diverse presentations. Some patients lack many posterior teeth and others lack anterior teeth.[468] The pattern of missing teeth is often bilaterally symmetrical. The frequency of oligodontia is low: about 0.1–0.5% people have seven to eight missing teeth.[1] [47] [219] [371] [485] [541] [594] [664]

Oligodontia occurs either sporadically in just one individual[26] [559] or it may be inherited without other anomalies.[583] It commonly occurs in association with Down's syndrome (trisomy 21[116]) and syndromes in which the epithelium or its derivatives are involved, such as ectodermal dysplasia with abnormal hair, nails and sweat glands (Chapter 11). When a larger number of teeth are missing or more "stable" elements, especially the maxillary central incisors,[468] are absent, the presence of a syndrome should be suspected. Conversely, three or more (inherited) skin conditions require investigating for dental agenesis,[517 518] but absence of "stable" teeth is not inevitably a sign of a general disorder.[572]

In *cherubism*, a hereditary (autosomal recessive?) painless disorder with oligodontia, the middle and lower part of the face become progressively more and more rounded.[335] The cherubic appearance may be enhanced by skin stretching and downward pulling of the lower eyelids, causing an upward directed look.[153] [467 616]

In *microsomia I*, agenesis and delayed maturation of teeth is related to the severity of the disorder. It affects the face unilaterally, with underdevelopment of the mandibular ramus and adjacent soft tissues, possibly caused by a vascular lesion of the first and second branchial arches.[113 175]

Hall (1983) mentions 34 syndromes and a number of clefts with isolated dental agenesis or oligodontia,[235] but the number is at least 120.[660]

In one study, some 60% of oligodontia patients had ectodermal dysplasia; the other 40% had intermediate severity eczema and asthma, and some experienced hyposalivation.[423] "Isolated" oligodontia patients had fewer sweat glands than controls.[218] Oligodontia (Figure 1.8) is, moreover, characterised by reduced tooth size[423] and morphology (conical crowns, short roots),[11 317] and underdevelopment of the alveolar processes.[80 222 317 480] The face tends to resemble that of an edentulous person, with protrusion of the mandible and pouting lower lip, and often a decrease in vertical dimension.

Heredity

Analysis of family trees suggests an autosomal dominant inheritance pattern in more than half of oligodontia patients.[187 213 517 572] Different mutations of the *PAX9* gene encoding the PAX9 protein appear to be associated with

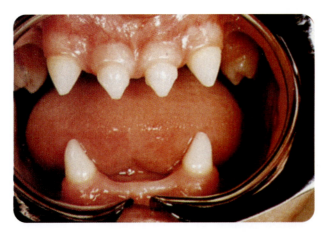

Figure 1.8 Oligodont dentition with hypoplastic and conical teeth. (Courtesy of Department of Oral Surgery, University of Groningen.)

specific oligodontia patterns, but other genes are most probably involved in specific combinations of multiple missing teeth. *PAX9* is expressed in the neural-crest-derived mesenchyme of the mandibular and maxillary arches. *MSX1* has been found to be associated with agenetic second premolars and third molars, but *PAX9*, on chromosome 14,[186] was associated with missing first and second molars.[327] A mutation in *MSX1* was found to be unlikely in family members who, to various degrees, had missing first, second and third molars, premolars and mandibular incisors.[213]

A *PAX9 nonsense mutation* changes a chain-termination codon from one that specifies an amino acid into one that does not,[633] which results in incomplete protein synthesis and oligodontia.[417] A *de novo deletion* of the proximal long arm at chromosome 14 resulted in developmental defects, but oligodontia was not mentioned in the report.[522] A deletion involving the *PAX9* locus was observed in a proband with absence of most deciduous and permanent teeth. A *frame-shift mutation* in *PAX9*[126] encodes an abnormal protein or disrupts the synthesis of the protein completely.[633] Identical twins have been found to have a frame-shift mutation and a premature stop codon.[125] A *missense mutation* in the *PAX9* gene was found in a family with a distinct oligodontia type.[342] The mutation changes a codon specific for one amino acid into a codon specific for another amino acid (an arginine to tryptophan change),[342] but the new protein maintains some biological activity.[633] Another oligodontia patient had a heterozygous missense mutation in the paired domain of *PAX9*: arginine was substituted by praline;[297] other substitutions also exist. *Allelic heterogeneity* in *PAX9* was found to be responsible for the autosomal dominant molar agenesis in one kindred, but in other families with a similar pattern of missing molars *PAX9* did not appear to be mutated.[187] A *de novo* mutation in *PAX9* has been confirmed in a patient with oligodontia. Other patients with oligodontia had no mutations in the coding regions of either *PAX9* or *MSX1*, indicating different genes must be responsible.[409]

Mutations of *PAX9* are associated with varying oligodontia patterns in the deciduous and permanent dentition, and missense mutations affect only the permanent dentition.[297] *MSX1* mutations have been found to be linked to isolated hypodontia and seldom to oligodontia.[150] *MSX1*, *PAX9* and *FGFA* (expressed during craniofacial development) have been suggested to interact and to play a role in non-syndromic tooth agenesis.[626] Recently, mutations in *AXIN2* have been found to cause severe oligodontia and a predisposition to colorectal cancer.[341] It has been concluded that oligodontia and anodontia are determined polygenetically.[80]

1.2.3   Anodontia

Anodontia is the rare congenital absence of all teeth, that occurs in serious, often fatal, syndromes. Anodontia is also reported as a representation of a homozygous state (autosomal recessive) of the gene responsible for peg or missing lateral incisors in heterozygotes. The deciduous dentition is not affected and no associated anomalies have been noted.[428]

Treatment of oligodontia and anodontia

Partial or full (over)dentures[165 460 548 644] with increase of the vertical dimension,[63] and implants and bridges are indicated for maintenance of the functional space and occlusion.[96] Because failure of an implant used as an abutment for a bridge may result in the loss of large amounts of bone, orthodontic realignment of the teeth, if present and possible, might be preferred,[630] but is troublesome.[280]

Due to psychosocial effects, anodontia and oligodontia in young children should be treated.[489 548] Extraction of retained[264 471] deciduous teeth must be delayed as long as possible.[632] Siblings must be examined for similar anomalies.[567]

1.3   Hyperdontia

Hyperdontia (or *hyperodontia*) denotes the presence of one or more extra teeth, that is a dentition with more than the 20 deciduous and/or 32 permanent teeth; the extra teeth may be morphologically similar to or dissimilar in size or shape compared with the normal teeth. The additional teeth occur singly, multiply and uni- or bilaterally. Their morphology may be similar to that of normal teeth (*eumorphic*), allowing recognition as a specific tooth. Such teeth are also called *supplemental* (or *supplementary*) teeth.[457] Other additional teeth are *atypical* or *dysmorphic*, rudimentary in size and form, with a peg-shaped crown or a reduced multi-cusp crown, and are alternatively called *supernumerary teeth*. Unerupted extra teeth within the jaws may be detected incidentally on radiographs, but a disturbed eruption pattern of the regular adjacent teeth may provide a clue.[178]

Extra teeth resemble odontomas to a certain degree. Odontomas belong to the group of benign odontogenic tumours and consist of epithelial and mesenchymal tissues. *Complex odontomes* are composed of dental hard tissues in a state of disarray and *compound odontomes* are tooth-like structures.[76 434 601]

Compound odontomes are more common than complex ones,[305] but several large studies did not find a significant difference.[579 601] Of 19 000 oral pathological conditions, 0.5% were odontomas.[432 601] and in another study, one-third of 349 odontogenic tumours were odontomas.[408]

The rare *ameloblastic fibro-odontoma* is thought to be a third type of odontoma, but may be a predecessor of the other odontomas. In *ameloblastic fibroma*, there is uncontrolled growth of epithelial and mesenchymal tissue, but without formation of real enamel. Dentine or enamel and dentine may be formed in the *ameloblastic fibro-dentinoma*.[617]

It has been questioned whether odontomes and hyperdontia are fundamentally different.[272] The term "odontoid structures" may therefore be preferrable.[257]

About half of odontomes are associated with unerupted teeth.[306] The argument that odontomes and hyperdontia are identical is weak. A relative difference is the age at which they develop. Odontomes develop at any age whereas in hyperdontia, the extra teeth rarely develop late.[210 452 456] Moreover, odontomes continuously increase in size.[368]

Teratomas are neoplasms made up of different types of tissue not belonging to the body part in which they develop. Benign tumours in the ovary contained one to nine elements resembling canines and premolars and amorphous teeth, which are randomly distributed.[155 373] As yet unexplained is why teeth developing side by side are morphologically of different tooth class/type.[123] It has been concluded that the morphology of these teeth is genetically determined independently from each other.[93]

1.3.1   Hypodontia with hyperdontia

Concomitant hypodontia and hyperdontia[31 100 159 177 206 421 501 538 561 627 638] occurs in 0.5% of the dentitions.[206] It has also been found to occur in children with conditions such as cleft lip or palate.[465]

Epidemiology
Hyperdontia is less common than hypodontia.

Primary dentition
Four radiographs are sufficient to detect hypodontia-hyperdontia in 2–6-year-olds.[495] Hyperdontia affects 0.5–1% of the deciduous dentition, but, interestingly, up to 3% are affected in many Asian populations.[60 94 158 112 169 194 257 278 283 300] The late development of additional teeth may be the reason that they do not occur in the deciduous dentition,[634] but they might not have been observed or could have been extracted prior to the patient being enrolled in a study.[278] Parents may overlook a eumorphic extra deciduous tooth, often an incisor, because the interdental spaces that are common between the deciduous anterior teeth allow good alignment teeth in spite of hyperdontia. Conical (peg-shaped) deciduous supernumeraries have also been observed.

Permanent dentition
The prevalence of extra permanent teeth is 0.5% to about 3% in different populations, with a few populations showing higher prevalence, for instance 10% in an isolated population in Alaska.[31 47 60 89 94 101 112 131 159 169 194 220 231 257 275 281 282 283 300 352 362 366 388 441 469 508 564 594 638] The varying prevalence may due to ethnic differences, age, use of radiographs, forgotten extraction of extra teeth, sample selection, etc. On average one extra tooth is present,[160] but more than one is present in a third to over 40% of patients.[174 361 379 463]

Ten per cent of dogs show hyperdontia, some breeds less frequently (huskies 2%) and others more often (spaniels 19%).[245]

Location

Extra teeth are classified based on their morphology and the tooth type which they resemble.[515] The two-digit FDI tooth identification system has been extended to a three-digit one in order to include hyperdontia.[337]

Three-quarters to more than 90% of extra teeth are found in the maxillary anterior region.[101 316 328 463] It is noteworthy that a third of the odontomes are situated in the premaxilla, twice as often in Caucasians as in people of African descent.[248 249] Another preferred region is the mandibular premolar region; only a quarter of the supernumerary premolars occur in the maxilla.[551] The third preferred region is the retromolar region. It is not clear in which of the two latter regions hyperdontia is more common.[519]

Multiple hyperdontia is rare,[149 209 302 444 353 463 496 564] unless a syndrome is present,[519] and is more likely to present in patients with relatives possessing supernumeraries. There are several reports of familial localised juvenile periodontitis occurring in association with multiple extra teeth.[426]

Sex, ethnicity

Males show hyperdontia twice as often as females[47 60 94 112 169 257 278 283 300 381 463 469 662] but a lower sex ratio has also been reported.[469] Extra premolars occur three times more commonly in males than females,[361 551] as does the maxillary mesiodens.[174] Higher sex ratios, up to 6.5:1 in children in Hong Kong[131] have been reported, as well as in some other Asian populations.[313 361 507] A difference between the sexes has not always been found,[220 366 388] and is absent in the deciduous dentition.[469] One paper reported a female predilection.[31]

Hyperdontia might be an ethnic trait, being less common in Caucasian than in Asian populations.[131 421 507] In Nigerians, extra anterior teeth are most probably rare.[484] Maxillary mesiodens are twice as common in Hispano-Mexicans than in Caucasians.[300] About 3% of Japanese and Hong Kong Chinese have mesiodens[131 421] whereas a prevalence of 0.4% was reported in a Finnish population.[290]

Syndromes

Hyperdontia is part of some syndromes (Chapter 11). Rare syndromes with hyperdontia, such as the Nance–Horan syndrome,[660] are not discussed in this book.

Non-syndromic multiple supernumeraries

Some 40 articles have reported cases with five or more non-syndromic extra teeth;[524 657] there are also a few reports of hyperdontia with up to 22 extra teeth.[478 549] Multiple hyperdontia occurs most frequently in the mandible,[656 667] predominantly in the premolar region, followed by the molar and anterior region.[657] Non-syndromic hyperdontia may be familial.[668]

Time of development

Extra incisors may develop simultaneously with the regular teeth in both dentitions,[563 651] but usually late, particularly extra premolars.[6 104 115 207 249 318 329 382 389 406 456 467 493 563 537 634 661] The development of extra premolars may lag 5–10 years behind the normal ones,[104 207 329] but they may develop more rapidly. A barely visible semicircular radiolucent band was noted to develop into an almost complete extra premolar within 9 months.[351] Five extra premolars, situated at the apices of adjacent teeth in two 13-year-olds were partially developed.[329 537] In addition, the regular first premolars may be located apically to extra ones.[302]

1.3.2 Supernumerary permanent teeth

Atypical extra teeth, sometimes called *rudimentary teeth*, are commonly peg-shaped; tuberculate (multiple cusps) forms may be barrel-shaped and invaginated. Examples are *mesiodens, distomolar* and *paramolar*. Other supernumerary teeth reported are, for instance, a rudimentary tooth germ of a lower canine in a girl with hyperdontia of the incisors.[31]

Mesiodens

The mesiodens is usually located between the maxillary central incisors; however, mandibular mesiodens also occur.[135 146 336] In cases of anterior (premaxillary) hyperdontia, the majority (75%) of teeth are conical in shape and around two-thirds are found in the central incisor region.[460] Tuberculate mesiodens are more incidentally reported.[251 379]

Mesiodens, the most common supernumerary tooth, may nor may not be conical in shape, and more than one mesiodens may occur in the same patient.[184 313 413 348 396] Up to about 75% of mesiodens lie in an inverted position,[174 257 313 463 580] and a few have a transverse orientation.[463] Further, 50–75% fail to erupt,[300 460 463 662] due to their or inverted[174] position. A conical mesiodens is more likely to erupt (Table 1.2) than a tuberculate one.[185 251]

Table 1.2 Characteristics of conical and tuberculate supernumerary teeth[251]

Conical	Tuberculate
Usually erupt between the maxillary central incisors	Commonly sited palatal to the upper centrals
Erupt commonly during childhood	Erupt rarely in childhood
Roots complete before neighbouring teeth	Incomplete roots
	Develop later than conical teeth
Rarely delay the eruption of neighbouring teeth	Often delay eruption of neighbouring teeth
May displace neighbouring teeth	May displace neighbouring teeth

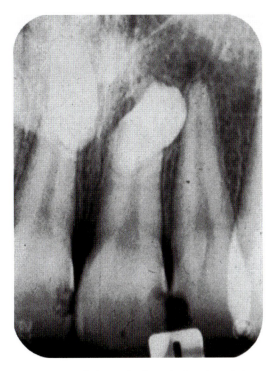

Figure 1.9 Two mesiodentes in the apical region of the permanent maxillary central incisors. They will not erupt because of their inverted direction.

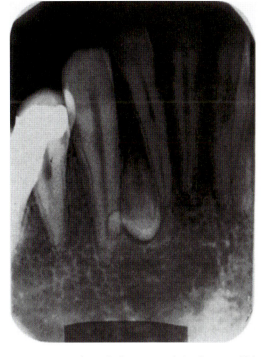

Figure 1.11 Inverted atypical extra tooth in the mandible. The small radiopacity visible on the root of the canine increased over time and resembled a late developing atypical extra tooth.

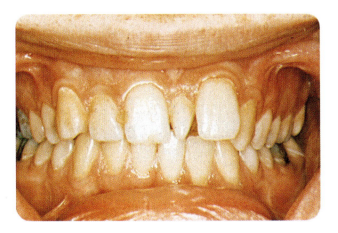

Figure 1.10 A mesiodens between the maxillary permanent central incisors.

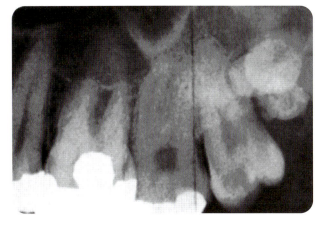

Figure 1.12 Distomolar situated behind the third maxillary molar.

Figure 1.9 shows two retained mesiodens, Figure 1.10 an erupted mesiodens, and Figure 1.11 an inverted mandibular supernumerary tooth.

Mesiodens may possess irregular enamel rods and dentinal tubules and contains more calcium and phosphate than the average tooth.[326]

Distomolar

The distomolar, typically situated distal to the third molar, is probably the second most commonly occurring atypical extra tooth (Figure 1.12). A quarter of 500 extra teeth were found to be distomolars, commonly with conical crowns. The more differentiated ones were smaller than their counterparts.[564] An atypical fifth molar with a few cusps has also been reported.[331]

Paramolar

The paramolar (*dens paramolaris*), an atypical extra tooth, may be attached (Figure 1.13) to the mesio-buccal surface of the second or third molar and sometimes the

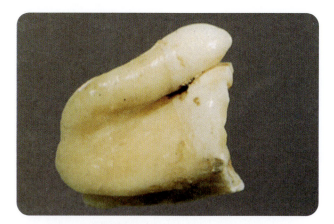

Figure 1.13 Paramolar (root and crown) attached to a decayed permanent second lower molar.

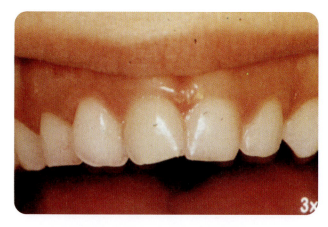

Figure 1.15 Supplemental incisor in the right upper quadrant.

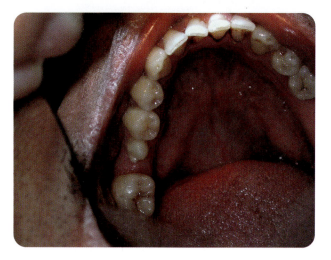

Figure 1.14 Paramolar or an atypical third premolar in the maxilla. (Courtesy of J.P. Nolte.)

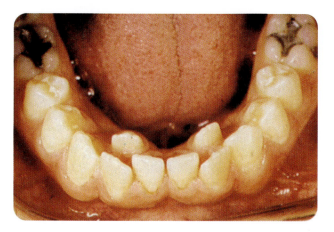

Figure 1.16 Two supplemental teeth in the mandible.

first permanent molar.[628] The tooth may manifest just as a cusp and/or a root (Chapter 2). When occurring as a separate entity, the paramolar may be situated next to, between (Figure 1.14) or possibly behind the molars. The distomolar may be a paramolar.

Among 500 extra teeth in one study, 11% were noted to be paramolars, a substantial number having multiple cusps.[564] Some 0.1% of the population possess one or more paramolars.[309 564]

1.3.3 Supplemental permanent teeth

The dentition may include extra teeth with recognisable forms: (lateral) maxillary incisors, mandibular incisors, third premolars, and fourth and sometimes fifth molars. Supplemental canines are rare.

Incisors
Among 500 extra teeth in one study, 45% were supplemental maxillary incisors,[564] commonly resembling a

lateral incisor (Figure 1.15).[483 564] A minority manage to erupt.[564] Among six maxillary incisors in a patient, one was a mesiodens, the other an extra lateral incisor.[624] Supplemental maxillary "lateral incisors" might be more common than mesiodens, followed by extra central incisors and then premolars,[366] but other frequency distributions have also been reported.[537]

Supplemental mandibular incisors (Figure 1.16) are not easily identified as first or second:[17 585] they are rare, especially lateral ones.[17] In the mandibular incisor area, 2% of the extra teeth are eumorphic.[102 564]

A supernumerary maxillary lateral incisor was present in adult *Australopithecus robustus*, living 1.7 million years ago.[477] Two eumorphic extra teeth were reported in the anterior mandible.[192] Early extraction of a temporary canine next to an extra lower incisor can enable the latter to erupt.[118]

Premolars
Premolars comprise around 10% of all extra teeth (0.08% of 48 550 patients,[564] although the numbers may be much higher[493]) (Figure 1.17); the majority are mandibular and

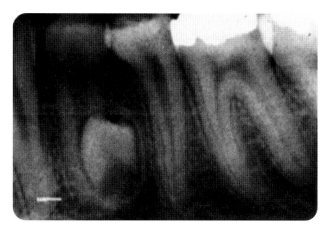

Figure 1.17 Late developing supplemental mandibular premolar.

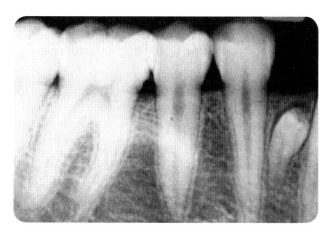

Figure 1.18 Extra premolar considered to be atypical because of its small size.

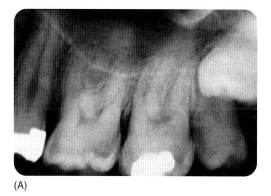

(A)

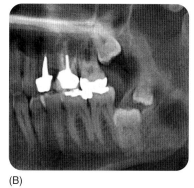

(B)

Figure 1.19 (A) A supplemental (fourth) molar. (B) Inverted eumorphic fourth molar in the ramus of the mandible.

often occur bilaterally. An extra premolar present at an early age increases the probability of developing more supernumerary premolars later; in one study, after removal of the extra premolar, a new one developed in 8% of the cases.[551]

Extra premolars are commonly supplemental,[36 68 168 239 253 393 406 452 456 467 479 536 663 655] but the tooth in Figure 1.18 should be classified as atypical. They may erupt, often lingual to the dental arch, and three-quarters are retained.[406]

Fourth molars

Having a fourth molar is not uncommon and fifth molars also occur.[444] One patient had seven "third" molars.[4] Bilateral maxillary and mandibular fourth molars and one fifth molar, and even three extra molars at one site have been observed.[642] Among 500 extra teeth, 25% were supplemental maxillary fourth molars, most of them unerupted.[564] In a study of 5000 military recruits, 14 had atypical or eumorphic fourth molars.[228] Eumorphic max-

illary fourth molars are often smaller than the third molars, but the one seen in Figure 1.19A was larger than the accompanying third molar. In the mandible, fourth and third molars are of equal size (Figure 1.19B).

Canines

Additional permanent canines have been described a few times,[24 293 513 564 570] but extra deciduous canines seem rare.[413]

Eruption issues related to hyperdontia

in some patients with hyperdontia, the teeth erupt far from the dental arch, such as within the maxillary sinus.[215] Extra teeth may also migrate to a different location after development (such as the fourth molar in Figure 1.19B?).

Aetiology

Various hypotheses have been proposed to explain the aetiology of hyperdontia. As yet, nothing can be concluded with certainty. Of patients with mesiodens, one-third showed a familial disposition. It may be worth mentioning that a permanent mesiodens has been found at the same side as a deciduous double tooth.[568]

Early splitting (dichotomisation) of the tooth germ into two buds produces two teeth (Section 1.4)[361] or a localised, independent hyperactivity of the dental lamina.[338 361 457] An extension of the dental lamina leads to formation of a supplemental tooth, whereas proliferation of the epithelial remnants of the lamina results in a supernumerary tooth.[457]

Phylogenetically speaking (phylogenetics is the science dealing with the evolutionary development of higher classes of animals from lower classes), the theory of splitting of teeth versus fusion of several tooth generations has had its adherents (Section 1.4). Arguments against phylogenetic fusion and splitting are based on embryology, fossil studies and comparative studies of the dentitions of animals. Supernumerary teeth would not be atavisms, because such evolutionary throwbacks occur predominantly in isolation instead of bilaterally, and with ectopic eruption.[457] Trauma, such as a jaw fracture, is an unlikely cause. Observations in animals lead to the supposition that a moderate or large outgrowth of the clone mass would lead to the development of an atypical or eumorphic fourth molar, respectively. An extra tooth could develop from a mesially extended anterior mass, but lack of mitotic activity would generally suppress its development.[527]

In animal experiments, it appeared possible to grow supernumerary teeth. Transplantation of the germs of the second and third molar into the eye of homologous animals developed in some cases into three molars.[311] Embryological ectoderm from regions other than the jaws assumed a bell shape when cells from the neural tube were added.[634]

Heredity

In view of a racial predisposition,[194 275 300 523] familial tendencies,[15 194 379 395 396 494 524 530 563] and gender predilection, heredity has once again been ascribed an aetiological role. Monozygotic twins have been found to have a concordant number of supernumerary tooth buds.[343] In a family with multigenerational consanguineous (next of kin) marriages, four individuals displayed five mandibular incisors,[102] two of which where fused to other teeth (Section 1.4).

Mutant genes appear to be a highly probable cause. Several inheritance modes are mentioned in the literature.[463] Whether the trait is autosomal dominant with eventual restricted or recessive penetrance needs further clarification. The higher frequency of extra permanent teeth in males has been attributed to an autosomal recessive gene with less penetrance in females.[421] The inheritance pattern deviates from a simple Mendelian pattern.[519] Supernumerary teeth as an isolated phenomenon may have a polygenic origin.[288]

Morphology

Knowledge about the determination of morphology in hyperdontia is increasing. Factors such as the location, cells originating from the neural crest, receptors, available space etc. play a role in determining the morphology in hyperdontia.

The tooth shape in mammals is possibly dictated by (1) a continuous shape-determining gradient from anterior to posterior or (2) various locations of the jaws. Each half of the jaws contains three clone masses of mesenchymal cells: the incisors, canine and the (pre)molars. As it extends due to proliferation, a clone mass progressively loses the potency/ability to determine the tooth shape. In each tooth class the most differentiated progenitor tooth develops first, closely followed by the less differentiated ones.[94 524]

Different receptors and/or different regulatory molecules play a role in the determination of the tooth shape. The level of activation of the ectodysplasin-A receptor (EDAR) appeared to control in the early stages, the cusp number and shape in transgenic mice. Less EDAR signalling results in few teeth with reduced cusps, more EDAR signalling results in more teeth with steeper cusps, and high EDAR signalling shifts the molar field distally, resulting in ectopic distal teeth, loss of the most proximal teeth, and many small cusps in the first and second molars.[607]

The cascade of events in the tooth germ is controlled by reciprocal induction. Regulatory genes tune on and off depending on the microenvironment. The fate of cells that become ameloblasts and odontoblasts is probably determined early, although transformation into the specific ameloblast takes longer. Already in the "cap" stage, the receptor for the epidermal growth factor in the cell membrane of the ameloblast is turned off; a "turning on" follows during maturation of the ameloblast. Other receptors (among which are Notch 1, 2 and 3) are also temporarily active.[592]

Consequences

The main immediate effect of hyperdontia is lack of space, delayed eruption of the extra or adjacent normal teeth, and crowding and malalignment once eruption takes place (Figures 1.20 and 1.21).[396] Mesiodens in particular may erupt quite early.[641] In children, one-third of supernumeraries erupt.[361] Hyperdontia is the most common cause for non-eruption of the normal maxillary incisors at age 8–10 years,[48 58] especially when the supernumerary tooth is tuberculate in shape and in a palatal position.[183 381] The predecessor may also be retained.[75] Extra teeth that form later in life are likely to have multiple cusps,[402] and tend to remain unerupted within the jaws.[225] Unerupted extra teeth may be the cause of diastema

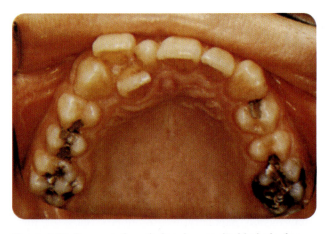

Figure 1.20 An erupted mesiodens has resulted in lack of space for the lateral incisor, which has erupted palatally.

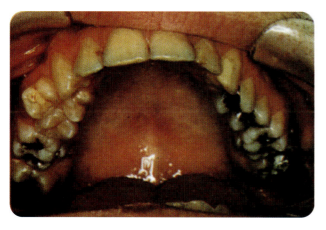

Figure 1.21 Malalignment of the teeth in the upper right quadrant as a consequence of an extra premolar.

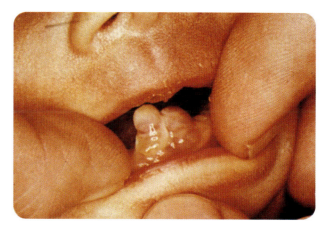

Figure 1.22 Neonatal teeth.

between the normal teeth[109] or lead to malpositions, such as rotation. They may also initiate resorption and follicular cyst formation.[382] Extra teeth may be conjoined with a regular neighbouring tooth (Section 1.4).[450]

Some evidence exists that premaxillary hyperdontia is associated with abnormalities such as dens invaginatus (Chapter 2), curved roots and delayed eruption after surgical removal of the supernumerary tooth.[241]

Treatment

Extra teeth should be extracted if (1) the eruption of the adjacent teeth is being obstructed, (2) envisaged orthodontic treatment will be compromised or (3) pathology, such as a cyst, develops. To prevent damage to the roots of the neighbouring teeth, the exact position of the extra tooth must be carefully determined. Early surgical removal could minimise interdental spacing and the need for orthodontic treatment,[661] but is not justified and is seldom indicated.[338] Complications of early removal are infrequent and minor in nature.[265 413] On one occasion an adjacent root temporarily resorbed (Chapter 7) and the situation returned to normal.[265] An extra tooth may be removed along with the deciduous predecessor when the permanent incisors roots are still incomplete.

As unerupted extra teeth may migrate,[569] it is not unwise to delay their removal until the tooth acquires a more favourable position and the roots of the adjacent teeth are fully formed. A conservative approach is warranted when the eruption of the regular teeth will not be hampered, pathology is absent, orthodontic treatment is not envisaged, and the removal of the extra tooth may compromise adjacent teeth.[202]

If the permanent incisors do not erupt into their normal position, a mesiodens is preferably removed between the ages of 8 and 9 years,[154] but pathology is extremely rare.[669] An erupted mesiodens is easily extracted, but the resulting diastema may persist.[328] A deeply situated mesiodens may

be left *in situ*, but requires regular radiographic review. Retained mesiodens may be fully resorbed.[236]

After the removal of extra teeth, the normal neighbouring teeth do not necessarily erupt spontaneously.[272] A quarter of maxillary central incisors with completed roots did not erupt after the removal of the (tuberculate) supernumerary[48 183] and required surgical exposure, in many cases followed by orthodontic traction.[183] Three-quarters of the latter teeth erupted subsequently within 16–18 months, and the rest needed exposure[58 202 381 402] and orthodontic traction. Surgical movement of a maxillary incisor situated labially is considered to pose a smaller risk than orthodontic movement.[454] Multiple hyperdontia may necessitate an interdisciplinary approach.[39]

1.3.4 "Extra dentitions"

Some sources mention more than two dentitions in humans, i.e. including teeth erupted around birth and teeth erupting after the loss of the permanent dentition.

Natal and neonatal teeth

Natal teeth are teeth which have erupted at birth and *neonatal* teeth refers to teeth erupting within the first month after birth (Figure 1.22).[383] The terms "extra dentition" is not appropriate for these teeth because the condition involves one tooth or a few teeth, although there are some reports of 11 and even 14 natal teeth.[389 447] Probably 90% of these, often the lower incisors, belong to the regular deciduous dentition.[13 43 59 197 302 504] *Dorland's Medical Dictionary* mentions "pre-deciduous teeth", a term applied to hornified epithelial structures without roots, which are not identical to natal/neonatal teeth.

In earlier times natal teeth were viewed with superstition. These children were thought to be witches or to become vampires after death, and also thought to bring about doom or blessings.[60] To prevent doom, the Basuto tribespeople in South Africa drowned such children or abandoned them elsewhere. Some famous people (Napoleon, Louis XIV) had neonatal teeth, which were believed to predict a glorious future.[139]

Epidemiology

Half as many natal/neonatal teeth are reported by hospital staff as by "specialised experts".[304] The teeth, the majority being natal ones,[383] are present in 1: 2000–6000 Caucasians. [8 20 43 13 121 304 598 504] Therefore, it is no surprise that in about 1000 newborns in Sweden no natal teeth were found.[182] Higher prevalence figures have been reported elsewhere: 10:1000 for Taiwanese newborns,[670] and 90:1000 for Tlingit Indians (Alaska).[386] The prevalence in children with cleft lip and palate is 50:1000.[14] The anomaly is possibly an ethnic trait.

A slight predilection for females seems likely,[6 20 219 304] but sex differences are not always reported.[43 363 523] The vast majority (59 of 62 natal/neonatal teeth in one study[23]) are mandibular central incisors. Natal/neonatal (bilateral) molars and canines have also been reported.[13 22 43 59 66 124 196 314 481 589]

Appearance

The crowns have either a normal size and shape or may be hypoplastic. In particular the lingual enamel is hypocalcified and incompletely formed,[148 250] lacking especially incisally[615] and cervically; the enamel may be thin (or absent), structurally abnormal and yellow in colour.[46 51 321 419 504 552] Amelogenesis arrests prematurely *in utero*.[51 552] There is abundant interglobular dentine (Chapter 3), irregular dentinal tubules and bone-like dentine, mainly cervically.[553] The roots may be barely formed or incomplete, covered with a thin layer of acellular cementum that is most likely not calcified.[20 111 148 196 237 304 380 447 553]

Aetiology

Reported causes include vitamin deficiency, endocrine disorders and fever. High levels of PCB (chlorinated bisphenyls) in food (Japan) may be responsible,[660] but in Finland no association was found with higher environmental levels (which have declined during recent years) of PCBs, PCDFs (dibenzofurans) and PCDDs (polychlorinated dibenzo-*p*-dioxins) in mother's milk. The prevailing levels of these substances are below the threshold reported to cause premature eruption.[8]

A hereditary,[237] superficially located tooth germ, above the alveolar bone,[419] seems more likely.[18 659] In some instances, the occurrence of the teeth is familial, both intergenerationally and in siblings, indicating a possible autosomal dominant trait.[13 18 23 43 59 237 304 383 386 540 659] Natal teeth may also occur as part of some syndromes and sequences, such as Ellis–van Creveld syndrome, Pierre Robin sequence, clefts, Wiedemann–Gautenstrauch syndrome,[120 660] in combination with a cleft tongue and deafness,[124] and the rare Pfeiffer syndrome type 3.[18]

Consequences

Natal teeth used to be removed for several reasons.

- Local mucosal infection.
- Mastitis, in a few cases, caused by nipple-biting during breast-feeding.[43 46]
- Ulceration of the underside of the child's tongue caused by contact with the natal tooth, which may lead to refusal to feed,[88 419 598] called Riga–Fedes syndrome[383] or Riga–Fedes disease.[211]

Risk of aspiration of a spontaneously shed natal tooth has been considered[252] but it has never been reported.[419] Around 30%[69] or even 60%[304] of the teeth are very mobile, being attached almost solely to gingiva,[504] which was the reason to remove half of them shortly after birth in one study.[304] Hertwig's sheath degenerates prematurely (Chapter 3),[556] but completion of the roots seems possible, at least partly. After early extraction or exfoliation, root-like structures may develop from remains of the cells of the dental papilla.[46 555 610] Such *residual natal teeth* may erupt. The root dentine is covered with an osteodentine-like substance and cementum.[610]

Left *in situ*, problems may arise in the longer term, but assumedly infrequently. One poorly developed neonatal molar became severely decayed, and impeded the eruption of the deciduous canine, disturbed the normal development and eruption of adjacent deciduous molar and caused osteomyelitis.[314]

Treatment

Natal and neonatal teeth belonging to the deciduous dentition must not be removed.[43 197 304] Curative treatment may not seem feasible,[88] but smoothing of rough incisal edges or adding composite to achieve a rounded, smoother surface has been proposed.[211] After extraction, gentle curettage is done to remove the papilla and Hertwig's epithelial root sheath.[88] No serious spatial consequences in the mandibular permanent dentition have been encountered after extraction.[304 598]

The majority of natal teeth may function well, like the other deciduous teeth,[197] but a third[54] (or two-thirds[271]) of the teeth exfoliate within the first year of life.

Third dentition

Occasionally the popular media will report a "post-permanent dentition", for example the eruption of 16 mandibular and 10 maxillary teeth in a 100-year-old Chinese person in 1983. Before 1875, reports on post-permanent dentitions were more common.[456]

The third dentition consists possibly of very late erupting regular and/or extra teeth. The eruption may be delayed considerably: in a 27-year-old woman none of the permanent teeth had erupted.[288] In cleido-cranial dysplasia, the multiple extra teeth erupt very late, because of abnormal bone remodelling owing to mutations in an osteoblast factor (RUNX2), which controls transcription of many bone and tooth-related genes,[671] and lack of acellular root cementum. Among the "teeth" of a third dentition might also be roots left behind during extraction.

1.4   Fusion and partial schizodontia

Fusion is the union of two discrete tooth germs at an early stage of the odontogenesis,[312 430 655] in which two teeth share part of at least the enamel and/or (root) dentine. In true fusion the teeth may show confluent dentine.[50 534] Synonyms include *synodontia*[143] and *connation* (born together).[261]

Fusion is not always complete. The extent and location of the union depends on the developmental stage at the time of fusion.[534] Three types have been described: total fusion (*fusio totalis*), partial fusion of the crowns (*fusio partialis coronaris*) and partial fusion of the roots (*fusio partialis radicularis*).[50 524] Clinically, a wide tooth or a wide crown with two roots is seen, particularly in the premaxilla,[254 274 355] or a single broad root with two crowns. The broad crown may show a normal morphology, an incisal notch or an inciso-cervical groove delineating the united crowns or it may be a bifid crown.

A *megadont* tooth (a large tooth of normal morphology) represents either macrodontia (Chapter 2) or complete fusion.[385] In one dentition a megadont tooth was accompanied by a contralateral double tooth.[71 81 142 163] Deciduous double teeth may precede permanent double teeth[30 35 47 65 71 81 83 116 142 163 191 425 451 507 640] or megadont/macrodont teeth, suggestive of fusion.[81 411]

Schizodontia denotes splitting of a tooth germ. If the split is complete, two teeth are formed (*twinning*, *gemination*) and hyperdontia results.[143 355] *Partial schizodontia* during early tooth development results in two partially conjoined teeth. Alternative names are "Siamese twin teeth" and "partial gemination". The appearance of a double tooth caused by partial schizodontia depends upon the timing of the splitting. Splitting may start at the incisal edge and stop before cleavage is complete. Such a division results in a mesial and distal crown components on a single root,[534] with either one or a partly divided pulp (pulpal bifurcation)[493] space.[74 312 355] A late incomplete split produces one crown on two roots.

Figure 1.23 shows schematically the hypothetical processes[586] of partial schizodontia, complete schizodontia, fusion and *concrescence* (teeth conjoined only via the cementum). Partial schizodontia and fusion may be viewed as morphological anomalies (Chapter 2), but as they may be associated with anomalies in the number of teeth, they have been included here. The knowledge of these two phenomena is based mainly on theoretical considerations and interpretation of the clinical outcome of the processes responsible. Although the nomenclature suggests an exact knowledge of the pathogenesis, this cannot be corroborated. Only one of the two processes may occur, therefore, the preferred name is "double tooth",[312 635] which simply indicates the tooth is mesiodistally wider than normal (Figure 1.24).

In sum, a *double tooth* is wider than a normal tooth and is the clinical manifestation of either fusion or partial schizodontia.

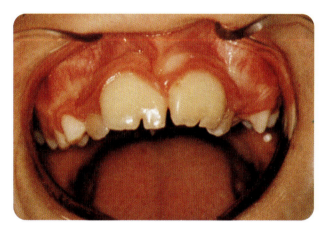

Figure 1.24 Two broad central double teeth; the incisal notches indicate existence of two components.

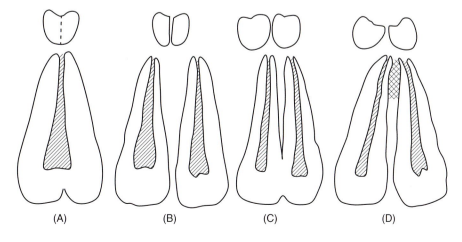

(A)   (B)   (C)   (D)

Figure 1.23 Schematic presentation (lower row) of partial schizodontia (A), complete schizodontia or twinning (B), fusion (C) and concrescence (D). The top panel shows a partially split tooth germ (A), a tooth germ split in two (B), two tooth germs pressed together, presumably resulting in fusion (C), and two tooth germs situated too close together (D).

1.4.1 Diagnosis

Diagnosis of a double tooth rarely poses a problem, but as mentioned above, there are no rigorous criteria to distinguish fusion from partial schizodontia (and hyperdontia from complete schizondontia?). Assumed fusion of a central incisor with a mesiodens (Figure 1.25) has been described a few times.[2 514 612]

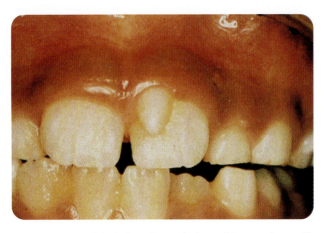

Figure 1.25 Possible fusion of a mesiodens with a regular maxillary central incisor.

Diagnostic criteria: fusion versus partial schizodontia

Many authors have diagnosed double teeth as products of fusion or partial schizodontia (correct or incorrect)[274 392] based on morphology, pulpal anatomy, location by jaw, crowding and number of teeth in the dentition.

Morphology

Incomplete schizodontia (and twinning)[50 369] (Figure 1.26) creates a mirror image (Figure 1.26A) of the coronal halves.[310 586] Manipulation of mice embryos resulted in twins which showed mirror-image teeth,[498] but this does not necessarily prove twinned teeth arise in the same way.

Fusion at an angle leads to a "crooked" appearance.[369] In fusion, one coronal part may be rudimentary,[49 493] usually the mesial component,[524] but malformed crowns may not allow classification into a tooth class.[49] These morphological differences are described *after* first giving the diagnosis fusion versus partial schizodontia although as mentioned above which of the two processes is responsible may not be clinically evident.

Anatomy

The pulpal anatomy and number of roots has been used for diagnosis of fusion/schizodontia.[56 70 74 107 130 147 164 188 189 242 301 312 355 356 438 442 443 449 499 502 582 584] Fused teeth have

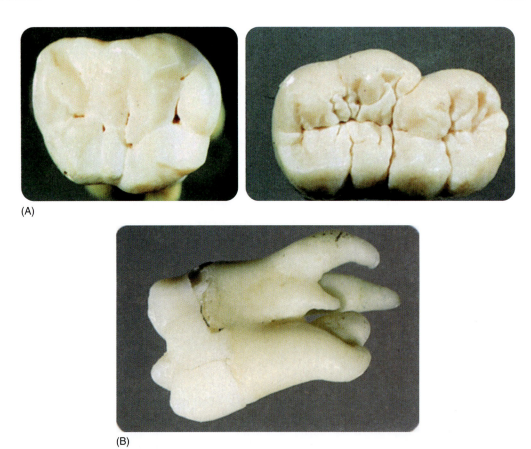

(A)

(B)

Figure 1.26 (A, B) Examples of permanent posterior double teeth from the upper and lower dentitions. The mirror image-like appearances of the occlusal left and right halves of the tooth (Figure 1.26A) possibly indicate partial schizodontia.

two pulp chambers and incompletely schizodont teeth have an undivided one,[355 586] whereas in fused permanent molars all root canals arise from one pulp chamber.[189] Some authors consider a vertical communication between the two pulps in double teeth as a criterion to classify these teeth as fused teeth[44 576] as well as partial schizodontia.[582] In both conditions the variability of the root canal system has been stressed,[130 189 312 355 369 586] which might preclude the diagnostic significance of anatomical[56 310] and pulpal features.

Location by jaw

Mandibular double teeth are almost exclusively considered to represent fusion but maxillary ones are occasionally thought to represent partial schizodontia.[143 164 640] Fusion with a supernumerary tooth seems to occur equally frequently in each jaw.[469] Half of the deciduous double teeth in the maxilla seemingly represent fusion between the central and lateral incisors.[655] Again, the morphological descriptions follow the diagnosis.

Crowding

Wide interdental spaces are common in deciduous dentitions with double teeth. Fused teeth require less arch length than normal teeth, leading to interdental spacing. Geminated teeth require more space, thus cause crowding,[369] as does fusion with a supernumerary tooth. Therefore, neither a diastema or crowding seems diagnostically decisive.

Number of teeth in the dentition

Two fused regular teeth counted as one unit reduces the regular number of teeth, unless there is concomitant presence of an extra tooth;[29] partial schizodontia does not affect the number of normal teeth.[312] Although fusion usually occurs as a singular anomaly,[112] the rare coexistence of hypodontia and hyperdontia (often in the same arch)[131 159 177 206 421 501 561 628 638] makes the number of teeth an invalid parameter for diagnosis. When an extra tooth is involved in fusion[67 81 469 645] the regular number of teeth is not reduced. Conversely, if a double tooth represents partial schizodontia, the number of teeth will be normal,[312] unless another tooth is agenetic.[81]

Fusion in the deciduous dentition is said to be associated with an agenetic successor,[233] but a double tooth due to partial schizodontia or fusion of a regular tooth with an extra one is not.[655] Deciduous double teeth are associated with a reduced number of teeth in both the deciduous and the permanent dentition[35 94 116 458 469 470 581 597 602 645] and with conical successor teeth.[655] In the literature, agenesis of 50–100% of permanent lateral incisors accompanied assumed fusion of the deciduous lateral incisors with the canines.[411 421 469 470 602] Assumed fusion of other deciduous teeth was less often associated with agenesis in the permanent dentition.[469 470] Hypodontia as a diagnostic crite-

rion is further compromised because deciduous "fusion with a supernumerary tooth" has been noted to be accompanied by hyperdontia in only four of 13 permanent dentitions.[83] Other maxillary deciduous central incisors fused with extra teeth were replaced by permanent normal and extra teeth.[599]

Counting a double tooth as one unit, the number of permanent anterior teeth was unaffected in a report of six deciduous anterior teeth. However, when five primary anterior teeth, including the double teeth, were present, the permanent dentition was noted to have five or even four anterior teeth.[205] The numbers of teeth in 367 children with double teeth corroborate the above findings.[655] All kinds of combinations of fusion, partial schizodontia, agenesis and hyperdontia may result in the presence of four to eight anterior teeth. Therefore, the number of teeth merely suggests a diagnosis.[576]

Conclusion

In sum, strict diagnostic criteria to discern fusion from partial schizodontia are lacking and it is difficult,[164] if at all possible,[312] to assign aetiological labels to "double teeth", the term that is preferred to the above-mentioned aetiological terms.[81 400 461 655] Diagnosis of fusion and partial schizodontia is said to be desirable in the deciduous dentition because of the expected probability of deviations in tooth number in the permanent dentition,[34] but the aetiological terms are merely of academic interest.[2]

1.4.2 Epidemiology

Double teeth have been frequently surveyed in Caucasian and Asian populations.[30 34 47 49 50 71 78 81 83 89 100 103 112 116 122 137 181 227 269 270 283 284 286 287 288 289 290 291 292 295 296 298 300 301 302 330 372 388 394 414 424 429 445 469 488 495 499 507 508 581 587 597 602 640 654] Many samples were randomly drawn, but some studies used selected samples or retrospective data or had other flaws. For instance, the 95% confidence interval for 3.7% of cases found in 107 Amerindians[122] is 1% to 12%, but in a random sample this may be doubtful because of the rarity and possible inherited nature of double teeth.

Double teeth are more often present in the deciduous than in the permanent dentition. It seems reasonable to conclude that double teeth in Caucasians are manifest in 0.6% of deciduous dentitions and in 0.1% of mixed/permanent dentitions, which is in line with an earlier estimate.[164] In Japanese and probably Chinese and Amerindian children, the average prevalence is 2.8% in the deciduous and almost 1% in the permanent dentition. The prevalence of deciduous double teeth in (western) India is 1.5%, a figure between that of Asian and European samples.[587] Among a sample of Jordanian adults, 0.42% had double teeth.[238]

Deciduous double teeth are mostly present in the anterior mandible (Figure 1.27).[655] About 90% is suggestive of fusion between incisor and canine.[655] Double teeth in adults may prevail in the maxillary incisor region and often concern the central incisors.[238]

Sex
Males and females might be equally affected.[81 116 291 469 507 524 602] Other studies point to a predilection in males.[49 470 654 655]

Syndromes
Double teeth are part of (or coincide with) a number of syndromes.[40 81 82 90 141 156 216 224 261 390 450 512 531 600 614 647 653]

Bilateral double teeth
Until 1987, some 30 bilateral double teeth had been reported,[164 405] but the number may have doubled since then. Around 50 (0.01%) were included in the surveys cited above. Another study estimated 0.02%.[164] In 372 double teeth cases, 1% were present in both the maxilla and mandible of the same individuals.[524] Bilateral double teeth were observed in both jaws and both dentitions of a Chinese girl.[418]

Posterior double teeth
In several hundred case reports reviewed,[526] 40–50 posterior double teeth (Figure 1.26) were described, mostly permanent ones.[27 44 81 105 106 109 130 136 144 145 157 179 189 204 212 221 225 229 245 256 259 266 273 298 301 400 407 461 492 503 520 523 524 525 539 558 562 573 606 620 658] Three double deciduous molars have also been reported.[3 95]

Triple and quadruple teeth
Occasionally triple teeth are encountered,[7 80 91 97 112 173 323 411 444 475 524 525 526 528 605 612] mostly deciduous ones. "Fusion" of two normal teeth with a supernumerary between them may be implicated.[7 81 91 173 323] In one report, one of two siblings had a triple and a double tooth, the other possessed two double teeth. Another patient had bilateral triple teeth. Two permanent triple teeth suggested fusion of the first, second and third molars.[524 528] A triple tooth may even consist of two deciduous teeth and one permanent tooth; the successor tooth being absent.[323] Another triple tooth was thought to represent a double tooth with a fused talon.[584] Figure 1.28 shows three triple teeth (previously unpublished).

Quadruple premolars (four conjoined teeth) have been reported twice,[523 524] but the reports may have concerned the same patient.

Solitary symmetrical median central incisor
A single maxillary symmetrical central incisor of normal size may be present across the midline (1:50 000 live births)[672] in both dentitions,[191 243 270 332 378 435 451] and less frequently in the mandible.[236] The phenomenon is linked to multiple genetic malformations, such as a short stature and midline defects (e.g. nasal defects and cyclopia, i.e.

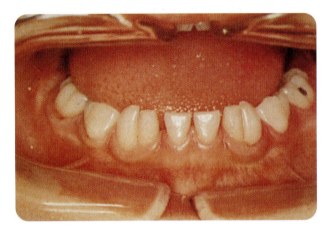

Figure 1.27 Bilateral mandibular fused anterior teeth, suggestive of fusion between the lateral incisors and canines (see text).

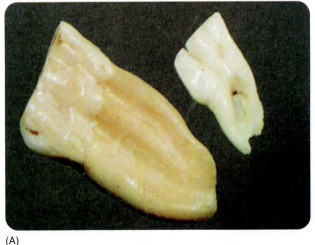

(A)

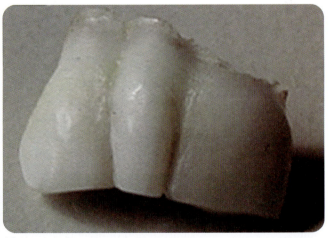

(B)

Figure 1.28 Two mandibular triple teeth (A). The maxillary triple tooth (B) was functional until its shedding. (Courtesy of M.A.C.J. Wevers.)

one eye).[82 171 193 216 243 270 378 435 510 639] The aetiology is uncertain.[672] Premature fusion of the right and left dental lamina has been assumed to prevent development of the medial halves of the central incisors, leaving the distal halves fused together.[247 378]

1.4.3 Aetiology

The manner in which and the reason why double teeth develop is still unresolved. Implicated factors are evolution, trauma, heredity and environmental factors. A multifactorial model comprising numerous genetic and environmental factors may present a unifying aetiological explanation for deviations in tooth number and size. An underlying continuous scale of the distribution of number and size with thresholds at each extreme has been proposed.[79] Double teeth may fit to such models.

Evolution Since the sixteenth century, the prevalence of both hypodontia and hyperdontia has increased distinctly, but that of fusion and partial schizodontia only slightly.[72] In Japan, the prevalence of double teeth has shown a tendency to rise.[654] An evolutionary trend might exist, which warrants a brief description of some evolutionary theories.[333 524 628]

Human (pre)molars represent fusion of haplodont (cone-like) teeth of the Mesozoical reptiles. Shortening of the jaw resulted in pressing of tooth buds of different generations together into triconodont teeth that would have separated later again into haplodont teeth when the jaw became again longer.[333 524] In evolutionary terms, both fusion and splitting would therefore be possible, but the theory seems implausible with respect to double teeth in humans.

Human teeth have also been considered to be the product of both fusion and differentiation.[62] Two triconodont teeth, like those of primitive reptiles, were "concentrated", and reduction of the triconodont character as well as differentiation and partial schizodontia may explain the morphology of the different human teeth.[333 524] This theory has become obsolete.

E.D. Cope and H.R. Osborn assumed that the (pre)molars came into being by differentiation of a haplodont tooth. Over a period spanning many centuries, a mesial and distal tuberculum conus, originating from a cervical thickening (cingulum), gradually developed into full cusps. In due time, the cusps adopted a triangular pattern. Later, the other cusps differentiated from an outgrowth of the cingulum. In spite of being criticised,[529] this (adjusted) theory is the most accepted one.[333 524]

Schizodontia has been assumed to be an evolutionary phenomenon,[214] but minor variations in tooth traits are considered of more evolutionary importance than major ones such as fusion and twinning.[529] Double teeth are viewed to lack phylogenetic significance.[333]

Trauma Development of supernumerary premolars has been ascribed to jaw fractures.[419] However, double teeth have been reported in cases with no history of trauma, which casts doubt on whether trauma may be

an aetiological factor in the development of these teeth.[56 163 176 547 578]

- Trauma and (incomplete) partial schizodontia: Root duplication and hyperdontia in the permanent dentition could result from a traumatic injury to the deciduous dentition,[21] as would the duplication of a permanent incisor crown.[453] A triple tooth was attributed to a traumatically geminated permanent tooth fused with a deciduous tooth.[97] Experimentally, schizodontia appeared possible. When 20-day rabbit tooth germs were cut into two, two supernumerary teeth were formed;[400 529] tooth germs cut on day 22 did not.[529] Complete labial and lingual incisors developed 1 month after mesiodistal splitting of the odontogenic organ of rats.[659] Collectively, intrusive trauma may cause partial schizodontia.

- Trauma, crowding and fusion: Anterior deciduous tooth buds in close proximity show the highest incidence of fusion,[655] the space between them diminishing gradually on bud enlargement.[429] Forced contact between two tooth buds may cause necrosis of the intervening tissues, whereupon the enamel organs and papillae unite.[236 364 534] However, the tooth germs are neither horizontally nor vertically arranged in a straight line. Supernumeraries developing simultaneously with regular teeth lead to crowding, yet fusion rarely occurs or is not mentioned.[60 272 275 281 366 413 478 563 564 590] Fluid incompressibility may not allow the germs to merge.[430] Additionally, it has been noted that remnants of the external enamel epithelium are absent in the fused area within the teeth.[430]

Environment A relationship between double teeth and fetal alcohol exposure has been suggested.[119] Thalidomide embryopathy has also been blamed.[444] In mouse embryos hypervitaminosis A and in induced exencephaly (the brain lies outside of the skull), fusion of the enamel organs of the maxillary incisors was observed, mostly as a total fusion.[324] Administration of retinoids, the active agents of vitamin A, in 9-day mouse embryo mandibles resulted in fusion.[529] Riboflavin deficiency and triptan-blue injection had the same effect but with a lower frequency, and cyclophosphamide in extra incisors.[325 350]

Heredity Epidemiological studies do not reveal a distinct inheritance pattern with double teeth,[655] yet heredity has been implicated.[163 364 534 646] The high prevalence of double teeth in Japanese children suggests an ethnic trait. No consanguinity effect has been demonstrated in familial double teeth.[421]

An autosomal dominant and a recessive trait have been suggested.[81 116 362 377 404 437 649] The penetrance of several tooth anomalies is 90% (collectively in the deciduous and permanent dentitions), double teeth being included in this group. Based on incorrectly interpretation of family trees,[324] a Y-linked trait has been reported.[158 507] Excluding twins, familial double teeth are cited in at least 25 case reports,[28 74 81 87 91 98 116 122 220 232 267 355 400 404 436 437 475 523 586 602] [652 655] but other reports explicitly mention their absence in family members.[95 115 142 177 203 322 418 436 472 473 533 539 547 557 558] [571 605 621 623] In one survey the absence of familial double teeth was highlighted,[388] and in others a familial occurrence seemed unlikely.[116 488 597] The majority of the cited epidemiological studies and case reports do not mention double teeth in parents, siblings and second- and third-degree family members. No report on heredity seems available for permanent posterior double teeth.

Relatives of Japanese children with "fusion" have been found to have a higher rate of tooth anomalies (peg-shape, hypodontia) than in the general population.[507] Among inbred dogs several tooth anomalies were present, including double teeth.[262] The presence of tooth number anomalies, such as hyperdontia, in family members of patients with double teeth[81 119] might be meaningful.

Twins The study of twins may help to disclose the relative contributions of heredity and the environment.[604] Assuming that double teeth are inherited, mirroring in a set of monozygotic twins might be explained by, for instance (1) asymmetry-determining genes, (2) late cleavage of the embryos,[560] and (3) differences due to a modestly incomplete penetrance of double teeth.[334] Monozygotic twins may differ as does a single child's left and right sides,[604] and may experience different prenatal environmental (different birth weight!) and perinatal circumstances, such as oxygen deficiency in the second-born twin.[334]

The nine reported monozygotic twins showed mirror-image and discordant double teeth.[116 334 418 420 521 526 581 559 602] In a tenth, one monozygotic twin had normal teeth, as did the relatives, and the other had a double tooth.[526]

1.4.4 Pathogenesis

Fusion takes place during the initiation-morphodifferentiation stage.[512] Inbred dogs have a variety of dental anomalies, among which are double, triple and macrodont teeth. When the interdental lamina splits near an adjacent tooth germ, a supernumerary (geminated) tooth develops from the remnants of the lamina.[263]

Hypothetically, mitotic activity in the dental lamina presses its cells together into bulging masses (primordia) within a confined space. Per quadrant, space exists for just five bulges, from which the deciduous teeth develop, leaving room for no more than the eight primordia for the permanent dentition.[462] After renewed mitotic activity in the primordial cells, epithelial strands extend into the direction of the mesenchymal cells,[492] which allows the development of enamel organs by reciprocal epithelial and mesenchymal interactions.[593]

On the anterior part of the lamina, the beginnings of an incisor and the canine appear first and, posteriorly the "cheek tooth" appears first. The development of the intervening teeth starts later.[93] In contrast with the continuous anterior–posterior field (Butler), Osborn states that the tooth primordia are pre-programmed to produce the different tooth classes.[114] Based on Osborn, Yuen *et al.* postulated that a decreased hereditary proliferation of the clone cells in the tooth class, which cluster together with an inhibitory zone around the tooth germ, is responsible for double teeth (=fusion). Such teeth are more frequently associated with agenesis of successors than double teeth resulting from partial schizodontia.[655]

In many instances the appearance of double teeth suggests that they originate from the incisor and canine tooth classes. Perhaps the tooth class boundaries in humans, like in many species,[529] are not as distinct as thought?

Speculatively, an extra bulge might develop if there is larger space and mitotic activity, leading to a double tooth or twinning. Lack of space might inhibit the formation of a regular tooth primordium, resulting in hypodontia. If in a narrow space the normal number of tooth primordia develop, the mesenchyme may not be able to condense between two of them, making fusion possible. It may be significant that two-dimensional area measurements show decreases in the size of the maxilla associated with tooth agenesis (cause or effect?), but relatively few age groups show significant changes in mandibular size.[588] Altogether, the origin and pathogenesis of double teeth remains enigmatic.

1.4.5 Consequences

Double teeth may not erupt or hinder the eruption of adjacent or successor teeth.[108] Malpositions and misalignment of the double tooth or adjacent teeth are frequent.[576] A secondary consequence is resorption of adjacent teeth.[105] Double teeth may interfere with occlusion and articulation or may show excessive wear.[248] The notch or groove in the crown may be susceptible to caries[108 307 398] or periodontal problems if it extends to the attached gingiva.[369 398]

Combinations of double incisor teeth and a protuberance on the premolars (dens evaginatus, Chapter 2)[152] and other morphological deviations may be coincidental.[399 636]

1.4.6 Treatment

Double deciduous teeth pose a transient aesthetic problem but some were treated endodontically.[32] If they are expected to affect the succeeding teeth, they must be extracted; a space maintainer is mandatory.[173] Erupted double permanent teeth are cosmetically unattractive, and together with space problems and malpositioning, demand intervention – if possible splitting, often preceded by endodontics and followed by orthodontics.[113 128 266 277 307] [391 486 650] Surgical splitting of a double tooth into two teeth is an option when the degree of "fusion" is mild[287 405] and when one wide crown is present on two separate roots (Figures 1.19, 1.20, 1.21, 1.22, 1.23, 1.24, 1.25, 1.26,

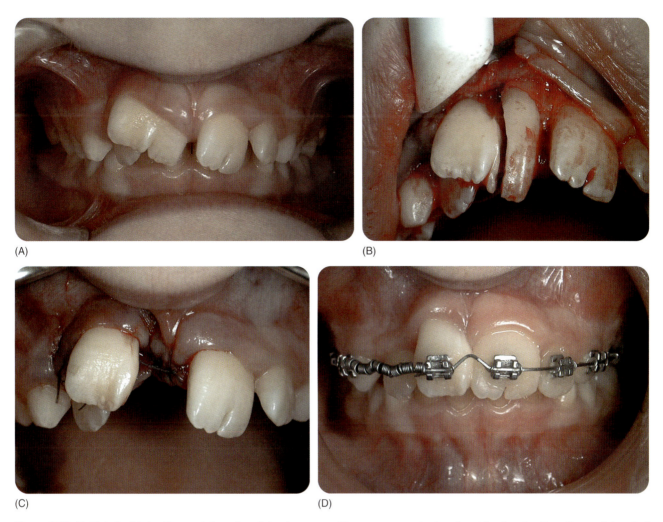

(A)   (B)

(C)   (D)

Figure 1.29 (A–D) A double tooth, consisting of conjoined crowns with a common pulp chamber. After hemisection, the mesial part of the tooth was removed and the exposed pulp was treated with direct pulp capping. The resulting diastema was closed orthodontically. (Courtesy of M.H. Ree.)

1.27, 1.28 and 1.29).[303] A double tooth was endodontically treated, extracted, split and one part was replaced.[611] A protuberance-like part of a double tooth may be reduced in size either before or after endodontics, followed by orthodontics.[303] If due to reshaping, part of the cementum is lacking, a pocket may develop or the root may resorb.[57] In the case shown in Figure 1.30, the components were separated without endodontic treatment, but the latter may be required.[247 514]

Other double teeth with a wide crown have been split and one part extracted. Treatment involving vital pulp amputation ensured completion of the root formation.[223 395] The root-to-crown ratio co-determines which part will be retained. Endodontic treatment is not required when two pulp cavities are present,[260 405] but the pulps may be horizontally connected,[557] or atubular dentine with blood vessels ("vasodentine") may connect two separate pulp chambers.[430]

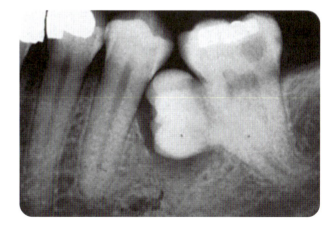

Figure 1.30 Crown of a first molar fused with a second lower molar.

The double molar crown in Figure 1.30 was removed without root canal treatment; the exposed pulp remained vital. In other cases guided tissue regeneration has been employed after splitting double teeth to promote periodontal healing.[427] Root canal treatment in permanent posterior double teeth may be complex.[606] Extraction may be required for a double tooth, but retaining the teeth seems acceptable when other treatment modalities are not suitable, as was the case with two maxillary double central incisors.[246] A multidisciplinary approach might be needed to achieve a satisfactory solution.[621]

1.5   Concrescence

Concrescence is a union of the roots of two adjacent teeth via their cementum only. Union of the cementum at the time of the odontogenesis is called *true* concrescence and that occurring post development is *false* concrescence, or alternatively "primary" and "secondary". In practice it impossible to distinguish between the two conditions.

Concrescence of two teeth (Figure 1.31) or even more has been reported.[259 312 360 370 444 534 487 534] Cementum may unite two roots when the alveolar bone between them is absent. Ectopically located tooth germs or a lack of space within the jaws seems an aetiological requirement.

Radiographs do not reveal concrescence, but it may be suspected when the roots of adjacent teeth are

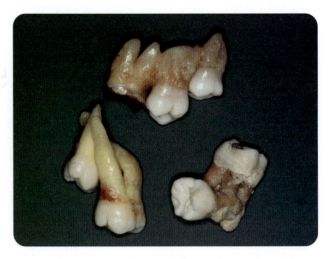

Figure 1.31 Concrescence of a second and third molar and a rare case of concrescence of three molars. The left maxillary first molar in the top panel was extracted because of extensive caries; but unexpectedly, the two other molars were extracted as well.

radiographically undistinguishable or projected on each other.[437] A consequence of this condition is that extraction, commonly of a maxillary second molar, results in removal of the conjoined tooth as well (usually the maxillary third molar). Vitality testing is difficult.[347] Prevalence data are lacking; it seems a rare phenomenon.

2

Deviations in Tooth Morphology and Size

2.1 Introduction

Morphological deviations such as *premolarisation* of the upper canines,[361] maxillary premolars resembling mandibular premolars (Figure 2.1), and *lobodontia* ("wolf teeth"), that is, enlargement of the middle labial lobe of the canine (Figure 2.2), are rare. Lobodontia may occur together with peg-shaped teeth and multi-cusp molars[344] and may also be seen in cases of renal hyperfunction.[154] Other morphological deviations are more common.

2.2 Compression

Compression is when a developing tooth cannot grow to its full size because of being pressed against a hard anatomical barrier.

2.2.1 Appearance and aetiology

Crown

The enamel organ of a compressed maxillary third molar cannot develop to its full size if it is squeezed between the tuberosity and the mineralised crown of the second molar, and the tooth therefore shows an impression of the second molar after mineralisation (Figure 2.3).[102 452] Compression of supernumerary teeth[102] is rare due to the relative position of the tooth germs in the jaws. However, diagnosis requires a certain degree of caution;[102 106] the small, mesio-distally and bucco-palatally elongated, rhomboid crown shapes of the maxillary second molar are not due to compression. Additionally, the canine fossa in the maxillary first premolar, which might guide the erupting canine into its correct place[107] is a normal characteristic of these teeth and does not represent compression.

Root

Factors assumed to cause development of excessively curved roots include anatomical constraints, ectopic location and tooth migration.[245 292 402 423 435] Angulation of

lower third molar roots has been attributed to idiopathic developmental disturbances[510] and to environmental factors and incomplete eruption, which is more prevalent in females.[501] The sickle-shaped root (Figure 2.4) is attributed to an eruption path circumventing around scar tissue during root growth. Furthermore, the lack of space and confinement within the hard tissues can supposedly lead to "corkscrew"-shaped roots (Figure 2.5), even in third molars that curve around the second molar during their eruption (Figure 2.6).

2.2.2 Epidemiology

Currently data on crown compression are scarce. Curved incisor roots are mostly caused by ectopic development,[435] but can sometimes represent *dilaceration* (Section 2.5).[423] A small disto-labial curve in the apical half of upper lateral incisor roots is a common occurrence.[77] Apical and mid-root curves are seen in 3–4% of (pre)molars.[97] In radiographic studies, 15–24% of mandibular third molar and 8–15% of the maxillary molar roots had at least a 90° mesial or distal curvature or a "bull's eye" appearance, implying a sharp buccal or lingual curvature.[179 511]

2.3 Dens invaginatus

Dens invaginatus is a developmental anomaly, a deep invagination of a portion of the enamel organ,[493] which results in deeply inverted lingual/occlusal enamel and dentine and often an unusually shaped crown. Other invaginations may originate on the apical and/or lateral tooth surfaces.

The coronally invaginated surface can be described as a deep foramen caecum, the small palatal blind pit that extends deep into the enamel (Figure 2.7). The maxillary lateral incisor is the most commonly affected tooth. The anomaly was (and still is)[224] named *dens in dente*, because radiographs portray an (additional) tooth (germ)

Pathology of the Hard Dental Tissues, First Edition. Albert Schuurs.
© 2013 Albert Schuurs. Published 2013 by Blackwell Publishing Ltd.

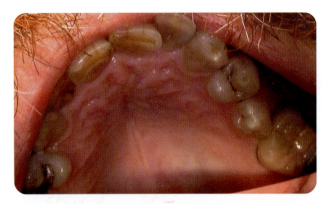

Figure 2.1 Underdeveloped lingual half (the "deuteromere") of a maxillary second premolar.

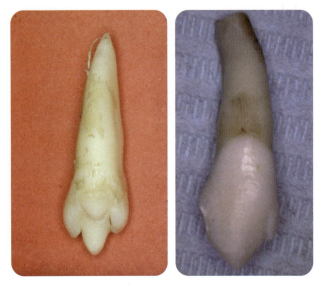

Figure 2.2 Palatal surface of a lobodont maxillary canine (lower panel) and another viewed from labial aspect (upper panel).

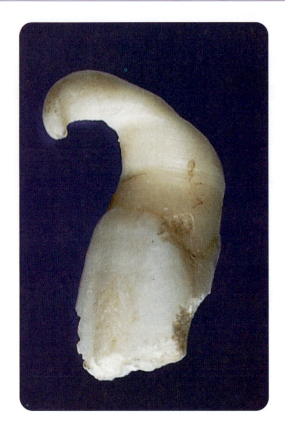

Figure 2.4 Sickle-shaped root of a permanent upper incisor.

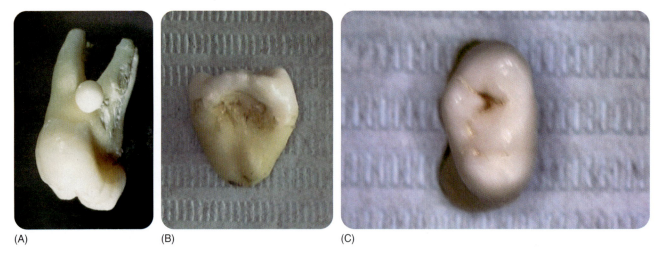

(A)   (B)   (C)

Figure 2.3 (A,B) Compression: a third molar with an underdeveloped mesial aspect due to the already calcified crown of the upper second molar being pressed against the uncalcified mesial side of the third molar during its development. Note the large enamel pearl. (C) The shape of this maxillary second molar crown – broad buccolingually but small mesiodistally – is not a result of compression, but represents the rhomboid crown type.

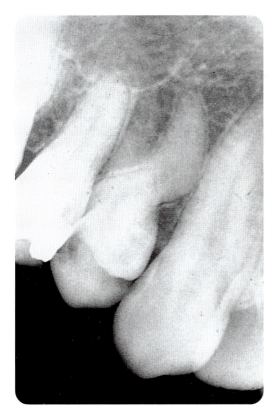

Figure 2.5 Corkscrew root form of a premolar.

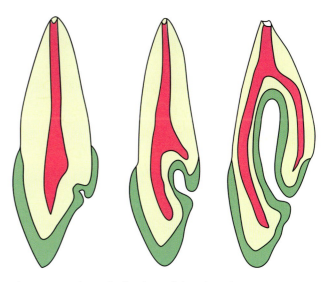

Figure 2.7 Schematic drawings of dens invaginatus: green represents the enamel, yellow the dentine and pink-red the pulp cavity. The left panel shows a lingual foramen caecum. A deepening of the foramen caecum leads to formation of dens invaginatus: if restricted to the crown of the tooth the anomaly is considered to be dens invaginatus type I (middle panel). The right panel illustrates a deep invagination (type II).

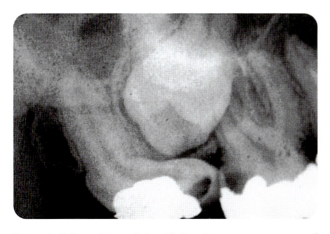

Figure 2.6 Curved root of the third molar as a consequence of erupting around the second molar.

embedded in a successor tooth,[490 496 636] that is, a "tooth within a tooth". Alternative names are *dilated composite odontome* and *gestant odontome*.

Prior to the availability of radiographic diagnostics, the maxillary lateral incisor was thought to be the only tooth affected. Other teeth seldom show this morphological aberration.[178 233 337]

2.3.1   Coronal

The invagination of the enamel and dentinal tissues creates a small palatal opening, leading to an internal pit lined with enamel.[338] The narrow entrance rapidly broadens to form the internal lumen of the invagination.[110] Other configurations also exist.

Type I invagination affects the most cervical portion of the tooth. Type II invaginations invade the root portion. Type III invaginations extend into the apex, as if it was a canal with its own apical foramen[456] with apical in-growth of cementum. A slightly different classification has also been proposed.[176] More than one type of invagination is possible on the same tooth.[333 402] Clinically, the crown is often barrel-like or tapers sharply towards the incisal edge,[154 338 400] with an unusually broad root.[40 193]

The enamel deep in the invagination is irregular, thin and poorly mineralised[319 337] with accessory canal-like channels communicating with the dentine;[174 337 392] these probably do not occur in type I invaginations.[111] The canals may be restricted to the enamel,[40 51 245] but the dentine may also show some patent defects or canals, although such structural irregularities here are few.[40 337] The pulp cavity and the lumen of the invagination most likely communicate, but this observation requires histological confirmation.[110 359] Figure 2.8 show a maxillary dens invaginatus *in situ* and the sectioned tooth and Figure 2.9 shows a mandibular invaginated tooth.

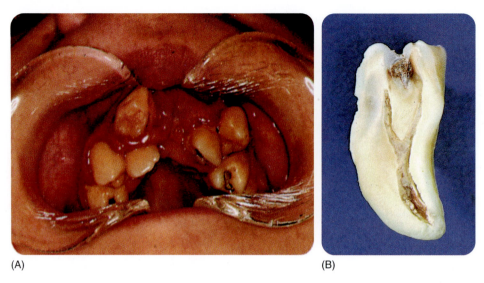

(A)   (B)

Figure 2.8 Dens invaginatus in a permanent maxillary right lateral incisor (A); and the sectioned tooth (B).

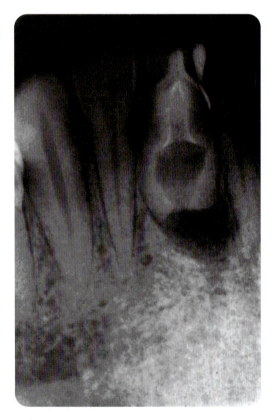

Figure 2.9 Dens invaginatus in the mandible.

Association with other anomalies
Dental invaginations are associated with double teeth,[115] [117 285 288 330 400] the presence of multi-rooted teeth,[509] shovel-shaped incisors (Section 2.9.1)[235] and the talon (Section 2.10.2);[159 339 375] the latter is sometimes referred to as dens evaginatus. Supernumerary teeth, such as the mesiodens,[512] may also have invaginations. Conversely, the invagina-

tions may also occur in normal, unaffected teeth in cases of hyperdontia.[44 51 213 392 456] Invaginations have been reported in cases of dentinogenesis imperfecta (Chapter 3),[232] in taurodontism (Section 2.12), and in cases with increased or decreased numbers of occlusal cusps, microdontia (Section 2.8) and short roots.[15 70 208 379] In some instances enamel is grossly lacking.[192] Invagination of maxillary lateral incisors is frequently associated with the bilateral presence of Carabelli's cusp on the maxillary first molars. The occurrence is less frequent with unilateral presence or total absence of the cusp[29] (Section 2.10.3). Bilateral dens invaginatus was reported in a young male patient with shovel-shaped incisors, talon and peg-shaped supernumerary incisors.[272] It has also been observed in some syndromes (Chapter 11).

2.3.2   Apical

An apical invagination can be considered as the true antipode of the coronal condition.[354] The defect is lined with cementum and it has an apical origin.[334] The longitudinally orientated, linear invagination has been considered as an anomalous counterpart of the snake's fang.[100]

2.3.3   Lateral

The lateral invagination arises in the cervical region of the tooth. It can be seen as a "tube" extending from the cervical crown surface, and is orientated towards the apex, as if it was an extra root canal.[85 105 339 401] The lateral invagination can also arise below the cervical area, on the root surface. In both cases the lumen may be lined with enamel, or also with cementum in the case of those that arise below the cervical area.[41] A lateral invagination starting below the cervix may also reach high into the crown.[424]

2.3.4 Epidemiology

Radiographs show that invaginations occur in 0.25–41% of patients.[15 24 27 137 167 170 176 177 178 202 205 234 235 259 260 331 352 365 384 395 458 476] The wide variation is largely due to the definition of this anomaly. The foramen caecum, which is present in 30–40% of the population,[249 476] should be distinguished from dens invaginatus. To date, arbitrary criteria have been used: (1) The invagination should be deeper than 1 mm[176] and (2) the broadened lumen must extend beyond the cingulum.[458] The age distribution of the sample may also skew the data due to the fact that many invaginated teeth are extracted early because of aesthetic reasons or pulpal complications. Yet, higher reported percentages seem an overestimation. The prevalence[458] of this anomaly may be as low as <0.1% in Western countries, but may be higher elsewhere. The role of familial traits and ethnic background must be recognised in view of the inherited nature of this anomaly.[41 170 171 338 379]

The coronal type II invagination was by far the most frequently encountered defect in patients referred to one university clinic.[375] Some premolars, and in one patient all of them, were invaginated.[11 59 178 225 473] Bilateral occurrence is also common,[178 375] in approximately 40% of cases.[213] Most cases occur in the maxilla, with a few in the mandible;[36 159 232 324 343] there is one report of its occurrence concurrently with agenetic incisors.[81] Invaginated lower premolars have been reported a few times.[30 52 181 225] Invaginated lower canines are very uncommon and an affected primary canine is a rare occurance.[162 194] A few deciduous invaginated teeth have been described and on one occasion, a deciduous invaginated molar.[122]

An invaginated third molar occurring with an ameloblastoma has also been documented.[238] Data on the radicular and lateral forms of invagination are scarce.[41 195 207 424] These anomalies may occur more often in patients of Chinese or Malaysian descent.[339]

2.3.5 Aetiology

The development of an invagination requires an infolding of the developing dental hard tissues prior to their calcification. The development of part of the (inner) enamel epithelium might be temporarily arrested or slowed down while the surrounding tissues continue to grow. Theories about focal growth acceleration and/or retardation[49 205 206] are merely speculative. Other factors such as localised external pressure fail to explain the occurrence of bilateral dens invaginatus.[122]

Different inheritance patterns may exist.[70 208] In one family, 43% of the parents and 32% of the children were affected.[170]

2.3.6 Consequences

Caries

The coronal entrance to the invaginated area may be predisposed to plaque accumulation, but surprisingly caries has been diagnosed in only a small proportion of cases.[167]

Pulpitis

Bacteria colonising the lumen pose a more serious threat to the pulp due to the canal-like defects that exist within the invaginated tissues.[381] The frequency of periapical infection has been said not to exceed that in normal incisors,[386] but in one study, almost 20% of invaginated teeth had periapical pathology and a further 10% became necrotic despite receiving preventive treatment.[375] Pulpitis may ensue not long after the eruption, before the apex has closed.[471] Conversely, at 18 years of age, a large proportion of the pulps are still vital;[178] this is especially true in type I invagination.[111]

Periodontal problems

Bacterial ingress into lateral invaginations that connect the oral cavity with the periodontal tissues leads to (apical) periodontitis.[41 85 207 451 456] One invagination located parallel to the root canal, and communicating with the periodontal space at the mid-root, caused a periodontal granuloma; the tooth was treated "endodontically".[168]

2.3.7 Prevention of complications and treatment

When a visible opening is noted and there is absence of pulpal pathology, sealing this entrance might suffice.[206] However, preventive measures often fail due to communicating channels with the pulp cavity, compounded by the fact that tissue present in the lumen of the invagination becomes necrotic post-eruptively. Failure of preventive therapy is not seen in type I invaginations. Preventive cleaning and filling of the lumen of the invagination appears to be the desired therapy, preferably undertaken immediately after eruption. Lining the lumen with calcium hydroxide may lower the chance of pulpal complications.[375]

The pulp cavity is very complex, with concavities, intracanal communications, inaccessible accessory canals and other anatomical irregularities,[111] and may require the complete removal of the invaginated tissues. The anatomy, and root canal(s) openings that are difficult to localise, complicate endodontic treatment, which is not always feasible.[49 59 202 383 445] Type II invaginations have been successfully treated with conventional endodontic therapy and apexification, and type III invaginations with surgical root exposure for cleaning and obturation.[45 53 111 136 153 159 266 418 450 469 503] Apical curettage or resection may have a favourable outcome[438] but success is dependent on many factors. Extraction was the favoured therapy in previous years,[205] but this fate – in some cases – may still be inevitable.[87]

2.4   Palato-gingival groove

The *palato-gingival groove*, a type of invagination, is a sharp, somewhat irregular, funnel-like groove, running from the palatal enamel of the crown and extending along the root. This particularly occurs in the permanent maxillary lateral incisors. Labio-radicular grooves also occur.

2.4.1   Appearance

The groove (Figure 2.10) commonly starts at the junction of the marginal ridge and the cingulum, and then continues along the proximal surface of the root, extending to the apical third of the root[251] or to the apex itself. The groove may be visible on radiographs as a narrow radiolucent line.[486] Internally, the pulp cavity contour may be altered, with sparse enamel and dentine and increased cementum thickness. Occasionally the pulp cavity may communicate with the periodontal space.[251] The groove may be so deep, that a bifurcation and a small, additional proximal root may be present.[251 402] Further, the cemento-enamel junction is irregular and distorted in the region of the palatal groove.

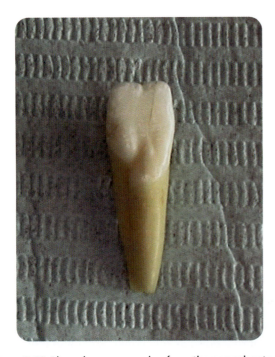

Figure 2.10 Lingual groove running from the enamel onto the root.

2.4.2   Epidemiology

Prevalence figures vary from some 2% to 8.5%. The grooves are mainly present in the maxillary lateral incisors.[228 239 356 494] Labio-radicular grooves occur mostly in the central incisors and are seldom deep or long. A groove may also be accompanied by dens invaginatus.[251 402]

2.4.3   Aetiology

The groove results from a superficial infolding of the tooth germ, the cause of which is not known, and parallels the pathogenesis of dens invaginatus, although it is less extensive. Suspected mechanisms include an undesirable location of the lateral incisor germ that is "surrounded" by the central incisor, canine and first premolar.[251]

2.4.4   Consequences and treatment

Plaque accumulates subgingivally in the groove, impairing periodontal health and disrupting the gingival attachment.[494] Flap reflection, removal of granulation tissue, grinding and flattening of the groove, followed by suturing of a polytetrafluoroethylene (PTFE) membrane has been shown to improve periodontal health.[16] Odontoplasty, that is, filling the osseous defects with hydroxyapatite, and additional use of medications (minocycline and chlorhexidine) also resolved the problem.[212] In the presence of exposed, patent dentinal tubules or lateral canals, the pulpal tissues may become infected,[251 486] possibly creating a combined endodontic-periodontal problem.[513] An abnormally shaped pulp canal will hinder endodontic treatment; and failure has been reported.[72]

2.5   Dilaceration

Dilaceration is a developmental tooth anomaly caused by mechanical trauma that tears away the calcified part of a tooth from the uncalcified part, following which ongoing mineralisation unifies the two parts at an angle to each other.

The dilacerated tooth often shows an abrupt labial change in the axial inclination between the crown and root[361 423] (Figures 2.11). The angle should be at least 20°.[510] A more apically situated dilaceration results in a tortuously curved root (Figure 2.12). A non-traumatically caused curved or bent root is considered to represent compression (see above).

2.5.1   Aetiology

Mechanical injuries that displace deciduous incisors may damage the tooth germ of the successor teeth, most fre-

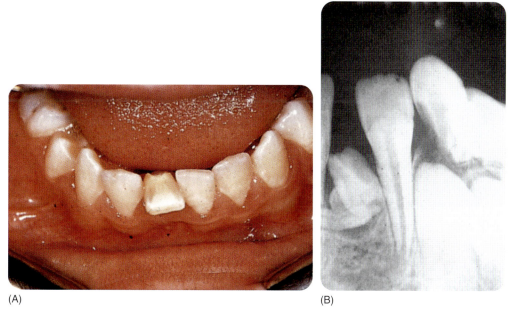

Figure 2.11 (A) Dilacerated crown of a mandibular permanent lateral incisor; the lingual surface is visible instead of the labial surface. (B) X-ray showing a dilacerated tooth.

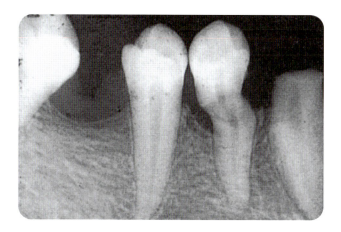

Figure 2.12 Dilacerated root of a lower first premolar.

quently the maxillary central incisors (Chapter 9). The crown may be partly torn apart from the developing root, but root growth may continue, with deposition of irregular dentine.[73 151 278] Traumatic extraction of a primary first molar caused crown dilaceration of the first premolar.[294] Direct trauma to an erupting permanent tooth may also cause this deformity.[274] Almost 60% of dilacerated teeth show disturbances in amelogenesis[484] (Chapter 3).

2.5.2   Prevalence

Among samples of Chinese and Nigerian children, 0.2% had dilacerated, unerupted teeth, assumed to be the consequence of trauma.[97 345] Following trauma in the primary dentition, 1% and 3% of the successors had dilacerated roots and crown, respectively.[17 18 179 483] In an Iranian sample, 15% had dilacerations.[514] Primary teeth are seldom dilacerated.[237] Bilateral dilaceration exists.[261]

2.5.3   Consequences

A dilacerated crown, if erupted, compromises the aesthetics and may show enamel defects (exposing the dentine, which hastens pulpal infection) and a distorted form. Dilacerated roots interfere with endodontic treatment, orthodontics and extraction.

2.5.4   Treatment

When the eruption is delayed, the tooth may be extruded orthodontically after surgical crown exposure.[121 264 328] A multidisciplinary approach may be needed[295] for cosmetic problems, problems with occlusion and articulation, and possible secondary pathology.

2.6   Enamel pearls and enamel extensions

2.6.1   Enamel pearls

An *enamel pearl* is a small oval to round enamel bulb, which may or may not have dentine and pulp tissue. It is typically found on/within the root, and sometimes on the crown. A "true pearl" consists of enamel, a "composite

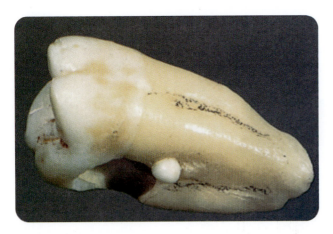

Figure 2.13 Enamel pearl.

pearl" contains dentine ("enamel-dentine pearl"), and rarely an "enamel-dentine-pulp pearl" may also occur.[321] Alternative names are enamel *nodules*, *globules*, *knots* and *exostoses*. The pearls are often small but some may be up to 4mm in diameter. They are commonly singular, but two or more pearls may be present on one (primary) tooth.[71 248 440]

A premolar of a Tibetan sheep was covered with approximately 60 pearls.[104 197] A political fugitive took the tooth to India in 1959 and was said to have belonged to a Tibetan saint and presumed to possess protective powers.

Epidemiology
Most pearls are microscopically small and covered with root cementum.[320] Larger pearls are obvious on radiographs and after extraction (Figure 2.13).

Of 2000 extracted teeth, 2.5% showed enamel pearls, a few embedded in the root and one in the crown.[71] In a radiographic study, pearls were present in about 5% of patients.[95] Macroscopically visible pearls were present on 1.6% of teeth, the majority of which were in the cervical area of the maxillary molars, especially distally. A stereo-microscopic study found enamel islets on 5% and enamel "drops" on 1.6% of multi-rooted teeth.[440] Enamel islets are exclusively located along the inter-radicular grooves, especially buccally and distally, and in the furcations.[440]

Considerably higher prevalence rates of enamel pearls have also been reported.[158] In a microradiographic study, enamel pearls were found in the furcation of one-third of deciduous molars.[21] In nine surveys, the mean prevalence was 2.7%.[321] They seem more common in people of Inuit decent (about 10%) than in other races.[321 361]

Histology
There are three types of enamel pearl: (1) pearls within the dentine that originate at the time of the dentinogen-

esis, (2) pearls on the root surface, which affect dentine formation, and (3) pearls on the root surface that do not affect dentinogenesis and easily break away.[71] The enamel structure is disorganised, but the chemical composition is normal,[21 377] although the enamel prisms running parallel to the surface are hypocalcified.[231] In contrast to larger pearls, small ones have a high content of residual enamel matrix and a low mineral content.[47] Hunter–Schreger bands are rarely visible and the striae of Retzius are irregular (Chapter 3). Pulp tissue forming in the pearls communicates with the main pulpal tissue.[231]

Aetiology
The cause and pathogenesis are uncertain. Hertwig's root sheath is suggested to preserve or recover local potential for cell proliferation and differentiation[103 321] and produce the enamel pearls. Amelogenins found in the dentinal tubules adjacent to the pearls suggest diffusion of the proteins towards the pulp,[47] but enamel protein synthesis by pulpal cells of mesenchymal origin seems possible too.[134]

The network of epithelial remnants (named after Malassez) of Hertwig's sheath could produce the pearls, but Malassez rejected this idea.[321] Perforation of the radicular pulp in young rats has been seen to cause migration of the root epithelium, which produced structures resembling the Malassez epithelial remnants. In contact with calcified osteodentine, the remnants in the pulp transformed into ameloblast-like cells that secreted amelogenin.[177] Secretory ameloblasts express over 1000 times the level of amelogenin mRNA than odontoblasts.[342]

Although beyond the scope of this book, *cementum pearls* are anomalies on the maturing enamel of continuously erupting guinea pig molars.[210] Enamel pearls should not be confused on basis of their name with *Epstein pearls*, which are keratin-filled cysts that occur in the mid-palatine raphe region close to the mucosal surface in about 80% of neonates. The cysts usually resolve within a few months.[188]

Consequences and treatment
Larger pearls may interfere with the removal of calculus and there is a risk of fracture of the tip of the scaler. Small pearls may show up on radiographs, resembling calculus.[412] Unless the pearls are associated with localised periodontal destruction,[86 155 321 422] treatment is not required.

2.6.2   Enamel extensions

An *enamel extension* is enamel running from the cervical region of the crown towards or into the furcation area of molars. Class III extensions reach the root furcation proper (Figure 2.14), class II run halfway, and class I are less deep.[293] Class III has been subdivided into IIIa, a long slender enamel projection into the furcation, and IIIb, an interrupted or discontinued projection.[506] The extensions may end in an enamel bulge (Figure 2.15), which might be considered a separate type.[401]

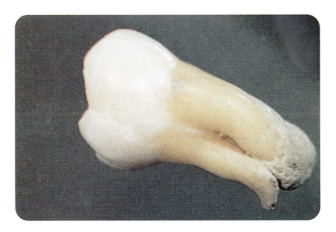

Figure 2.14 Cervical enamel extension.

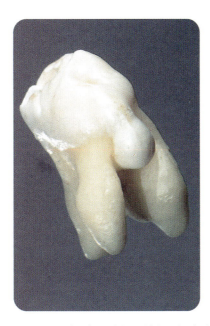

Figure 2.15 Enamel projection with a thick spherical end.

Epidemiology

The extensions occur particularly on the buccal side[190 507] in 8.3–33.6% of cases in different populations.[43 171 172 256 293 376 440 442 466 507] Mandibular second molars are particularly affected. In Asian populations, 40–78% molars have enamel projections, as do two-thirds in the Inuit population.[506] Observational studies including magnified examination (×15) show that the majority of molars possess enamel extensions. The occurrence of enamel pearls and extensions concurrently has been reported.[196] In some studies, class III extensions represented a large minority of the cases with extentions.[171 257 293] An extension on a maxillary incisor was reported to emerged through the overlying gingiva.[22]

Aetiology

The cause is either bulging out of the enamel organ or the Hertwig's sheath together with the inner and outer epithelium, the stratum intermedium and reticulum stellare, creating locally favourable conditions for amelogenesis.

Consequences

The gingiva cannot attach to the enamel and the extensions allow dental plaque to accumulate subgingivally, predisposing to periodontal disease. This may happen near or within the root furcation.[43 171 198 199 281 442] Not all researchers report extensions related to pocket formation.[256] Presence of extensions is reported in 22% of periodontal furcation problems.[43] In a group of molars, 60% had furcation problems,[488] of which more than 80% possessed extensions, generally long ones.[199 281] Pearl-like extensions encouraging local plaque stagnation can be removed after raising a flap.

2.7 Fused roots

Fused roots occur when, in principle, multi-rooted teeth share part of their root dentine. Here, root grooves essentially indicate that more roots exist and several root canals are present.

2.7.1 Aetiology

Either incomplete invaginations of Hertwig's sheath[4] or lack of space are said to underlie root fusion, although both have the same end result. Also, the more distal the teeth, the higher the probability of roots being fused.[380] Compression of the upper third molars against the maxillary sinus and the maxillary tuberosity may lead to fusion and/or distal inclination of the roots of these teeth.

2.7.2 Epidemiology

About a third of the wisdom teeth are single-rooted,[380 482] which is probably linked to ethnicity. Proportionally, more females than males have fused roots,[201 380] possibly due to smaller cranial dimensions. Single-rooted molars, in particular the third molars, are present in 3–8%[380] or 30% of European Caucasians, usually bilaterally. In Chinese populations, the roots of 30–50% of the mandibular second molars are completely fused,[200 201 485] and in 5% in North Americans.[393] Complete root fusion occurs in 1–5% of maxillary first molars in Chinese populations.[200 201] Complete and incomplete root fusion is common in China.[200 201 502] Elsewhere, fusion of the two buccal roots of the maxillary second molar was present in 2% of cases.[393] In the USA, 0.5–3% of maxillary second molars are two-rooted and 6–12% are single-rooted.[263]

2.7.3 Consequences

Teeth with fused roots show marginal periodontitis significantly more often than those without root fusion, possibly because of the root grooves.[200 201]

2.8 Macro- and microdontia

Teeth may be comparatively large (macrodontia) or small (microdontia). To define aberrant tooth measurements, statistical analysis of data may need to be done, using the mean score in the population and the standard deviation.

2.8.1 Normal tooth size

The normal variability in tooth size is not formally defined.

Tooth measurements (essentially the mesio-distal tooth width) are ethnically determined.[38] Inuit have larger teeth than European Caucasians and Australian Aboriginals. Some Native American tribes and African Americans have even larger teeth.[25] Whether females have smaller teeth than males is open to debate.[38 143 317 364 403] The mesio-distal size of the teeth is significantly larger in Swedish and Japanese boys than in girls,[279 346] but others have not found such a difference.[409] The effect of the tooth size growth-promoting factors on the Y-chromosome exceeds that of factors acting on the X-chromosome.[13] Females with only one X-chromosome have smaller teeth than those with two, this being due to thinner enamel,[478] and men with two X-chromosomes also have larger teeth.[29 461] The relationship between sex and tooth size might be indirect because body length and tooth size seem associated,[357] although this is not the case in Pygmies.[131] However, tooth length and body size might not be related.[419]

Tooth size has varied through the centuries.[135 253] In the past the size decreased, possibly due to polygene mutation,[300] and additive effects of marriage, diet, and so on. In European males the reduction has taken place over the last 15 000 years and over about 12 000 years in females. The "feminisation" (less in African Americans) of men's teeth might represent a regression to the mean.[419] The crown size of the permanent teeth of Norwegian children living between the fourteenth and eighteenth centuries were smaller than present day, possibly related to improved nutrition and reduced morbidity. Prenatal conditions such as premature birth, short birth length and low birthweight are associated with smaller teeth (decreased crown dimensions in white girls and black boys).[515] Teeth might not develop to their maximum genetically determined size through interference from exogenous chronic stress factors.[267] Fluorosis illustrates the effect of environmental influence (smaller teeth, fewer obvious pits and fissures),[2 163 215 273 500] in the same way as tooth asymmetries and variations in monozygotic twins.[83 413 415] However, tooth sizes in monozygotic twins are remarkably similar compared with those in dizygotic twins and controls.[222]

Tooth size in part is inherited[462] and seems polygenetically determined. The mesio-distal and labio-lingual measurements of the incisors are likely independent from each other, in contrast to those of the (pre)molars.[144 241 463] Within a tooth class, incisor and (pre)molar measurements are highly correlated.[235] In short, there are conflicts between the various theories.[182] The presence of a small element in a tooth class is compensated by enlargement of another tooth in that class,[182] and some "compensation" for an agenetic tooth has been established,[141 426] recognising environmental influences.[425]

2.8.2 Macrodontia

Macrodontia implies that either one dimension of a tooth, the whole tooth, several teeth or the whole dentition exceed(s) the mean measurements considerably. Average-sized teeth in small jaws are common: the teeth seem large and the condition is called *generalised relative macrodontia*. The difference between the cumulative mesio-distal crown widths and the available space depends on the dental arch dimensions (length, width and perimeter) and determines the degree of primary crowding of the teeth.[370]

Generalised true macrodontia exists when all teeth are "objectively" large in general, without any other morphological aberrations. Statistical criteria are rarely used. Macrodontia, which is defined separately in males and females, has been considered as exceeding the mean mesio-distal length plus 3.5 times the standard deviation. It has been reported in about 2% of the deciduous and permanent teeth of Japanese people.[356] On the one hand, only one tooth or some (bilateral) teeth may be too large.[382 412] On the other hand, only one measurement of a single tooth may be excessively large,[412] for example, overall length.

Aetiology

The rare generalised true macrodontia is probably caused by genetic and environmental factors. Causative factors are: pituitary gigantism in which the tooth size is proportional to the enlarged jaws,[412] pinal hyperplasia, otodental syndrome, XYY karyotype in males (Chapter 11) and type 1 (insulin-resistant) diabetes.[382] *Segmental odontomaxillary dysplasia* (overdeveloped half of the face (about 250 patients)[234] is now called *hemihyperplasia*.[165] This syndrome, in association with soft-tissue disorders (*hemi-maxillofacial dysplasia*), shows macrodont teeth at the affected site, in particular the canines, premolars and first molar. Additionally, the crowns and roots of the maxillary primary molars are enlarged on one side; the primary teeth have a tendency to exfoliate early,[19 35 93 116 348 363] but not in all cases.[369] Unilateral angiomas, which are tumours made up of blood or lymph vessels, may be accompanied by macrodontia.[391] Unilateral macrodontia also occurs without facial hypertrophy.[361]

Macrodontia may occur independent of other abnormalities in development. Macrodont mandibular third molars with unerupted second molars[52] were seen in a patient with other macrodont teeth, multiple cusps, occlusal central cusps and invaginations.[124] "Multiple macro-

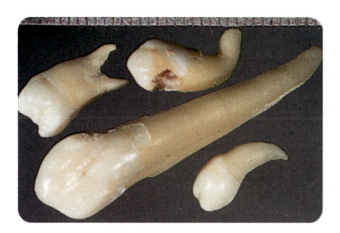

Figure 2.16 Macrodont permanent upper canine (38 mm) and some microdont third molars.

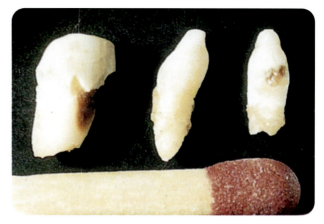

Figure 2.17 Microdont teeth (the partly visible matchstick is of regular size).

dontic multi-tuberculism" is called *Ekman–Westborg-Julin syndrome*,[289] although is not a syndrome.[37]

Macrodont second deciduous molars and first permanent molars which had a wrinkled appearance have been reported in a 5-year-old, fifteenth-century child of native American origin (Virginia, USA). In addition, large shovel-shaped maxillary central incisors, dens invaginatus, agenetic teeth and other dental anomalies were also reported.[289] Patients today also show the same aberrations or variants.[37 326 378 505]

The aetiology of an isolated macrodont tooth (Figure 2.16) is unknown. The relationship with supernumerary teeth in males[54] may be misleading, since macrodont teeth might be considered double teeth. However, to diagnose a double tooth as macrodontia[145] is incorrect. A few examples of individual macrodont teeth have been published, including a 50 mm long canine and lower premolars with a mesio-distal length of 10–15 mm,[74 118 189 275 368 388] some with multiple cusps and tapering roots, all of unknown aetiology.[412] A broad central incisor with a normal crown and two root canals might be macrodont[60] or a double tooth. Among 1000 Chinese patients, 1% had one or more macrodont teeth,[97] but among about 3000 Turkish orthodontic patients only one possessed a macrodont maxillary central incisor.[516]

As mentioned above, in macrodontia, only one tooth measurement/dimension may exceed the normal reference standard. For instance, two excessively broad lateral incisors have been reported.[101] Exposure *in utero* to anticonvulsant drugs for epilepsy is associated with a significantly increased mesio-distal crown diameter of specifically the primary molars.[347]

Rhizomegaly refers to a very long root in an otherwise normal-sized tooth.

2.8.3 Microdontia

Microdontia is a considerable diminution in the tooth size and often morphology, and comprises reduction of either one tooth dimension, one or several teeth, or the whole dentition. *Generalised true microdontia* is rare and occurs as part of some syndromes. The teeth may be conical in shape as in oligodontia.[398] *Generalised relative microdontia*, that is, large jaws with small teeth, is not the same as true microdontia. Just a few teeth may be microdont (Figure 2.17), such as conical or peg-shaped upper lateral incisors and small third molars – the teeth that are also often agenetic.[154]

Aetiology

Microdontia is a solitary autosomal dominant trait[432] with variable gene expression or incomplete penetrance, and other modes of inheritance.[349] A probable X-linked combination of microdontia, taurodontism and dens invaginatus has been reported.[70] Microdontia and macrodontia were found to manifest simultaneously in one female patient with agenetic teeth and persisting deciduous teeth, of which four were peg-shaped. The dermatoglyphs were also abnormal in this patient. It may be an autosomal recessive genetic disorder in females; in this report, the patient's sister had hypodontia and microdontia.[327]

Replacement of natal teeth with unusually small successors suggests a mutual cause.[291] Small teeth with a diminished number of occlusal cusps were noted on the affected side in a patient with hemifacial microsomia, which is caused by a vascular aberration in the early embryonic development of the first and second branchial arches or due to altered neural crest cells.[129] In some hereditary types of amelogenesis imperfecta (Chapter 3) the teeth with thin enamel are also small in size. Microdontia also occurs in several syndromes,[23] and inherited anaemia due to hypoactive bone marrow is another cause.[213]

The distal element within each tooth group develops only after the first element within the group has started to develop. Microdontia of solitary teeth, like the maxillary lateral incisors might be explained by environmental influences, interaction with other tooth germs, and anatomical constraints. When a tooth within a given group is large, the next developing tooth may be small or absent,[425] but such compensations are denied.[236]

Microdontia is not necessarily inherited.[302] Hypopituitary dwarf growth, hypothyroidism and gonad hyperfunction are associated with retarded tooth development and generalised microdontia.[154 412 416] In premature, low birthweight children, the mesio-distal and bucco-lingual measurements are 6–11% smaller than in children born at term. The maxillary lateral incisors on the left side are more severely affected than the right.[409] Treatment of a neoplasm with radiotherapy (and/or chemotherapy) can cause microdontia (see Rhizomicry below),[226 334] for example children treated at age 6–8 years with 10 Gy prior to transplantation of bone marrow.[92]

Epidemiology

The prevalence of conical upper lateral incisors varies by country and ethnicity,[54] and is associated with morphological deviations in other teeth, like a lower number of lower molar cusps.[254] One or more microdont or conical teeth have been found in 0.1–4.3% of ethnically different populations.[6 12 69 97 331 346 395] Microdontia, defined as the average mesio-distal length minus 3.5 times the standard deviation, is present in about 2% of the permanent and deciduous teeth of Japanese children.[346]

In women, inherited microdontia and hypodontia appears to be linked. Conical central incisors and mandibular premolars[6 475] are very rare. For example, 0.07% of the mandibular lateral incisors were reduced in size and 1.5% were peg shaped in an orthodontic sample.[516]

Rhizomicry

Rhizomicry, a specific tooth anomaly,[214] means "short-rooted" (crown-to-root ratio 1:1.6). Notably, the roots of the permanent maxillary central incisors may be shorter than the crowns (Figure 2.18). The maxillary central

incisor has an average length of 23.6 mm (range 16.5 mm to 32.6 mm).[498]

Short blunt-rooted posterior teeth, in particular the premolars, were present in 1.3% of cases in one study, often occurring in pairs.[20] Rhizomicry was seen in 10% of a sample of Japanese children and in about 2% of Swedish children; the roots were short and plump.[459]

Heterogeneity in eight pedigrees with short roots and other dental aberrations, such as hypodontia and taurodontism, do not allow definitive conclusions to be made about the mode of inheritance.[20] A patient with short roots in nearly all permanent teeth had experienced a severe attack of erythema multiforme (Stevens–Johnson syndrome).[109] Short roots on small teeth with large pulp canals were present in a hypodont dentition of a mentally retarded girl with a short height.[32] The combination of a short height with short roots and taurodontism has been reported several times.[140 208 397 497] Short roots are also reported as a trait in several generations of two families.[265]

Short, plump roots may resemble an onion, which in architectural terms is called "ogee", thus *ogee roots* (Figure 2.19). Ogee roots (autosomal dominant) were present in a family with hypodontia, rhizomicry and microdontia.[459]

Aetiology

Rhizomicry (and microdontia) after radiotherapy at a young age includes root blunting and mandibular hypoplasia.[133 226] Radiotherapy arrests the root growth through early apical closure or atrophy of the odontoblasts.[55 56 58 63 120 123 166 191 298 360 390 446 447 474 491] In extreme cases, irregular dentine covered with acellular cementum is formed at the bottom of the pulp chamber.[446] In one study it was not clear whether radiotherapy or chemotherapy caused the short roots.[349] Markedly short roots were observed after treatment with 27 Gy at the age of 3 years.[61] Chemotherapy at age 1–6 years of age was noted to have affected the dentition of more than half of the children in another study, and in around 25% at 6–12 years, causing microdontia, shortened roots, and delayed dental develop-

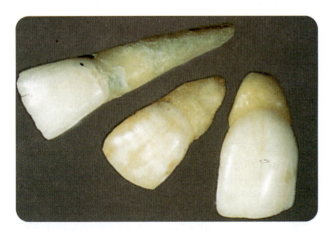

Figure 2.18 Permanent upper central incisors with microdont roots (rhizomicry) and an incisor (top) with average root length.

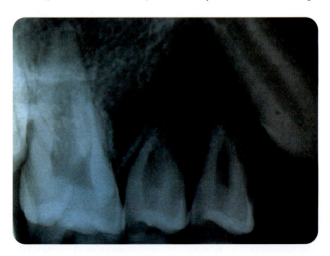

Figure 2.19 Radiograph of upper premolars with "ogee" roots.

ment.[314] Doses larger than 20 Gy damage the tooth germ, but dental anomalies may already appear with a dose exceeding 4–5 Gy.[61] Rhizomicry can also be idiopathic.[190] [258] [323] [446] Shortened, blunt roots may also occur as a consequence of orthodontic treatment (Chapter 7).

Short roots are seen in a number of syndromes and in dentinogenesis imperfecta, radicular dentine dysplasia, (pseudo)hypoparathyroidism (Chapter 3),[79] [417] [439] [497] herpes zoster[420] (in which the chicken pox virus remains in various ganglia, and causes repeated eruptions of cutaneous vesicles), circumscribed scleroderma (locally thickened skin) and dwarfism.[32] Short, thin ("spiky") roots are reported in thalassaemia.[517] [366] In homozygotic β-thalassaemia (Chapter 3) the middle part of the face, especially the maxilla, has a tendency to prognathism.[99] Not much is known about the effect of gene mutations on root development. Only one pathway that regulates the root development has been identified. Gene disruption in experimental mice compromised molar root growth and the development of the incisors.[431]

Treatment

Crowding as a consequence of generalised macrodontia is an indication for extraction therapy and orthodontics. Nevertheless, the individual circumstances should dictate the treatment in cases with few macrodont teeth.

Peg-shaped microdont lateral incisors may be treated cosmetically. In patients with indications for premolar extraction, one may extract microdont incisors, orthodontically move the canines into their place and reshape them to resemble the incisors. An alternative is to build up small teeth with composite resin after creation of additional space.[68] Relative microdontia is not treated "per se".

2.9 Other developmental anomalies of the tooth crowns

2.9.1 Shovel-shaped incisor

*Shovel-shaped incisor*s are characterised by thickening of the lingual aspects of the proximal ridges and an enlarged cingulum, with sometimes two cingula. The thick enamel makes the crown resemble a shovel (Figure 2.20). The diagnosis requires exact measurement of the depth of the lingual fossa above the cingulum: shovel-shape incisors have been classified from 0 (absence of enamel ridges and cingulum) to 3 (pronounced ridges and cingulum).[465] A labial shovel shape is uncommon.[79]

Epidemiology

No effect of "racial inbreeding" in an isolated Inuit population has been established,[1] but the anomaly is ethnically linked. Shovel-shaped incisors have been noted in a large

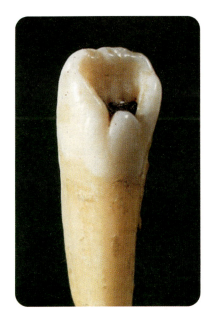

Figure 2.20 Shovel-shaped maxillary lateral incisor with a central amalgam filling.

majority of Chinese, Inuit, Pima Indian, Japanese and many Polynesian subjects,[310] predominantly in the maxillary lateral incisor. The prevalence of shovel-shaped incisors in Chinese people living in southern Taiwan is about 80%.[204] Although not a typical Asian ethnic trait, there are indications that it once was, and that migration and racial inter-breeding underlie its dissemination from Central Asia.[106]

A dichotomy exists in Asian dental traits. The sinodont pattern in northeast Asia is distinct from the sundadont pattern in the southeast. Thought to have evolved from the sundadonts (not in Thailand),[287] the teeth of the sinodonts, are more complex than those of the sundadonts, which are in turn more complex than the teeth of Caucasians. In particular, shovelling is seen more often in the sinodont pattern.[197] Prehistoric skulls show shovelling in 60–70% of the Inuit, 80–90% of Native Americans of the West coast and 90–100% of all other prehistoric Indians, which sustains the idea that America became populated via three successive migration waves, the first wave being some 15 000 years ago, the second 12 000 years ago and the third much later.

Shovel-shaped incisors have been reported in several populations: Syrian (5%), Jordanian (5%), Pakistani and Saudi Arabian (9%), Indian (12%), Sudanese and Yemenite (20%), and Egyptian (24%).[157] The occurrence is less frequent and less apparent in some other populations. Depending on the subjects studied, 1–10% of Caucasians in the USA show shovel-shaped incisors.[23] [63] [136] [203]

In view of the variability of the anomaly and a poorly correlated occurrence in parents and children in regions where shovel-shaped incisor prevalence is infrequent, the cause may be polygenetic.[173] There is a discontinuous distribution and it is also probably influenced by environmental factors.[23]

Treatment
Caries at the site of the anomaly is easily treated or prevented.

2.9.2 T-shaped, Y-shaped and stellate incisors

The *T-shaped incisor* has an outgrowth of the cingulum to the extent that is horizontally connected to the incisal edge. The *Y-shaped incisor* has an extension arising from the labial cervical region, again to the extent that it is horizontally connected to the incisal edge. The *stellate incisor* is a combination of the T-shape and Y-shape. It cannot be excluded that the T-shape (Figure 2.21) and Y-shape (Figure 2.22) crowns are the result of fusion with a conical additional tooth,[338] as shown in Chapter 1, Figure 1.25. The rare stellate incisor – an incisor with palatal and labial extensions – has been described, for instance, in a girl with Down's syndrome (Chapter 11).[175]

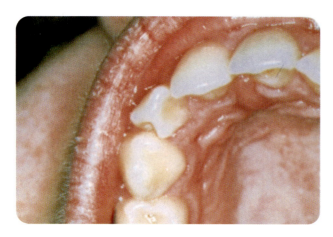

Figure 2.21 T-shaped permanent maxillary lateral incisor.

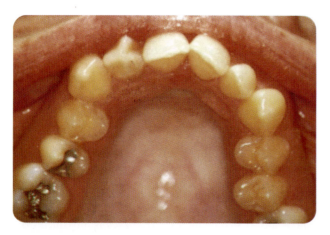

Figure 2.22 Y-shaped permanent maxillary lateral incisor. The combination of the T- with the Y-shape results in a crown resembling a crosshead screwdriver.

Treatment
Treatment depends on the problems being caused by the anomaly. If occlusion and/or articulation are compromised, the interference should be removed. The labial Y-shape is more of a cosmetic concern, which can be improved by removing the excess tooth substance and restoring the normal shape of the crown with composite.

2.10 Extra cusps

Additional cusps are in some teeth the rule rather than the exception, for instance maxillary first molars with Carabelli's cusps (Figure 2.23) in Caucasians and mandibular second premolars with two lingual cusps. Interestingly, 10% of the mandibular second premolars have three buccal cusps (triconodont), which represents not so much an anomaly but a normal variant.[107] Occurring less frequently is the third lingual cusp (*tuberculum intermedium*), which is found in the lower first molars between the two lingual cusps, and a sixth cusp (*tuberculum sextum*), which is located at the marginal ridge between the distal and the disto-lingual cusps. Such interstitial, extra occlusal cusps are of paleontological importance.

2.10.1 Dens evaginatus

Dens evaginatus in a (pre)molar describes the presence of an extra occlusal, often slender, conical cusp, consisting of enamel, dentine and a pulpal extension about half way up into the projection (outfolded enamel organ).[496]

Dens evaginatus is also known as Leongs' premolar (after M. Leong), Mongoloid or Oriental premolar (because of the occurrence in east and southeast Asia), odontome of the axial core type, simplest type of composite dilated odontome, occlusal enamel pearl, evaginated odontome, interstitial tubercle and tuberculated premolar/premolar.

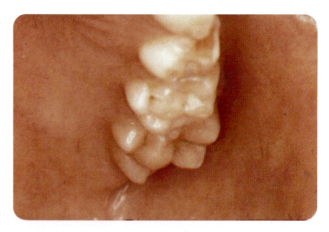

Figure 2.23 Carabelli cusps on the mesio-palatal surface of the permanent maxillary first and second molars.

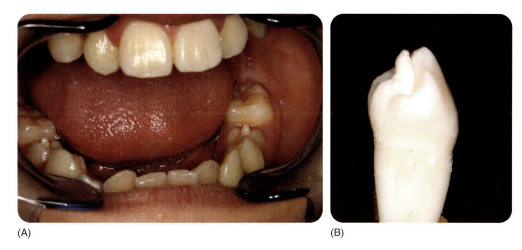

Figure 2.24 (A) Bilateral dens evaginatus. (B) A conical evagination.

Appearance

Dens evaginatus (Figure 2.24) has two subclasses: one group where projections arise from the central fissure and another group with projections arising buccal or labial to the fissure.[309] Anterior teeth with palatal projections have been classified as dens evaginatus,[94 139 148 518] but may represent a different deviant morphology (talon, Section 2.10.2).

After fracturing or wearing away, hardly any sign of the conical projection is left.[374] As the occlusal pit present may be very small,[78] pain due to pulp exposure then poses a diagnostic challenge.[430] A substantially large tubercle does not tend to break away.[402] The average height of an intact tubercle is 3 mm, with a 1.5 mm diameter at its base. In 50%, pulp extensions reach into the enamel. Dens evaginatus usually occurs bilaterally.

Epidemiology

Dens evaginatus presents, in particular, on the mandibular premolars.[34 88 252 309 402 504] In order of decreasing prevalence, projections are found on maxillary premolars, molars, canines (?) and incisors (?),[251 367] and to a lesser extent on the mandibular canine.[9] This aberration is also present in the deciduous dentition.[346]

Dens evaginatus is most common among Asian populations, with a prevalence of 1–6%,[33 88 252 309 346 374 436 504 519] more frequently in females than in males, and seldom occurs in Caucasians or Africans.[350 355 444] Due to migration from Asia, the incidence in other countries may be increasing.[146] Reported prevalences may be compromised because the teeth may have been extracted soon after their eruption due to caries, pulpal complications or other reasons.

Pathogenesis

Proliferation and evagination of the enamel organ is necessary for this anomaly to occur[88 296 437] but the reasons

are not known. Families with an autosomal dominant and X-linked inheritance have been reported.[296 436]

Consequences

The tubercle or projection may break off or wear away soon after the eruption, owing to the contact with an antagonist tooth. The rate of pulp necrosis, which usually happens before complete root formation, is 3–40%.[34 75 309 421 504] Cessation of root growth has been observed.[322]

Treatment

Prior to contact with an antagonist, a stepwise grinding of the tubercle[227] to promote the formation of reparative dentine in the pulp extension will prevent unpredictable pulp exposure.[518] In the first session the apex of the tubercle is cut away just into the dentine; in following sessions, at intervals of approximately 2 months, grinding is repeated until the tubercle does not interfere anymore with occlusion.[75] Grinding may, however, contribute to secondary infection of the pulp.[146]

The treatment option depends on the stage of root formation. When fracture/wear or treatment leads to exposure of the pulp, endodontic therapy can range from direct shallow pulpotomy using a layer of mineral trioxide aggregate, which induces hard-tissue formation more predictably than calcium hydroxide, to extirpation with apexification.[455 518] Partial pulpotomy with trioxide aggregate has been successful[240] and may secure the root growth.[296 297]

One-visit removal of the evagination followed by an occlusal amalgam filling after (in)direct pulp-capping[493] was found to result in pulpal complications 5% of the time, whereas a similar procedure with a shallow composite restoration had a failure rate of 0.5%. No treatment has had a better outcome than treatment with composite.[421] Alternatively the evagination may be covered with acrylic resin,[227] but the reliability of this method has been questioned.[221 252 296 322 373] Also, as the base of the tubercle may be enclosed by a layer of bonded composite, the disadvantage is that this prevents wear of the tubercle and the tooth remains infra-occluded.[449 499]

A dens evaginatus is the primary candidate for extraction when orthodontic treatment is indicated. Orthodontic treatment may be delayed when an unerupted dens evaginatus is suspected,[296] but pre-eruptively, the anomaly is rarely visible on radiographs.[296]

2.10.2   Talon

The *talon* is an accessory, curved cusp on, or outgrowth of the cingulum of, incisors and canines, consisting of enamel and dentine, with or without a pulp extension. The name derives from its resemblance with the eagle's talon.

Appearance

Talons occur most frequently on the permanent maxillary incisors.[173 448 467] The often horn-like beak (Figure 2.25A) projecting away from the tooth, consists of enamel and dentine and may[173 220 283 303] or may not[284 339 394] contain a thin pulp extension. A talon on a deciduous tooth showed a radiographic pulp extension that could not be detected clinically after grinding.[305]

A talon is identical to dens evaginatus,[303] and is also called "dens evaginatus of anterior teeth".[94 139 148 299 406 407] Here, dens evaginatus and talon cusp are described separately because their aetiology may differ. Several labial talons are reported,[3 220 299 470] but a figure in one of the reports[3] suggests "fusion" of a mesiodens with a regular central incisor (Figure 1.25). One patient had a tooth with a labial and palatal talon,[3] and another patient a palatal talon on one maxillary central incisor and a labial talon

on the contralateral tooth.[112] Incisal wear of a long talon might transform the tooth into the T-shaped incisor.[283 412] A labial talon in a child[470] may also be confused with a Y-shaped incisor.

In order to call the "protrusion" talon, its height must be at least half that of the crown height.[98] A talon seldom reaches above the incisal edge. Deep grooves exist laterally at the point where the protrusion originates.[283] A smaller "protrusion", named a *semi-talon*, is minimally 1 mm high, and does not extend beyond half of the coronal height (Figure 2.25B). Minimal "protrusions" are called *trace talons*.[185] The latter two do not posses the typical talon form. Bifid talons (a cusp split in two) also occur.[46]

Aetiology

The aetiology of the anomaly is not known. The presence of the talon in two members of one family suggests an inherited origin,[307 405] as do talons in the deciduous maxillary incisors in female twins.[268] Epidemiological data also point to an ethnic trait.

A talon could be the result of either fusion with an extra peg-shaped tooth, or an outward folding of the enamel organ (Chapter 3), or a focal hyperplasia of the mesenchymal dental papilla. The talon may originate lingual to the cingulum[284] or represent an outgrowth of the cingulum itself.[140] In some patients with a talon, the dentition showed hyperdontia,[113 325] supporting the idea of fusion as aetiology.

Epidemiology

With lesser strict criteria, the talon is certainly not an exception. In the deciduous dentition, it affects primarily the central incisors.[94 98] Formerly, reported patients only numbered in dozens,[185 467] often Chinese adults and children,[76 97 98] but it has been suggested the anomaly is not

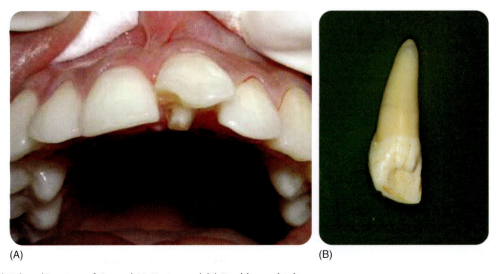

(A)   (B)

Figure 2.25 (A) Talon. (Courtesy of Gregori M. Kurtzman.) (B) Double semi-talon.

rare.[271] Indeed, prevalence of talons have been reported as 0.6–5.2% in different, especially east Asian, populations.[93 286 389 404 414 465] In an eleventh-century Hungarian population 40% had talon versus 2.5% at present.[520]

Talon appears twice as frequently in males than females,[94] but in a Malaysian population, a sex difference was not observed.[389] One-fifth of talons are bilateral and 75% of cases are seen in the permanent dentition. Talons show a predilection for the maxilla, with two-thirds of cases affecting the lateral incisors and a quarter affecting the central incisors.[76 184 185 405]

Talons are seen in some syndromes with hypodontia and hyperdontia and disorders of eruption.[157 371] They were present in two siblings with Ellis–van Creveld syndrome[186] (a coincidence?). There is an association with variations in tooth number without the presence of a syndrome,[329] seemingly in the majority of cases.[185] Talon may be associated with other dental aberrations,[98 283 329] such as shovel-shaped incisors and three-rooted deciduous and permanent mandibular molars.[5] Talon has been observed in an individual with an odontoma, dens invaginatus, exaggerated Carabelli's cusps and microdontia.[173] Another combination that has been reported is talon with dens invaginatus, short-rooted central incisors and premolars, and pyramidal roots of second molars.[301] Further, a lateral incisor with two root canals and a canine with three root canals showed a talon.[126 467] Hyperdontia and double tooth both may also present with a talon.[187 508]

Talon has been observed in a supernumerary deciduous tooth, with another one in a mesiodens, while a second mesiodens was reported to have an exaggerated cingulum.[394]

Consequences

The grooves promote caries and, if extending to the root, periodontal problems could ensue. Tooth mobility is caused by premature contact. The talon may irritate the tongue, and interfere with biting and chewing,[184 306 340 362 407] and lead to displacement of teeth.[306] On radiographs of unerupted teeth, the talon may give the impression of an odontome or an extra tooth, which may lead to overzealous surgical intervention.[303] A long talon may delay the eruption of the tooth.[76]

Treatment

The treatment, if necessary, consists of gradual grinding down of the talon. In one report, 1 mm of talon that was interfering with the occlusion was removed during each of three consecutive appointments, 6 weeks apart, without exposing the pulp. The residual projection was covered with resin composite.[407] Others have removed 3 mm in one session without pulp exposure or pulpal complaints.[84]

[85 86 87 88 89 90 91 92 93 94 95 96 97 98 99 100 101 102 103 104 105 106 107 108 109 110 111 112 113 114 115 116 117 118 119 120 121 122 123 124 125 126 127 128 129 130 131 132 133 134 135 136 137 138 139 140 141 142 143 144 145 146 147 148 149 150 151 152 153 154 155 156 157 158 159 160 161 162 163 164 165 166 167 168 169 170 171 172 173 174 175 176 177 178 179 180 181 182 183 184 185 372] Capping of the exposed dentine is recommended.[18]

2.10.3 Carabelli's cusp

Carabelli's cusp is an extra cusp (or pit) on the mesial site on the palatal surface of the maxillary molars. The cusp presents as either a real protuberance (positive expression), a groove, a pit or groove (negative expression),[216] classified as type 0 (no trace), types 1 and 2 (small line or pit, no cusp), and types 3–5 (a cusp,[465] up to a height of 5.5 mm).[308]

The primary dentition possibly shows more frequent negative expression of the cusp than the permanent dentition,[423 457] but in India the reverse has been seen.[223] The prevalence is 50–90% in European Caucasians, in particular in the maxillary first molars, and generally bilaterally equivalent,[14 62 128] both in the negative and positive forms.[14 308] Japanese children have the cusp solely on the maxillary first permanent molar in 8% of the times and 12% at deciduous molars.[346] More than half of the maxillary deciduous second molars of Chinese children show the cusp, the "pit" type prevailing by far.[209 223] In a Nigerian population, a positive cusp is present in 70% of the maxillary molars.[128] The positive form is less frequent in Native Americans than Europeans. Inuit people of east Greenland grossly lack the cusp. The cusp is considered an inherited trait, but the mode of inheritance is uncertain.[160 164 246 255] Studies of monozygotic and heterozygotic twins show factors other than inheritance to play a role.

The chances of equal presence of the cusp in homozygotic twins are small,[42] however, the association is large in both dentitions.[219] The prevalence of the cusp, varying in size and expression, in mono- and di-zygotic twins was found to be 90%, determined by inheritance.[464] Phylogenetically, the tubercle is an outgrowth of the cingulum and represents a progressive and early evolutionary trait. A well-developed cusp would compensate for wear of the crown and would therefore be of evolutionary significance.[114] Whether the increase in volume of the crown is significant, is arguable.[142 230 242] Both the crown size and its form seem to be expressed, independent from Carabelli's cusp.[142] Further, the association between agenetic third molars and the cusp is thought to negate an evolutionary trend.[230]

Treatment

The groove between the cusp and the palatal surface of the molar may be at risk of a carious attack. Grooves or fissures which are caries free can be sealed with unfilled, light-cured resin.

2.10.4 Paramolar tubercle/cusp, paramolar roots, paramolars

The paramolar tubercle or cusp (*tuberculum paramolare*) is an extra cusp occurring on second and third molars and incidentally also in premolars. The tubercle is usually mesio-buccally located. A rudimentary or fully formed root, the paramolar root (*radix paramolaris*), may or may not accompany the paramolar tubercle. Presence of an extra root may be more likely when the tubercle is lobulated. In other instances, the crown and root may occur as a singular entity. This is known as a paramolar (*dens paramolaris*; see Chapter 1).

The paramolar tubercle (Figure 2.26) may manifest "positively" or "negatively":[216][465] type 0 (no sign); type 1 (a pit or wrinkle); type 2 (small cusp without a groove); type 3 (cusp without groove); type 4 (small, but positive elevation); and type 5 (well-defined cusp,[465] which may be lobulated).

Data collected on this anatomical anomaly are scarce and incomplete. The reported prevalence is between 2% and 3% in Malaysians,[249] somewhat lower in the Japanese population,[346] and surprisingly exceeds 30% in some Native American tribes. Approximately half of the wisdom teeth of Caucasians possess the tuberculum. Mesial to the third molars, the frequency becomes rare in the first molars and very rare in premolars.[216] The tuberculum tends to be present unilaterally and might be manifest in 0.1% of maxillary first molars, 0.4–2.8% of maxillary second molars and in 0–4.7% of maxillary wisdom teeth.[341]

Paramolar roots (*radix paramolaris*) are always connected with the distobuccal root and root canal of maxillary molars, at various levels.[341] In a collection of maxillary molars with paramolar roots and/or distomolar roots, approximately 70% of the supernumerary roots were identified as paramolar roots, half of them clearly separated from other roots. Where fusion was observed, the grooves were indicative of the presence of a paramolar root. Of the maxillary paramolar roots seen, 92% were in third molars, 7% in second molars and only 1% in first molars.[66]

Paramolar (*dens paramolaris*), which is an entity on its own, is associated with hyperdontia. Paramolars are not exclusively situated mesio-buccally. A solitary paramolar with a bifid crown form was located between the permanent maxillary first and second molars.[269] Distomolars may also be considered as paramolars. See Chapter 1 for epidemiological data and images of paramolars (Figures 1.13 and 1.14).

Treatment

Treatment is not necessary unless caries develops in the groove between the tubercle and the buccal surface. The tubercle may contain pulp tissue, which may or not communicate with the (disto-buccal) root canal at various levels.[341]

2.11 Supernumerary roots

Supernumerary roots is when there are one or more roots on a tooth in excess of the regular number. Anomalies in the number of roots are (assumedly) the consequence of a root cleft or an additional root.

2.11.1 Bifid roots

Bifid roots (*radix bifida*) are supernumerary radicular structures resulting from cleavage of a regular root (Figures 2.27 and 2.28). Maxillary first premolars often show two diverging buccal roots, more or less bifid-like (Figure 2.28).[256] Bifid roots probably manifest in every tooth, but some roots seem to have a predilection for cleavage (Table 2.1). Other teeth show more incidental

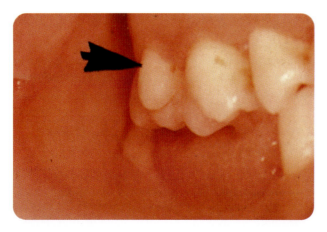

Figure 2.26 Paramolar tubercle (arrow) at the mesio-buccal surface of the permanent upper second molar.

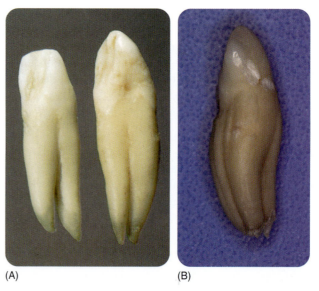

(A)   (B)

Figure 2.27 (A) Permanent upper lateral incisor (left) and lower canine (right) with bifid roots. (B) Deciduous lower left canine with three roots (in microsomia type I).

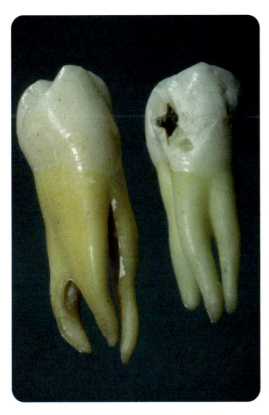

Figure 2.28 The buccal roots of these second upper premolars are split into mesial and distal parts.

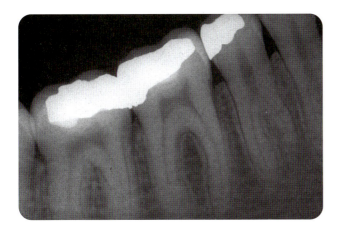

Figure 2.29 A lower second premolar with a root split into mesial and distal parts.

cleft roots, in the assumed descending order shown in Table 2.2. Besides those already mentioned, other molar roots may also be cleaved. This can manifest as a mandibular premolar with two roots (Figure 2.29) and as molars with four, five and six roots, but in some cases may just concern fusion of two teeth (Figure 2.30).

The uncommon extra root in the permanent maxillary central incisor in Figure 2.31 may represent a cleavage. A similar (or additional?) root at the lingual side of the distal root in the mandibular first molar on a radiograph

Table 2.1 The proportion of teeth with cleft roots

Tooth	Per cent	Details
Mandibular canines	8	Labial and lingual part[482] (Figure 2.27A) and three-rooted canine (Figure 2.27B)
Mandibular second premolars	7	Mesial and distal part, right side more often than left[410]
	21–46	In 45,X/46,XX women[a]
Maxillary first premolar	3	Bifid buccal root: a mesial and distal root[480] (Figure 2.28)
Mandibular first premolars	0.7	Mesial and distal root[6] (Figure 2.29)
Mandibular first premolars	29	Women with abnormal number of X-chromosomes[479]
Maxillary molars[b]	0.4	Bifid palatal root in a mesial and distal root[263]
Maxillary second premolars	0.3	Buccal and palatal root[482]

[a]Instead of the common 46,XX; the mandibular first premolar often shows a bifid root.[478 479]
[b]Rarely at the maxillary first molar and with increasing frequency at the second and third molars.[66]

Table 2.2 Teeth showing incidental bifid roots

Tooth	Details
Maxillary lateral incisors	Labial and palatal root[150 441 481] (Figure 2.27A)
Mandibular incisors	Labial and lingual root[107 315 443 489 509]
Maxillary canine[13 24 31]	Labial and palatal root, also primary canines[57 353]
Mandibular premolars	Two buccal and one lingual root[101 454]
Maxillary first molar[67]	Bifid palatal root in mesial and distal (also second and third molar)[71 354]
	Bifid mesio-buccal root in buccal and palatal part (Figure 2.30)
Mandibular first premolar	Bifid mesial root in buccal and lingual part[107]
Maxillary second premolar	Three buccal roots[127]

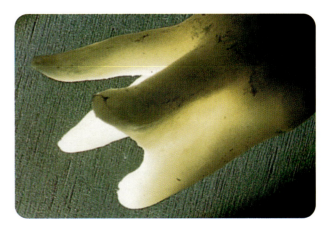

Figure 2.30 Permanent first upper molar with two mesio-buccal roots, united by a thin sheet of dentine.

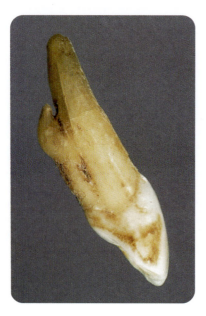

Figure 2.31 A permanent upper central incisor with an additional small-sized root.

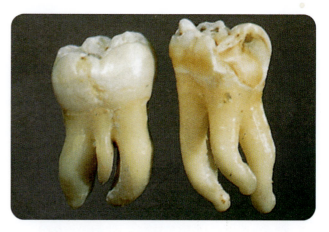

Figure 2.32 Paramolar root (left) and a lingual molar root (right).

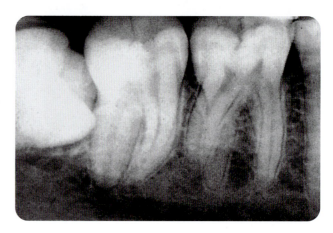

Figure 2.33 X-ray of first molar with a lingual molar root, originating distally.

was initially thought to represent a root fracture.[247] A second root on a maxillary central incisor (with dilaceration) was attributed to trauma to the deciduous predecessor.[228]

Treatment

Bifid roots do not require treatment. Endodontic treatment is expected to be more complex. Radiographs do not necessarily reveal a bifid root. One may suspect two-rooted lower anterior teeth and therefore two root canals when an endodontic file's position relative to the root is off-centre. A radiograph taken at a mesial or distal angulation may help confirm whether there is a single root with a canal that is off-centre (and hence the unexpected position of endodontic file) or there is more than one root or root canal.

2.11.2   Additional roots

Additional roots are supernumerary roots that probably represent autonomous outgrowths at the level of the crown. Additional roots may be either fully developed or rudimentary. If fused to other roots, they are difficult to detect on radiographs and sometimes even on extracted teeth. In Brazil, 3% of the population of African origin have three-rooted mandibular first molars like the Senegalese,[429] as is the case with 4% of Caucasians and 11% of Asians.[429]

The previously described paramolar roots are additional roots (Figure 2.32). Others mentioned in the literature are distomolar roots *(radix distomolaris)* and *lingual*

molar or entomolar roots (radix entomolaris or *radix praemolarica* as they can also occur in premolars), based on the belief that the root was a manifestation of a premolar that had "disappeared" in the course of evolution.

When fusion of the root is restricted to the crown only, the seemingly "extra root"[48] is essentially different from an additional root, albeit being considered an entity on its own.

Radix distomolaris

Around 25% of maxillary molars possess distomolar roots, with more than half being fused with the regular roots. Most distomolar roots occurring in the maxilla have been found on third molars, a few on the second and only one on the first molar.[66]

Radix entomolaris

Lingual (pre)molar roots originate from the lingual of the distal root, particularly in mandibular first molars and tend to curve towards the mesial (Figure 2.33). The roots have been observed in the mandibular first and third molars,[270] but may be present in any of the mandibular molars and rarely at the second premolar.[101] The two buccal roots of the mandibular second premolar are considered to be homologous to the mandibular molar roots and the lingual one represents radix entomolaris.[108] The rare third root of a mandibular second molar[492] may also be lingual molar root.

In general, the root manifests itself only in a small proportion of Caucasians, in 5–42% of Asians, and in 55% of the Aleuts.[89 90 112 270 372 427 428 432 472 482 487] The root plays a role in determining the origin of Native American tribes.[472] A lingual molar root is inconspicuous when fused with the regular roots, which may lead to an underestimation of the prevalence. Taking root fusion into account, extracted mandibular third molars showed lingual molar roots four to five times more often than the first and second mandibular molars.[64] Regardless of root fusion, radix entomolaris was found on two-thirds of mandibular third molars, almost one-third of mandibular second molars and 2.5% of mandibular first molars.[65] The root may be difficult to see on radiographs, therefore if it is not recognised, it could jeopardise endodontic treatment. During extraction the risk of root fracture is also increased.

Accessory roots

An accessory root (*radix appendiciformis*) is a small, thin root next to the regular root of, for instance, a maxillary central incisor.[10 402 482] They may also occur elsewhere along the length of the root.[10 402] In the latter case it could be a variant of lingual molar root[64] or the paramolar root.[65] In the tooth seen on the left in Figure 2.31, the small root between the two regular roots may be a paramolar root or an accessory root. An accessory root may also be present underneath the sixth cusp between the two lingual cusps (see Chapter 1) of the mandibular first molar.[429]

2.12 Taurodontism

Taurodontism is characterised by a cylindrical root, an enlarged pulp cavity, and when it involves multi-rooted teeth, an apically situated furcation and pulp chamber floor. In taurodont teeth, the root canal system resembles that of multi-rooted teeth. This differs from teeth with pyramidal roots where the root canal system often has one apical foramen.[256] The name taurodontism (*taurodontia*) is based upon a superficial resemblance with the molars of cattle.[217]

2.12.1 Appearance

The vertically enlarged pulpal canal has a cylindrical form. The cylindrical root is thick and plump. The cervi-cal area is not constricted. In multi-rooted taurodont teeth the furcation lies much further towards the apical end of the root, so that there is rudimentary separation of the roots (Figures 2.34).

"Taurodontism" is the term used when the height of the coronal pulp is equal to or larger than three-tenths of the crown length (the average plus two times the standard deviation of the ratio of the heights of the pulp and crown).[218] Other criteria state that the pulp chamber floor has to be at least 2.5 mm below the cemento-enamel junction and, the distance between roof and pulp chamber floor divided by the distance from the roof to the apex (=Taurodont Index) must exceed 0.2 mm, and, alternatively, the distance from the bottom to the cemento-enamel junction is greater than 2.5 mm.[420] However, some teeth with anomalous pulp configurations seem taurodont, but do not meet the criteria.[385]

Taurodontism is subdivided into hypo-, meso- and hypertaurodontism,[311] the first and last being considered the most "extreme" on a continuous scale of pulp size.[82 217] Taurodont molars are recognised as hypotaurodont (Taurodont Index value 20–29.9%), mesotaurodont (Taurodont Index value 30–39.9%) and hypertaurodont (Taurodont Index value 40–75%).[420] The use of such discrete categories may be misleading in comparative studies.[82]

Determination of criteria is important to avoid a subjective diagnosis: without the use of these criteria the diagnosis of taurodontism made by experienced researchers showed poor agreement.[218]

2.12.2 Epidemiology

The molars are the mostly affected,[386] in particular the second maxillary molars,[96 318 460] followed by the premolars[262 282 453] and lastly the anterior teeth. Taurodontia occurs in the deciduous and the permanent dentitions[3 27 147 277 316] and can occur uni- or bilaterally. A few teeth or a single tooth in a dentition may be involved.[147 411]

Isolated taurodontism has been described,[7 119 156 244 277 290 310 313 371] but in these cases a genetic basis is still likely, which does not hold true in children treated for cancer (15% taurodontism).[521] A family trait has been reported,[39 156 304] in some cases in three generations.[130 365] Taurodontism, which is often mild, is far from uncommon in Inuit, Australian Broad-beach Aboriginals, Iranian, Yugoslavs and Maltese populations.[125 180 304 310 401 495 514] An ethnic trait seems likely, increasing from west to east, and affecting up to 50% of Senegalese and Chinese subjects.[8 27 50 96 97 132 142 195 217 218 280 318 387 420 470]

Whether the anomaly is sex-linked is not clear.[195] A predilection for males is reported.[514 336] In Senegal, no difference between the sexes was found.[460] The lack of sex differences in (the expression of) taurodontism[82] is in accordance with the findings of others, the only exception being a higher prevalence in Chinese females (56% versus 46%).[280]

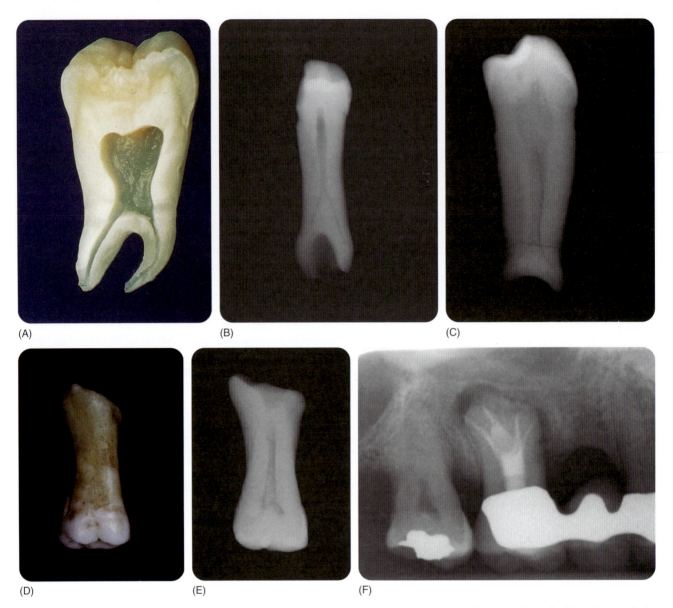

Figure 2.34 (A) A sectioned taurodont molar. (B) X-ray of an extracted taurodont upper premolar. Note the cylindrical form and the broad apex. (C) X-ray of an extracted taurodont lower premolar. (D) An extracted taurodont upper molar. (E) X-ray of the tooth shown in (D). (F) Endodontically treated taurodont upper molar.

None of the first molars in a Zulu population was taurodont. However, 3% and 24% of second and third molars, respectively, were taurodont. In prehistoric Khoisan in southern Africa, these values were 30%, 53% and even as high as 90%.[82] The posterior teeth of Australian Aboriginals (Broad-beach excavation in Queensland) showed meso-taurodontism in over 10% of the molars,[125] although it has been reported that earlier the majority were mesotaurodont.[304]

The anomaly may have been a distinguishing feature of the Middle Palaeolithic populations,[311 495] such as Neanderthals and the Heidelberg man, presenting in relatively high frequencies, although it was not ubiquitous. The Neanderthals inhabited Europe and Western Asia approximately between 30 000 and 200 000 years ago. Their large anterior teeth were shovel-shaped. The posterior teeth were taurodont and tended to possess extra

occlusal fissures and cusps.[28] This anomaly is of importance in the study of the ancestry of modern humans.[276] The deciduous teeth of Neanderthal children were taurodont too.

Because taurodontism was more frequent in ancient times, the anomaly was thought to have an impact on survival. An example of this was the greater ability to tear animal hides with their teeth: the consequent formation of extensive reparative dentine does not easily obliterate the pulp canal in taurodont teeth.[495]

2.12.3 Aetiology

Various modes of inheritance have been established, with varying expressivity and incomplete penetrance.[4 70 149 208 217 495] A patient with taurodont and supernumerary teeth had characteristic dermatoglyphs.[149] Factors other than inheritance might be involved:[195] children who have received radiotherapy were more frequently affected than their siblings.[334]

Taurodontism is related to an abnormal number of X-chromosomes, such as the most severe variant of the Klinefelter syndrome (Chapter 11).[183 229 478] Taurodontism, missing teeth, sparse hair and some characteristics of ectodermal dysplasia are reported in siblings.[434] In ectodermal dysplasias, taurodontism is often overlooked.[336] Taurodontism is a manifestation of, among others, trisomy 21 (Down's syndrome)[211] in 60% of the patients,[217] in microcephaly with extremely short roots,[397] possibly in osteoporosis[138] and other syndromes.[336] Taurodont teeth were present in almost 30% of oligodont patients with short roots versus 10% of controls.[389 399]

In mono- and dizygotic twins with (palatal) clefts, taurodontism was equally frequent (about 40%). In half of the twins examined, both showed taurodontism and hypodontia outside the cleft region, this being a reason to suspect a common aetiology.[249 250] Taurodontism is often present together with other inherited tooth anomalies and in patients without physical deformities. Its presence is presumed to be either interdependent or coincidental.

Taurodontism occurs together with hypodontia,[408 433] dens invaginatus,[15 70 208] amelogenesis imperfecta[80 84 351 372] (Chapter 3), microdontia, multi-cusp teeth,[70] dentine dysplasia,[243 312 358] thalassaemia[517] (Chapter 3) and severe vitamin D-resistant rickets[161] (Chapter 3).

2.12.4 Pathology

Taurodontism originates as a developmental disturbance in Hertwig's sheath,[180 217] but the pathogenesis is uncertain. The condition must result from a failure of the epithelial sheath to fold inwards and taper towards the apex.

The enamel is usually normal. In some taurodont teeth the dentine has very short tubules, much inter-globular dentine and disorientated odontoblasts.[316] The apical dentine may resemble reparative dentine and many pulp stones may be present.[96 316 335]

2.13 Consequences

Cavity preparation is not associated with particular risks.[119] However, endodontic treatment is hampered by the more apical location of the openings of the root canals in the low floor of the pulp chamber, making them hard to find and clean.[468] This problem can be compounded by the presence of pulp stones and calcifications. Fortunately, periodontal furcation problems are less likely than in normal teeth. The taurodont roots are less able to withstand lateral chewing forces than normal multi-rooted teeth and may be less fit to serve as abutments.[335]

2.13.1 Pyramidal roots versus fused roots

Pyramidal roots refer to conical roots with an enlarged pulp chamber and one root canal; they are found in molars or premolars. They are presumed to arise due to a lack of potential in Hertwig's sheath to invaginate, resulting in the development of one root instead of a root stem with two or three roots.[402 477] An explanation for the conical form is lacking. An alternative name is *cuneiform*.[402] There are reports of subjects with generalised (skin) aberrations, pyramidal premolars and taurodont molars with a single root canal and the presence of evaginations. The canines may be lobodont.[332]

Pyramidal molars are probably an ethnic trait. They were reported to be present in almost 5% of a Senegalese population,[396] and in 5% of mandibular second molars and 9% of mandibular third molars of contemporaneous Zulu populations of South Africa and in the Khoisan, a prehistoric Southern African population.[82] The proportion of single-rooted first molars retrieved from an old graveyard was very low. Second molars exhibited a single root in 15–25% and third molars approximately 33% of the time, but it is not clear whether this involved fused or pyramidal roots.[402]

3

Developmental Structural Anomalies of Enamel and Dentine

3.1 Introduction

A variety of causes are responsible for the developmental structural anomalies of enamel and dentine. For better insight into these anomalies, the development and structure of the teeth are first briefly reviewed here.

Odontogenesis starts with development of outgrowths from the oral epithelial band that lines the (future) jaws, from which the tooth buds develop. The tooth bud is initially cap shaped, which then grows to form the bell-shaped enamel organ. The enamel organ surrounds the mesenchymal dental papilla and has four layers: the outer epithelium, stellate reticulum, stratum intermedium and inner epithelium.

Enamel

After predentine formation by specialised cells of the papilla (the odontoblasts), cells from the inner enamel epithelium transform into ameloblasts (Figure 3.1). These ruffle-bordered cells: (1) produce the organic enamel matrix, (2) resorb the greater part of the matrix and (3) mineralise (through mineral deposition) the remaining matrix. The enamel production proceeds in an incisal/occlusal to cervical direction. Next, the ameloblasts disappear and the as-yet partly mineralised enamel[825] undergoes "maturation", a process that starts before and continues after eruption.

The enamel matrix consists mainly of two proteins: the amelogenins and, to a lesser degree, the enamelins. The amelogenins regulate the formation of the hydroxyapatite crystallites. During the calcification, the amelogenins are split step-wise by proteases secreted by the ameloblasts,[517] and new proteins are added until early maturation, when few new proteins are formed.[825] Two groups of enamel proteases exist: a matrix metalloprotease called enamelysin and a serine proteinase. The amelogenins are cleaved by enamelysin, from the inner to the outside side of the crown, and disappear totally during the maturation of the enamel. The enamel matrix contains several amelogenins, as a result of their destruction and differences in transcription.[517] The mineralised enamel undergoes final calcification as the remaining proteins are removed,[825] but the acidic enamelin concentration increases.[218] The loss of matrix protein creates pores, which are subsequently filled with mineral. The enamel crystals slowly expand, filling the spaces formerly occupied by the proteins, and the local pH changes from mildly acidic to near physiological.[823] The longer the developing enamel remains partially mineralised, the greater the likelihood that the tissue will be damaged, which might explain why the incisal edge shows anomalies more often than the cervical region.[219] There is a time-dependent difference in enamel maturation in males and females.[1]

The enamel is composed of almost parallel, about 1 mm long rods (enamel prisms) with diameter of about 4 μm, composed of small hydroxyapatite crystals. In a cross-sectional view, the rods resemble keyholes. Their direction is perpendicular on the outer surface of the enamel, and occasionally at an angle of 30 degrees and in the cervical region it is almost greater than 45 degrees.[121] The minimal spaces between the prisms are filled with interprismatic material, which consists of very small hydroxyapatite crystals, water and organic components.

The enamel surface of newly erupted teeth shows numerous fine horizontal ridges (the perikymata) separated by very small grooves ("imbrication grooves of Pickerill"),[738] which correspond to the growth lines within the enamel. The growth line that marks birth is named after Retzius. A lower premolar shows some 30 perikymata/mm at the cervical site, gradually declining to 6–7/mm near the occlusal surface.[848]

Dentine

The odontoblasts first produce fibroblasts and extracellular collagen fibres. Collagens consist of microfibrils of some 20 protein families. Type I collagen constitutes 85–90% of the mass of the dentinal framework.[209] Collagen type V is associated with type I collagen molecules that have formed into fibrils[209] and is present in small amounts.[6] Type III collagen is found in the predentine.[209] In cross-sections, the bundles of collagen fibres (the Korff fibrils) become orientated perpendicularly on the basal membrane (the basal lamina situated between the mesenchyme and inner enamel epithelium) that separates the papilla from the inner enamel epithelium. The Korff fibrils constitute the matrix for the first-formed dentine, the mantle dentine (this is 150 μm wide, lacks phosphoryn, and is less mineralized than the later formed dentine). Mineralisation of the matrix, which until then is called predentine, occurs in the form of round deposits of calcium salts after the basal lamina is removed. Dentine forma-

Pathology of the Hard Dental Tissues, First Edition. Albert Schuurs.
© 2013 Albert Schuurs. Published 2013 by Blackwell Publishing Ltd.

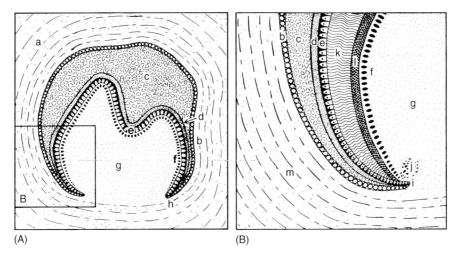

(A)   (B)

Figure 3.1 (A) Schematic of the bell stage of development of a tooth. (B) Magnified view of the inset in (A).
a: Enamel organ.
b: Outer enamel epithelium.
c and d: Stellate reticulum and stratum intermedium.
e: Ameloblasts (developed from the inner enamel epithelium).
f: Odontoblasts.
g: Dental papilla, which becomes the pulp.
h and i: Cervical loop (consisting only of the inner and outer enamel epithelium).
j: Cells undergoing mitoses and meioses above the cervical loop.
k: Enamel matrix.
l: Dentine (with predentine at the pulpal side).
m: Connective tissue.

tion thereafter takes place in the absence of Korff fibrils. Dentine contains a much higher proportion of organic substances than enamel. Many uncertainties still exist in regard to the inherited anomalies of dentine.[107]

A very large number (up to some $18\,000/mm^2$ and locally even thousands more) of dentinal tubules run from the pulp to the enamel and cementum (Figure 3.2) and are filled with fluid and, within about the proximal half, extensions of the odontoblasts. In the axial parts of the dentine, about 10% of the extensions of the odontoblasts within the tubules are accompanied by nerve endings. The tubules are surrounded by peritubular dentine, which is more calcified than the intertubular dentine, and are interlinked by transverse connections. Imperfect calcification of the dentine, in particular near the enamel, results in many regions with abundant organic material, called interglobular dentine.

The tooth root and cementum
Cell division above the "cervical loop", which consists of only the inner and outer epithelium of the enamel organ (Figure 3.1B), moves the cervical loop apically, leaving a shaft, the "sheath of Hertwig" of inner and outer epithelium surrounding the mesenchymal papilla. On the inside of Hertwig's sheath, the outer cells of the dental papilla transform into odontoblasts, which produce the root dentine. Next, the sheath becomes a loosely connected network, which in cross-sections is visible as the "islands of Malassez". The mineralised dentine induces migration of the

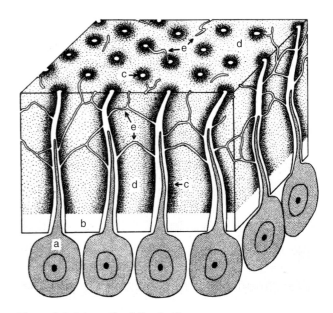

Figure 3.2 Schematic of the dentine.
a: Odontoblasts – columnar cells with extensions (Tomes' fibres) lying in the proximal parts of the dentinal tubules.
b: Predentine (uncalcified dentinal matrix).
c: Peritubular dentine.
d: Intertubular dentine.
e: Anastomoses between the dentinal tubules.

nearby mesenchymal cells of the follicle (a loose connective sac) through the network, which become cementoblasts. These cells produce a collagen cement matrix, which becomes calcified to form cementum.

The first-formed cementum is acellular. Induced by the cementum, connective tissue fibres develop and transform into Sharpey's fibres, the ends of which are embedded on one side in the cementum and on the other side in the alveolar bone. These fibres form the periodontal ligament that attaches the tooth to the alveolar bone. Cementum produced afterwards contains interconnected cells (cellular cementum). The production of cementum is a life-long process.

The pulp

The odontoblasts are located in a neatly ordered fashion along the predentine. Dentine production continues steadily after the eruption (secondary dentine), although slowly. External stimuli, such as caries, evoke tertiary/reparative dentine formation (Chapters 5 and 8). The contents of the pulp include nerves, blood vessels and connective tissue.

3.2 Developmental and acquired structural anomalies of the enamel

Anomalies in the enamel structure may arise during enamel matrix formation or its resorption and subsequent calcification. *Hypoplasia* is a quantitative developmental defect caused by failure of matrix production or insufficient deposition of proteins on the outside of the developing enamel surface, whereby the normally smooth enamel surface becomes pitted or lacks in substance in large parts – it may be very thin or totally absent. *Hypocalcification* is a qualitative developmental deficiency that arises due to interruption of the resorption of the organic enamel matrix or a deficiency in the active calcium transport through the ameloblasts, and/or failure of maturation.

In both conditions the enamel is imperfect, but the term *(hereditary) amelogenesis imperfecta* is reserved for a group of inherited enamel abnormalities that occur in the absence of other tissue or systemic anomalies[999] (and as a phenotypical feature in some syndromes, for instance with renal calcification),[1032] although an association with biochemical changes elsewhere in the body may exist.[21] When the enamel of a solitary tooth or a few adjacent teeth exhibits structural anomalies, a local cause is likely. A temporary systemic disturbance will lead to a chronologically linked disturbance in enamel formation of the (homologous) teeth formed at that time. More generalised defective structure of the enamel is due to systemic causes which are active during the whole period of tooth formation.

Appearance

Hypoplasia is manifested locally as reduced enamel thickness, occasionally as pits arranged in rows and columns, especially in the buccal mid-third crown region[235 326 327] of the permanent incisors and first molars (the lower canines in Western India).[538] The defects may be microscopic in size.[315] In more severe cases, the enamel is missing in some areas of the tooth (Figure 3.3).

Hypocalcification presents as localised abnormalities in tooth colour, called *opacities*, which may be:

- Diffuse, non-demarcated chalky-white spots
- Well-demarcated spots, often white (Figure 3.4), and otherwise cream, yellow or brown.

The diffuse opacities are often less than 150 μm deep. The depth of demarcated areas varies. The white "spots" are softer[547] than normal, translucent enamel, and the coloured opacities are even softer.[857]

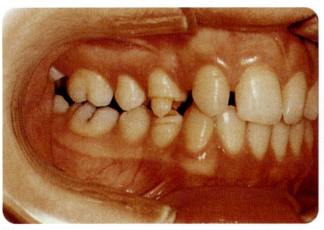
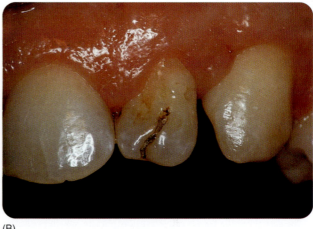

(A)   (B)

Figure 3.3 (A) Hypoplasia of the enamel (attributed to tuberculosis). (B) Hypoplasia due to trauma of the deciduous predecessor leading to its intrusion.

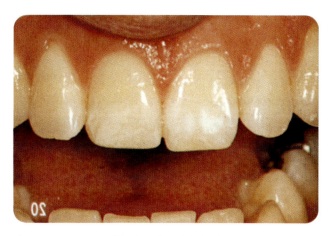

Figure 3.4 Hypocalcification (opacities) of the enamel of the upper central incisors.

The defects represent events in earlier life and may testify to fetal insults.[438] Because the ameloblasts cease to exist after completion of amelogenesis and the enamel lacks blood vessels and an active metabolism, natural repair cannot take place. With time, the lesions may undergo alterations and tooth wear might make them less obvious.[2]

Prevalence

The prevalence of hypoplasia and hypocalcification varies widely from country to country and from time to time. For instance, children born in Sweden in 1970 showed more opacities in the deciduous dentition than those born before and after that year.[471] Operationalisation of the definition of hypocalcification and hypoplasia is difficult. A carious "white spot" lesion and a developmental opacity may be diagnostically mixed up.[346 963 1031]

Opacities

The percentages of opacities in the permanent dentition varies between different countries, regions and towns from 30% to 75%:[50 168 179 234 262 471 619 842 854 858] 99% of 12-year-old Hong Kong children[461] versus 2% of rural Chinese[518] have been found to be affected. A few to some 20% of the deciduous dentitions show opacities.[471 619 628] In an Irish study, 37–52% of cases had demarcated and 11–23% had diffuse opacities.[248]

Hypoplasia

Among 9–21 year-olds, 8–15% possessed hypoplastic enamel but reported rates for different populations[70 234 248 461 518 531 755 628 919] vary tremendously – even up to 100%,[718] whereas one small study reported a rate of only 3%.[692]

In the period AD950–1300 the proportion of hypoplasia increased in the Illinois area of the USA from 45% to 80%, in association with a change in lifestyle (with a decreased life expectancy) from hunting to agricultural-based settlements.[327]

Hypocalcification Index

In 1982, the Féderation Dentaire Internationale proposed the Developmental Defects of dental Enamel index (DDE)[178 179] to quantify the type, number and localisation of the defects (but not their aetiology, which in many instances cannot be determined).[178] According to the DDE index, a mean of 7.5–12.7 teeth/person have such defects.[179]

Causes

More than 90 causes of structural enamel defects have been noted, divided into local, systemic and inherited ones,[404] for example, genetic abnormalities and syndromes, hormones, medicines, and infection and allergy.[404] The presentation of enamel hypoplasia is rarely cause-specific. The location of the defects and distribution over the dentition are indicative of time the disturbance occurred (see chronology in Appendix I), which helps to determine the cause and predict which of the, if any, unerupted teeth will be affected. For example, the deciduous teeth and permanent incisors/first molars show signs of fetal and postnatal insults.

The calcification times (see Appendix I), determined with the help of radiographs, are possibly underestimations. Examination of fetal material has showed the initiation of calcification to occur earlier, in the twelfth fetal week[477] or between week 5 and 13.[870] The age of fetuses is difficult to ascertain and lethal conditions possibly influenced the calcification times.

The appearance of opacities also is not cause-specific. The enamel organ responds to the wide spectrum of insults in a limited number of ways and the threshold levels of many aetiological agents are unknown. The aetiology may therefore be difficult to determine, more so in the case of diffuse opacities.[797] One main cause of enamel opacities is too much fluoride (Section 3.2.5), but other causes also underlie more or less clinically identical defects.

A low serum calcium level would explain hypoplastic enamel and a deficiency in phosphate the presence of a large amount of interglobular dentine,[292 635] but other mechanisms also exist. For instance: non-degraded amelogenins attached to the apatite crystals prevent their growth, but the affinity of the later-formed amelogenins for the crystals is diminished due to their lower molecular weight.[133 499 518 825] In cystic fibrosis (see below), the disturbed pH regulation affects amelogenin processing negatively, causing defects in enamel structure. Fluoride does not affect the uptake of calcium from the diet, but inhibits enzymatic degradation of the amelogenins and affects the ameloblasts.[45]

3.2.1   Pre- and perinatal causes

Incisor-molar-hypomineralisation (IMH; "cheese molars")

This condition occurs when one or more first permanent molars show occlusal or larger areas of demarcated yellow

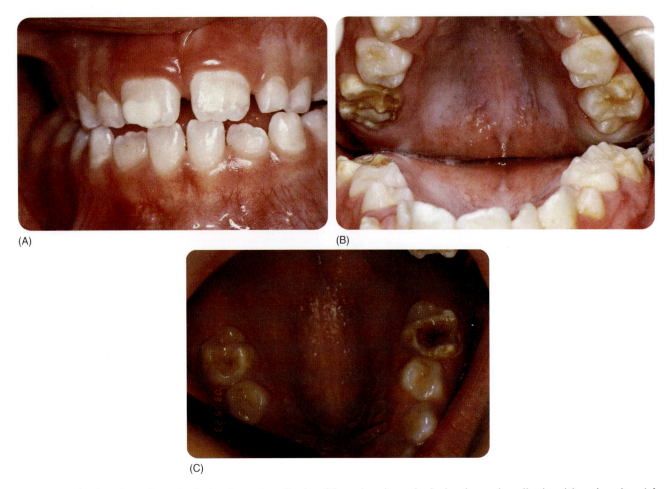

(A)

(B)

(C)

Figure 3.5 (A–C) Incisors in molar-incisor-hypomineralisation (A), molars in molar-incisor-hypomineralisation (B) and molars (of another patient) in molar-incisor-hypomineralisation (C). (Courtesy of K. Weerheim.)

to brown hypocalcified enamel. In the past they were called *cheese molars* because their colour and consistency resemble aged Dutch cheese. Post-eruptively, the enamel wears rapidly. The more yellow-brown the colour, the more porous is the enamel.[426] The anomaly is named *molar-incisor-hypomineralisation*[960] because the permanent incisors may be involved, the maxillary incisors more often than the mandibular incisors (Figure 3.5). IMH is, however, also observed in deciduous second molars, permanent second molars and the canines.[958] A disturbance in enamel maturation is suspected,[957] and the enamel is hypersensitive to cold stimuli.

No change in the function of the more cervically located ameloblasts indicates a temporary insult.[426] The causes of hypocalcification include many well-known systemic health problems that occur around and up to 3 years after birth,[911 1033] such as high fever, digestive tract disorders[910] and problems related to birth (oxygen deficiency), and respiratory diseases[427 911] such as asthma and bronchitis[446] (the latter has been found to occur in regions with drinking water containing higher levels of fluoride).[856] Other causes include: renal insufficiency, hypoparathyroidism,

dioxins, diarrhoea and malabsorption.[446] IMH in two siblings was ascribed to dehydration due to an intolerance of cow milk. Duration of breast-feeding might be associated with IMH,[427] but birthweight and length at birth, problems around and during birth do not seem to be associated.[92 426] IMH is seen in about 5 to >10% of children.[220 428 446 470 959] A more extreme range has also been reported: from 3.5% to 25%.[956 957]

Small affected areas can be treated with fissure sealants. Somewhat larger areas may be restored with glass ionomer cement. Composite resins seem better,[272] but the restoration fails frequently,[1033] although crowns with two sound surfaces on follow up after 4 years were still satisfactorily restored (one-third remaining hypersensitive for 1 week and a few teeth for 1 year).[539] The hypomineralised enamel shows unusual etching patterns, either because the defective enamel is not uniformly removed,[547] or because of deviations in the prism boundaries[857] or because the tissue underneath the sound enamel may be hypocalcified.[426 428] Larger affected areas require onlays, stainless steel crowns,[272] or adhesive copings.[1023] To avoid a repeated cycle of restorations, extraction of a severely affected first molar should be considered,[985] ideally at age 8–9 years, when radiographs show complete calcification of the crown of the second molar or when its bifurcation is visible, which minimises the need for orthodontics. Following late extraction of the first molar, the second molar will show less forward movement, with mesial tipping and lingual rolling.[986] If the first molar is extracted too early, the second premolar will drift distally. To prevent a centre line shift, a non-compromised contralateral molar may be removed too.[986]

Congenital syphilis

Intra-uterine infection with the spirochaete *Treponema pallidum* causes among other defects, deafness, blindness and a typical enamel hypoplasia: the "triad of Hutchinson" (English physician, 1820–1913).

Evidence of venereal syphilis in European skeletons post dates Columbus' discovery of the New World, but the disease has been noted in skeletons in the Dominican Republic from the pre-Columbian time, which is why it is considered that the disease spread from the New World.[746]

Hutchinson's incisors are small and barrel shaped. They are called "screwdriver teeth" because the approximal surfaces converge towards the incisal, the vertical middle third of the labial surface being absent. The incisal edge shows two mamelons flanking a deep crescentic notch (Figure 3.6). Only two pulp horns are present. Alterations in blood vessel walls, oedema and degeneration of the centrally situated ameloblasts in the papilla account for the decreased central growth. Wear of the dirty-greyish incisors subsequently eliminates the notch.[122 208 391] A hypoplastic, incisal constriction in the permanent canines is not likely to be "syphlytic".[746]

The rounded permanent first molars with a large number of small occlusal cusps, with pigmented areas in between, resemble a mulberry ("mulberry molars",

"Moon's molars" after Henry Moon). Parts of the enamel may break away.[391] Hutchinson's triad is fully present in 1% of the patients: about 30% have screwdriver teeth and mulberry molars.[122 283 391 706] For unknown reasons the incisors are not always bilaterally anomalous. The deciduous dentition is free from defects: the spirochaete does not penetrate the tooth germs before the fourth (or fifth) month *in utero*, when the placental Langerhans layer disappears,[941] but crown growth might be disrupted after birth (unlikely) rather than before.[391]

Owing to the inadequate treatment alternatives prior to the Second World War, almost all incisors and first molars in such cases were hypoplastic.[564] From 1943, syphilis declined,[932] but its incidence increased again around 1960,[283 941] a trend that has persevered;[605] it continues to be seen in the USA and Europe especially among males not using condoms, who are at a higher risk.[489] Antibiotics control the disease effectively. If left untreated, the primary effects disappear spontaneously, but the patient enters the next stage(s) of the disease.

Though the dental features are considered to be distinctive,[391] the diagnosis of syphilis cannot be based on the morphological features of the teeth, which are also seen in Nance–Horan syndrome.[330 658] The microorganisms must be demonstrated, and serological examination should show an increase in the titre of antibodies.

Cystic fibrosis

This is an inherited pancreatic disease, which affects the chloride channel that regulates salt and water excretion in exocrine cells. Both cystic fibrosis and long-term administration of tetracyclines for airway infections are associated with disturbances in enamel formation; they are described later in the chapter.

Cytomegalovirus (CMV)

This virus is a member of the herpesviruses group and causes severe morbidity congenitally (e.g. pneumonitis). Intra-uterine infection, in 0.3% or 2%,[607 1021] affects the DNA, but 90% of the children are asymptomatic.[1021] Of prematurely born infants, 13% are infected.[238] If moderate, mucosal lesions mimic other ulcerations (e.g. aphthous ulcers, herpetic stomatitis).[105] The more severe the infection, the more severe are the dental anomalies, ranging from opaque deciduous enamel to yellow discoloration and considerable hypoplasia.[102] Hand washing by pregnant women and the patients' caregivers effectively prevents acquisition of the virus.[659 1021]

Gestational diabetes

Diabetic mothers may give birth prematurely in the 36–37th week or before, or deliver a child by caesarean section, who is often overweight.[339] Deficient insulin production (type 1) alters the metabolism of carbohydrates (hyperglycaemia with glycosuria), proteins and lipids. In type 1 diabetes, the body makes antibodies against the

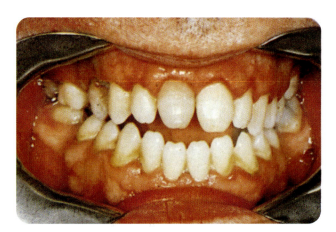

Figure 3.6 Screwdriver teeth in congenital syphilis. Note the characteristic central notches in the lower incisors. (Courtesy of Department of Oral Surgery, University of Groningen.)

Langerhans cells in the pancreas: less and less insulin is produced. Uncontrolled diabetes causes among other conditions, vascular and kidney disease and blindness.[819] Tongue burning and *Candida* infection are also likely.

Children of diabetic women show deciduous enamel hypoplasia more often than other children,[337] about 40% versus 15%, respectively.[339] The enamel matrix amelogenins are insufficiently resorbed,[648 817] even after insulin supplementation. Children born prematurely have a broad neonatal line in the permanent teeth and in 77% the postnatal subsurface enamel is hypomineralised.[638]

The neonatal line is found in teeth that start to develop *in utero*, the deciduous teeth and the permanent first molars and central incisors,[991] and is a lasting testimony of the environmental changes at the time of birth.[774 980 990] Enamel prisms crossing the line have an altered orientation and are less densely packed in postnatal enamel.[981] Neonatal hypocalcaemia in the children may be the result of fetal hypoparathyroidism (Section 3.1.5).[641 902] A high proportion show hypocalcified permanent incisors despite correction of the hypocalcaemia.[691] However, every neonate has some hypocalcaemia,[851] which is corrected on breast-feeding (which influences also mandibular growth).[969] In children of diabetic mothers the calcium content at birth is comparatively low and later it decreases more than in others.

Breast milk contains too little calcium and phosphorus for pre-term children, but cow's milk cannot be given because of its high phosphate level, which further increases the hypocalcaemia between days 2 and 5.[318] Children with clinical signs of neonatal hypocalcaemia may show a groove in the enamel surface instead of the neonatal line,[508] more so when the hypocalcaemia is severe and of longer duration.

Dioxins

High dioxin concentrations in breast milk owing to environmental contamination (until 1987) caused enamel hypomineralisation and hypoplasia and dentinal defects in the permanent first molars and incisors of many children.[13] No child with enamel defects in a sample of Finnish children had been breast-fed for less than 8 months.[14 15] Dioxins are by-products of the manufacture of phenols and combustion of chlorine-containing waste. Near such factories, dioxins may be present in cow's milk and in pigs due to food pollution. After an explosion in one chemical factory, the 5-year-olds who lived nearer the factory and therefore had greater exposure to dioxin were more likely to have hypoplastic enamel.[13] Environmental dioxin levels (cow's milk) currently are probably of minor or no account with regard to dental defects, but little is known about synergistic effects with other chemicals.[1034]

The placenta transports dioxins. High concentrations have been found in adipose tissue of children who died in the early neonatal period.[474] The most toxic chemical compound in the dioxin group caused depolarisation of odontoblasts and ameloblasts in cultured embryonic molars. The dentine matrix failed to mineralise and the enamel matrix was not deposited. Dioxin affects epidermal growth factor receptor (EGFR) signalling and thereby odontogenesis.[677]

Erythroblastosis fetalis and ABO incompatibility

Congenital haemolytic anaemia (erythrocyte destruction) is caused by the presence of incompatible proteins in the cell membrane of the fetal and maternal blood cells: the *Rhesus factor* (Rh) (the rhesus monkey possesses the same factor).

When a Rhesus negative (Rh−) woman (probability 15%) becomes pregnant from a Rhesus positive (Rh+) man (probability 85%), the fetus has Rh+ blood, unless the father is heterozygote (which occurs mostly): then the child has a probability of 50% of having Rh+ blood.[809] Cells from the child (antigens) leak into the mother's blood at term and during delivery. Antibodies developed in the mother cross the placenta during the next pregnancy, whereupon the second fetus develops haemolytic anaemia with hyperbilirubinaemia, manifested as jaundice (formerly called icterus gravis neonatorum).

For neonatal jaundice appearing between day 4 and day 7 of life, breast milk is the most common cause.[78]

The haemolytic product *bilirubin* (e.g. porphyrin remnants after degradation of the erythrocytes) and its oxidation product *biliverdin* circulate in the blood. The child's liver cannot process large amounts of bilirubin, which is therefore deposited in the body tissues. Bilirubin causes jaundice, damages the basal ganglia in the brain (kernicterus) and discolours the dentine. Jaundice is not a disease but a symptom and is treated by exposing the child to a blue – nowadays a green – light, which transforms the bilirubin into a form that the child's liver can process.

If the Rh− mother has not been treated with immunoprophylaxis, Rh+ blood needs to be transfused to the second and any other children. Only 1:200 neonates experience the above symptoms,[92 809] because not all mothers form antibodies, and the antibodies do not always cross the placenta and immunisation could occur.[809]

Structural anomalies

About 0.1% to 30% show enamel hypoplasia in the teeth formed at birth.[56 383 692] Tooth germs in stillborn and deceased neonates demonstrate vacuoles in the regions of the odontoblasts and ameloblasts, corresponding to structural defects in the permanent teeth.[383] The hypoplasia depends on the albumin to bilirubin ratio; the amount of unconjugated bilirubin determining the level of damage to the ameloblasts.[56] Rh− incompatibility may also affect the dermatoglyphs of the hands and feet.[56]

Discoloration

In hyperbilirubinaemia, soft tissue turnover removes the bilirubin deposited throughout the body, but it remains semi-permanently entrapped in the teeth.[952] Tooth discoloration is also possible without signs of kernicterus.[971] Bilirubin in the dentine discolours the teeth in 10–70% of the deciduous dentitions green (incorrectly called "chlorodontia"),[952 972] blue, grey, yellow and brown.[329 383] [563] The discoloration disappears spontaneously after some years.[692 779 809]

Bilirubin (as a green line parallel to the incremental lines) has been found also in the deciduous teeth of patients with a history of severe *liver dysfunction*.[952]

ABO incompatibility

The erythrocytes contain the blood group antigens A, B, AB or O. During pregnancy, a woman may become sensitised against a blood group antigen present on the child's erythrocytes. The mother's IgG anti-A and anti-B antibodies (not the IgM antibodies) cross the placenta. Depending on the mother's IgG titres,[907] a severe haemolytic reaction follows, though less often than in erythroblastosis fetalis.[383] Symptoms include anaemia due to excessive destruction of the erythrocytes, kernicterus and icterus gravis. In children of A and B blood group mothers, the incidence of significant hyperbilirubinaemia is not increased.[671] Children of O blood group mothers and non-O fathers have a 5–10 times increased chance of needing exchange transfusion due to hyperbilirubinaemia,[372 906] in addition to treatment with phototherapy. Haemolysis is seen in 0.03%.[575]

Serum bilirubin measurement at the sixth hour of life is used to predict whether a newborn will develop hyperbilirubinaemia (critical level 4 mg/dL) and/or a haemolytic reaction (critical level 6 mg/dL).[767]

Reports of dental effects of ABO incompatibility are lacking, except one case of discoloured deciduous anterior teeth.[77] Most children receiving blood transfusion after birth have hypocalcaemia for at least 3 days. Their deciduous dentition shows hypoplasia and hypocalcification near the neonatal line.[715]

Infantile encephalopathy (central paralysis, cerebral palsy, other neurological disorders)

Improved neonatal care has enlarged the numbers of surviving, prematurely born children and the survival of those with brain damage through asphyxia (deficient oxygen) or ischaemia (insufficient blood). Larger numbers of children with delayed psychomotor development and, later, spasticity now survive. The probability of development of cerebral palsy, a motor disorder caused by brain damage, increases with antenatal complications, such as infection of extra-embryonic membranes, and delays in caesarean section decisions (unless carried out at the expected delivery time).[616]

Cerebral palsy and enamel hypoplasia are associated,[315] but many of these children experience other pre- or perinatal disturbances such as asphyxia and fever,[438] which may be the real cause of the enamel defects. The likelihood of hypoplastic deciduous enamel increases if premature babies have cerebral palsy:[600] in one report about 30% had enamel pits, vertical or horizontal grooves or coloured enamel opacities[102] and 45% had enamel hypo-

plasia when cerebral palsy occurred in combination with hereditary developmental defects of the central nervous system.[475]

In a study of mentally retarded children, almost half of the central incisors exhibited isolated white opacities and more than one-quarter of the teeth had several white diffuse opacities; these children had suffered significantly more bacterial diseases than other children.[566] Children with minimal brain dysfunction show a broad neonatal line and hypocalcified prenatal enamel,[640] but Rh incompatibility could also be responsible.[4 565 919 920]

The prevalence of hypoplasia varies in reports from 0% to 35% and 68%.[565 600 919] The children's age at the time of the study may be a factor. In a follow-up study, the number of hypoplastic lesions reduced within 6 months, owing to wear, fractures and so on.[103] Inconsistent associations may be a result of methodologically limitations of older studies.[102]

Intolerance to cow's milk

Non-allergic hypersensitivity to cow's milk affects amelogenesis, by interfering with the activity of vitamin D (Section 3.2.3) and leading to calcium and phosphate deficiency.[794]

Hypoxia

Maternal or neonatal hypoxia (oxygen deficiency) causes defects in the enamel structure and is closely related to prematurity. The occurrence of enamel defects was similar in children with and without history of neonatal asphyxia,[341] but later a significant difference was found. [342 433]

Central cyanosis and hypoxia was noted to result from transposition of the great arteries, in 1:5000 births, and may recur after surgical treatment.[610] Suffocation almost to death in experimental animals influenced the structure of the enamel.[921]

Orotracheal intubation

An orotracheal tube used for oxygen administration to premature babies was excluded as a cause of incisor damage,[433] but there are indications that the tube, by compressing the alveolar processes,[176] is associated with enamel hypoplasia in 50–95% of children undergoing tube placement. The deciduous and permanent incisors particularly on the right side are affected, due to the securing of the tube.[39] Laryngoscopy causes defects on the left side,[802] but a right-left difference has not always been reported.[268] The longer the treatment, the greater the number of maxillary deciduous teeth that show hypoplasia.[10] Preterm children with *osteopenia* (undermineralised bone) may require laryngoscopy.[803] Intubation with a tube pressing on the alveolar bone may lead to dilaceration.[39]

The teeth are yellow-brown,[268] and opacities are observed outside the area affected by the tube, e.g. in deciduous first and second molars,[801] and also in cases with perinatal hypoxia.[754]

Errors of metabolism
Phenylketonuria
Chiefly seen in Caucasians, this is an inherited absence of a liver enzyme (phenylalanine-hydroxylase) or a co-enzyme (apo-enzyme) that inhibits the transformation of the amino acid phenylalanine into tyrosine and phenylalanine accumulates.[167 937] Without dietary therapy, a consequence is brain damage (mental retardation, convulsions). The disorder may cause enamel hypoplasia and brown discoloration.

Ochronosis
An inheritable deficiency in the enzyme homogentisate oxidase underlies the faulty degradation of phenylalanine and tyrosine.[693] Consequently, homogentisine accumulates in the body causing *ochronosis*. The colour of the connective tissues and teeth is blue to black,[693] and occasionally dark brown, and the enamel might be hypoplastic.

Galactosaemia
Galactosaemia occurs when the galactose metabolism through absence of enzyme activity (galactose-1-phosphate-uridyl-transferase) results in hepatocellular injury and developmental delay.[94] Continued consumption of galactose and lactose (milk) in early childhood leads to enamel hypoplasia in the permanent teeth.[94] Mild untreated galactosaemia does not interfere with amelogenesis. A subsequently severe course is associated with hypoplasia of the enamel formed at that time.

Rubella (German measles/rubeola) during pregnancy
The neonate of a mother affected with the viral disease rubella before week 13 of pregnancy[348] has many congenital disorders due to transplacental transfer of the infection. The virus can be demonstrated until 3 years after birth.[348] General developmental abnormalities include abnormalities of heart, eyes, ears, brain, bone, low birthweight,[615] and even death may occur.[102] Congenital dysfunction of the salivary glands[1022] promotes caries and tooth wear.

Some decades ago, tooth defects were not viewed to be associated with rubella. In the absence of rash in the mother (pink macular exanthema), the disease was overlooked. Grahnén in 1958 concluded that it was not possible to assess whether the disease had dental consequences,[336] but later a relationship was established.[348 349] Retrospectively, 82% of children with rubella embryopathy showed enamel defects against 9% of controls.[356] The eruption is delayed, which is not associated with either birthweight or length at birth.[535]

Segmental odontomaxillary dysplasia (Chapter 2)*
In this condition, the deciduous molars are hypoplastic or atypical.[51 91 228 305 597 964] In cases of hypodontia,[216 330] the

---

* The opposite of facial hemiatrophy, with retarded formation and eruption of teeth at the affected side.[758]

eruption is delayed or teeth remain unerupted.[91 201 597 974] Unusual external resorption of such deciduous molars has been reported.[51 91 672 703] The pulp shows fibrous enlargement and a deficient odontoblastic layer, and there are tubular defects in the coronal dentine.[51]

Sickle cell anaemia
This disease belongs to a group of autosomal recessive inherited disorders of haemoglobin formation with icterus, and occurs almost exclusively in persons of African origin and in the south and east Mediterranean regions. The relatively short-living red blood cells are sickle shaped.

In haemoglobin, haem is coupled to polypeptide chains of the globulins α, β, γ and δ. In sickle cell anaemia, β-globulin is chemically abnormal (while in β-thalassaemia, β-globulin is normal but formed in insufficient amounts although the other globulins are increased). In heterozygotes, periods with few complaints alternate with periods of sickle cell crisis. In homozygotes the disease is fatal.[204] Patients with the "Mediterranean disease" (thalassaemia major) usually require blood transfusion to normalise their haemoglobin level in order to prevent hypoxia. The transfusions may lead to iron overload and haemosiderosis, causing morbidity and mortality. Instead of management with transfusions, bone marrow may be transplanted.[369]

Sickle cell anaemia is associated with hypocalcified enamel and accentuated perikymata, poorly mineralised dentine, obstructions in the dentinal tubules, denticles, and hypercementosis.[831] The size of the opaque crowns and roots is reduced.[369]

Vitamin D deficiency in pregnancy
Vitamin D deficiency in the mother influences pre- and perinatal amelogenesis.[705 822] The deficiency leads to maternal hyperparathyroidism, which suppresses fetal parathormone production (Section 3.2.4).[705] The baby shows signs of tetany (tonic and clonic muscle spasms) due to hypocalcaemia. Enamel hypoplasia develops postnatally, due to the transiently inactive ameloblasts.[508]

Weight at birth and preterm children
Low birthweight, in particular in prematurely born children, is associated with enamel defects,[273 338 518 743] and intubation and hypoxia may be responsible.[268 273 295 433] Failing postnatal (intravenous) feeding, hypocalcaemia and systemic disturbances that underlie the low weight are co-factors.[273 518 637 801 796] The relationship between prematurity, hypocalcaemia and hypoplastic enamel appeared insignificant in one report,[691] but these conditions all have mineral deficiencies in common.[796] Children with a low birthweight may show subnormal growth[934] and develop idiopathic epilepsy more often than others, along with hypoplastic, orange-coloured enamel.[580 581]

In 1990, 7% of the neonates in the USA weighed <2500g due to reasons including maternal smoking.[934 935] Almost all neonates weighing 2000–2500g, 50% of those weighing 700–800g and 10% of those weighing 500g survive.[796 936] The sequelae of a very low birthweight include long-term general health problems, poor physical growth, behavioural disorders, etc.[936] Low birthweight children consume less maternal milk in the first weeks after birth; the few but more severe dental defects are worsened by seasonal deficiencies in calcium and vitamin D.[588]

Discoloration

A few cases show horizontal yellow bands in the deciduous teeth, presumably due to a high bilirubin serum level or a low calcium level.[295] Opacities are less common than hypoplasia.[802]

Enamel defects

A high proportion of symmetrical enamel hypoplasia cases are associated with low birthweight.[102 841] Generalised hypoplasia affects 40–70% of the deciduous dentition[796] and 10–20% of the permanent first incisors and molars.[273 295 518 794 795] The high prevalences have been corroborated by other studies,[356 518 842] for children with and without kernicterus.[600] Prematurity (odds ratio 2.6) and no breast-feeding (odds ratio 3.2) are associated with developmental defects in the enamel of primary teeth.

In spite of supplementation of breast milk with minerals and vitamin D, in one study enamel structure was impaired in 84% of preterm children (weight <2000, gestational age <37 weeks), versus 36% in controls.[10] The lower the birthweight, the higher the frequency, especially of hypoplasia.[802] In the absence of macroscopic anomalies, the enamel contains microscopic pits.[804]

The deciduous molars of very low birthweight children, in particular, in extremely low birthweight infants, are comparable with those of controls who are smaller in size.[296]

Other conditions

Several conditions, such as nephrosis, spina bifida, meningitis and dermal disorders are incidentally reported to be associated with structurally deficient enamel. Half of children with congenital cardiovascular disorders (patent ductus arteriosis, cardiac failure) are reported to have deciduous enamel hypoplasia.[357 796] Stillborn children and neonates dying upon birth have more or less severely anomalous enamel.[478] In defects of the biliary ducts (1:10 000–14 000) and end-stage liver disease, the green discoloured postnatal deciduous enamel shows hypoplasia.[805 1024] Congenital allergic conditions, such as asthma,[722] affect the enamel structure.[919] Haemangiomas of the lip may indirectly cause hypoplastic enamel, but this hypothesis has not been confirmed.[58]

Curvilinear hypoplasia on especially the labial surfaces of the deciduous mandibular canines is present in one-third of (African American?) children in Mississippi, USA.[236] Local thinned cortical bone is assumed to protect insufficiently against minor injuries.[796]

It has been hypothesised that anomalies of both the brain and the enamel may have identical causes. But *learning disabilities* at school were found to be unlikely to be associated with the hypoplastic enamel of deciduous teeth.[509]

3.2.2 Postnatal infectious diseases

Several infectious diseases cause structural enamel anomalies.[822]

Exanthematous diseases

The viral infectious exanthematous diseases such as measles have been stated to cause hypoplastic enamel,[271] but most seem at the most associated with it.[422 873] A causal relationship is unlikely, but a very sick child with minimal resistance might develop dental hypoplasia.[692] There is no evidence of an effect of the exanthematous diseases on the teeth,[292 338 422 535 693 858 982] except for rubella, high fever lasting for longer periods and varicella infection in the third year of life.[422 883] A short bout of high fever will not affect the ameloblasts that are resting at that time, which might explain why some children are free from enamel anomalies and others are not. In some studies, the majority of children had an exanthematous disease after the enamel anomalies had already developed.[422 982]

Cells damaged by viral diseases are replaced by proliferating neighbour cells.[941] Skin eruptions, for instance, in measles, are for a large part allergic in nature. In how far other tissues of epithelial origin are directly or indirectly affected by viruses, is not known.

Other postnatal infectious diseases

Non-exanthematous infectious diseases affect amelogenesis: whooping cough, pneumonia,[836] tuberculosis, diphtheria and gastrointestinal illness[317 826 883] with diarrhoea that disturbs the calcium metabolism and causes dehydration, vitamin D deficiency,[102 292] urinary tract infections,[858 883 982] especially in the second year of life,[883] otitis media[842] in the third year of life,[883] convulsions[982] and malaria (Figure 3.7).

The relationship between diarrhoea (*Salmonella* infection) and hypoplasia requires confirmation.[826] Parasitic diarrhoea was found to cause enamel hypoplasia in animals, attributed to hypocalcaemia. The ameloblasts showed vacuoles.[855]

These diseases have in common high fever with dehydration, which causes inadequate kidney function, and which in turn alters the calcium:phosphate ratio of serum. Diseases of the kidneys, such as "nephrotic syndrome"[423 653 814] are associated with enamel hypoplasia. The tooth

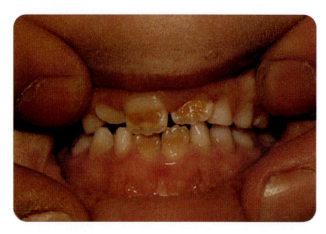

Figure 3.7 Malarial fever was assumed to have resulted in the hypoplasia and brown discoloration of the enamel of the permanent central incisors seen here. The permanent first molars were likewise affected.

Table 3.1 Factors related to the prevalence of developmental enamel defects in deciduous teeth[751]

Cause	Risk factor	Odds ratio
Generalised defects		
Birthweight	<2.5 kg	5.0
Enteropathy	Disease	3.7
Oral trauma	Trauma	3.0
Nutritional status	Measured with height for age	2.6
Toothpaste swallowed		2.4
Area	Urban low class-rural low class	2.2
Bronchial disease	Disease	2.0
Distinct defects		
Birthweight	<2.5 kg	3.0
Nutritional status	Measured with height for age	2.8
Bronchial disease	Disease	2.5
Hypoplastic defects		
Birthweight	<2.5 kg	2.2
Nutritional status	Measured with height for age	1.9

defects may also be caused by medicines such as the tetracyclines.

3.2.3 Malnutrition and systemic-nutritional disorders

A sufficient supply of calcium and phosphate, the building blocks of hydroxyapatite ($Ca_{10}(PO_4)_6(OH)_2$), and an adequate nutritional supply of vitamins and trace elements are essential for enamel and dentine matrix formation.

Nutritional deficiencies
Severe and chronic malnutrition causes (chronological) enamel hypoplasia,[102 256 415 750 751 874] with black stained teeth.[770] The substandard diet and health status in children and adolescents whose remains were excavated from a sixteenth- to eighteenth-century graveyard in London had caused severe enamel hypoplasia and molars with multiple additional cusps (resembling the mulberry molars).[1035] White or otherwise discoloured band-like constrictions encircling the deciduous incisors, called *odontoclasia*, were more frequent and severe whenever malnutrition was more evident. The occurrence of enamel hypoplasia and hypocalcification has been found to be race-related/dependent, as is malnutrition.[361 362] Nutritional status is a factor, but birthweight and enteropathy and child's stature[531] seem of more importance (Table 3.1).[751]

The supply, for instance, of vitamins will also continue to be low in malnourishment.[874] Among a sample of severely malnourished children, 73% had hypoplastic deciduous incisors versus 43% with moderate malnutrition.[874] Of less well-fed children, about 20% showed hypoplasia against none with a good diet.[256] Similar results were found in another study.[586 770]

Minerals
Calcium The dry weight of calcium in the enamel is 34–40% and in the dentine 26–28%. To affect the teeth, the calcium deficiency must be extreme.[193] The combined action of parathormone, calcitonin and vitamin D maintains very stable calcium and phosphate blood levels, even when the mineral intake is suboptimal. When the bone shows signs of deficiency, the enamel will be normal, but the dentine seems more vulnerable.

At birth, the calcium level suddenly decreases. A very low level, 7.5 mg/100 mL and less (at which neonates experience tetany) is associated with enamel hypoplasia and abundant interglobular dentine.[777] An experimental study found that diet-induced chronic hypocalcaemia in rats probably interfered with cellular and extracellular events during enamel maturation,[624] and caused hypocalcification of the enamel of the incisors, with many residual enamel proteins.[116] While human teeth are formed in a different way, dietary hypocalcaemia may affect development of human enamel.

Pregnancy and lactation alter the maternal skeletal metabolism to accommodate fetal skeletal mineralisation and milk production.[668] Rats nursed and weaned after 30 days on a diet low in calcium had hypocalcified enamel. Pups fed the first 10 days on a normal and the next 20 days on a low calcium diet had normally calcified enamel.[116] In a similar experiment, low birthweight offspring were weaned on a calcium-free diet: the enamel matrix was hypocalcified and the reduced dentine matrix was normally calcified. When restored to a calcium-containing diet, the enamel became completely mineralised and the dentine thickness and mineral apposition increased.[527] A diet low in calcium caused variable and heterogeneous distribution of amelogenins in the enamel, with albumin leakage into the enamel organ.[624]

Phosphate The dry weight of phosphate in the enamel is 16–18% and 12% in the dentine. Phosphate deficiency is commonly not due to insufficient supply, but due to other causes, such as vitamin D-resistant rickets.[719]

Trace elements

Magnesium (0.4% dry weight of the dentine and the enamel)[777] appears essential in odontogenesis,[407] but teeth with higher levels of magnesium are more vulnerable to caries.[777] Insufficient iron causes enamel hypoplasia through enzyme damage.[701]

Fluoride is also essential for odontogenesis.[322 632] Other trace elements (which are not similarly distributed within the enamel and dentine) include: zinc, silica, and to a lesser degree copper, chromium, manganese, molybdenum and tin. Very small quantities of selenium, vanadium and cobalt are also present. Their importance in odontogenesis is largely unknown. Strontium in the crystal lattice may cause diffuse opacities.[195] A diet may not contain all the above elements.

Proteins

Diets with variable ratios of sucrose and casein, fed to female rats during pregnancy and lactation, resulted in smaller molars (due to reduced amounts of dentine) in the offspring. When a diet low in protein was given, many of the offsprings' third molars lacked cusps, that is, small amounts of protein deficiency at different times during the perinatal period resulted in abnormal cuspal patterns of the third molars.[626]

Protein deficiency in animals increases the risk of enamel hypoplasia[874] and caries,[46 642] and hypoplasia may enhance caries progression. Malnourished children, however, show hardly any dental caries, possibly because of the lack of sucrose in the diet. Prenatal malnutrition causes hypoplasia of the deciduous enamel, which was found to associated with caries development in Native Americans living in 100BC to AD500.[183]

Vitamins

The average diet in Western industrialised countries guarantees roughly an adequate supply of vitamins.[240 384] Deficiencies are apparent in various groups including older people, vegetarians, alcoholics and persons with other addictions, immigrants, young people, ill or cancer patients, etc.[240 778 780]

Vitamins B and E are water-soluble, and A, D, K and E are fat-soluble. Excess amounts of B and C have a low potential for toxicity, because they are rapidly excreted with the urine.

Vitamin A

Vitamin A in its active form is present in meats and as pre-vitamin in vegetables and fruit. The vitamin is stored in the liver and is mobilised from there, and is essential for embryogenesis, growth and epithelial differentiation.

Deficiency of vitamin A, *hypovitaminosis A*, causes night blindness, and if this is long-lasting, corneal keratinisation develops, with furthers alterations in the mucosa and the brain. Severe hypovitaminosis A causes disturbances in the formation of the (pre)dentine and enamel (matrix).[366 586]

Hypovitaminosis A was found to alter collagen synthesis and the calcium:phosphate ratio in molar tooth germs in rats. The ameloblasts atrophied and dentinogenesis was delayed.[627] Hypovitaminosis A during the first postnatal month resulted in pitted enamel in many rats.[873] Infants with hypovitaminosis A were found to have atrophied tooth germs. In less severe cases, the stellate reticulum was condensed, the dentine was poorly mineralised, and the predentine was widened.[221] Another study found that vitamin A-deficient rats lacked odontoblast differentiation, and retinoic acid supplementation reduced this effect.[704]

The incisors of rats fed for 200 days on a diet poor in vitamin A showed marked morphological changes; the enamel was folded in an accordion-like fashion.[182] In another study, the inhibition of intra-uterine growth of the rat tooth germ due to vitamin A deficiency was transient, although the enamel remained less dense.[290]

Hypervitaminosis A, through its toxic effects, also impedes the growth and development of the tooth germ, differentiation of the odontoblasts and possibly the ameloblasts.[157 410] Where odontoblasts are formed, predentine development is disrupted. Hypervitaminosis A also causes gingivitis, fissures at the angles of the mouth, and generalised symptoms (irritability, headache and fatigue).[280]

Injected radio-labelled vitamin A has been found to be taken up by the liver, kidneys and ameloblasts active at that time, but not by the hard tissues.[818] These finding might be related to the decreased stratum intermedium volume in hypervitaminosis A.[182]

High-dose vitamin A supplementation in pregnant women results in fetal defects, although exact amounts are not known.[745 967] A range of 700–1000 µg vitamin A/day has been advised; 3000 µg/day may be the upper limit in post-menopausal women to alleviate the risk of hip fractures,[279] but this dose certainly seems too high for the unborn child.

Vitamin C

This vitamin is present as ascorbic acid in (plant) foods. Children up to the age of 3 years need 20 mg vitamin C/day, increasing to 30–35 mg/day in 7–9-year-olds. A large kiwi fruit contains about 70 mg of vitamin C.[749] *Hypovitaminosis C*, also called scurvy, causes weakness, anaemia, subcutaneous and gingival bleeding and loss of teeth (scurvy was formerly fatal in sailors on long sea voyages).

Deficiency of vitamin C at the time of the odontogenesis causes pitted enamel and reduces the height of the odontoblasts, which also become disorganised. Bleeding is seen in the pulp and in the enamel organ.[692] *In vitro* explanted/

excised tooth germs appear to need vitamin C for the synthesis of collagen[131 380] and the incorporation of proline (and lysine) into the collagen molecule.[940]

Vitamin D

This vitamin is formed from a provitamin (7-dehydrocholesterol) in the skin under the influence of sunlight. The vitamin is present in some foodstuffs as ergocalciferol or cholecalciferol and is transported to the liver and hydrolysed into $25(OH)D_3$, which is metabolised in the kidneys into the active, functional "vitamin D_3 hormone", i.e. $1,25\ (OH)_2D_3$. D_3 hormone is of importance in the resorption of bone,[552] but its role and that of the other vitamin D metabolites has not been fully elucidated,[282] partly because the consequences of a deficiency are compensated for by normalisation of the plasma level of calcium,[712] or a direct effect on ameloblasts.[884]

Vitamin D together with parathyroid hormone (Section 3.2.4) regulates the serum levels of calcium and phosphate, even when the supply is irregular. Hormonal D_3 regulates the serum concentrations of calcium and phosphate, stimulates the uptake of these minerals in the small intestine, promotes the transport of calcium within the skeleton, and directs the reabsorption of calcium in the kidneys.[282] Kidney malfunction reduces the excretion of phosphate, which causes hyperphosphataemia and formation of calcium–phosphate complexes, which in turn induce *secondary hyperparathyroidism*.[708] Hypoplastic, hypocalcified and discoloured enamel and pathological root resorption is present in children with chronic renal failure.[162] Severe chronic renal failure results in reduced synthesis of D_3 hormone, which then leads to increase in the synthesis and secretion of parathormone; this is also a cause of secondary hyperparathyroidism (Figure 3.8).

Hypovitaminosis D causes rickets in children; nowadays rickets is rarely seen in the developed Western countries, but it continues to occur in countries such as Yemen and Saudi Arabia[243 906] where children's and women's skin is not exposed to the sun (even after emigration to countries in the temperate zones). Children born to mothers with vitamin D deficiency in sunny Crete (Greece) were found to respond favourably to treatment with calcium and vitamin D.[30] Breast-fed children may have vitamin D deficiency if the mother is a strict vegetarian.

In rickets, the skeleton does not ossify completely and the osteoid tissues hypertrophy. Under normal loading, the bones become distorted, and the clinical features include lateral bowing of the legs and scoliosis. The dental hard tissues are affected, particularly the dentine: irregular tubules, atubular globular areas, and a large amount of interglobular dentine are evident.[80 163 587 635] With more severe rickets, the defects noted in the teeth also increase.[244 340]

Steady-state levels of amelogenin and enamelin mRNA, which regulate the tooth proteins, were reduced in the incisor epithelium of vitamin D-deficient rats, which also showed a dramatic decrease of interprismatic enamel.[675]

Calcium deficiency is more serious than a reduced supply of vitamin D.[587] Vitamin D deficiency alone has less impact on the teeth than on bone, but a combined deficiency of vitamin D and calcium affects the teeth and bones to the same extent.[277] With such a deficient diet, the calcium serum levels are reduced,[255] the predentine layer is widened[255] due to accelerated protein production,[252 254] and odontoblastic enzyme activities are also affected.[252 255 256 455] However, the deficiency state must be sustained for a longer period to cause enamel defects.[714] Whether the hypocalcaemia or the increased synthesis of parathormone enhances the activity of the odontoblasts is unknown.[253] The secreting ameloblasts are also affected directly.[885] Severe rickets is accompanied by significant enamel hypoplasia in some regions, but not in others.[271 692] The pulp chambers and horns are large.[635] Rachitic deciduous dentitions exfoliate early[635] and children often show a vertical open bite.[810]

Calcium (900 g/day) and fluoride (50 mg NaF/day) supplements have been used to treat osteoporosis in post-menopausal women in whom oestrogen production has dropped. If not complemented by a huge supply of vitamin D (50 000 units/week), large amounts of unmineralised bone matrix are formed.[437] Fluo-

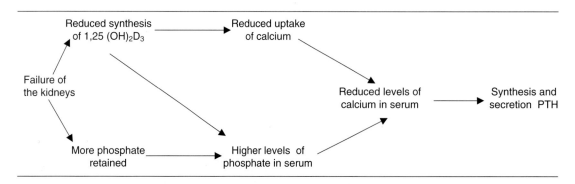

Figure 3.8 Renal failure promotes the synthesis and secretion of parathormone (PTH).[162]

ride supplementation via milk (calcium) in vitamin D-deficient women does not alter the (subclinical) signs of rickets.[845]

Hypervitaminosis D is rare and leads to hypercalcaemia. Symptoms include calcium deposits in the kidney, weakness, gastrointestinal distress and deranged fat metabolism.[280] Enamel hypoplasia (depressions) corresponds to the time of the hypervitaminosis. Dogs had hypermineralised enamel.[320 692]

Vitamin E

This vitamin stabilises the unsaturated fats against autooxidation, thus protecting the cellular membranes against damage. Vitamin E supplements are given to prematurely born children as prophylaxis against hyperbilirubinaemia, but study results are contradictory.[104] *Hypovitaminosis E* leads to oedema in the enamel organ of rats.[692] In *hypervitaminosis E*, the calcium and phosphate levels in teeth are increased, but the consequences of this (in humans) are not known.

Other vitamins

Hypovitaminosis K could in principle underlie enamel defects as it lowers the calcium levels in plasma. Effects of a deficiency state of other vitamins are not described in the literature.

Systemic disorders due to decreased uptake of dietary substances

Malabsorption or the inability to respond to a regular supply of a nutritional component may also cause enamel defects. Due to lack of data, diseases such as necrotising enterocolitis, a common medical complication of preterm infants, are not discussed here.[796]

Coeliac disease This inherited digestive disorder is an allergy involving a selective lack of T cell tolerance for gluten (proteins in grains), which leads to atrophy of the small-bowel villous mucosa. Coeliac disease is the most common cause of malabsorption in the industrialised countries.[8] Patients do not tolerate gluten in wheat, oat, rye and barley, but they can tolerate other proteins. Glutamine is enzymatically (transglutaminase) transformed into glutamine acid, to which gliadin is linked. The complex consisting of the two proteins sensitises and provokes the allergic reaction.[908]

In patients with coeliac disease consuming gluten, the absorption of other dietary substances is deranged. Clinical features include diarrhoea, weight loss, anaemia (iron deficiency), spontaneous fractures (due to deficient vitamin D and calcium), dermatitis herpetiformis, sometimes in only one location (elbow), diabetes mellitus and delayed puberty. Today, the clinical picture of the disease often is atypical.[9 11]

In the Netherlands, the prevalence of coeliac disease is approximately 2: 100000, varying by region and city due to diagnostic reasons and dietary differences. In the UK, the prevalence is twice as high.[429] One paper estimates 1% of the population may be affected.[584]

The teeth (70–75%, mainly incisors and molars, in any quadrant) of most patients (80–95%) show defects that are chronologically distributed (Figure 3.9). The tooth defects may be the only sign of the disease; a gluten-free diet reduces the risk of development of enamel defects. Seemingly healthy family members may also show dental lesions, which is an indication to screen them for the disease. In coeliac disease, it is the immunological response, and not the hypocalcaemia, that causes the defects in the enamel.[8 9 11 549 559]

The patients typically have leucocyte antigens (DR3 and DQ2),[8] while DR5,7 seems to protect against enamel defects.[539] The coeliac-type enamel defects are classified into:

I: Enamel discoloration
II: Mild hypoplasia: horizontal grooves
III: Hypoplasia: deep horizontal grooves and large vertical pits
IV: Severe hypoplasia: altered tooth morphology.

The teeth of both dentitions are severely hypomineralised with shortened, irregularly distributed prisms and decreased interprismatic substance.[1036]

The diagnosis is based on biopsy of the mucous membrane of the small intestine, and is confirmed with a second biopsy 1 year after start of treatment and a gluten provocation test to exclude patients who have a temporary intolerance. The provocation test is not performed before the age of 6 years in patients presenting with tooth defects suspected of having coeliac disease.[721] An immunochromatographic assay for IgA and IgG antibodies to transglutaminase may be used instead of the biopsy.[833]

Late detection of coeliac disease in adults, owing to an atypical course of the disease, may have serious consequences: some 10% of unexplained osteoporosis cases are ascribed to the disease, and about 5% develop T cell lymphoma.[584]

Hypophosphataemic vitamin D-resistant rickets (hypophosphataemia) *Vitamin D-resistant rickets* ("refractory rickets") resembles hypovitaminosis D, notwithstanding a normal vitamin D status. An autosomal dominant[292 316] ("hypophosphataemic bone disease")[788] and a X-linked form[381 793] ("familial hypophosphataemia")[4] exist. Additionally, an autosomal recessive form has been reported.[282 291 292 293]

Hypovitaminosis D is rapidly remedied with small amounts (up to 50 µg/day) of the vitamin, but vitamin D-resistant rickets requires large doses, hence its name.[108 215] Several forms of the disease exist.[98] Adults show active and inactive hypophosphataemia with and without post-rachitic deformities. Another form is the vitamin D-resistant hypophosphataemia, which requires treatment with large vitamin D doses (but there is risk of hypervitaminosis).

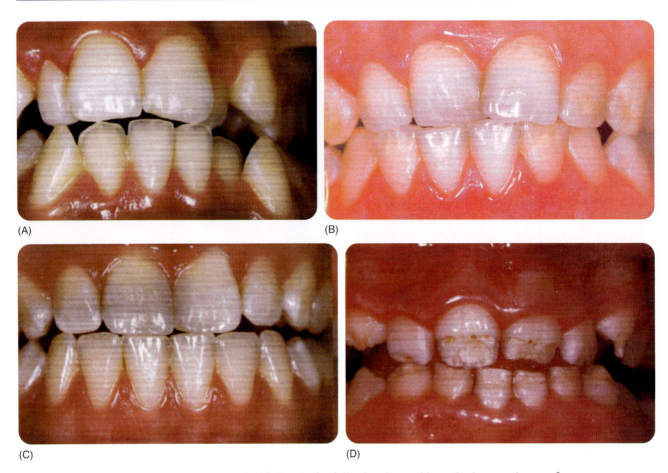

(A)   (B)
(C)   (D)

Figure 3.9 (A–D) The teeth in coeliac disease, classified on basis of discoloration and hypoplastic enamel as I–IV.[9]

In spite of treatment at an early age, some rachitic skeletal effects, such as a mild bowing of the legs, invariably remain.[174] The first symptom may be a delay in walking caused by deformed legs (bowing) at approximately 2 years of age,[681] but osteomalacia is often so mild that the dental manifestations are the first indication of presence of the disease.[793]

Dental manifestations Some patients show few or mild effects but others develop severe anomalies.[806]

- Alveolus development and calcification is poor in untreated patients and leads to loss of the lamina dura and periodontal ligament.[174] Chronic periodontal disease may be present.[1025]
- The enamel may be normal,[4] but is mostly hypoplastic, thin and yellow,[924] with clefts.[49 300 328 355 365 561 670 981] The enamel may be free of caries even when microorganisms have penetrated the dentine.[390] Enamel hypoplasia and diffuse hypocalcification seem more frequent in the autosomal than in the X-linked form.[788] At the time of its maturation, the enamel of vitamin D-resistant pigs was found to contain large amounts of non-degraded

amelogenins.[520] Various degrees of enamel fractures and wear have been reported.[174] In the hypovitaminosis D form of rickets the incisal and occlusal enamel is hypoplastic more frequently as well as to a greater extent than in hypophosphataemia.[108]

- The amelodentinal junction is histologically quite normal.
- The dentine is primarily affected. The mantle dentine is normal,[390] the deeper dentine is hypoplastic, thin, globular and poorly mineralised.[154 174 799 806 981] The more severe the disorder, the greater is the amount of globular dentine,[4 126 807 924] which is graded as (in deciduous teeth); I (<50% globular); II (>50% globular); and III (almost 100% globular).[807] The predentine is wide and there is extensive reparative dentine formation.[39] Although a diet rich in calcium and phosphate lead to increase in the serum phosphate level in vitamin D-resistant mice, the amount of interglobular dentine did not decrease,[3 387] which is indicative of genetic influences.[387] The dentinal calcium:phosphate ratio in rickets is increased.[4] The teeth contain more sodium and magnesium than normal, and the interglobular spaces contain more zinc than other parts of the

tooth, but the significance of these findings remains unexplained.[387]

- Tubule-like extensions (or microcracks) in the dentine around the pulpal extensions connect the pulp horns of the large pulp chamber[4 520 788] with the amelodentinal junction and enamel clefts, with fissures linking the enamel subsurface to the pulp horns.[540] The pulp may become necrotic without any sign of caries,[4 126 681 924] or even when any decay has been adequately treated.[154] In severe cases, periapical abscesses are common.[381 793 807] Sinus tracts may be the first sign of the disorder, especially in the deciduous dentition.[806 799 1019]

- The cementum has also been found to be abnormal: there is less cellular cementum and irregular calcification.[174] Root completion and eruption are delayed.[316 365 520 561]

Taurodontism has been observed in more severely affected males.[328] In hypovitaminosis D, the prenatal dentine is abnormal[900] and interglobular dentine develops postnatally.[355 561] Angle's Class III malocclusion is frequently seen in the X-linked form.[788]

Epidemiology Vitamin D-resistant rickets (prevalence 1 : 20 000) affects more girls than boys,[108 788] although the reverse has also been documented.[583] Boys show more severe anomalies.[300 799]

A substantial number of (untreated) patients have multiple periapical abscesses in the deciduous and/or permanent dentition, even in caries-free and clinically normal teeth,[48 174 328 583 710 1037] especially in the deciduous dentition.[583] The medication dose is an unreliable predictor of abscess occurrence.[583] The younger the patient when the first abscesses occur, the more severe the dental manifestations of the disease.[799] Wear of the enamel and the defective dentine accounts for the microbial invasion of the pulps of deciduous teeth, but the reason why the pulps of permanent teeth become necrotic remains unexplained in a number of cases. In the absence significant wear, enamel infractions may provide a route of entry for the microorganisms.[328]

Aetiology The tubular reabsorption of inorganic phosphate in the kidneys and the gastrointestinal uptake of calcium is below normal, and this affects women more than men.[4 300 355 456 550] In X-linked rickets, the availability of calcium is the main problem, although some researchers have implicated phosphate. The calcium level is, however, normal.[788] The disorder is attributed to the inability to form hormone D_3 due to a deficiency in the enzyme 25(OH)-D-1-hydroxylase.[291 292 293 1025] Hypocalcaemia due to insufficient D_3 hormone leads to hyperparathyroidism, which partly corrects the calcium plasma level, but impairs the reabsorption of phosphates in the

renal tubules, causing hypophosphataemia.[154 292 293] The mineralisation of bone is thus defective.[550]

In autosomal dominant rickets, the amount of D_3 hormone is sufficient; but the hormone D_3 receptors in all kinds of cell are abnormal.[456] In the X-linked and autosomal dominant disorder the serum values for phosphate are similar.[788] In the autosomal form, the alkaline phosphatase and D_3 hormone levels are persistently high.[456] The deficiency in phosphates caused by other diseases and syndromes may be expected to result in dental anomalies, but not much is known in this regard.[998] For instance, hypophosphataemia caused by an inherited excessive renal excretion of phosphates increases the production of D_3 hormone.[889] Effects on the teeth are not reported, but might exist via a vitamin D-dependent calcium-binding protein in the ameloblasts.[885]

Prevention and therapy The dentist may play a key role in identification of the disorder because of the presence of dental abscesses. Prevention lies is in the hands of the physician. The tooth anomalies in the X-linked form may be prevented by early administration of D_3 hormone or 1-α-(OH)D_3 with phosphate supplements,[154 282 550] which also alleviates the bone or joint pain in adults.[864]

Standard treatment with D_3 hormone followed after 1 year by supplementation with 24,25(OH)$_2$D$_3$ corrects hyperparathyroidism.[147] The improvement in rachitic symptoms is greater when the treatment is started earlier than after the first year of life, but it does not completely normalise skeletal development.[550] Oral phosphate and calcitriol effectively prevent skeletal abnormalities, but prolonged high-dose treatment is associated with secondary and occasionally tertiary hyperparathyroidism (i.e. with hypercalcaemia).[551]

In partial nephrectomy, intestinal calcium absorption is not influenced by treatment with D_3 hormone, nor when this is combined with 24,25(OH$_2$)D$_3$. In one study, in rats with normal renal function, 24,25(OH$_2$)D$_3$ enhanced the hypercalcaemic effect of D_3 hormone, whereas in rats with chronic renal failure, 24,25(OH$_2$)D$_3$ suppressed hypercalcaemia.[748]

Autosomal rickets is treated with long-term supplementation with phosphate[868 889] and various forms of vitamin D. Children treated from infancy with these agents have been shown to develop a normal dentition, although with prominent pulp horns and enlarged pulp cavities.[154]

Any endodontic treatment required may be jeopardised[1020] because the defective dentine obstructs mechanical endodontic cleaning.[799] Preventive treatment with temporary crowns is advisable,[800 1020] but passage of microorganisms through microcracks in the dentine increase the risk of pulpitis. Tooth separation with orthodontic elastics before crown placement to minimise tissue removal is recommended.[126 799] The least biologically damaging luting cements must be used.[126] Prophylactic formocresol pulpotomy and a stainless steel crown resulted in 75% failure rate; however, the shorter the time between eruption and treatment, the higher is the success rate.[813] The dentine cannot support restorative posts for crowns.[799]

3.2.4 Endocrine disorders

The neurosecretory cells of the hypothalamus, the part of the brain located under the thalamus, produces and secretes in concert with the demands of the body several hormones that act as signalling molecules for the anterior part of the pituitary gland.

Pituitary gland

The pea-sized pituitary gland lies underneath the hypothalamus and regulates other endocrine glands by secreting hormones. Deficient production of the thyroid-stimulating hormone (TSH) by the anterior part of the pituitary leads to hypothyroidism.[611]

Thyroid gland

The thyroid gland lies at the front of the neck and produces two hormones: thyroxine and calcitonin. Thyroid disease, which predominantly occurs among women, affects an estimated 15% of the population in the USA. General anaesthesia for uncooperative or phobic dental patients may be contraindicated in those with hypothyroidism and hyperthyroidism.[610 611]

Thyroxine (thyroid hormone) regulates the metabolic rate of most cells in the body, the body temperature, growth and development. Deficiency in childhood causes cretinism, a condition characterised by physical and mental underdevelopment as well as extensive enamel hypoplasia.[473] The pituitary gland produces TSH in response to a low thyroxine level. High levels of thyroxine inhibit TSH production and therefore of thyroxine itself.

Hypothyroidism may for several reasons be present even before birth. Anti-thyroid treatment during pregnancy for hyperthyroidism (also known as Graves' disease; goitre with exophthalmia) prevents malformation and intrauterine death of the fetus, but may lead to reversible fetal hypothyroidism,[188] and thereby enamel hypoplasia. The thyroid may be aplastic or absent. Other reasons are maternal iodine deficiency, severe iron deficiency, chronic thyroiditis, tissue resistance to hormones, use of pharmacological agents such as lithium and radioactive iodide for the treatment of goitre, or it may be idiopathic.

Deficiency of growth hormone may result in enamel hypoplasia and hypocalcification of the deciduous teeth and delayed eruption; the latter is the most frequent anomaly.[392] In permanent teeth the lines of Retzius are broader than normal. These anomalies might represent a direct or a secondary effect.[181] In half the children with congenital hypothyroidism the enamel formed both pre- and postnatally is hypomineralised and hypoplastic and the crowns are malformed. Pore size in enamel is increased, in particular when thyroxine deficiency com-

mences before birth.[638] Dentine development is retarded.[82 392 639] Early recognition, in which the dentist may play a role,[695] and treatment of juvenile hypothyroidism prevents development of dental abnormalities to a degree.

In one report, removal of the pituitary gland and administration of thiouracil resulted in enamel and dentine defects,[83] probably because thyroxine deficiency caused secondary hypothyroidism. In another report, hypothyroidism due to deficiency in TSH resulted in deciduous teeth with structural defects.[197] Severe enamel hypoplasia and delayed eruption may follow hypothyroidism (or renal acidosis) due to congenital disease of the renal tubules (glomerulopathy). Reabsorption and retention of calcium is severely reduced in acute and chronic renal acidosis.[317]

Hyperthyroidism, caused for instance by abnormally high secretion of TSH, is associated with increased susceptibility to caries and periodontal disease.[353]

Parathyroid gland

Parathormone (PTH) is produced by the parathyroid gland, which consists of four small compact collections of cells at and in the posterior region of the thyroid gland. Together with its antagonist *calcitonin* (from the thyroid gland) and vitamin D, PTH regulates the serum levels of calcium and phosphate. The peptide calcitonin inhibits calcium release from the bone.

Calcium ion sensing cells in the parathyroid and elsewhere (brain, kidney) detect minute perturbations in the extracellular calcium concentration and respond by adaptive mechanisms, for instance rapid increase in renal tubular reabsorption of calcium, inhibition of renal blood flow and glomerular filtration.[135] The effect of vitamin D metabolites on the production of PTH is neither direct nor acute.[546] In case of (pseudo)hypoparathyroidism symptoms do not arise, or they disappear after administration of vitamin D.[432]

PTH deficiency results in insufficient absorption of calcium from the bowel and reduced urinary excretion of phosphate, resulting in tetany. Insensitivity of the target cells of PTH may have a similar effect. PTH deficiency can be part of a syndrome or it is idiopathic, with tetany and physical and mental retardation. Parathyroid hypofunction is rare and starts, unless familial,[304 696] around the age of 1.5 years.[781] Hypofunction can also occur inadvertently due to removal of the glands at thyroidectomy or trauma to the neck at birth. This hypofunction may be transient.[651]

Parathormone-related protein (PTHrP) and its receptor (PTHR1) regulate fetal epithelial–mesenchymal interactions , for example, in the skin and teeth. In PTHrP knockout mice, osteoblasts lining the inner aspects of the alveolar bone produced bony spicules that penetrated the enamel organs, partially destroying them, but morphological abnormalities were absent in cells of the tooth germ proper.[468] Loss-of-function mutations in PTHR1 did not suppress tooth development, but the teeth, being enclosed in the bony crypts, did not erupt.[1017]

PTH enhances the action of vitamin D in the uptake of calcium by the enamel organ in its secretory stage.[84] Effects of PTH and calcitonin on odontogenesis are not exactly known.[763] In idiopathic[294] and familial[629] (X-linked)[996] *hypoparathyroidism*, the enamel is hypoplastic, due to either the ectodermal effects of the hormone deficiency or as a direct consequence of the low calcium serum level.[304] Dentine defects correspond closely with the calcium level, which varies depending on the type and timing of treatment of the disorder.[466]

In *pseudohypoparathyroidism*, a congenital and inherited disorder, the patient does not respond to supplementation with PTH; the condition is also known as osteodystrophy or Albright's disease. Hypoparathyroidism and pseudohypoparathyroidism are differentiated by measuring the phosphate level in urine after administering PTH. Vitamin D therapy influences the results of the measurement of the phosphate levels.[1018]

More patients with pseudohypoparathyroidism than those with hypoparathyroidism are reported to have enamel hypoplasia (Figure 3.10); all exhibit hypodontia and delayed eruption.[432 865] Pseudohypoparathyroidism results in short roots and yellow discoloured, hypoplastic and thin enamel,[739 865] and defective dentine.[466] The large pulp chamber contains pulp stones. Caries is another sign. The fourth and fifth fingers are not well developed and calcifications are found in the femoral muscles.[865] Family members showing all symptoms except dental symptoms are said to have *pseudo-pseudohypoparathyroidism*,[739] which presently is regarded to differ only in severity from pseudohypoparathyroidism.[765]

In patients on *haemodialysis*, the renal failure alters vitamin D metabolism, which in turn lowers the intestinal absorption of calcium. The consequent secondary hyperparathyroidism may result in decalcification of cortical bone, specially of the mandible, which also reduces in width at the gonion, and is used a measure of renal or

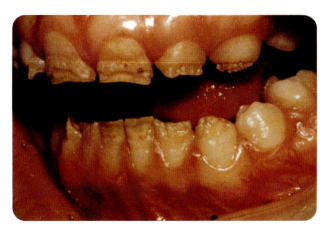

Figure 3.10 Hypoplasia and discoloration of the enamel caused by hypoparathyroidism.

dialysis osteodystrophy.[123 162] The predentine in adults with renal failure or undergoing haemodialysis is thickened and shows irregularities.[162] A patient with renal failure had lesions resembling internal resorption (Chapter 7) which, remarkably, disappeared after the patient recovered.[413]

Pancreas (islets of Langerhans)
The pancreas produces digestive enzymes, which are excreted into the small intestine, and endocrine hormones are produced by the islet cells. Insulin is formed by one type of islet cells (Langerhans cells). Failure of production of insulin causes type 1 diabetes mellitus, which, as has already been described, affects the developing teeth in the fetus. In diabetic children in whom the disease is well controlled, the mean number with enamel hypoplasia will match the population mean.[339]

Gonads and adrenal glands
Dysfunction of the gonads leads to accelerated or delayed development of bone, but rarely affects odontogenesis.[765] Ovariectomy in rats increased the rate of the bone metabolism, leading to osteoporosis, and activated the odontoblasts, which produced more dentine, in particular in young animals.[388]

There are no reports of any effects of adrenaline, noradrenaline or the corticosteroid hormones produced by the adrenal glands on odontogenesis.

3.2.5 Chemicals/medicaments
Fluoride
Dental fluorosis includes structural anomalies of the enamel that manifest as white or brown discolorations and hypoplasia, caused by overconsumption of fluoride during odontogenesis. Around 1900, Frederick McKay, an American dentist, noticed stained teeth in individuals who had grown up in Colorado Springs (called "Colorado brown stain", later "mottled enamel") that were free of caries. McKay presumed the drinking water was responsible. Some 30 years later, a chemist, H. V. Churchill, found that the water contained significant amounts of fluoride: 13.7 parts fluoride per million parts of water.[618] [632] The term "endemic dental fluorosis" is preferred to "mottling" and "mottled enamel".

Later studies showed that water in other areas also appeared to have high fluoride levels and supplementation of water with fluoride produced – proportional to its concentration – mottling in animals.[630] Fluorosis also occurs in animals in the wild.[454]

General health aspects
Fluoride is essential for general health. The reproductive ability of female mice on a low fluoride diet was found to progressively decline over two generations and was restored after the rats were given additional fluoride.[595]

Water, mostly from deep wells worldwide, contains 6–10 mg fluoride/L or even more. Ingestion of fluoride at such high levels, for at least 10 years (*chronic high doses*),[949] is associated with endemic dental fluorosis and in (sub)tropical regions with "crippling" fluorosis.[977 1005 1006 1007] Children may already show slight clinical signs of skeletal fluorosis in the legs.[689] Skeletal fluorosis results from calcifications of ligaments causing rigidity, hyper-mineralisation and exostoses of flat and long bones, and other deformities in the body.[1005 1006] The disorder has not been observed in the USA despite high fluoride concentrations; presumably predisposing factors such as dietary deficiencies also need to be present.[977] Increased fluoride intake may increase the calcium demand, and the effect of calcium deficiency on the skeleton might be enhanced by fluoride surplus.[689] Fluoride has been, as said, administered to prevent osteoporosis in menopause and thereafter, when loss of bone tissue and calcium predisposes women to fractures.

Calcium, 50–75 mg NaF/day, and vitamin D supplementation, and eventually female hormones, have been shown to reduce the number of fractures,[237 556] but some research has also found an increase.[389] Negative effects of fluoridated water have been questioned because no association with water fluoridation has been established.[504 700 977 1005] Bone resistance against compression increases, but not against torsion.[237]

Chronic low fluoride ingestion does not cause, in contrast with statements made by anti-fluoridists, disturbances in the immune system, a higher incidence of cancer or cardiovascular disorders, genotoxicity or teratogenicity, a higher rate of trisomy 21, or increased mortality.[112 150 184 632 977] Anti-fluoride supporters have pointed out the difference in death rates between life-long residents of two towns with high and low fluoride levels, but they failed to mention that the average age in the former town was much higher.[949]

In one Chinese study, the IQ of children ingesting 4.12 mg fluoride/L drinking water was lower than in a neighbouring town (0.91 mg/L) under otherwise identical circumstances.[1030] These findings are yet to be confirmed. The evidence for issues raised by the anti-fluoridation lobby is based mainly on low-quality studies. For example, the inclusion criteria in a review were less stringent for papers reporting an adverse effect than for papers with positive findings.[901] In people who assumed that their drinking water was artificially fluoridated, (which, however, was not the case) and reported subjective complaints, such as headache, diarrhoea and constipation,[487] the complaints were most likely psychological in origin rather than biological.

An *acute high fluoride* dose is toxic and causes nausea, vomiting, abdominal pain and even death by cardiac or respiratory failure; a decline in plasma calcium and a rise in potassium concentration cause pathological changes in the muscles. Reported fatal doses include 32–64 mg, 15 mg and 5 mg fluoride/kg bodyweight; 5 mg fluoride/kg requires emergency hospitalisation.[949 977 978] *Sensitisation* to fluoride salts has not been reported since the past many

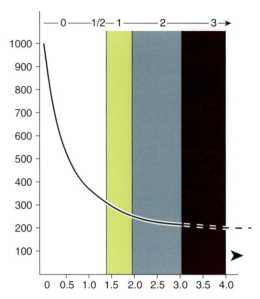

Figure 3.11 Relationship between fluoride concentration in the drinking water, caries and fluorosis. The scores on the Dental Fluorosis Index (Dean) are given at the top of the graph and the fluoride concentration (parts per million) at the bottom. The higher the fluoride concentration, the fewer is the number of carious teeth per 100 12–14-year-olds (X axis). The curvilinear line shows that an increase in the fluoride concentration is accompanied by a decrease in caries as well as more severe signs of fluorosis (opacities, brown discoloration and eventually hypoplasia).

years, in spite of the use of fluoride by tens of millions of people.

Dental fluorosis indices

Lustreless, narrow, parallel white lines, corresponding to the perikymata and caused by hypomineralisation of the enamel subsurface, characterise the mildest form of dental fluorosis.[895] When merged together (Figure 3.11), the lines constitute diffuse (cloudy, feathery, lacy, fleecy) white spots or flecks, without a clear border demarcating them from the unaffected enamel.[276] The prevalence of diffuse opacities increases with higher fluoride levels in water.[37 854 858 892] More severe fluorosis is manifested as brown stains and hypoplasia.

Dentists' views with respect to "mild fluorosis" have been found to differ from those of the public, who showed fewer aesthetic concerns. Parents were concerned when their children's teeth showed large white areas.[861] The aesthetic effects of fluorosis need to be determined in more detail bearing in mind the differences in risk of developing fluorosis in different countries and differences in dental health policies.[976]

Dean (1934) developed an index for classifying endemic fluorosis defects: the Dental Fluorosis Index (DFI, Table 3.2).[206] Summed scores for each individual are divided by

Table 3.2 Indices of dental fluorosis

Score	Dean[206]	Thylstrup and Fejerskov[896]	Horowitz et al.[403]
0	Normal	Normal after drying	Normal
0.5	Normal?	–	–
1	White flecks <1/4 of surface	Small white, parallel lines <1/3 of surface	White spots
2	White flecks <1/2 of surface	Broader white lines Occlusal small white spots	White spots >1/3 and <2/3 of surface
3	Brown All surfaces	Melting white lines Occlusal white demarcated spots Occlusal wear	>2/3 surface white spotted
4	Brown Pits, wear	Whole surface white Occlusal white and wear Soon after eruption	As above plus brown
5	–	Whole surface white + pits <2 mm	Discrete pits
6	–	Pits in horizontal bands Occlusal hypoplasia <3 mm of surface	Pits plus brown
7	–	Hypoplasia <1/2 of surface Occlusal morphologic changes	Melting pits or hypoplasia
8	–	>1/2 of surface hypoplastic	–
9	–	Larger part enamel absent	–

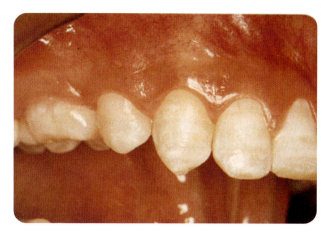

Figure 3.12 Fluorotic opacities are not very obvious in the enamel of the primary teeth.

the number of the subjects to achieve the score for a group.

Group scores (ordinal level of measurement) do not provide information about the distribution of the defects and are rather insensitive with respect to the severe forms of fluorosis.[141][165] A group may be assigned a score of 2 because all the children had score 2 or because it was the mean of different scores.

Since then, other researchers have also devised indices.[22][106][248][264][403][619][896] The Tooth Surface Fluorosis Index (TSFI) is useful to determine the problem of fluorosis at a community level.[401][403] The Thylstrup–Fejerskov Index (TFI), frequently applied in epidemiological studies, is more sensitive than Dean's DFI,[335] and reflects the fluoride content of the enamel[729] and correlates well with the degree of enamel hypomineralisation[165][852] (Table 3.2).

Dean et al. (1941–1942) studied 12–14-year-olds from 21 towns, calculated the DFI for each town and scored caries by counting, per individual, the number of carious

(Decayed), missing (Missed) and filled (Filled) teeth, to estimate the mean caries score, the DMFT index. The fluoride content in the drinking water per town was expressed as parts per million (ppm), which equals mg/L. More sophisticated is the DMFS (surfaces) index, in which the tooth surfaces instead of the teeth are scored, however, such subtleties reduce the reliability and reproducibility of the index.[89]

Dean's results[589] led to the conclusion that an increasing fluoride level in the drinking water is associated with higher DFI scores and reduces the DMFT scores in a curvilinear fashion (Figure 3.12). Other studies in areas with different concentrations of fluoride in water (ppm) and in different climate zones confirm Dean's findings.[38][152][263][266][288][344][406][470][525][747][792][966]

The "optimal" fluoride concentration in water in *temperate* zones is 1–1.2 ppm, at which level caries is reduced considerably and fluorosis is almost absent. At higher fluoride levels, more and more children show fluorosis of increasing severity. When the optimal concentration is exceeded considerably, the caries prevalence should increase again,[230][288][344][414][558] but this, however, is doubtful.[12][37][373][516] In *tropical* zones, children drink more water, which requires adjusting the optimal concentrations.[732] In, for instance, South Africa, Senegal and Chile, the optimum level is 0.7 ppm.[923] Despite much fluorosis being found in regions with a hot, dry climate,[946][1005] a decrease from 1.0 to 0.6–0.7 ppm in Hong Kong and Singapore still caused considerable fluorosis.[156][266] Fluoridation cessation decreased fluorosis scores in Canada.[1047]

McLure (1943) estimated water consumption from the amount of calories absorbed per day and the volume of dietary liquids.[579] Factors that were difficult to measure, such as salt consumption, and assumptions about the levels of liquid in foods, influenced the estimation. It appeared (at least in the UK) that children consume half of the estimated amount of water.[752] Moreover, the decline in water consumption and increase in that of carbonated beverages and juices had reduced the difference (USA) in water consumption between the climate zones.[377] Thus the guidelines for the fluoride concentration in drinking water need to be re-evaluated.[830]

In (warm) countries, drinking water is defluoridated if its level is high.[732] Yet, in tropical, subtropical and temperate zones with an (sub)optimal fluoride level, many children show mild mottling, likely caused by the fluoride.[37] [151 156 230 373 378 504 620 876 942 944 945 946] It seems a factor of 0.3 needs to be subtracted from the DFI score before it can be concluded that fluorosis is present in a community.[480] For the sake of caries reduction, mild fluorosis may be viewed to be acceptable.[515]

When optimal fluoride levels in drinking water were estimated, other sources of fluoride, such as toothpaste, were not available to the population.[504] Presently, fluoride is absorbed from several sources, including regions with optimally fluoridated water, which causes more frequent and more severe fluorosis.[418] The current prevalences of fluorosis and caries in regions with and without water with fluoride do not differ as much as in the past.[514]

Fluorosis may also result from the preparation of baby foods with water containing fluoride, even no more than 0.4 ppm.[259 498] Some mineral waters are rich in fluoride (Table 3.3) and should not be used to prepare baby foods.

Preparation of baby food powder with water low in fluoride decreases the fluoride content of the food from 3.7 μg F/g to 0.25 μg F/g.[816] Enfamil powder (Hong Kong) contains well over 1 ppm.[370] Manufacturers (USA) had promised to reduce the fluoride content in baby foods,[434] nevertheless, in 1997, baby food with chicken contained some 8 μg/g fluoride. This food alone would provide the recommended daily fluoride dose.[375]

The fluoride level has been more successfully reduced in baby foods based on milk than on soya products, making the daily dose too high.[286 577] Powdered milk dissolved in fluoridated water resulted in more fluorosis than did the consumption of pasteurised milk.[494] Processed cereals produced using fluoridated water contain 30–40 times more fluoride than those produced using non-fluoridated water. The daily intake from such formulas varies from several tens to some 100 μg/kg bodyweight.[286] The fluoride content in baby foods also varies by country.[142] None of the 113 tested baby foods in the UK were considered a risk for fluorosis.[926]

There is no established specific threshold below which fluorosis will not occur,[275] but it might be considered to be 0.1 mg/kg bodyweight.[872] The maximal safe daily dose suggested is 0.05 (to 0.07) mg/kg bodyweight,[839 960] which includes dietary and non-dietary fluoride.[512] Half of the optimal dose in a Hong Kong-based study was absorbed from food.[370] Low birthweight did not explain the higher prevalence of dental fluorosis in African American children.[483] Because of the relatively large levels of consumption of seafood, the mean daily uptake is somewhat higher in Japan[45] than in the USA (unless the water is fluoridated).[458]

Table 3.3 Fluoride contents (ppm) of some spring and mineral waters[574 782 839 899 961]

Brand	Country	ppm
Vichy-Celestines	France	5.8
President's Choice	Canada	4.8
Birgy Bronn	Germany	3.8
Christinen Brunnen	Germany	3.5
Hardenstein Brunnen	Germany	3.3
Redinger Mineralbrunnen	Germany	3.1
Überkinger Mineralwasser	Germany	2.9
Saint Yorre	France	2.8
Astra Quelle	Germany	2.8
Schwarzwald Sprudel	Germany	2.2
Zwestener Löwensprudel	Germany	1.6
Kellerwald-Quelle	Germany	1.5
Badoit	France	1.4
Fortuna (Rhön)	Germany	1.4
St. Maria Brunnen	Germany	1.4
Lavaredo	Italy	1.4
A & P	Canada	1.25
Ramlosa	Sweden	1.25[a]
Förstina Sprudel	Germany	1.2
Hirschquelle	Germany	1.2
Montclair	Canada	1.2
Kronthal-Quelle	Germany	1.0
Selters-Mineralquelle	Germany	1.0
Teinacher	Germany	1.0
Saint Leger	France	1.0
San Pellegrino	Italy	0.80[b]

[a]Identical to the Swedish with 3 ppm.[370]
[b]Toumba et al. 1994.[898]

Epidemiology

The term "fluorosis" has been used to indicate opacities that are not all fluorotic in origin.[822] To discern white fluorotic enamel defects from other lesions may be difficult.[665] To reiterate: enamel containing *strontium* mimics mild fluorosis.[779] In a region with optimally fluoridated water, the strontium content of the water varied locally between 0.02 and 33.9 mg/L and mottling varied accordingly.[195] Chronic acidosis and hypoxia (rats) have the same effect.[45] The carious white spot is more homogeneous and distinct than the fluorotic fleck. In 1961, Russell proposed some diagnostic criteria.[760] Drying the teeth and taking magnified photographs of the spots help to discern fluorotic lines.[247 507]

The question arises whether it is warranted to use specific fluorosis indices instead of the DDE.[250 665] There is no consensus with respect to the possibility of diagnosing fluorosis solely on the basis of its clinical appearance. The diagnosis "fluorosis" is warranted only if the patient history reveals a chronic, high intake (and the enamel defects are symmetrical), "chronic" meaning minimal of 3 months.[379] In one study, exposure to water containing almost 8 ppm of fluoride up to 11 months after birth had no effects, but exposure up to the age of 11 years caused many children to have scores of 3 and 4 on the DFI.[417] A shorter period with high fluoride peak levels in the plasma can also lead to fluorosis.[40] Release of fluoride from the bone around the tooth is possibly responsible as well.[41] [730] Fluorosis scores are also influenced by the age (wear) at which the children are studied.[213] Different measurement methods makes comparison between studies difficult and assessments of trends in fluorosis prevalences unreliable,[976] which can also be because of differences in water consumption per area, climate, nutrition and availability of fluoride sources other than drinking water.

Fluorosis in regions/countries with optimal/high fluoride levels

In regions with optimal fluoride levels in the water, children in various age categories have more diffuse opacities than children with fluoride deprivation.[166 224 249 358 396 644 645 955] Clearly demarcated opacities are more frequent in regions with a low level of water fluoridation,[22 54 247 249 287 396 631 733 986 1031] although not always.[334 620 854 965] In studies, the incidence of diffuse opacities increased with use of topical fluorides[504 570] and the total number of opacities decreased somewhat,[954] presumably due to a reduced number of carious white spots.

A review based on more than 50 studies in 13 countries concluded that nowadays fluorosis of greater severity than expected is seen because of the higher fluoride concentrations of potable water.[620] The mean prevalence of mild fluorosis in 1945 was 16%, and increased in 1992 to a minimum of 33% and even as high as 60% in some reports.[64 515] This is in part likely due to the use of more sensitive fluorosis indices and consumption of fluoride from additional sources.[396]

In the Republic of Ireland, DFI scores from 1984 for three age categories in regions with 0.8–1.0 ppm fluoride in water were compared with those in 2002: the prevalence of fluorosis had increased. The same age categories without fluoridated water also showed more fluorosis in 2002, but not as severe. The data suggest an excessive use of fluoride supplements by both groups.[975] In seven European countries the prevalence of diffuse opacities ranged from 28% in Athens (Greece) to 61% in fluoridated Cork (Ireland), that of demarcated opacities from 16% to 25%, and of hypoplasia from 0 to 3%. Prevalence figures based on photographs of dried teeth were substantially larger: DFI scores of 1, 2 and a few higher ones were found for 51–89% of the children.[170]

Some fluoride is absorbed from the air (factory emissions and dust in, for instance, phosphate-mining areas, such as in Morocco),[354] pesticides and insecticides,[827] the diet (in particular fish, and wholemeal and rye bread), beverages (tea from volcanic soil),[654] and certain anaesthetic gases. Immigrants from Africa and Asia have dental fluorosis due to too much fluoride in the drinking water and eventually in their diet.[1006]

Fluorosis in "fluoride-poor" regions/countries

The UK, Belgium, Germany, France,[975] the Netherlands, and some states in the USA are among the many regions of the world where the fluoride content of water is in general very low. Fluoridation of tap water provides an excellent source of delivery alternative, though in many developing countries access to piped water is not universal. In the USA, 40% and in Canada more than 50% of the population receives fluoridated water,[949] but elsewhere water has not been fluoridated because of objections by the public.

Legal and sociological aspects of water fluoridation have been analysed for the USA.[32] Arguments against water fluoridation concern costs, effectiveness, harm to general health, and water pollution, although water all over the world, including the seas and oceans, contains fluoride. Water fluoridation is claimed to violate individual autonomy, because it makes it difficult to consume water without fluoride. However, the protection of vulnerable populations, who often have no voice during the decision making, against dental caries, may be of greater value.[582]

The dental profession has sought alternatives to water fluoridation. Use of fluoride tablets enables controlled administration, but not all parents cooperate. Weekly school rinse programmes with a fluoride solution can reach many children. Local application of fluoride gels in disposable trays, and twice-yearly application in the dental office of fluoride varnishes/lacquers are other modes of administration. Fluoridated salt (250–350 mg potassium fluoride/kg table salt)[949] was introduced in Switzerland and in Central and South American countries (and greatly increased the risk of fluorosis). Fluoride has also been added to milk.[845 847] Of major importance was the introduction of toothpastes containing fluoride, the sales of which increased sharply. In addition, topical fluoride therapies in countries without fluoridated water account for fluorosis in 25–40% of the children.[164]

In Switzerland, where fluoride was added to bread, fluorotic opacities were present in 28% of the children and 13% had opacities through other causes. In an area with no availability of fluoridated bread (but having access to fluoridated tablets and toothpaste) the proportions were 13% and 19%, respectively.[843] Fluoride in milk had an anti-caries effect of almost 50%;[845 847] 16% of children (Chile) developed questionable and 8% mild fluorosis.[560]

Swallowing fluoride intended for topical application introduces the risk of fluorosis,[737] as does foods and drinks produced in fluoridated areas that are transported to other areas ("halo" effect). The dental profession has assumed that in countries without fluoridated water too much fluoride is ingested from all artificial sources.

Topical fluorides

- *Local (half-yearly) application of fluoride gels* in disposable trays is not without risk.[88] Fluoride from swallowed gel is quickly absorbed in the digestive tract and the plasma level soon peaks,[241 501 571] followed by a slow decrease back to normal after several hours.[241] Much of the gel is swallowed.[241 371] Per application, 7–8 mg gel stays behind in the mouth, equal to maximally 0.5 mg F⁻/kg bodyweight.[491 947] Application of a 0.4% fluoride gel gives a plasma concentration of 0.1–0.5 mg F⁻/L.[7] A daily plasma peak value of 0.1 or 0.2 mg F⁻/L causes fluorosis.[40 288] The gels of most concern are the acidulated 1.23% F gels, which delivered a 1% free F⁻ ion concentration (resulting in transient damage to the gastric mucosa and kidneys)[913] and used to be advocated to maximise caries reduction.[947] Fluoride solutions are applied in smaller quantities.
- *Mouthrinses (weekly)* may be ingested by young children, generally in volumes up to 25–35%. A maximum of about 9 mg fluoride can be swallowed from the recommended mouthrinse amount of 10 mL NaF.[512]
- *Fluoride toothpaste* (daily) is epidemiologically of greater importance. Children may swallow (and eat) the toothpaste.[87 93 114 226 262 397 511 735 984] About 60% of the children swallow the paste, 10% almost all of it, but this decreases with time.[87 363 511] Per episode of tooth brushing, a mean of 0.33 mg (range 0–1.16 mg[512]) fluoride is absorbed, or more, depending on the fluoride concentration of the paste,[76 511 512 726] which differs between countries.[171] A mere 10% of toddlers rinse and spit after brushing and the proportion varies considerably between countries for somewhat older children.[172 914] In Europe, many children use(d) toothpastes with 1200 ppm and more.[170] An average of 0.5–1.5 g toothpaste is applied on the brush, often 2–2.5 g,[194 226] as promoted in advertisements.[226] The majority brush twice a day.[171] Very young children in European countries swallow 0.01–0.04 mg fluoride/kg bodyweight daily.[172] When using toothpastes with 500 ppm fluoride, a maximal of 5–20 µg/kg bodyweight is ingested.[914]

Thus use of fluoride toothpaste as well as fluoride tablets may lead to fluorosis.[115 491 515] Swallowing of toothpaste has not been proven to increase the risk of fluorosis in regions with low water fluoride levels,[262 472 568 877 944] yet much of the increase in fluorosis is attributed to dentifrice swallowed at a young age,[950] that is, before the age of 3 years[680 1038]/14 months.[944] Use of 1500 ppm fluoride toothpastes accounts for 80% of the total ingested fluoride in a child, which is too much.[1038] Findings are diverse, owing to, for example, different study designs.[678 852]

Higher levels of fluoride in urine are associated with fluorosis.[915] In one study, the daily urinary excretion of fluoride was within acceptable limits,[453] yet parents were advised to supervise the amount of toothpaste applied on the brush by their children, preferably limiting it to the size of a pea.[93 231 263 515] However, peas come in different sizes and the advice may not be heeded,[656] but an amount less than the size of pea may compromise the cariostatic effect.[1039] Brushing after meals results in less absorption of fluoride.[232]

The US Food and Drug Administration advises seeking professional help or visiting a toxicological centre if a child "swallows more than is used during tooth brushing",[594] which suggests that the desired small doses of fluorides endangers the health and makes its use suspect.

Fluoride has also been detected in the nails. However, toenails, clipped twice after growth of 15 day, did not reflect the fluoride plasma level.[510] The relationship between the fluoride concentration in nails and total fluoride intake was not found to be significant.[1038] After 16 weeks of brushing with a 1500 ppm fluoride toothpaste, the fluoride concentration in the nails of a sample of children peaked, although already after 4 weeks a small, unexplained increase was seen in some children.[185]

Special 0.025 g fluoride dentifrices are marketed for children younger than 5 years.[42 285 785] The fluoride content of these toothpastes and the age categories for which they were intended, are not always indicated. The remineralisation potency of such "safe" toothpastes is less than that of preparations containing 0.10–0.15% fluoride,[210 399 472] although some have found them just as effective.[515 1040]

Of 101 toothpastes from developing countries, 25% were found to have less than half of the fluoride indicated on the labels in an available active form.[916] Nearly all Chinese fluoride toothpastes tested in the laboratory were less efficacious than Crest toothpaste, despite consisting of theoretically equivalent formulations, due to variations in the quality of the raw materials.[269]

- *Fluoride tablets* are intended for local effect and are swallowed after they dissolve in the mouth. The number of fluoride tablets to be taken daily is still a point of dicussion,[227 229 492 784 960] because of additional fluoride sources. The expected risk of fluorosis (in the Netherlands)[784] has been confirmed in surveys: scores 0.5 and 1 on the DFI were recorded.[441 442 986 1004] Parents forgetting to give the fluoride tablets according to the schedule (four times/day) often administered them all at once. The risk of fluorosis exceeds 50% when between the age of 3 and 7 years one tablet of 0.5 mg F is ingested daily.[493] In one study, children using fluoride tablets until the age of 6 years had more opacities than who did not and taking the tablets until the age of 9 years resulted in a higher percentage opacities.[212] The tablets tripled the prevalence of enamel defects to 40%,[987] but some studies did not find a significant difference or at most found a weak trend.[775 875] In 22 studies the prevalence of mild fluorosis due to tablet use varied over a considerable range.[418] Unexpectedly, one tablet/day with 2.2 mg NaF (=1 mg F) did not result in fluorosis.[27]

- *Silver fluoride* has been used to arrest caries "atraumatically" (non-invasively) in deciduous teeth. A 40% solution was expected to contain 6% fluoride (60 000 ppm), but levels of 100 000–140 000 ppm have been found. As the result of the manufacturing process, the solution contained a mixture of ammonium fluoride, sodium fluoride or potassium fluoride, silver difluoride and hydrofluoric acid. Severe fluorosis developed in rat incisors given a single topical application of 4% AgF. To avoid toxicity, children should be treated with very small quantities of 4% AgF,[332] but further research is required.

Mechanism of action

In adolescents the uptake of fluoride by the enamel does not result in fluorosis.[686] Dental fluorosis develops before a tooth erupts. In one experimental study, 7 mg F/kg body-weight (in rats) caused vacuolisation within the ameloblasts; 3 mg did not induce significant alterations.[481] An excess of fluoride initiates development of cysts between the ameloblast layer and already formed enamel, particularly at the sites of actively secreting ameloblasts.[636] The enamel thus becomes fluorotic, the deciduous teeth in the first year of life.[513] Fluoride sensitivity of ameloblasts differs from person to person.[276] Some questions remain:

- Fluorosis could develop during the transformation of the ameloblasts from the matrix-secreting to the mineralising phase. An excess of fluoride counteracts resorption of the matrix.[812] The failure in breakdown of the amelogenins is followed by decreased production of proteases or low protease activity.[214 519] Fluorotic enamel contains more low-molecular proteins than normal.[1013]
- It is during the maturation stage rather than the secretory stage[45] that fluorosis begins to develop.
- The permanent maxillary incisors are most susceptible at 15–24 months in males and at 21–30 months in females,[265] or during the 2-year period extending through the second and third years of postnatal life,[45] or in the first year of life.[419] The odds ratio for development of a fluorotic maxillary incisor in children exposed to fluoride before 2 years of age versus later was about 7 in one study; a significant factor was the start of the exposure during amelogenesis.[75]
- The subsurface hypomineralisation of fluorosed enamel in animals has been ascribed to disturbances in maturation,[454] and in human maxillary central incisors it occurs during the maturation stage at 22–26 months.[267]

    One study found that one 0.5 mg F tablet/day during the late secretory and mineralising phases resulted in hypomineralisation of the outer enamel.[493] Experimental studies have demonstrated damage to the ameloblasts in their secretory phase,[859] leading to the formation of pits in the enamel.[860] The World Health Organization stated in 1994 that with levels higher than 1.2 ppm in a moderate climate the incisors are at risk, in particular between 18 and 36 months of age.[1006]

- No specific period of odontogenesis is most critically susceptible. Fluorosis can develop at every stage of tooth development, including the pre-eruptive maturation of the enamel,[267 276 308 402] but further evidence is needed.[402]

Regardless, an increase in severity of fluorosis directly reflects an increase in fluoride concentration in the enamel.[45] The fluoride levels in developing enamel are directly related to the fluoride plasma levels, and are not under the control of ameloblasts.[835] Ionic fluoride is incorporated into the growing enamel crystals. An excess of fluoride affects the ameloblasts and mineralised enamel becomes hypermineralised at the expense of newly formed enamel, because insufficient calcium is available. Nucleus formation in the enamel crystals, crystal growth and the calcium metabolism are all affected.[276] The deficiency in calcium increases the production of PTH, but an increased plasma fluoride level does not affect the calcium level,[31] unless the calcium supply is low.[689]

The deciduous teeth are not spared,[60 186 257 288 308 334 576 608 633 653 663 891 948 951] but the defects are less pronounced, because the deciduous enamel is whiter and thinner, the maturation period shorter, and only a part of the supplemented fluoride is transported from the mother to the fetus.[308] A Kenyan study found that the second deciduous molars and the first permanent molars were affected similarly by 9 ppm fluoride in the drinking water, but 0.7 ppm affected the deciduous[513] and permanent first molars more than the deciduous second molars.[663] Fluoride ingested prenatally was associated with fluorosis of the deciduous teeth, but was more strongly associated when ingested during the postnatal 6–9 months, and the deciduous second molars appeared most affected.[510]

Fluorotic deciduous enamel may have a "marbled" appearance.[948] In the deciduous dentition, fluorosis is more severe in the molars than in the incisors. Deciduous tooth fluorosis has likely increased during the past decades.[948 951] Use of amoxicillin during infancy for 6 weeks to 3 months and 3 months to 6 months seemingly increased the risk of fluorosis, but administered for a longer period did not. After controlling for fluoride intake, the risk was not increased and other antibiotics also did not increase the risk.[400] Opacities in the deciduous teeth signify that fluorosis might be present in the permanent dentition,[603 948] and the fluoride regimen must then be adjusted.

Fluorotic permanent incisors draw the most attention,[12] but the premolars[965] and second molars are affected more severely.[589] The later the tooth is formed, the more fluorotic it will be.[494 643] This finding is not universal,[12] perhaps more in areas with an altered fluoride supply over time. One study found progressive worsening from anterior to posterior, at 6 and 21 mg F/L in water. At 3.5 mg F/L the premolars were the worst affected.[895] At a relatively small concentration, no anterior–posterior difference was noted.[633]

The severity of fluorosis is also influenced by environmental factors. The climate and a poor diet may play a role.[643] Tanzanian children consuming water with 3.6 mg F/L scored moderately higher on a fluorosis index than children consuming water with 0.2 mg F/L, who consumed, however, "magadi"-containing food, a natural sodium bicarbonate with up to 1750 mg F/L.[57]

Prenatal fluoride

The effect of fluoride ingested by a pregnant woman on the fetus is not well known. Because fluoride is quickly excreted in the urine and incorporated in the bones of the mother, only a small amount is incorporated into the fetal enamel.[308] The placenta also acts as a partial barrier,[307] but equal concentrations in fetal and maternal blood have been established.[52] Conflicting findings are based on flawed fluoride measurements.[308]

The cariostatic effect of prenatal fluoride uptake is significantly smaller than that of postnatal fluoride supplementation.[308] At least 2 mg F/day should be ingested during pregnancy for good-quality development of the baby's teeth and more tightly packed crystals in the tooth enamel.[322]

The fluoride content in prenatal enamel of guinea pigs increased in accordance with a higher supply to the pregnant animals, but was considerably lower in the fetus than in maternal blood.[85] High doses given to their mothers caused fluorosis in young mice,[284] and hamster incisors became longer.[322] A human study did not lead to any clear conclusions.[321] More recently it has been found that the fetal ameloblasts and odontoblasts are surprisingly well developed with prenatal fluoride availability. Severe deciduous primary tooth fluorosis is caused by both high pre- and postnatal exposures.[948] Prenatally formed crowns in animals exhibited at most moderate fluorotic enamel, while later formed enamel showed fluorosis.[454]

The fluoride content in breast milk is lower[61 242 258 632] or equal[497] to that of water, but increases when the water intake is high. The fluoride content of enamel of breast-fed children, living in areas with 1.2 mg F/L of water, is two to three times lower than that in the enamel of bottle-fed children.[256 942]

Fluorotic enamel

Replacement of a hydroxyl ion by a fluoride ion results in a tighter enamel crystal lattice and improves the lattice stability. However, fluorotic enamel is less hard than unaffected enamel.[632] In mild fluorosis, the subsurface enamel is hypocalcified and porous, which is most probably due to non-degraded matrix proteins.[45 1009] The more porous the enamel, the whiter its colour. In more severe fluorosis, the surface itself is porous.[310 731] The pore volume may be larger (10–15%).[859 896] Mildly fluorotic enamel is fully

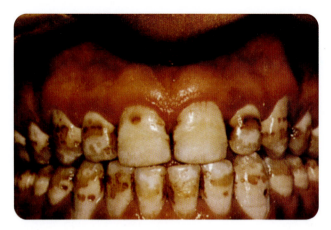

Figure 3.13 Severe fluorosis: brown discoloration and hypoplasia.

functional, but severely fluorosed enamel is prone to wear and fracture.[975]

The fluoride content of fluorotic enamel is relatively high,[136 345 776] particularly in the outermost layer,[196 1009] and is more so with increasing severity of fluorosis.[731] The fluoride distribution in fluorotic enamel resembles that of sound enamel, but the concentrations are higher throughout its thickness.[729] The fluoride content decreases locally due to wear of the outer enamel.[880 947 953] Fluorotic enamel may be thinner than normal,[896] with an irregular prismatic pattern and more pronounced interdigitation at the amelodentinal junction.[617]

Opacities are present at the time of eruption of the tooth. The cause of the brown discoloration is not known,[692] but post-eruptive penetration of dietary pigments into the tooth tissues has been implicated.[45] The discoloration (Figure 3.13) is often restricted to the superficial enamel layer. Brown staining depends on post-eruptive influences, therefore it cannot be a criterion for diagnosis.[255] The symmetrical enamel lesions[557 643] (90% identical in homologous pairs of teeth),[897] exclude local causes, such as trauma.

Pits develop post-eruptively through wear (and/or pressure),[893 896 965] even years after the eruption.[71 213] At 2 ppm fluoride in drinking water, 50% of Kenyan children showed pits in more than half of the teeth.[557] In teeth with more severe fluorosis, there are larger areas of post-eruptive mechanical destruction of the enamel and therefore it does not represent true hypoplasia.[45] Ongoing wear may obliterate the pits.[2]

Prevention

In the Netherlands, the recommended number of fluoride tablets (four 0.25 mg NaF tablets/day)[59 405] has been re-evaluated twice,[421 753] taking into account the concomitant use of fluoride toothpaste.[913] Presently, after the emergence of the first deciduous tooth, parents starts to brush the child's teeth once a day with a 500–750 ppm fluoride toothpaste. From the second birthday, the teeth are brushed twice daily, and from the fifth year with a 1000–1500 ppm dentifrice. If caries still develops, one has to question compliance with the regimen. Eventually, additional fluoride is recommended, such as one or two 0.25 mg NaF tablets daily. Two tablets should not to be taken together, or on an empty stomach, and not immediately after brushing. Children must be asked to suck the fluoride tablets to enhance local remineralisation. If a child has swallowed too many tablets, they should be given milk, which slows down the absorption in the digestive tract; if the dose ingested is very high, the child must be encouraged to vomit and hospitalisation may be needed.[62] Alternatively, a fluoride varnish or a gel can be applied to the teeth in the dental office.[421]

In the UK where the drinking water contains less than 0.3 ppm F/L, 1–3-year-old children should use one fluoride tablet (0.15 mg/day), 3–6-year-olds two tablets and older children four tablets.[130] In view of the availability of fluorides from a variety of sources, fluoride supplementation in Canada is considered to be required only in high dental caries risk patients.[146] Dental fluorosis declined in Australia following discouragement of the use of fluoride supplements and ingestion of toothpaste, which now contains 400 mg F/L instead of the 1000 (up to 1500) mg F/L previously. The rate of dental caries did not increase with these changes.[736] Some remarks should be made at this juncture:

- Additional sources of fluoride should be avoided if the water is optimally fluoridated.
- Local application should be reserved for children over the age of 5 years who either have caries or did not use any additional source of fluoride until now. A fluoride solution is a good choice, but 0.4% gel (not 1.23%) in a disposable tray may be applied. The patient must bow their head while sitting in an upright position and a salivary ejector must be used. If the patient applies a gel at home, they must bend over the washbasin. A maximum of 40% volume of the tray is filled with no more than 2 g of gel. Advise the patient to spit for 30 seconds after the application.[500 1006]
- (Strong) tea from volcanic regions may contain much fluoride.[233 713 834]
- The fluoride contents of spring and mineral waters (Table 3.3) may be high, but is not always mentioned.[961] In the USA and Canada most mineral waters contain <0.3–0.7 ppm fluoride, but some have a higher fluoride content.[949] The waters with a higher fluoride concentration should neither be ingested by children nor used to prepare infant food.

As mentioned above, the halo effect is an additional risk when fluoride supplements are given in areas with fluoridated water.[903]

Tetracyclines and cystic fibrosis

Soon after the introduction of the tetracyclines (1947), it became clear that they are deposited in bones and teeth[699] [755 938] and cause enamel discoloration[598] and hypoplasia. New-generation tetracyclines, except minocycline, do not in general discolour the teeth. Tetracyclines, having few side effects, used to be prescribed for long periods and to premature infants during the first week(s) of life.[698] *In vitro* studies showed that the antibiotic penetrated the dentinal tubules and was bound, in a concentration-dependent manner, non-specifically and loosely to fully mineralised dentine.[159 160]

Presently, minocycline is used against inflammatory acne vulgaris in adolescents and for long-term treatment of *rosacea*, infections such as *Chlamydia* (sexually transmitted), and rheumatoid arthritis. Minocycline discolours already erupted teeth. The other second-generation drugs may discolour teeth mildly if used for longer periods during odontogenesis.[698]

Cystic fibrosis ("mucoviscidosis") is an inherited disorder in which tetracyclines are administered for long periods to children with infectious bronchitis. The *CFTR* gene encodes a protein that functions as a channel for the transport of chloride in and out of the cells. One mutated gene, either from the father or the mother, makes half of the channels ineffective and two mutated genes make all of them ineffective. The disease causes generalised exocrine gland dysfunction, whose characteristics include pancreatic duct blockage, sweat containing too much chloride, and thickened mucous secretions in the lung that threaten respiration and makes the bronchial airways susceptible to infection. The upper (nasal) and lower (trachea, bronchi) airways hyper-absorb sodium, which is thought to contribute to the thick, sticky mucus whereby the mucociliary clearance decreases and the airways become predisposed to infection.[319]

Treatment nowadays includes physiotherapy, mucolytic agents and antibiotics, and pancreatic enzyme replacement, and an appropriate fat diet.[625] Dentists are likely to encounter more of these patients since their life-expectancy has increased.[904] The majority still die in early adulthood, unless they undergo lung transplantation.[451] One in 1800–2000 neonates is affected, in particular among Caucasian populations.[904]

The sublingual and submandibular glands in particular may be enlarged in children with cystic fibrosis with higher than normal Ca^+ and Na^+ concentrations, causing calculus formation, obstruction of the salivary ducts, and reduced salivary secretion.

Enamel

Tetracyclines affect the deciduous teeth *in utero*, and also the permanent teeth.[435 482 667 786] They are diffusely incorporated into the enamel.[101 829] The prevalence of enamel hypoplasia in cystic fibrosis patients receiving the older tetracyclines ranged from 24% to 100%. Discoloration was observed in 6–64%. [113 424 702 786 871 935 938 1027] In other studies, 1–20% (hypoplasia?) and 4–13% (discoloration?) children were affected.[125 724 905 945]

Higher doses of older tetracyclines per kg/bodyweight, led to greater discoloration and more severe enamel hypoplasia,[101 936] but this was not documented consistently.[871] Some cystic fibrosis patients exhibited hypomineralised enamel similar to that in cystic fibrosis mice, but many of the enamel defects in humans with cystic fibrosis might be associated with tetracycline therapy, which confounds their exact aetiology.[319] Were the anomalies caused by cystic fibrosis,[653 814 936 1027] premature birth,[599] or tetracycline treatment?

Most (80%) premature neonates treated with tetracycline in one study had hypoplastic enamel, versus 10% without tetracycline.[599] Hypoplasia was located at the site of the discolorations. That tetracyclines damaged the enamel was confirmed in a comparative study of teeth of cystic fibrosis patients with those of patients with other respiratory disorders.[625] The tetracyclines affected the ameloblasts,[968] and the enamel was hypocalcified.

CFTR is involved in the pH regulation of the enamel matrix.[863] In cystic fibrosis patients the pH regulation may not be adequate. Acidic conditions inhibit most enamel proteinases,[824] leaving the matrix proteins undegraded.[823] The ameloblasts transport bicarbonates into the enamel, which buffer the massive amounts of hydrogen ions released during maturation.[823] *CFTR* lowers the bicarbonate transport, and the pH remains low, leaving many proteins in a matrix with low mineral content.[101 1011] Cystic fibrosis mice show soft, chalky-white enamel of normal thickness. The ameloblasts degenerated prematurely after the secretory phase and the amelogenins were insufficiently resorbed.[1013] In homozygous cystic fibrosis mice, the hypomineralised enamel contained less calcium and had an altered iron and potassium content,[53] which explains the white colour of the teeth.[306] An altered pH secondary to respiratory acidosis caused by exposure to air with 10% carbon dioxide (CO_2) during odontogenesis also resulted in enamel hypomineralisation.[979]

Dentine

Hypomineralised areas and extensive interglobular dentine is observed in the dentine of deciduous teeth[47 101 588 925] and teeth of experimental animals.[44 101] Tetracycline is incorporated in the dentine matrix.[159]

The incorporation may take place through chelation.[101 590] In dentine the tetracycline binds to calcium-orthophosphate[938] on the crystal surface or to calcium and the organic matrix.[771] A fully mineralised tooth does not take up tetracycline,[488] which does not hold true for minocycline.

Tetracycline has been found at the dentinal growth lines,[101] visible as a bright-yellow lines. Others have observed identical lines in the dentine, associated with a globular mineralisation pattern.[360]

Cementum

Tetracycline is incorporated into the cementum. A single dose, visible as a thin fluorescing line under ultraviolet (UV) light, marks cementum formed before and after administration of the drug. For instance, the start of dietary changes can be marked and the effects studied by comparing the new and the previously developed and mineralised cementum.[623 660 661] The normal phosphorescence of teeth is altered by tetracycline.[994]

Caries and periodontal disease

The caries prevalence is lower than in controls, especially in deciduous dentitions that are discoloured by tetracycline,[124 444 464 465 495 496 702] however, others have reported conflicting findings.[725 871 973] The reduction is ascribed to the antibiotic action on the oral bacteria,[496] and to altered salivary properties,[465] i.e. a higher pH and buffering capacity of stimulated saliva.[685] The long-term use of tetracyclines may confer some protection, but reported differences in the rate of caries in cystic fibrosis children versus those with other respiratory disorders are not significant.[625]

The antibiotics have a favourable effect on periodontal health,[113 465] but contrasting findings have also been reported.[424] Calculus has been found to be more common in cystic fibrosis because of the high salivary calcium content.[465]

Discoloration

The first tetracyclines caused yellow discoloration of the teeth (first reported in 1954).[787] That bones also discolour was already known. The yellow teeth of young children became brown as they grew older.[936] One half of a split yellow tooth stored in the dark remained yellow while the other half became brown due to oxidation caused by exposure to daylight.[936] Additionally, grey-black and brown-black[1028] and cream-white stains[667] have been reported (Figure 3.14, 3.15 and 3.16), depending on the

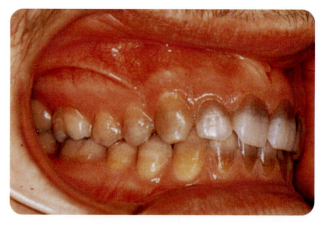

Figure 3.14 Yellow (and brown) tetracycline discoloration (the upper incisors were bleached rather unsuccessfully). (Courtesy of Department of Pedodontics, University of Utrecht.)

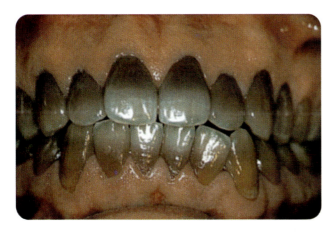

Figure 3.15 Green-grey discoloration caused by chlortetracycline.

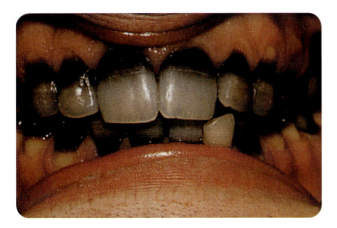

Figure 3.16 Brown oxytetracycline discoloration.

type of tetracycline and the duration of the therapy.[972] The permanent teeth in particular discolour grey (63%), yellow (28%) and brown (10%).[702] Both the affected enamel and dentine fluoresce under UV light.[666] In one study, while 15% of the first permanent molars and 7% of second deciduous molars were stained, much higher proportions of these teeth typically fluoresced.[849] Without investigating for UV fluorescence, tetracycline discoloration may be diagnosed as fluorosis.[425]

The newer tetracyclines hardly stain the teeth:[602] prolonged use discoloured the teeth in 1 of 36 patients.[86] However, modern tetracyclines must still be avoided during pregnancy due to the risk of enamel dysplasia with brownish discoloured deciduous teeth.[117] Long-term, and even short-term, use of minocycline has been found to stain bones, nails and oral mucosa (blackish-blue because of pigmented alveolar bone underneath); in 3–6% of adolescents affected, the (middle of) the erupted teeth were

blue-grey or the crowns and developing roots were much darker in colour.[145 155 173]

The pigmentation is due to accumulation of insoluble quinone, which is produced during the degradation of the aromatic ring of the drug,[173] but the actual process of staining remains an enigma. Minocycline binds poorly with calcium. Minocycline in combination with phenothiazine therapy caused black galactorrhoea. The discoloured tooth tissues do not fluoresce.[155]

Epidemiology

In the 1960s (and the 1970s), some 50% of the children and 75% of the youngest ones treated with tetracyclines showed traces of the drug in their teeth,[476 849 850] as physicians did not give preference to the least discolouring drug.[850] Thereafter, the use of the severely discolouring tetracyclines declined.[73 476 702] In one Hong Kong (1989)-based study, almost one-fifth of 12-year-olds showed discoloured teeth, mostly tetracycline stains.[462] Native Americans did not have access to the newer medicines for years and continued to present severely discoloured teeth for a long time.[724] In some other countries, tetracyclines associated with severe discoloration have been in use until recently (and possibly are still prescribed).

Extrinsic stain

Tetracyclines stain the tooth surface extrinsically,[927] which involves adherence of the antibiotic to the pellicle, followed by oxidation and growth of a bacterial flora in which chromogenous microorganisms predominate. Enamel immersed in an aqueous solution of (chlor)tetracycline (pH 2–3) became etched and large yellow crystals tightly settled on the surface.[110] In an *in vitro* study, tetracycline became superficially incorporated into the enamel,[111] possibly by chelation.[112]

Prevention

Tetracyclines causing discoloration should not be prescribed before the age of 8 years, but because in older children the drug is still taken up in the dentine, the least discolouring types are to be preferred. The newer drugs cross the placenta and are excreted in breast milk, because of which the child's teeth may become slightly stained. Abstaining from breast-feeding may be a sensible choice. The newer tetracyclines (e.g. doxycycline (Vibramycin)) are effective in lower doses and cause lesser discoloration, if at all, than the older types. Because minocycline may stain teeth that erupted a long time ago, other therapies for acne are warranted.

Other medicaments and materials

- *Chemotherapy* can cause enamel hypocalcification, expressed as broad growth lines, sometimes hypoplasia,[199 604 794] and other tooth anomalies (Chapter 2) whose development coincides with the time of the therapy.[479] The formation of the dentinal matrix might be (slightly) disturbed.[199 794] The crowns of all the teeth in children with leukaemia receiving chemotherapy were found to have more white-cream and yellow-brown opacities and fine discoloured horizontal lines compared with controls. Children with other cancers (sarcoma) showed anomalous enamel in the permanent teeth in the mixed dentition.[673] Chemotherapy at the time of odontogenesis is associated with enamel discoloration and root malformation,[652] but neither the colour nor the kind of malformation developing has been reported.

- *Radiotherapy.* Paediatric oncological patients frequently receive both chemotherapy and radiotherapy. Dental anomalies arise when the dose exceeds 4–5 Gy.[144] Radiation affects not only the tumour cells but also physiologically active cells. Tooth germs irradiated at an early stage were found to either not produce enamel at all or produce an insufficient amount of enamel.[222]
- *Radium* was used as a luminous paint to read the numerals on watches at night. Women workers who painted the radium on the digits pointed the brush between their lips. The radium thus swallowed might have affected the dentition of their children during pregnancy.

  Intraperitoneal injection[24] of radium in mice caused alterations in the teeth, including hypoplastic, grooved enamel and pulp obliteration.[408]

- *Phenytoin* (Dilantin), which is used in the treatment of epilepsy, is associated (in rats) with deviations in tooth size and root abnormalities.[741] The drug has been suggested to cause *pseudohypoparathyroidism*.[740] *In utero* exposure to phenytoin is associated with decreased height and length of the maxilla and length of the mandible. Prevalence of agenesis of teeth was found to be 12% lower than the prevalence in a reference population, but exclusion of the wisdom teeth "normalised" the figure. Hyperdontia prevalence was similar to that in the general population.[664]
- Prenatal exposure to *thalidomide* (Softenon). Thalidomide is a sedative and antiemetic agent with an analgesic effect, and enhances the efficacy of other painkillers. The drug was used in the past to prevent abortion and to fight nausea in the first weeks of pregnancy. However, it was shown to be teratogenic. The fetus was severely malformed, in particular the upper extremities. In a Swedish study, half of the deciduous dentitions had hypoplastic enamel.[58] In Germany several thousand children were affected, and up to 12 000 children worldwide.[569 690] The drug has been recently reapproved in the USA for the treatment of painful leprosy-associated erythema.[117 569 690] Because of its favourable properties,[690] thalidomide is presently used in various dermatological, oncological, gastrointestinal and oral conditions.[452 569 690]

3.2.6   Trauma

Local trauma directly effecting the teeth needs to be distinguished from generalised trauma, which acts indirectly through alterations in metabolic pathways.[788]

Local factors
Local factors affect, in general, a single tooth or a few adjacent teeth.

Infection
Deciduous tooth pulps may undergo necrosis due to deep carious lesions. The consequent periapical, and in molars, inter-radicular, infection (via accessory canals in the furcation area) endangers amelogenesis in the succedaneous tooth germ, resulting in development of "Turner teeth" or "Turner's hypoplasia".[351 443] Premolars are twice more prone to Turner's hypoplasia than incisors.[443] The severity of the infection and the developmental stage and location of the successor tooth determine the degree of damage,[894] which is more often manifest as opacities than hypoplasia;[524] the altered mineralisation is not evident on radiographs.[33] One study found that the permanent anterior teeth are mainly affected on the labial aspect, and the premolars occlusally, but eventually the damage extends to other surfaces.[443] Due to their timing of development, the premolars are damaged due to infections occurring at the age of 6–9 years.[572]

On a five-point scale, lesions vary from slightly discoloured and minor loss of substance to gross loss of the crown. Turner premolars have been observed in 0.7% of the population, the mandibular premolars being affected more frequently than maxillary,[352] but a prevalence of 6% has also been reported.[443] Almost a quarter of deciduous teeth with abscesses have defective successors.[572]

In the first few postnatal weeks, *acute osteomyelitis of the maxilla in the newborn* may cause malformed deciduous Turner-type teeth and jaw deformation.[697]

Mechanical trauma
Mechanical trauma to erupted deciduous teeth may injure the tooth germ of the successor, resulting in impaired hard tissue formation; the teeth most frequently affected are the maxillary incisors (Figure 3.17).[32 34 853 857] Pre-eruptive injury to the deciduous teeth is caused by orotracheal intubation, intraoral laceration on the labial aspect of the maxilla,[176] etc.

A 2.5-year-old girl lost a maxillary central incisor in a car accident. The permanent successor erupted partially at 7 years. The "lost" deciduous incisor appeared to be embedded in the labial alveolar bone and the permanent incisor had a small zone of hypoplastic enamel.[612]

Trauma to deciduous teeth results in defects in the successor teeth in 6–12% or more cases.[26 32 422 593 929] The direct successor of the traumatised deciduous tooth and the germs of adjacent teeth may be involved.[854] Trauma

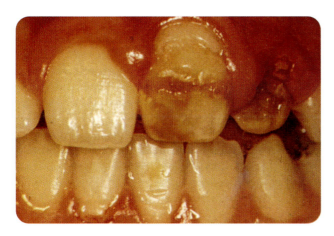

Figure 3.17 Discoloration and hypoplasia of the permanent incisors following trauma to the primary predecessors.

to a deciduous tooth before the age of 4 years is associated with the greatest risk of visible damage to the successor tooth.[36][95] An intrusive force is most damaging to the unerupted tooth germ,[882] resulting in a deformed crown/root[1041] either before or during thickening of the matrix before it starts to calcify;[882] thereafter[88] localized enamel hypoplasia develops.[2]

After *mild* trauma at age 2–7 years, 25% of permanent successors in one study showed yellow to brown discoloration. After *moderate* trauma at age 2, 12% of the successors showed white to yellow-brown discoloration, mainly incisal, and grooved enamel.[95] The discoloration is caused by break down of haemglobin.[35] Even slight intrusion can cause hypoplasia of the labial enamel of the successor.[928] *Severe* trauma at age 1–5 years may result in root dilacerations, odontome-like malformations, disruptions in eruption time and site, double roots and cessation of root formation. If the trauma occurs in the early stages of tooth development, sequestration of the tooth germ is possible. Discoloration, either in or not in combination with mild hypoplasia (grooving) is, however, the most frequent sequela.[32][33][3][35][96][129][572][613][779][928] If the alveolar bone fractures, the dental consequences are severe. Cementum may be deposited on the enamel upon contact with the dental follicle.[609] In fully developed crowns of non-erupted teeth, trauma causes development of opacities; extrusion of an intruded tooth increases the risk of further damage.[894]

The degree of root resorption of a traumatised deciduous tooth is unrelated to hypoplasia in the successor tooth,[32][95] presumably because the distance between the two teeth may not alter.

Uncommon causes of local trauma

- *Electrical burns* to the lips and mouth may happen at a young age, when children explore the world by way of the mouth through chewing and sucking. For example, a child may put the female end of a live extension wire in their mouth. Early oedematous tissue makes it difficult to delineate the extent of the injury. Burns to soft tissues result in contractures, microstomia and malformed teeth that acquire a lingual inclination. Bleeding (6–20%) from the labial or lingual blood vessels starts after 1–2 weeks following loss of non-vital tissue.[24][223][436] Use of a symmetrical oral acrylic appliance may prevent unilateral contraction of the lips.[744] Microstomia might be prevented with an appliance exerting light pressure on the oral commissures.[679]
- *Gunshot wounds* can cause serious damage.[692] Teeth directly hit by a bullet can fracture into multiple fragments. An indirect hit can cause complete loss of the crown.[29]
- *Ritual extraction* (mutilation) of deciduous canines in Uganda led to anomalies in 16% of the permanent succcessors.[693]

Generalised metabolic causes

Some of these have already been described above. In *hypophosphatasia* (Chapter 4), the enamel may be hypoplastic.[246]

3.2.7 Miscellaneous causes

Ankylosis, the direct contact between alveolar bone and root, of the deciduous molars is in one-third of cases associated with opacities, hypoplasia and abnormal crown morphology of the permanent teeth.[754]

3.3 Hereditary amelogenesis imperfecta

Hereditary amelogenesis imperfecta consists of heterogeneous structural and morphological enamel defects of genetic origin occurring in the absence of systemic disorders. The condition is subdivided in various classes depending on the defect present: hypoplasia (type I), hypomaturation (type II), hypocalcification (type III), and the combination of hypomaturation-hypoplasia with taurodontism (type IV).

The name hereditary amelogenesis imperfecta was suggested by Weinmann *et al.* in 1945.[962] Formerly, the terms aplasia and hypoplasia were used, either with or without the addition of "hereditary".[28] Hypoplastic and hypocalcified types had been distinguished,[962] with clinical and genetic subtypes. Schulze in 1970 distinguished between seven hypoplastic and three hypocalcified subtypes.[783] Around the same time, the hypomaturative type was discovered and around 1975, the hypomaturative-hypocalcified type with taurodontism.[992]

Hereditary amelogenesis imperfecta is considered as a solitary anomaly (no other epithelial disorders),[64 992] but as the complex interactions of both the genetic and biochemical components are further revealed, hitherto unknown relationships may become evident.[21]

Deviations in the dermatoglyphic patterns on the palms of the hand and soles of the feet have been found to be associated with hypodontia or amelogenesis imperfecta.[55]

In a number of syndromes the enamel is poorly developed or absent (Chapter 11). Light yellow, abraded teeth and delayed or absent eruption is found in nephrocalcinosis, possibly due to a common cause, but the exact relationship is as yet unclear.[211]

The location of acquired enamel defects helps to determine their period of development, but in hereditary amelogenesis imperfecta there is no chronological pattern to the manifestation of the defects. The predentinal areas show irregular canaliculi and there is resorption of the pulp tissue,[808] but the enamel is the main target.

3.3.1 Classification

The classification[999 1000 1001] shown in Table 3.4 is a modification of older ones[992 1002] and other classifications also exist.[867 868] Each of the four types is further subclassified, based upon the mode of inheritance, clinical features and histological characteristics.[992 1002] Variable gene expression may confound the clinical diagnosis of the (sub)types,[217 868] which, together with the few, small family trees available, lead to indecisive diagnoses.[794] "Borderline cases" have also been reported.[868]

Hypoplasia and hypocalcification may both present in one and the same tooth, independent of clinical appearance and mode of inheritance.[65 66 67] Conversely, hypoplasia and hypocalcification have also been separately observed in different members of the same family.[66] While the ultrastructural findings may not correlate with the clinical features,[69] one type of defect usually predominates.[64] Hereditary amelogenesis imperfecta can also differ in severity in the deciduous and permanent dentitions of the same person.[65] The variable phenotypes found both within families and within the different teeth of the same person do not warrant a phenotypical classification as lack of consistent findings make a classification based on phenotype, molecular defects and biochemical composition of the enamel unrealistic.[19] Yet, classification and subtyping may be forthcoming, based on the mode of

Table 3.4 Classification of hereditary amelogenesis imperfecta (AI)

Type of AI + subtypes	Mode of inheritance	Enamel features
I Hypoplastic		Localised or generalised thin, normal radiodensity
IA	AD	Small pits in rows or columns with brown discoloured bottom
IB	AD	Pits and grooves in horizontal bands on especially the middle third of the crowns
IC	AR	Like IB, but more severe + local hypocalcifications
I.D[a]	AD	Smooth, glossy, generally thin, no approximal contacts, white-brown, 50% anterior open bite
I.E	X – males	Smooth, shiny, uniformly thin, no approximal contacts, (yellow)-brown, anterior open bite
	X – females[b]	Alternating thin and normal vertical bands (ridging), 33% open bite
I.F[a]	AD	Rough, granular, glassy, universally thin, no approximal contacts, hard, 50% anterior open bite
I.G[a]	AR	Rough, granular, yellow-brown, hard, universally thin or absent, anterior open bite
II Hypomaturative		Mottled, softer than normal, lowered radiodensity, breaks away
II.A[a]	AR	Pigmented agar-brown, relative soft, normally thick, chips away, often anterior open bite
II.B	X – males	*Deciduous teeth* ground-glass white
		Permanent teeth mottled yellow, thin, smooth
	X– females[b]	*Deciduous teeth* alternating vertical white and normal bands
		Permanent teeth alternating vertical white/yellow (mottled) and normal bands, soft (probe penetrates)
II.C	X	"Snow-capped" (1/4 to 1/3 incisal/occlusal part is opaque white)
II.D	AD	"Snow-capped"
III Hypocalcified		Very soft, normal thickness, radiodensity lower than of dentine, enamel disappears
III.A	AD	Yellow-brown to orange becomes (through food stains) brown-black, very soft, sensitive
III.B	AR	Like IIIA, but more severe
IV Hypomaturative- hypoplastic with taurodontism		
		(Localised) thin areas, mottled, soft, radiodensity similar to that of dentine
IVA	AD	Soft, mottled yellow-brown and opaque white, with pits
IVB	AD	Thin and soft with hypomaturative areas

AD, autosomal dominant; AR, autosomal recessive; X, X-linked.
[a]Also delayed eruption and secondary intra-alveolar resorption.
[b]Due to lyonisation (visible with transillumination).[142]

inheritance, locus of the mutated gene and type of mutation, the biochemical outcome and phenotype.[21]

Taurodontism, an inherited anomaly of the dentine, is considered to be a feature of hereditary amelogenesis imperfecta type IV. Therefore, the mutant genes in hereditary amelogenesis imperfecta could affect cells other than the ameloblasts or several modifications in genes may be involved.[177] According to Seow, taurodontism cannot be considered a consistent feature of any type of hereditary amelogenesis imperfecta; taurodontism of the mandibular first permanent molar has never been reported in patients with hereditary amelogenesis imperfecta. Defects in enamel with taurodontism occur, however, in the tricho-dento-osseous syndrome (TDO), which may be misdiagnosed as hereditary amelogenesis imperfecta.[798]

Varying expressions of taurodontism have been found in three kindreds with TDO.[1014] Nowadays, TDO can be distinguished from hereditary amelogenesis imperfecta, because the responsible gene in TDO has been identified in a region of chromosome 17 that includes members of the "homeobox" gene family,[700] the *DLX3* gene.[1042] The prevalence of taurodontism in patients with hereditary amelogenesis imperfecta and controls is considered to be similar.[177]

3.3.2 Hereditary considerations

The mutated gene coding for amelogenin is X-linked.[64 484 460]

In several types of hereditary amelogenesis imperfecta, the protein content of enamel is higher than normal.[1012] A mutated amelogenin gene on the X-chromosome (*AMELX* gene) more or less destroys the encoding role of amelogenins,[485] which is only partly compensated for by the amelogenin gene on the Y-chromosome because of the 10 times smaller number of transcriptions.[764]

An X-linked subtype of hereditary amelogenesis imperfecta, with several clinical expressions, has been reported.[502] The amelogenin gene *AIH1* is located on the short arm of the X-chromosome,[9] but at least two critical disease loci exist, one of which – *AIH3* – is on the long arm.[17 502] Currently, 14 different *AMELX* mutations have been identified, including missense and nonsense mutations and deletions, resulting in different phenotypes. The relationships between genotype and phenotype have started to be understood.[367 368 457 459 1043]

Both X-linked recessive and dominant forms of hereditary amelogenesis imperfecta have been reported;[63 997] however, some authors consider it unwarranted to distinguish between the dominant and recessive forms in X-linked hereditary amelogenesis imperfecta.[18 193] Sexual dimorphism in the X-linked types are based on lyonisation.[63 66 997] Genes encoding proteins other than amelogenins are responsible for the autosomal forms of hereditary amelogenesis imperfecta. The subtypes might be explained by the varying gene expressions.

Of the autosomal dominant forms of hereditary amelogenesis imperfecta, which represent about 85% of all cases, two forms (local hypoplastic and smooth hypoplastic) have been linked to two proximal gene clusters on chromosome 4q21 (ameloblastin).[543]

A gene responsible for the autosomal dominant hypoplastic hereditary amelogenesis imperfecta subtypes IA and IB is located on the long arm of chromosome 4, but not in all families.[64 289] The mutation concerns enamelin or tuftelin.[820] In some instances, the genetic locus is known, but the mutation and the biochemical outcome are unknown.[19] Autosomal recessive amelogenesis imperfecta has been associated with mutations in the genes encoding kallikrein, enamelin, metalloproteinase, etc.[1043]

More recently, two enamel proteins (ameloblastin and enamelin) have been mapped to the critical regions. Four loci for inherited dentinal disorders are located nearby on the long arm of chromosome 4.[543] In male mice in which mutations were chemically induced, homozygotic mutants of the offspring had total enamel aplasia and heterozygotic mutants had a significant reduction in the enamel thickness. The dentine showed a reduction in mature collagen cross-linkages. The ameloblastin gene is also located on part of chromosome 4 along with other genes.[791]

3.3.3 Prevalence

The prevalence of hereditary amelogenesis imperfecta is largely unknown. A few families may account for the differences in the prevalence in small populations (Table 3.5). Consanguineous marriages are considered responsible for the high ratio in Västerbotten County in Sweden.[68]

Of 425 000 Swedes, 105 had hereditary amelogenesis imperfecta, 63 the hypoplastic and 42 the hypocalcified type.[867] Rough enamel was found in 9% of 165 patients.[63] Hypomaturative hereditary amelogenesis imperfecta is rarely encountered.[68] The autosomal dominant (hypocalcified) subtypes dominate.[655 743]

Early diagnosis of the type of hereditary amelogenesis imperfecta is important since delays in tooth eruption may require clearing the eruption path, particularly in the autosomal recessive hypoplastic rough subtype.[828] The development of dental caries and calculus deposition are also type-dependent;[866] timely rehabilitation of the dentition in some subtypes is a major consideration in hereditary amelogenesis imperfecta.

The following brief descriptions of the types and some features of the subtypes are based mainly on research by Witkop.[995 997 999]

Table 3.5 Prevalence of amelogenesis imperfecta

First author	N studied	Prevalence per 1000 individuals	Country
Witkop[995]	96 417	0.06 : 1000	Michigan
Sundell[867]	425 000	0.25 : 1000	Sweden[a]
Chosack et al.[158]	70 359	0.50 : 1000	Israel
Bäckman[68]	56 663	1.30 : 1000	Sweden[b]

[a]Mid Sweden.

[b]Västerbotten County.

3.3.4 Types of hereditary amelogenesis imperfecta

Hereditary hypoplastic amelogenesis imperfecta
Some hypoplastic subtypes are characterised by vestibular pits, occasionally of pinpoint size, often arranged in bands, but the enamel in other subtypes is uniformly thin and there are no interdental contacts, even when the enamel is not fully absent (Figure 3.18). The density and calcification of the reduced enamel is normal.

Subtype 1.A Hypoplastic autosomal dominant pitted amelogenesis imperfecta
The enamel of this most common subtype[868] is locally absent in the deciduous dentition and to a greater extent in the permanent dentition. The expression and penetrance vary in family members. The lines of Retzius are bent backwards under the pits; the floor of the pits shows signs of hypocalcification or contains much organic material that discolours brown to black post-eruption (Figure 3.19).[67]

Subtype 1.B Hypoplastic autosomal dominant local amelogenesis imperfecta
Pits and grooves run in horizontal bands across the (facial) middle third of the teeth (Figure 3.20), varying in expression and penetrance. The premolars, and often more severely, the deciduous molars, are most frequently affected.

The enamel prisms are disorientated. Deeper enamel is better mineralised than superficial enamel, which shows pits and craters on its surface.[769]

Subtype 1.C Hypoplastic autosomal recessive local amelogenesis imperfecta
The enamel of nearly all deciduous and permanent teeth is usually more severely hypoplastic than in subtype 1.B.

Subtype 1.D Hypoplastic autosomal dominant smooth amelogenesis imperfecta
The smooth enamel has frequently a quarter or less of its normal thickness. The conical crowns lack interdental contacts (Figure 3.21) and are opaque to translucent yellow-brown at eruption,

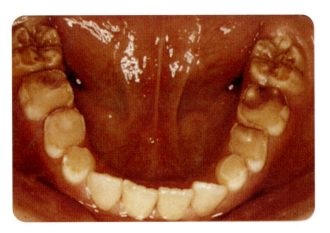

Figure 3.18 The enamel is absent on the larger part of the crowns of the posteriors teeth in this case of autosomal recessive hypoplastic amelogenesis imperfecta.

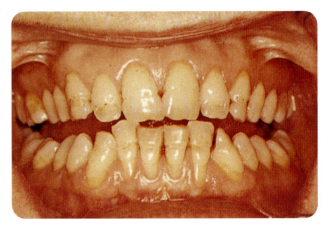

Figure 3.20 Autosomal dominant hypoplastic amelogenesis imperfecta; the defects are arranged in horizontal bands.

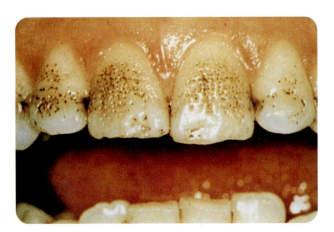

Figure 3.19 Autosomal dominant hypoplastic amelogenesis imperfecta; note the secondary discoloration (brown) in the base of the characteristic pits.

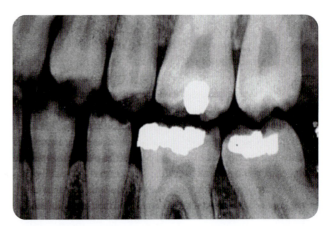

Figure 3.21 Autosomal dominant hypoplastic amelogenesis imperfecta with smooth, thin enamel; there are no approximal contacts between the teeth.

which may be delayed or absent with secondary intra-alveolar resorption. Hypodontia may be present. The subtype has a high penetrance.[139]

The smooth enamel is porous[762] with short prisms and thick interprismatic sheaths. A large part of the enamel is covered by a 1mm thick layer lacking the normal ultrastructural features. In the interdental spaces, proliferating, calcified epithelial remnants are indicative of early loss of the ameloblasts. The calcium concentration at the dentino-enamel junction is low.[1016]

Subtype 1.E Hypoplastic X-linked smooth (males) and thin-thick (females) amelogenesis imperfecta

Males have smooth, brown enamel, a quarter to an eighth of the normal thickness, and interdental contacts are absent. The tooth surface is glossy and shiny. The enamel is very homogeneous; prisms are often indistinct or lie close to each other. If eruption fails, there is intra-alveolar resorption.

Females have alternating vertical bands of normal thick and thin enamel, as alternating groups of ameloblasts are under the influence of the mutated and the normal gene (lyonisation), with "subsurface" hypocalcifications.[203] The deciduous tooth with rough enamel in Figure 3.22A is from a female (sixth generation) of a family with this subtype.

Subtype 1.F Hypoplastic autosomal dominant rough amelogenesis imperfecta

The rough enamel surface is thin (a quarter to an eighth) without interdental contacts. Failure of eruption is less common than in the smooth subtype (subtype I.E). Unerupted teeth may show resorption. Half the patients have an anterior open bite. The subtype has been noted in five generations of a family, manifested chiefly in the females.[886]

The enamel does not show prisms[695] and the dentino-enamel junction is smooth. If the enamel is present as a thick layer, the prisms bend in all directions and the enamel–dentine interdigitation is exaggerated. The lines of Retzius are malformed.

Subtype 1.G Hypoplastic autosomal recessive rough amelogenesis imperfecta

The rough, granular enamel is generally thin or absent. On eruption the enamel is yellow-brown (Figure 3.22B), and affected individuals also have an anterior open bite. Many teeth remain embedded in the jaws, with secondary crown resorption, which may progress into the pulp chamber,[1044] or they erupt late.[622]

The dentino-enamel junction is smooth rather than interdigitated, so the enamel breaks away. The coronal dentine is either covered with granular cementum, or is lamellar or globular and covered with remnants of the enamel follicle.

Hypomaturative hereditary amelogenesis imperfecta

The normally thick enamel matrix is poorly mineralised. Under pressure, a sharp explorer will penetrate the enamel, which also wears and tends to chip. The colour of the crowns is mottled brown-yellow.

Subtype II.A Hypomaturative autosomal recessive pigmented amelogenesis imperfecta

The incisal/occlusal enamel shows rough pits. Newly erupted teeth are uniformly or mottled agar-brown to yellow-white or milk-white (Figure 3.23),[991] and the soft enamel chips off. The radiographic contrast between enamel and dentine is reduced. The saliva may be rich in minerals leading to extensive calculus formation.[1001]

The enamel closest to the dentine is the best mineralised. On the surface, the mineral content of the interprismatic sheaths is decreased. Brown pigment is found in the middle of the enamel. A thick layer of organic material surrounds the crystallites.[1015]

Subtype II.B Hypomaturative X-linked recessive amelogenesis imperfecta

Males exhibit opaque-white or mottled white deciduous teeth and a mottled dark-yellow permanent dentition. On radiographs the soft enamel resembles the dentine.

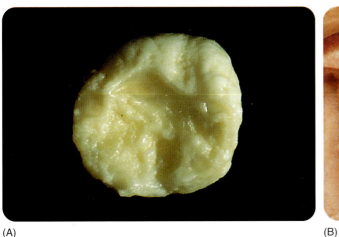
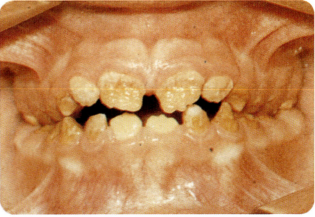

(A)   (B)

Figure 3.22 (A) Rough hypoplastic X-linked amelogenesis imperfecta (deciduous tooth) in a female member of a large family. The male family members had smooth and thin enamel. (B) Rough and yellow discoloured teeth in autosomal recessive amelogenesis imperfecta.

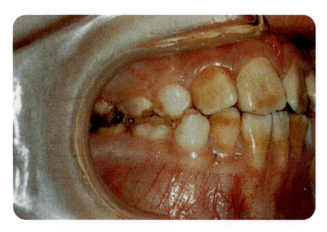

Figure 3.23 Autosomal recessive pigmented hypomaturative amelogenesis imperfecta. (Courtesy of Department of Pedodontics, University of Nijmegen.)

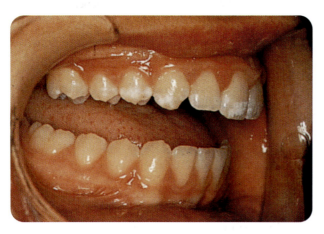

Figure 3.24 Mild form of "snow-capped" hypomaturative autosomal dominant hypoplastic amelogenesis imperfecta. (Courtesy of M.J. Walvis.)

In the female deciduous dentition, vertical opaque white bands alternate with normal coloured enamel, and in the permanent teeth with yellow and normal coloured bands. One family showed absence of a father-son transfer and daughters had mildly expressed amelogenesis imperfecta. The bands represent lyonisation[443] and are best detected with transillumination.[193] Radiographs show normal contrast between enamel and dentine in females.[1000]

The enamel contains large residues of organic material. The axial and superficial enamel layer is the best mineralised.[578]

Subtype II.C Hypomaturative X-linked "snow-capped" amelogenesis imperfecta

The incisal/occlusal parts of teeth are opaque white, like the tops of mountains covered with snow (Figure 3.24). It was first described by Witkop and Sauk in 1976.[1002] In one study, in some patients the anterior teeth were affected but in their family members the posterior teeth or all teeth were affected.[1000]

Chosack *et al.* in 1979 describe a local hypoplastic autosomal recessive type that closely resembled the snow-capped form.[158] An identical phenotype, but X-linked, has also been reported.[261]

The white enamel contains many pores.

Subtype II.D Hypomaturative autosomal dominant "snow capped" amelogenesis imperfecta

The subtype is based upon the presentation in a father and his son and daughter.[1000] A few other reports have also described this form,[63 193] but the existence of the X-linked subtype II.C is doubtful.[193] An autosomal recessive subtype could also exist.[63]

Hypocalcified hereditary amelogenesis imperfecta

The irregular enamel surface is very soft and easily removed with a relatively blunt instrument. On eruption, the enamel is of normal thickness, but subnormal mineralisation eventually leads to an eroded appearance and promotes severe wear. The enamel contains about 10% organic material. Hypoplastic bands may be present in the middle of the labial/buccal surfaces.

Subtype III.A Hypocalcified autosomal dominant amelogenesis imperfecta

On radiographs, the barely translucent enamel has a moth-eaten appearance; irregular dark areas are visible in the enamel, which is less opaque than the dentine. The cervical enamel may be better calcified. Teeth may not erupt, which together with a possible anterior open bite, is characteristic of the condition. On those that do eventually erupt there are abundant calculus deposits.[311] The yellow-brown to orange-coloured crowns becomes brown-black through dietary staining. The enamel chips away.

Empty interprismatic spaces are found in the poorly calcified enamel. The superficial enamel prisms are thin and disoriented.

Subtype III.B Hypocalcified autosomal recessive amelogenesis imperfecta

The recessive subtype is clinically and histologically similar to, but more severe than, the dominant form.

Hypomaturative-hypoplastic hereditary amelogenesis imperfecta with taurodontism

The soft and mottled enamel is thin and pitted. The molars are taurodont and other teeth may have enlarged pulp cavities.[1000] The two rare subtypes may be different expressions of the same mutation.[17] This type was reported in a boy whose sister and mother had only taurodont teeth.[17]

Subtype IV.A Hypomaturative-hypoplastic autosomal dominant amelogenesis imperfecta with pits and taurodontism

This subtype has been described in some families, with an autosomal dominant mode of inheritance;[190 192 541 991 992 993 997] however, taurodontism in a female with X-linked amelogenesis (yellow-brown rough teeth with vertical ridging due to lyonisation) has also been reported.[540]

The combination of more or less symmetrically yellow-brown discoloured and pitted enamel (incorrectly diagnosed as "fluorotic") and taurodontism probably belongs to this subtype. An explorer is able to penetrate the enamel, which appears to chip away.[991] The dentinal tubules are reduced in number and the root morphology is anomalous. The pore volume of the enamel is enlarged by 25%. The porosities do not correspond to the growth lines usually seen in the enamel.[993]

Amelogenesis imperfecta, classified as "hypomaturative", reported in a case of dizygotic triplets was more severe in the monozygotic twin than in the (third) heterozygotic child,[398] and was most likely the hypomaturative-hypoplastic subtype.

Subtype IV.B Hypoplastic-hypomaturative autosomal dominant amelogenesis imperfecta with smooth surfaces and taurodontism

This subtype was first described by Crawford in 1970,[190] and was mentioned as a separate subtype in the classification by Winter and Brook in 1975.[992] However, it could involve (like in some other cases)[180 676] the dental abnormalities present in the TDO syndrome. Witkop considered the data insufficient to warrant a new subtype.[1000]

In four generations of a family with the subtype, considerable variation in the phenotype was seen inter- and intra-individually. The teeth differed in the nature of the discoloration and wear.[20]

3.3.5   Anterior open bite and deep overbite

Insufficient occlusal enamel leads to reduced vertical dimension, worsened by chipping and wear, and a deep overbite. The open bite has been used as a criterion to distinguish the subtypes in hypoplastic amelogenesis imperfecta (Figure 3.25),[783] but it may not be specific to the condition. For example, it could be a consequence of tongue/jaw posturing[1002] or a coincidental feature.[193] [260] How far the open bite is skeletal or dental[633] in origin, or a consequence of facial deformities,[683 429] remains to be determined.[148]

3.3.6   Pathogenesis

The *hypoplastic* types develop due to a ameloblasts transforming too early from the secretory to the next phase.

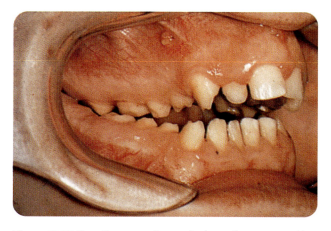

Figure 3.25 Hereditary amelogenesis imperfecta: open bite. (Courtesy of Department of Pedodontics, University of Nijmegen.)

The enamel organ degenerates too soon.[962] In one report, the whole crown of the impacted tooth was covered with enamel cuticle, normally found only at the cervix.[523] Total absence of enamel might be evidence of failure of differentiation of the inner enamel epithelium.

Hypocalcified subtypes result from inadequate initial mineralisation. Alterations in the enamel matrix[1002] or disturbances in matrix protein degradation during the maturation phase both inhibit sufficient calcification.[878] The hypocalcified enamel contains considerable amounts of amelogenins. Albumin is a major constituent of the protein fraction.[878]

In *hypomaturation* types the organic matrix between the individual crystallites is insufficiently resorbed,[1008 1045] and there is poor pre-eruptive enamel maturation.

3.3.7   Treatment

The treatment of amelogenesis imperfecta depends on the type. The dentine is normal, as is the pulp, although a considerable amount of secondary (?) and tertiary dentine is deposited in the hypoplastic rough form.[933] The hypocalcified subtypes are more prone to caries than the hypoplastic ones.[866]

Pitted *hypoplastic* hard enamel can be restored with composites, after cleaning out the pits. Atypical etching patterns have been reported in the smooth enamel and in males with X-linked amelogenesis imperfecta.[800] Before restoring severely hypoplastic enamel with composite, reduced posterior vertical dimension and excessive overjet, if present, should be corrected (Chapter 8).[538] Crown preparations risk exposing the pulp when there are spaces between the teeth with thin or absent enamel.

Teeth with *hypomineralisation* and *hypomaturation* require wear prevention. Treatment in the deciduous dentition aids the treatment in the permanent dentition[313 486] with (if needed) temporary crowns (such as stainless steel on the molars and polycarboxylate crowns on the anterior teeth)[119] or overdentures to maintain the vertical dimension. In the mixed dentition, semi-permanent provisions may be made. Depending on the type of amelogenesis imperfecta, the permanent teeth may be crowned. If the enamel is already lost, the vertical dimension must be restored with temporary crowns posteriorly, thus reducing the overbite and providing an intermediate occlusal scheme;[23] any permanent treatment may need to be postponed until the second permanent molars have erupted.[120] Adhesive cast crowns placed without tooth preparation on the permanent first molars in the mixed dentition may increase the vertical dimension by up to 3 mm. The teeth with casts intrude and the others erupt further into occlusion within 3 months and can be treated next. Full occlusion is restored by replacing the cast crowns at intervals of between 10 and 54 months, which gradually increases the total face height.[364] Poor retention of crowns on

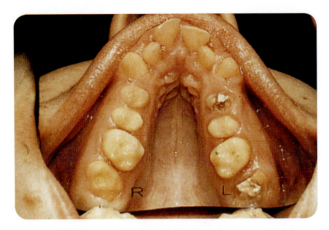

Figure 3.26 Hereditary amelogenesis imperfecta: constricted, omega-shaped, maxillary arch. (Courtesy of Department of Pedodontics, University of Nijmegen.)

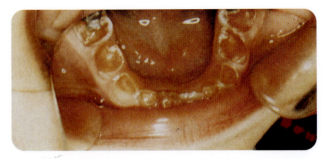

Figure 3.27 Deciduous dentition with type I dentine dysplasia exhibiting markedly abraded crowns. The dentine is amber coloured. (Courtesy of Department of Pedodontics, University of Utrecht.)

chipped and worn enamel/dentine warrants the use of extra- or intrapulpal pins. The crown preparations must extend subgingivally if the cervical enamel is absent.

Orthodontic treatment can be used to upright tilted teeth and treat malocclusions, thus reducing the interdental spaces. Periodontal therapy may be needed in older patients with severe defects.[853] A multidisciplinary approach with surgery is advocated when the dental arches, as is often the case, are constricted (Figure 3.26) and correction of the sagittal and vertical open bite and low alveolar ridges is necessary.[217 918]

3.4   Developmental structural anomalies of the dentine

The two main inherited dentine disorders are dentine dysplasia and dentinogenesis imperfecta. The genetically altered formation, composition or organisation of the dentine matrix is to be distinguished from defective mineralisation, which is most often a consequence of acquired disturbances.[301] Other extremely rare dentine disorders include, for instance, *fibrous dysplasia of the dentine*.[999] In *pulpal dysplasia* (large pulp chamber, pulp stones) the dentine of the permanent teeth is normal,[719] and the pink deciduous teeth show alternating bands of normal and almost atubular dentine.[532]

3.4.1   Dentine dysplasia

Dentine dysplasia is an inherited dentine structural anomaly, which manifests in both dentitions as:

- *Type I* or *radicular dentine dysplasia*, featuring normal crowns on (very) short roots with pulpal obliteration.[811 999]

- *Type II* or *coronal dentine dysplasia*, featuring short, bulbous, yellow-brown crowns in the deciduous dentition with pulpal obliteration, and commonly crowns of normal colour in the permanent dentition, with abnormally large pulp chambers, which are later obliterated, and more or less normal roots.

A third type of dentine dysplasia showing the radiographic findings of both types I and II has also been proposed.[161]

Dentine dysplasia was earlier called "Capdepont's teeth" (after a French dentist), "hereditary brown teeth", "opalescent teeth", "rootless teeth" and, interestingly, "opalescent non-opalescent dentine".

Characteristic features
Coronal dentine dysplasia (DD type II)

- In the deciduous dentition the crowns have a translucent, amber colour.[137 312 430 505 591 719 840] The pulp chambers are obliterated, starting from the floor upwards[430] The crowns are often severely worn (Figure 3.27); the denuded dentine becomes brown. The dental tubules are irregular in shape.
- In the permanent dentition, the colour of the normal[127 922] or short bulbous crowns[734] is occasionally grey or brown.[343 719 811] Pulpal obliteration makes the initially large pulp cavities of the anterior teeth flame-like in shape, or resembling a "balloon on a string" with the root canal being the string.[347 496] In the (pre)molars, the pulp chambers are reduced in width and often contain pulp denticles.[707 717] The roots may be short and conical with, in most instances, a sharp apical constriction. The teeth are often mobile and are susceptible to trauma, even to minor injuries.[132 312 343 395 530 591 719 734 840]

In dentine dysplasia, the dentino-enamel junction is flat,[591] allowing the enamel to break away, or shows defective interdigitation.[137 430] The normal dentino-enamel junction is scalloped,[225] and some researchers have observed a normally scalloped junction in dentine dysplasia.[343 395] Enamel fractures and excessive wear are common.[717]

The circumpulpal dentine in permanent teeth is irregular and consists partly of atubular dentine. At the cemento-enamel junction, an abrupt transition exists from regular into irregular dentine with few and irregular tubules.[430 591 717 734] In the deciduous teeth the mantle dentine is normal.[717] There is abundant interglobular dentine peripherally and relatively large areas near the pulp are not calcified.[395]

Deciduous and permanent teeth with irregularly oriented, up to 140 nm thick (normal is 50 nm), collagen bundles in the atubular dentine, have been reported.[941] "True" denticles, which probably start to grow at the apical end of the pulp chamber, contain irregular tubules (Chapter 8).[137 430 811] The root dentine may contain enamel-like structures.[395] Apically, cementicle-like structures have been infrequently observed in embedded in cellular cementum.[395] The cementum is reported to be normal,[430 591] albeit with some empty spaces. A molar root covered with an extremely thick layer of cellular cementum has been reported.[717]

Radicular dentine dysplasia (DD type I)

The crowns, which are most often slightly yellow-brown[72 811 840] or opaque white, are associated with (very) short and bulbous roots that taper towards the apex.[99 811] Eruption may be delayed.[440] Variations in root presentations – normal or underdeveloped, stunted, short and blunted, conical or sharply tapering, or absent – in both dentitions have led to further subcategorisation.[646 650 790] Four subcategories are noted in dentine dysplasia type I: (a) absent roots, total pulp obliteration and periapical radiolucencies in relation to many teeth; (b) and (c) have better developed roots, less pulpal obliteration with crescent-shaped radiolucent areas in the pulp chamber, and less frequent periapical radiolucencies; and (d) shows pulp stones in the coronal part of the root canal (where the root bulges) in more developed roots and few or no periapical radiolucencies.[650]

The crown morphology is unremarkable.[299 646] The teeth fracture easily, are malaligned,[596] and if mobile, they tend to migrate and to exfoliate. The apically located furcation of the deciduous and permanent molars is suggestive of taurodontism.[43] In the deciduous dentition, dentine dysplasia type II shares features with both type I dentine dysplasia and dentinogenesis imperfecta type II.

The pulps of the deciduous teeth are obliterated pre-eruption.[526 573 781] The permanent teeth show cervical crescent-shaped (bow-tie) remnants of the pulp chamber at the cemento-enamel junction, which may also include denticles.[239 526 573 687 781] Total obliteration and semicircular-shaped remnants of the pulp chamber have been described.[646 647]

Epithelial cells, breaking off from an "abnormal" Hertwig sheath, migrate to the dental papillae and induce odontoblast differentiation, which may be responsible for dysplastic dentine formation.[1000]

The mantle dentine seems rather normal, although the tubules may run irregularly.[526] The later-formed dentine has abnormal ultrastructural features and contains whorled tubules. Denticle-like spherical structures (globules) suggest multiple attempts to form (root) dentine.[769 922]

The denticle-like dentine contains vascular elements.[682] The dentinal and pulpal disorganisation increases in an apical direction.[408 580] The dentine resembles a structure with a head and shoulders: above the head the tubules are obliterated.[765] This structure is similar to osteodentine and the inner side of a shark's tooth.[682] The dentine in three deciduous teeth was reported to differ: for instance, the tubules in one of them were arranged in the shape of a ring.[592]

In view of the pulpal obliteration and the abnormal dentine structure, apical abscesses and cysts are to be expected,[134 175 528] although their origin is unclear. The periapical lesions are typically granulomas.[128]

Epidemiology

The anomaly is rare. In 1991, almost 200 cases were reported,[647] some 50 cases of type I dentine dysplasia.[43] In one study, one in about 10 000 children had type I dentine dysplasia.[995] Type I occurs incidentally and information on familial occurrence is grossly lacking.[685]

Aetiology and pathogenesis

Cases of dentine dysplasia without a direct cause[922] or of unknown aetiology, have been reported, and possibly are the result of maternal genetic mutation.[596] Both types are autosomal dominant,[430 591 734] but the mutated gene(s) are unknown.[239 573 646 717 790 995] One of the genes coding for collagen is probably involved. The candidate region for dentine dysplasia type II is on chromosome 4q21, and although the precise location is not known, it probably overlaps location of the defective gene in dentinogenesis imperfecta type II,[207] which may be allelic.[207 709]

Dentine sialoprotein (DSP) and dentine phosphoprotein (DPP), which are cleavage products of a single protein (DSPP), encoded by DSPP, have a major role in dentinogenesis.[1029] A missense change in DSPP was the underlying cause of dentine dysplasia type II in one family. The mutation caused loss of function of both DSP and DPP, with concomitant defective dentine mineralisation.[709] The gene locus of DSPP on chromosome 4q21 is situated in the same region as genes that cause some forms of amelogenesis imperfecta and dentinogenesis imperfecta type II and III.[542]

Gene MEPE/OF45 is also located in the same cluster on chromosome 4q21. MEPE expression has been shown in dental tissues, in particular in the odontoblasts, and is considered responsible for disturbances in the protein component of the dentine matrix.[544] One paper reported that in five generations of one family, the male:female ratio was 1:1, with a penetrance of 100%.[646]

A disorder resembling radicular dentine dysplasia has been reported in a case of *generalised calcinosis*[100] (multiple calcifications in the skin and muscles and in the soft oral tissues).[409]

In *coronal* dentine dysplasia, the formation of irregular dentine occurs under enzymatic influence.[840] Type I collagen, found in normal bone and dentine, consists of two α_1 chains and one α_2 chain interwoven into a stable triple helix. Any alteration to this form or the presence of collagen other than type I may cause structural abnormalities in the bone and dentine.[298]

Collagenous proteins constitute more than 85% of the organic content of the dentine, the remainder being proteins such as sialoprotein. Collagen type I plays a key role in the mineralisation process of the dentine. Abnormal dentine may contain a high level of collagen type III (normally absent),[768 1000] which inhibits mineralisation,[140] but in one study, the dentine of affected teeth was neither detected with the aid of specific antibodies nor with the analysis of procollagen.[717]

In *radicular* dentine dysplasia, multiple degenerative processes in the dental papilla finally lead to pulp canal obliteration and the development of denticles.[526] Another hypothesis is that epithelial cells penetrate into the (mesenchymal) papilla, initiating formation of dentine there.[769 995] An epithelial defect underlies type I dentine dysplasia.[1000]

Invagination of the radicular sheath early in development and a futile attempt at correction leads to the curious root morphology with whorled dentine in the pulp chamber.[769]

It has been questioned whether the pulpal calcifications interfere with the activity of the odontoblasts and the root morphology. Radio-opaque nodules in the central part of the roots could force them to grow around these obstacles, causing a bulbous root shape.[838]

Consequences

The coronal type of dentine dysplasia shows excessive wear.[127 312 430] During extraction, there is a risk of fracture at the level of the pulp chamber.[128 134 251 682 685] Type II dentine dysplasia is associated with delayed eruption.[840]

Prevention and treatment

In radicular dentine dysplasia, pulp necrosis and apical granulomas/cysts may be present pre-eruptively.[281] Post-eruption, abscesses are common because of bacterial ingress into the pulp through the dysplastic dentine after the loss of the enamel.[799] Surface protection with crowns may prevent pulp pathosis and excessive wear. Abscesses may also be the result of endo-perio lesions. Meticulous oral hygiene has been shown to be effective.[799]

Endodontic treatment is problematic; in one study, 20 months after pulpal extirpation, periapical bone loss had increased.[888] Curettage and resection of the apex resulted in healing after 2 months.[183] Several authors favour apical resection and retrograde pulp closure in view of the difficult conservative treatment,[281 716] but success is not guaranteed. The alternative is extraction. When periapical radiolucencies were left untreated in teeth that were asymptomatic and the lesions were not related to periodontal or pulpal disease, none of the teeth exfoliated in 2 years of follow-up after diagnosis.[440]

3.4.2 *Dentinogenesis imperfecta*

Dentinogenesis imperfecta is an inherited anomaly of dentinal structure, which presents with and without osteogenesis imperfecta, with bulbous crowns of an opalescent (translucent) soft brown (amber or opal) colour (Figure 3.28), thin and short, often transparent, roots, and pulpal obliteration after tooth eruption.

Shields *et al.* distinguished three types:[811]

- Type I, "*hereditary opalescent dentine*"[416] associated with osteogenesis imperfecta;
- Type II, *dentinogenesis imperfecta* without osteogenesis imperfecta;
- Type III, *Brandywine isolate hereditary opalescent dentine* – reported to occur in a mixed population of Native Americans, African Americans and Caucasians in the town of Brandywine (Maryland, USA), involves pulpal obliteration as well as large pulp cavities in the deciduous teeth.

Dentinogenesis imperfecta was recognised as early as in 1882, but Capdepont (1905) presented the first adequate clinical description. Fargin-Fayolle and Malassez made the first histological sections.[757]

Osteogenesis imperfecta is an inherited bone disorder (fragile, deformed bones) caused by mutation in genes for

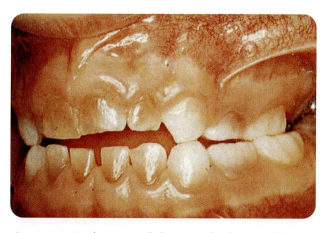

Figure 3.28 Opalescent teeth in type I dentinogenesis imperfecta. (Courtesy of J.A. Baart.)

collagen type I.[529] Dentinogenesis imperfecta types I and II are genetically different,[995] but the dental phenotypes are similar. Dentinogenesis imperfecta type III may show different characteristics in the deciduous dentition, but there are indications that types II and III are different expressions of the same mutated gene, which was the reason to combine them;[376 1000] however, other authors have distinguished four types of dentinogenesis imperfecta morphologically and biochemically.[297] Currently Shields' categorisation is used.

Dentinogenesis imperfecta occurring in combination with amelogenesis imperfecta is called *odontogenesis imperfecta*. Another reported combination is "interradicular dentinogenesis imperfecta with amelogenesis imperfecta (hypoplastic type)", in which the cementum is thickened.[622]

Characteristic features
Shields' dentinogenesis imperfecta types I and II
The types of osteogenesis imperfecta that are accompanied by dentinogenesis imperfecta show dentinal aberrations very similar to type II dentinogenesis imperfecta.[473] [506 522 718 811 869 939] However, the features in type I dentinogenesis imperfecta are more variable than in type II both in a single dentition and between families.[811] For instance, in one patient with osteogenesis imperfecta all the deciduous teeth were affected macroscopically, while the permanent dentition showed only large denticles.[529]

Type I shows greater variation, according to type and form of osteogenesis imperfecta. In patients in the osteogenesis imperfecta group but with histologically subtle and clinically undetectable dentinal changes* should not be diagnosed as having dentinogenesis imperfecta.[555]

A striking feature is the light to dark greyish-blue mother-of-pearl or amber-brown (opalescent) colour of the crowns. The bulbous crowns often show cervical constriction, resulting in a bell-shaped crown on frequently thin, short and blunt roots (Figure 3.29) that appear transparent after extraction.[998 999] The large gamut of colours is because of deposition of different minerals in the dentine and which are reflected through the enamel. The discoloration, which is minimal on eruption, worsens with time. The translucency of the teeth is associated with the decreased number of dentinal tubules.[757]

All types of dentinogenesis imperfecta show pulpal obliteration. The teeth may show severe signs of wear soon after the eruption.[202 562 728]

Enamel The enamel is normal,[110 420 521 718] although a prismatic structure is not always visible,[602] and the enamel of one-third of the teeth is somewhat hypoplastic or hypomaturative[772 999] and fragile.[411] Alternating bands of normal and abnormal enamel have been reported.[970] Near

---

* See 195 (GAGE JP) in Chapter 1 reference list.

the dentino-enamel junction, the prisms bend or become discontinous.[1010] Deciduous tooth enamel is slightly more irregularly mineralised than that of the permanent teeth.[521] No association has been found between enamel morphology and the types of osteogenesis imperfecta.[521]

Dentino-enamel junction The junction is smooth, but not cervically.[420] Starting at the occlusal/incisal edges, enamel pieces break away[26 602 898 998 999] during chewing and on biting.[728] The fractures occur either within the enamel[602] [1010] or within the dentine under the scalloped dentinal surface.[869 881]

There are some reports of normal dentino-enamel interdigitation,[533 811] and others of small high "peaks",[602] variable scalloping,[521 869] a flat junction,[869] and some deciduous teeth show a scalloped to smooth junction while in other deciduous teeth it is smooth.[521]

In spite of normal interdigitation, enamel easily breaks away along the pronounced lines of Retzius,[1010] which does not happen in normal circumstances.[720] The question remains whether the enamel breaks from the dentine or whether the fracture line lies within the enamel. A thin layer of enamel may be left after the fracture,[602 1010] but the fractures may also be located in the dentine.[869 881] The denuded mantle dentine has been reported to have been mistakenly diagnosed as the dentino-enamel junction.[869]

Dentine The 20–30 μm thick mantle dentine is (almost) normal,[16 324 385] but later formed dentine is biochemically and (ultra)structurally abnormal, coarse and fibrous,[324] although the mantle dentine might be abnormal too.[90 757] [1010] The tubules under the mantle dentine are wide, peripherally branched,[740] few in number, and irregularly oriented.[381 386 533 772 811 869 999] The dentine closer to the pulp has fewer tubules,[110] or it may even be atubular.[718] Remnants of blood vessels are present in the dentine and in the tubules. The dentine contains cells, probably former odontoblasts.[81 110 324 718 811 983 998 999] Large areas are poorly calcified or not at all and nodes of crystallisation are either absent or do not increase in size.[110 394 420 757 832 999] The tissue hardness is half that of normal.[394]

Hodge *et al.* found the soft dentine had a normal mineral ratio.[394] The red-brown dentine is cut easily.[420] A high dentinal calcium : phosphate ratio exists in carbonate-containing apatite; the number of crystallites is decreased.[448] The water content of the dentine is high.[394 448]

The collagen fibres in the dentine run parallel with the tubules and are thickened in cross-section (80–120 nm versus normal 50 nm).[385] The collagen in the dentine of dentinogenesis imperfecta type I patients has an abnormal composition, which is also seen in seemingly normal teeth.[298]

After the break up and loss of the enamel, the exposed dentine wears away rapidly.

Pulp The pulp contains bundles of collagen,[324] and an abnormal protein-carbohydrate ground substance, which does not calcify, has also been suggested.[138] The collagen

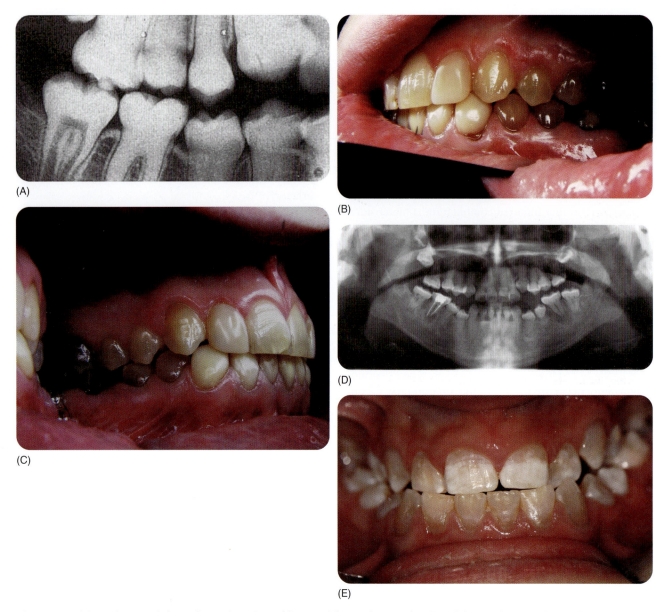

Figure 3.29 (A) Dentinogenesis imperfecta: the pulp cavities are obliterated except for that of the newly erupted second molar and the crowns are short and bulbous. (B–D) Another case with the permanent dentition showing dentinogenesis imperfecta. (E) A deciduous dentition with dentinogenesis imperfecta.

fibrils are structurally and biochemically aberrant.[879] The first formed collagen is not replaced by other collagen,[768] perhaps due to the wrong configuration,[297] which implies a deficient predentine. Structural aberrations and disturbances in epithelial–mesenchymal interactions are mentioned in the literature.[1010] Other authors have reported absence of phosphorylated protein in the dentine of dentinogenesis imperfecta type II.[880]

The oval odontoblasts are normally arranged in the early phases of development, but after the formation of the mantle dentine they become disorganised[533] and angular in shape.[324] Dentine formation continues in a

deficient form. Mesenchymal cells differentiate into odontoblasts, produce predentine, degenerate, and are incorporated in the dentine matrix. Successive generations of pulpal fibroblasts assume the task of the odontoblasts and cause pulpal obliteration,[534] which almost totally occurs pre-eruptively[412] and indicates an internal cause.[79 110 533 998] Any remaining pulp often undergoes necrosis, owing to infection via the wide "canals" in the dentine.[97]

Cementum The cementum is normal,[90] but thickened in the root furcations.[169 420 772 832] The amount of cellular cementum is relatively increased,[772 832] which may indicate degenerative changes. The cemento-dentinal junction might be blurred.[970]

Shields' type III
This type was reported in 1956 in 166 persons belonging to 14 intermarried families in Brandywine, USA (4000–5000 inhabitants). The patients showed enamel hypoplasia. In general, only the mantle dentine was normal.[411]

The bulbous crowns wear soon after the eruption. The pulp becomes exposed after spontaneous hard tissue fractures, in particular in the deciduous dentition. Both dentitions are affected. The teeth of the permanent dentition resemble those of dentinogenesis imperfecta types I and II. Phenotypes differ largely in the deciduous dentition. Some young children do not show pulpal obliteration; their deciduous teeth resemble "shell teeth".[169 411]

Shell teeth The enamel and mantle dentine are normal, but the rest of the dentine is absent with a large pulp cavity (resembling a shell). The enamel tends to break away and dentinal wear soon results in pulp exposure.[297] [463] The pulp contains thick bundles of collagen fibres, attached to dentine. The root formation lags behind.[756 757] Isolated shell teeth have been reported[720 756 773] in the Brandywine population.[998] Shell teeth are also seen in homozygote dentinogenesis imperfecta types II and III.[297]

Epidemiology
Dentinogenesis imperfecta type I is present in 80% of the deciduous and 35% of the permanent dentitions in patients with osteogenesis imperfecta tarda (see below),[331] [533] and is more severe in the deciduous than in the permanent teeth.[109 649] Osteogenesis imperfecta tarda occurs in 1:5000–10 000 births[431] and osteogenesis imperfecta congenita in 1:100 000.[205] In 1971, 2200 cases were described.[998] There is almost 100% penetrance of the familial anomaly in each generation.[998] Dentinogenesis imperfecta type II is as severe in the permanent dentition as in the deciduous dentition.[109] Dentinogenesis imperfecta type III was found in 6% of the population of Brandywine, that is, in 14 intermarried families.[411]

Aetiology
Dentinogenesis imperfecta type I In the past, two forms of osteogenesis imperfecta were distinguished. The autosomal recessive congenita (sub)lethal form (10%), which may be diagnosed *in utero*, and late osteogenesis imperfecta, the autosomal dominant tarda form (90%). Genes on chromosomes 7 and 17, respectively, are considered to be responsible.[1000] The terms "congenita" and "tarda" are, however, incorrect because bone fractures may be present at birth in both.[330 331] Characteristics include short stature, blue sclerae (in 82–90%, absent in mild forms) (Figure 3.30), fragile bones (60%), joint hypermobility,

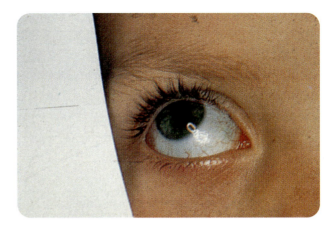

Figure 3.30 Light-blue coloured sclera in osteogenesis imperfecta. (Courtesy of J.A. Baart.)

scoliosis, and abnormal dentine (50%).[331 431 614 649] Excessive bleeding during surgery has been reported.[614]

Presently four groups, most with subtypes, are distinguished in osteogenesis imperfecta, based upon the clinical features and mode of inheritance (Table 3.6).[302 330 331 394 431 529 789]

The autosomal dominant forms are the most common, and the recessive types are the most severe. Reports that the teeth in one form are always normal and in another discoloured,[505] seem incorrect.[533] Recently, dentinogenesis imperfecta was found in 80% of the deciduous dentitions of patients with osteogenesis imperfecta I and IV,[649] and in another study two-thirds of patients with osteogenesis imperfecta I and IV had visible dentinogenesis imperfecta.[684]

Osteogenesis imperfecta IV comprises heterogeneous disorders. A group of children with moderate to severe bone fragility, calcification of interosseous membranes, and white sclerae may represent a new type (osteogenesis imperfecta V). The autosomal dominant disorder is not associated with collagen type I mutations.[323] (Table 3.6)

The generalised collagen disorder affects the bones and the teeth, but it is not clear why the penetrance and expression of the tooth anomalies vary so much, even within the same dentition.[789] In clinically normal teeth of osteogenesis imperfecta patients the chemical composition of the collagen also deviates from normal.[298]

All the members of three osteogenesis imperfecta families had dentinogenesis imperfecta while all the members of three other osteogenesis imperfecta families had healthy dentitions. It was hypothesised that dentinogenesis imperfecta develops at a later stage than osteogenesis imperfecta, assuming that both have a common origin. An alternative metabolic pathway, however, cannot be excluded.[109]

A study of unrelated patients with different types of osteogenesis imperfecta revealed that dentinogenesis imperfecta type I was present in 40%, and that it was more common in osteogenesis imperfecta III than in

Table 3.6 Features of the various types of osteogenesis imperfecta[330]

Type of osteogenesis imperfecta	Mode of inheritance	Teeth	Sclerae	Bone[b] fragility
I. Mild				
I. A[a]	AD[c]	Normal	Blue	+/++
I. B[a]	AD	Opalescent	Blue	+/++
I. C	AD	(Like dentinogenesis imperfecta type II)	Blue	+/++
II. Perinatal lethal				
II. A,B,C	AD/AR	Does not apply	Blue	++++
III. Serious, progressive, deforming				
III. A,B	AD/AR	Normal/opalescent	Blue	++/+++
IV. Moderately severe				
IV. A[a]	AD	Normal	Normal[d]	++/+++
IV. B[a]	AD			

[a]It has been proposed to change the descriptions in osteogenesis imperfecta type IA and IB and type IVA and IVB into "with dentinogenesis imperfecta" and "without dentinogenesis imperfecta".[684]
[b]+ = mild fragile; ++ = moderate fragile; +++ seriously fragile; ++++ severely fragile.
[c]Heterogeneity is reported.
[d]In some, light blue when young.

osteogenesis imperfecta I and IV and in patients with a severe form of the disease. Agenetic teeth and taurodontism were quite common. Second permanent molars tended to remain impacted.[554] Class III dental malocclusion was present in 70–80% of the patients with osteogenesis imperfecta III, with a high prevalence of crossbites and open bites.[649]

Dentinogenesis imperfecta or a phenotype without osteogenesis imperfecta may be present in Ehlers–Danlos syndrome type II and rare syndromes such as Goldblatt's syndrome, Schminke's immuno-osseous dysplasia and skeletal dysplasia with opalescent and rootless teeth.[445]

Dentinogenesis imperfecta type II This type has been recorded in five generations of one family and even more generations in other families.[79 109 376 553 562 602 740 757] None but one[109] of the cited publications mentioned osteogenesis imperfecta. All family trees point to an autosomal dominant trait. The mutation grade was assessed to be low.

To reiterate, dentinogenesis imperfecta type II and III may represent different expressions of the same gene.[1000] The responsible gene is located on the short arm of chromosome 4.[74 189] A candidate gene for dentinogenesis imperfecta type II should also be considered a candidate for dentinal dysplasia type II. Both anomalies might be allelic.[207]

The odontoblasts secrete the collagenous and non-collagenous proteins that form the dentine matrix. Among the non-collagenous proteins, DSP and DPP play a crucial role in mineralisation.[837] Mutated genes involved in protein production may cause, for instance, premature termination of such proteins.

The dentine phosphoryn gene (DMP2) on chromosome 4 might be involved in dentinogenesis imperfecta type II,[891] but some authors did not find the gene localised on chromosome 4, suggesting that dentine phosphoprotein is not directly associated

with dentinogenesis imperfecta type II and III. Other proteins might be responsible.[545] A cluster of genes on chromosome 4q21 contains the loci for dentinogenesis imperfecta types II and III and dentine dysplasia type II. Located within an overlapping segment is a dentine/bone cluster.[542] Dentinogenesis imperfecta type II has been found associated with a nonsense mutation encoded by *DSPP*. The minor component of the extracellular dentine matrix consists of DSP, and DPP is the major non-collagenous protein: both are cleavage products of the single protein DSPP. DPP binds a large amount of calcium and has a major role in dentinogenesis. A mutation in the DPP portion of *DPSP* might disrupt normal dentine formation, leading to dentinogenesis imperfecta type II, whereas DSP will have a minor effect (unless it is a nonsense mutation).[1029] Deletion of the entire *DSPP* coding region in mice resulted in the development of tooth defects similar to human dentinogenesis imperfecta.[837]

Transgenic mice that overexpress active "transforming growth factor" (TGF-β1) from embryonic day 17 had teeth with dentinogenesis imperfecta features. TGF-β1 induces secretion of dentine matrix proteins, but overexpression of TGF-β1 down-regulates the expression of the sialophosphoprotein gene.[890]

Dentinogenesis imperfecta type III In all probability, dentinogenesis imperfecta type III is autosomal dominant.[411] The expression is variable, more so in the deciduous dentition.

The locus of the mutant gene (*DMP1*) of dentinogenesis imperfecta type III is on chromosome 4q21, which overlaps the critical region of dentinogenesis imperfecta type II, which is either an allelic variant of dentinogenesis imperfecta type III or the result of mutations in two tightly linked genes.[543]

Characteristic features
The teeth are often lost prematurely. Full dentures at the age of 16 are common,[562] but overdentures may also be used. Early wear of the teeth, quickly down to the gingiva, reduces the vertical dimension. Class III malocclusion and

posterior crossbites are common.[789] In one study of patients with osteogenesis imperfecta III and IV, 90% had class III or class II malocclusions, often with an anterior or posterior open bite and crossbites. The molars tend to erupt ectopically (Chapter 4).[649] A patient with dentinogenesis imperfecta had dens in dente,[450] but this could have been a coincidence.

Prevention and treatment

Early loss and excessive wear of the teeth may be prevented with use of stainless steel crowns on the posterior teeth in the deciduous dentition and composite crowns on the anterior teeth, or alternatively, overdentures.[149 313 412 548] Objectives of early treatment of the deciduous dentition are maintenance of the dentition (vitality, form, size), aesthetics, prevention of loss of vertical dimension, maintenance of arch length, and normal growth of facial bones and the temporomandibular joint. The advantages of treatment outweigh the disadvantages, such as risk of general anaesthesia and the technical problems associated with the as yet wide pulp chambers.[766] Care must be taken to minimise an increase in the posterior vertical dimension to avoid untoward development of an anterior vertical open bite.[412]

In the mixed dentition (prefabricated) crowns are placed as soon as possible on the severely affected permanent molars; if the teeth are worn down, an overlay denture may correct the vertical height of occlusion. An overdenture requiring minimal preparation of the maxillary teeth and porcelain-gold crowns in the lower jaw has been reported to be effective.[846] Elastics may be required to separate the teeth.[799] Malocclusions require orthodontic treatment.[649]

Multiple surgical procedures may sensitise the osteogenesis imperfecta patient to latex.[649] These patients are prone to bleeding, secondary to platelet and possible vascular disorders. Thus haemorrhage after orthognathic surgery and extractions is a likely serious complication.[459]

The use of crowns possibly prevents periapical pathology. However, dental abscesses are also thought to arise due to disruption of the pulpal vascular supply in association with the abnormal pulpal calcifications, which leads to pulp necrosis.[799] Sequential radiographs are therefore desirable. Endodontic treatment in case of pulpal pathosis is difficult if initiated after pulp canal obliteration,[688] and may make extraction unavoidable. The outcome of endodontic treatment may be unfavourable and short roots are a contraindication for endodontic surgery.

3.4.3   Regional (or segmental) odontodysplasia ("ghost teeth")

Regional odontodysplasia is a rare developmental disorder of, in general, a few teeth, where the enamel and

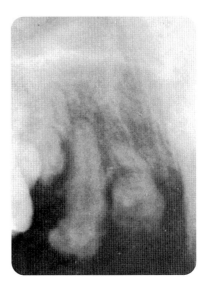

Figure 3.31 Ghost teeth (photonegative). (Courtesy of I. Van der Waal.)

dentine are hypomineralised, hypoplastic, thin and discoloured, and the pulp cavity is wide.

The teeth are seen on radiographs as vague images (Figure 3.31); the term "ghost teeth" has been generally adopted. The cementum is involved, and many teeth do not erupt. The disorder was probably described for the first time in 1934.[374] A variant without the typical radiographic appearance and affecting all the teeth is *dentino-enamel dysplasia*.[606]

Characteristic features

Many ghost teeth do not erupt (about 40%).[887] The teeth are poorly calcified and most of the X-rays pass through them when a radiograph is taken. That is, the radiodensity of the enamel, dentine and pulp is more or less similar, resulting in the indistinct image. The pulp cavity is large and the roots are relatively short. With time, the teeth may become more calcified,[309] and the root may fully develop.[1046] The gingiva covering the teeth may get infected (50%)[887] and enlarged (as does the alveolar crest), and consists of dense collagenous fibrous tissue with focal aggregations of calcified bodies and many islands of odontogenic epithelium.[309 567] Unerupted ghost teeth are often detected incidentally because of the associated gingival infection, swelling[153 299 601 630 862 909 917 1003] or delayed or absent eruption, leading to radiographic investigation.[5 278 359 490 537 657 674 694 1003] Odontodysplastic deciduous predecessors have been reported.[143 274 439 585 630] The jaws and the face on the side of the ghost teeth may be underdeveloped.[314 350 674 711]

Enamel

Erupted teeth have a rough surface, and seem to be brittle as they "crumble", and have a distinct morphology, which

is co-determined by the crumbly nature of the enamel.[25]
[303 382 393 469 503 634 924] Surgically removed teeth are small with chalk-like yellow to brown crowns. The enamel surface is very irregular, rough and soft on probing.[118 153 191 301 393]
[449 537 601 727 742 759 1026] The enamel contains degenerated globular calcifications and is hypocalcified.[340] Areas with both disorganised and normal prismatic structure have been observed,[191 314] but without a chronological basis for the location of the defects.[887] The enamel may be covered with cementum, which could hinder eruption.[198]

Two "kinds" of enamel have been observed: prismatic enamel with large spaces between the crystals and hypoplastic enamel consisting of relatively small crystals that are closely packed together. Round structures, which may or may not be hypocalcified, on the enamel surface consist of even smaller crystallites originating from the reduced enamel epithelium.[449] The enamel is covered by a glasslike mixture, consisting of the calcified enamel organ and other calcified structures[143 303 314 333 386 469 630 694] which may induce gingival swelling.[5 270 630 912]

Dentine
At the dentino-enamel junction the interdigitation is variable. Under the thin dentine is a broad layer of predentine. The coronal dentine contains many spaces and wide tubules, which are reduced in number and run irregularly[439 694] in a poorly formed matrix.[303] The mantle dentine may show a normal structure,[274 449 467] just like the dentine near the pulp cavity.[467] About half of the little dentine that is there is interglobular dentine.[467 537] Collagen-free dentinal matrix,[303] in which enamel may be present, may extend to the pulp,[301] leading to communication between the pulp and the oral cavity.[274] More severe cases exhibit cellular dentine, amorphous areas or loose connective tissue.[303 314 694] In short roots, the dentine has few tubules but these follow a more regular course.[694]

Cementum
The cementum is less abnormal,[301] yet hypoplastic.[989]

Pulp
The large pulp cavity contains round and oval calcified structures, bulges of dentine and free or dentinal wall-bound denticles, or tertiary dentine.[191 274 301 393 467]

Epidemiology
The number of case reports has increased slowly over the years,[191 270 490 537 694 759] to some 140 cases in 2003.[887] Ghost teeth are present 2.5 times more often in the maxilla than in the mandible,[191] but a ratio of 1.6:1 has also been reported.[887] Most frequently it involves the permanent maxillary central incisors, followed by the lateral incisors and the canines, predominantly on the left side. Every tooth may be involved, including the deciduous teeth, in which case the succedaneous teeth are also affected. In

around half of the cases, both dentitions are involved.[887] However, in other patients, the deciduous teeth may have erupted and succumbed to caries.[669] The anomaly is generally confined to one quadrant, but not crossing the midline is not an absolute rule, as it has even been reported to occur in all four quadrants (*generalised odontodysplasia*).[153 299 325 761 844 909 943 999] Incidentally, ghost teeth may occur on both sides of a normal tooth,[278 537 723] which may be aetiologically important. There is a slight predilection for females (1.4:1 or 1.7:1).[191 887]

Aetiology
The aetiology is not known. Several causes have been suggested.

Trauma and local infection are mentioned,[98] but radiotherapy is not causative.[1026] The presence of ghost teeth in all four quadrants may point to a more general genetic problem or (local) mutation[761 1026] involving part of the epithelial dental lamina.[759] If the latter is correct, the more distally situated teeth will be inevitably involved but will be the least affected.[118] Dietary deficiencies, trauma, etc. are unlikely causes. A latent viral infection of the odontogenic epithelium was suspected, but no evidence of the presence of the virus was found.[621 759] A neural origin was also proposed, based upon the combination of odontodysplasia in the deciduous and permanent dentition with hydrocephaly[198] and early maternal hypoxia.[988] Local hypocalcaemia,[815] teratogenic drugs and neural crest cell defects have also been implicated,[887] whereas Rh incompatibility and hyperpyrexia have also been considered causative.[669]

Resection of the inferior alveolar artery in rabbits, creating prolonged local ischaemia of the continuous erupting mandibular incisors, produced changes similar to ghost teeth.[536] Hypoplastic teeth and ghost teeth have been observed in patients with "birthmarks", other haemangiomas, and even with locally red skin,[331 350 439 447 821 844 941] but absence of cutaneous vascular abnormalities has also been stressed.[630 909] Vascular disturbances due to maternal use of medicines (diuretics) are mentioned too; if this were true, it is not clear why the anomaly generally occurs unilaterally.

The gingival tissue around the follicle of a ghost tooth contains highly fragmented collagen fibres and shows an increase in gingival matrix metalloproteinases, which could be the origin of the aberration. In some pathological conditions and inflammation, the secretion of some metalloproteinases and their inhibitors from stimulated tissue cells is increased. Such an imbalance might be associated with a breakdown of connective tissue in the ghost teeth.[187]

Treatment
The therapy consists of extraction or surgical removal of the teeth because of the weak roots, followed by space maintenance. Facial development may be deficient if the teeth are removed prior to cessation of active skeletal growth.[200] Despite the possible presence of abscesses

related to pulpal necrosis in the absence of an obvious cause,[309 537] the teeth have been crowned in an attempt to preserve them.[528] If the teeth erupt (aided by surgery) and abscesses are absent, pulp complications might be prevented with timely composite resin restorations or (temporary) crowns.[191] Ghost teeth that retain vitality upon eruption often demonstrate a thickening of the dentine and develop a normal root complex.[309] The alveolar

fibrous tissue adjacent to erupted ghost teeth may need to be trimmed.[567]

A ghost tooth was utilised as an abutment for a bridge, the prosthetic tooth replacing a surgically removed adjacent ghost tooth.[989] In view of the pulpal abnormalities, endodontic treatment is not advised.[930] After extraction, autotransplantation of normal teeth to the affected region may be an option.[931]

Section II
Anomalies of Eruption

4

Deviations in Timing and Site of Eruption

4.1 Eruption

4.1.1 The eruption process

Eruption is defined as the act of emergence of any part of a tooth into the oral cavity. However, in practical terms, eruption includes the entire axial movement of a tooth, from the movements during odontogenesis[267] in its crypt to when it makes contact with its antagonist(s), and the axial movement thereafter to compensate for tooth wear. The eruptive process is influenced by several factors including the growth of the face, jaws and alveolar height.

Pre-eruptive movements start after initiation of root formation, even prior to calcification. Previously, root growth was incorrectly[43 63 220] considered to deliver the eruptive force. However, teeth without roots or those with extremely short roots due to radiotherapy,[197 481] congenital kidney disease[63] or due to surgical root removal also erupt. The developing root even penetrates 2–4 mm further into the surrounding bone, without any eruptive movement.[271]

It has been suggested that the eruptive force could be delivered by the periodontal ligament itself.[284] The ligament fibres are rapidly renewed and remodelled by the local fibroblasts[267] and might be responsible for eruption. However, in humans, this might hold true after emergence,[271] but before that time the tooth–alveolus connection is incomplete and there are too few fibres,[240] and thus the mechanism of eruption may be different from that of rodent incisors which erupt continually throughout life.[72] Microtubules in the periodontal ligament may be involved in eruption,[33] but evidence is lacking and results of experiments are conflicting.[72]

Cells in the dental follicle and possibly in the periodontal membrane are targeted by the epidermal growth factor and other hormones (such as growth hormone), which initiate several cellular processes including cell differentiation and DNA synthesis in the ligament fibroblasts.[385 416] A pushing force, instead of traction, is generated in the periodontal ligament, due to a hydrostatic pressure gradient in the periodontal ligament and the interstitial fluid. Blood vessel permeability is altered under the influence of growth hormone, which controls the secretion of insulin-like growth factors.

The pre-eruption path of the tooth lies within the *gubernaculum dentis*, a narrow sheath of soft tissue within the bone.[72] Resorption of bone and eventually the roots of the deciduous teeth broadens the path. Increased secretion of enzymes such as hyaluronidase and gelatinase,[352] cytokines such as interleukin-1[430] and other regulatory molecules for osteoclastogenesis[501] are required for the breakdown of the tissues ahead of the erupting tooth.[72 220 271] Calcitonin inhibits osteoclastogenesis and may have anti-eruption properties.[502] The dental follicle contains monocytes and chemotactic molecules necessary for the formation of osteoclasts, the bone resorbing cells.[486]

The number of monocytes in the coronal part of the dental follicle increases proportionally to the number of the osteoclasts.[487] Tooth germs transplanted to elsewhere in the jaw erupted when the dental follicle was left intact in experimental studies but if there was follicular damage the teeth did not erupt.[224] Thus the dental follicle may be essential for eruption,[71] but signalling molecules in the stellate reticulum may act as factors controlling the timing of eruption through their interaction with the dental follicle, and may also possibly initiate the eruption.[486]

After emergence into the oral cavity, the eruptive movement continues until the tooth makes contact with its antagonistic(s). The tooth moves at night in the direction of the antagonist(s), about 4 mm within 14 weeks. During the daytime, in particular during breakfast and the midday meal, a small apical movement takes place.[240] Risinger *et al.* found that from 20:00 to 24:00 hours, premolars moved 65 μmm orally, in cyclic eruptive rhythms of 20–50 seconds, and between midnight and morning they intruded 33 μmm.[385]

Shifts in the position of the teeth and their sockets occur to compensate for the growth of the face. For example,

Pathology of the Hard Dental Tissues, First Edition. Albert Schuurs.

between the ages of 9 and 25 years the permanent maxillary incisors move some 6 mm downwards and 2.5 mm labially.[195] After the age of 16, vertical movement diminishes and the displacement occurs mainly in the horizontal plane.[196] An active spurt of movement occurs during puberty.[425] As mentioned above, minimal eruptive movements continue to occur after establishment of occlusal contact to compensate for tooth wear.[482] In the absence of involvement of a tooth in mastication, eruption continues, whereby the epithelial attachment of the tooth comes to lie on exposed cementum.[302]

4.1.2 Timing of eruption

Most teeth emerge when half to three-quarters of the final root length is achieved.[29] [155] There is marked variation in the timing of eruption of individual teeth with respect to chronological age. Mean eruption times can be determined retrospectively or prospectively. With the case–control method, large groups of children of different age cohorts are examined to record which teeth are erupted, although a cohort effect or a period (calendar year) effect may introduce bias.[328] The *physiologic* eruption timespan of a tooth may be arbitrarily defined, for instance as the mean $\pm 3 \times SD$ (standard deviation). An eruption time outside this is by definition delayed[380] or accelerated. The standard deviations for the emergence times of individual teeth differ.[189] In practice, the time periods and eruption sequence shown in Table 4.1 may be used, although these will differ considerably by country and population.

Deciduous dentition

A sex difference is absent in the maturation and the eruption times of the deciduous teeth.[215] [297] Earlier eruption both in boys[111] [323] [441] and girls[104] has been recorded, but may apply only to the maxillary lateral incisors and mandibular canines.[160] One has to take into account that eruption patterns vary between individuals as they are (weakly) correlated with factors such as birthweight, increase in weight after birth (in boys), birth order, mother's age at time of conception and body length (in girls). Maternal smoking in particular has been shown to retard dental maturity and eruption.[194] [210] [215] [323] [440] A weak association between head circumference and number of emerged teeth increased greatly when comparing children below the 25th percentile with those above the 75th percentile (Yule's coefficient of association (Q) = 0.6 for boys and 0.4 for girls).[194] Hypodontia is clearly accompanied by delayed development of the dentition,[34] [147] [179] [356] as are congenital clefts of the lip, jaws and palate.[355] [376]

"Teething", i.e. the eruption of especially the deciduous mandibular and, to a lesser degree, the maxillary central incisors (23%), and occasionally other teeth,[91] is accompanied by several symptoms. Parents reported gingival itching (85%), agitation (74%), dribbling (70%), fever

Table 4.1 The sequence of eruption and time periods within which the deciduous and permanent teeth erupt

Eruption sequence	Tooth	Time period	Tooth	Time period
Primary dentition				
1	Central incisor	6–8 months		
2	Lateral incisor	8–10 months		
3	First molar	12–18 months		
4	Canine	16–20 months		
5	Second molar	24–30 months		

	Maxilla		**Mandible**	
Permanent dentition				
1	First molar	6–7 years	First molar	6–7 years
2	Central incisor	7–8 years	Central incisor	6–7 years
3	Lateral incisor	8–9 years	Lateral incisor	7–8 years
4	First premolar	10–11 years	Canine	9–10 years
5	Second premolar	10–12 years	First premolar	10–12 years
6	Canine	11–12 years	Second premolar	11–12 years
7	Second molar	12–13 years	Second molar	11–13 years
8	Third molar	17–21 years and later	Third molar	17–21 years and later

(46%), disturbed sleep (39%), diarrhoea (35%) and runny nose (26%). Proteins of the degrading enamel matrix act as antigens and cause an auto-immune response.[343] However, systemic symptoms such as fever and diarrhoea are absent.

Permanent dentition

The eruption times of the deciduous and permanent teeth correlate moderately (in the order of $r = 0.40$), but more so between first permanent molars and the second deciduous molars (in the order of $r = 0.70$).[260] At observations made at three different ages, a sample of Finnish girls had more erupted teeth than boys;[327] the tooth-dependent difference ranged from 0.1 to 1.0 year.[475] In a longitudinal study, the difference in eruption times of the individual teeth was 2.5–14 months.[160]

The interval between two check-ups in a longitudinal investigation may, for instance, be 1 year. [475] If a tooth erupts between check-ups, one only knows that the tooth emerged within that year, which is not very accurate. One may then assume that the tooth erupted at the midpoint of the yearly interval, but such an assumption may give rise to bias. This disadvantage may be overcome by use of appropriate statistical methods.[328]

Variations in the mean eruption times in different studies are due to sex, sample, age and country differences at the time of observation.[358] A variation of 15 months related to sex has been found for all permanent teeth.[170] It has been shown that at 5–6 years of age sexual dimorphism is absent.[245] Per tooth, girls aged 6–12 years are a few months in advance of boys, more so for the (mandibular) canines.[151 152 245 260 264 327] At 8 years, tooth mineralisation in girls is ahead, reaching its peak at 13 years,[186] but the third molars erupt earlier in boys.[245] According to some researchers, there are no sex differences in the eruption times of the individual teeth.[67 251]

As mentioned above, eruption times also vary between individuals,[67 169] ethnically and geographically. A 1.5-year advance in eruption noted in sub-Saharan Africa may have been due to errors in the data,[352] but more recently the mean eruption times of third molars in Nigerian females was noted to be 13 years and in Nigerian males it was 15 years.[322]

The eruption of the permanent dentition is also influenced by presence of caries in the deciduous teeth,[1 449] but this effect is now seen less often due to the general decline in the prevalence of caries. In the 1980s, permanent teeth erupted 4–5 months earlier than in 1934,[185 256] and in 1965 (in Denmark) earlier than in 1913,[178] a secular trend comparable to an increased body length and earlier onset of the menarche (which, however, weakly correlates with eruption times).[207] In France, a trend has been noted for later eruption of the maxillary premolars and earlier emergence of permanent second molars.[391] Today, many children mature at a younger age than 50 or 100 years ago, they are growing faster and have increased stature, all of which seem to be associated with accelerated eruption.[186 328]

Sequence of eruption

Several sequences of eruption have been reported (Table 4.2), deviating from that presented in Table 4.1.[170 251] The eruption sequence of the maxillary second premolar and canine is changing (Denmark, USA, France).[328 391 478] In a sample of boys in New York, the mandibular second premolar was found to erupt after the second molar.[478] In Finland, the mandibular central incisors presently emerge before the first molars in 68%.[311]

Chronological age, dental and skeletal maturity

The intellectual and physical burden in, for instance, orphans will be too heavy if their age is estimated to be older than they actually are and they will lack exposure to appropriate challenges if estimated to be too young. Age when not known is estimated on the basis of the degree of ossification of the bones such as the hand and wrist. Another possibility is to use the level of dental maturation. One scoring method (Demirjan, 1973) is based upon eight stages of calcification seen on radiographs of the seven left mandibular permanent teeth (the third molar is excluded).[110] The eight stages are related to skeletal development. For example, in stage eight the mandibular canine root apex is closed and the epiphyses of the long bones are fused with the diaphyses.[90] With the seven tooth scores, the dental age is determined, using conversion tables for sex,[109 110] because a French-Canadian study noted that after the age of 7 years, girls were more dentally mature than boys.[111] The reference group data appeared invalid for other populations. A modified method has resulted in a better fit.[445]

Correlation between the skeletal age and dental maturation in different age categories is reported to be low ($r = 0.2$–0.4).[108 177 358] Even in one study which showed high correlation ($r = 0.59$), this was not high enough to substitute the age determined by skeletal maturity with that determined via dental estimation.[396] The calcification of the mandibular canines probably correlates better (and that of other teeth less) with specific ossification areas in the hand bones.[90 418] In a few towns or countries, some children of known age were estimated to be older based on dental estimates and others younger,[121 249 269 308 310 446] whereas use of skeletal maturity led to more correct estimates.[269] A large impact of environmental factors on dental maturity may explain differences between children with the same ethnic background. Genetic factors may

Table 4.2 Sequence of eruption of some permanent teeth[170]

Eruption sequence							
Maxilla				Mandible			
First	Second	Third	Frequency of occurrence	First	Second	Third	Frequency of occurrence
P_1	P_2	C	51%	C	P_1	P_2	86%[a]
P_1	C	P_2	35%	C	P_2	P_1	8%
C	P_1	P_2	7%	P_1	C	P_2	4%
P_2	P_1	C	3%				
Other sequences			4%	Other sequences			2%

[a]Also 50%; consequently the percentages for the other orders become higher.[251]

explain racial differences.[338] The remains of eighteenth and nineteenth-century British children of known age were used for dental estimation. Several of the younger children were dentally delayed, their dental age being below the lowest limit of the scale (2.5 years).[250]

Other dental-based methods have been developed,[288] requiring the assessment of fewer teeth.[57 257 290] A study of one of these methods[288] in monozygotic and dizygotic twins revealed that variation in dental age was best explained by additive genetic influences (43%), environmental factors common to both twins (50%) and specific environmental factors that were not shared by both.[338]

Age estimation via different dental-based methods by different observers using identical radiographs had very diverging/differing results.[382] One method led to age estimations that were too high and two others to age estimations that were too low. The 95% confidence interval (for Demirjian's method) for individual age estimation exceeded 15 months,[100] 2 years,[290 308 421] and 3 years.[121]

Compared with Caucasians, the eruption is accelerated in the Bantu and delayed in autochthonous Australians.[345] Dental maturity[110] and eruption times[136] show varying degrees of correlation.[358] Methods to assess dental maturity are not interchangeable.[311] The independent physiological determinants[177] "dental age" and "skeletal maturity" are used to find as precise as possible the age of war orphans and adoptive children.[137] Some researchers prefer solely the use of skeleton maturity for age estimation[177] while others prefer dental maturity. Marked differences between individuals and populations make the estimation of the chronological age based on the dental development precarious.

4.2   Abnormal eruption times

Beyond the physiological variations, the eruption of the deciduous and permanent dentition may be accelerated or retarded and teeth may not erupt or only partially erupt. Eruption delays are more common than acceleration.[430]

4.2.1   *Pathologically accelerated eruption*

Pathologically accelerated eruption occurs when one or more deciduous or permanent teeth emerge at a younger age than expected on the basis of eruption times or the stage of root development.

Deciduous dentition
Local factors

- *Natal and neonatal teeth.* Teeth erupted at or around birth are described in Chapter 1. A superficially located tooth germ seems the likely cause.

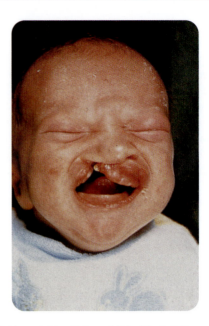

Figure 4.1 Neonatal tooth in a child with cleft lip and palate.

- *Early teething (dentitio praecox).* Many or all deciduous teeth erupt prematurely, probably again due to superficially located germs. The precocious dentition may be familial.[345]

General factors

- *Fever.* Infectious diseases with fever may be associated with early eruption of some teeth, but some teeth may erupt later than normal.[345]
- *Syndromes.* Premature eruption is linked to a number of syndromes (Chapter 11), including oral clefts (Figure 4.1).

All deciduous teeth had erupted (except second molars) in a child aged 11 months with three copies of chromosome 8,[342] and in a 4-month-old child with Letterer–Siwe disease (involves proliferation of the macrophages that is fatal).[9]

Permanent dentition
Local factors

Early loss of deciduous teeth   When a deciduous tooth is lost *earlier* than its normal exfoliation time, for example due to caries requiring extraction of the tooth,[185] accelerated root resorption[345] or trauma, the successor tooth's eruption is accelerated. There are reports of premolars having emerged prematurely when the predecessors were extracted less than 2 years before their exfoliation time.[93 351] Others have found both delayed and accelerated premolar eruption,[73] except in the mandibular premolar-canine region.[207] Early eruption requires that the space available for the successor is of normal proportion. Delayed eruption of usually the mandibular second premolar and the maxillary canine occurs when the space is too small,[207] due to drifting and tilting of the adjacent teeth into the space.[306]

Rural Maasai (Africa) traditionally removed the tooth buds of the deciduous canines, because febrile illnesses in childhood are believed to be caused by the swelling over the canine region, which was thought to contain "worms". The removal did not affect the eruption time of the successors, which may, however, be damaged.[171]

Emergence of the premolars was reported to be accelerated by 4–8 months and 2–4 months in boys and girls respectively, when their predecessors were decayed and restored.[244] Pulpotomy of a deciduous molar may accelerate the emergence of the successor,[239][320] but delayed exfoliation is reported too. Caries, pulp necrosis and pulpotomy hasten the resorption of the deciduous roots, but not the rate of root growth of the succedaneous teeth.[164] However, in a 6-year-old with erupted mandibular canines, root development was similar to in a 13–14-year-old,[303] while erupted premolars in other 6-year-olds were reported to be mobile because of insufficient root development.[73]

Extraction of deciduous molars with abscesses and resorbed alveolar bone accelerate the emergence of the succedaneous tooth regardless of its developmental stage,[73] in a buccal or lingual direction, with the tooth taking the path of least resistance.[189]

Prepubertal periodontitis Deciduous teeth exfoliate prematurely due to aggressive (formerly called early-onset pubertal)[503] periodontitis,[325][463] which is not necessarily followed by an accelerated eruption of permanent teeth.[22] Extraction of the very mobile teeth and scaling with subgingival chlorhexidine irrigation of other teeth in a 5-year-old girl was followed, until the age of 13, by mobility and root resorption that led to extraction of all permanent teeth.[463]

Juvenile periodontitis may be present in otherwise healthy patients. Curettage and antibiotics have been advised if the process starts at the age of 4 years around a few teeth. Symptoms are local gingival recession and bone resorption, but without root resorption and gingival inflammation. A generalised, rapidly progressive process starts early in the mixed dentition with acutely inflamed gingiva. Abnormal leucocytes are also reported. Afterwards, the permanent dentition may show severe periodontitis.[325][326] The pulp cavities of the teeth may be large, with abnormal cementum and root resorption.[326]

The roots of deciduous teeth in "prepubertal" periodontitis show bacteria within the dentinal tubules or in the cementum. The cementum is either normal, wider than normal or hypoplastic, and both resorption and repair are evidenced. Suprabony root surfaces exhibit resorption lacunae, calculus and colonies of heterogeneous bacterial populations.[45] Permanent teeth of subjects with prepubertal periodontitis had thicker cementum and were infiltrated by microorganisms compared with the teeth of 50-year-old healthy controls. A cuticle may cover the cementum in prepubertal periodontitis, which is not seen in adults with periodontitis.[255]

General factors

- *(Facial) hemihypertrophy.* Eruption is advanced by 4–5 years on the side of the face showing overgrowth.[34]
- *Mercury poisoning.* Early exfoliation of deciduous teeth and breakdown of periodontal tissues was described in a 15-month-old child exposed to mercury in the house of a former gold miner. The miner routinely used mercury to extract gold from ore and boiled away the mercury condensed on the walls and floor.[272] Mercury is still used to extract gold from sand obtained from rivers. In the past, mercury caused early loss of permanent teeth in mercury miners, mirror makers and workers in the felt-making industry ("mad as a hatter").
- *Precocious puberty (pubertas praecox).* When puberty starts prematurely due to central or peripheral disturbances, all permanent teeth erupt early. Central disturbances may have several causes including idiopathic ones and premature activation by tumours of the hypothalamus. An example of a peripheral cause is a gonadal tumour. Medroxyprogesterone medication for idiopathic precocity is associated with accelerated root development and eruption.[77] Slightly advanced tooth development[148] and definitely advanced root formation has been confirmed in cases of precocious puberty not on medication.[205] Odontogenesis is retarded in idiopathic precocity and but proceeds normally when other causes underlie premature puberty.[388]
- *Syndromes.* Eruption is accelerated in cases with syndromes (Ellis–Van Creveld, Hallerman–Streiff, pachyonychia congenita, Sturge–Weber, etc.). In the Klippel-Trénaunay syndrome (which includes unilateral bony and soft tissue hypertrophy) the permanent teeth erupt prematurely on the affected side of the jaw.[293] Although dental maturity seemed to be delayed by more than 12 months in about 20% of patients with osteogenesis imperfecta type III and accelerated in as many of those with osteogenesis imperfecta type IV, the eruption times of the deciduous and permanent teeth were normal, but in some subjects the permanent second molars emerged late.[314]
- *Systemic diseases. Hyperthyroidism* leads to thyrotoxicosis, which is accompanied by tachycardia, hypertension and accelerated tooth eruption.[346] In advanced cases the deciduous teeth are lost from atrophied alveolar bone and the permanent teeth erupt early.[408] Well-controlled *diabetes* does not influence eruption. In

uncontrolled diabetes, there is accelerated exfoliation of the deciduous teeth and eruption of the permanent teeth, but long-standing diabetes delays the eruption of permanent teeth.[2][56] The effect in the mixed dentition period is probably mediated by the pituitary gland, which is stimulated in the initial stages of the disease but in then becomes exhausted in juvenile diabetes of longer duration, the reasons for which remain unclear.[56]

- *Systemic diseases and syndromes with juvenile perio-dontitis.* Premature loss of a few or all deciduous teeth, possibly followed by accelerated eruption (and loss) of permanent teeth, may occur in many diseases[168][281][285] that compromise the host response and cause peri-odontitis. Examples are acute lymphocytic leukaemia (leucocyte proliferation and hyperplasia of lymphoid tissue), cyclic neutropenia (decreased number of neu-trophilic leucocytes), histiocytosis X (abnormal macro-phages), acatalasia (absence of the enzyme catalase), haemangioma and lymphangioma.

Several syndromes are associated with prepubertal periodon-titis and early tooth loss. *Chediak–Higashi syndrome* is charac-terised by oculocutaneous albinism, abnormal neutrophils, respiratory system and skin infections, and severe gingivitis.[168][285] Antibiotic treatment proves ineffective.[504]

Papillon–Lefèvre syndrome is characterized by hyperkeratosis of palms and soles and early, rapid, destructive periodontitis. The prematurely lost deciduous teeth are replaced by the earlier erupting permanent teeth.[174] Antibiotics and extraction of the deciduous dentition followed by a period of edentulism seem effective in preserving the permanent dentition.[138] Extraction of teeth with poor prognosis and conventional periodontal treat-ment improve the condition,[359] although edentulism in a 12-year-old affected child has been reported.[174] The crevicular fluid may not show clear-cut pathognomonic expression of cytokines and matrix metalloproteinases.[459]

- *Tumours, inflammation.* Accelerated loss of the decid-uous teeth, even starting at the age of 1 year, may be caused by malignant and benign neoplasms and osteomyelitis.[22]

4.2.2 Pathologically delayed eruption

Pathologically delayed eruption is the emergence in the mouth of one or more teeth of the deciduous or perma-nent dentition at a later age than expected on the basis of published mean eruption times. Delayed eruption is more common than early eruption and has many more causes. Alternative terms are *late, retarded, depressed, impaired, (primary) retention, primary/idiopathic failure of erup-tion, impaction, embedded teeth,* and *pseudoanodon-tia;*[430] some terms have a specific meaning and will be defined later.

Deciduous dentition
Dentitio tarda occurs when a deciduous tooth erupts 6 months later than it does on average.[166][171]

Local factors

- *Gingival fibromatosis and hyperplasia.* After dental trauma/surgery, the follicle of an erupting deciduous tooth may not merge with the overlying mucosa, which also does not break down (or this is delayed). Gingival hyperplasia with dense connective tissue may act as a barrier: hormonal and hereditary causes, vitamin C deficiency and use of drugs such as phenytoin are underlying causes. In general, mucosal barrier will be more likely to cause delayed eruption of permanent rather than the deciduous teeth.[430]

- *Hyperdontia.* In hyperdontia, the eruption of the regular teeth may be delayed (Chapter 1). *Odon-tomes,*[163] tumours and morphological aberrations such as double teeth occasionally delay the eruption of deciduous teeth, and this may be the first sign of the underlying abnormality.[430]

- *Prematurely born children.* Low birthweight is related to eruption delay of the deciduous teeth,[404][405] and the permanent dentition lags 3 months behind. However, the differences between these children and children born at term are negated when age adjustments are made for prematurity: that is, 6-month-old children born 2 months too early must be compared with chil-dren aged 4 months.[406] Subsequently, there are no differences in between the groups in "teething" or maturation of the permanent teeth.[24] Eruption seems delayed until 18 months after birth. Thereafter, during infancy, catch-up is observed. By age 9 the delay has been compensated.[405][406] Significantly accelerated erup-tion of permanent incisors and first molars is possible in the prematurely born due to the influence of catch-up growth and related factors.[165]

General factors

- *Dietary deficiencies, inclusive hypovitaminoses.* Nutri-tional influences on eruption are minor compared with other factors, but extreme nutritional deprivation and intra-uterine growth retardation markedly delay the general development of teeth and eruption.[3][64][127][381][399][430] Vitamin C deficiency causes scurvy, a "gingivitis" that results in premature shedding of the deciduous teeth. Insufficient vitamin D causes retardation;[379] dietary intake of minerals or vitamin D in very young children does not affect the maturation of the decidu-ous dentition.[24]

- *Endocrine disorders.* Growth retardation in familial *hypoparathyroidism,*[146][347] *cretinism* (hypothyroidism in infancy) and *hypopituitarism* is associated with retarded dental development, and that of the skeleton lags even further behind; (over)treatment also has an impact.[148][296] Due to absence of functional "type 1 par-athyroid hormone related protein" and its receptor during tooth development, the whole tooth becomes enclosed within a bony crypt because of lack of bone resorption around the tooth crowns, and non-eruption.[489]

- *Heredity.* The deciduous and permanent dentition emerged late in siblings in one family despite normally developed teeth. The family reported the condition in previous generations.[379] *Ethnicity* also has an impact on the eruption times.[345]

- *HIV.* Paediatric human immunodeficiency virus (HIV) infection is accompanied with eruption delay. The mean number of erupted deciduous teeth is normal up to the age of 2, but it then plateaus and thereafter decreases in both dentitions depending on the clinical symptoms of the disease.[374] In one study, the severity of clinical symptoms but not that of T-lymphocyte depletion appeared strongly associated with a retarded eruption in children aged 5 months to 13 years.[175]

- *Hypophosphataemia.* Eruption is possibly delayed, but deciduous teeth also exfoliate early, at the age of 18–28 months,[168] because of rapidly destructive periodontitis.[503] At what age the permanent teeth erupt in these cases has not been reported.

- *Hypophosphatasia.* In this condition, the paediatric skeleton fails to mineralise properly and the eruption of the deciduous teeth is delayed.[262] It is a rare (1:1 000 000, an underestimation), autosomal recessive and dominant metabolic disorder with alkaline phosphatase deficiency, reduced phosphatase activity in the cells and increased urinary excretion of phospho-ethanolamine. Deposition of bone following resorption is defective. Phosphate ions precipitate on the tooth roots due to supersaturation.[32] Alkaline phosphatase protein may be abnormal.[187] The (anterior) deciduous teeth shed very prematurely, with or without root resorption following resorption of the alveolar bone and gingival recession. The permanent teeth may also be lost early. In neonatal hypophosphatasia, the cementum is hypoplastic or aplastic in young children, if they survive to this age.[52 58 66 168 187 243 257 319] In one family, children with exfoliation of the deciduous incisors and canines as early as at 1.5 years of age had symptoms of hypophosphatasia, but localised prepubertal periodontitis could not be ruled out.[22] Some children reported to have prematurely lost part of the deciduous dentition had normal dentitions 15 years later,[243] with large pulp cavities and possibly hypocalcified enamel;[58 262] in one report the enamel was reported to be black.[262] When the disorder manifests after infancy, the first symptom is loss of the teeth, followed later by bone fractures.[52] The roots of the lost teeth are resorbed.[126] In patients requiring extractions in the deciduous dentition, a more conventional approach could be attempted.[285] Adults with the disorder may be either asymptomatic or have osteomalacia, like in vitamin D deficiency, with soft bones due to impaired mineralisation. Collagen fibres may not attach to the defective cementum,[66] but more recently, cementum resorption has been considered responsible for the early exfoliation. The timing of onset and the length of time the disorder remains untreated determine whether a patient has generalised or local juvenile periodontitis.[52] Any permanent tooth root resorption may be caused by factors other than hypoposphatasia.[320]

- *(Benign/malign) osteopetrosis.* This inherited bone sclerosis condition, *marble disease,* is characterized by concentric areas of very dense bone, in particular in the hands, because of reduced resorption. Odontome-like tooth masses are formed. The eruption of the deciduous dentition is delayed, with ankylosis. Malformed teeth, enamel hypoplasia and hypomineralisation, and disturbances in dentinogenesis are other features.[115 191 339 434 496 505] In osteopetrotic rats, the teeth were gradually replaced with bone.[340] In mice with osteopetrosis the bone around the teeth was not resorbed, which prevented them from erupting with development of short, dilacerated roots.[434] Tooth germs of the mice in the early stage of mineralisation explanted in a culture medium without bone developed normally; tooth germs explanted with bone were cervically invaded by the alveolar bone. The abnormal development of teeth is therefore secondary to the congenital lack of bone remodelling. Osteoclastic differentiation fails owing to the absence of the "functional macrophage colony-forming factor" (M-CSF) in the dental follicle.[190] The invasion of the tooth germs by bony trabeculae divides them into odontomes.[191] After daily administration of M-CSF to adult mice, pre-osteoclasts fused together to transform into osteoclasts.[460]

- *Maternal rubella, cerebral palsy, hypoxia.* The 15-month-old children of mothers who had rubella during pregnancy were found to have on average 1.3 fewer erupted teeth than controls.[258] In another study, in children with cerebral palsy, more deciduous and permanent teeth remained unerupted compared with controls. The first permanent molar erupted significantly late.[350] Other conditions at birth such as hypoxia, anaemia and renal failure are associated with delayed eruption.[430]

- *Syndromes.* Syndromes such as trisomy 21 and Prader–Labhart–Willi are associated with delayed eruption. An 11-year old patient with *cleidocranial dysplasia* had almost no erupted permanent teeth. Unerupted supernumerary molars were present. Like in hypophosphatasia, alkaline phosphatase activity was below normal and urinary phospho-ethanolamine levels were elevated,[461] but the disturbances in eruption were attributed to another mechanism (see Chapter 11).

- *Idiopathic delayed eruption.* Teeth may develop slowly and erupt late for unknown reasons. One such patient had a sister with Down's syndrome.[44]

Table 4.3 The number of days (mean (SD) and range) between shedding of the deciduous teeth and the eruption of the successors[312]

	Mandible			Maxilla		
	Mean	SD	Range[a]	Mean	SD	Range[a]
Central incisor	14	28	−51–188	42	70	−48–329
Lateral incisor	44	61	−21–221	133	173	−5–852
First molar	43	66	−29–1022	139	139	−48–955
Canine	6	12	−29–73	6	15	−58–41
Second molar	5	8	0–16	0	6	−34–12

[a]The first figure in the range is negative because successors sometimes erupt prior to the exfoliation of the deciduous teeth.

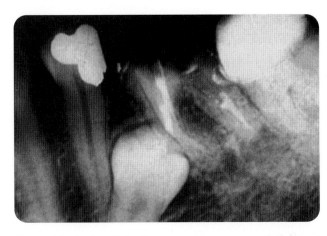

Figure 4.2 The distally inclined second premolar could not erupt because of mesial movement and tipping of the (maltreated) first molar following extraction of the primary second molar at a young age.

Permanent dentition

The general causes of delayed eruption of the deciduous teeth also apply to the permanent dentition. Table 4.3 shows the mean times between the exfoliation of the deciduous teeth and the eruption of the successors.[312] In this regard, sexual dimorphism is absent.[309 312]

Local factors

- *Ankylosis*. In the (local) absence of the periodontal ligament, the deciduous tooth is retained, which delays the eruption of its successor. Partially failed resorption of the deciduous molar roots is due to alteration in the direction of eruption of maxillary premolars and small crowns of the mandibular second premolars; the retained deciduous molars prevent the eruption of the succedaneous teeth.[362]
- *Root dilaceration and extremely curved roots* may retard eruption of the pertinent teeth. Delayed eruption of dilacerated maxillary incisors has been treated successfully with surgical exposure or repositioning.[81 247 453 458] Third mandibular molar tooth germs start to develop in the ramus of the mandible, the occlusal surface facing mesially. The impacted tooth descends below the occlusal plane and rises gradually.[383 433] The root growth continues while the tooth does not erupt or erupts ectopically and the roots may therefore become curved. Erupted mandibular third molars may show root curvatures of up to 90°.
- *Fusion/partial schizodontia, concrescence*. Double teeth may erupt late or not at all.[193] Concrescence of the second and third maxillary molars prevents eruption of the third molar.
- In *hyperdontia and odontomes*, the eruption of the extra teeth or their neighbours is frequently delayed or completely prevented. In reports of supernumerary

teeth in the anterior maxilla, one-quarter showed eruption delay,[258 279 422 442] but many more mesiodentes are permanently unerupted. Odontomes, which are likely to present in particular in the premaxilla,[322] that is compound ones,[317] may delay the eruption of adjacent teeth.[397] After removal of an odontome, a mandibular first molar is reported to have erupted.[203]

- *Pericoronal hamartomas* are embryonic disturbances in which the organ components develop in abnormal proportions. Odontogenic tumours, such as ameloblastic fibro-odontoma,[341] within the opercula (the loose flaps of gingiva overlying the crowns) of first and second permanent molars delayed their eruption.[495]
- *Prematurely lost deciduous teeth*. A consequence of early loss of deciduous teeth is often delayed eruption of the permanent successors (Figure 4.2) and malalignment after eruption.[15] If the primary tooth is lost *long* before its exfoliation time, before half of the root of the permanent successor has developed,[425] the eruption of the successor is delayed.[15 93 253 351] Extraction of deciduous molars at 7 years resulted slightly more often in accelerated than delayed emergence of the permanent teeth and at 9 years in accelerated eruption.[351] Scar tissue impedes the eruption mechanically[132] but according to one study there is little evidence of changes in the connective tissue and thick, fibrous gingiva.[430] The reported eruption of a permanent mandibular canine at the age of 5 years, with a genetically absent deciduous canine, may have been associated with the absence of scar tissue.[456] Gross dental decay and premature extraction of the deciduous molars permits the first permanent molars to move into the premolar space,[178 307 357 389] leaving insufficient space for the eruption of those teeth. Figure 4.3 shows a premolar erupted lingually due to lack of space.

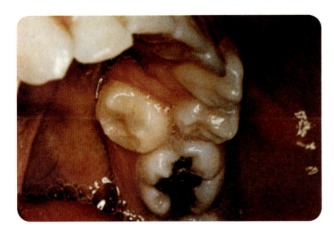

Figure 4.3 A palatally erupted second premolar.

- *Trauma to the deciduous teeth.* The rare damage to the dental follicle may preclude or delay eruption of permanent teeth.[224 287] The delay amounts to about 1 year.[15]
- *Ectopic or deep location of tooth germ.* When a developing tooth is located deep within the jaw or encounters a neighbouring tooth in its path of eruption because of incorrect orientation, it may fail to erupt. Rotated mandibular premolars may also show delayed eruption.[141]

General factors

- *Cystic fibrosis.* A delay in odontogenesis of 4–8 months has been reported in cystic fibrosis.[265]
- *Dentine dysplasia, amelogenesis imperfecta.* The first signs of dentine dysplasia may be spontaneous premature exfoliation of the teeth with defective roots, and delayed[204] eruption in both dentitions. In subtypes ID, IF, IG and IIA of hereditary amelogenesis imperfecta eruption is delayed. Early loss of deciduous and permanent teeth showing dentinal dysplasia (not the same as dentine dysplasia I and II) has been reported in patients with *Singleton–Meten syndrome* (which includes skeletal deformities, ligament rupture, short stature, osteoporosis).[168]
- *Diseases and systemic disorders.* One-third of a sample of children with chronic *renal failure* treated by haemodialysis showed delayed eruption, while two-thirds exhibited delayed bone maturity; half had enamel defects.[388] Renal failure has many causes.[86 400]
- In *hyperimmunoglobulin IgE (hyper-IgE) recurrent infection syndrome*, the deciduous teeth and the first permanent molars erupted normally, but most other teeth appear late. Bone resorption is enhanced, but that of the deciduous tooth roots fails. Once the deciduous teeth are extracted, the successors erupt.[314]

- *Endocrine disturbances. Hypothyroidism* affects the closure of the root apices and the eruption of teeth.[168] [182 216 252 446] In cretinism there is delayed dental maturation and deciduous teeth exfoliation and eruption of permanent teeth is delayed by more than a year. In *hypopituitarism*, skeletal development is delayed more than dental development.[296] In pituitary dwarfs, there is timely enamel development but root development is delayed. The deciduous teeth persist and the permanent teeth erupt late,[42 217] in particular the premolars, which have small crowns on roots of normal dimensions.[88] Teeth of animals without a pituitary gland did not reach the occlusal plane in a timely fashion and apical root closure was retarded.[27 220 452] Children with idiopathic short stature are similarly affected;[214] other dental abnormalities are microdontia and dental crowding with facial retrognathia.[214 415] In a sample of Belgian boys, *constitutionally delayed puberty* was related to a significant retarded dental development.[143] The teeth of patients with *(pseudo)hypoparathyroidism* have been reported to erupt late, with yellow, hypoplastic enamel,[200 386 391] although this feature is not consistent.[139] Progressive loss of cellular potential to specialise has been blamed for the disorder. Apically, osteodentine is formed.[429] A slight eruption delay of the permanent teeth is reported in *diabetes*, except for the molars.[144 273]
- *Fluorosis.* The eruption of the permanent teeth is delayed in regions with too much fluoride in drinking water.[475] Increase in fluoride levels decreases the number of active osteoclasts in the bone overlying the erupting teeth. Toxic effect on cell enzymes and secondary effects on calcium and phosphate metabolism are responsible.[251]
- *Hemifacial atrophy.* Localised scleroderma, a rare disease with chronic hardening and shrinking of the connective tissue, which leads to underdevelopment of part of the skin, muscles and jaws, and becoming manifest in the first and second decades of life, results in hemifacial atrophy. The roots of the teeth on the affected side do not develop and the crowns may be small with atypical morphology.[483]
- *Macrodontia.* The dental arch length must be large enough to accommodate the last erupting teeth: the maxillary permanent canines, mandibular second premolars and the wisdom teeth. In one 18-year-old, macrodont maxillary canines were still present within the jaw as were many other teeth of normal size,[176] which suggests the presence of another causative factor. The combined widths of the mandibular permanent incisors reliably indicate the size of the teeth in both arches, allowing the compilation of prediction tables.[241] In females, the size of the teeth can be used to predict whether the third molar will erupt or not. This may not be true in males (except the size of the maxillary second molar).[140]

- *Radiotherapy.* An eruption delay is reported with radiotherapy in children, attributed to poor root development.[179 481] Caries, which is exacerbated by the xerostomia caused by radiotherapy, has also been implicated (Chapter 5).[180] In contrast, radiotherapy in adolescents was found to accelerate eruption, besides causing microdontia, rhizomicry and accelerated mineralisation.[65 457 481]
- *Regional odontodysplasia.* The poorly developed teeth in regional odontodysplasia do not erupt or erupt late;[162] this is called "focal delayed eruption".[95]
- *Segmental odontomaxillary dysplasia.* Delayed eruption of the maxillary premolars and first molar on the affected side has been reported.[31 112 118 324]
- *Syndromes.* Eruption delays are part of the features of Apert's syndrome and pyknodysostosis, in which defects in bone resorption may be causative, and in syndromes with multiple cysts or tumours that cause a generalised delay in eruption.[430] In microsomia I development, including that of the teeth, is retarded, progressively in a caudal (distal) direction.[133]
- *Idiopathic.* For unknown reasons none of the permanent teeth of a 27-year-old woman erupted.[196]

4.2.3 Prevention and treatment

It is essential to take a family and medical history in patients with disorders of eruption. Treatment of delayed eruption is not always possible and prevention, if possible, is commonly in the hands of the physicians or surgeons; for instance, control of hypothyroidism or tumour removal may prevent delays in eruption.

Suri *et al.* described three treatment options:[430]

1. Delay with defective tooth development. If severe, the teeth should be removed, unless a permanent tooth may need to serve as an abutment.
2. If a tooth's development and location in the jaw are normal, a wait and watch approach is indicated. When a local factor delays eruption of a permanent tooth, interventions such as removal of deciduous teeth, surgical exposure of the crown of the delayed tooth with or without orthodontic traction and eventual space creation may be tried. The consequences of hyperdontia and macrodontia may be alleviated surgically and with orthodontics. A space maintainer may be used to maintain the space created by premature loss of a deciduous tooth. Circumstances dictate the therapy when causes such as fusion and concrescence affect eruption.
3. When systemic disorders are associated with generalised delayed eruption, a variety of possible management options have been suggested, ranging from no treatment, elimination of obstacles to eruption, exposure and traction, to autotransplantation.

4.2.4 Retained and impacted teeth (retentio dentis)

Retention or *impaction* is the persistent absence of emergence of a tooth. A retained tooth has a normal path of eruption while an impacted tooth has an abnormal path of eruption (with evidence of a physical barrier in the eruption path). Here, the terms are used interchangeably. Systemic factors, syndromes, genetic disposition, and local factors such as inadequate arch space, a deeply situated or misdirected tooth germ, regional odontodysplasia underlie retention. In view of the sequence of eruption, the third molars, maxillary canines and mandibular second premolars are the main candidates for retention if insufficient space is available. (Multiple) retention occurs in hyperdontia.[490]

Deciduous dentition

Retained deciduous teeth are exceptional, and in particular, the second deciduous molars are involved.[14 99 321] Odontomes, odontogenic tumours, traumatic injury, myxofibromatous hyperplasia, dentigerous cysts, inverted position or ectopic location and other unknown causes are associated with the condition both in the anterior and in the posterior region.[17 23 59 99 162 238 321 462 493] Multiple retention of deciduous molars with fully developed roots is an inherited anomaly.[379 380] With regard to prevalence, in one radiographic study, three retained deciduous teeth were observed in 30 000 panoramic radiographs.[38] A normal course of eruption may follow surgical exposure of the teeth.[55] Retained deciduous teeth may be associated with defective development and eruption of the successors.[321]

Permanent dentition

In Thilander *et al.*'s study, about 5% of children showed retention: 41% were maxillary canines, 27% were maxillary second premolars, 23% were mandibular second premolars and 9% were other maxillary anterior teeth.[448] Similar prevalence rates were reported in a sample of university students.[94] A cumulative percentage of 18% has been found too.[222] In other studies, two-thirds to 98% of adolescents showed impaction,[157 291] mainly of the third molars, with a preference for the maxilla. The second most often retained tooth was the maxillary canine,[157] followed by the mandibular second premolar.

Third molars

Reviews quote not only large but also greatly varying prevalence rates of retained wisdom teeth,[16 277] with a predilection either for the maxilla[94 172 222 277] or the mandible.[6 85 188 366 373] Retention of wisdom teeth has been found to be more common in women than men[277 366] but some studies did not find a sex predilection.[161 172 222] The age of the subjects included in a study affects the reported

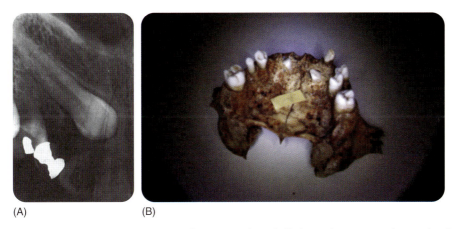

(A)   (B)

Figure 4.4 (A) Palatally situated canine. (B) This jaw bone from an ancient skull shows the upper canines to be situated in the palatal vault. Note the conical tooth in the place of the second premolar; it is either a paramolar or microdont premolar.

prevalence, because many third molars do not erupt before the age of 17–21-years. In one sample of Hong Kong Chinese aged 17–89 years, 28% showed impacted third molars.[85] Two-thirds of subjects had at least one and a quarter had up to four retained wisdom teeth.[291]

Retained wisdom teeth may move into an upright position with time,[383 433] and erupt: some 10–30% retained at age 18–20 years had erupted by 26 years,[225 470 473] but higher percentages at somewhat higher ages have also been reported.[506] After the age of 20 years, sagittally (the majority mesio-angularly)[85 366] oriented wisdom teeth in particular are still tilted distally.[407] Mesially inclined wisdom teeth often change to 0° inclination and erupt if the initial angle did not exceed 25°.[173] Mollaoglu et al. found that the retromolar space in cases with impacted third molars was smaller and the teeth showed a greater angulation than erupted teeth.[286] After the age of 25, retained third molars are unlikely to erupt in a functional position,[145] although 10% may erupt to reach the occlusal plane.[507] They may erupt in older adults, following recession of gingival tissue behind the second molar,[145] or after extraction of the adjacent tooth.

Are retention data from the past still valid today? According to the literature, around 1950, 20% of the third mandibular molars were partially erupted versus 30% in 1990. The prevalence figures for fully erupted wisdom teeth fell by 10% in the same period. Decreased wear of the interdental contacts through dietary changes (Chapter 8) has led to reduction of arch space,[261 315 373 403] to the disadvantage of the third molars. Moreover, over time, the human jaws may have reduced in size.[419] The mineralisation of retained third molars is less advanced than that of fully erupted wisdom teeth, especially in women.[432]

Maxillary canines
The maxillary permanent canines are 20 times more likely to be retained than the mandibular canines. The eruption path of these teeth is the longest and they are often the last to replace their predecessors, but the eruption sequence is said to be changing.[478] The distance between bilaterally impacted canines is smaller than in controls,[275] but insufficient space may not be the reason for retention.[480] Obstacles in the path of eruption may force the canine to erupt palatally instead of labially.

The prevalence of canine retention is 0.8–3%. Retained canines are twice as common in females than in males, and occur more frequently on the left side than the right side.[6 30 94 185 354 423 448] In Europeans and Americans, canine retention is twice as often encountered palatally than in a transverse orientation to the lateral incisor or labially (Figure 4.4),[275] but among Asians the ratio is reversed.[192]

Agenesis or underdevelopment of the lateral incisor seemingly encourages the condition:[30 336] guidance of the canine's eruption by the lateral incisor might be important.[30 242] Approximately 1:10 people will have a palatally displaced canine if the lateral incisor is small or peg-shaped and 1:20 if the lateral is missing.[62] The impacted canine belongs to the spectrum of dental abnormalities related to hypodontia.[344] However, the occurrence in mainly Europeans may be genetically linked,[48 197 336 480 500] rather than because of lack of eruption guidance due to an anomalous or missing lateral incisor.[197] The male to female ratio, population differences and bilateral occurrence (10%) point to a hereditary cause.[336] Others suggested causes are trauma, presence of a cyst or neoplasm and ankylosis.[192]

Second mandibular premolars
Mesial tilting of mandibular first molars[184] after extraction of the deciduous second molars, lack of space or deep location in the jaw[85] are causes of retained mandibular second premolars. Occasionally, the apex of a retained premolar is directed toward the oral cavity.[226] In a sample of Hong Kong Chinese, 0.2% mandibular second premolars were impacted.[85]

Maxillary incisors

Local factors such as supernumerary teeth, odontomes, trauma and dilaceration are the principal causes of retained maxillary permanent incisors, and which may affect the position of the ipsilateral lateral incisor and canine.[79] The canines are relatively more often displaced, many in the mesio-labial direction and overlapping the lateral incisor (*pseudo-transposition*, see Section 4.3.3). The apex of the lateral incisor may be displaced some 5 mm distally and become an obstacle in the path of eruption of the canine. Retention of a maxillary central incisor has been reported to follow the eruption of an odontome.[11] Impacted maxillary incisors must be exposed surgically and most will need orthodontic alignment; it may take 3 years before they reach the occlusal level.[29]

Other teeth

Teeth other than those mentioned above are rarely impacted, including the mandibular canines;[48 436] causes include odontomes[436] and endodontic treatment of a deciduous predecessor.[437] Second molars may be impacted owing to a mesial inclination, because of which they get trapped under the distal surface of the first molar.[361] The orientation and position of third molars may lead to retention of the second molars (Figure 4.5).[43 377] Mandibular first molar retention has also been reported.[417] A deeply located, retained mandibular first molar with an upward-curving distal root erupted after exposure.[213] Another report featured retention of both a mandibular lateral incisor and canine in one quadrant,[26] and a primary molar.[454]

Multiple retention

Idiopathic retention of the six mandibular anterior teeth with persisting deciduous predecessors has been reported.[142] Systemic causes of retention are malnutrition, congenital syphilis, tuberculosis, osteopetrosis, and pseu-doparahypothyroidism, and a few subtypes[398] of hypoplastic amelogenesis imperfecta.

Two brothers with multiple retention in the permanent dentition and persisting deciduous teeth showed all the characteristics of amelogenesis imperfecta and dentine dysplasia, but the anomalies were absent in other family members.[484] Multiple retention of different teeth, in three generations of one family, without any symptoms of a general disorder pointed to inheritance as a cause. The third and fourth generations showed infra-occlusion of several teeth.[365] In cleidocranial dysplasia, progeria (syndromic accelerated ageing) and achondroplasia multiple teeth are retained.

Consequences of retention

Teeth may erupt in spite of incorrect orientation, as is the case with a substantial number of third molars. Growth of the jaws or extraction of a nearby tooth also enables retained teeth to erupt. An inverted second premolar erupted after the extraction of its neighbouring teeth.[289]

Most patients do not exhibit symptoms other than persisting deciduous teeth, usually the mandibular second molar and maxillary canine. However, the pressure from a retained tooth on the root of a neighbour tooth may initiate resorption, which may be painful.[451]

Mandibular wisdom teeth

In one sample of patients older than 23 years, about 5% of retained mandibular wisdom teeth caused pain or infection (2%)[492] and about 15 showed some pathological changes, which were often innocuous.[5] Retained teeth may resorb and one-quarter of retained third molars are responsible for resorption of the distal root of the neighbouring second molar.[301] Other complications include follicular cysts (4%), loss of bone distal to the second molar,[125] displacement of other teeth and neuralgic pain. The reduced thickness of the jaw bone due to the impacted teeth increases the risk of fracture from blows or punches (contact sports).[125 274] The above rates are high compared with the 3% of resorbing second molars and 0.8% cysts found in almost 11 600 patients.[424] To correctly diagnose resorption of adjacent teeth, a computed tomography (CT) scan is needed.[223] Evidence for the view that retained and erupting third molars promote (tertiary) crowding of the anterior teeth is scant.[467] Retention itself could be the consequence of crowding.

Prevention and treatment

Third molars

One-quarter of Norwegian dentists undertake prophylactic removal of retained third molars,[94] often on the request of the patient,[37] but dentists and oral surgeons disagree with regard to the need to extract those without symptoms.[218 419 508] Surgical removal may have complications[82]

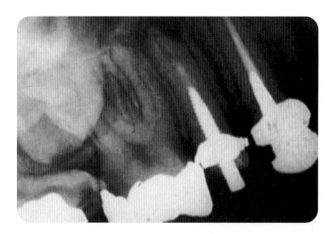

Figure 4.5 A third molar (partly visible) inhibiting the eruption of the second molar.

and leaving them *in situ* may lead to development of secondary pathology. Treatment may be unnecessary when secondary pathology is absent. But removal of third molars at older ages increases the risk of complications,[83] [105] which encourages removal in young adults,[83 492] all the more since older patients may also have comorbid medical problems that increase the risk of complications.

Prophylactic removal of retained wisdom teeth introduces the risk of damage to the mandibular canal (risk >0.5%),[428] antral perforation if the teeth are situated high in the maxilla, and damage to the second molars. The reported rates of complications are in the range of 5–10%.[47 61 261] Disturbed wound healing, alveolitis and decreased sensation are the most frequently encountered problems after surgical removal of the mandibular third molars.[401] Therefore it is desirable to be able to predict whether a third molar will remain impacted, which depends on the retention type.[469] The probability that a mandibular third molar will erupt is 0.72 if the distance between a line passing through the distal surface of the third molar and a perpendicular to the line passing through the tip of the cusps of the first and second molars and extending to the ramus exceeds 14.5 mm and it is 1.00 if it exceeds 16.5 mm.[471]

Retained third molars are common in clinically edentulous individuals.[5] These teeth may erupt after extraction of the second molars, migrate into the extraction spaces, and may become aligned rather well, notwithstanding a previously tipped position.[384] Third molars can be used as abutments after loss of the second molar.[419]

Permanent canines

If the canines are retained, they may remain impacted in edentulous people.[491] Canines retained in the palate rarely erupt spontaneously,[447] unless the deciduous canine is extracted at age 10 years or before, as long as sufficient space is available.[197 275 353] The tooth may be situated far to mesial, above the permanent lateral incisor,[353] or far to distal. Denudation of the maxillary canine crown may be followed by eruption, and if not, it often enables orthodontic extrusion.[134] Lack of space prevents successful alignment of the tooth.[499] Orthodontic extrusion following crown exposure is debated because a second surgical intervention is often unavoidable.[331] Surgery introduces the risk of root resorption and damage to the periodontal ligament,[209] but the risk may be (almost) absent in appropriately selected cases and with careful treatment.[276]

Labial impaction is due to inadequate arch space.[198] A labially retained canine may not be palpable at age 9 years due to late odontogenesis, yet it may erupt normally without early extraction of the deciduous canine.[129] Active management of retained canines may be required at a later age due to mobility/exfoliation (40%) of the deciduous canine, resorption of a neighbour tooth (25%) or other pathological conditions (33%).[305]

Before root completion, transplantation of a maxillary canine into its proper place is possible. Alternatively, the bone around the tooth may be removed and the tooth shifted within the enlarged alveolus into its correct position (transalveolar transplantation).[395]

Mandibular second molars

When tilted mesially, the tooth may be forced into an upright position after removal of the distal bone (and third molars).[361]

4.2.5 *Partially erupted teeth* (dentitio difficilis)

Partially erupted teeth that remain in that position because of a physical barrier (*dentitio difficilis*),may be partially covered with gingiva (operculum). All teeth undergo a transient phase of partial eruption. But some teeth, usually the mandibular third molars, with a deflected eruption path or due to insufficient space, remain partly erupted. A distally directed path of eruption increases the risk of partial eruption.[472]

Consequences of partial eruption

Collection of food debris under the operculum of the mandibular third molars leads to pericoronitis with trismus, swelling and pain, in particular in adolescents and young adults.[304] Professional irrigation of the space under the operculum with hydrogen peroxide is recommended for treating the infection, which, however, may recur.

Among a sample of partially erupted third molars, 15% of maxillary and 37% of mandibular were associated with a cyst;[94] but lower rates have also been reported.[291] A long-lasting chronic infection or (enlargement of a) cyst creates deep infra-bony pockets, in particular distal to the second molar.[261] Other sequelae include resorption of (the distal root of) the second molar. Caries was observed in a fully impacted tooth, supposedly caused by a transient exposure to the oral environment after extraction of a neighbouring tooth.[21] The risk of developing caries is greatest in mesially inclined, partially erupted mandibular third molars.[364]

Surgical removal might be required because of recurring pericoronitis. Orthodontic movement (eventually with a post in the root canal) of third molars prevents periodontal damage to the second molars and minimises the risk of damaging the inferior alveolar nerve.[183]

4.2.6 *Infra-occlusion*

Infra-occlusion refers to the permanently arrested eruption of a tooth once it has emerged. It is caused by ankylosis, and the tooth remains in a position below the occlusal plane of the adjacent teeth, which continue to erupt. In ankylosis, the root may not always be replaced by bone, even when a sharp and solid percussion sound is suggestive of it.[371] In such cases, radiography cannot confirm ankylosis and histological examination is required.[96 371] Osteoid tissue is found in the furcation area and the inner side of the roots of most deciduous molars in infra-occlusion with a successor,[181 233 371] but it is found apically when the successor is absent.[221] The anomaly is also called *secondary retention/impaction*.[369]

Occasionally, failure of the eruptive mechanism (unilaterally) occurs in the absence of ankylosis; this is called *primary (or idiopathic) failure of eruption*, and is partly familial.[360 365 380 408 509 510] Characteristic features are: enlarged dental follicles and crypts of the concomitantly affected deciduous and permanent molars.[360] Upon surgical exposure, the unerupted molar can be moved freely within the crypt.[35]

Ankylosis may commence at any time during eruption. Occlusal wear facets provide evidence of previous occlusal contacts.[96] The degree of infra-occlusion depends on the time at which ankylosis develops: the earlier it does, the more severe is the infra-occlusion. Infra-occlusion is classified as follows: slight (the occlusal surface is approximately 1 mm below the occlusal plane), moderate (level with the interdental contact points); and severe (level with or below the interproximal gingiva).[61 443] Almost two-thirds of ankylosed deciduous molars showed slight and almost 10% severe infra-occlusion.[61]

Aetiology and clinical features

During root resorption of deciduous teeth, periods of rest and deposition of bone are normally interspersed; excessive bone deposition may cause infra-occlusion.[181] Trauma, local metabolic disturbances, premature or ectopic eruption of an adjacent maxillary permanent first molar, facial morphology, abnormal tongue pressure, local infection or a deficient eruptive force with degenerative changes in the periodontal ligament are inconsistently present in cases with infra-occlusion and are unlikely causes, as is insufficient arch space.[41 61 181 234 276 371 375 443] Intrinsic factors (genetics) seem possible.[443] Affected children are more likely than controls to present with at least one other dental anomaly, notably cleft lip/palate.[511] In one family, infra-occlusion of deciduous teeth was present in 44% of siblings. Bilateral and familial deciduous molars in infra-occlusion (Figure 4.6) suggest an autosomal dominant and a recessive trait. In some monozygotic twins all second and third molars were found to be involved.[48 60 61 114 179 228 318 368 370 387 474 485] In one sample, infra-occluded deciduous teeth in two-thirds of the cases were associated with taurodont succedaneous teeth.[485] A genetic association with mesiodens has been suggested.[18] In dentitions with infra-occlusion, progressively additional teeth are likely to become involved.[61] Deciduous molar involvement is associated with infra-occlusion in one-third of the related permanent dentitions.[371 372]

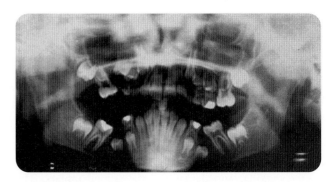

Figure 4.6 Infra-occlusion of deciduous second molars.

The alveolar bone around the affected tooth is underdeveloped.[232] The adjacent teeth tend to tilt towards the infra-occluded tooth,[235 477] causing food impaction and inhibiting continued formation of the succedaneous tooth root.[270] The local gingiva may grow over the infra-occluded tooth and the antagonists overerupt. The pulps of the teeth may show degenerative changes.[233]

The alveolar bone is not always underdeveloped and may even grow, so that the tooth in infra-occlusion is situated below the level of the alveolar crest. Some "infra-bony submerged teeth" (*reinclusion*) had been previously restored.[36 466]

Epidemiology

The deciduous mandibular second molar is most frequently infra-occluded,[21 39 40 61 221 234 371] or perhaps it is the first molar (Figure 4.7)?[107 219 237 292 426] In young children the deciduous first molar is most often affected and in older children it is the deciduous second molar.[116 221 228] Infra-occlusion of the maxillary deciduous molars occurs less often[61 367] or at an equivalent rate to that in the mandible.[368] Severe infra-occlusion of second deciduous molars has been noted to occur equally often in both jaws.[367] Multiple submerged deciduous molars occur as frequent as singly occurring ones.[61] The age-dependent[221 227 234 426] reported prevalences of 0.5–27.5% ankylosed deciduous molars[228 237] seems more likely to be closer to 1.5%.[61]

In the permanent dentition, the first molar in particular shows infra-occlusion.[39 101] In some patients mandibular second molars remained retained, probably as a consequence of an infra-occluded first molar.[372] The frequency of ankylosed second molars is increasing.[131] Occasionally other teeth are infra-occluded, for example the mandibular canine.[294] Multiple infra-occluded permanent teeth are also reported.[51]

The succedaneous tooth

The successor of an infra-occluded deciduous tooth may be agenetic (15%), ectopic or in the normal location.[107 368]

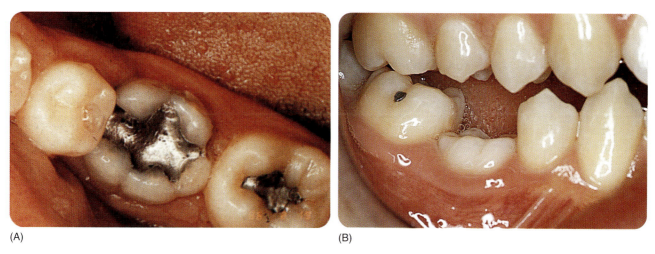

(A)   (B)

Figure 4.7 (A) Infra-occlusion of the first permanent molar. (B) Infra-occlusion of a deciduous molar, situated between two permanent teeth.

Agenetic succedaneous tooth The roots of the deciduous infra-occluded tooth are very slowly resorbed,[49 141 235] possibly initiated by erupting adjacent teeth.[268] Such resorption led to, over a 10-year period, to a 25% rate of loss of the retained deciduous teeth.[392] The degree of infra-occlusion increased on an average 0.5 mm/year, and less so in older children.[235] At ages 19–20 years, about half of the retained deciduous mandibular molars are infra-occluded by 0.5–4.5 mm.[47 49] Late onset of ankylosis with little resorption and mild infra-occlusion allows the deciduous tooth to function for many years.

Ectopic position of the succedaneous tooth Not every root of the persisting deciduous molar is resorbed. The successors may either or not erupt, erupt partially, or erupt outside the dental arches.[40]

Normally situated succedaneous teeth Ankylosis in these circumstances is not permanent.[117] The eruption of the succedaneous tooth is delays by about 6 months.[232 234] When a premolar replaces an infra-occluded deciduous molar, the underdeveloped alveolar bone recovers.[228 371 427] The premolar's root development may be delayed when the mandibular deciduous first molar is ankylosed.[299] The successor may erupt ectopically.[28 40]

Consequences As mentioned already, the consequences of infra-occlusion include delayed exfoliation with retarded eruption of the successor, tipping of adjacent teeth, overeruption of antagonists and malocclusion. The arch length on the affected side is slightly increased with deviation of the midline, the deciduous molars being larger than the premolars. Denudation of the root surface of adjacent teeth and caries in neighbour teeth may be observed.[443]

If the first molar is infra-occluded, the second and third molars will almost certainly be affected.[360] Extraction of an infra-occluded maxillary first molar, which was not ankylosed, resulted in migration of the maxillary second molar mesially and downwards.[365]

Prevention and treatment
Some advise extraction or, when this is not possible, surgical removal[369] of the infra-occluded tooth to prevent malocclusion, caries[299 477] and periodontal problems. Others have advocated dislodgement of the ankylosed teeth.[8] The removal of a severely submerged mandibular deciduous tooth may damage the inferior dental nerve and the developing adjacent teeth. The risk of surgery must be weighed against the benefits of removal, and the risks may often outweigh the benefits.[443] Extraction also has the risk that part of the root(s) may be left behind in the jaw.[228]

A panoramic radiograph in a patient showed a deciduous molar in severe infra-occlusion (together with a second premolar partly underneath the apex of the first permanent molar). Cross-sectional tomography demonstrated local structural weakness of the mandible, implying the risk of mandibular fracture during a complicated extraction. The path of the inferior mandibular nerve was unclear because the canal lacked cortical bone. Magnetic resonance imaging showed the submerged tooth to be close to the neurovascular bundle. Once the patient was made aware of these problems, he declined treatment.[87]

Age at onset of ankylosis and at diagnosis, the rate of progression of the condition and the speed of root resorption determine how to manage the problem. Late diagnosis of rapidly progressive, early-onset infra-occlusion increases the risk of complications. If the premolar is present, normal eruption is aimed for, which demands early extraction when the adjacent tooth is tipping toward the infra-occluded tooth.[229] Extraction of ankylosed deciduous molars must be avoided until the first permanent molar erupts,[371] unless the infra-occlusion is causing tipping of the adjacent teeth or there is insufficient space for the premolars,[228 232] or orthodontic problems arise. When an infra-occluded deciduous molar is extracted at about 9.5 years and a space maintainer is fitted, the majority of the succedaneous teeth erupt spontaneously. Extraction at age 11.5 years is too late.[367] It is recommended that an ankylosed deciduous tooth with an ectopic successor is removed[229] and that it is removed at an early age when the successor is agenetic.

Composite build-up of a deciduous molar is desirable when the onset of the infra-occlusion is late and its progression and root resorption are slow.[123] As eruption of the adjacent teeth continues, a new build-up (or extraction) will become necessary,[371] which will prevent tipping of the adjacent teeth over a moderately submerged deciduous tooth[444] and may also stimulate resorption and exfoliation.[117]

An ankylosed permanent tooth cannot be extruded and dislodgement of the tooth does not or rarely results in re-commencement of eruption. A luxated and orthodontically extruded ankylosed maxillary lateral incisor became ankylosed again.[74] Crown lengthening with composite when ankylosis starts late[368] prevents tilting (and is easily redone to adjust for the ongoing eruption of the neighbouring teeth). Extraction is proposed if ankylosis commences before the growth spurt or when the infra-occlusion becomes worse. The locally arrested bone growth around the ankylosed tooth may be a reason to remove the tooth.[427] An osteotomy in which the ankylosed tooth along with the surrounding bone is repositioned in a vertical direction is an alternative.[282] Orthodontic extrusion of a tooth with "primary failure of eruption" will result in ankylosis.[360]

4.3   Anomalies of site of eruption

Deviations in the site of eruption may occur to a lesser (dystopia) or more (heterotopia) severe degree. Slightly displaced teeth are present in all dentitions. Cosmetic aspects influence the choice of whether to treat or not to treat trivial deviations. If deviations remain untreated, the chances of developing secondary pathology, e.g. caries and periodontal disease, are increased; even small deviations are to be considered at least as harmful.

4.3.1   Dystopia

Dystopia is a relatively small deviation in the site of eruption of a tooth, which may be redressed with simple

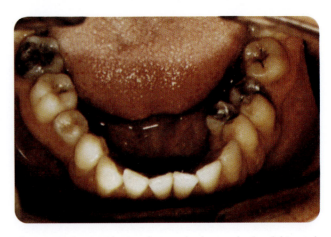

Figure 4.8 A rotated second premolar is seen in the right quadrant. In the left quadrant, two extra premolars have erupted lingually in a rotated position.

orthodontic treatment.[476] Insufficient space within the dentition is often the cause.

Rotation

The mandibular premolars, especially first premolars, are often slightly rotated (mean 13°).[280] Especially in females, the mandibular second premolar may show idiopathic rotation of 90° to mesial. A mesial diastema exists, the root apex is bent mesially, and eruption is delayed.[141] The larger size of the second deciduous molar leaves room for the smaller second premolar to rotate 90–180° (Figure 4.8). A relationship with space shortage is unlikely, although a genetic influence is possible.[345]

The maxillary incisors (2.3%) may be rotated 60° and even 180°.[236 448] The permanent maxillary first molar often erupts with a mesio-palatal rotation, thereby reducing the space available for the more anterior teeth.

Eruption site close to the dental arch

In a sample of 9–10-year-olds, the mandibular second premolars erupted next to the dental arch in about 1% of the time.[300] The maxillary permanent canines erupt palatal or labial to the dental arch in an ectopic position if there is a lack of space (Figure 4.9).[307] Extraction of a labially erupted canine is not indicated, unless root resorption or other pathology is present.[46] In almost 2% of maxillary canines, eruption is delayed or ectopic, in general in the palatal direction.[128 130] Other studies have found about 10% of 9–10-year-olds have incorrectly positioned maxillary canines.[128 300] Early treatment of an ectopic canine is recommended, because the eruptive movements may induce incisor root resorption.[128] Labial ectopic canines can be diagnosed early with X-rays and by palpating the buccal sulcus: normally the canine is palpable 18 months before its eruption, at 9–10 years of age.[229]

The maxillary permanent first molars may erupt mesially due to a combination of factors,[363] including (relative) macrodontia and an abnormal eruption path. The tooth becomes locked under the distal bulge of the deciduous second molar crown and induces early resorption of the distal root of that tooth,[231] while the other roots remain intact: the deciduous tooth thus remains *in situ*[149 498] (Figure 4.10). Consequences of this condition are periodontal abscess formation, tilting of the partially impacted first molar, and lack of space for the premolars and canine. Particularly predisposed are patients with cleft of the lip and palate,[40 75 97 375] osteogenesis imperfecta types III and IV,[313] and an underdeveloped midface (Crouzon's syndrome). The overall prevalence is 2–6%. Unless the deciduous second molar is lost prematurely, the teeth must be separated[149] or the deciduous tooth extracted early.[48 80 94 203 204 205 206 207 208 209 210 211 212 213 214 215 216 217 218 219 220 221 222 223 224 225 226 227 228 229 230 231 363 497] The variation in reported prevalences is partly due to differences in the ages of the children studied. No differences have been found between Caucasians and African Americans in the USA or between the sexes,[211] yet ectopic eruption of the maxillary first molar is perhaps genetic in origin, with greater penetrance in boys than girls.[230] A syndrome has been proposed because ectopic maxillary canines seem to be related to infra-occlusion of deciduous molars and agenetic premolars.[8 48]

There are two types of ectopic eruption of the first permanent molars.[47] One type is reversible: in two-thirds of the cases the tooth frees itself from its locked position and erupts into a normal position,[149 497] which warrants only observation. Self-correction may be possible between the ages of 6 and 7 years.[229] In children with clefts, self-correction occurs in a minority.[75] The other type is irreversible.[497] The tooth continues to erupt in a mesial direction, unless treated in a timely fashion by distalisation. Extraction of the deciduous second molar due to extreme resorption and impaction is indicated, eventually followed by transverse maxillary expansion. In milder cases, the teeth are separated with elastics, orthodontic bands, removable orthodontic appliances, brass separating wires (the least preferable)[158] or cervical headgear (by distalisation of the permanent first molars).[439] The lateral incisors are the most frequently ectopic teeth in the mandible.[98] Ectopic eruption of the permanent second molars occurs in 1.5% of the population.[512]

Diastema

Diastemata are common in the deciduous dentition, but not in the permanent dentition, unless there is

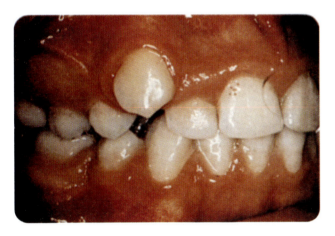

Figure 4.9 Ectopic permanent canine.

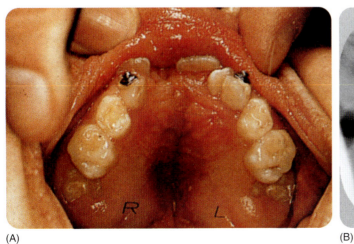

(A)

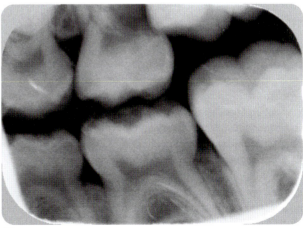

(B)

Figure 4.10 (A) Both maxillary permanent first molars have partly erupted in an ectopic (mesial) position. (B) Radiograph showing an ectopic first maxillary molar causing resorption of the deciduous second molar.

microdontia. In a small study, no relationship was found between hyperdontia and diastema,[135] but concomitant occurrence of diastemata and malpositions seem common (Chapter 1).

4.3.2 Heterotopia

Heterotopia is the eruption of a tooth far from its intended place, that is difficult or impossible to treat orthodontically. In general, a wrongly positioned tooth germ, lack of space, trauma, migration and possibly others still unknown causes are responsible.

Maxillary canines

Heterotopic maxillary canines erupt occasionally into the palate, but more often remain retained. Heterotopia may cause resorption of the root of another tooth, as do maxillary canines erupting in the lateral incisor region.[153]

Third molars

Third molars may be occasionally, unilaterally or bilaterally, located too far caudally, high up within the ascending ramus and even farther away,[4 25 69 70 84 206 277 431 435 455] or they may migrate into these areas.[50 337] The tooth germ may not move mesially from its original position in the inferior part of the ascending ramus.[206 383] Lack of space is not necessarily a prerequisite: a patient with severe hypodontia had third molars impacted in the coronoid process.[19] Impacted ectopic third molars may be associated with a dentigerous cyst.[69 70 435 455]

More extreme examples

Distal migration of impacted supplemental mandibular premolars high into the ascending ramus was followed radiographically.[254 431] Such migration may cause pain because of involvement of the mandibular nerve. The maxillary third molars have been reported to migrate to a horizontal position above the apices of the second and first molars. A third molar, an odontome[113] and other teeth have erupted in (the roof of) the maxillary sinus or into the nearby part of the nose.[124] Complications are dentigerous and follicular cysts, infection (sinusitis), obstruction pain and facial deformities.[227] One such lesion was initially interpreted as a malignant neoplasm.[122]

A primary mesiodens erupted palatally.[246] Other extra and regular teeth have erupted in the nose. Some 50 cases of intranasal teeth have been reported, one by the poet Goethe,[420] with or without unilateral nosebleeds.[12 76 152 278 283 298 465 485 488 494] A traumatically intruded deciduous molar was reported to have erupted in an inverted position into the nose.[390] Intranasal teeth may induce rhinorrhoea and speech problems. They are removed surgically, but may be loosely attached to the nasal mucosa.[159] Endoscopy is used to prevent comorbidity.[283] Radiographic evaluation is required at the minumum.[212 420]

Causes are infection, osteomyelitis of the maxilla and squamous cell carcinoma,[316] and cleft lip and palate.[159 212]

Figure 4.11A and B show heterotopy in eighteenth-century jaws and Figure 4.11C shows a tooth erupted in the nose. More extreme cases exist: when a patient tried to extract their own maxillary molar, it was displaced and thereafter migrated in the direction of the lateral pharyngeal space.[53] Extra teeth have been found in the pituitary gland[259] and a mesiodens in the soft facial tissues.[246] Twelve extra teeth were reported in the face and orbits in one patient.[106] Two incisor-like teeth erupted in the lower eyelid[345] and a third molar reportedly erupted behind the ear.[431] After an accident, a mandibular canine emerged on the underneath of the chin.[266] Lateral permanent incisors have been known to erupt in the place of mandibular deciduous first molar.[64]

4.3.3 Transposition (translocation)

Transposition (Table 4.4) refers to the situation in which the position of two teeth is interchanged. Transposition most frequently involves the maxillary canine and the first premolar, and this is labelled $Mx.C.P_1$; transposition involving the canine and second premolar is noted as $Mx.C.P_2$[103 333] and that involving the canine and lateral incisor as $Mx.C.I_2$.[102 263] Other recorded transpositions are between the second premolar and first molar ($Mx.M_1.P_2$) and the central and lateral incisors ($Mx.I_1.I_2$).[333 394 414]

The prevalence is 0.25%[335] in India and Hungary it is reported to be 0.4%.[78 119] Bilateral $Mx.C.P_1$ transposition has also been reported.[334] Both a female[334 349] and a male predilection has been reported.[78] Mandibular transpositions are more rare.[78 248 333 393] Lower canines are known to have erupted in the place of the lateral incisor ($Mn.P_2.I_2$), which remained retained or erupted at the place of the second premolar.[248 378 448] The prevalence in the mandible is about 0.03%.[199 335] Transposition of the lower first and second molars, with the third molar developing between them, is as rare as a positional change between the upper second and third molars.[513] In the deciduous dentition, the $Mx.i_1.i_2$ transposition has been described; the teeth were "fused".[120] Palatally displaced maxillary canines and transpositions are associated with tooth agenesis (Table 4.5).

Table 4.4 Transpositions (N = 201) in the maxilla[333]

Transposed teeth	Unilateral	Bilateral
	N (%)	N (%)
C and P_1 ($Mx.C.P_1$)	143 (71)	38 (19)
C and I_2 ($Mx.C.I_2$)	40 (20)	2 (1)
C and M_1 ($Mx.C.M_1$)	8 (4)	–
C and I_1 ($Mx.C.I_1$)	4 (2)	2 (1)
I_2 and I_1 ($Mx.I_2.I_1$)	6 (3)	2 (1)

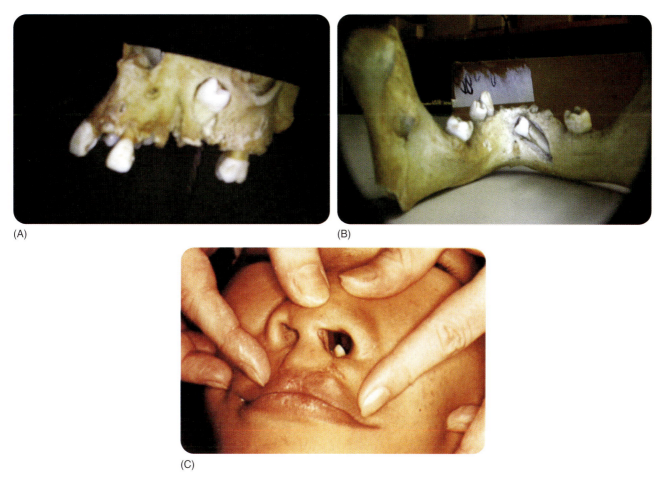

Figure 4.11 (A) Heterotopy: inverted upper premolar in the upper jaw of an ancient skull. (B) Heterotopic premolar in an ancient mandible. (C) Heterotopy: tooth erupted into the nasal cavity.

Table 4.5 Palatally displaced maxillary canines (PDC), mandibular transposition of lateral incisors and the canines (Mn.I$_2$.C) and maxillary transposition of the canines and first premolars (Mx.C.P$_1$) occurring concomitantly with tooth agenesis[335]

	Agenesis of:	Maxillary lateral incisors	Mandibular second premolars	Third molars (maxillary and mandibular)
	n			
PDC	58	3%	14%[a]	40%[a]
Mn.I$_2$.C transposition	60	2%	8%[a]	37%[a]
Mx.C.P$_1$ transposition	43	26%[a]	12%[a]	19%
PDC + Mn.I$_2$.C transposition	4	–	–	50%[b]

[a]There is a significantly higher frequency of displacement or transposition of the canine when other teeth are agenetic.
[b]Sample was too small.

Mn.I$_2$.C is associated with agenesis of the third molars, Mx.C.P$_2$ with agenetic lateral maxillary incisors in patients with clefts,[378] and canine displacements with agenesis of mandibular second premolars.[334 335] Mx.C.P$_1$ is often observed with peg-shaped or agenetic lateral incisors (also in Down's syndrome)[78 410 438] and with hyperdontia.[334 349] Mx.C.P$_1$ may be a polygenic trait, and other transpositions may have additional local causes (trauma).[333] A

preference for Mx.C.P$_1$ in Caucasians is mentioned.[34] A prevalence of 0.5% in some African samples[68] and 0.4% in India[78] suggests an ethnic influence. Many cases are isolated, but a (bilateral) familial occurrence is noted,[10 330 334 402] which supports the role of genetic influences within a multifactorial inheritance model.[334]

A canine–lateral incisor transposition after premature loss of the central incisor (Figure 4.12A) has been described

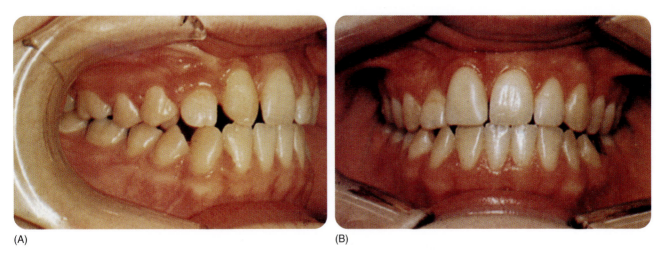

(A)   (B)

Figure 4.12 (A) Transposition of lateral incisor and canine. Note the absence of the central right incisor. (B) Dentition of the patient in (A) after curative treatment of the canine and orthodontics.

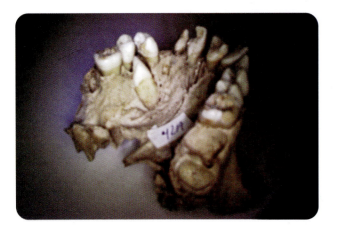

Figure 4.13 Transposition of an unerupted canine in the maxilla of an ancient skull.

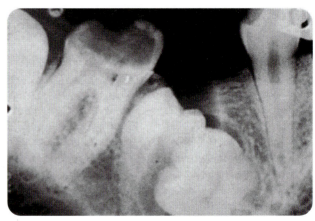

Figure 4.14 Transposition and retention of the second premolar and first molar.

a few times;[92] [150] treatment was restricted to placement of a crown on the canine (Figure 4.12B) after orthodontics. Figure 4.13 shows an eighteenth-century skull with an incomplete transposition of a maxillary canine into a site between the premolars. An uncommon combination of transposition and retention is shown in Figure 4.14, which is also reported for a maxillary first molar and second premolar, though with no retention.[329]

The anomaly is important mainly from the aesthetic point of view. Transposition is probably the consequence of migration of the developing tooth germs; the tooth erupting last is forced to follow a faulty eruption path.[263] [348] If Mn.I$_2$.C is detected at the age of 6–8 years, orthodontic repositioning of the mandibular lateral incisor into its correct place can be achieved.[413] When the condition is detected late, no attempts should be taken to correct

the position of the teeth, which holds true for maxillary transpositions as well.

Pseudo-transposition or incomplete transposition is described under maxillary incisor impaction earlier in the chapter.[412] The first premolar may show intraosseous migration, usually in a distal direction.[332] A mandibular third molar moved from a position underneath the roots of a mandibular second molar to a horizontal position beneath the roots of the mandibular first molar.[450]

4.3.4 Transmigration

Transmigration is a mesial migration of one half or more of the length of a permanent *canine* across the midline.[198] Persistence of the deciduous canine is a clinical sign; usually there are no other symptoms (Figure 4.15). Teeth

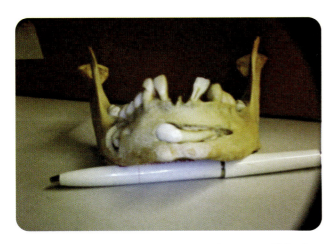

Figure 4.15 Transmigrating lower canine in the mandible of an ancient skull.

other than the mandibular canines have not been reported to transmigrate[409] but in 2003 the first case of a transmigrated maxillary canine was claimed to have been seen;[20] however, a search of the literature revealed that previously (1980) among 11 cases of canine transmigration, there were some maxillary ones.[411] A mandibular canine and its adjacent incisor were once reported to have transmigrated in a dentition with a supplemental premolar.[514] Bilaterally transmigration of mandibular canines with ectopic eruption has been reported.[7 13 142 198 201 295]

Transmigration is documented with serial radiographs.[89 154] The phenomenon implies that, if anaesthesia is needed for treatment, it must be given at the place of origin.[412 464] The transmigrated teeth are commonly (80–95%) retained in the bone,[198 202 295 332] underneath the apices of the contralateral incisors, premolars and first molars,[7 202 312 409] but they may emerge either in the midline between the central incisors or mesial or distal to the opposite canine.[295] The mesioangular inclination of the tooth determines whether transmigration (larger deflection) or transposition (smaller deflection) occurs. Trans-

migration patterns have been classified in five types, based upon the position in the bone, angulation and eruption of the teeth.[295]

Possibly some 100 cases, among them 15 in 4500 patients, have been described.[295 515 516] More females (80%) than males (20%) are affected and the left canine is most frequently (60 %) involved.[83 201 295 334] More recent data from 2011 found 90 transmigrant mandibular teeth in 87 persons out of a sample of 112 873, of which two were lateral incisors and three were premolars. The male:female ratio was 1:1.41.[518] The anomaly has been associated with a (follicular) cyst,[13] a horizontal eruption path,[202] and an odontome.[201 409] Transmigration is said to be "unhypothetical due to the presence of symphyseal cartilage",[208] and due to an "abnormal displacement of the tooth bud in embryonic life".[201]

4.3.5 *Prevention and treatment*

Orthodontic treatment combined with surgery, if needed, may prevent and correct dystopia, such as ectopically erupting permanent maxillary first molars.[156 167 468] Heterotopia requires surgery, if possible, though slight transmigration has been corrected with orthodontics.[479] A possible consequence of transposition is delayed shedding of the deciduous predecessors. If detected early, the removal of these deciduous teeth is desirable, followed by orthodontic correction of the obliquely located successors. When Mx.C.P$_1$ is detected early, prior to eruption, the cusp of the canine must be positioned superior to the root of the first premolar, which is then tipped distally, thus correcting the transposition.[54] The shapes of transposed canines may be altered to resemble an incisor by grinding of the cusp tip and use of composite to build up the crown.

In the absence of secondary problems in cases of heterotopia, treatment is often unnecessary and prevention is in most cases not possible. Transposition may be managed with orthodontic treatment in young patients.[517] Transmigrated teeth have been occasionally transplanted.

Section III
Post-eruption Hard Tissue Physiological Changes and Pathological Conditions

5

Caries

5.1 Introduction

Caries is a progressive, localised, destructive process in which:

- First, the mineral component of the dental hard tissues (enamel, exposed dentine and cementum) dissolves due to repeated disturbance of the equilibrium between the oral environment and the teeth, as a consequence of a localised decrease in pH because of microbial acid production in the presence of appropriate substrate (Section 5.3).
- Second, the organic component is destroyed. Unless the lesion becomes arrested, in time cavitation results.

If the 1–1.5 L of saliva produced daily (pH ~7) was not supersaturated in calcium, phosphates, carbonate and OH^-, the main constituent of the hard dental tissues, hydroxyapatite $(Ca_{10}[PO_4]_6OH_2)$, would dissolve gradually.

The tooth crowns are covered with *plaque*, a slimy biofilm that harbours bacteria within numerous micro-environments.[14] Some bacteria produce acids from the substrates present in the plaque, but the buffering action of saliva prevents a pH drop, until the acid production becomes excessive. At a pH of about 5.5 the environment is undersaturated with respect to hydroxyapatite, which then dissolves. Once the available substrate is used up, acid production stops, salivary action neutralises the pH and remineralisation starts. Repeated periods of demineralisation during the longer periods required for remineralisation result in a net loss of minerals from the enamel, leading to formation of the carious lesion. Initially, such a carious lesion consists of widened intercrystalline spaces,[49] or "pores", which manifest clinically as a chalky, opaque *white spot*. Cavitation starts after numerous prolonged acidic attacks.

Chemists describe caries in terms of the relationships between pH and mineral solubility. Microbiologists stress the interactions

between bacteria and the food substrates. Psychologists and sociologists emphasize the role of the socio-economic status of patient/parent(s), dental anxiety,[217 335] use of snacks and educational level,[508] lifestyle,[160 259 510] long-lasting conflicts in infancy, and low self-control.[379]

The essential description of the carious process in this chapter is, unless otherwise indicated, based on material drawn from several books and reviews.[80 166 167 275 387 405 406 423 425 431 432 597 610 611 637]

Genetics and caries

Exogenous factors, such as fluoride, interfere with any genetic influences on caries. The frequent occurrence of caries obscures the contribution of genetics, which contributes to, among other factors, the morphology of the teeth.[249 423 586]

Studies on twins have revealed that the influence of genetics is smaller than that of the environment.[542] Such twin studies often have weaknesses, such as small sample sizes and absence of surface-specific caries rates.[95] Genetic screens of large populations have not been performed.[542]

The genetic make-up appeared decisive in animals:[294] a difference in the immune response to specific bacteria is assumed,[586] but the relationship between caries and immunity remains unclear.[148 311] Caries susceptibility of rats seems to be genetically co-determined.[503] Major host genes for susceptibility to caries may be located on chromosomes 1 and 2, and on 7 and 8 for caries resistance.[429] Proline-rich saliva, an inherited trait, promotes the adherence to the teeth of early colonising streptococci (but *not* of *Streptococcus mutans*) and *Actinomyces*. Salivary immunoglobulins, another inherited trait, are bactericidal. Differences in dermatoglyphic patterns in persons with and without caries may also point to a heritable influence.[36]

5.2 Bacteria in caries

5.2.1 Plaque development

Soon after polishing a tooth, a biofilm of negatively charged salivary glycoproteins, the *salivary pellicle*, is seen to adhere to the tooth. Salivary bacteria (~2.10^8/mL) are attracted towards this pellicle, and the sparse, reversible colonisation of the pellicle with a few species soon stabilises: microcolonies develop, which produce an interbacterial matrix that encloses other bacteria which do not have a capacity to adhere to the pellicle. The complexity of the plaque microbial population strongly depends on the salivary properties, crevicular fluid, mechanical factors, the substrate and other plaque-related factors (e.g. age of the plaque). It takes a few days for newly formed plaque to become cariogenic.

5.2.2   Composition of plaque

Already at birth, the mouth is colonised by bacteria. The oral epithelium is in a state of continuous replacement; thus, bacteria that need to adhere to stable surfaces to multiply (e.g. *S. mutans*) only colonise the oral cavity permanently after tooth eruption.[88] The then more complex plaque that forms contains bacteria associated with caries. Bacteria comprise 70% of plaque; the remainder 30% is composed of intercellular material derived chiefly from the bacteria, salivary proteins and epithelial cells, and also plaque fluid with calcium and phosphate, and, rarely, food remnants. The amount and rate of plaque formation varies between individuals due to differences in tooth brushing, sugar consumption, antimicrobial features of saliva, etc.

In experimental studies, germ-free animals fed on a cariogenic diet developed caries only after transfer of microflora from other animals. Long-term use of antibiotics or chemotherapeutic agents restricted the oral microflora and reduced the frequency of occurrence of carious lesions. Certain genera of oral bacteria can produce carious lesions *in vitro*. Huge numbers of *S. mutans*, *Streptococcus sobrinus*, some strains of *Streptococcus mitis*, *Streptococcus sanguis*, *Streptococcus milleri*, *Lactobacillus* and *Actinomyces* species have been isolated from *in vivo* carious lesions. Streptococci isolated from carious lesions were given the name *Streptococcus mutans* because of their oval shape, which seemed a *mutant* form.[365]

The plaque may contain several hundred bacterial species and the visible white layer (*materia alba*), which forms a diffusion barrier, particularly for substances with high-molecular weight. The barrier creates chemical gradients between the different layers of the plaque, which co-determine the kinds of bacterial species that may exist, and their activity, in the different plaque layers. There is a:

1. *Diffusion limit.* A fermentable substrate does not penetrate the entire depth of a plaque because it is either totally metabolised or absorbed, or chemically blocked before it reaches the deeper parts. Consequently, the deeper layers of plaque are inactive: the "reaction-free zone". The substrate concentration in the saliva is low in such cases.
2. *Reaction limit.* A fermentable substrate with a sufficiently high salivary concentration penetrates the plaque totally, but is only partly metabolised.

The plaque composition thus depends on the diffusion and reaction limits, on the type and supply of substrates and local oxygen tension. Strictly anaerobic areas exist next to aerobic ones. Water channels enable transport of bacterial products and nutrients between microenvironments within plaque.[14] The plaque composition determines its pathogenicity and this is different for different types of tooth surface.

- *Pits and fissures* harbour many bacterial genera, but 80% are Gram-positive cocci, among which are large numbers of *S. mutans*, *S. sanguis* and *Lactobacillus* strains. *Actinomyces* species are also present. *Candida albicans* and other yeasts adhere to and dissolve *in vitro* hydroxyapatite to a greater extent than *S. mutans*,[434] but usually few yeasts are present in the mouth, and mainly on the tongue; *in vivo* their cariogenic role seems small. After progression of the carious lesion into the dentine, *S. mutans* remains important (Table 5.1),[449] but many other bacteria are also present.
- *Approximal.* Plaque accumulating underneath the contact points has a more varied and locally different composition.[40] In particular it contains actinomycetes, followed by fewer numbers of Gram-negative bacteria and even fewer streptococci, but the numbers of *S. mutans* increase when caries develops. Because sound contact points also harbour all these microorganisms, plaque composition is a poor caries predictor.[547]
- *Free smooth surfaces.* Here, the mechanical action of the cheeks, tongue, mastication and tooth brushing restrict plaque growth. Only bacteria that are able to strongly adhere to the teeth initially become established. *S. mutans*, preceded by *S. salivarius* and *Actinomyces*, are important in smooth surface caries.
- *Cervical.* The most complex and thickest plaque is found cervically. The crevicular fluid and saliva maintain the plaque, which consist of more than 50 species, including *Actinomyces* and strict anaerobic bacteria in large quantities. Some of these play a role in root caries. In children, as the rate of crevicular fluid flow is low, the cervical plaque resembles the approximal plaque.
- *Subgingival plaque* differs from *supragingival plaque* and has a high percentage of anaerobes.

As stated above, the quality and quantity of the microflora (plaque) at a site that may be considered vulnerable to caries determines whether the disease develops or not.

Table 5.1 Frequency (%) of occurrence of various bacteria in the proximal[a] carious dentinal lesion[449]

Bacteria	Lesions in		
	Pits/fissures	Smooth surfaces	Roots
Streptococcus mutans	100	100	71
Streptococcus sobrinus	56	54	17
Streptococcus sanguis	81	77	63
Actinomyces viscosus[b]	50	69	92
Lactobacillus casei	63	54	21
Lactobacillus plantarum	63	62	33
Peptostreptococcus micros	56	54	29
Eubacterium alactolyticum	63	62	42
Propionibacterium acnes	50	31	38
Streptococcus aureus	25	15	13
Fusobacterium nucleatum	31	39	8
Porphyromonas endodontalis	6	8	0

[a]The numbers of bacteria decrease with increasing depth of the dentinal lesion.
[b]*A. viscosus* serotype II later classified as *A. naeslundii* genospecies 2.[91]

5.2.3 Caries-specific bacteria?

In cross-sectional studies, plaque composition was moderately associated with caries. The majority of plaques are not cariogenic because they are insufficiently thick, contain few virulent bacteria, with little carbohydrate substrates, etc. Comparison of caries-free with caries-active subjects shows a strong association of caries with specific microbial species. Longitudinal studies of plaque compositions and caries show that caries progression in the enamel is strongly associated with persistently high numbers of *S. mutans* and, additionally, lactobacilli in dentinal lesions.

Until the 1960s, lactobacilli were considered to cause caries. However, it was shown that the consumption of varied diets, with or without cariogenic sweets between meals did not lead to any differences in the numbers of lactobacilli compared with a control group, which had less caries.[432]

Presently, the mutans streptococci in particular are thought to be the main culprits. Prior to the first sign of decay, the number of *S. mutans* in the area increases. The numbers of lactobacilli increase after caries initiation.[144] [390 547] Incremental caries progression, in particular on smooth surfaces, appeared associated with *S. mutans*,[607] but was found to be greatest when *S. sobrinus* were present in greater numbers than *S. mutans*.[248] Two-thirds of approximal surfaces did not show signs of caries when both *S. mutans* and *S. sobrinus* were present. This does not point to bacterial specificity of caries, but to the large production of acids by these bacteria.[40] In "open" lesions, *S. sobrinus* prevails while in "closed" lesions with a less complex microflora, *S. mutans* predominates.[138] Older plaques on healthy enamel also contain *S. mutans*,[318] which may not be present in plaques overlying newly developing lesions.

The numbers of *S. mutans* are only weakly associated with the risk of development of caries.[564] In one study, children with high sugar consumption and caries rates had lower *S. mutans* counts than many of the caries-free children with low sugar consumption.[105] Most of the mutans streptococci in plaques of caries-free children were, however, *S. rattus* instead of *S. mutans* strains.[365] In one town, caries prevalence in children was associated with mutans streptococci and in another town with lactobacilli.[204] Caries has been found to develop in the fissures of rat molars even in the absence of *S. mutans* and sugar.[597] In Europe, Africa and North America, at least 70% of children less than 7 years of age harbour mutans streptococci: differences in the caries prevalence are due mainly to differences in the cariogenicity of the diet,[647] and fluoride use.

The findings show that caries is not uniquely associated with one bacterial species. At least 300 species (possibly 1000) are indigenous to the mouth, but not many of them are dental pathogens. *S. mutans* and lactobacilli are significantly related to the onset and progression of caries and circumstantial evidence shows that they belong to the principal group of aetiological agents.[365]

In root caries, large numbers of anaerobic bacteria are present in addition to *S. mutans*, including some with proteolytic activity. Anaerobes assumedly play a role in caries progression. Weak positive correlations have been established with *Actinomyces*. The microflora consists of *Actinomyces viscosus*, *S. mutans* and *S. sanguis*, but *S. sobrinus* predominates, and in leathery root lesions, it is the lactobacilli.[88 159 180 368 373]

Experimentally, *Actinomyces* has been shown to produce root caries:[158] high levels have been found to be associated (co-dominating with *S. mutans*) with greater numbers of root lesions.[60][195] *Actinomyces naeslundii* forms 10% of the plaques on both healthy and carious roots,[91] but has been, like other filamentous rods, ascribed an aetiological role. On caries-free roots, *S. sanguis* was found to predominate.[195] The presence of both *S. sobrinus* and *S. mutans* was associated with more root caries than *S. mutans* alone.[368] Aamdal-Scheie *et al.* found that plaques on healthy and carious roots were identical[2] and had the same levels of *S. mutans* and lactobacilli.[195]

When carious dentine is lost, the root becomes recolonised.[530] In case of "arrested caries", the amount of plaque decreases.[529]

These findings do not point to a bacterium-specific aetiological basis for root caries.[650]

5.2.4   *Transmission of cariogenic flora*

Oral infection in children is related to frequent contact with large numbers of bacteria from the mother ("cuddle effect") and other caregivers[108][135][319] within the discrete period between 18/19 and 31 months (the "window of infectivity").[108][596] But the presence of caries testifies that children aged 9–10 months are also already infected[630] and *S. mutans* was detected in 25% of one sample of pre-dentate children.[413] Caries prevalence rates in children follow those in mothers more than those in fathers.[89] Maternal caries best predicts caries in 11–12-year-olds.[621]

A study of mother–child dyads during the first 7 years of life revealed that two-thirds of the children had acquired *S. mutans* and one-quarter had acquired *S. mutans* plus *S. sobrinus*, while all the mothers possessed both species.[356] The correlation between numbers of mutans streptococci in maternal and children's saliva is low:[498] 70% of 3-year-old children harboured *S. mutans*, compared with 40% when mothers' microflora was suppressed for a period spanning a few years. If 15-month-olds harboured *S. mutans*, the probability of caries at the age of 3 years was 75%.[319] In one study, children free of mutans streptococci until age 5 had more sound teeth at age 11 than children who acquired the bacteria earlier.[581]

When the number of *S. mutans* in a mother is reduced permanently, her child's mouth is colonised at a later stage or not at all. Bacteria newly introduced in the mouth are more likely to get established in children than in adults with their highly colonisation-resistant, optimally adapted flora. In adults, a new bacterium rarely spreads from the inoculation site and becomes undetectable within a few weeks. In contrast, tooth eruption creates conditions favourable for colonisation. In 19–31-month-old children a new bacterial colony is established relatively easily.

5.2.5   *Virulence factors*

The amount of acids, the rate of production and the time for which they remain on the tooth surface co-determine the cariogenicity of plaque. In the presence of sugar, plaques with larger numbers of mutans streptococci quickly produce much acid. Virulence factors of such plaques are as follows.

- *Intracellular polysaccharides* formed from sugars within *S. mutans* (in *S. sobrinus* these sugars are largely absent)[597] are fermented after exhaustion of the external sugar supply, thereby prolonging periods of low plaque pH.
- *Extracellular polysaccharides* make the plaque stick to the smooth tooth surfaces. *Mutan*, produced exclusively by *S. mutans* from saccharose, and *glucan* produced by *S. sobrinus*, are important components of this system. Glycosyltransferases from the saliva, new pellicle and *S. mutans* catalyse the synthesis of glucan linkages from sugars. Interactions between glucan linkages leads to the formation of extracellular polysaccharides, which adhere to the teeth and then incorporate other bacteria.[500]
- Sucrose-independent surface protein antigens I/II (PAc) participate in the initial adherence of *S. mutans*:[212] these bacterial proteins interact with lectins in the pellicle.[560]
- *S. sobrinus* excretes a virulence-associated immunomodulatory protein (VIP), which inhibits the host's response.[140]
- High catabolic activity, manifest at a low pH, of notably *S. mutans* and *S. sobrinus*, ensures a high concentration of acids.
- *Autoselection.* Acid-producing bacteria are aciduric and multiply at a low pH, which adds to the process of bacterial selection that alters the plaque composition.

The cariogenic bacteria absorb and ferment sugars, form acids, secrete H^+ through their cell walls and take up K^+, thus maintaining their electrochemical equilibrium and preventing acidification of the bacterial cytoplasm. At lower pH, some of the plaque acid does not dissociate and this acid is taken up in the bacteria. Within the somewhat less acidic bacteria, the acids dissociate and H^+ is released. Ultimately the capacity to release H^+ fails, the internal pH drops and the metabolism of the bacterium stagnates, which prevents the pH in the plaque from become lower than about 4.[107] *S. sobrinus* produces more acids at a low pH than *S. mutans*.[136]

Acid formation and secretion of H^+ by *S. mutans* is governed under anaerobic circumstances by fluoride, which behaves as a non-dissociated acid: the degree to which this occurs is determined by whether the bacterial species thrive in an acidic or neutral pH environment.[195]

Because of bacterial resistance to acids, erosion (Chapter 6) may alter the plaque composition. Some research indicates in such circumstances *S. mutans* and *S. sobrinus* are present in proportionately high numbers, but this has not, however, been confirmed.[251]

None of the virulence factors are unique properties of *S. mutans*, with the exception of *mutan* production, which supports the non-bacterial species-specific aetiology of caries. However, if *S. mutans* are present in substantial numbers, which depends on the diet, carious lesions may develop relatively rapidly. The group of related oral bacteria known as mutans streptococci, which include *S. rattus*, *Streptococcus cricetus*, and *S. sobrinus*, is implicated as the primary aetiological agent of caries, and within this group *S. mutans* and *S. sobrinus* are the species most commonly isolated from carious lesions.[137 365]

5.3   The substrate

Many plaque bacteria survive on a diet of salivary glycoproteins, but the rate of plaque formation in humans on parenteral nutrition increases quite rapidly on resumption of oral feeding. The plaque swiftly assimilates low-molecular compounds (sugars, peptides) and a small proportion of proteins and polysaccharides after enzymatic breakdown. Substances other than carbohydrates, fluoride, calcium and phosphate seem to be of minor importance as far as direct uptake by plaque is concerned.

Sugars may be consumed a number of times daily, and then in high concentrations. Consequently, the plaque synthesises polysaccharides and produces acids, which promote plaque growth, auto-selection of mutans streptococci, and caries. Frequent sugar consumption results time and time again in acid production and shortens the remineralisation periods: under these circumstances carious lesions then develop or progress.

5.3.1   Sugars

Polysaccharides, such as starches, usually remain too briefly in the mouth to be sufficiently transformed into sugars that can diffuse into the plaque. The buffering capacity of the saliva and plaque fluid easily neutralise the acids thus formed. In contrast, free dietary sugars immediately penetrate the plaque and are absorbed by the bacteria and hydrolysed. These mono- and disaccharides are: saccharose (=sucrose = "sugar"), glucose, fructose, maltose, lactose and galactose. Pollard showed that the plaque pH fall was largest after sugar consumption, followed respectively by pasta, ripe banana, white bread, cornflakes and the sweetener sorbitol.[469] The pH drop is smaller and shorter lasting in children than in adults.[589]

5.3.2   Saccharose

Sucrose provides 15–20% of the dietary caloric value, other saccharides a few per cent. Caries development therefore depends mainly on the consumption of sugar, although glucose, fructose and lactose are almost as cariogenic. Sucrose, a disaccharide of fructose linked to glucose, is refined from the juice of sugar cane and beet. Hydrolysis of the molecule frees the energy from the fructose–glucose bond, which the bacteria use to synthesise the extracellular polysaccharides, mediated by the glycosyltransferases which direct the glucose to the growing polysaccharide.

Sucrose is used rapidly and effectively:

- For synthesis of extracellular polysaccharides. Without sugar, adherence of plaque to the tooth is reversible; with sugar the bond becomes insoluble in water.
- As an intracellular substrate, after splitting and uptake, which serves as an energy source when the external food supply is exhausted.
- For intracellular synthesis of cell membrane material, etc.

The hetero-fermentative bacteria in "resting plaques" (i.e. in times where there is nothing else other than saliva and crevicular fluid in the mouth) form acetic, lactic, propionic, butyric and formic acid, alcohol, carbon dioxide, and other products. In the presence of rapidly fermentable sugars, the concentration of lactic acid increases quickly, more than that of other acids.

In one study neither the amount nor the frequency of sugar consumption differed between children with and without caries,[341] which stresses its multifactorial character; but generally the main distinction between individuals with and without caries is more frequent consumption of cariogenic food, that is sucrose, between meals.[267]

5.4   The initial lesion (enamel)

5.4.1   The carious process[167]

With respect to the enamel at a pH of 7, saliva is supersaturated with calcium and phosphate. Enamel closely resembles hydroxyapatite, but contains a variety of impurities.

Some impurities (fluoride, zinc) are mainly superficially located; others (sodium, carbonate) are far from the enamel surface or are distributed evenly (strontium, vanadium). Many impurities are soluble, but when they form part of the crystal lattice they are not easily dissolved, for example fluoride which has substituted for the hydroxyl group during odontogenesis.[431] Post-eruptive administration of fluoride may lead to formation of calcium fluoride, or fluorhydroxyapatite, which is somewhat less soluble than hydroxyapatite.[340] Aluminium makes the enamel less soluble in acid,[313] but a fluoride toothpaste was found to be more effective than an aluminium paste.[234] Copper, strontium and barium reduce the risk[125 126 127 145 502 668 701] and magnesium, zinc and selenium increase the risk of developing caries as well as progression of developed lesions.[126 442] The knowledge of the action of trace elements such as lead, iron, and molybdenum in the teeth is incomplete.

Bacterial acids at the plaque–enamel junction make the environment of the tooth undersaturated at the "critical" pH of 5.5 (a pH below 6 is potentially harmful).[613] After a sugar solution rinse, the pH underneath plaque drops to about 4.0, and remains low for 0.5–1 hour,[348] or even longer at sites protected from salivary flow.[280] The pH depends on the buffering capacity of saliva, which is determined mainly by the bicarbonate (HCO_3^-) system:

$$HCO_3^- + H^+ \rightleftharpoons H_2CO_3 \rightarrow H_2O + CO_2$$

The HCO_3^- concentration increases considerably on salivary gland stimulation. The buffering capacity of the phosphate system is insufficient because of its low concentration.[275]

Under acidic plaque, the enamel demineralises when the buffers are depleted and H^+ ions from the acids penetrate the interprismatic substance. First the intercrystalline spaces enlarge due to partial dissolution of the individual crystal periphery. Later the thin overlapping portions of the perikimata dissolve with further enlargement of the intercrystalline spaces. The process advances along the prisms into the deeper layers of the enamel. The mineral dissolution creates pores in the enamel, which act as transport channels through which dissolved minerals diffuse to the outside of the enamel and are carried away with the flow of fluid from the pulp.[28]

Dissolved minerals from the surface are replenished with minerals from the subsurface layer, which becomes poorer in minerals.[405] The superficial (30–50 μm) enamel therefore remains largely intact and provides surface protection, also due to the formation of macromolecules under the influence of proline-rich saliva and other salivary inhibitors, which cannot penetrate the deeper parts of the enamel, although up to 5% of it consists of pores; but underneath, mineral loss is greater. Explanations have also been offered for why the surface is, at large, unaffected.[98] The surface is thought to be protected by absorbed proteins, which would contain more minerals than the deeper layers and contain more fluoride and less carbonate, making it less soluble.[349] Or a gradient may exist in solubility rate, and low fluoride concentrations considerably affect the solubility gradient.[606]

The mineral loss described above makes the lesion visible as a "white spot" after blowing air on the tooth surface in the earliest phase of caries development; this is because fluid within the pores maintains the translucency of the enamel. Later, the white spot is clearly visible without air-drying the tooth (Figure 5.1), signifying an enlarged subsurface pore volume. Microcavities may develop.[167] The pores encourage progression of the process, chiefly along the enamel prisms and the lines of Retzius.[606]

Fluoride-containing apatite dissolves at a pH lower than 5.5, which implies that the enamel is less frequently exposed to an harmful pH (the pH must be lower than 5.5 to be critical) and because the pH returns slowly to neutral, the critical period is shorter. The margins of the white spot and plaque correspond. In the interdental

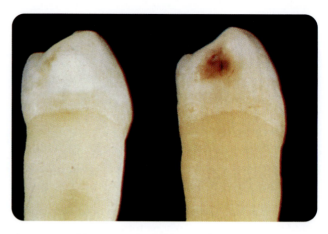

Figure 5.1 White spot caries (initial lesion) and brown spot (discoloured white spot).

contact areas, the white spot is oval and resembles cervically a half moon. The enamel is most porous at the centre of the subsurface lesion, following the direction of the enamel rods from the surface to the deepest point.

When the external sugar supply and the intracellular polysaccharides are exhausted, the salivary buffering mechanisms slowly raise the plaque pH to neutral, aided by the rinsing of the tooth surface by saliva and dilution. Pellicle proteins promote the remineralisation by attracting salivary calcium ions.[645] The local environment becomes saturated and minerals precipitate superficially into the pores. Demineralisation is retarded in concert with the concentration of calcium and phosphate ions in saliva and plaque fluid. A sucrose rinse increases the plaque calcium concentration by a factor of 2.5 and also increases the phosphate concentration. Ions released from the enamel slow down the demineralisation by saturating the plaque fluid with ions.[595,645] The fluoride concentration in plaque remained unaltered, indicating supersaturation.[595]

Half an hour of demineralisation requires several hours for complete remineralisation. Under laboratory conditions, equilibrium was found to be established when the pH was lowered no more than six times for 30 minutes each per day.[600] Passive transport of salivary and plaque Ca^{2+} and $H_2PO_4^-$ ions down the concentration gradients into the lesion is the main driving force for remineralisation, but solubility constraints limit the mineral ion concentration in the remineralising fluid.[113] Moreover, a mineral shortage exists, because during the acid attacks ions from the enamel are lost to the oral cavity.[275]

In vitro, five factors limit the remineralisation within the depth of the lesion:[339]

1. Even supersaturated saliva does not contain much calcium and phosphate.

2. The concentration gradient of the remineralising fluid in the enamel lesion is small.
3. Calcium and phosphate are incorporated so rapidly in the enamel that they do not reach the deeper layers.
4. The enamel surface itself acts as an obstacle for mineralisation underneath the surface.
5. Nucleation of new apatite crystals does not take place.

During remineralisation, pigments from dietary components may become incorporated into the lesion. The white spot then becomes a *brown spot* (Figure 5.1). The amount of mineral that can dissolve depends on the saturation of the solution, and is governed by the thermodynamic ion activity product of a given solution.[113] The extent to which fluorapatite is dissolved, in a given solution, is less than that of apatite. If the hydroxyl ions in the enamel were systematically replaced by fluoride ions during its formation, a small percentage of the enamel would consist of more tightly formed fluorapatite.[431] The local effect of fluoride by far exceeds this systemic effect.[691] Fluoride in the plaque and saliva enhances the precipitation of CaF_2 and some fluorapatite is formed. Precipitation of minerals including pH-resistant CaF_2 plugs the entrance to pores, which inhibits the remineralisation of deeper parts.[600] With dissolution, the CaF_2 provides a slow-release fluoride depot.[501]

Enzymatic[612] destruction of the *organic* component starts after mineral dissolution. Collagen, which forms a small proportion of enamel (10 times less than dentine), must be free of minerals before it can be destroyed. The enamel lamellae are organic (hypomineralised) linear defects that cross the enamel. Contrary to the notion that these lamellae are pathways along which caries can easily progress,[460] they are quite resistant to acids.[71] The exact role of proteases in enamel caries is not known.[82 115 652] Enamel cracks (Chapter 9) may visually resemble the lamellae, but they allow ingress of cariogenic bacteria.[670]

5.4.2   Histology and chemistry of the initial enamel lesion[167 432 549 551]

Initially, the enamel pores are about 20–50 μm deep. Fresh acid attacks enlarge the pore volume: the crystallites become smaller and hollowed out lengthwise, the enamel rods dissolve peripherally, and the pores become deeper. "Focal holes" (micropits) and small areas with irregular destruction develop.[216]

In the presence of acids, the hydroxyapatite $(Ca_{10}(PO_4)_6(OH)_2)$ dissolves into Ca^{2+} and $H_2PO_4^-$ and H_2O. Other reactions also occur. Brushite $(CaHPO_4.2H_2O)$ is formed, which in the presence of fluoride is rapidly converted into fluorapatite. Phosphate as a tooth mineral exists in the basic form of PO_4^- but under mildly acidic conditions, dissolved phosphate ions are predominantly in a more acidic form.[113]

An acid concentration gradient exists in the enamel from the outside to the inside. The deeper, less acidic but weak bacterial acids dissociate at a relatively high pH and may therefore be active in the deeper layers. Dissolved calcium and phosphate ions diffuse to the outside, where they precipitate as acidic calcium phosphate, thereby maintaining the surface integrity.[275]

Smooth surfaces
The initial lesion is conical, with its base towards the surface (Figure 5.2). Demineralisation is worst in the centre, the oldest part of the lesion, and becomes gradually less deeper within the lesion, away the periphery. The deeper the central pores, the wider is the lesion peripherally.[80]

Fissures
White spots develop back to back in both walls of the fissure (Figure 5.3). The shape of the occlusal fissures

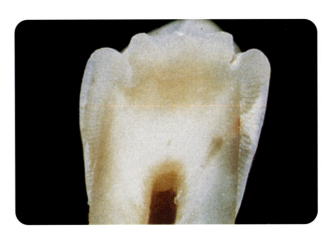

Figure 5.2 Initial carious lesion in a smooth tooth surface; the demineralisation defect (white) at the right side is conical in shape, with its base towards the surface of the tooth. The dentine is just involved, visible as a small, brown discoloured area.

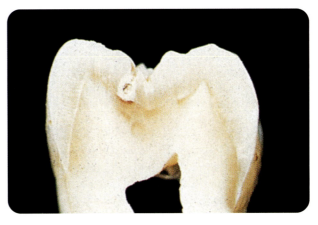

Figure 5.3 Initial carious lesion in a fissure; the defect is present on both walls of the fissure. Again, the dentine is involved.

varies and the direction of the enamel rods is not always perpendicular towards the dentino-enamel junction; but the shape of the fissural carious lesion is principally conical. After some time, the two demineralised areas merge underneath the fissure. In small, artificially created grooves, less mineral was lost from the walls than in broader grooves, which might have been because the diffusion of acids to the inside and that of the mineral ions to the outside was restricted.[332]

Bacteria are absent in the initial enamel lesion: the result of a demineralising acid front.[92] Microscopically, four zones are distinguishable:

1. The surface is not much different from unaffected enamel: the pore volume increases from 0.1% (normal) to 1–5%.
2. Underneath the surface lies the "core of the lesion", the broadest zone. At the periphery the pore volume is 5%, centrally it is 25% or greater. The internal cohesion of the enamel is still adequate to prevent cavitation, but after substantial subsurface loss of minerals, application of an external force may cause the surface to collapse, resulting in cavitation.
3. Next follows the "dark zone", which has a pore volume of 2–4%. Young teeth lack this zone.[302]
4. Still deeper a "translucent zone" may be present. The initial demineralisation process preferentially dissolves some magnesium and carbonate. The pore volume is 1%.

The deepest enamel layer may be normal.

5.5   Progression of the carious lesion[167]

- *Enamel.* Demineralisation advances little by little towards the dentine (Figure 5.4). Cavitation, in general, does not start before the dentine is involved,[7] and is not seen when, on radiographs, the demineralisation front extends to and even beyond the dentino-enamel junction. In a sample of caries-active patients, the approximal surfaces with demineralised areas on radiographs showed discontinuity of the enamel.[367]

Many *cervical* white spots remain unchanged in the long term.[610] Backer Dirks found that within 7 years, 10% of initial lesions on *smooth surfaces* of children cavitated, 40% remained unchanged, and 50% became indistinguishable from the surrounding enamel. Considerably more *fissure* lesions cavitated and the process was faster.[42] A minority of *approximal lesions* reaching the dentine, and brown discoloured fissures, healed within 1–5 years. The rate of progress of the approximal lesions was slow, particularly when confined to the outer enamel.[461] In another study, within 3 years, 15% of approximal enamel

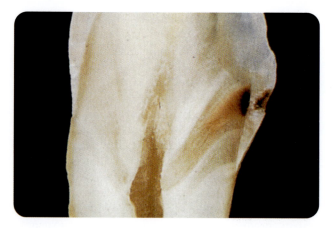

Figure 5.4 Smooth surface caries lesion showing progression in all directions. The defect in the enamel is conical in shape with its base towards the surface. The width of the lesion in the dentine is the same as that of the lesion at the enamel surface. The two light brown areas in the dentine represent sclerotic tissue.

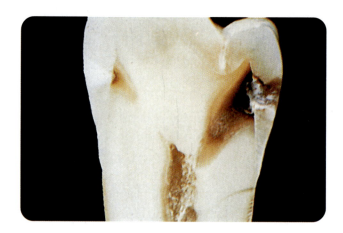

Figure 5.5 The carious lesion has reached the pulp.

lesions had healed after application of preventive measures, 35% had stabilised, and 50% had progressed.[266]

- *Dentino-enamel junction.* Before the lesion reaches the junction, dentinal changes occur. Deposition of minerals causes narrowing of the tubules, creating a hypermineralised zone. At this stage, the pulp becomes involved via communications with the tubular fluid and the odontoblastic processes (Figures 5.5 and 5.6). Thereafter, bacterial products penetrate through the enamel and reach the dentine. The critical pH for the dentine is 6.0–6.5 and freshly exposed dentine does not contain much fluoride.[158]
- *Dentine.* The connections (anastomoses) between the tubules have been considered to be pathways for lateral

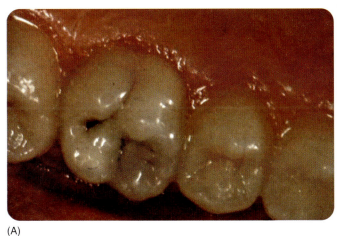
(A)

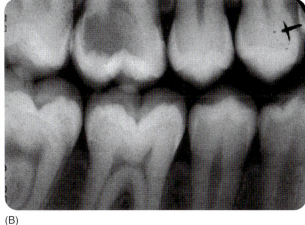
(B)

Figure 5.6 (A) The occlusal surface shows a discoloured distal fissure, but seems otherwise more or less intact. (B) An X-ray of the same tooth showing a large carious lesion ("hidden caries") in the dentine underneath the small occlusal entrance of the lesion.

expansion of the demineralisation process along the dentino-enamel junction. However, in the *precavitated* stage, the width of dentine lesion does not exceed that of the enamel surface lesion,[76] and demineralisation does not spread along the dentino-enamel junction,[48] but follows the tubules.[80]

The process, at first a demineralisation front, progresses in the direction of the pulp. The hypermineralised zone protects against lesion progression, but the tubular blockade fails if the (repeated) attack is strong enough. The base of the conical, truncated lesion is at the dentino-enamel junction. An enamel cavity is commonly still absent. At this stage the odontoblasts produce tertiary dentine (Section 5.5.3).

When the process extends beyond the dentino-enamel junction and an enamel cavity has developed, the dentinal lesion spreads along the junction, undermining the enamel. At this stage the deeper dentinal layers are already demineralised. Lateral spread is also observed in microcavitated lesions, which are invaded by bacteria. It is associated with softening of the dentine, which depends initially on the way in which the bacterial acids penetrate the enamel prisms.[155] By this stage demineralisation has reached the middle third of the dentine.

Once there is frank cavitation, the inner half of the dentine is demineralised and the outer half infected.[155] Proteolytic enzymes degrade the collagen matrix that is denuded by demineralisation.

Once exposed by the acids, the organic matrix is destroyed by non-specific proteases after breakdown of the electrostatic bonds of the side chains.[314 315] Demineralised dentine shows considerable loss of collagen, unrelated to specific bacterial species. Great numbers of *Actinomyces* have been found to be present in dentine with largely exposed organic component.[650]

The non-collagenous organic dentine components may counteract remineralisation: their removal with sodium hypochlorite *in vitro* was found to promote remineralisation.[265]

Among the proteolytic enzymes are matrix metalloproteinases that are capable of degrading native and denatured collagen type I and might be activated by bacterial acids. Metalloproteinases are also present in plaque, saliva and crevicular fluid. Metalloproteinase activity is seen in extracts from demineralised dentine, but appeared unrelated to the collagen loss. Activity of a cystein proteinase (cathepsin B) which degrades collagen in mildly acidic conditions, correlated positively with activity of metalloproteinases.[651]

5.5.1 Histology of dentine caries

The dentinal lesion comprises six zones:

1. An outer layer of *destruction*. Here, the structure of the dentine is lost as proteolytic enzymes destroy the dentinal matrix, and bacteria produce acids. The denatured and infected dentine cannot remineralise.
2. A layer of *infection:* the tubules contain bacteria, and are widened and confluent.
3. A layer of *demineralisation*: a narrow zone ahead of the zone of infection, in which the peritubular dentine in particular dissolves.[92]
4. A transparent layer of *sclerotic* (hypermineralised) dentine. This acts as a barrier against bacterial and acid progression,[51] and is important in dentinal resistance to caries progression. The peritubular dentine widens at the cost of the tubules, by mineral precipitation during the periods of varying pH gradients. The mineralisation may also be the result of activity of the odontoblasts.[185] Necrotic teeth lack this layer.[183] *In vitro*, perfusion of the pulp with a simulated dentinal fluid resulted in less deep lesions than with

non-perfused pulps,[450] [540] but the rate of flow of the fluid does not correlate with the rate of demineralisation.[450] Others claim that the transparent layer undergoes an intermediate phase of softening due to demineralisation of peritubular and intertubular dentine.[441]

5. An *opaque* layer. The parts of the dentinal tubules nearer the pulp contain lipids, originating more superficially from the bacteria and deeper from the degenerated Tomes' processes (though the odontoblast processes may not degenerate)[176] or from demineralised peritubular dentine.[432]

6. *Tertiary* (reparative) dentine in the pulp.

Bacteria penetrate the dentine only after cavitation. Layers 3, 4 and 5 are absent where the carious process has penetrated very deep into the tooth.[551]

5.5.2   Macroscopic appearance

In enamel, white and brown spots and cavitation are the macroscopic signs of caries. Carious dentine is more or less discoloured. Before restoration, the layers of destroyed and infected dentine are removed (Section 5.12.2). The remaining demineralised dentine layer must be hard enough to support the restoration.[185]

5.5.3   Pulpal reactions

The relationship between clinical caries and the histopathological condition of the pulp has not been "classified" for a variety of reasons,[80] [559] including: marked variations in pulpal reactions,[337] lack of information on caries activity, and artificial loss of enamel prior to pulp examination. The organic and inorganic phases are difficult to study simultaneously.

Yet, some conclusions seem warranted.[80] The pulpal reaction starts when white spots develop. The odontoblasts are smaller in size underneath any *active* caries lesion extending to the dentino-enamel junction and cellular proliferation is seen in the cell-free zone of the pulp. These changes have not been seen underneath arrested caries lesions,[80] implying that they are reversible.

The pulp–dentine complex shows different responses that interact in a complex way. Their relative contributions are critical for determining the fate of the pulp–dentine complex.[559]

- *Injury responses.* The dentinal matrix and solubilised minerals buffer the hydrogen ions, but the odontoblasts underneath active enamel lesions show cytoplasmic changes and decreased activity, and dentinogenesis may cease.
- *Defence reactions.* A defensive inflammatory pulpal reaction is followed by reactions that determine the

degree of healing and repair; tertiary dentine modifies the permeability of the dentine. As bacterial ingress progresses, the inflammatory pulpal reaction becomes more pronounced and acute and can compromise pulp survival.

- *Repair reactions.* Odontoblasts secrete focally *reactionary* dentine in milder (active)[77] carious attacks. When the odontoblasts do not survive, a new generation may arise from differentiation of other pulpal cells and form *reparative* dentine.

Bacterial acids and other metabolic products are, as irritants, directly responsible for *tertiary* dentine formation, hence named *irritation* dentine. Growth factors (which have a limited diffusion distance) and cytokines present in the dentine matrix stimulate the odontoblasts and presumably the progenitors of second-generation odontoblasts.

Tertiary dentine is already formed in non-cavitated caries, somewhat apical of the enamel lesion in relation to the direction of the tubules.[551] In some cases irritation dentine is absent there, but large amounts of it are formed in the vicinity.[337] The more active the carious process, the more irregular is the reactive dentine. Under slowly progressing caries, tertiary dentine resembles secondary dentine. When lesions progress rapidly, the odontoblasts are damaged and no tertiary dentine is formed.[80]

Inflammatory and immunological pulpal reactions follow the ingress of microbial antigens, toxins, allergenic bacterial agents and bacteria through the tubules. When pulpitis develops, it may be symptomless.[80] [337] [559] In one sample of deciduous teeth with exposed pulps, one-third showed transitional pulpitis, but two-thirds of deep carious teeth without pulp exposure had a normal pulp or transitional pulpitis.[151] The pulp becomes significantly diseased when caries invades the tertiary dentine.[479]

The degree of both reversible or irreversible pulpal inflammation cannot be assessed non-invasively,[80] necessitating complete removal of affected dentine. The status of the pulp is no indication of the severity of the caries process, unless the pulp is severely infected or necrotic.

5.6   Root caries

Gingival recession exposes the cementum to the oral environment: root caries may then develop (Figure 5.7). Dentine has a lower mineral content and crystallinity than enamel and is therefore more soluble. Bacterial invasion occurs along the direction of the Sharpey's fibres, which are degraded, and causes a rather wide subsurface than deep lesion,[256] [528] in relation to dentine sclerosis in older persons.

Multiple small demineralisation foci[528] and mini-channels or clefts reaching into the cemento-dentine junction are character-

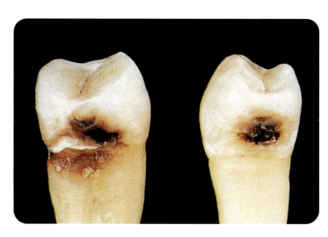

Figure 5.7 Root caries (plus approximal caries, left panel) and approximal caries (right panel).

istic. Hypomineralised areas allow an exchange of fluid between the dentine and oral cavity. Underneath, a thin hypermineralised surface layer contains areas with destroyed collagen. The lesion spreads and undermines the cementum.

A brown-coloured lesion signifies a slowly progressing lesion whereas a light colour indicates an active lesion.[373] Coronal and root caries may be considered different entities because the latter is present: (1) sometimes almost exclusively on roots of teeth free of coronal caries; and (2) to the same degree in persons with and without fluorosis.[201] Root caries correlates moderately with coronal caries ($r = 0.60$).[180]

Root caries accounted for some half of the carious lesions in the Middle Ages, including in the deciduous molars.[299 448 653 663] There is a strong relationship with periodontal disease, as found in tribes of New Guinea, where coronal caries is uncommon.[516]

Gingival recession is a precondition, but it does not explain the prevalence of root caries.[214] Medical, socioeconomic and behavioural variables partly explain lesion development.[58] Alterations in the oral condition also play a role. The salivary buffering capacity is reduced when the salivary flow decreases (see Section 5.7.3). Bacterial production of acids and enzymatic proteolytic activity of the anaerobic bacteria cause root caries.[2 147 528] Host-derived salivary proteases are also involved. The collagen fibrils must be almost free of mineral before they are degraded but for remineralisation sufficient mineral must be present on the fibrils.[314 315]

Ongoing eruption of the teeth and recession of the gingiva shift the area covered with plaque apically: thus alternating sound and carious zones may exist.

5.7 Some risk factors

Several groups are especially vulnerable to caries, including people with mental and physical disabilities and anxious patients. Several other factors may exert a large influence on the development of caries, and these are described in the following subsections.

Anxiety lowers the salivary flow rate or alters the salivary composition,[507] which decreases its rinsing and buffering actions, and concentrations of anti-bacterial enzymes.[432] Emotional stress reduces the serotonin level in the brain, which is restored by consumption of cariogenic carbohydrates. Children with caries have higher urinary levels of catecholamines, a measure of emotional stress.[636] Whether anxious people develop more caries than others is questionable.[59]

5.7.1 Chronic malnutrition

A shortage of proteins and fats during growth may permanently reduce the amount of stimulated salivary flow and buffering capacity, impair calcium and protein levels in *stimulated* and decrease immunological and agglutination defence factors in *unstimulated* saliva.[282 283] Malnutrition may result in caries if xerostomia (Section 5.7.3) is a consequence.[282] Anomalies of enamel structure as a result of malnutrition, such as in coeliac disease,[473] are associated with increased risk of caries.[353 413]

5.7.2 Inborn errors of metabolism and other diseases

Some rare disorders of amino acid metabolism require consumption of cariogenic diets for normal growth or can lead to chronic xerostomia.

Phenylketonuria (PKU)
PKU is uncommon (1:10 000). The amino acid phenylalanine needs a liver enzyme (phenylalanine hydroxylase) to convert it into tyrosine. When this enzyme is lacking, phenylalanine accumulates in the body fluids, with consequences such as progressive mental retardation and epilepsy.

PKU patients are treated with a diet poor in proteins and rich in carbohydrates, and with a mixture (drink) of amino acids, free of phenylalanine. The acid and therefore sweetened drinks are consumed at least twice a day. To guarantee full energy intake, snacks and sweetened beverages must be consumed, often every 2 hours.[118] The artificial sweetener aspartame (a dipeptide of phenylalanine) is contraindicated.[420] Phenylalanine in the diet reduces likelihood of plaque formation but the risk of caries development might be increased: the literature is inconclusive.[118] However, children with PKU receiving fluoride had markedly less caries, an effect absent in unaffected siblings.[671]

Enamel hypoplasia is associated with PKU, but dietary improvements may have reduced the risk of development of enamel defects.[118]

Other inborn errors of protein metabolism

Several very rare disorders are due to lack of various enzymes. Abnormal accumulations of the (intermediates of) amino acids necessitate a low protein and a high carbohydrate intake.[118]

These disorders include maple syrup urine disease (urine has a caramel smell), organic acidaemias (patients may require dialysis), urea cycle disorders (ammonia accumulates because no waste nitrogen is formed), homocystinuria (homocystine and methionine accumulate), and tyrosinaemia.[118]

Glycogen storing disorders (four types of protein and/or carbohydrate disorders) cause excessive storage of glycogen in liver/muscles and hypoglycaemia. Extra glucose is needed. There are few anecdotal reports of high caries rates in affected children. Administration of cornstarch supplement results in sticky debris on the teeth.[118]

Diabetes

In diabetic people in whom hyperglycaemia is prevented[295] and dietary precautions are taken, the caries prevalence is similar to the population average. However, samples of people with diabetes were found to have more restored tooth surfaces than controls.[10 397] Poorly controlled patients may develop more caries, associated with the increased presence of oral fungal microorganisms.[295] Hyperglycaemia strengthens the association between caries and mutans streptococci and lactobacilli.[588] In non-insulin-dependent diabetes, there is no effect on the caries and yeast prevalence, despite the protective effect of saliva being partly lost.[119] In older people with diabetes, a tendency for more active caries may exist, but an increased prevalence has not been reported.[359]

Diabetic rats develop root caries despite a diet poor in carbohydrates. The crevicular fluid might contain much glucose.[483] Compared with controls, people with diabetes were found to have both more and fewer cavities.[609] Unless diagnosed late, people with diabetes do not have more (root) caries than other people, owing to the insulin therapy and consumption of a (probably) non-cariogenic diet,[188 203 397 422] perhaps with the exception of lingual caries.[468] The number of cariogenic bacteria is "normal".[609] Saliva parameters may be identical to those in people without diabetes and those with well-controlled diabetes.[587] However, in people with diabetes, the saliva may contain more fructose[609] and, at the start of the disease, more glucose and IgG.[61]

People with diabetes may also have a reduced stimulated salivary flow due to use of antihypertensive medication.[609 698]

Fructose intolerance

The inherited intolerance lowers the risk of caries, because patients quickly learn to avoid fructose and sucrose, which cause abdominal discomfort.[118 432]

Graves' disease

The disease is the most common form of hyperthyroidism and makes patients (with mild xerostomia?) more suscep-tible to caries. Routine dental treatment may evoke a sudden onset of a thyroid storm (muscle weakness, confusion, psychosis, cardiovascular collapse and shock). The thyroid condition must be under control prior to dental treatment. The use of local anaesthetics with vasoconstrictors is contraindicated.[215] Hyperthyroidism promotes periodontal disease.[215]

5.7.3 Xerostomia

Xerostomia is a subjective complaint of oral dryness, not necessarily implying a reduced (sympathetic) amount of, and a more viscous, saliva.[211] Saliva moistens and softens, dilutes and aids in swallowing of foods in the mouth. Mucins lubricate the teeth and proteins such as lysozyme inhibit bacterial growth. Electrolytes together with proteins prevent growth of cariogenic bacteria and promote remineralisation.[211] Insufficient saliva increases the risk of development and the rate of caries spread and fungal growth (candidiasis). In xerostomia, patients feel an urge to suck candies and to keep sweetened or acidic liquids in the mouth for longer periods, which promotes plaque formation and auto-selection of aciduric bacteria.[365]

An estimated 80% of xerostomia patients with low salivary flow of <0.1 mL/min (unstimulated normally 0.22 mL/min)[478] develop at least one cavity/year.[565] Caries typically occurs as cervical lesions and on "self-cleansing" tooth surfaces that are normally free from decay.[661] In one study, people with xerostomia had almost 50% more decayed/filled tooth surfaces and nine times more root caries than in controls.[478]

Causes of xerostomia

There are several causes of xerostomia, but salivary duct stones are rarely implicated.

Medicaments

Xerostomia is indirectly associated with old age.[69] Elderly people, in particular, use one or more of the more than 250 pharmaceutical agents that can cause xerostomia, such as antihypertensives, analgesics, anticonvulsants, antidepressives, antihistaminics, antinauseants, antispasmodics, sedatives, anti-anxiolytics, psychotropic drugs and antiparkinsonian agents.[200 211 660] A quarter of elderly people have xerostomia,[252 541] and half of medically compromised older subjects.[363]

Smoking cannabis habitually[130] and alcoholism[658] cause xerostomia. Drugs for asthma (Chapter 6) may influence the composition and flow of the saliva: some studies point to an increased caries risk but others do not.[83]

Radiation

Radiotherapy of the head/neck region can damage the salivary glands.[347 432 662] The severity of hypofunction, which recovers slowly,[286] is related to the radiation dose.

The reduction in salivary flow and increase in viscosity due to destruction and fibrosis of the salivary glands[200] add to the caries susceptibility of the smooth surfaces and incisally/occlusally exposed dentine, which gradually undermines the enamel.[189] Without an adequate preventive regimen, rampant caries may develop, at a rate of >2 new lesions/month,[704] although new lesions can develop despite following an adequate fluoride regimen.

The numbers of *S. mutans*, lactobacilli and *Candida* increase.[97] [189] Use of a bactericidal unguent and parenteral antibiotics has been found to reduce *S. mutans* counts but not of lactobacilli.[286]

Radiotherapy might reduce the solubility of the dental hard tissues. If true, other factors must be responsible for the increase in caries.[287] Unbrushed radiated enamel did not show deeper lesions than non-radiated enamel; brushing with fluoridated toothpaste counteracted new lesion formation, but there was no effect on lesion depth.[309]

Sjögren's syndrome

The syndrome, named after the Swedish ophthalmologist Sjögren, is a chronic autoimmune disease that is mainly seen in females, affecting, in some,[399] the exocrine glands, with xerostomia, dry eyes and vaginal dryness. The rate of salivary secretion falls considerably at an early stage,[87] and is one-sixth in the intermediate stages.[661] In patients in later stages, the unstimulated secretion rate is 0.006 mL/min. The stimulated flow rate is proportionately less affected.[478]

Diagnostic criteria differ[129] and the severity of the symptoms changes over the time.[399] Viral infections (Epstein–Barr) could be causative.[357] The presence of xerostomia in postmenopausal women is associated with lowered hormonal levels.[592] Mouth dryness results from lymphocyte infiltration of the salivary glands. In secondary Sjögren's syndrome, there is an underlying connective or collagen disease that is causative (rheumatoid arthritis etc.). Rapidly progressive caries and candidal infection are observed in one-third of patients,[87 129 399 538] and also in children.[430] In some patients, there are increased numbers of *S. mutans* and lactobacilli.[190 321] The number of *Candida* species may not differ from non-Sjögren patients with xerostomia.[312] The susceptibility to periodontal diseases is probably not increased in this condition.[619]

Syndromes

Caries thrives in people with some syndromes. In the Prader–(Labhart)–Willi syndrome (Chapter 11), xerostomia, the diet, or "dysplastic" enamel may be responsible.[511]

5.7.4 Crohn's disease

This recurrent intestinal disease may require intestinal resection, which can lead to malnutrition. With a diet poor in fat and rich in carbohydrates, the salivary flow is probably decreased.[65]

5.7.5 Nursing-bottle caries

Nursing-bottle caries involves the presence of extensive carious lesions (Figure 5.8) of especially the incisors in very young infants, and is also called "nursing-bottle syndrome".[421] Causes are: (1) bottles with (sweetened) milk or sweet drinks such as Rose Vicee and (unsweetened) fruit juices given at sleeping time and at any time of the day/night the child desires; (2) bottle-feeding past the age of 1 year, and (3) prolonged night breast-feeding (Figure 5.9), in which the child holds the nipple in their mouth just before and while sleeping. Causes 2 and 3 are disputable (Section 5.11.9).[224]

In one study, mixing saliva with breast milk lowered the pH to 4.6 and with cow milk to about 5,[360] yet children breast-fed for a longer period had less caries than bottle-fed children.[496] Acid is formed from lactose in cow milk, but the mineral content

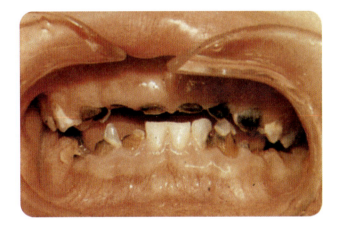

Figure 5.8 Extensive nursing bottle caries.

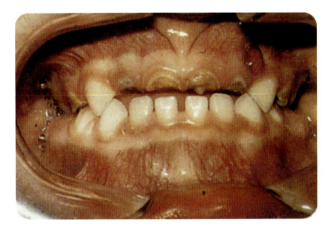

Figure 5.9 The crowns of the deciduous upper incisors destroyed by caries: the child was breast-fed throughout in the night for 3 years. (Courtesy of Department of Pedodontics, University of Nijmegen.)

of cow milk is four to five times higher than mother's milk, and is harmless, unless given very frequently.[323] Neither the duration nor the frequency of breast-feeding, but sleeping with the nipple in the mouth was associated with "nursing bottle caries".[395] Despite an absent relationship between prolonged breast-feeding and caries, it was advised to restrict breast-feeding to 12 months.[445] Breast-feeding combined with sweetened bottle-feeding at the age of 3 years seemed to cause more damage than solely sweetened bottles.[548] Acids are present in unsweetened fruit drinks.[146]

One sample of children with nursing bottle caries had relative large numbers of *S. mutans*.[328] Despite prevention, 4-year-old children developed new cavities, which points to an increased susceptibility,[537] or frequent consumption of sweets. The effect was still observable at age 10.[548]

A pacifier might be worse than a nursing bottle at night.[445]

5.7.6   Cleft lip/palate

Children with a cleft lip or palate tend to have more caries than controls[128] and, in one study, at 18 months of age, higher levels of *S. mutans* and lactobacilli.[84] Children wearing an acrylic plate from shortly after birth for obturation of a palatal cleft are colonised earlier with cariogenic bacteria (increasing with age) than children with other oral clefts, but at the age of 18 months the bacterial counts were similar and comparable with those in control children.[641] At 2.5 years of age, children with clefts show markedly more decay[85] due to poorer oral hygiene.[128] *S. mutans* counts in cleft patients seem to be associated with level of snacking.[641] One sample of children with clefts aged 6–16 years had higher plaque scores compared with children without clefts; their oral clearance time was longer and they had higher levels of sucrose and starch-derived saccharides. Longer clearance times contribute to higher caries scores.[4]

Like other children, 2-year-olds with an oral cleft going to bed with a nursing bottle had more decay than those who did not.[359]

5.7.7   Thalassaemia

Several studies point to a larger caries risk in thalassaemia major patients (Chapter 3), but data vary considerably. The patients may have swollen parotid glands and reduced IgA levels,[227] but it is unclear whether these features are responsible for the higher risk.

5.8   Identification of carious lesions[455 456]

5.8.1   Smooth surface caries

On the buccal and lingual surfaces the white and brown spot lesions and cavities are clearly visible directly or using a mouth mirror.

5.8.2   Occlusal caries

Demineralised occlusal dentine may produce dark shadows through the enamel.[465] Underneath a normal or brown discoloured but seemingly intact fissure, a lesion may be present, sometimes a large one. Disagreements have been found between dentists relating to the diagnosis of occlusal caries.[109] Opening the fissures offers the opportunity to ascertain whether caries is present, but non-invasive methods are needed to avoid unnecessary cutting of tooth material.

Radiographs can show (extensive) radiolucencies underneath "intact" fissures,[20 680] (and approximally), called *hidden caries* (Figure 5.6B) and *closed cavities*, which are more frequently seen nowadays.[465] The remineralising effect of fluoride does not affect the size of the enamel lesion, which means that a small enamel lesion leads into a much larger dentinal lesion and delays enamel cavitation, but this notion is disputable.[676] In a non-fluoridated-water municipality, more hidden caries was present than in a fluoridated town,[488] but in the former other sources of fluoride would have been available. Whether hidden caries is a distinct entity, reflecting a particular fissural topography or a different bacterial aetiology, is not known:[488] several bacterial species are associated with caries.[365] Hidden caries is a problem in 15% (range 3–50%)[488] of visually healthy molars of 6–18-year-olds. If detected late, the pulp is threatened.[675]

Caries may not be detectable with clinical methods even when it is proved to be present in histological sections (= the "gold standard"). Diagnosis, using a clinical method, as "sound", is a *false-negative diagnosis* if the gold standard method shows caries. The **"sensitivity"** of a method is the ability to diagnose caries when the gold standard shows caries. A tooth clinically diagnosed as "carious" while the histological picture does not show caries, is a *false-positive diagnosis*. **"Specificity"** is the ability of a clinical method to diagnose teeth as being sound, when caries is absent according to the gold standard.[208 233] False-positive diagnoses lead to unnecessary restorations. False-negative diagnoses imply that caries is left untreated.

Visual inspection
The limited value of visual inspection of occlusal surfaces becomes more reliable using criteria based upon translucency (after 5 seconds of air drying), opacity and brown discoloration.[154 156] Prior to air drying, the surface is cleaned with a rotary brush. Such visual diagnosis by trained observers was found to be highly sensitive (92–97%) and specific (85–93%).[154]

Probe
A sharp probe sticking in a sound fissure is suggestive of caries. Use of force may damage the enamel and prevent an initial lesion from remineralising.

Transillumination (FOTI)

Fissures may be inspected with a cold-light source.[16] Fibre-optic transillumination (FOTI) of molars revealed deeper dentine caries moderately successfully.[632 680 681] Combined with visual inspection, FOTI is useful for the assessment of occlusal lesion depth, and performs better than electric conductance method (ECM) and DIAG-NOdent (see later).[124] Digitised transillumination with a camera and computer (DIFOTI) seems promising.[523]

Radiographs

Radiographs of molars show small, non-cavitated occlusal lesions if extending into the dentine.[300 633] Based on radiographs, many histologically severe carious molar fissures were falsely declared sound.[154] The sensitivity of radiographic assessment in one study varied from 0.41 to 0.94.[162] Radiography by itself may be "inaccurate and non-sensitive",[656] but in combination with visual inspection it may be highly sensitive (0.90) and reproducible.[369] Larger dentine lesions are easily detected, but "false-positives" are sometimes a problem.[162] Repeat radiographs can provide evidence of lesion progression.

Electric current

Sound enamel is a good electrical insulator. Demineralised, porous enamel takes up fluids, which increases electrical conductance. ECM performs well, but is time consuming and difficult.[20 34 154 487 656] Sensitivity of ECM is high (up to 0.96)[490 656] if the air flow used to dry the surface is strong enough.[489] Compared with visual examination, FOTI and bitewings, ECM was *in vitro* more sensitive and specific in diagnosing initial occlusal caries.[34] The specificity of ECM means that, however, about 13–23% of sound teeth may be restored.[370 656] On the one hand, studies show that visual inspection outperforms ECM,[154] but on the other hand, studies show that ECM over a period of 2.5 years was a better predictor of occlusal caries than visual inspection and FOTI, but there were only small differences between the results obtained with the various methods.[169]

In the presence of brown spot lesions and staining, different cut-off points may be required for ECM and DIAGNOdent.[124]

False-positives, for instance fissures without enamel at the bottom, may decay with time. ECM has been found to aid prediction about whether freshly erupted molars should be sealed 1.5 years later.[263]

The Electronic Caries Monitor incorporates a probe, the tip of which touches the enamel, and measures the site-specific resistance of the tooth, while the surrounding enamel is dried with air. With this less time-consuming technique, the entire occlusal fissure system is covered with a conducting medium; experimentally, the reproducibility has been found to be good.[261] Caries Meter L has a solid probe (wet with saline), which is placed on air-dried occlusal enamel. The sensitivity of the electrical methods has been shown to be higher than that of bitewings and visual inspection, but the specificity of visual inspection was higher.[260]

Other detection techniques

Laser fluorescence (DIAGNOdent®)[123] is based upon the difference in fluorescence of sound and carious enamel.[371] Red light from a laser diode directed to a tooth surface with a probe penetrates the outer 1.5 mm of thoroughly cleaned and dried occlusal enamel. The scattered, reflected light is measured. The emitted fluorescence is displayed as a numerical value and differs between sound and carious enamel and dentine containing fluorescent material (either with or without bacterial contamination).[584] The high reproducibility of DIAGNOdent may enable monitoring of lesions.[428] The sensitivity is 0.76–0.87 for non-cavitated occlusal lesions in enamel and/or dentine.[26]

DIAGNOdent outcomes have been confirmed against the gold standards "histology" and "transverse microradiography". The technique has been demonstrated to measure remineralisation of small white spot lesions as well as longitudinal mineral loss along amalgam restorations,[220] and gives more true positive diagnoses than bitewings.[50] High rates of bacterial ingress in dentine increased the DIAGNOdent readings,[271] as did in fissures that changed from sound to carious. Anttonen *et al.* found that DIAGNOdent values at baseline were higher in teeth that became carious than in teeth that remained sound.[23]

Problems associated with the use of DIAGNOdent include effects of extrinsic staining, distinguishing between carious and developmental hypomineralisation, and access to interproximal surfaces.[220]

DIAGNOdent appeared a useful adjunct to visual examination of occlusal caries, but use of sealants leads to lower values;[255] however a clear sealant may not affect the DIAGNOdent measurements.[22] Compared with visual inspection, pressure probing and bitewings, DIAGNOdent has been found to perform better (in deciduous teeth) for detecting caries in the inner and deeper occlusal enamel. In particular the sensitivity exceeds that of conventional methods.[371] However, diverging results for the various methods are reported.[497 655] Polishing the teeth may increase DIAGNOdent values.[255]

The *Er:YAG (erbium:yttrium aluminum garnet) laser* was found to be excellent (sensitivity 0.96 and specificity 0.97) in detecting *in vitro* occlusal caries, if reaching beyond the dentino-enamel junction.[634] The validity of assessment of the extent of natural intrinsic fluorescence in carious dentine with an *argon ion laser* is doubtful.

The relative mineral content of carious dentine as seen with backscattered scanning electronic microscope correlates with the autofluorescence, but the depth of the lesion was greater according to confocal laser scanning microscopy.[47]

The newer methods of caries detection need further development and *in vivo* validation. They are often time-consuming, expensive and impractical,[461] but may be adequate for research projects, such as the quantification of demineralisation and remineralisation.[12 18]

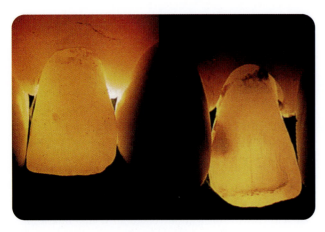

Figure 5.10 Transillumination facilitates caries detection, specially in the anterior teeth. The lesion is visible as a dark spot.

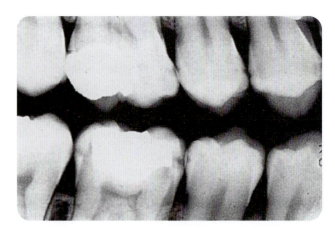

Figure 5.11 Caries on the approximal surfaces seen on a bitewing radiograph; the lesions are of varying severity.

5.8.3   Approximal caries

Visual inspection of anterior teeth often suffices to detect approximal lesions, enhanced by transillumination (Figure 5.10).

FOTI (preferably from buccal aspect)[546]

On the posterior teeth, FOTI discloses only those lesions that extend into the dentine as dark areas, that is lesions restricted to the enamel are not revealed.[465] Sidi *et al.* found that FOTI revealed 75% of radiographically established lesions.[546] FOTI, while equally effective as radiographs for detection of dentine caries *in vitro*,[453] appeared inferior for detection of caries in the permanent (pre) molars *in vivo*. The sensitivity was very low. In another study, bitewings were moderately sensitive (the "gold standard" was inspection of the teeth after forced separation).[247]

In order to decide whether approximal caries needs curative treatment and to evaluate whether preventive treatment has been successful, the depth and the rate of activity of the carious process must be known. In this regard FOTI might be preferable to repeated radiographs. Efforts have been made to improve the diagnostic capability of FOTI by use of a specific wavelength and application of a red dye on the enamel surface; the dye is taken up by the lesion,[628] and carious dentine.[696] This method has been found to be equally effective as radiography *in vitro*.[628]

Radiographs

It has been shown that visual examination without radiographs may leave 75% or more of approximal lesions of the permanent posterior teeth undetected.[161 238 577] However, radiographs show far from all approximal dentinal lesions; the sensitivity ranged from 0.56 to 0.69, the specificity exceeded 0.90.[247] In populations with a low caries prevalence many diagnoses are false positives.[161 208 461] Omitting radiographs results in a considerable loss of information, even if teeth overlap, which hinders assessment of all surfaces.[139]

Dependent on the age of the patient, one-quarter to two-thirds of approximal surfaces of the deciduous dentition cannot be inspected visually.[570] The presence of lactobacilli and mutans streptococci in the saliva and three discoloured fissures in the deciduous dentition warrants further investigation with radiographs because clinically unobservable dentine caries may be present.[499] Bitewings taken in one sample of 5-year-olds doubled the number of visually carious surfaces, which were often cavitated.[558] However, when a deciduous dentition is (almost) free of decay, one may consider delaying radiographic investigation.

Diagnosis of approximal caries in the (pre)molars requires the use of radiographs, on which demineralisation is depicted as dark areas (Figure 5.11). In deciduous teeth separated for 1 week, far more initial approximal lesions were visible to the eye than were evident on radiographs.[465]

A dentine lesion is only manifest radiographically after a certain amount of mineral loss. Technical factors, the mass of the enamel and lesion, the angle of the X-rays, etc. co-determine the visibility of the lesions on the radiograph.[208] In sections of carious teeth, the lesions may be 40% larger than they appear on radiographs.[571] Disagreement has been found among dentists with regard to the diagnosis of approximal lesions on bitewings,[405 410 470] the lesion stage and the type of restoration needed.[134 409 470]

The diagnostic problems associated with detection of caries of the posterior approximal surfaces on radiographs[411 412 464 631] can be overcome by use of computerised caries detection on digitised radiographic pictures, which increases the accuracy.[172] Reproducibility of grading of radiolucency size is shown to be more consistent with image analysis than on visual assessment.[467]

One software program using image analysis correlates image features with a database of known proximal caries problems. In one study, compared with visual diagnosis using radiographs, this method increased the sensitivity of the diagnosis from 70% to 91%; the specificity, however, remained unchanged.[187]

Two more diagnostic indicators

- Discoloured carious dentine may shine through sound enamel. If an (amalgam) filling is already present, the abnormal colour may be due to the filling or corrosion products.[306 506]
- Dental floss drawn between the (pre)molars will fray if it comes in contact with sharp cavity walls.

5.9   Rate of progression of the carious process

Underneath undisturbed plaque on sound enamel, a white spot develops within 2–3 weeks.[318] In deciduous teeth, lesion progression through the outer half of the enamel takes about a year and through the inner half somewhat lesser time. During the first 1.5 years, 3% of the initial enamel lesions in permanent teeth and 20% of the dentinal lesions with an intact surface on radiographs cavitate.[682] A white spot in children's permanent teeth cavitates on the average within 1.5 years,[452] in 15-year-olds within 2 years, and in 21–24-year-olds in about 3 years.[699]

In approximately 3 years, an untreated approximal enamel lesion reaches the dentine, more slowly in buccal and lingual caries, and the majority do not extend beyond the outer half of the dentine for about another 5 years.[404] During a 3-year period, preventive measures (fluoride application, professional plaque removal, hygiene instructions) in children halted the progression of 86% of approximal enamel and 63% of dentine caries.[67] In areas with low fluoride water, approximal carious lesions progressed through the permanent enamel of Swedish adolescents in 85 months versus in 43 months in American adolescents. The difference was attributed to a superior dental care system in Sweden.[543]

The median survival time of initial caries in Swedish adolescents was more than 5 years, the progression rate being highest in the first 2 years. The median survival time of manifest caries was 3.2 years, with a 5-year survival of 33%.[213]

Caries commonly progresses more rapidly in younger than in older teeth. Probable causes are:

- Incomplete maturation in the newly erupted teeth. Particularly in the first posteruptive year, the enamel continues to acquire significant amounts of minerals, including fluoride.
- The diameter of the tubules in young teeth is so large that the reactive blockage reaction in the tubules is inadequate to stop the caries from progressing.

- Remineralisation may fail to occur in youngsters due to frequent consumption of sweets.

Xerostomia, and, in the elderly, decreased buffering capacity and increased proteolytic activity increase the rate of progression of caries. A lesion in enamel may become permanently arrested and even heal under favourable conditions (see also Section 5.5). Lesions that continue to progress in spite of preventive measures, e.g. brushing twice a day with fluoride toothpaste may take 5–6 years before restoration is needed.[80]

The rate of progression of the caries process determines the time interval between taking radiographs. Both minimising the exposure to radiation and timely detection and monitoring of a carious lesion are desirable, particularly in children and adolescents.[209] Six-monthly radiographs are not recommended, unless severe xerostomia is present or a regular exposure to fluoride is absent.[545] Even in children at high risk or when approximal initial enamel lesions are present, a half-yearly radiographic examination seems unwarranted.[330 436]

Shwartz et al. found that radiographs showed less than 5% of the lesions in a sample of 8–20-year-olds extended within half a year into the inner half of the dentine and about 20% did so within 2 years. Over a period of 12 years, on average 11 lesions developed, of which six reached the dentine.[544] Bitewings every 2.5 years is warranted if enamel lesions are absent in fluoride users.[545] The time interval between routine radiographic examination should be based on individual carious risk assessment.[682] (Enamel) lesions nowadays progress slowly, if at all, and even regress,[463] except in patients at risk. Lack of regular exposure to fluoride (poor prevention) and a cariogenic diet (e.g. consumption of sweets between meals) are the main risk factors, others are older patients with existing cavities, restorations, extractions.[466]

Rapidly progressive dentine caries (acute caries, florid caries) is macroscopically (Figure 5.12) characterised by

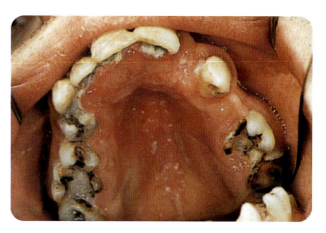

Figure 5.12 Acute caries (see text) in a severely affected and mutilated dentition.

a (light) yellow, sometimes light-brown colour and wet, decayed dentinal tissue (*caries humida*), which can often be removed layer by layer with an excavator. Slow progression is associated with dark-brown to black dentine that is dry and leathery or hard (*caries sicca*) (Figure 5.13). The dentine in the progressing lesions in Figure 5.14 is wet. A brown spot may remain unchanged for many years (*caries insistens, arrested caries, consolidated caries*).

5.10   Epidemiology

5.10.1   Indices

The D(ecayed) M(issing) F(illed) index was introduced in Chapter 3. The DMFT index is used for teeth and the DMFS index for tooth surfaces. For deciduous teeth the lower cast letters dmft and dmfs are used.[55]

Instead of M, A is used to indicate absence due to agenesis, trauma and extraction for orthodontic or periodontal reasons. Deciduous teeth may be spontaneously exfoliated or extracted because of caries; e indicates "extracted" in deft and defs.

When a carious tooth is irreparable, the letter I (in the deciduous dentition i) is noted instead of D (and d).

Teeth that cannot be inspected, for instance due to presence of orthodontic bands, are excluded, indicated with X.

The indices do not provide information about the severity of the lesions: scores from D1 to D4 indicate the lesion depth.[385] D is sometimes estimated twice, once including initial lesions and the second time without.[268] In the CSI (Caries Severity Index) scores 1, 2 or 3 for each surface of the deciduous teeth denote the degree of the decay. The scores are added per tooth.[112]

The extent of root caries is expressed as the percentage of affected/filled roots of the number of denuded roots.[158]

5.10.2   Some prevalence data

In the past, as the cost of sugar went down it became easily affordable for most people. At the same time, in particular during the twentieth century, the prevalence of caries increased enormously. Thereafter, thanks to use of fluoride, caries declined considerably, as is illustrated in Table 5.2.[21]

In 1911–1915, 40% of 25-year-old Dutch men had caries in their posterior teeth and women in 53%.[75] In the Second World War, sugar was scarce: the incidence of caries was low, an effect

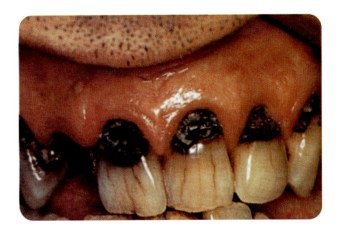

Figure 5.13 Slowly progressive cervical caries in an older person: caries sicca.

Table 5.2 DMFT in Finnish army recruits by year[21]

Year	1919	1965	1976	1981	1986	1991
DMFT	5.2	13.9	15.8	14.5	11.2	7.3

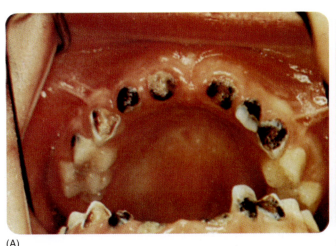

(A)

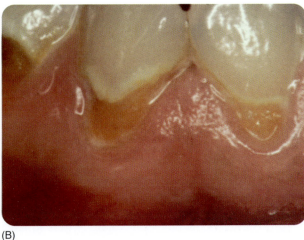

(B)

Figure 5.14 (A) Active caries affecting the whole dentition. (B) Another example of active caries: the lesions are light brown and wet.

lasting to 1979.[9] Epidemiological data show a very substantial decline in dental decay in Dutch children since 1975.[257 258 612 616 618 683]

Some decades ago, 80–90% of (young) West European children had caries,[66] which thereafter decreased in many countries.[202 482] For instance, the DMFS index in 14-year-old Swedes fell from 34 in 1959 to 7.5 in 1984.[72] Also, it halved in a Brazilian community between 1991 and 1997 (fluorosis increased by 80%).[457]

Despite unchanged consumption of sugar from 1960 to 1985, caries prevalence declined.[74] And in dentate persons who consumed sweets[659] caries declined[482] in both the deciduous and mixed dentition,[168] a trend also noted in older age categories.[293 618] In particular Danish and Dutch children scored well in an international comparison of seven countries, but the DMFS in 35–44-year-olds was 13–22.[152] In some countries, the majority of cavities are present in relatively small groups of children and adolescents.[26 205 617] Nationality, socio-economic status, cultural background, environment and age are important factors in the caries experience.[46 293 257 617]

Caries in youngsters is often present in the pits and fissures.[293 485] In western Europe, the dmft has tended to stabilise at 1.3–1.6, but in the former Warsaw Pact countries much higher values are found. At 12 years, the DMFT value may be stabilised at 1.0. Nearly 70% of all countries have achieved the World Health Organization (WHO) goal of a DMFT score 3 for 12-year-olds: In Nepal it is 1.1,[694] but in Puerto Rico it is 6.5.[157] Only a few countries report DMFT scores between 1.1 and 2.1 for older children. European values for the middle-aged range from 13 to 21.[393] In many developing countries, such as Kenya, the prevalence of untreated deep carious lesions is high, though the majority of the lesions are present in a minority of the population.[385] In a sample of 11–12-year-olds, 70% of the approximal surfaces were caries-free and at 21 years about 30%.[404] The scores for second molars were considerably lower than for the first molars. In subsequent years, more and more approximal caries affects the premolars.[485]

Statements that approximately 75% of caries is present in 25% of the population[26 209] are only accurate when applied to a specific age range at a given time.[374] DMFT scores do not reflect the skewed distribution in the population. The significant caries index (SiCI) reveals more, i.e. the mean DMFT of one-third of the individuals having the highest caries values in a population. The SiCI of 12-year-olds varies from 13.7 in Costa Rica to 2.8 in Jamaica.[435] Caries, although far from extinct, has generally declined in children because of the use of effective preventive methods, in particular the use of fluoride.

Nursing bottle caries

Almost 10% of a sample of babies and very young children had nursing-bottle caries; use of fluoride toothpaste reduced the incidence.[677] The proportion of children with nursing bottle caries is not exactly known because published data are derived from selected groups.[421] The reported prevalence varies from 6.8% (Tanzania), 12% (Virgin Isles) and 27% (Riyadh)[690] to 53% (some groups in the USA.).[297 298 537]

Tee found that 5-year-old children with extensive caries were bottle-fed for longer periods than children with few cavities.[599] Immigration has been implicated as a factor.[421] The maxillary central incisors are the most frequently affected teeth, but a great majority of these children have caries in the posterior teeth too.[690]

Root caries

Root lesions are especially found in the elderly population: the age-dependent prevalence increased from 10% to 80%.[164 210 693] DFS scores in elderly Americans were found to decrease with time because of extractions, but the root caries frequency increased.[414] Older people with many natural teeth do not have much root caries,[57] probably because of the composition of their microflora, behaviour, etc.

Studies of selected groups, such as institutionalised patients, may result in overestimation, but population studies may underestimate root caries because of absence of older people with comorbidities in the samples studied.

In different countries 57–95% of older people have been reported to have at least one cervical lesion/restoration.[56 177 180 181 201 364 414]

The Dutch Root Caries Index increased in the 1980s from 7% in 30–34-year-olds to 24% in older people,[290] a trend also noted elsewhere.[322] During a 3-year study, almost two defects developed yearly in 100 denuded roots of older people in rural Iowa, USA.[221] Within 5 years, 2.5% of denuded roots of 60-year-old Swedes became carious compared to 10% in 80-year-olds.[178] Caries and fluorosis were present together.[57] A group of hospitalised elderly people, average age 79 years, developed caries in 0.3 roots in the first year and 1.3 in the second.[375] In another study, the incidence in older people was 0.7 lesions over 3 years, somewhat more in the Caucasian than in the African American group.[343] The ethnic difference was explained by restoration of abrasions, extractions, etc.[344]

Root caries frequently occurs buccally in the mandibular molars, in association with a dry mouth,[32] but also approximally and lingually.[343] The mandibular anterior teeth are least affected.[58] No differences by jaw and between premolars and molars have been noted.[343] Because posterior teeth may be extracted earlier than anterior ones, the distribution of root caries over the dentition does not tell much about the caries experience.[344]

Extractions

Around 30 years ago, caries was the main reason for extracting teeth before the age of 35 years,[526] and it was responsible for half of all extractions in France and the UK[102 355] and for one-third of all extractions in

28–80-year-old men in the USA.[111] Presently, caries and periodontal diseases both account for some 40% of the extractions in Japan.[724] In other studies, extractions decreased the numbers of decayed and filled teeth with age, but the ratio between the decayed, filled and healthy surfaces did not change much until the age of 65 years.[19] [290] [615] From 1983 to 1995 the Dutch DMFT index scores fell only for those younger than 35 years, but the number of edentulous dentitions also fell.[291] From 1978 to 1998, the average number of decayed teeth in the UK dropped because older adults had more filled teeth.[437]

5.10.3   Distribution through the dentition

Caries develops at plaque stagnation sites. Black (1908) classified cavities according to the site of caries as:[82]

- Class I: fissures and pits
- Class II: approximal surfaces of the (pre)molars
- Class III: approximal surfaces of the anterior teeth
- Class IV: Class III including the incisal edge
- Class V: gingival third of the vestibular and lingual surfaces.

In every class, the treatment of the cavity required a specific form of preparation.[455] The composites, which are increasingly replacing the older restorative materials (e.g. amalgam) does not require following strict preparation rules, e.g. extension for prevention.

Caries tends to develop bilaterally and symmetrically,[55] in association with the mirror image morphology of the teeth in the two halves of the dental arches. The mandibular first permanent molars are most frequently carious. Least affected are the mandibular anterior teeth; the maxillary anterior teeth in general are affected more often. The mandibular premolars show relatively few (occlusal) carious defects. The distal surfaces of maxillary teeth, in particular the premolars and lateral incisors, are frequently carious,[55] [403] as are the approximal molar surfaces.

5.11   Prevention

Lesion initiation may be prevented and progression may be arrested or postponed.[466] [598] Caries management includes prevention of demineralisation, promotion of remineralisation, suppression of bacterial growth, acid neutralisation and dietary recommendations. As mentioned above, despite abundant sugar consumption, caries prevalence has decreased, mainly due to the increased in daily exposure to fluoride.[165] [391] Approximately 60% of radiolucencies in the outer half of the dentine are non-cavitated; efforts must be made to promote remineralisation.[24]

One has to diagnose whether a carious lesion is active or passive. The depth of active lesions and the possibility of arresting the process determine whether a preventive or curative intervention is desired, unless aesthetics is an issue. Currently, many dentists are inclined to leave enamel caries untreated,[149] and to avoid creating a cycle of re-restorative treatment.

Risk assessment of individual patients (Section 5.11.9) determines the optimal preventive regimen. Daily fluoride use for primary and secondary prevention and sometimes weekly use of chlorhexidine,[24] counselling and application of fissure sealants are the cornerstones of preventive dentistry. At baseline, the size and extent of all lesions are recorded and the lesion behaviour over time is established with radiographs.[465] High-risk patients must be seen at least four times a year, until lesion arrest is documented for a longer period.

5.11.1   Removal of plaque

Perfect tooth cleaning prevents caries effectively,[318] but many people do not remove all the plaque. Probably owing to the – albeit imperfect – tooth cleaning, a relationship between regular tooth brushing and caries has either not been found[5] [6] [37] [62] [235] [492] [508] [585] or was weak.[64] [568] [620] However, it has been reported that more teeth are preserved by brushing twice rather than once a day, which in turn is better than a lower frequency.[654] Fluoride accounts for a preventive effect both via and not via tooth brushing.[318]

Variations in caries experience are related to the presence of gingival bleeding, which is suggestive of infrequent or insufficient tooth brushing and therefore an infrequent contact with fluoride.[45] [396] *Professional* plaque removal once every fortnight has been shown to prevent caries effectively,[62] [259] [365] which together with intensive patient education has been found to result in a remarkable reduction of visible plaque and active lesions.[106]

5.11.2   Counselling

Caries scores were almost identical in some Dutch municipalities with and without community dental health education (DHE) and counselling.[289] However, since some information is also provided by the mass media in the Netherlands, this may have confounded the effects noted due to DHE. DHE in a Dutch community was found to increase dental knowledge and result in lowered frequency of consumption of sweets,[593] but behavioural changes were only weakly related.[505] However, *intensive* individual DHE, together with use of fluoride, has been found to minimise childhood caries.[593] A dietary history may lead to recommendations, for example regarding the consumption of "hidden sugars" in food and (fruit) drinks and in/around antacids, cough drops, sore throat lozenges, corn syrup, yoghurt and use of (sticky) sweets between the meals.

Marthaler suggested that parents must be warned about transmission of bacteria by kissing the children on the mouth (although it seems unrealistic) and not putting the child's pacifier into their own mouth.[391]

5.11.3 Diet

Sugar in liquid form, consumed *as part of* a meal, is innocuous, but frequent consumption of sweets *between* meals promotes caries, as does that of crisps[301] and other snacks containing starches with a long clearance time; frequent contacts with fluoride make these attacks less damaging.[433] Chronically ill children often consume sugary medicines and/or diets over long periods of time. However, sugar-free alternatives are available.[380]

A pH drop can be neutralised by chewing on neutral food stuffs. Paraffin stimulates the salivary flow, but cheese, peanuts, urea-containing chewing gum and eggs neutralise the pH more rapidly.[263 432] Urea is rapidly converted in ammonium.[311]

After consumption of a doughnut with a sweet jelly, 10 minutes of chewing paraffin raised the pH to 6.2 and of sorbitol gum neutralised the pH.[278] Even a sucrose-containing gum chewed for 20 minutes enhanced remineralisation.[219]

Cheese seems better.[243] In one study, Edam cheese, 5 g chewed over 1 minute in a 2 year intervention study of school children, lowered the caries incidence by one-quarter,[191] and nullified the difference between xerostomia patients and controls.[539] Cheese inhibited (root) caries in animals with inactive large salivary glands.[329] The effect is attributed to casein (which contains a high level of glutamate), calcium and phosphate in the cheese.[240 243 539] Casein inhibits glucan production *in vitro* and thereby bacterial adhesion.[629] Notably, glutamate is present in resting plaque, but the concentration decreases when the plaque acidifies: cheese counteracts this effect.[243]

Use of fluoridated milk, in which CaF_2 does not precipitate since a fraction of the calcium is in the form of free ions, has been found to remineralise root caries under pH cycling conditions *in vitro*. Milk alone also increases mineral deposition and reduces lesion progression.[270]

Apples do not have a substantial positive or negative effect on the pH.[192] Apple polyphenols (tannins) were found to inhibit the activity of bacterial glycosyltransferase *in vitro*, but had no significant effect on the growth of cariogenic bacteria.[692] Grobler *et al.* reported that regularly eating apples influenced the caries experience negatively compared with eating grapes.[206] Ongoing cultivation of sweet apples may have a negative impact on the dental health.

The numbers of *S. mutans* and *S. sobrinus* in the saliva and plaque fell when subjects abstained from consuming sugar over a period of weeks. After the experimental period, the numbers of bacteria increased again, to their original values.[681]

5.11.4 Fluoride

The plaque bacteria are vulnerable to many chemical substances,[517] including components of filling materials[38] and antibiotics. The risk of sensitisation and bacterial resistance makes the use of antibiotics unsuitable.

Fluoride is the most important preventive chemical agent,[165] because it promotes remineralisation. (Aside, fluoride was unsuccessful in preventing postmenopausal hip fractures, as were high doses of vitamin D.[170]) Suggested fluoride regimens (if absent in drinking water) are presented in Chapter 3. Exposure to low doses of fluoride at least a few times a day counteracts the effects of daily pH drops better as opposed to weekly or half-yearly application with higher concentrations.[96]

Some *herbal dentifrices* inhibit the growth of a few microorganisms *in vitro*: *S. mutans* and *S.sanguis*, *A. viscosus* and *C. albicans*, but their antimicrobial properties vary greatly. Some of these dentifrices are contaminated and can promote bacterial growth. Their efficacy and safety (killing of bacteria may disturb the oral ecological balance) requires evaluation.[346]

Caries is not caused by fluoride deficiency, though in fluoride-deficient situations caries does thrive. There is strong evidence that fluoride is effective in early caries management.[96] The anti-caries effect of fluoride is described in various reviews, books and published meta-analyses[45 165 386 505] with regard to administration *via* drinking water,[44] milk,[686] salt,[392] tablets,[196] toothpaste,[664] rinses,[73] and professional gel and solution application.[99]

In Tanzania, children living in low-fluoride areas consume *magadi*, a natural sodium bicarbonate, which has up to 1750 mg fluoride/L.[39]

Fluoridation of drinking water is desirable, but other methods are effective too,[143] such as use of fluoridated toothpastes, which reduces caries by some 25%.[386] Steiner *et al.* found that a 1000 ppm fluoride toothpaste was slightly more effective than one with 250 ppm, developed for pre-school children, for the former concentration increases the risk of fluorosis.[574 672] One systematic review found the strength of evidence to be fair for fluoride varnishes and insufficient for chlorhexidine and agents such as an antibiotic and chewing gum. Use of fissure sealants, acidulated phosphate fluoride, stannous fluoride and silver nitrate reduced the progression of the lesions.[45]

The effect of fluoride is largest for smooth surfaces and relatively small for pits and fissures.[43 44 610 684] In an experimental study, the efficacy of fluoride toothpaste was greater in artificially prepared broader grooves than in narrower grooves, being greatest halfway inside the broad grooves and least at the bottom.[333] The plaque pH is neutralised by mineral dissolution, the resultant action of the acid production. Fluoride reduces enamel solubility, thereby reducing the capacity for pH neutralisation by dissolved minerals, implying that the bacterial acids may diffuse deeper into the fissures.[700] To reiterate, the preventive action of fluoride is based on several mechanisms.

- After demineralisation, the incorporation of fluoride during remineralisation creates acid resistance:[602] a lower pH is needed for demineralisation to occur and the exposure time to the critical pH is shortened. The OH^- ion activity in cariogenic plaque fluid is about 4000 times lower than that of F^- ion activity.[113]
- Small amounts of fluoride during periods of undersaturation reduce the rate of mineral loss from the enamel because the enamel crystal surface absorbs fluoride ions, which acts as a barrier.[602] Fluoride liberated from enamel by the action of the bacterial acids possibly provides temporary protection.
- Antimicrobial effects[424] are doubtful, although rinsing with amine fluoride/stannous fluoride (SnF) moderately inhibits plaque,[481] and brushing with stannous fluoride lowered the plaque index more than brushing with sodium fluoride in a sample of elderly people.[705] Neither the plaque bacterial composition nor the acid production by mutans streptococci are altered by use of fluoride toothpastes.[642]
- Systemic fluoride incorporated during amelogenesis makes the enamel crystal lattice tighter and may prevent caries to a small extent,[391] but the effect is no longer seen in people who move to live in areas without fluoride in the drinking water or after discontinuation of water fluoridation;[116 351] the differences in these people were subtle because of other fluoride sources.[398]
- The local effect is the most important.[30] Fluoride catalyses the precipitation of dissolved calcium and phosphate, which therefore are not lost to the saliva.[601] Small amounts of fluoride (some 1 ppm) influence reaction rates with dissolution and transformation of various calcium phosphate mineral phases within the tooth and plaque.[242] In an *in vitro* study, a remineralising fluid containing calcium and phosphate enhanced the caries resistance effect of 1.23% acidulated phosphate fluoride.[706]

Precipitation partly takes place within the enamel pores and is promoted by the anti-cariogenic potential of casein phosphopeptide-amorphous calcium phosphate nanocomplexes. Incorporation of such complexes in lozenges has been found to significantly enhance remineralisation of the carious subsurface lesions.[103]

The level of free Ca^{2+} ions in the plaque fluid is low. A dicalcium phosphate dihydrate in a fluoride toothpaste increases Ca^{2+} activity in the plaque fluid and thus remineralisation.[583]

It has been noted that the decrease in caries experience is only partly due to the increased use of fluoride[289 393] because the decline started before the widespread use of fluoride.[207]

Fluoridated drinking water

The specific effectiveness of water fluoridation has reduced from 50–70% to 20–30% because of the availability of other fluoride sources.[673]

Fluoride tablets

The use of fluoride tablets (dose: four 0.25 mg tablets taken together every day) can prevent development of caries,[70] but it may increase the risk of fluorosis, more so when the tables are taken once a day. Taking the "motivation of the mother" into account, which determines the number and kinds of all home preventive measures, Kalsbeek et al. did not find any relationship between the use of tablets at age 1.5–6 years and caries at the age of 15.[292] Not all tooth surfaces benefit alike from the use of tablets, and fissures in the least. The fluoride concentrations differ substantially in the left and right site of the mouth and in the upper and lower jaws.[133]

Fluoride toothpaste

Fluoride toothpaste seems the best alternative for fluoridated drinking water[228] and in many populations it is the principal fluoride source. Its use diminished the prevalence of caries in children and adolescents by 20–30%,[386 664 685] but increased the fluorosis scores.[457]

Which form of fluoride is preferred in toothpastes?[152] Studies have shown that sodium fluoride (NaF), within 2–3 years, reduced the prevalence of caries by 6% more than sodium mono fluorophosphate (MFP);[285] after 10–20 years the difference was 10–12%.[578] The fluoride uptake by demineralised enamel is not necessarily highest from a toothpaste with the highest fluoride concentration. A combination of different fluoride formulas may be best.[707]

Rinsing once after brushing, 1 minute with 10–15 mL water, may leave (more) fluoride behind in the mouth and plaque.[554 556]

Almost no fluorosis was found to develop when subjects rinsed three times after brushing, each rinse lasting 2 seconds.[557] Thorough rinsing diminishes the local effect of the fluoride.[554] Sjögren et al. found that compared with three rinses with 15 mL water, a 1-minute rinse with 10 mL water resulted in 26% fewer approximal carious lesions,[555] but these results need confirmation.

Lower and higher concentration fluoride toothpastes are almost equally effective.[13 366 495] In one study, the efficacy of a topical fluoride gel (12 500 ppm) plus a toothpaste (1450 ppm) in lesion reduction was similar to that of use of toothpaste only.[334] Children at risk should brush with toothpastes containing 1000–1500 ppm fluoride.[250] Prescription toothpastes with 1.1% NaF are available for high-risk patients.[704] Addition of magnesium or triclosan may improve the efficacy of fluoride toothpastes.[171]

The bactericidal *triclosan* has not been found to add to the efficacy of a sodium fluoride toothpaste,[233] although plaque was reduced by almost 20%. Triclosan does not remain long in the mouth, but a NaF paste with triclosan plus an essential oil was found to have a positive effect in patients with periodontitis during a 28-week period,[100] and therefore possibly on caries.

The abrasive silica in a NaF dentifrice improves the anti-caries activity of a NaF paste, whereas trimetaphosphate does not.[446]

The depth of artificial lesions reduced after 3 months brushing with a paste containing Mg^{2+} and MPF compared with a NaF paste. Magnesium may enhance the repair of initial lesions, change the fluoride distribution in the lesions and reduce interprismatic pore clogging.[29]

An analysis of toothpastes found that one-quarter of toothpastes from developing countries had less than half of the fluoride available in the free ionised or active form.[646] An established toothpaste showed superior properties to Chinese toothpastes with comparable formulations *in vitro*[163] and a Korean child dentifrice.[708] The abrasive dicalcium phosphate in toothpastes decreases the total fluoride concentration and increases the soluble fluoride concentration over time.[225]

Fluoride rinses

Fluoride preparations are available (USA) as 225 ppm non-prescription rinses for daily use, and 900 ppm for weekly use, as well as 1000–1500 ppm rinses.[272] Rinsing at school ensures that fluoride-deprived children are exposed to fluoride. The effects have been questioned,[141] but neutral 0.2% NaF in countries where dental caries has already declined substantially[480] had an efficacy of 20–50%. High-risk individuals, including those with orthodontic appliances,[193] may benefit from daily rinsing with 0.05% NaF solution.[480]

Rinse formulas, for instance containing SnF, have proven effects. Other active agents in rinses are chlorhexidine, triclosan and thymol, sanguinarin and menthol. Rinses containing alcohol (cancer!) cannot be prescribed to children and those with detergents cannot be used by patients with a dry mouth, because they worsen the oral condition.[480]

Fluoride rinses partly prevented lesion development in enamel slabs from deciduous teeth and completely in slabs from permanent teeth placed in the same mouth.[117]

Root pieces treated for 1 minute with 4% titanium tetrafluoride (TiF_4) were placed in the mouth of volunteers not using fluorides. A dense surface coating formed on the pieces, which partly reduced mineral loss and lesion depth. TiF_4 (pH 1) was also found to reduce caries around orthodontic brackets.[101]

Professional flossing with SnF_2, but not with NaF, reduces caries.[505]

Fluoride gel application

Topical, half-yearly application of a fluoride gel should be reserved for groups at risk and its use in most people is superfluous.[525] Progressive caries in xerostomia requires rinsing twice a day with a fluoride solution, but severe hyposialosis requires two applications per day of a stronger neutral fluoride gel in disposable trays.[274 661]

When the population caries incidence is low, the fraction prevented by professional and self-applied gels containing >1% fluoride is about 20% in permanent teeth. The associated costs though are high.[494 505 649] Evidence that caries-active or high-risk individuals benefit from the applications is insufficient because of flaws in study designs.[45]

Fluoride containing varnishes

Substantivity (the slow release of molecules) of drugs in the mouth demands sustained-release devices, which include varnishes. Topical varnishes differ in their polymeric matrix,[572] additives, therapeutic agents and behaviour. Some adhere to the tooth surfaces by their resin fluoride carrier for a longer time than the other fluoride products.

A fluoride varnish was found to be more effective for enamel than some chlorhexidine formulations in an *in vitro* situation; dentine was protected better by the latter.[643] Use of 2.6 w% fluoride and other varnishes, for instance, chlorhexidine, reduces caries in the permanent dentition on the average by almost 40%. The evidence for caries reduction in deciduous teeth is limited.[505] For people with special needs living in optimally fluoridated communities, fluoride varnish is preferred to an acidulated fluoride gel and a 0.2% NaF rinse, but sealants are preferred when occlusal surfaces are at risk.[679]

In a Chinese study, carious deciduous teeth were treated annually with 38% silver diamine fluoride (SDF with 44800 ppm fluoride). A second group was treated every 3 months with a fluoride varnish (22600 ppm). The SDF group developed fewer new caries lesions and more existing lesions became arrested. Prior removal of carious tissue did not enhance the effect. A black-stained impermeable, caries-resistant layer on the tooth surface consisted of yellow silver phosphate that discoloured black under sunlight.[362]

Varnishes are suited for high-risk patients, if compliance with the other topical fluoride regimens is difficult.[272] Fluoride varnish (or topical fluoride gel) application at 6-monthly intervals for patients at a moderate risk, and when older than 6 years, every 3 months for those at high risk seems in order.[709] An intraoral fluoride releasing system that can be worn continually and is attached to the upper molars has shown encouraging results in radiation-induced xerostomia.[704]

Prenatal fluoride

Fluoride tablets taken by the mother during pregnancy (Chapter 3) does not have a substantial effect on the deciduous teeth of the child.[352]

Unexpected findings

Villa and Guerrero reported that equal amounts of fluoride do not protect all to the same degree.[657] In regions with optimally fluoridated water, the caries prevalence in women has been reported to be higher than that in men.[684]

5.11.5 Other preventive chemical agents

Strontium in drinking water reduces caries,[125] maximally at 5–6 mg/L.[127] Lithium may also prevent caries.[126] These findings require further confirmation; in addition, these studies did not suggest practical measures for using these chemicals.[126]

Chlorhexidine

Chlorhexidine (bisguanide) after rinsing adheres for 8–12 hours to the mucosa and possibly the pellicle, and is an effective anti-plaque agent (the more so with zinc).[197] Its substantivity is dictated by the balance with free molecules. Of the anti-caries varnishes, some penetrate deeper into demineralised dentine and block the pore entrances.[31]

Caries reduction

Fissure caries is reduced with chlorhexidine risining,[284] but not approximal caries, in high-risk and in older children.[229 567] Evidence of an effect is "inconclusive" for caries-active schoolchildren and adolescents with regular fluoride exposure, but the varnish may prevent fissure caries in children with low fluoride exposure. Effects on white spot lesions are doubtful, although it may be beneficial in root caries,[626] but regular rinsing with 0.12% chlorhexidine did not substantially affect the preservation of sound coronal and root tooth structure in older adults.[710]

A positive preventive effect of 46% has been estimated,[649] but more recent studies provide mixed and insufficient evidence of preventive effects.[505] Semi-annual application of a mixture of a fluoride varnish and 1% chlorhexidine was not found to have any additional effect on approximal caries incidence compared with the fluoride varnish alone.[458]

Bacteria

A 15-minutes application of a 40% chlorhexidine varnish on interproximal plaque suppressed mutans streptococci growth for 4 months.[514] A single 7.5-minute application suppressed the growth of salivary mutans streptococci and lactobacilli and reduced lactic acid production in sucrose-challenged plaque, but the effect was not sustained in the long term and was not seen in all the study participants.[711] After a single application of 40% chlorhexidine, the mutans streptococci were still absent after 2 weeks, although the original levels of *A. naeslundii* and *Streptococcus oralis* were rapidly restored.[515] Growth of other bacteria may suppress that of, in particular, *S. mutans* and may account for the long-lasting antimicrobial action of intensive treatment with chlorhexidine.[244 638]

Chlorhexidine inhibits glycosyltransferases, and thus extracellular polysaccharide production,[500] and is thus bactericidal.[196] The hydrophilic properties affect the cell membranes, namely of *S. mutans*.[324] In older people rinsing once a day with 0.12% chlorhexidine there was almost no effect[114] – in fact *in vitro* even 0.2% did not provide sufficient protection. In dentine substrates, the numbers of streptococci declined, but not those of *Actinomyces* or lactobacilli.[650]

Applications (four times at weekly intervals and then every 6 months up to 36 months after birth) of a 10% chlorhexidine varnish could not prevent transmission of *S. mutans* from mother to baby and did not alter maternal caries increments,[132] but the 10% concentration is too low. In another study, levels of *S. mutans* reduced in the mothers, but the oral cavities of their children became colonised with *S. mutans* at the age of 23 months, which was similar to the controls (22 months).[132]

Half-yearly application of 40% chlorhexidine varnish in fissures of permanent molars lowered the incidence of caries in subjects in whom 1 mL saliva contained >10^6 mutans streptococci.[168 678] There was greater suppression of *S. mutans* with thrice-weekly application than application than three times per month.[623] Six-monthly applications over 2 years of a 40% chlorhexidine varnish on the deciduous molars less than halved the caries increment, which was more than with the use of a placebo varnish.[712]

Three applications of a chlorhexidine-gel with 0.2% NaF was less effective than of a varnish with 40% chlohexidine.[459] In another study, use of a fluoride varnish suppressed *S. mutans* growth for 3 months.[624] After 3 months, the numbers of mutans streptococci in saliva were lower after daily brushing with a 0.4% chlorhexidine-fluoride toothpaste than after three applications of a 1% chlorhexidine gel. The number of mutans streptococci in interdental plaque reduced only slighly.[625]

Use of toothpicks impregnated with chlorhexidine, three times a day for 23 days, affected neither the number of mutans streptococci in saliva nor the plaque pH after the first 2 days.[296]

Chlorhexidine, as mentioned above, reduced the number of bacteria and the number of new carious lesions in children and adults,[589] but was not effective against post-radiotherapy acquired Gram-negative bacteria.[566] In other studies, two daily rinses with 0.2% chlorhexidine solution in addition to tooth brushing reduced the plaque and caries increment.[94 354]

Sodium lauryl sulfate, present in toothpastes, may inactivate chlorhexidine,[277] but this claim is unfounded.[713] Zinc ions improve the action of chlorhexidine.[195]

Patients complain about a bitter taste, loss of taste, a burning sensation, occasionally swelling of the parotid gland, and tooth discoloration.[354 459 644] On the whole a single or several chlorhexidine applications do not seem effective in the long term.

Listerine

This bactericidal phenol with essential oils (and alcohol) seems to have a smaller effect on plaque than chlorhexidine,[214] possibly because of lower substantivity, but its use is still promoted in the Netherlands.

Triclosan

The bacteriostatic bisphenol triclosan is added to toothpastes (and mouthrinses) together with a copolymer (vinyl methyl ether)[230] or zinc citrate.

Triclosan is incorporated in soaps, deodorants and cosmetics.[703] Phenols in higher concentration damage bacterial cell membranes and in a lower concentration inactivate bacterial enzymes[517] and interfere with the bacterial uptake of nutrients.[703] *In vitro*, triclosan is bacteriostatic against cariogenic streptococci.[517] Triclosan (0.2%) and zinc citrate (0.5%) added to a sodium lauryl sulfate toothpaste did not result in an additional inhibition of plaque growth. Higher concentrations might be active.[276]

In vitro, triclosan also decreased the number of *S. mutans* and *S. sanguis* in mixed cultures. The effect was larger with added zinc citrate[389] and NaF;[703] 0.3% triclosan was found more effective against plaque than a fluoride toothpaste.[355] Many dentifrices contain 0.3% triclosan, which combined with calcium carbonate, prevents the pH drop after a sucrose rinse to a greater extent than carbonate alone.[590] Because of the differences in the results of various studies, these issues require further investigation.[626]

Triclosan in chlorinated water forms chloroform. However, the amounts are low and not proven to be harmful (i.e. non-carcinogenic). Drinking water contains up to 200–300 mg chloroform/L due to a reaction of hypochlorite with natural organic material.[726]

Tannin
Tannins, phenol-like substances, are present in, for example, wines and some teas. The tannins precipitate proteins and affect the action of glycosyltransferases.[517] Drinking black tea was found to attenuate the development and progression of caries, but was less effective than fluoridated water.[614]

5.11.6 Sugar substitutes

Caloric sugar substitutes (xylitol, sorbitol) are slowly fermented by the oral bacteria and do not lower the plaque pH appreciably. Non-caloric sweetening agents (aspartame, saccharin, cyclamate, stevia) are not fermented and are added to food and drinks to inhibit the development of caries.[420 432 517] The cariogenicity of combinations of such agents is lower than the added cariogenic effects of all the agents separately .[420 517]

Use of chewing gums containing xylitol and sorbitol or urea sodium bicarbonate increases the oral pH.

Xylitol
Xylitol, a sugar alcohol, is obtained from, for example, birch trees and coconut shells. Most plaque bacteria do not ferment xylitol,[150 317 520] but ultimately adapt to it,[563] which seems of little clinical significance. After discontinuation of use, rapid de-adaptation has been noted.[35]

The growth of xylitol-sensitive strains of mutans streptococci is inhibited, which promotes growth of natural xylitol-resistant mutans streptococci, which lack sugar transport mechanisms and phosphorylation. The genes involved have been identified.[63]

In a 2-year experiment (Turku, Finland), all dietary sugar was substituted with xylitol: the caries reduction was almost 100%.[317 520] Use of xylitol gum lowers the bacterial acid production from sugar and reduces counts of *S. mutans* and lactobacilli, while use of sorbitol gum

increases both.[3 90 288 381 382 383 522] However, although xylitol and sorbitol as such were associated with reduced amounts of visible plaque, the number of salivary mutans streptococci was not altered with sorbitol.[714]

Xylitol chewing gums are used in particular by adolescents.[253] The market share of such gums in some countries is 80%.[420] Xylitol gum chewed over several years had the same effect as sealants;[8] children attending daycare centres were found to have a slightly better oral status than those who only brushed their teeth.[326] Söderling *et al.* found that mothers using xylitol-gum during 21 months from the third month after delivery transmitted fewer mutans streptococci to their offspring than mothers treated with fluoride or chlorhexidine.[562] Such a maternal regimen followed for 2 years resulted in 70% lower dmf scores at age 5 years than three half-yearly applications of chlorhexidine varnishes.[269] Xylitol in an enzyme-containing toothpaste decreased the number of *S. mutans* in saliva and plaque; a 10% concentration was more effective than 5%.[273]

The majority of 250 publications have demonstrated xylitol to be effective,[15] but the claims of anti-caries effects and superiority of xylitol over other sugar-alcohols still need confirmation.[518] Gum-chewing data indicated that use of xylitol by young adults with low caries experience altered neither the formation nor the features of plaque.[519] The protective effect remains inconclusive.[361] Xylitol may reduce the numbers of *S. mutans*, but the relevance is not clear. Chewing sugar-free gum three times/day over prolonged periods may reduce caries irrespective of the type of sugar alcohol, due to salivary flow stimulation and mechanical cleaning.[232 376] An antimicrobial effect is not excluded, but evidence is lacking for a therapeutic effect with regard to caries.[640] Indeed, use of a low-dose xylitol tablet did not have a caries preventive effect in preschool children.[715]

The slow absorption of xylitol and sorbitol draws water osmotically into the bowel. High dosages may cause diarrhoea.[432] Chewing a xylitol gum five times a day for 5 minutes caused diarrhoea in 10% of the subjects. The maximum daily dose is set at 4 g xylitol,[518] half of the beneficial dose in persons with (many) carious lesions.[519]

A chlorhexidine-xylitol gum did not stain the teeth, but existing discolorations worsened.[552]

Sorbitol
Sorbitol, manufactured from glucose, is slowly fermented by *S. mutans* and *S. sobrinus*. Use of sorbitol chewing gum promoted enamel remineralisation,[345] more so with addition of 0.1 mg fluoride to the gum.[336] Caries reduction is less than that seen with xylitol chewing gum. After frequent use, the production of bacterial acids from sorbitol increases steadily, but remains relatively small. In patients with diabetes mellitus or xerostomia, sorbitol

gum may be contraindicated.[420] In sum, the anti-caries effect of sorbitol is disputed.

Aspartame

This artificial, non-fermentable, sweetening agent is commonly used in low-calorie diet drinks. In rats infected with *S. sobrinus* fed on a diet containing aspartame, the bacteria were exterminated. As more sucrose was added to the diet, more caries developed in relation to a return of the bacteria in increasing numbers.[131]

5.11.7   Sealant

Fissure sealing, i.e. filling the fissures of the (pre)molars with a resin after etching, is efficient, but expensive. Enamel is, in particular, susceptible to caries during eruption. Fluoride chiefly prevents caries of the smooth surfaces, which means that fissure caries proportionally increases.[205]

Use of fissure sealants additionally reduces the numbers of *S. mutans* and lactobacilli in the saliva.[41]

In 1987, use of fissure sealants was almost absent in Dutch 11- and 17-year-olds; in 1993, an average of two sealed teeth were reported in the same age groups.[293] Since then, 0.5 sealants per year per child are placed in the Netherlands.

Sealants are effective, even where caries is an endemic problem.[268] Rozier found that use of auto-polymerising resins prevented caries in around 70% of teeth, but light-activated resins might be as effective.[505] The reduction seen with second-generation resin sealants ranged from 86% at 12 months to 57% at 48–54 months.[716] A resin sealant seems more effective than a glass ionomer cement,[564 716 717] which is, however, useful when one cannot keep the tooth dry during sealing.

McLean found that in wide fissures, 78% of glass ionomer sealants were retained after 2 years.[402] Two-thirds of the sealants were lost within 2–3 years and after 5 years, only about 10% were fully or partially retained. However, unsealed first molars were twice as much more likely to develop dentinal lesions.[591] Use of glass ionomer sealants may postpone the need for a composite sealant by several years. In one follow-up study, after 7 years, 24% of glass ionomer-sealed occlusal surfaces became carious versus 17% of resin-sealed fissures.[174] The cement is less resistant against wear than a resin sealant.[491] Diluted glass ionomer flows more adequately into narrow fissures.[491] Newer, less viscous glass ionomer materials penetrate and seal the fissures more adequately than the older ones; however, their role in protection against caries needs evaluation.[695]

The protection afforded depends on the retention of the sealant. Irrespective of the dentition and methods used, full retention of resin sealants after 1 year has been found to be 98%, and after 3 years about 95%.[198 667] In other studies, after 4.5 years, 60% of the sealants on molars and 86% on premolars remained,[408] and after 7 years, 45% of sealants were completely and 20% partially retained.[174] The auto-polymerising sealants are probably preferable to the light-activated, because of larger proportion that is retained.[401 493 550] However, according to a systematic review there is no difference in retention between the two types of resin-based sealant, but if the sealant contains fluoride, the retention is decreased.[718] Flowable composites with dentine adhesives may perform equally well as other materials.[719] Loss of the sealant affects the reduction in caries.[493] Re-sealing is possible.

Is sealing cost-effective?[550] In a fluoridated area (re) sealing over a period of 10 years appeared cheaper than (re)restoration,[553] but a recent longitudinal 6-year study showed caries development in as many sealed as unsealed fissures.[471] Sealants must be applied only in fissures at risk, in particular when deep and sharp. The benefits of sealing decline when the caries incidence decreases in the population.[153] Candidates for sealants are patients with caries in the deciduous teeth. High dmfs scores at the age of 6 years are indicative of higher DMFS scores at age 15,[292] and the higher the dmft score, the greater is the number of first permanent molars with carious fissures.[477] However, these associations ($r = 0.50–0.70$)[237 393] do not allow prediction on an individual basis. Early identification of caries with ECM may be an improvement.[262]

One may decide to seal a fissure at the first sign of caries. The preparatory etching reduces the bacterial counts in the fissures by 75%,[605] and a further reduction is due to the sealant application, which prevents substrates from entering the fissure.[303] Underneath 1-year-old sealants in slightly carious fissures the microflora was reduced by 99%,[279] but where caries has extended into the dentine, progression is not excluded.[674]

When a decision is made to seal, the permanent molars should be protected as soon as possible, because occlusal caries usually develops in the first year after eruption, later followed by the second molars and premolars. A fissure must not be sealed where 1 year after eruption the mixed dentition is free of caries, unless the circumstances become less favourable. Exceptions are newly erupted teeth with deep fissures and pits; ("deep" refers to when the point of a probe applied without pressure sinks >1 mm into the fissure).[401]

Evidence-based sealant application

Like all treatments, the decision to seal must be evidence based. To start with, a question is formulated in PICO format: Problem, Intervention, Comparison and Outcome (Table 5.3). Unsealed fissures may remain sound (utility = 100) or become carious (utility = 0). A sealed fissure might have remained sound *without* the sealant, in which case sealing was not desirable (utility = 50). But the sealant may have protected a fissure that would have cavitated otherwise (utility = 100).[639]

In 10–12-year-olds, 40% of fissure caries progresses further.[440] Therefore, one has to decide first whether the carious process in the fissure is active. When every fissure

Table 5.3 Question in PICO format[63]

	The question, divided in 4 parts, states
1. **P**roblem	If a 10–12-year-old patient presents with likely caries in a fissure
2. **I**ntervention	would then the application of a sealant
3. **C**omparison	compared with no treatment
4. **O**utcome	result in less caries?

with active caries is sealed, the probability that the decision to seal is correct equals 40% (utility = 100), but the probability changes to 60% when a fissure that will not become cavitated is sealed (utility = 50). Bearing in mind the utilities and probabilities mentioned above, the outcome of the decision to seal is *actually* estimated to be: $(100 \times 0.4 + 50 \times 0.6) = 70$. The outcome of the decision *not* to seal is: $(0 \times 0.4 + 100 \times 0.6) = 60$. The decision to seal has a higher (70) value than not-to-seal (60), when the caries is active.[639]

Approximal caries was in the past a contraindication to seal, because the "extension for prevention" method required including healthy fissures in the preparation. This principle of preventive extension of the preparation is now obsolete.[456]

5.11.8 Mouthrinses

Mouthrinses may be effective if they contain chlorhexidine or fluoride. Efficacy claims of other rinses are probably inaccurate,[513] and they may even be harmful (Chapter 6).

5.11.9 Identification of groups at risk

Children especially at risk must be identified, so that restorative treatment may be postponed and preventive measures are directed towards those who benefit most from prevention.[26] The combined knowledge about diet (sweets), microflora, hygiene, use of fluoride, cavities and/or restorations enables one to classify the level of risk in a child.[569] The diagnosis of caries should reflect the individual's caries activity, based upon development of new and extension of existing lesions.[20] The "San Antonio Caries Risk Assessment" uses a set of data to classify patients as at low, moderate or high risk. The assessment includes evaluation of the presence of incipient and frank lesions along with co-indicators of caries activity, such as the number of filled surfaces, fluoride exposure, sugar/diet history, the time of the last filling, *S. mutans* counts in saliva, and the unstimulated salivary flow rate.[582]

Prevention of caries occurring as a consequence of xerostomia after radiotherapy is essential,[689] because of the risk of osteonecrosis induced by extractions. Frequent fluoride application at home with a gel and use of artificial saliva are necessary when the rate of stimulated salivary flow is low.

Caries experience

Past caries experience in children may strongly correlate with new caries lesion development,[472] but whether caries in deciduous teeth can predict caries in the permanent teeth is not certain.[209 393 477] Steiner *et al.* found that a low number of sound deciduous molars was the best and most consistent predictor of a high caries increment, followed by "high numbers of pre-cavity lesions on permanent first molars".[573]

Caries of especially the deciduous incisors is the best predictor, and in the mixed dentition the dmfs. At the time of eruption of the permanent second molars, the DMFS of first permanent molars is the best predictor. In adolescents, presence of incipient smooth surface lesions is most indicative.[472] In somewhat older children, the presence of approximal carious lesions or restorations predicts new caries.[358 576]

In 11–13-year-old children without approximal caries, about 2 approximal lesions/subject were present by age 21 years , and those with 3 lesions at baseline had about 7. The risk of new approximal lesions was highest in the first 2 years of the study.[576]

Bacteriological (see below, section on 'Bacteriological test to predict caries development') and behavioural factors, tooth morphology, and cultural background may not add appreciably to the level of prediction.[472 648] The DMFS score represents the most powerful predictor of caries increment in high-risk patients.[26] That is not to say that factors such as smoking are harmless (root caries). In Switzerland the "Dentoprog-method" was developed to estimate the probability of a child's future risk of caries. It involves an equation including the variables: number of sound deciduous molars, non-cavitated but discoloured pits/fissures, and white spots in the smooth surfaces of the permanent first molars.[264 573]

The Dentoprog has been validated against another caries detection method, in other age groups and in groups with different caries experience.[648]

To identify the risk factors in children up to the age of 6 years, an electronic literature search was performed. Altogether, 106 factors were found related to the prevalence/incidence of caries, but because of different study designs only a few risk factors could be identified. Children are most likely to develop caries if they acquire *S. mutans* when young, which is (partly) compensated for by good plaque control, use of fluoride, a non-cariogenic diet and use of xylitol chewing gum by the mother. Bottle and breast-feeding appeared unimportant, while consumption of sugary liquids in bottles appeared a risk factor.[224]

Bacteriological tests to predict caries development

Information on caries development may be gained at the chairside with semiquantitative measurements of

S. mutans and lactobacilli in the saliva, and salivary buffering capacity. *C. albicans* (xerostomia) levels also can be measured.[93 484] It may be argued that presence of active caries makes the tests redundant, because the risk clearly exists, but it has been found that based upon additional test results, dentine lesions can be detected[499] and these tests have helped to predict development of root caries in older people[521] and enabled evaluation of the effect of prevention.

The tests are performed with saliva. However, while bacterial counts in saliva may indicate the degree of colonisation on teeth, the reliability of these tests is doubtful.[603 625] In many patients the number of mutans streptococci and lactobacilli appeared to vary considerably at tests conducted at three timepoints.[281] The sensitivity of the separate and combined tests (75%) is insufficient to detect groups at risk.[604] The differences in counts is the reason for using a broad classification of the counts: presence of 10^3, 10^4, 10^5 or 10^6 bacterial colony-forming units. Monoclonal antibodies with a fluorescent marker can be used to identify specific serotypes of *S. mutans* and other pathogens and provide a reasonably accurate prediction in individual caries-active children.[14 608]

5.11.10   Immunisation

Absence of tooth decay does not *per se* indicate immunity, and the correlation between level of antibodies and caries experience varies.[148 311] Since mutans streptococci are among the primary aetiological agents[365] and caries is an infectious disease, impeding colonisation in early childhood via immunisation may be beneficial. Secretory IgA is the principal immunoglobulin in the saliva.[560]

IgG from the crevicular fluid and IgA from the salivary glands together make up 5–15% of the salivary proteins. These immunoglobulins inhibit bacterial adherence to and colonisation of the teeth. Other antimicrobial salivary proteins are enzymes, such as lactoperoxidase and lysozyme, and non-enzymatic proteins like lactoferrin. Lactoperoxidase inhibits bacterial glycosyltransferases *in vitro*.[325] Antimicrobial peptides (histatins, defensins) might be used as templates to develop a new generation of antibiotics with negligible cytotoxicity.[645]

Enhancement of IgA activity might be the primary effector of adaptive immunity against caries. Targets for immunological intervention could be the virulence factors of the cariogenic bacteria. Antibodies may block either the initial colonisation or the glucan binding of *S. mutans* or inactivate the glycosyltransferases. Another possibility is modification of the bacterial metabolism.[560]

Secretory immunoglobulin A (sIgA) in the saliva reduces the opportunity for *S. mutans* to get established. The serum immunoglobulins IgG and IgM are secreted in insufficient quantities into the crevicular fluid.[14] Children showing developing caries were found to have lower levels of serum IgG antibodies against *S. mutans* than children without caries, but effects of antibodies on caries activity have not been proven.[1 327 604] Extra IgA antibodies from immunised animals or transgene tobacco plants were transferred into the oral cavity (passive immunisation),[310 509 580] which was successful for 4 hours.[226]

Rats orally infected with *S. sobrinus* were immunised intranasally with virulence-associated immunomodulatory protein (VIP; Section 5.2.5) and 3 weeks later they were reimmunised, which inhibited oral colonisation and reduced the number of carious lesions through inducement of salivary immunoglobulin A specific to VIP.[140]

Notably, no relationship exists between the levels of IgA in breast milk and maternal saliva. Active and widespread caries has been found to be associated with only a slight tendency to relatively low IgA levels in breast milk.[104]

In animals, vaccination seems to be effective against caries caused by a *single* microorganism. Parenteral immunisation also seemed possible. The aim is to develop antibodies in the saliva by injection of, for instance, attenuated *S. mutans*.

Immunisation against caries may be promising. Different approaches and delivery systems have been considered.[509 560] Problems include research on animals instead of humans, and that parenteral immunisation might cause side effects and cross-sensitisation. Mucosal immunisation of mothers or children may be safer.[509]

Rats on a cariogenic diet developed less caries after immunisation; the animals were subcutaneously injected with an anti-caries DNA vaccine with inhibited glycosyltransferase (HTF-I) and PAc (protein antigens) which belong to the group of virulence factors of *S.mutans*.[212]

5.11.11   Introducing modified bacteria into the mouth

To establish a less cariogenic flora, modified bacteria have to compete with others already residing in the oral cavity.[597] The plaque is remarkably stable, an outcome of the immune responses of the host and the balance between synergism and antagonism between the various bacteria.[388] Recently, a bacterium has been "engineered", which might be successful in replacing the cariogenic bacteria.

An effector strain must persistently colonise the mouth, prevent colonisation by wild-type strains and growth of other indigenous pathogens to harmful levels, and replace them. *S. mutans* produces alcohol from sugar instead of lactic acid by switching off (with molecular techniques) the gene coding for the enzyme lactate dehydrogenase. If the modified bacterium is implanted at a young age, it survives and caries will be prevented.[580] Recombinant DNA methods yielded a new effector strain of a naturally occurring strain of *S. mutans*. The genetically stable clone produced less acid and more alcohol, appeared less cariogenic, and had a selective advantage in colonising the mouth. A single application of the strain to the patient or mother should result in a permanent protection.[245 246]

Clinical trials, preferably with children at risk, are needed to substantiate the claim that the new bacterium permanently replaces the noxious bacteria.

5.11.12 Ozone therapy

Ozone (three oxygen atoms) is an unstable oxidising and toxic agent that inactivates microorganisms and might in principle be used to prevent and treat caries. *In vitro*, exposure of carious root dentine to ozone for about 10 seconds reduced the microorganism counts to less than 1%. An effect on *S. mutans* and *S. sobrinus* has been demonstrated.[53] *In vivo*, ozone treatment reduces "dramatically" the levels of most microorganisms without side effects. In one study, half of 65 lesions became hard after 3–5.5 months, 27 became less severe and 5 remained unchanged.[53 54] Open carious lesions become harder after 4, 6 and 8 months and laser fluorescence values may be reduced immediately after the therapy.[720]

The literature on ozone therapy to the occlusal pits and fissures and to roots has been reviewed.[486] Of the trials, three met criteria such as randomisation and outcomes measured after 6 months. The risk of bias in the studies was high and the effect on caries inconsistent. It was concluded that there was no reliable evidence that ozone application stops or reverses decay.[486] Approximal caries and deeper cavities cannot be treated with ozone. The therapy might be useful for initial caries on occlusal and buccal surfaces, but good-quality studies with long-term follow-up are needed before the treatment can be considered acceptable.

5.12 Curative treatment

Caries is curatively treated to arrest the process and to replace the lost tissues. Enamel caries must not be treated invasively, yet many dentists still select operative intervention.[594] Cavitation may necessitate restoration to preclude plaque accumulation in and progression of the cavity, but it is preferable to arrest the process with preventive measures.

Criteria have been developed to distinguish active from inactive caries.[439] Active, progressive dentine caries is light coloured, soft and wet. An active lesion becomes arrested within 1 week if plaque is systematically removed.[438] If a closed cavity is exposed, for instance due to enamel fracture, active dentine caries may arrest. In the same vein, Gruythuysen has recently shown that caries treatment in primary molars can be restricted to simply exposing carious dentine by removing just the affected enamel so that the cavity can be kept clean by the patient.[725] This means a consolidated, open dentinal lesion (dry, hard or leathery, brown to black) does not need curative treatment, unless (1) the cavity cannot be cleaned, (2) the cavity is unaesthetic, (3) it has sharp walls that may damage soft tissues, or (4) food becomes impacted between the teeth. To enable maintenance of hygiene, one may cut away enamel that has been undermined by caries of the dentine.

Table 5.4 Classification of carious lesions according to the management options[465]

Management option	Code	Description of caries status
No active care (in low-risk patients)	–	Subclinical (suspected) lesion in state of progression or regression (requires use of additional diagnostic aids)
	–	Lesions detectable only with additional diagnostic aids (e.g. FOTI, bitewings)
Preventive care	D1	Clinical obvious but closed lesions
	D2	Cavities limited to enamel
	D3	*Stable* lesions in dentine, open or closed
Preventive + operative care	D3	*Progressive* lesions in dentine, open or closed
	D4	Lesions involving the pulp

FOTI, fibre-optic transillumination.

Curative treatment involves removal of at least part of the infected dentinal tissues (Section 5.12.2). Active caries is characterised by progression on sequential radiographs. There are systems available to classify and record the depth of caries (progression over time), for example the caries lesion depth classification system.[2] Table 5.4 shows the management options based on the level of caries activity.[465] Curative treatment has been proposed for a D1 lesion.[26] A visual and tactile scoring system (Table 5.5) is used for smooth surface caries.[439]

To validate "active" and "inactive" scores, Nyvad *et al.* re-evaluated teeth after 3 years. The probability that an active non-cavitated lesion cavitates is 1.24 times greater than for an inactive one, but both behave in a similar fashion if children brush with fluoridated toothpaste under supervision.[440]

The preparation and restoration of cavities has been described elsewhere.[455 456] Modern restorative materials and new insights have brought about considerable changes in the principles and methods of cavity preparation and restoration.

5.12.1 Extension of the preparation outline

G.V. Black's (1908)[82] principle of "extension for prevention" has became outmoded because of improved preventive measures. Nowadays, preparation is direct to minimizing tissue removal: the cavity opening has to allow access for removal of infected dentine (but see Section 5.12.2) and insertion of the restorative material. Undermined enamel is removed, however, because restorative materials provide less support than dentine,[342] but occlusal enamel overlying carious dentine is not always likely to collapse, being stronger than was believed in the past.[407]

Table 5.5 Score system for smooth surface carious lesions

Score	Category	Description
0	**Sound**	Normal translucency and texture of enamel; sound fissures may be stained
1	**Active** caries (with intact surface)	Whitish-yellow enamel surface, opaque with loss of lustre; feels **rough** when a probe tip is gently moved across surface. No visible loss of substance
		Smooth surfaces: lesion is typically located close to the gingival margin
		Fissure/pit: intact fissure morphology; lesion extends along the fissure walls
2	**Active** caries (with break in the surface)	Same criteria as for score 1. Localised surface defect (microcavity) in enamel only
		No undermining of enamel surface or softened floor detectable with explorer
3	**Active** caries (cavity)	Enamel/dentine cavity easily visible with naked eye; surface of cavity feels **soft** or **leathery** on gentle probing. Pulp may or may not be involved
4	**Inactive** caries	Whitish, brownish or black enamel surface, that may be **shiny**, and feels **smooth** and hard when the tip of the probe is moved gently across the surface. No visible loss of substance
		Smooth surfaces: lesion is typically located some distance from the gingival margin
		Fissure/pit: intact fissure morphology; lesion extends along the fissure walls
5	**Inactive** caries (with break in surface)	Same criteria as for score 4. Localised surface defect (microcavity) in enamel only
		No undermining of the enamel or softened floor detectable with explorer
6	**Inactive** caries (cavity)	Enamel/dentine cavity easily visible with naked eye; surface of the cavity may be **shiny** and feel **hard** on probing with gentle pressure. No pulpal involvement

Scores 7–9 for fillings with and without active/passive caries omitted.[439]

5.12.2   *Removal of infected dentine*

After removal of all soft dentine, bacteria have been found in the tubules of healthy dentine.[337] However, microbial invasion seems restricted to the outer soft, discoloured dentine; under this layer is a soft, discoloured layer without bacteria, followed by soft dentine of normal colour. These observations imply that with the removal of discoloured dentine, either black-brown, brown, brown-yellow, yellow or light yellow, all infected dentine is removed.[186]

There are some problems in regard to excavation. Demineralisation of dentine precedes microbial invasion. Soft dentine cannot support a filling and must therefore removed. However, assessing the hardness of the dentine with hand instruments is subjective, inconsistent and unreliable,[186 310] and the degree of hardness does not differentiate between infected and non-infected demineralised dentine.[527] Discoloration may be a better guide for the removal of infected dentine than hardness.[185] Discoloration of dentine, which precedes bacterial invasion, does not extend as deep as the demineralised dentine; but it may not be a valid guide for tissue removal because of several reasons, including that the discoloration may be light and indistinct.[186]

Caries indicators

Caries indicators, 1% acid red or 0.5% basic fuchsin dye in propylene glycol (the latter believed to be carcinogenic)[184] may stain infected[514] (Figure 5.15), but not uninfected decalcified dentine.[16 17 183] These dyes have been

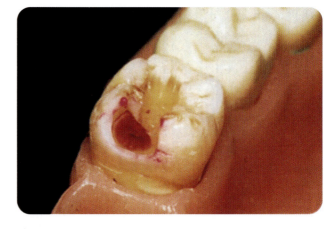

Figure 5.15 After rinsing away of the caries indicator dye (red) the infected dentine remains discoloured and this must be removed. Currently, when a two-step treatment method is used such discoloured tissue is left behind, unless it is present at the dentino-enamel junction (see text).

shown to be reasonably reliable indicators for dentine that must be removed,[182 504 697] although some studies shed doubt on their reliability.

In one study, only half of the microorganisms in dentine underneath old amalgam restorations were stained by red acid.[86] Bacteria, admittedly not many, were present in non-stained (fuchsin) dentine areas.[17] Stained and non-stained areas in hard, normal coloured dentino-enamel junctions were equally infected.[305] The caries indicator showed lesions to be less deep than the polarising microscope and micro-hardness measurements.[310] The untangling of collagen fibres due to irreversible breakdown of the intermolecular cross-linkages might permit penetration of the dye and the discoloration may therefore not be related to demineralisation.[184 331] The non-specific protein dyes stain carious dentine, the organic matrix of less mineralised dentine, circumpulpal dentine and sound dentine at the dentino-enamel junction.[400 697] Use of a dye may therefore result in unnecessary tissue removal.[304] With the use of another (blue) dye, some infected dentine was left behind, but sound dentine was seldom removed.[316]

Lennon *et al.* found that fluorescence-aided caries excavation was more effective in removing infected dentine compared with use of caries detector dyes.[721]

Softened dentine may recalcify completely.[182] The need to remove all infected dentine has been challenged. This is because one may over-prepare a cavity and open up non-obliterated tubules in unaffected dentine, which may lead to pulpal reactions.

Stepwise excavation

In this method, deep carious dentine is removed in two sessions, in an attempt to arrest an active process, and to prevent damage to the fragile dentine layer covering the pulp to avoid pulp exposure. In the first session, centrally located infected dentine is left behind and covered with a layer of calcium hydroxide ($Ca(OH)_2$) base and a temporary filling. Weeks to (many) months later, the cavity is re-opened and the remaining soft dentine is excavated, which at this stage often is possible without pulp exposure: hard, dry, dark dentine is left behind.[81 350 378] Maltz *et al.* found that provisional sealing led to hardening of the dentine in 80% of the teeth and a leathery dentine layer in 17% (the dentine remained unchanged in 3%).[384]

Some authors therefore propose not to re-open the cavities.[384 394] In one study of deciduous molars the stepwise method failed to produce a significant reduction in the risk of pulp exposure compared with one-step excavation.[236]

$Ca(OH)_2$ sealing decreases the bacterial counts,[17 236 384] which no longer represent a typical cariogenic microflora.[78 236] Long-term sealing with $Ca(OH)_2$ reduced, sometimes completely, the number of bacteria in the carious dentine left behind.[79] Hydroxyl ions from $Ca(OH)_2$ may suppress infection.[451] Bacterial counts indicated that only soft and wet dentine at the dentino-enamel junction must be completely removed.[308]

Also, in a 10-year follow-up study, soft, wet dentine sealed with composite restorative materials or amalgam fillings did not progress during the follow-up period, as nutrients were unable to reach the lesion.[407] Application of sealants on occlusal dentine caries also inhibits caries progression.[222]

5.13   Preparation/excavation techniques

More recent techniques for the removal of the dental hard tissues and carious dentine are listed in Table 5.6. When using burs, it is difficult to discriminate between irreversible and reversible demineralised dentine; even sound dentine may be removed. Hand excavators are more self-limiting, and only denatured and demineralised dentine may be removed.

Carisolv, composed of sodium hypochlorite (0.51% w/v; pH 11) mixed with a red gel (containing three amino

Table 5.6 Relative efficacy of various preparation techniques used on sound as well as carious enamel and dentine[49]

| Category | Efficacy on[a] | | | | Notes |
| | Enamel | | Dentine | | |
	Sound	Carious	Sound	Carious	
Mechanical, rotary					
High-speed air turbine burs	3	3	3	3	Pain, unable to discriminate between sound and carious dentine
Slow speed handpiece burs	2	3	3	3	Pain, unable to discriminate between sound and carious dentine
Mechanical, non-rotary					
Hand excavators	0	0	1	2	Less pain, unable to discriminate between sound and carious dentine
Air-abrasion	3	3	2	1	Depends on abrasive
Air-polishing	1	1	1	0	Requires hard surface
Ultrasonics	1	1	1	0	Retrograde root cavity
Sono-abrasion	1	1	1	0	Under-preparation
Chemo-mechanical					
Caridex	0	0	0	?	Expensive/large quantities required
Carisolv	0	0	0	3	Mechanical access needed
Enzymes	0	0	0	1	Need more research
Photo-ablation					
Lasers	1	1	1	1	Expensive/type dependent

[a]Score 3 = very effective. Score 0 = no effect.

acids and sodium hydroxide), decomposes the framework of degraded collagen; the unsupported mineral is easily scraped off with specific hand instruments. The treatment is continued until a hard surface is left.[48][49] Denatured and demineralised dentine dissolves completely in the sodium hypochlorite.[223] The longer treatment time with Carisolv is compensated by the reduced need for anaesthesia. Drilling and injections are among the most feared dental procedures: use of Carisolv may be preferred in anxious patients.[179] However, neither children nor dentists in one study found a direct advantage in using Carisolv compared with traditional caries removal methods in lesions with minimal cavitation.[722]

Lasers cannot be used to shape a cavity, but they are painless. In contrast to earlier findings, enamel irradiated with erbium lasers *in vitro* appeared to be more susceptible to acid cycling than a cavity prepared with a diamond drill, and is therefore less resistant to secondary caries.[27]

5.13.1   Side effects of commonly used restorative materials

The choice of the restorative material is dictated by objective and subjective considerations. Patients prefer tooth-coloured fillings for cosmetic reasons over dental silver amalgam that is allegedly toxic. However, every restorative material has its own disadvantages.

Amalgam fillings continuously release some mercury vapour ($Hg°$) and possibly mercuric ions (Hg^{2+}). Part of $Hg°$ is absorbed (lung, gastrointestinal tract) and circulates with the blood. Before $Hg°$ is oxidised, it diffuses through the cell membranes and is then oxidised into Hg^{2+} and as such stored in tissues, including the brain, with the main target being the kidneys. Part of the absorbed mercury is excreted with the urine and in other ways.[687]

In spite of dissenting opinions and poorly substantiated claims of toxicity,[462][579][702] there remains a lack of convincing evidence that mercury from amalgam fillings is toxic to patients.[120][121][122][194][218][254][377][531][627][688][725] Any adverse effect on human reproductive function is unlikely, even in the dental team, which is exposed to higher mercury concentrations than patients.[533] Incidentally, doses higher than the commonly ingested 5–9 µg/day may be reached, in particular, with excessive use of chewing gum.[52][190][338] [377][512] Oral lichen planus (there are several variants of this persistent mucosal disease) is possibly of allergic origin. Removal of amalgam fillings in contact with areas showing lichen planus often results in remission, also in case of a negative skin test.[535]

Composite restorations and sealants release minor amounts of pseudo-estrogens (especially bisphenol-A)[443] [444] of low potency,[534][561] but large doses of leached out components have been found to lead to reduced fertility in male mice[11] Although several composites based on bisphenol-A-dimethacrylate (bis-GMA) do not contain detectable quantities of bisphenol-A.[669] composites based on bis-GMA dissolved up to 100 ng bisphenol-A/mg saliva.[723] Leached out photo-stabiliser, photo-initiator and an inhibitor with an oestrogenic effect were identified *in vitro*, but the amounts of these very weak oestrogen mimicking agents seem too small to cause any adverse effects.[669]

Composite may release components like bisphenol-A and bis-DMA.[443][474] In saliva and with esterases bis-DMA may be converted into bisphenol-A.[522] High doses of bisphenol-A (37.5–150 mg/kg) caused molecular changes and cell proliferation in the uterus and vagina in ovariectomised rats. A continuous dose over 3 days (300 µg/kg/day) induced differentiation and hypertrophy of epithelial tissues in oestrogen-sensitive rats. Bisphenol-A dissociates slowly from the oestrogen receptors.[575] Exposure of rat fetuses to high doses of oestrogens inhibited prostate development, but low doses induced a twofold increase in the number of prostatic androgen receptors[666] and prostate enlargement with reduced sperm efficiency.[427][665] The findings have not been confirmed.[33]

Altogether, it is premature and unnecessary to bar use of composite resins because of an oestrogenic action,[725] but as yet not all questions have been resolved.[561] Sensitisation (delayed or type IV or contact allergy) may be a problem, but with the exception of dentists (dermatoses of especially the fingers), few individuals are reported to experience allergic problems.[239][536]

5.13.2   Longevity of common filling materials

The lifespan of all restorations is limited. Two-thirds of restorations placed are re-restorations.[688] Half of the *amalgam* fillings placed every year are replacements of existing ones, the majority because of secondary caries.[415] Recurrent caries along the margins of restorations,[175] bulk fracture of the restoration, marginal failure, dimensional defects, size of the filling, and type of alloy affect the longevity of amalgam restorations.[241] Corrosion products fill the space between the amalgam filling and cavity wall; slight marginal failures do not lead to recurrent caries.[454]

Secondary caries may be masked by the amalgam restoration. For detection of secondary caries under a composite restoration a 10° vertical angle of the X-ray tube is best; under amalgam the angle is unimportant.[622] Secondary caries shows up as radiolucent areas but must not be confused with a thick layer of bonding agent applied on the floor of the cavity and underneath composite restorations.

Secondary caries usually consists of an outer lesion, caused by plaque and carbohydrates that are trapped or diffuse through the restoration margins, and an inner lesion in the walls along the tooth–restoration interface.[307] A marginal defect about 50 µm (or >250 µm)[418] wide between tooth and filling might suffice for initiation of secondary caries.

Use of a fluoride varnish was found to slow down secondary caries progression but a placebo varnish tended to do the same.[173]

Radiopaque areas on radiographs underneath amalgam restorations do not represent active caries,[635] but are assumedly related to metals that have penetrated demineralised dentine.

Most of the factors responsible for failure of amalgam restorations also account for failure of *resin-composite* restorations, in particular secondary caries due to accumulation of plaque in gaps in the cavity walls, a consequence of setting shrinkage.[241] However, microleakage in the gaps may not be significant.[532] Main disadvantages of composites are discoloration and wear, but modern materials have greatly improved properties. Fracture of the filling (less frequent with hybrid composite) and tooth fracture/infraction are other problems.[241]

In the 1980s, half of the resin-based composite restorations failed within 6 years, and in permanent teeth of children within 2 years.[475] At that time, half of the amalgam restorations were replaced after 8 years.[476] However, in three Australian dental offices, half of the composite fillings survived for 16 years (amalgam 22 years).[231] Small composite restorations were in 1997 assessed to last 4 years and large ones 3 years,[419] but in a 5-year clinical evaluation, 28% of class II composites failed.[320] Between 1986 and 1997, composite restorations lasted fewer than 5 years to more than 14 years, and amalgam restorations lasted 5 and 11–12 years, respectively.[142]

More recently, the median survival of amalgam restorations in adults was found to be 11 years and of composite restorations 8 years, and in adolescents 5 and 3 years, respectively.[417] According to a meta-analysis, the median annual failure rate of stress-bearing posterior fillings in permanent teeth was 1.1% for amalgam, 2.1% for resin-based composites and 7.7% for glass-ionomer cements.[241] Many of the factors affecting the longevity of fillings could not be confirmed; the multiplicity of study designs makes meta-analysis impossible.[110]

The longevity of amalgam restorations still seems to exceed that of composite resin ones by almost a factor of two,[175] but if carried out under ideal circumstances the annual failure rate of composite and amalgam fillings would be similar.[524] The longevity of *glass-ionomer cement* (GIC) fillings in stress-bearing situations is the least, often because of bulk fracture, but research into improvements in the material's properties is ongoing.

In developing countries, carious lesions are excavated and successfully filled with viscous glass ionomer (atraumatic restorative treatment). Retention rates in deciduous teeth are not impressive. Materials and methods that yield greater success are needed.[25]

The rate of wear of GIC is high, but as the wear progresses, the rate declines. Despite relatively poor mechanical properties, GIC offered new perspectives for treating root caries,[68] especially the release of fluoride, which may prevent caries in the surrounding areas of the tooth.[426] Compared with a fluoride-releasing dentine-bonded composite, a conventional GIC with its replenishable fluoride content performed better in a short trial.[199] However, secondary caries is a main reason for failure of GIC fillings.[241] GIC, resin-modified GIC and glass ionomer modified composites (the compomers) are useful as semi-permanent fillings in deciduous teeth and in cervical lesions.

In a Swedish study, 50% of GIC fillings were replaced after 3 years, 50% of composite fillings after 6 years, and 50% of amalgam restorations after 9 years.[416]

S. mutans counts in plaque near brackets bonded with either GIC or composite did not differ. *S. sobrinus* was present close to the composite bonding material in a few patients, who subsequently developed caries.[447]

More recent developments include *giomer* cements (pre-reacted glass ionomer technology to form a stable phase of glass ionomer in the restorative) and orcomers.

6

Erosion

6.1   Introduction

Dental erosion is an often painless, progressive, irreversible loss of hard tooth tissue, first the enamel and denuded cementum and subsequently the exposed dentine. Erosion occurs due to chemical dissolution of these tissues by mechanico-acidic or idiopathic processes.

In material science, erosion is viewed as wear caused by flow of fluid with abrasive particles.[243] "Corrosion" is a physico-chemical or electrochemical process.[116 117] Hence, erosion is also called "corrosive wear".[192]

Enamel dissolves in distilled water,[169] but not in saliva, which, at pH 7, is supersaturated with respect to the teeth, unless chelation takes place,[75] i.e. organic molecules bind calcium ions bivalently.[47] At a pH ~5.5 (or <6)[305] saliva is undersaturated and dissolves the enamel: the more acidic the environment, the greater is the enamel surface loss and softening.

Rinsing with 2% citric acid (pH 2.1) makes the saliva undersaturated for 2 minutes. As the acid is washed away and neutralised by the saliva[216] the oral environment returns to a state of supersaturation.[27]

Erosion versus caries (Figure 6.1)
Under the plaque layers, bacterial acid production leads to carious white spots (Chapter 5). As with composite etchants,[118 292] the amount of minerals dissolved by the strong exogenous acids from the superficial tooth surface layer is too large to be adequately replaced with materials from the deeper subsurface layers; in vitro studies show that the enamel tissue loss increases linearly with time.[139 303] The pellicle covering the teeth, regardless of its age,[125] protects the enamel somewhat against acids, as does the plaque, which helps to neutralise the acids with calcium and phosphate.[142 209 288] The thickness of plaque varies between individuals after a short time of its initiation and is inversely related to the degree of erosion.[10] Eroded enamel does not have plaque and high-erosion patients accumulate less plaque than low-erosion individuals.[155] In contrast with the dull surface that is produced after etching, eroded enamel is usually shiny, because the softened enamel wears away.[65]

Erosion and mechanical factors
Miller (1907) attributed erosion to tooth brushing,[215] but later research showed that acidic dissolution initiates erosion (Figure 6.1) rather than wear and salivary characteristics.[231] Acidic dissolution leads to loss of a thin surface layer and makes the demineralised, and thus softened, superficial enamel more susceptible to wear,[26 80] in particular, immediately after the exposure to the acids.[65 116 188] Surface loss through tooth-to-tooth contact and tooth brushing (Figure 6.2) are co-responsible for further development of the erosive lesion,[4 28 65 75 195 205 258] as is repeated contact with the lips, cheeks and tongue,[112 192] and also prosthetic materials.[43 258] At the bottom of the erosive lesion is a zone of highly softened enamel, which is a few micrometers deep.

Concerning wear, some studies show interesting findings.

- In an in vitro study, more enamel wear was seen in neutral than under acidic conditions, owing to a smoothing and flattening effect of erosion on the contacting surfaces (but periodontal stress relief and salivary lubrication of the teeth were lacking).[79]
- When enamel slabs demineralised with citric acid were fixed to the teeth and exposed to saliva for 0, 30 or 60 minutes and then brushed, there was loss of 0.26, 0.22 and 0.20 μm of the superficial layer, respectively:[144] that is, the longer the enamel was exposed to the saliva, the lower was the amount lost. The loss due to brushing was 10–27 times greater than that from the control enamel.[144 184] Demineralised dentine is also more susceptible to abrasion.[18]
- The shape of the occlusal lesions in teeth of people living in the Medieval times caused by severe wear

Pathology of the Hard Dental Tissues, First Edition. Albert Schuurs.
© 2013 Albert Schuurs. Published 2013 by Blackwell Publishing Ltd.

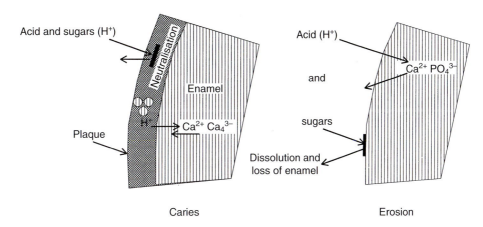

Figure 6.1 Diagrammatic comparison of the reactions occurring on the tooth surface in caries and enamel.

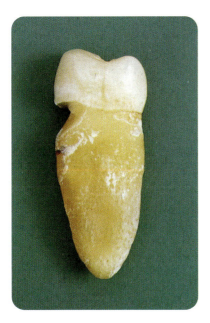

Figure 6.2 Defect in the cervical part of the root with undermining of the enamel, a consequence of the combined effect of tooth brushing, the toothpaste and, presumably, acid.

associated with a coarse diet closely resembles the defects produced by acids in individuals consuming a contemporary "normal" diet: however, whether a lesion was caused by erosion or wear was not distinguishable on the basis of the lesion shape.[95]

• In another *in vitro* study, at pH 5 maintained over a period of several days, the undersaturated environment with a low fluoride concentration was associated with softening of the enamel surface. A somewhat higher fluoride concentration in a more saturated environment led to formation of white spot lesions.[304]

Role of saliva

In erosion, there is insufficient dilution, buffering and washing away of the acids by the saliva. Stimulated saliva has a higher buffering capacity than unstimulated saliva. Van Nieuw Amerongen reported that the buffering capacity and the stimulated salivary flow rate seemed normal in 75% of a sample of erosion patients, but in some patients the small amount of the stimulant citric acid lowered the oral pH to less than 5.5.[316]

Saliva stored in experimental conditions was found to protect the enamel to a greater degree against an erosive challenge than deionised water. The salivary protection *in vivo* is greater with a greater quantity of saliva and with the deposition of an organic pellicle on the specimen, and varies with different chemical compositions of saliva.[123]

6.2 Aetiology

6.2.1 Acid erosion

Several studies show erosion is associated with exogenous acids.[8 14 64 74 76 82 89 119 128 134 135 149 172 174 204 207 210 235 254 281 321 341] Variations in effects of acids in rats have been attributed to differences in individual characteristics.[135] Tests for determining the validity of these findings are being carried out.

Laboratory techniques

Several techniques are used to assess the effects of acids on the enamel.[23]

Scanning electron microscopy[114] and *digital image analysis*[226] are used to measure erosion *in vitro*.

Microindentation reveals the hardness of the enamel surface before and after contact with acid. The greater the indentation produced by a diamond upon loading, the softer is the enamel.[23] In another study, the elasticity of enamel and dentine was not reduced after 10 minutes of immersion in erosive beverages.[191]

Nanoindentation is sensitive to the initial stages of erosion. The displacement of the registering tip as a function of the applied load is continually monitored and enables calculating the enamel hardness and the plastic and elastic deformation. The technique has been applied to determine reduction in the erosive potential of fluids after addition of calcium and phosphate.[23]

Profilometry is performed with a stylus that scans a surface partly exposed to an acid. The surface is scanned before and after the exposure. The amount of material lost and the erosive potential of agents are determined from the scan trace.[23 210] More recently, *laser profilometry* has also been used.

Microradiography. A beam of X-rays is directed to an enamel block. The degree of blackening on a photographic plate is used to record the amount of penetrating radiation; the mineral density of the block is mapped.

Chemical analysis measures the concentrations of dissolved calcium and phosphate.[23]

6.2.2   Dietary erosion

Fruits

The pH of citrus fruits is in the range of 2.0–3.8.[4 8 32 76 306 307] Citric acid in fruits has greater capacity to chelate and demineralise enamel than other acids,[83] including dietary phosphoric and hydrochloric acids.[330] Citric acid with a pH 5.9 is erosive and malic acid with a pH 5.9 is not.[210] Chelation is irrelevant at pH 2, but not at a higher pH.[17] Most fruits, which have a pH 3–4, contain tannic, tartaric and other organic acids.[318] Oranges contain 75% citric and 17% malic acid, apricots 55% citric and 35% malic acid, apples 95% malic acid and 24 other acids, and grapes contain 50% tartaric acid.[119] Enamel immersed for 6 minutes in fruit juices was found to show differing "etching" depths:[216]

- 5.5 μm in apricot juice
- 3 μm in grape juice
- 1 μm in apple juice.

Commercial fruit juices are six to eight times more erosive than homemade juices. Children drinking fruit juices from nursing bottles are easily exposed to acids for 6 minutes or for more time.[119]

Drinks

The pH of a fluid is exponentially related to its erosive potential.[169] Meurman *et al.* found that the pH of commercial sports drinks was low and all of them dissolved enamel,[210] although another study found that dental erosion in athletes (37%) did not differ with the use of different sports drinks.[201] Moreover, 85% of a sample of cyclists using sports drinks had palatal erosion.[224] The pH of most sport drinks is <4.[210]

Frequent consumption of wine, cider, acid herbal teas, iced teas with fruit aroma, carbonated beverages, fruit juices and other acidic drinks is associated with erosion.[14 74 110 134 152 221 252 317] Carbon dioxide in carbonated beverages forms carbonic acid.[78] Ascorbic acid is present in many (sport) drinks and candies.[330] Some phosphoric and citric acid is present in nearly all soft drinks, including (<0.1%) colas.[257 226 330] The consumption frequency of carbonated drinks and (diluted) fruit juices has been

shown to be significantly higher in children with erosion than in those without.[239] Frozen fruit juices "on a stick" (Popsicles) are worse, as they are sucked slowly.[308] Cider (pH 3–4) seems to be as erosive as orange juice.[252] Wines may be very erosive[110] and induce a greater loss of tooth minerals than Coca-Cola and apple juice.[337]

Nowadays, large quantities of soft drinks and fruit juices are consumed, for instance in the UK (160 L/person/ year in 1996),[234 274 326] and Saudi Arabia.[153] The consumption by children and adolescents in particular, has increased in the past 50 years from 2 cans/week to 2 cans/ day. Presently, Dutch teenagers consume daily, on average, 7 glasses of acidic drinks, some 100 g of fruit, and 3 glasses of dairy-based drinks.[320]

The desire for a healthy life influences the diet.[192] Slimming and health diets may be dentally unhealthy because the consumption of fruit drinks is encouraged.[185] Substitution of sugar-containing drinks by fruit juices fortified with vitamin C prevents caries but makes the teeth vulnerable to erosion.[280]

Other food

There are "hidden" acids in commercial food products, masked by sugar. For instance, sweets such as sourballs,[286] salad dressings, yoghurts and tomato ketchup are acidic.

In some tribes (Burma) the teeth are coloured black with a tree resin, citron juice and iron (Chapter 10).

Factors modifying the effects of dietary causes of erosion

Modifying factors include the amount of drink consumed, frequency and manner of consumption,[154 155] dietary constituents, tooth brushing, use of chewing gum, fluoride exposure, the quantity and quality of the saliva, the pellicle and the plaque.[123 219 352]

Holding a cola-type drink in the mouth for some time rather than swallowing immediately was found to lower the pH to ~4; a less pronounced pH drop, but lasting for 20 minutes, was recorded with slow sipping. Gulping decreased the pH minimally. The method of drinking strongly determines the risk of erosion.[154] A patient with severe erosion had a habit of swirling every swig of cola throughout the mouth. Abandoning the habit arrested the process.[127] Swishing acidic drinks (agitation) dissolves more enamel than just holding in the mouth.[143 202 238] As elsewhere, wines in Sweden are tested (wine tasting) before they are marketed. Within a few hours 20–50 wines are swirled through the mouth. Sessions take place four to five times/week. In one study, three-quarters of about 20 tasters demonstrated erosion, against 5% of controls.[336] Other studies have also shown that frequent wine tasting is associated with extensive erosion.[56 110 269]

The moment of consumption has an impact: about 60% of a sample of children with severe erosion drank fruit juice just before sleeping, versus about 30% with modest and around 15% with minimal erosion.[217] In contrast, tooth wear in the deciduous dentition was not found to be related to the consumption of fruit juices and soft drinks.[328]

The adherence of different soft drinks to the enamel is different. Coca-Cola and (low sugar) blackcurrant drinks are retained longer on the enamel than distilled water and saliva.[143] Desorption of the salivary proteins from the enamel reduces their protective ability and renewal of the protein coat takes time. Sipping is therefore more damaging than gulping.[353]

Studies have found that contact between the teeth and a cola for 1 hour softened the enamel, which became harder again after 5 minutes of chewing cheese (Cheddar, Edam). However, these findings should be viewed with caution because the chewing action may have resulted in loss of the softened superficial enamel layer. Drinking milk also hardens the enamel. Chewing on paraffin, to stimulate the salivary flow, lacks a beneficial effect.[97][98][99]

Titrability

The total amount of *titrable* acid is important.[29][32] Titrability signifies the hydrogen ion availability, i.e. the acid's erosive potential,[349] and is a measure of the degree of resistance against a pH rise. Acids that resist buffering act for a longer time and are more destructive than fluids that are quickly neutralised. The buffering capacity of soft drinks has a greater effect than their initial pH.[118] The type of acid and temperature are also co-factors. Organic acids are able to maintain the pH below the dissolution threshold for a long time because of their buffering capacity.[326]

Precipitation of brushite prevents saturation of the eroding solution with dissolved tooth minerals and maintains the enamel dissolution as long as the pH is low.[169]

Table 6.1 shows the pH of and the amount of the alkaline sodium hydroxide (NaOH) needed to buffer some beverages.[188] Other studies have confirmed these values.[78][261]

Acidic drinks requiring lower amounts of NaOH for buffering are associated with less enamel hardness

changes.[186] Therefore, "old" Coca-Cola is, despite its lower pH, less erosive than grapefruit juice.[188] However, others have found pure fruit juices to be most erosive. Fruit-based carbonated drinks lead to more tooth erosion than carbonated drinks. Plain mineral waters are harmless. Parry *et al.* found very low dissolution with still and sparkling mineral waters and slightly higher dissolution with carbonated waters, but this was still 100 times less than with orange juice and cola drinks.[245] Regular and diet versions of the same drink show fewer differences in erosive potential than different brands.[78] "Light" drinks with sugar substitutes may be as erosive as the sugar-containing regular versions,[315] but in view of titrability, Diet Coke is less erosive than regular Coca-Cola.[257][261]

Erosion caused by fruit drinks correlates with pH, but not titratable acidity.[354] Fruit particles in citrus drinks enhance the buffering capacity.[29] The erosive potential of soft drinks is co-determined by their composition, such as the calcium concentration.[186][354] Acidic drinks with calcium and phosphate do not erode if they are supersaturated with respect to apatite.[169]

Most wines (pH 3–3.6)[336] and beers (pH ~4) are relatively easily neutralised.[314] Orange and blackcurrant concentrates used for preparing drinks demonstrated, in a variety of dilutions, higher titrability than citric and hydrochloric acid and were neutralised faster as the dilutions increased.[49] Vinegar and salad dressing (pH 3.5) required remarkably large amounts of NaOH for neutralisation.[314] Grapefruit and kiwi fruit juice require smaller, yet also substantial, amounts.[185] The pH of most vegetables is >5.5. Asparagus, beets, cabbage (sauerkraut) carrots, olives, rhubarb, spinach, and tomatoes are more acidic.[318]

Table 6.2 shows the weight lost from enamel blocks immersed for 14 days in a range of beverages. Different amounts of enamel was lost in some soft drinks of almost equal pH. Colas caused 50 times higher enamel weight loss/cm^2 than tap water; some non-cola drinks dissolved much more mineral. Bearing in mind the salivary buffering capacity, this 14-day immersion period can be considered equivalent to 13 years of normal soft drink consumption.[326]

Contact with acids does not have to last long to soften the enamel, but the contact time differs by acid, for instance lemons erode faster than grapefruit.[4] Erosion does not require very frequent contact with acids. A comparison of patients with and without erosion showed the risk to be increased:

- 37 times when citrus fruits were consumed more than twice daily
- 10 times when apple vinegar was used weekly
- 4 times when soft drinks were consumed daily
- 4 times when sport drinks were consumed weekly.[149]

Table 6.1 Acidity (pH) and buffering capacity of some beverages[188]

Beverage	pH	Volume of base (NaOH, 0.1 N) required for neutralisation (mL)
Coca-Cola (fresh)	2.4	3.9
Coca-Cola (old)	2.4	0.9
Isodrink	3.0	10.0
Apple wine	3.2	8.6
Grapefruit juice	3.2	22.0
Rivella Marathon	3.4	4.0
Orange juice	3.6	12.4
Isostar	3.7	4.0
Isostar Light	3.7	4.0

Table 6.2 Acidity (pH) of some soft drinks and the loss in weight of enamel from enamel blocks immersed in the beverages for 14 days (% and mg/cm²)[326]

Beverage	pH	Enamel weight loss	
		%	mg/cm²
pepsi (cola)	2.4	1.4	3.3
Coca-Cola	2.5	1.4	2.8
Diet pepsi	2.9	1.5	3.2
Dr Pepper	2.9	1.7	3.2
Canada Dry Ginger Ale	2.9	3.5	6.3
Arizona Iced Tea	2.9	4.9	9.0
Diet Dr Pepper	3.0	1.5	3.0
Mountain Dew	3.1	6.2	14.3
Diet Coke	3.2	1.5	3.1
Diet Mountain Dew	3.3	8.0	14.8
Sprite	3.3	3.9	8.6
Diet Sprite	3.3	3.7	6.4
A&W Root Beer	4.8	0	0
Brewed black tea	5.4	0.2	0.4
Brewed black coffee	6.3	0.2	0.3
Tap water	6.7	0	−0.1

Dietary groups at risk

- People with *diabetes* consuming large amounts of fruit juices are at higher risk.[86]
- *Antihypertension* (and other) medicaments cause xerostomia,[325] which increases consumption of acidic sweets (and possibly acidic foods) and acidic drinks.[29]
- Some sports, occupations and environments leading to *dehydration* promote the consumption of (sports) drinks in large quantities. Although intended for athletes for rehydration, electrolyte replacement and energy replenishment, children and adolescents consume these drinks as well. Moreover, dehydration through strenuous exercise reduces the salivary flow and buffering capacity.[349]
- *Ecstasy* use combined with vigorous dancing results in life-threatening hyperthermia. Xerostomia is exacerbated by dehydration. Thirst is relieved by soft drinks, but the sugar enhances drug absorption.[72]
- *Cocaine* causes erosion.[158 164]

Cocaine is synthesised from coca paste (Bazooka) and contains hydrochloride, which dissolves in the saliva and lowers the pH to 4.5.[164] The occlusal and buccal surfaces of cocaine addicts are glass-like and smooth.[34] Regular application of cocaine to the buccal gingiva results in necrotising ulcerative periodontitis and erosions.[158] Nasal insufflation erodes the whole dentition.[164] Cocaine introduces the risk of cardiovascular complications with local anaesthetics and retraction cords, which requires postponing the dental treatment for 6–24 hours after application of the cord.[34]

Medicaments

Acidic medicines are erosive, for instance iron medications taken for longer periods,[147] regular chewing of aspirin[44 105 298] and vitamin C,[63] and hydrogen peroxide rinses.

Enamel placed in a 1% acetylsalicylic acid solution (pH 2.40) became rough within 30 seconds and the superficial enamel disappeared within 15 minutes.[126] Chewing aspirin tablets, 90–130 mg/day/kg body weight, for juvenile rheumatoid arthritis (250 000 children in the USA) causes severe occlusal erosion; immediate swallowing of the tablets does not.[298] If not fully swallowed, aspirin taken just before sleeping causes the formation of a mucosal white slough that gradually rubs off, leaving red, ulcerated and painful lesions.[199]

Dissolution of 500 mg vitamin C in saliva lowers the pH to 4.4, lasting 5 minutes or longer.[129]

Hydrochloric acid medications for achlorhydria (in patients with lack of gastric acid production) are erosive[7 200] (but non-erosive substitutes exist[293]), as was the acid formerly used to dissolve small renal calculi.[141]

Studies have found that children with asthma had more erosion than controls,[7 203 272 273] and explanations included more frequent vomiting,[7 279] heartburn,[7] reduced salivary flow after prolonged use of medicaments, altered salivary composition, and pH of the medication,[35 203 273] although the latter seems unlikely.[305] Asthma medicaments are smooth muscle relaxants that act on the oesophageal sphincter and are associated with gastro-oesophageal reflux and xerostomia in the long term. The drugs may promote consumption of acidic drinks.[273]

Dry powder inhalers have a pH of 5.06 and pressurised metered inhalers a pH of 6.45; the titrability of the former is twice that of pressurised inhalers, but Tootla *et al.* found that neither the salivary nor the plaque pH dropped below 6 with their use.[305] Other studies have shown that the (un)stimulated salivary pH and buffering capacity of children with erosion is lower than in controls,[238] as is the case in children using asthma medicines, who also secrete less salivary proteins.[260] However, these findings have not been substantiated.[7]

Mouthcare products are not medicaments.[349] The pH of some mouthrinses used against halitosis (offensive breath) is <5.5, but neutralisation requires only a small amount of NaOH. The alcohol content varies from 0% to 27%.[30] *In vitro*, alcohol is cytotoxic to the fibroblasts.[296] Frequent rinsing introduces the risk of oral cancer[30 91] and softened the surface of composite restorations.[121] In bedridden patients with insufficient self-care, the mouth is sometimes cleaned with cotton swabs impregnated with citric acid (pH ~2.7).[212]

Industrial and environmental erosion

Industrial workers are exposed to, for instance, hydrochloric or sulphuric gases in the electrolytic zinc galvanising, battery, fertiliser, munitions and beverage industries.[117] The concentration, exposure time and mouth breathing, which is prompted by the fumes, determine the lesion severity.[44 193 280] Other factors, such as not using a commercial toothbrush (e.g. using *dattun sticks* instead), also have an effect.[309]

Swimmers, especially competition swimmers, swimming in water disinfected with chlorine may exhibit extensive erosions if hydrochloric acid is formed under the influence of light.

In chlorinated (Cl_2) water, the disinfectant hydrochlorous acid (HOCl) is formed. Hydrochloric acid (HCl) is an unwanted by-product. Supplementation with calcium or sodium carbonate (Na_2CO_3) neutralises the acid. Some 40% of a sample of swimmers training more than 2 hours/day were found to exhibit erosion.[54]

Disinfection with sodium hypochlorite (NaOCl) results in a high pH, at which little HOCl is formed, and which is neutralised with sulphuric acid. At pH >7 the teeth of competitive swimmers are yellow-brown in colour, because the disinfecting chloride (or bromide) products denature the salivary proteins on the surface of the teeth.[355 356]

An Israeli study found that the pH in swimming pools varied from 3.6 to 7.8. Teeth immersed for 1–2 hours in water with pH 3.6 became etched.[90] In the USA, the pH of water of a swimming pool treated with chlorine was 2.7. In the Netherlands, of 3600 samples of swimming pool water, five had a pH <5.5.[182]

Jockeys occasionally try to lose body weight by frequent vomiting (and use of laxatives): in the last 2 days before a race, up to 10 kg weight may be lost. Severe erosion is a consequence.[33]

Endogenous erosion (perimylolysis)

Regurgitated gastric acid in the mouth is erosive. Vomiting once a week is as erosive as consuming 2 citrus fruits/day. In one-quarter of a sample of erosion patients, gastric juice was the cause of the erosion, in another quarter it was exogenous acids and in half it was endogenous plus exogenous acids.[149]

In *chronic regurgitation*, the gastric acid that is regurgitated has a pH 1–1.5. Peristalsis clears the oesophagus, followed by salivary neutralisation. The pH of vomit is ~3.8. Vomiting caused the extensive lesions shown in Figures 6.3, 6.4 and 6.5.

In a sample of children with gastro-oesophageal reflux disease (GORD), about 15% had more frequent and severe erosion than their siblings (10%).[179 240] Others have found a trend for severe erosion.[24] Half of a sample of patients referred for gastro-oesophageal disease met the criteria for GORD; they exhibited more erosion than the other half.[113] In GORD patients with erosion, 24-hour monitoring of the oesophagus revealed a pH <4 for 12% of the time, versus 1.5% of the time in controls. The hoarse (oesophagitis) patients reported heartburn; some had asthma. Salivary buffering capacity was poorer than in controls, but not in general in all patients. The unstimulated salivary volume and bicarbonate content were normal.[228]

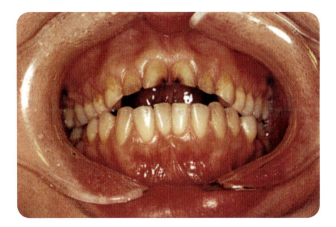

Figure 6.3 Labial view of the dentition of a patient with frequent vomiting. Note the shortened incisors and the bucco-cervical defects in the maxillary teeth (which are more difficult to discern).

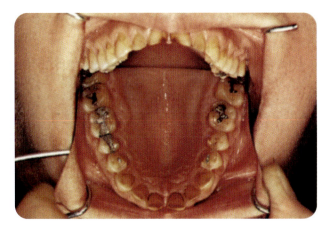

Figure 6.4 Note the eroded lingual and occlusal surfaces of the teeth in the same patient as in Figure 6.3.

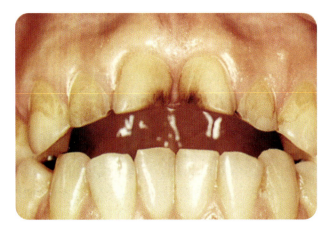

Figure 6.5 Magnified view of the anterior teeth of the same patient as in Figure 6.3. The incisal edges of the central incisors are severely affected.

In one study simultaneous measurement of the pH in the oesophagus and mouth over 24 hours in reflux patients indicated that the gastric juice did not enter the mouth. Nevertheless, the oral pH appeared to fall slowly to 4–5.[120] But another study found the gastric juices do reach the mouth.[26]

- *Provocative meals.* A curry meal with alcohol shortly before going to sleep caused belching and an oral pH <5.5 for 3% of the time, against 0.1% after a neutral meal.[25] Low salivary production when sleeping washes the gastric acid away slowly.
- *Vigorous exercise* with much body agitation induces reflux, in particular postprandial reflux, proportional to the exercise intensity. Weightlifters experience most reflux.[59 62]
- *Rumination.* Extensive erosions in half of a sample of mentally retarded subjects, were caused by reflux and rumination (re-chewing of the gastric contents). A pH <4 for more than 4.5% of the time caused 65% of the erosions.[36]
- *Voluntary reflux.* Some stressed people find comfort in regurgitating and holding the gastric contents within the cheeks before they swallow or spit it out. Erosion develops on the surfaces against which the vomit is held.[26]
- *Tooth clenching* in 10% of people is secondary to a low oesophageal pH.[227]
- *Myodystrophia fetalis deformans* (congenital skeletal disorder), where one or more of the extremities and the lower jaw are deformed with movement restriction, is associated with frequent vomiting.[92] Vomiting is common in *pyloric stenosis* (obstruction of the stomach orifice),[335] pregnancy,[273 329] and a *defective oesophageal sphincter* with or without *hiatus hernia of the oesophagus*, i.e. the stomach extends above the congenitally weak and progressively weakened diaphragm.[138] Gastric and duodenal ulcers and cancer are associated with reflux,[9] but gastric ulcers may not be.[148] Scleroderma (an autoimmune rheumatoid factor positive disease) causes reflux.[357]
- *Use of medicaments* such as antihistamines, β-blockers, cytotoxics, digitalis, diuretics, oestrogen, non-steroidal anti-inflammatory drugs, opiates, tetracyclines, and oncolytics may lead to vomiting.[263 273]
- *Chronic alcoholism* is associated with regurgitation and vomiting.[277 284 285] Even young adults indulge in alcoholic binges, which often end in vomiting.[160] The erosion prevalence was almost 50% in a sample of alcohol abusers.[13]
- *Other causes* of vomiting include neuralgic disorders, such as migraine, and metabolic and endocrine disorders, such as uraemia and hyper(para)thyroidism.[263]
- *Anorexia nervosa* and *bulimia.* Self-induced vomiting, often coupled with a low resting salivary flow, seems

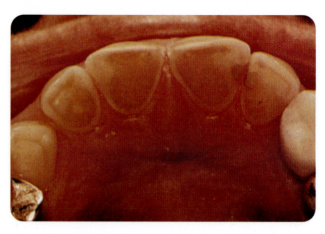

Figure 6.6 Lingual surfaces of the maxillary incisors in an anorexia nervosa patient. The denuded dentine (centrally) is surrounded by a thin white line, representing the approximal enamel.

the most important cause of erosions in these patients.[1] [12 38 45 46 60 74 108 131 132 157 214 223 229 255 256 259 262 263 264 291]

Patients with anorexia nervosa (loss of appetite) and the more frequent bulimia (obsessively increased appetite) try to hide their disorder.[214] The dentist may suspect their presence because of presence of erosion (Figure 6.6). The lesions may reach (in)to the pulp cavity.[157 278] These conditions are discussed in more detail below.

During vomiting, the salivary flow increases greatly because the medullary centre that controls vomiting is connected to the salivary nuclei. In non-vomiting patients with eating disorders, the stimulated salivary flow might be normal or lowered. In purging and non-purging patients with erosion, the salivary bicarbonate level may be reduced and the salivary viscosity increased, secondary to structural changes in the glands.[220]

Anorexia nervosa

The disorder consists of an identity problem, insecurity, low self-esteem, pathological body awareness and rigid self-discipline. The aetiology is unknown, but it is possibly somatic in origin.

Pre-anorexic children meet parental (mothers') over-expectations by working hard, showing an eagerness to please and perfectionism. They do not go through periods of negativism and stubbornness and do not develop autonomy. The decision to diet is an attempt to control at least their body.[327]

The patients starve themselves to lose weight, viewing themselves as too fat.[131 255] Anorexic patients are often young, affluent white females of at least normal intelligence,[327] who camouflage muscle wasting with loose clothes. A lean face with pronounced cheekbones, eventually shortened lower face height due to loss of occlusal enamel, and the thin lips are indicative of the condition.[264]

The patients are pathologically preoccupied with the constant struggle to overcome hunger to achieve the desired thinness.[327] They encourage each other via the internet. The disorder is not a problem of a specific age, social class or sex,[38] although males are under-represented.[262] Symptoms include decreased sex hormone secretion, smaller ovaries and absence of at least three consecutive menstrual cycles, unless, for example, oestrogen is administered.[180] Anorexics may lose 25% body weight within a few months, feel cold, and often have stomach complaints. The arms and back show fine hair ("lanugo hair") and dry skin.[229 255 264] An estimated 25–50% of anorexia patients purge frequently.[256] Some half of ex-patients do not recover their weight and/or the normal menstrual cycle.[220] About 20% of emaciated patients die within a few years[173] due to development of cardiac myopathies or by committing suicide.[180]

Most of the physical and endocrine abnormalities in anorexia are also seen in starvation secondary to other conditions: gastrointestinal diseases (Crohn's disease), endocrine disorders, e.g. hypopituitarism, Addison's disease, hyperthyroidism, cancer, chronic infections such as tuberculosis, and psychiatric disorders, such as depression and schizophrenia.[327]

Bulimia

Patients who binge eat (mainly carbohydrates) have minimally twice a week periods of uncontrollable voracity, an excessive, often hurried, secret gluttony indulged in chiefly at night, but not with the purpose of gaining weight. After such periods of indulgence, a minority stimulate the vomiting reflex,[131 180 223 256 262] and some administer emetics, laxatives an/or diuretics.[180 229] The body weight of bulimic patients alternates between high and low, but they are rarely lean,[1 214] because throwing up is never 100% effective.[255] About 80% of bulimic patients recover versus 50% of anorexics.[220]

The patients experience hypokalaemia, muscle weakness, sometimes heart palpitations and other symptoms. Hurried feeding and vomiting stimuli may cause mucosal trauma.[259] One-third to half have enlarged parotid glands, unilateral or bilateral, of unknown aetiology.[255 256 291] The angles of the mouth may be red due to dietary deficiencies or trauma.[259]

6.2.3   Idiopathic erosion

In a number of cases, erosion may not seem to have an explainable cause.[73] In the past, half of erosive lesions were thought to be idiopathic,[137 149] but careful history taking may uncover the most likely cause in nearly all patients.[149]

Salivary factors have been implicated. Briefly,[249] patients with idiopathic erosion may have: increased citric acid concentration in stimulated saliva; highly mucous saliva; and a low pH in the vicinity of the erosive lesions. The pH of (un)stimulated saliva is 6.7–7.4, but occasionally it may be acidic.[292 318] Lussi *et al.* found that saliva with low buffering capacity was present in about 20% of persons with a high risk of erosion progression and in 5% of those with a low risk.[187]

Theories of idiopathic erosion have now lost most of their relevance and are therefore just briefly described here.

- Drinking water (pH 5–7.5) with citrate was found to cause erosion in rats: the calcium–citrate complexes[249] formed in the post-eruptive enamel dissolved easily.[109] The citrate in human saliva was assumed to result in local demineralisation, but outcomes in follow-up studies were inconclusive.[275 351]

Chelation by citrate may play a role, but this is speculative.[85] Citrus fruit juices increase the salivary citrate concentration,[84] but have not been found to cause dissolution of the enamel at pH 5–7.5.

- Precipitation of salivary minerals may result in repair of extremely small scratches in the enamel caused by tooth brushing, unless the saliva is very mucous.[195 196 197] The salivary viscosity may indeed play a role in erosion.[222] Enamel without perikymata and with incidental scratching showed a clearly visible prismatic structure.[196] The pattern seen in idiopathic erosion involves scooping out of the centres of the heads of the enamel prisms by the action of the acids.[194] The saliva of a sample of patients with idiopathic erosion was found to be rich in mucins, versus in 28% of controls without erosion. The groups were similar with respect to the amount of saliva, salivary pH and calcium and phosphate. Questions remain though. For instance, why were 28% of the controls with highly mucous saliva free of erosion?[196]

For completeness, it is worth noting that in erosion the flow of fluid from the pulp through the dentine may prevent penetration of the acids into the tooth, whereas in caries, the fluid flow may be suppressed, allowing acid penetration.[294 295]

Saliva

Weak acids have been found to cause erosion in rats without saliva.[135] In Sjögren's syndrome, erosion is worsened.[268 342] An insufficiently buffered, locally acidic environment is thought to be caused in the night, for instance by lactobacilli, in the then dry mouth.[335 339 340] The viscosity of the saliva is substantially increased in Sjögren's (also in hyperthyroidism) and the salivary secretion rate is decreased.[318 342]

Comparison of a group of lacto-vegetarians, 75% with erosion, with a control group consuming less acidic berries and vinegar, revealed that increased salivary flow and, to a lesser degree, the salivary buffering capacity prevent erosion: 78% of the variance was explained by these factors.[178]

A low salivary buffering capacity allows acids to exert long-lasting erosive action.[120] The buffering capacity of the stimulated saliva allowed discriminating between patients with a high risk of erosion progression and those with a low risk.[87] However, in a multifactorial model, low unstimulated salivary flow was associated with erosion but not the calcium and phosphate levels.[149 339]

The pH of stimulated saliva has been found to contribute to toothbrush abrasion of enamel that was exposed to citric acid.[184] In other studies, the oral glucose clearance time of erosion patients was longer than in controls,[339] and their saliva was richer in mucins.[222 249]

Idiopathic (?) cervical lesions

Usually occlusal and cervical enamel are almost equally susceptible to erosion.[124] Occlusal forces transmitted to the cervical region of teeth in malocclusion could underlie erosive cervical defects, previously considered to be idiopathic.[171] Under occlusal loading, the crown bends laterally on the firmly fixed root. The crown flexure results in alternating compression and tensile stress in the cervical region. Enamel withstands compressive forces adequately, but the interprismatic substance is more susceptible to tensile forces.[66] The prisms become separated, especially bucco-cervically in the premolars and first molars. The disrupted bonds between the crystals cannot be repaired and penetrating water, acids and other ions increase the mechanical deterioration.[171] The enamel fractures locally. Loss of cervical enamel changes the two-"body" process into a three-"body" process (that is, penetration through the surface into the deeper layers). The action of acids and tooth brushing worsen the destruction by dissolution and abrasion. The V-shaped lesions develop at the fulcrum, the region of maximum stress.[171] Because mechanical forces seem to be primarily causative in these situations, the process is described further under "abfraction" in Chapter 9.

6.3   Epidemiology

6.3.1   Acid erosion

Epidemiological data may be compromised because "grading systems . . . [cannot] be used specifically for erosion . . . as most enamel loss is multifactorial",[231] erosion and wear being partly interdependent.[195] Assessment methods are insufficiently sensitive to record small changes in longitudinal investigations.[231]

Some 20 years ago the prevalence of erosion was determined to be 2–9%.[149] In the past few decades, in general, substantially higher proportions have been reported.[37 139 188 217 234 275 282 287 320 338 344 345 351 358] The age at which the first signs of erosion of the permanent dentition are reported varies considerably,[74 132 178 234] although even young children are affected.[234 280 282 320] In a UK-based study, half of 5–6-year-olds had eroded deciduous incisors.[139] Across various studies, some 15% of 5–9-year-olds, 50% of 11-year-olds and nearly all 14-year-olds had erosion in the permanent dentition, occasionally extending into the dentine.[5 70 146 218 234 282] In a sample of 46–50-year-olds, some 80% had occlusal erosion of at least one tooth.[188 189] One-third of occlusal erosive lesions in a large majority of Swiss subjects were associated with exposed dentine, and in one-fifth, buccal defects were present.[145] In another study, cervical erosion of at least one tooth increased proportionally with age.[266]

Not all patients with erosion have serious problems. The chemical composition and morphology of the teeth helps explain differences in severity of the symptoms. In addition, improved oral hygiene removes the protective plaque.[231] As mentioned, although frequent consumption of acidic drinks is blamed, lesion severity may not relate to the quantity, frequency and period of fruit and fruit juice consumption.[76 320] Appreciable tooth erosion/wear in half of British 14-year-olds, in particular from lower socio-economic backgrounds correlates up to a point with the increased consumption of soft drinks.[5 6 234]

The incisors and premolars are most frequently eroded,[344] but in a number of cases tooth wear predominates over erosion.[234] The prevalence of erosion seems higher in maxillary than mandibular teeth.[352]

6.3.2   Industrial erosion

One- to two-thirds of workers in acid-processing factories (1–5 mg acid fumes /m^3 air) have been found to have erosion.[44 310] More than half of employees in a car battery factory had "sharp, thin" and one-third "shortened" teeth.[248] In one study, the age of the workers did not influence the differences in distribution of erosion in the anterior and posterior oral regions among those of Finnish origin, but in older Tanzanians posterior erosion was more likely.[309] In a Jordanian sample of industrial workers, erosion and general health were associated.[11] Factories in poorer countries (and photographers working from home) may lack scavenging apparatus.

6.3.3   Anorexia nervosa and bulimia

An estimated 5% of women and 12% of adolescent girls in the USA and 20% of Australian young women have an eating disorder at one time or another.[229] For UK and West Germany the figures are lower.[108 255] Among students in the USA, 2–35% have bulimia.[46] Altogether within different Western populations, 2–8% have/had eating disorders.[45]

The observation that dehydration occurs in bulimia due to the vomiting was deduced from the excessive use of (acidic) drinks, which caused buccal erosion, in addition to the lingual damage caused by the gastric acid.[108] Xerostomia is not uncommon in these patients.[291] Carbohydrates may promote tooth decay in bulimia patients,[132 256] but some studies did not find higher caries rates in bulimics compared with controls and people with anorexia.[157 223] Palatal erosion of the maxillary anterior teeth has been observed in 33% of anorexia and bulimia patients.[256] However, the duration of the disorder must be taken into account,[262 263] and mouthrinsing versus brushing after purging contributes to differences in the extent and depth of the lesions.[60 109 262] Milosevic et al. found that bulimics with erosion had a mucous saliva whereas those without erosion had more viscous saliva, and lower salivary bicarbonate levels and secretion rate.[222] Like in pregnant women, the serum amylase level is elevated in 45% of bulimia patients.[180]

6.4 Appearance and diagnosis

6.4.1 Macroscopic appearance

Early erosion is confined to the enamel. In *late* erosion the dentine is also involved.[267] Erosion is often diagnosed late because the initial appearance is unremarkable, and there are no clear-cut criteria for diagnosis. In the earliest stages, the perikymata and imbrication lines disappear, leaving a smooth, silky, glazed surface,[74 359] but a dull enamel and "white spots" may also be signs of erosion.[44 195 349] Air drying the teeth helps to detect such signs. The lesions do not become stained.[293] One method of monitoring progression of erosion is by comparing serial casts made of high-density die stone.[348]

Later in the early stages, the convexity of the labial surfaces of the tooth crowns and the occlusal cusps level off. A peculiar sign, already seen in adolescence, is occlusal "cupping" (Figure 6.7) and grooving.[359] Cupping

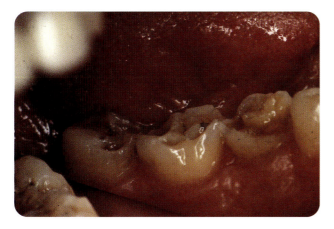

Figure 6.7 One of the first signs of erosion on the occlusal surface is cupping. The present case shows excessive occlusal erosion; note the cupping of the buccal cusp of the first molar.

starts as a pit near the apex of the mesio-buccal cusps of the first molars because there the dentine is locally denuded and wears more readily than the surrounding enamel.[75 174] The combined action of hydrochloric acid and the proteolytic enzyme pepsin in the gastric juice plays a role in cupping,[117] but other acids and occlusal stresses also cause abfraction of invaginated enamel prisms.[241]

In later stages, decisive erosive lesion (other than cupping) develop. Labial lesions are smooth, concave, ovoid shaped with an irregularly outline, and in the intermediate stages there is uneven erosion. The incisal edges may show grooving. Tissue loss may go unnoticed until the more yellow dentine is exposed: then, acids, sweets and thermal and tactile stimuli may elicit pain in a rapid process.[268] Pain is absent when dentine sclerosis (Chapter 8) and tertiary dentine formation (Chapter 5) match the rate of erosion.[108 188] Usually the enamel(-dentine) lesions are shiny, translucent and smooth, but the surface may be irregular,[73] sometimes with "islands" of enamel left standing within the dentine lesions.[109] An irregular enamel surface may be seen before the dentine is denuded. The organic dentinal smear layer and the matrix act as a diffusion barrier and provide some protection. However, the acidic environment and tooth brushing remove the smear layer.[334]

Scanning microscopy shows the incisal wear facets as flat planes with well-defined margins and as step-like areas in the palatal surfaces of the anterior teeth, while erosion is seen as hollowing out of the tissue. These two specific patterns do not seem to be reliable indicators to distinguish between bruxists (Chapter 8) and non-bruxists, although erosion is strongly associated with perceived bruxism.[161] In active erosion, the transition between enamel and dentine is smooth and becomes indistinguishable if a probe is gently passed over the tooth surface to detect the junction. In the passive or resting phase the enamel rim close to the dentine is relatively thick.[232]

Erosion is not progressive in all affected dentitions.[44] In resting phases remineralisation occurs.[194]

Scoring of erosion

Classifications of erosion are based upon the aetiology, severity of lesions, i.e. which tooth tissues (enamel, dentine, pulp) are involved, and pathogenic activity.[44 73 106 141] Table 6.3 presents a guide to scoring lesion severity.[73 76]

In extensive palatal erosion of the maxillary incisors (3b in Table 6.3; Figure 6.6), the dentine is bordered by a rim of approximal, whiter enamel.[75 76] The incisal enamel seen from the labial side is glass-like and dark.[179] Severe occlusal erosion on the (pre)molars, and extending onto the palatal surfaces, makes the morphology unrecognisable.

Table 6.3 Erosion scores and description[73 76]

Score	Lesion description
0	Shiny enamel, no perikymata
1	Loss of enamel only, with a satin sheen
2	Localised dentine lesions, <1/3 of the surface lacks enamel
3	Extensive dentine lesions, >1/3 of the surface lacks enamel
3a	Labial/buccal surfaces
3b	Lingual surfaces
3c	Incisal edges/occlusal surfaces
3d	Labial and lingual surfaces + sometimes other surfaces

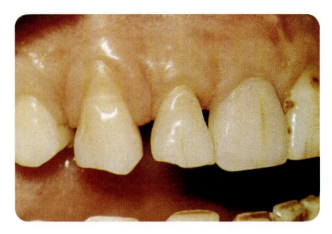

Figure 6.8 Bowl-shaped cervical erosive lesions restricted to the enamel.

Some authors have used modified versions of the scores shown in Table 6.3:[183 188]

- "1/3 of the surface" may be replaced with "1/2"
- Scores of 0–3 have been used for the buccal/labial surfaces and 0–2 for the occlusal and lingual surfaces.

The lesion depth determines the scores in the "Tooth Wear Index" (TWI, Chapter 8). The TWI adjusted for children[217 284] is also used to score erosion. Acceptable levels of "wear" have been determined for different age categories.[284] Smith *et al.* found that acids were co-responsible for tissue loss in 60% of patients with high TWI scores, 10% had tooth wear without erosion and 30% of the lesions were idiopathic.[283]

Restorations

Restorations may protrude above (stand proud of) the eroded tooth surface,[172 192 293] which seems indicative of ongoing erosion.[73 192] However, composite and amalgam also erode, albeit less than the tooth tissues,[65 121 131] and some researchers view wear as the cause.[286]

In one study, at pH 1.2, composites were least prone to wear, followed by resin-modified glass ionomer cement, conventional glass ionomer cement, and enamel, which was most prone to wear. At pH 3.3 the wear rates were much lower, but the order of likelihood of wear of the materials did not change.[271]

A higher current may selectively dissolve the most electro-active amalgam components, promoting corrosion and thereby wear. Rinsing with Coca-Cola and orange juice did not increase the magnitude of the galvanic current between contacting amalgam fillings.[322]

Rate of erosion

Xhonga *et al.* found that 1 µm enamel is lost daily, with large individual variation.[346] Erosion becomes evident within 6 years (minimum 2 years),[346] when 500–1000 µm has been lost.[76] Deep lesions develop within 3–10 years.[268] The rate of progression of the process is higher in the inner enamel, which is less resistant.[89] Immersion of bovine enamel for 4 hours in cola caused 26 µm deep lesions, in sports drinks 14 µm lesions, and "light" cola

9 µm lesions.[261] Extrapolating these findings to human enamel, 0.5–2 µm/h is lost, but humans are not continuously exposed to erosive agents for 4 hours and modifying factors also have a role.[213] Enamel immersed in citric acid for 5 minutes six times a day and placed in the mouth showed a loss of 40 µm in the absence of fluoride.[93] During etching, depending on the acid and its concentration, the "lesion depth" is ~5 µm to >25 µm.[80 122] However, etchants are applied once in a while in operative dentistry but erosive attacks occur frequently.

An acid attack demineralises dentine to a depth of 100 µm.[286] The acidic action widens the orifices of the tubules within 30 seconds. The peritubular-intertubular dentine is demineralised after 60 seconds of immersion in acid; the tubules become hollowed out.[208 213] Lussi *et al.* found that within a 6-year period, erosion in dentine in 46–50-year-olds progressed more markedly than in 26–30-year-olds; one-quarter of the sample accounted for 60% of the total progression.[187]

Some 10% of a group of patients with severe erosion showed near or frank pulp exposure.[279] Rapidly progressive palatal defects caused by vomiting may result in pulp necrosis.[162]

6.4.2   Sites of erosion

Erosion can be distinguished by its location as follows:

- Labial bowl-shaped defects (Figures 6.8 and 6.9)
- Bucco-cervical defects (Figure 6.2)
- Extensive labial defects (Figure 6.10)
- Approximal defects
- Occlusal defects (Figure 6.7)
- Extensive lingual defects (Figure 6.11), often with crumbling incisal edges and severe occlusal erosion.

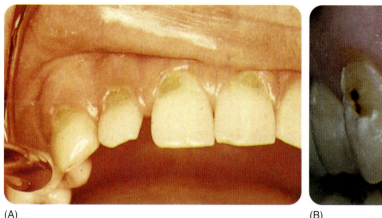
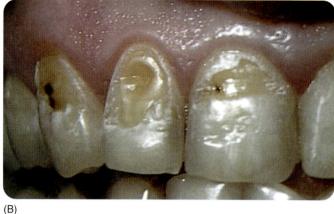

(A)   (B)

Figure 6.9 (A) The bowl-shaped lesions are more clearly visible once they have progressed into dentine. (B) Severe erosive lesions. Note that a large part of the remaining enamel of the lateral and central incisors is rough, which may be observed before the dentine becomes denuded: the enamel is clearly not universally prone to the acid effects.

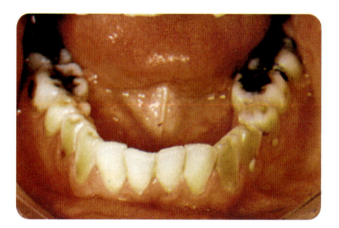

Figure 6.10 Extensive labial and buccal erosive lesions.

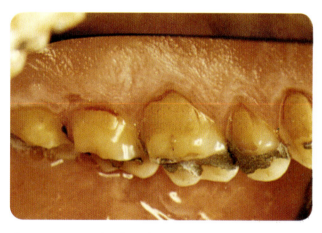

Figure 6.11 Extensive lingual and occlusal erosive defects.

The cause of erosion cannot be deduced reliably from the location of lesions. Both extrinsic and intrinsic acids attack the labial/buccal and lingual surfaces,[150] the incisal edges and the occlusal surfaces. The above mentioned labial lesions (bowl-shaped and extensive labial lesions) may be particularly ascribed to the action of extrinsic acids, but with caution. The manner of consumption is a co-factor.[118]

The lingual defects are frequently deep,[157] and are more common in the maxilla than in the mandible,[108] with the lower incisors being least affected.[113] Main causes are gastric acid regurgitation, use of medicaments and dietary factors.[75] Although in regurgitation the gastric acids are not forced hard against the tooth surfaces like in vomiting, the duration of acidic attack may be more prolonged. Erosion occurs on the lingual surfaces and at other locations where the gastric acids pool, especially during sleep.[117] Related to the head position, the acidic action of vomiting is directed to the palatal surfaces of the maxillary anterior teeth.[323]

Tooth brushing is an important aetiological co-factor in bucco-cervical erosive defects. Wedge-shaped, small lesions may represent abfraction, while wide open lesions (Figure 6.2) may be wear caused by tooth brushing along with erosion.[9 75 130] Local acidosis in the periodontal tissues has been implicated in approximal lesions,[117 324] but the pH of crevicular fluid is neutral and alkaline in periodontitis.[31]

6.4.3 Microscopic appearance

The perikymata and imbrication lines disappear and scratches are incidentally seen. Debris is absent.[195] Next, the prismatic sheaths are attacked, followed by the destruction of the enamel prisms.[109] The enamel surface shows pores with a diameter 6 μm, arranged in a honeycomb-like pattern in concordance with the enamel prisms. Aprismatic enamel (deciduous teeth) dissolves irregularly and may be pitted.[209 213] As the prism boundaries contain fluorapatite, they firstly lose material from the cores.[122 213] The active phase can be microscopically discerned from the resting phase.[194 196 267]

Citric acid with pH 2.54 caused lesions in dentine about 2 μm deep; after buffering, with the pH at 6, the lesions were 0.5 μm deep. The acid-stable dentine matrix is unable to halt lesion progression sufficiently. The lesion depth in dentine increases non-linearly in relation to the duration of exposure.[321]

At pH 4.4, enamel erodes less than dentine. Enamel may remineralise as long as it structure has not been lost but demineralised dentine does not.

6.5   Prevention

The dietary history should include questions on consumption of drinks and information on occupational exposure to acids. The general medical history may reveal the causative factor(s). Patients must be made aware of dietary and "hidden" acids and those with erosion should restrict their intake of acids to once or twice a day, but inducing changes in lifestyle/habit is difficult. Drinking with a straw may prevent worsening of labial defects. The straw must not be pressed against the lingual surfaces of the teeth;[190] placement in the back of the mouth prevents contact of the drink with all teeth.[77] Patients must not swirl erosive drinks in the mouth.

6.5.1   Tooth brushing

The type of toothpaste used is important.[201 311] Patients must use a small amount of low-abrading toothpaste and a soft toothbrush.[73 107] A "whitening" and a regular toothpaste (Chapter 10) were found to be equally abrasive on acid-treated enamel,[311] but use of whitening toothpaste was one of the predictors of erosion in people consuming sport drinks.[201] Use of a hard toothbrush enhances progression of cervical erosion.[187] Rotary-oscillating and (ultra)sonic power toothbrushes abrade demineralised dentine more than sound dentine and have been found to be worse than manual toothbrushes.[360]

After vomiting, gentle tooth brushing with a desensitising or bicarbonate toothpaste has been advised,[20] but abstaining from tooth brushing for 1 hour is better,[77 144] as it permits the enamel to mount its own defence by remineralisation.[16] Use of larger numbers of tooth brushing strokes was associated with a linear increase in enamel loss. Unbrushed samples lost the least enamel.[81 361] However, brushing with a fluoride toothpaste and rinsing with a fluoride mouthrinse immediately after an erosive attack was slightly better than abstaining from any action.[361] Bovine dentine, demineralised 10 times and then stored in saliva for 120 minutes, was more prone to toothbrush abrasion than undemineralised dentine.[16] Patients must be dissuaded from brushing more than twice a day, even without a dentifrice.

6.5.2   Perimylolysis

Patients with perimylolysis must consult a physician. Meanwhile, the dentist may suggest ways to neutralise the oral gastric acid. Antacids held in the mouth for some time can raise the pH from 4 to neutral.[211] Antacids containing bicarbonate (Na_2CO_3) have become obsolete. Patients can be advised to rinse with a small amount of dissolved baking soda ($NaHCO_3$)[142] and to brush the tongue. Alternatives are a night guard filled with $NaHCO_3$ and rinsing with milk.[273]

6.5.3   Fluoride

Meurman et al. concluded that use of fluoride in erosion lacks a good scientific base, but they "intuitively" assessed it as desirable,[213] preferably as varnish.[172] Daily fluoride rinses have been advised.[60] An acidulated NaF solution[135] and fluoride toothpaste[64] may be protective, but findings are not consistent. Fluoride has limited effectiveness in severe erosive conditions, unless intensively applied and in high concentration.[15 93 96 135 151 168 170 172 233 261 288 289 343] Application of acidulated fluoride would be the best choice.[142] Jones et al. found that acidulated phosphorous fluoride (APF) 1.23% performed better against repeated attacks than a neutral 2.2% NaF gel.[156]

Another study found that fluoride slightly modified the effects of citric acid (-based) drinks on enamel, but the clinical benefits were small.[140] A single 30-second rinse with amine/sodium fluoride did not prevent toothbrush wear of softened enamel.[184] Enamel slabs immersed in citric acid 6 times/day for 5 minutes for 5 days were then placed in the mouth. Lesion depths after brushing 3 times/day were:

- 49 μm, using a toothpaste without fluoride
- 35 μm, using a toothpaste with fluoride (0.15% F^-)
- 19 μm, using a fluoride toothpaste, a fluoride mouthrinse (0.025 F^-) and a gel (1.25% F^-).[93]

The combined regimen was better at protecting the dentine.[96] High amounts of fluoride protect the dentine as long as the organic material is present.[94] Dentine exposed to a drink with pH 2.9 abraded in a brushing machine more than non-exposed samples, but recovered its hardness after exposure to 2000 ppm NaF.[18] Pepsin may counteract the beneficial effect of fluoride on tissue loss from the dentine.[362]

The buffering capacity of fluoride dentifrices/gels and the pH influences the abrasion values of the substance.[334] *Sodium hexametaphosphate*, recently included in a SnF_2 toothpaste, was found to provide greater erosion protection than a conventional fluoride toothpaste, by being incorporated and remaining in the pellicle for hours and, probably, binding to free calcium sites on the enamel surface.[363] *Titanium fluoride* (4% TiF_4) may inhibit erosion to a greater extent than other fluorides.[364]

6.5.4 Chewing gum

Salivary urea protects against erosion.[155] Chewing gums containing urea or bicarbonate neutralise acids. The enzyme urease hydrolyses urea: the release of ammonia (NH_4^+) increases the oral pH to about 8 within a few minutes. A bicarbonate gum was found to buffer the longest.[318] However, chewing gum (or eating cheese) after contact with acids[97 98 220 318] worsens loss of softened tooth tissues.

6.5.5 Treating malocclusions and cervical dentine protection

"Idiopathic" cervical erosive defects require correction of premature contacts and malocclusion. Application of a (filled) composite-based adhesive cervically creates a protective dentinal hybrid layer, but due to wear and fracture of the adhesive the effect may be temporary.[19]

6.5.6 Manufacturers of drinks

Manufacturers should add preventive constituents to erosive drinks.[22 115 136] Calcium and phosphates, citrate (stimulates saliva production) and calcium-citrate-malate are most commonly used. However, addition of calcium and phosphate to acidic drinks was found to lack a noticeable effect,[169] unless they were added in concentrations >120 mM; moreover, the relationship between enamel dissolution and degree of saturation is complex.[2]

Blackcurrant juice (pH 3.8) with calcium has an erosive capacity eight times greater than orange juice (pH 3.8) with calcium.[139] A blackcurrant drink with more calcium is less erosive.[332] A drink with calcium plus maltodextrin was hardly erosive.[333] Calcium and xanthan gum (polysaccharide gum) in a blackcurrant drink were equally protective, but the drink with xanthan was more acceptable to consumers.[333]

6.6   Treatment

In the presence of acids, erosion continues to occur in the enamel surrounding restored lesions. Existing composite

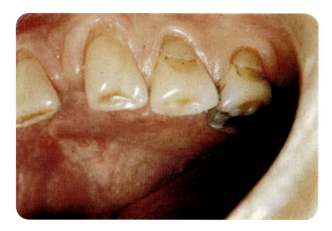

Figure 6.12 The enamel around the restored erosive lesions has disappeared because of ongoing erosion. The restorations are not or only slightly affected and are protruding from the enamel surface.

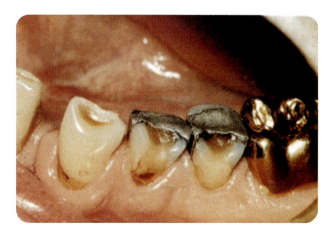

Figure 6.13 Occlusal and buccal erosion; the amalgam fillings are standing "proud" of the teeth.

or amalgam restorations (in the past cohesive gold was used)[137] may require substitution with larger ones within half a year (Figures 6.12 and 6.13). Glass ionomer cements disintegrate in an acidic environment.[347]

Extensive destruction requires crowns,[162 214] also to restore the vertical dimension. The crown margins must be situated subgingivally, when acid attacks are expected to continue. Restorations of "idiopathic" cervical lesions are subjected to flexure stresses, which may overcome the adhesive and marginal integrity of composite. A flexible microfilled or hybrid composite is indicated in a V-shaped preparation with an angle <135° and a cervical retention groove, after heavily loaded contacts with the antagonistic teeth have been corrected. The occlusal load on the tooth must not exceed that of adjacent teeth.[166 319]

6.7   Alleviation of cervical hypersensitivity

Patients with denuded cervical dentine may respond with a sharp, briefly felt pain upon chemical, thermal, osmotic, evaporative or tactile stimulation.[53] The diagnosis is made on basis of exclusion of other causes of pain, experienced by 15% to over 50% of patients.[55 76 88 104 181 188 253 270 300]

The term sensitivity is nowadays used to indicate pain associated with periodontal disease and its treatment.[3] In erosion the term hypersensitivity is proposed.

Cold is the most common stimulus eliciting dentine hypersensitivity. More females than males complain of pain.[104] Which teeth in particular are involved is not clear.[55 181] Aδ nerve fibres at the pulpal wall,[42] activated via the tubular hydrodynamic system, are responsible for the pain.[39 40 41 100 246] Under the influence of heat, the fluid in patent dentinal tubules moves rapidly inwards and cold causes an outwards movement, exciting the nerve endings.

The peripulpal dentine tubules contain nerves.[48 100 177] A difference in pain perception between coronal "sharp" and cervical "dull", is ascribed to the distribution of nerves.[176]

Kapila et al. reported that presence of plaque on dentine did not stop the fluid movements within the tubular hydrodynamic system, thus the pain continued;[159] however, the plaque caused the orifices of the tubules to increase in size by 400% within 3 weeks. Mechanical and chemical (chlorhexidine) cleaning decreased the width of the orifices.[159]

Absence of hypersensitivity has been linked to covering of the tubules orifices by the smear layer.[20] Surfactants in toothpastes remove the smear layer and open the tubules, but the abrasive constituent of a silica-based paste occluded the orifices.[331]

Patients may avoid tooth brushing and cold because of persisting pain. On teeth not very sensitive to thermal or tactile stimuli, an air blast was painful.[51] Not all denuded roots are hypersensitive though. Prerequisites for hypersensitivity are: erosion/wear of cementum, patent tubules and absence of smear layer.[20] Spontaneous occlusion of the tubules or degenerative changes in the odontoblastic layer leads to desensitisation.[247] The number and diameter of open tubules per unit area seem to have an influence.[2] The fluid flow in the tubules may be 100 times greater in sensitive than non-sensitive teeth.[53]

Desensitising systems aim to achieve:

- occlusion of the tubules
- coagulation of the tubular contents
- tertiary dentine formation
- blockage of the neural responses in the pulp.

It is not possible to say which treatment regimen is best,[270] because of the number of factors involved, placebo effects and lack of adequate experimental models.[313] None of the methods has been found to be consistently effective and their efficacy seems limited.

6.7.1   Fluoride

Sorvari et al. found that pain caused by consumption of a sports drink (pH 3.2) diminished after addition of fluoride to the drink as the tubules became partly occluded.[290] No difference in pain relief was found between use of toothpaste with 1400 ppm amine fluoride or 1400 ppm NaF or a toothpaste without fluoride, all with the same composition.[250] Use of amine fluoride for 4 weeks resulted in moderate reduction in cervical pain.[350] A commercial solution of 0.7% fluoride applied twice, each time for 1 minute, with a light rubbing motion, did not prove to be more effective than water used as a placebo.[230]

Potassium salts in toothpaste/gel/mouthwash
More rapid pain reduction has been attributed to occur with a monofluorophosphate toothpaste with potassium nitrate (KNO_3).[53 276 301] Potassium citrate may be more effective, and superior to potassium nitrate, but toothpastes with fluoride have also not appeared inferior.[237] Compared to non-potassium toothpastes, dentifrices with potassium nitrate had a significant treatment effect, but only after being used for 6–8 weeks.[251] Dentifrices with either KNO_3 or KCl (potassium chloride) have been assessed to be more effective than those not containing these chemicals, but other constituents may contribute to the desensitisation and placebo pastes also reduce pain substantially.[237]

- KNO_3, which is the most often used potassium salt, delivers K^+ ions which implement sustained depolarisation of the pulpal nerves and thereby interrupt the transmission of the pain signal to the brain.[53 198 237] KNO_3 does not change the permeability of the dentine,[111] but with silica the tubules are blocked. Use of stannous fluoride led to deposition of an insoluble tin hydroxide in the dentinal tubules, which inhibited the outward fluid flow from the pulp, but allowed increased pulpal potassium ion influx:[302] hypersensitivity 4 and 8 weeks later was better controlled than with a dentifrice with potassium nitrate.[265]
- *Potassium oxalate* is converted into insoluble calcium oxalate, which occludes the tubules.[236 237] Some 60% of teeth rubbed for 15 seconds with a potassium oxalate solution became less sensitive compared with 30% with a placebo. Inflammation may prevent the teeth from responding to treatment.[51] Aluminium and ferric oxalates, silica and calcium-containing agents also occlude the dentinal tubules.[53] Oxalate-containing agents precipitate crystals on the tooth surface.
- *Other potassium salts*, e.g. citrate. Trials of several potassium salts in solutions, gels, mouthwashes and toothpastes delivered varying results.[237] A nitrate and a citrate mouthwash with NaF reduced hypersensitivity, but no more than the effect of a placebo rinse.[237]

- *Strontium chloride* and *strontium acetate* occlude the tubule orifices and leave a heavy deposit covering the dentine.[20 53] Potassium carbonate with calcium chloride does not effectively block the tubules.[111] Consumption of water and orange juice decreases tubular occlusion, in particular that caused by a fluoride toothpaste.[20]

In the long term, strontium toothpastes may be efficacious,[225 312] but the literature is equivocal.[206] *In vitro* application of strontium chloride for 5 minutes formed a barrier within the orifices of the dentinal tubules.[165] Although a strontium chloride toothpaste may only cover the surface,[331] 10% strontium chloride + calcium carbonate abrasive occluded the tubules more than 3% monopotassium oxalate, 2.26% sodium fluoride, and strontium chloride with potassium nitrate.[242] No difference in pain reduction was found between two strontium toothpastes and a fluoride toothpaste.[247]

Sodium lauryl sulfate, a detergent found in many dentifrices, may reverse the blockage. The main question is whether use of these toothpastes opens or occludes the tubules.[331]

West *et al.* investigated four pastes containing:

A. Strontium acetate, NaF, hemihydrate, silica;
B. Strontium chloride, diatomaceous earth;
C. Potassium chloride, sodium monofluorophosphate, dicalcium phosphate;
D. Dicalcium phosphate, sodium monofluorophosphate.

By etching the dentine, the authors demonstrated that the degree of occlusion achieved was different between the four toothpastes. After 2 minutes, toothpaste A occluded the tubules significantly more than the other pastes. Toothpaste B was second best. The smear layer on unetched dentine was altered after brushing with the toothpastes and made the tubules visible, but toothpaste A occluded the tubules with silica after 1 minute of brushing.[331]

Despite the absence of strong evidence supporting the efficacy of potassium-containing toothpastes, there is no reason to advise against them,[137] because they may have a placebo effect.[329] Blockage of tubule orifices with "anti-sensitive" pastes may be reversed by new acidic attacks. Patients with erosion should not use a dentifrice that is very abrasive,[107] although such a paste[21] appeared to counteract hypersensitivity.[103]

6.7.2   Other desensitising agents

Application *in vitro* of either Gluma (hydroxymethacrylate, glutaraldehyde, mequinol) or MS Coat (polystyrene sulfonic acid, polymethylmethacrylate, oxalic acid) had no immediate effect on the hydraulic conductance of previously etched dentine. After 1 month storage in deionised water, the controls showed the same hydraulic conductance as treated dentine samples. However, Ms Coat relieved pain immediately *in vivo* in almost 100%

of the samples and may have the same effect as calcium oxalate.[52] Application of Gluma 2000 Conditioner (with oxalic acid) had a temporary desensitising effect[68] and probably coagulates the proteins in the fluid in the dentinal tubules.[52]

Calcium phosphate occluded the outer half of the tubules of vital teeth (dogs).[297] In the long-term, factors such as tooth brushing may modify the efficacy of the paste, because the abrasives may remove the coating on the root or a layer of dentine with blocked tubules, and by denuding dentine that was covered with gingiva.[52] Application of oxalic acid (2 minutes) blocked the tubules, which did not persist when rinsed for 1 minute with a water spray.[163]

A variety of other substances has been used to manage cervical pain, such as (black staining) silver nitrate, (para) formaldehyde and cocaine. Arsenic coagulates the proteins in the tubules, but damages the pulp.[133] Professional application of formaldehyde, tin fluoride and calcium hydroxide diminished hypersensitivity.[206] Glutaraldehyde superficially (10–20 μm) occluded the tubules *in vivo*.[69]

Incubation of etched dentine, four times in a buffered supersaturated calcium phosphate solution with fluoride, reduced the dentine conductance by 75%, presumably with fluorapatite. The authors suggest chewing gum as the vehicle.[57] Topical application (at day 1, 7 and 28) of aqueous calcium chloride followed by potassium phosphate resulted in the formation of amorphous calcium phosphate, which reduced hypersensitivity more rapidly than a placebo.[101]

6.7.3   Bonding systems

Bhatti *et al.* found that application of adhesives used for amalgam and composite restorations did not provide relief in all cases.[30] Composite adhesives relieved hypersensitivity,[87] but lost their efficiency over a period of some months.[244]

A one-bottle adhesive system when applied infiltrated (with and without etching) the dentinal tubules. In two-thirds of the teeth the bonding agent had to be re-applied 1–2 weeks later. Hypersensitivity returned gradually. After 3 months, the protective layer was partly present on etched dentine, but even after 1 month it was no longer present on non-etched dentine.[87] A light-cured resin occluded the tubules, whereas fluoride agents applied for 2 minutes lacked an effect.[163] Compared with a fourth-generation dentine adhesive, use of two fifth-generation adhesives reduced pain more effectively, but after 3 months the number of patients reporting "no improvement" increased. The fifth-generation adhesives were less likely to peel off than the fourth-generation adhesive.[244] One layer of a single-bottle dentine adhesive alleviated cervical pain immediately and the pain reduction remained significant 24 weeks after the treatment.[299]

Different bonding agents (adhesives) are not equally effective. After 3 months, a bonding agent with methacrylates and silica reduced pain more effectively than four other agents with different compositions, although there was loss of some effect with all with time.[71] An amalgam bonding was effective.[50] An *oxalate-containing pre-polymerised resin solution* provided immediate relief after a single application, but was found to reduce cervical pain no more than water or a 0.7% fluoride solution.[230]

6.7.4   Lasers

The effect of an neodymium:yttrium aluminum garnet (Nd:YAG) laser after 16 weeks did not differ from that seen with a placebo treatment. A drop in hypersensitivity was recorded, but pain diminution was also recorded after treatment with a switched-off beam.[175]

One 2-minute session with a Ne:He (neon-helium) laser may have an effect lasting for at least 3 months, as does the combination of Ne:He and Nd:YAG (neodymium: yttrium aluminum garnet).[102] *In vitro*, the Nd:YAG laser obliterated the dentinal tubules over a distance of 5–7 μm,[67] and clinically the blockage in the tubules was still present after 6 months.[58] Scanning electron microscopy has shown laser treatment to be effective.[167]

6.7.5   Occlusal equilibration

Selective occlusal grinding of cusps has been shown to result in long-term resolution of cervical hypersensitivity due to flexing of the tooth crowns on their roots.[61]

7

Tooth Resorption

7.1 Introduction

Tooth resorption is the destruction of the hard dental tissues by osteoclasts. Bone is continuously being resorbed (broken down) by the osteoclasts and re-formed (deposited) by osteoblasts. The resorption of the roots of the deciduous teeth is a *physiological process*. Pathological tooth resorption includes *external transient resorption*, which arrests spontaneously, and *progressive resorption*, which starts from within the tooth in the walls of the pulp cavity or on the external surface of the tooth.

The multinucleated (>20 nuclei) osteoclasts likely develop from haemopoietic, pluripotent stem cells circulating within the blood,[83 284] which first transform into mononuclear precursors, and which then fuse together,[84] possibly under the influence of colony-stimulating factors.[305] The osteoclast precursor cells attach to the bone and remain dormant until they are signalled by the osteoblasts to proliferate and fuse to form the osteoclasts.

Factors released by the osteoblasts, such as the receptor activator of nuclear factor κB ligand (RANKL), regulate the functions of the osteoclasts.[330] Pre-osteoclasts treated with RANKL transform into osteoclasts. Osteoprotegerin (a member of the tumour necrosis factor (TNF) receptor superfamily) suppresses the resorption activity of the osteoclasts.[376]

The tooth-resorbing cells, the odontoclasts, may be smaller than the osteoclasts, with a maximum of 10 nuclei.[105 160] The existence of specific odontoclasts is not confirmed but if they do exist they have the same origin as the osteoclasts.[397] Cementoblasts may transform into cementoclasts.[55]

The ruffle border of the osteoclasts, which consists of a system of canals, is the active site of resorption. The osteoclasts secrete factors that lower the extracellular pH, resulting in dissolution of the mineral bone phase, and attack the organic matrix with enzymes.[22 46 284 313 330]

Antiresorptive factors

A healthy periodontal ligament prevents migration of alveolar bone components towards the root,[139 295] but when the ligament is compromised, osteoclasts spread over and resorb the denuded cementum and dentine.[69 436]

Pre-cementum (a 3–8 μm thick, chiefly organic layer on the cementum)[46] appears to be protective,[244] as osteoclasts cannot bind to such non-mineralised tissues.[162 314 369 422] The predentine is also protective.[162 194] The circumpulpal dentine, which is less mineralised than the mantle dentine[184] and richer in acid polysaccharides,[447] protects the pulp from cervical resorption for a considerable period of time. The dentinal destruction proceeds and encircles the pulp cavity, but the pulp itself remains vital.[146 396 447] Collagen-rich predentine is supposedly formed in response to the eventual resorption.[146] Macrophages seeded on predentine and demineralised dentine remain attached and do not migrate. The organic, non-collagen component of dentine may contain an inhibitor against macrophages and osteoclasts.[435 436] Research is ongoing to discover inhibitors, for instance a collagenase or protease,[168 258] and to understand the processes by which cells disperse over the surface.[434]

Cementum and dentine contain mucopolysaccharides that are active in the ligament of resorbing deciduous teeth, but these substances have not been found when these teeth are ankylosed.[8]

Denervation of the inferior alveolar nerve was found to result in ankylosis of the second molars. It was proposed that the microscopic epithelial islands of Malassez (see Chapter 3)[267 329] may help maintain the width of the periodontal space. Denervation results in loss of the islands of Malassez, which may then allow an increase in the number of osteoclasts in the periodontal space.[139] However, this idea of protection provided by the network of epithelial islands has not gained support,[422] and nor has the notion of protection by Sharpey's fibres in the cementum.

Pathology of the Hard Dental Tissues, First Edition. Albert Schuurs.
© 2013 Albert Schuurs. Published 2013 by Blackwell Publishing Ltd.

7.2   Physiological external root resorption: deciduous teeth

Physiological resorption is the breakdown of the roots of the deciduous teeth by osteoclasts. Resorption of the deciduous roots, which is necessary for exfoliation, starts soon after root completion on the linguo-apical aspect of the deciduous anterior teeth roots and at the inner side of the molar roots. Pressure exerted by the succedaneous tooth damages the cells lying in the path of eruption, which secrete chemical mediators such as prostaglandin E_2, hormones, neurotransmitters, cytokines and monokines (including interleukins), and proteinases.[22 75] During resorption, the cementoblasts adjacent to the osteoclasts continue to regularly deposit small amounts of cementum and bundles of collagen fibres;[377] this "remodelling" process activates the osteoclasts. If there is agenesis of the succedaneous tooth, the root of the predecessor may or may not be resorbed.[288]

While a deciduous root is being resorbed, any permanent root in the vicinity is not resorbed. This is because of the differences in the spatial pattern of expression of two extracellular matrix proteins (osteopontin and bone sialoprotein) which influence osteoclast adhesion and activity.[251]

7.3   Transient external root resorption: both dentitions

Transient resorption is limited osteoclastic resorption of cementum and the adjacent superficial dentine, with apposition of cementum in the repair phase. Transient resorption arrests spontaneously. This innocuous[289] process occurs in almost all dentitions.[183] The minute apical shortening and lateral defects caused by transient resorption are often not visible on radiographs. A localised absence of periradicular space allows the alveolar bone cells to come in contact with the root. The normal renewal of the periodontal ligament may underlie the transient destruction,[44] but other causes have also been suggested.

7.3.1   Trauma

Mechanical injuries to the teeth cause transient external resorption when a *small* part of the periodontal ligament is lost as a consequence of a local, sterile inflammatory response.[14 22 421] Transient internal resorption at the apical end follows more severe injuries and allows ingress of a vascular network, which aids pulpal healing.[14] The process arrests spontaneously[14 15 18] in the absence of ongoing stimulation.[141] Symptoms may include short-term crown discoloration and temporary loss of pulpal sensibility.[14]

Healing depends on the outcome of the competition between the bone cells and periodontal cells.[22 260] Renewal of the ligament via differentiation of adjacent ligament cells occurs when only a small area (up to a few square millimetres) of a generally healthy periodontal ligament is involved.[351] In contrast with transient resorption, bone cells invade the ligament space permanently when larger areas are damaged.[141] Healing involves deposition of cellular cementum.[171 245 246 297] When the resorptive phase ends, repair is accomplished within a few weeks.[38 141 259] In experimental root cavities, macrophage-like cells from the blood stream have been observed after 24 hours. Three days later lacunae were formed by the osteoclasts, which were attributed to activity of cells with a ruffle border, and fibroblast-like cells from the periphery started to colonise the cavities. Six weeks later the cavities showed formation of reparative cementum.[209 210] Receptors for the epidermal growth factor in the cell membrane of the active cementoblasts in the neighbourhood of the resorption lacunae are "switched on".[397] The periradicular space regained its normal width.

7.3.2   Orthodontics

Orthodontic tooth movement may cause transient external root resorption.[104 288] At the site where the orthodontic force is directed, the periodontal ligament becomes compressed and the pressure is transmitted to the adjacent bone. The pressure exerted by the orthodontic force interferes with the metabolism of the ligament and its cells secrete the mediators already mentioned above, whereupon osteoclasts residing in the bone marrow resorb the bone. As the cementum is more resistant, when bone is resorbed, the tooth moves and the hyalinised tissue (sterile necrosis) is replaced by newly formed vital tissue.

When the orthodontic force is applied, regardless of whether is it heavy or light, the blood supply within the periodontal ligament is compromised when the hydrostatic pressure exceeds the capillary blood pressure.[452] The necrotic ligament tissues stimulate cellular activity that degrades these tissues, and the root is no longer protected from the osteoclasts.[108] On the pressure side,[282] root resorption is seen in relation to the hyalinised zones.[237]

Healing

After the pressure from the orthodontic force is relieved, the necrotic tissue is cleared. Cementoblasts lay down cementum in the resorptive lesions,[108 334] followed by the renewal of the periodontal ligament. The process (in rats) takes about 3 weeks.[80] Root resorption arrests either during the late phase of active orthodontic treatment[171] or in the retention period.[93] In the post-treatment period, sharp root edges become rounded.[357] In one-quarter of a sample of adolescents undergoing orthodontic treatment, repair started 1 week after the placement of retention appliances, and in the remaining sample after 8 weeks.[334]

Prevalence and degree of orthodontic root resorption

The reported prevalence of tooth resorption caused by orthodontic treatment varies between 3.5% and 100%[75] [130] due to differences in identification criteria and treatment methods used in the various studies. The maxillary central incisor is most frequently affected, followed by the mandibular incisors.[108 213 292 357] "Blunting" (shortening) of the root apex is often the only sign of orthodontic root resorption, in general a few millimetres, and occasionally reported to be much as 5–6.5 mm.[3 16 168 240 264 269 281 299 345 357] Maxillary lateral incisors with abnormal root morphology become more blunted than the central incisors.[373] Treatment involving extraction of first premolars leads to greater blunting of the central incisor roots than non-extraction therapy.[374] Full-grown roots show more resorption than incomplete ones, and this is a reason for early orthodontic treatment,[181] but whether adults undergoing orthodontic treatment show more resorption than adolescents is doubtful.[264 299]

Blunting up to 3 mm leads to loss of tooth attachment as much as that caused by 1 mm loss of cervical bone in periodontitis. When the apical resorption is progressive, the greater root circumference increases the amount of attachment loss disproportionately.[214]

Factors

- Studies show either a weak or no association between treatment duration and degree of blunting.[50 95 181 264 298 345 412] A pause in treatment leads to cessation of resorption,[256 282] but Owman-Moll et al. found that the effects of orthodontic appliances exerting a continuous force were no worse than those of a discontinuous force.[333]
- *Appliances*: Begg's orthodontic treatment is accompanied by resorption,[240] but use of intermaxillary elastics with other appliances may often cause more resorption than seen with Begg's or use of magnets.[76] Other studies have found similar degree of resorption with the edgewise and Begg's techniques.[255 358] Edgewise appliances might generate stronger forces than the "straight wire" appliance, which involves using pre-formed archwires, which are deformed on insertion into the brackets attached to the teeth. These archwires then slowly attempt to recover their original shape, and in the process the teeth are moved into the desired arch form. Orthodontic tipping movements may be less damaging than bodily movement with fixed appliances.[130]
- The *distance* over which the tooth is moved is related to the severity of root resorption.[108 282 298] The larger the apical displacement of the incisors, the more severely blunted are the roots.[374]

- The *strength* of the force may not be a factor,[108 282] but this is an oversimplification.[374] A fourfold increased force, from 50 to 200 g, indeed may not cause more frequent or more severe resorption,[336] but higher force magnitudes may be detrimental. A light force may initially seem more detrimental than a stronger one,[335] just like a light force has been shown to move a tooth initially over a greater distance than a stronger force.[225 335] However, the cementoid tends to decrease in thickness on the side of compression, where more resorption occurs than on the tension side, and this has been shown to be more with a heavy force compared with a light force.[453]
- The degree of resorption has also been found to vary regardless of the above factors.[7 239 292 333] The bone quality and effects of medicaments and diseases also co-determine whether resorption occurs.

Hypocalcaemia in cats undergoing orthodontics was associated with an increase in the number of osteoclasts and root resorption.[120] Hyper(para)thyroidism promotes alveolar bone remodelling. After parathormone therapy, the intercellular space between the osteoblasts is widened, thereby offering the osteoclasts the opportunity to colonise the bone surface; the cementoblasts do not do the same.[261]

Medicaments such as thyroxine that increase alkaline phosphatase activity, affect bone metabolism.[349] In one study, administration of 0.5 g thyroxine/day arrested initial resorption during orthodontic treatment.[266] However, before this can be used clinically, it needs to be clarified which patients may be treated in this way.[90 350] Administering prostaglandin E_2 stimulated bone resorption and initially speeded up tooth movement, though inconsistently.[65] Indometacin counteracts the action of prostaglandins and tooth movement.[148] Bisphosphonate, a potent blocker of bone resorption, affected tooth movement (and also tooth eruption) negatively.[203] Phenytoin (anti-epileptic) reduces the number of osteoclasts in the bone walls on the pressure side and thereby delays tooth movement.[216]

Ultrasound may be preventive.[117] Low-intensity ultrasound has an anti-inflammatory action and when it was applied for 20 minutes/day to premolars that required to be tipped, the numbers and areas of resorption lacunae decreased and healing with hypercementosis was seen.[117]

- *Direction of tooth movement*. Intrusion, torquing (rotating) and bodily tooth movements are, in this order, the most likely to cause orthodontic root resorption.[108] *Torquing* immediately caused resorption. Continuous torquing of premolars resulted in formation of many resorption lacunae.[89 206] Resorption is frequently seen after *intrusion*,[50] but a light force caused, in 4 months, only a slight blunting of the roots.[95] The duration of intrusion may be more influential than the degree of intrusion,[268] specially in maxillary incisors versus the mandibular ones.[292] However other studies did not report a significant effect of duration.[103] In adults, *retraction* has been found to be most damaging.[47]

- *Anatomical features*, such as the proximity of nasal floor may be a limiting factor for intrusion of the maxillary incisors.[103] The risk of severe resorption is increased 20-fold for roots situated close to the cortical bone,[213] however, others have suggest that the amount of tooth movement was more important.[298] Severe resorption occurs when the apex is moved outside the bone.[164]
- *Predisposing factors* are overjet, anterior open bite (tongue thrusting), mouth breathing, thumb sucking and nail biting (which also leads to blunts in the absence of orthodontic treatment), trauma prior to orthodontic treatment, deviations in root morphology and gender.[75] [76 168 169 255 264 326 366 373 413] In adults, treatment duration and the degree to which the apex was moved were found to be related to resorption, and this was more in men than in women;[47] however, this was not the case in a study of brothers and sisters.[170] Teeth with *blunt* and pipette-shaped roots might particularly be at risk.[254] Resorption on the prominent sides of the root during rotational movements emphasises the importance of the root morphology.[206]
- In asthmatic people, the incidence, but not the amount, of root resorption may be increased.[293] Vital teeth may be resorbed more than endodontically treated teeth,[298] [299 357 405] but others have not found a difference.[454] A Class III molar relationship increases the risk of severe root resorption.[213]

7.3.3   Chronic periodontitis

The more severe is the periodontitis, the greater is the amount of resorption of the root surface in the gingival third of the roots and apically.[172 361] The transient resorption may become progressive. Repair with cementum has been observed after improvements in oral hygiene.[109]

7.3.4   Other causes

Blunting has been reported in 7–10% of patients with occlusal overload after extraction and loss of periodontal attachment.[169] An experimental study found that occlusal overload results in resorption of the cementum without ankylosis.[367] The distal root of mandibular permanent second molar may become blunted as part of ageing.

7.4   Progressive resorption: both dentitions

In progressive resorption, the continuation of the process depends on ongoing stimulation of the osteoclasts.[141] Several types of internal and external resorption exist.

7.4.1   Internal resorption

Internal resorption is progressive breakdown caused by osteoclasts, starting at the internal (pulpal) walls and

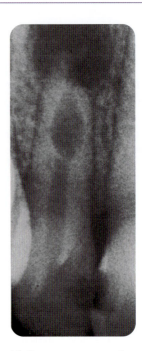

Figure 7.1 Internal inflammatory resorption.

progressing to the periphery of the tooth, sometimes with formation of bone-like dentine.

Types and macroscopic appearance
A vital pulp is needed for the initiation and progression of internal resorption.[18] The anomaly is commonly detected incidentally on radiographs. Clinical symptoms are absent or may not be noticed by the patient or the dentist. There are three types of internal resorption:

- *Internal inflammatory resorption* (more recently termed *radial pulp enlargement resorption*). Radiographs show an oval to round and rather smooth edged radiolucent widening of the pulp cavity (Figure 7.1) or apically. Unless the lesion has advanced to the root surface (Figure 7.2), dentine (and continuous forming[53] cementum) separates the lesion from the periradicular space.
- *Internal replacement resorption (metaplastic pulp resorption)* (Figure 7.3) is associated with irregular, radiolucent pulpal widening with radiopaque areas where osteodentine is formed. A well-demarcated lesion may distinguish internal from external resorption,[144] but which as such is probably not true.
- *Internal tunnelling resorption*. This process of tooth tissue breakdown after an injury is characterised by the formation of a "burrow" or tunnel behind the predentine layer, along the pulp chamber, occasionally extending into the root. Ultimately the tunnel and the pulp chamber are obliterated.[22]

On radiographs, areas of external labial/buccal and lingual resorption are projected over the pulp cavity and

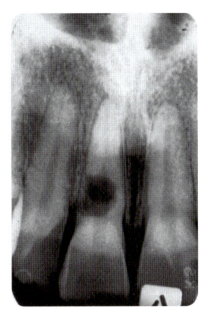

Figure 7.2 Internal inflammatory resorption perforating the root.

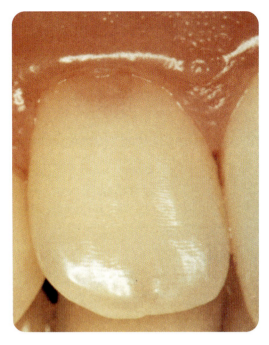

Figure 7.4 The pink spot is the result of either internal resorption in the crown or cervical resorption starting in the root.

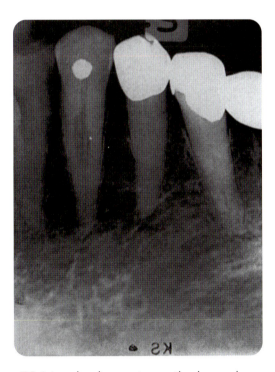

Figure 7.3 Internal replacement resorption in a canine.

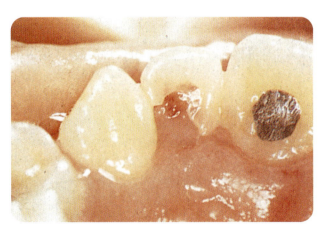

Figure 7.5 A pulp polyp formed due to progression of an internal resorption lesion from within the crown towards the tooth surface.

may mistakenly be diagnosed as internal resorption. If on taking radiographs at an angle (from mesial and distal) the lesions are projected outside of the pulp contour, they are external, and if not, they are internal.[22] The ligament/alveolar bone is normal, unless the root surface is involved.[67]

Internal defects are stated not to perforate the external root surfaces, because it is unlikely that both the predentine/odontoblastic layer and the cementum/cementoblasts are involved in the same lesion.[271]

When internal resorption reaches the dentino-enamel junction, the pulp shines through the enamel: this is called *pink spot (of Mummery)* (Figure 7.4).[310] A pulp polyp, a proliferation of pulp tissue, is seen (Figure 7.5) when the process breaks through the enamel.[392]

Microscopic appearance and associated findings
The resorptive lesions are filled with proliferating granulation tissue. Irregular *lacunae (of Howship)* in the pulpal walls contain macrophages in the predentine and osteoclasts in the dentine.[435] Resorbing cells showed strong acid phosphatase activity, similar to osteoclasts.[437]

The predentine is resorbed locally by the action of the macrophages/enzymes but new predentine is not laid down because of the death of the odontoblasts. The osteoclasts or their precursors are thus no longer prevented from reaching the dentine. However, it is only after the granulation-like tissue comes in contact with mineralised dentine that the osteoclasts attack the dentine. The internal resorptive activity usually occurs in relation to an infected vital pulp, but the pulp may also be necrotic coronal to the resorptive defect.[418] Root predentine may also undergo physiological "resorption", as part of ageing, starting apically.[408]

In replacement resorption, bone-like dentine is formed within the lesion, by odontoblast-like cells. Phases of clastic and blastic activity are interrupted by intermittent resting periods.[152]

Aetiology and epidemiology
The prevalence of internal resorption in the permanent teeth is 0.1–1.6%;[346] it is lower in the deciduous dentition.[392] In general, only one tooth per dentition is involved. The causes of internal resorption can be divided into three groups: inflammatory, systemic and idiopathic.

Inflammation-related causes
Replacement resorption accompanies moderate pulpal inflammation and inflammatory resorption is seen in more severe pulpitis.[275]

Deep caries (caries profunda) Rarely, pulpitis caused by deep carious lesions results in internal resorption.[415] The resorptive lesions always contain inflammatory cells.[275] Inadequate caries removal is considered another cause.[228]

Trauma Within a few weeks after tooth injury, internal resorption may start as a consequence of pulp inflammation. After luxation (traumatically displaced tooth) about 1.5% of deciduous and permanent teeth undergo internal resorption.[22 221] Pulpitis may also develop due to microleakage through a crack in the tooth.

Iatrogenic Restorative dental materials may elicit an inflammatory pulpal reaction, as does microleakage along the cavity walls. Insufficient water cooling during cutting procedures in the permanent teeth[309] has been implicated. With cooling, cavity preparation with a coarse diamond bur results in rise in the pulpal temperature of about 3 °C,

which does not lead to pulpal damage. Despite this, short intervals of rest during preparation are advised.[332] A temperature rise during external bleaching of newly erupted teeth could lead to internal resorption.[389]

Brief heat application to the enamel to several hundred degree Celsius has been shown to cause reversible pulpitis.[136] A rise in temperature of 42.5 °C and 47 °C led to irreversible pulpal damage in 15% and 60% of the pulps, respectivley.[450] A gradual increase to 49 °C also led to irreversible pulpal damage.[10]

In an *in vitro* study, application of heat at 60 °C to amalgam and composite fillings with para-pulpal pins elevated the temperature in the pulp to about 45 °C.[33] Most people consume coffee and tea that is at a temperature of 55–68 °C,[102] which elevates the temperature in pulps under amalgam fillings by just a few degrees.[296] In another study, heat application to the teeth until the subjects reported pain and thereafter maintained for 30 seconds did not affect the pulp.[40]

In an *in vivo* study, light curing of a composite increased the mean temperature of the filling and surrounding tissues by 11.7 °C maximally.[198] Finishing composite restorations with flexible, coarse discs was found to raise the pulp temperature to a mean of 45 °C (maximum 50 °C); which may endanger the pulp.[77] There are no reports of development of internal resorption after these procedures.

Direct pulp capping/vital amputation Direct pulp capping/ vital amputation with calcium hydroxide $(Ca(OH)_2)$ and glutaraldehyde (7%),[140] formocresol,[185] and zinc oxide-eugenol cement[276] is a major cause of internal resorption in deciduous teeth.[275 385 415] Ferric sulfate medication was found to be worse than sodium hypochlorite.[455] A blood clot between the vital pulp and the $Ca(OH)_2$ dressing[384] or an operative procedure such as aggressive amputation technique,[22] have also been implicated. Mineral trioxide aggregate (MTA) may be as effective as $Ca(OH)_2$ or superior[456] as it has better qualities, and is increasingly used in place of calcium hydroxide.

After pulpotomy with $Ca(OH)_2$, 80% of one sample of deciduous molars showed internal resorption within 0.5–2 years.[275] Other studies have reported rates of 20–33% after 1 year.[385] Removal of the blood clot from the pulp surface prior to application of the dressing markedly reduced the likelihood of resorption.[386]

Formocresol, a controversial medicament, has been found to induce internal resorption in some 10% of cases,[185 194] but only in 2% of permanent teeth with acute pulpitis.[194] Similar clinical and radiographic success has been reported with pulp capping with formocresol and the non-toxic ferric sulfate.[457] Half of one sample of pulps with zinc oxide-eugenol cement dressings showed internal resorption on radiographs,[276] but histological examination revealed that all teeth were affected.[276 277]

Orthodontics Orthodontic treatment in adults and traumatic occlusion occasionally cause internal resorption;[71] [228 353] this is because movement of teeth with small apical foramina may lead to pulpal inflammation due to the reduction in blood supply.

Systemic disease

Internal resorption lesions in the lower incisors of a patient with end-stage *renal disease* resolved after kidney transplantation,[200] but in a study of patients with chronic renal failure no internal resorption was found.[2] Internal and external resorption was seen in patients with *hypophosphatasia*.[66] *Herpes zoster* (shingles) seems causative[403] and some systemic diseases may lead to internal resorption in multiple teeth.[353]

Reactivation of latent varicella virus (chicken pox virus) leads to herpes zoster: neuralgia is followed by vesicular eruptions on the part of skin that is innervated by the nerve fibres of the infected ganglion. In about 20% of cases, the disease affects the trigeminal nerve and has been implicated in internal resorption.[403]

Idiopathic causes

In many patients, none of the conditions mentioned above are present.[88 156 323] Long-forgotten trauma or bruxism may be causative.[189] Internal resorption in some deciduous teeth has been reported to be idiopathic,[189 372] as was internal resorption in non-erupted teeth[71 431] and an erupting premolar.[78] In a sample of impacted third molars, about 0.4% had internal resorption.[36] Pre-eruptive resorption of the hard tissues surrounding the pulp chamber[390] may leave just a shell of enamel. In these cases, the osteoclasts are thought to reach the dentine via a break in the enamel.

Treatment

Internal resorption in a deciduous tooth is not treated, unless the child is in pain. Endodontic treatment of a permanent tooth arrests progression of internal resorption.[310] Experimental studies have shown that the process may be transient in the absence of pulp inflammation.[435] However, this is rarely reported to be the case in humans,[200] so a "wait and see" approach is not recommended. Endodontic treatment has predictable outcomes.[141] However, the files may not reach the lesion walls and filling of the lesion cavity using the lateral condensation technique usually results in incomplete obturation (Figure 7.6). One solution is cleaning the pulp cavity with a Gates Glidden drill by hand, ultrasonic irrigation with sodium hypochlorite and obturation with warm gutta-percha (Figure 7.7). Çaliskan *et al.* found that internally resorbed teeth without perforation were asymptomatic 4 years after endodontic treatment.[85]

A perforated root is filled with $Ca(OH)_2$,[135] which must remain *in situ* for 2 months.[419] When the surrounding bone is not involved, a period of 2–4 weeks is sufficient.[409] Alternatively, a surgical approach may be used. A buccogingival flap is raised, the bone is removed, and the perforation is curetted and closed with a retrograde or antegrade filling.[145 247]

$Ca(OH)_2$ application results in resolution of the inflammation and it induces closure of the perforation with hard dental tissue.

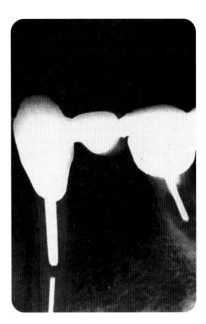

Figure 7.6 Unfilled internal resorption defect associated with an intracanal pin. The lesion will not progress because the pulp is non-vital, but apical microleakage is possible.

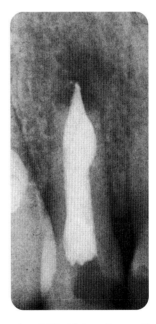

Figure 7.7 Cleaned and filled internal resorption defect 8 years after endodontic treatment. The root canal filling was overextended apically.

In this way, later endodontic manipulation of the root canal will not lead to bleeding and the root canal can be obturated adequately. Çaliskan *et al.* suggested using root-end (retrograde) fillings or extracting the teeth because of the low success rate.[85]

Internal coronal resorption that is encroaching the pulp may require surgical exposure of the unerupted tooth.[390]

7.4.2 Progressive external resorption of roots(/crowns)

Progressive external resorption refers to ongoing osteoclastic breakdown, starting on the outside of the tooth, either with or without replacement of lost tissue with bone.

Types and macroscopic appearance

Based upon macroscopic appearance, the cause and location, three or possibly four types are distinguished:[18] external inflammatory resorption, external replacement resorption, cervical resorption and (?) multiple cervical resorption. A large increase in mobility after resorption of most of the root is a consequence of external inflammatory resorption. In case of external replacement resorption, as the root and bone are in close contact and bone replaces the root, the tooth becomes immobile. A pink spot is indicative of a cervical or internal process. Other clinical symptoms are commonly absent.

External inflammatory root resorption

The periradicular space is locally widened. Bowl-shaped proximal and more often apical root lesions are seen on radiographs as radiolucencies (Figure 7.8). A large apical granuloma may be present. A large part of the root may be resorbed within a period of months. Radiographs sometimes show remnants of a root canal filling in the bone (Figure 7.9). Tooth mobility increases as the process progresses.

External root replacement resorption

There is local absence of the periodontal space and the alveolar lamina dura on radiographs and bone replaces the root progressively,[421] with interdigitation of the bone and root tissues. Gradually the whole root is replaced to the level of the alveolar bone crest, when the resorption halts. The process is slower than inflammatory resorption.[27 29 418] *Ankylosis* (immobility) develops within 4–8 weeks, but is detectable earlier with the use of Periotest, an instrument that measures tooth mobility. Ankylosed teeth cannot erupt further, leading to infra-occlusion (Chapter 4), which renders extraction more difficult or impossible, with increased risk of root fractures.

Radiographs show replacement resorption as angular, somewhat vague lesions (Figure 7.10) within 8 weeks after the start of the process on the proximal surfaces or at the apex.[13] Labial and lingual lesions may not be visible before 12 months have elapsed.[22] After replantation of avulsed teeth, external inflammatory and replacement resorption may be radiographically evident within 2 months but often go undetected for about 6 months. The risk of resorption is markedly reduced if it is not evident radiographically up to 2 years.[22]

The percussion sound is dull when <10% of the root surface is ankylosed and becomes metallic, high and clear when a larger part of the surface is involved.[13] The change in sound can be heard before the lesion is visible on radiographs.[18]

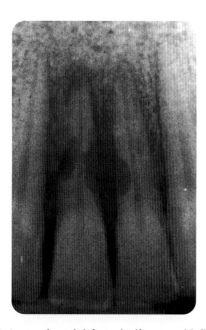

Figure 7.8 Saucer-shaped defects signify external inflammatory resorption; the periodontal space is enlarged.

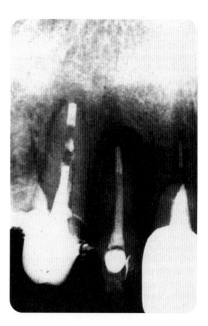

Figure 7.9 The root of the front teeth shows external replacement resorption; the old root canal filling material is visible within the bone that has replaced the root. The lateral incisor shows a granuloma with apical inflammatory resorption.

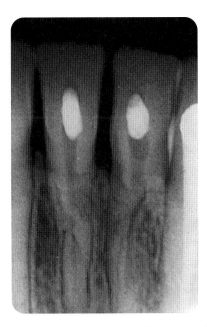

Figure 7.10 External replacement resorption. Due to the absence of the periodontal ligament, the bone is in intimate contact with the root dentine. The replacement dentine has a "ghost-like" appearance.

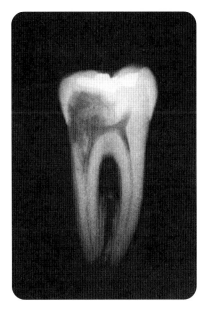

Figure 7.11 Cervical resorption seen on an X-ray of an extracted molar. The defect shows some resemblance with a carious lesion, but it is not uniformly black.

Cervical resorption

Progressive cervical resorption is inflammatory in nature,[420] with replacement starting underneath the epithelial attachment, probably after injury to the precementum and bacterial stimulation from the gingival sulcus.[141] The process results in hollowing out of the root dentine and may extend into the coronal dentine. The hyperplastic invasive resorption, i.e. resorptive tissue, invades the tooth lesion contains patchy areas of reparative remineralisation, resembling osteodentine.[346 420] Radiographs may show a mottled image with radiolucent and radiopaque zones (Figure 7.11). The periodontal space and the bone may be spared,[134] or the alveolar bone may be involved.[418] Numerous, loosely organised blood vessels and a fibrous mass are present within the lesion, a granulation-like tissue with inflammatory cells,[177] which bleeds abundantly upon touching.[46] Eventually the enamel is resorbed,[146 193] and the lesion may perforate the enamel.[177] External cervical resorption is more likely the underlying cause of a "pink spot" than internal resorption.[417 420 429]

A thin radiopaque line separates the pulp from the lesion, but several radiographs may be needed to clearly visualise the line, which is important as it distinguishes cervical from internal resorption. The lesion encircles the pulp, which is protected by the undermineralised dentine. The pulp thus remains vital,[177 193 447] and the process is thus also termed *invasive extra-pulpal resorption*.[134] When pockets are present, the resorptive lesion may be situated close to the apex. The lesions may be infra-osseous (at the height of the retracted bone crest) or supra-osseous,[134] and have alternatively been termed *invasive radicular resorption* and *invasive coronal resorption*, repectively.[177]

The rate of progression of the process is not well documented. Mock *et al.* estimated that in 1.5 years a new lesion becomes significantly large.[300]

Multiple cervical resorption

Multiple idiopathic cervical lesions may represent a separate condition.[270] It occurs in the permanent teeth, but one case has been reported in which all the deciduous teeth showed triangular cervical defects.[223] The few reported patients are mostly females, often in the second or third decade of life.[222] The lesions expand considerably within a few months.[270]

Microscopic appearance

External inflammatory resorption Lymphocytes, plasma cells, polymorphonuclear (PMN) leucocytes and granulation tissue are present in the periradicular space. The dentinal wall shows Howship's lacunae with osteoclasts.

The process proceeds as follows. A minor trauma causes transient surface resorption, which exposes the orifices of the dentinal tubules, whereby (and at the apical foramen and the openings of additional pulp canals) microorganisms and/or their endotoxins (from an infected or necrotic pulp) reach the periradicular space.[18 20 22 162]

Because of the continuous infectious stimulus, the transient process becomes progressive.[18 22 259] The role of the granulation tissue and proliferation of capillaries in the granulation tissue has been emphasised; the bone is also resorbed.[37 195 327]

External replacement resorption Traumatic non-bacterial necrosis of the periodontal ligament precedes replacement resorption.[18] The necrotic area is too large for cells from the intact, surrounding ligament to replace; osteoclasts and osteoblasts thus reach the root.[19 30] The newly formed bone extends into the resorption lacunae in the root, leading to ankylosis.

Sometimes bone is deposited on non-resorbed cementum.[13] After removal of bone and periodontal ligament from one half of the root, Melcher *et al.* found that bone callus filled the periodontal space and ankylosis developed. On the root half without bone but covered with ligament, callus formed on the outside of the ligament.[295]

Transient replacement resorption is not necessarily accompanied by ankylosis, and thus the tooth may regain mobility after repair of the lesion.

External cervical resorption Initiation and progression of the lesion requires a steady blood supply, which also originates under the attachment of the periodontal ligament. Hence it is also called *subepithelial external root resorption*. Osteoclasts penetrate the root through a small area lacking (pre)-cementum, leading to breakdown of the inorganic component and exposure of the dentinal matrix. Peritubular dentine and, in particular, the dentine closest to the pulp are the tissues most resistant to resorption.[70 418] The lesion shows numerous tunnel-like areas and islands consisting of rarefied connective or fibrous tissue, fibroblasts and collagen fibres, inflammatory cells and many blood vessels.[146] Cervical resorption may cause ankylosis.[418]

Aetiology and epidemiology
The causes of external resorption may be divided into six groups.

Inflammation
Pulpitis/pulp necrosis Pulp infection/necrosis initiates and maintains progressive external inflammatory root resorption.[141] Lateral and/or apical lesions have been noted to develop (Figure 7.12) in few to almost half of permanent teeth with a necrotic (or infected) pulp[211 218 287] and incidentally in deciduous teeth.[221] The longer the inflammation exists, the more severe is the resorption;[391] and the greater the periapical bone destruction, the higher the probability of resorption.[211] Teeth with filled root canals resorb less often and less severely than those with unfilled roots.[211] Young teeth with their wide dentinal tubules are more frequently resorbed than older teeth.[162]

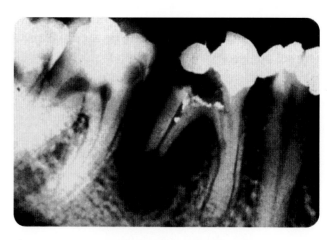

Figure 7.12 External inflammatory resorption of the distal root of a first molar. The root canals in the mesial root are obliterated, which may have inhibited the toxins from reaching the apical region and thereby may have prevented resorption of the mesial root.

Gingivitis/periodontitis Gingivitis/periodontitis is associated with cervical resorption,[172 279] also termed *external granuloma (granuloma externum)*. Peripheral giant cell granuloma of the gingiva, a benign tumour, is a rare cause.[319] Osteoclasts and granulation tissue penetrate the dentine.[382]

In view of the frequent occurrence of gingivitis and periodontitis, cervical resorption should be common. Indeed, Schroeder *et al.* reported the presence of numerous 30–80 μm deep resorption cavities in roots near resorbed alveolar bone.[383] Macroscopic cervical resorption is, however, rare and demands a predisposing (absent cementum) and continuous presence of the aetiological factor.[69 369 418 429] Mandatory prerequisite conditions are long-term periodontal infection, combined with trauma to the ligament, such as due to excessive usage of toothpicks leading to formation of blood clots in the periodontal space,[300] periodontal surgery,[418] damage due to extraction of an adjacent tooth, etc.[46 130 308] Severe cervical resorption has been reported to develop after guided tissue regeneration,[62] and near pockets filled with autogenous bone grafts,[109 147] ceramic implants substituting bone,[140] hydroxyapatite particles in infrabony pockets,[204] and after orthognathic surgery.[188]

Brösjö *et al.* found that lacunae filled with granulation tissue and osteoclasts developed in foil-covered cervical dentine cavities while an epithelial layer developed on uncovered cavities.[79]

Trauma (Chapter 9)
Trauma causes progressive inflammatory, replacement and cervical resorption. After tooth transplantation, cervical resorption may develop in the long term.[56]

Concussion Minor trauma without tooth displacement and mobility leads to periodontal injury with a small risk external replacement resorption.[346]

Luxation Intentional traumatic luxation in animals and luxation occurring accidentally in humans causes progressive external replacement resorption.[16][367] Depending on the luxation type (lateral, palatal/lingual or labial/buccal displacement of a tooth), resorption is observed in 1–18% of cases.[22] *Intrusion* (inward displacement) is most frequently associated with resorption and *subluxation* (mobile, but not displaced teeth) and *extrusion* (partial outward displacement) least frequently.[23][287] The root development stage and the severity of the intrusion determine whether the pulp will survive, and thereby the probability of external inflammatory resorption. Al-Badri *et al.* found that permanent incisors in children with <3mm intrusion had good prognosis, while teeth intruded >6mm resorbed. Neither spontaneous nor orthodontically mediated re-eruption influences the prevalence and rate of resorption.[6] Figure 7.13 shows resorption (and dilaceration) following trauma.

Stabilisation of luxated teeth with a rigid splint (Chapter 9) and splinting for longer than 1–2 weeks promote internal and external resorption and ankylosis.[17][22] Non-rigid splinting for 4–6 weeks does not lead to resorption.[115]

Root fracture Resorption leads to rounding off of the sharp edges of fractured root fragments, but tunnelling or external inflammatory or replacement resorption develop

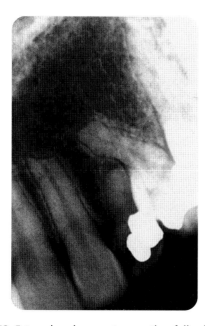

Figure 7.13 External replacement resorption following trauma to a lateral incisor and canine (and a first premolar with a curved root).

in 60%.[22][346] The processes may last several years or may be self-limiting. Fracture of the alveolar process is implicated in external inflammatory resorption in 3–30% of traumatised teeth.[22] A crushed alveolus requires repositioning of bone fragments and splinting for up to 6–8 weeks.

Crown fracture External root resorption occurs in 0.2% of teeth with a crown fracture[22] and rarely cervical resorption. The force from the trauma damages the periodontal ligament and/or apical the blood vessels.

Avulsion (exarticulation) and replantation An avulsed tooth can be replanted. Greater insight into the resorption process has been gained by studying replantation of avulsed teeth and autotransplantation (implantation of a patient's own tooth in the place of another absent tooth).[175][283] The probability of injury to the periodontal ligament is greater in the case of replantation than in autotransplantation. In animal experiments under ideal circumstances, complete healing occurred after replantation,[22] but in a prospective real-life study about 25% of teeth, and in a retrospective study 50–90% of teeth, survived.[22][27][219]

Avulsion leads to tearing of the periodontal ligament and the blood supply to the pulp is severed. A few studies with large sample sizes have looked at the aforementioned aspects.[25][26][27] Replantation is successful when periodontal fibres are able to re-attach the tooth to the alveolar bone and resorption is absent. The factors determining the likelihood of resorption are: vitality of the pulp and periodontal ligament,[163] presence of contamination and the method/duration of splinting.

Resorption often occurs within a few months of replantation, but sometimes it may be manifest after years. An observation period of 3 years is adequate to monitor for resorption.[68] Inflammatory resorption starts sooner and its rate of progression is greater than replacement resorption,[106] but in the first year superficial resorption is seldom visible.[26]

Pulp vitality Pulp revascularisation and survival after transplantation is most likely when the apex is still wide open,[210][235] with a diameter of at least 1mm.[32][210]. Blunting occurs in a minority[22][236][312][400] and is rarely the reason for extraction. Immature teeth that have been transplanted and subject to normal function soon after may undergo pulp obliteration.[302] Transplanted and endodontically treated teeth with fully formed roots undergo (almost) no resorption.[119][212] Endodontically treated teeth transplanted along with the surrounding alveolar bone did not become ankylosed,[253] but replacement resorption has been also reported.[236]

In studies, in half of exarticulated teeth with an open apex that were stored in wet conditions and replanted within an hour, sensitivity returned, usually within 6 months, but pulp obliteration often occurred.[426 239] Revascularisation (monkeys) was not found to depend on the width of the apical foramen, but on the presence of bacteria in the pulpal lumen. Immediately replanted teeth had fewer microorganisms in the pulp and a higher likelihood of complete pulp revascularisation than teeth replanted after a delay.[97] Replantation in germ-free rats was followed by replacement resorption and in conventional rats, it was associated with pulpal problems and inflammatory resorption.[324]

Although a dry-stored tooth is prone to replacement resorption,[21 331] one may, considering the circumstances such as available space in the dentition, replant such a tooth, which may function for years.[174] Because of the risk of ankylosis, replantation, unless done immediately, must be considered carefully for teeth with a wide open apex.[21 26 239] Ankylosis impedes local alveolar growth and eruption. Fractures of avulsed teeth and advanced periodontal disease are contraindications.

Deciduous teeth are not replanted because the mechanical manipulation may damage the successors germs. Pulp necrosis and immobilisation also pose a problem. However, Filippi et al. have reported successful replantation of avulsed deciduous teeth with retrograde calcium hydroxide filling after apex resection.[128]

Use of antibiotics following transplantation/replantation
Intramuscular injection of broad-spectrum antibiotics immediately after replantation, followed by oral antibiotics for at least 2 weeks, is recommended to prevent resorption.[1] For patients under 12 years, penicillin is preferred to avoid tooth discoloration but in case of patients allergic to penicillin, aztreonam may be used.[1 464] In experimental studies, pulp revascularisation and presence of bacteria in the pulpal lumen in monkeys were, however, not influenced by antibiotics administered before and after extraction and replantation.[97] When extracted teeth of dogs were soaked with doxycycline (1 mg/20 mL saline) for 5 minutes, 60% showed pulpal revascularisation and continuation of root development versus 30% of teeth which were stored under dry conditions for 5 minutes.[448]

In the case of teeth which are treated endodontically prior to replantation or transplantation, antibiotics are applied directly within the pulp cavity to prevent inflammatory resorption.[161] Bryson et al. filled root canals of extracted teeth immediately with either Ledermix (which consists of corticosteroid and tetracycline) or calcium hydroxide. The teeth were replanted after an extraoral dry time of 1 hour. The Ledermix group performed better than the calcium hydroxide group 4 months later.[81] However, immediate replantation without sealing in Ledermix had better results than replantation after 1 hour of dry-stored teeth with Ledermix, which was also noted in another similar experiment.[445]

Findings of human studies regarding the effect of antibiotics on pulpal and periodontal healing in replanted teeth are conflicting,[161 229] and some animal studies do not

support their use.[81 97] In addition, endodontically treated teeth with cementum defects coated with minocycline and stored under dry conditions for 1 hour did not fare better than uncoated roots.[82]

Due to the risk of sensitisation and bacterial resistance, it has been recommended to avoid using antibiotics, unless their use is imperative, such as in high-risk patients (juvenile rheumatism, endocarditis, etc.).[207 243]

Age of the replanted/transplanted tooth Ebeleseder et al. compared three groups of permanent replanted teeth: (1) immature teeth, (2) mature teeth in children and adolescents and (3) mature teeth in adults. Pulp revascularisation/healing was best in group 1 and poorest in group 3. Root resorption was greatest in group 3. Local gingivitis with epithelial down-growth was more likely in group 2. In adults, the bone proximal to the replanted teeth was resorbed while in children alveolar bone growth arrested. Cervical root resorption was the reason for extraction. The authors concluded that replantation should be considered in children and adolescents.[114]

- *Immature teeth.* Root development after replantation may continue if Hertwig's root sheath is preserved,[31 236] but the degree of root completion is unpredictable. Pulp necrosis stops root growth. The pulp remains vital in about one-third of teeth with an open apex,[25 229] provided the teeth are stored under wet conditions, replanted within 5 minutes, and the pulp length is <17 mm.[25] Endodontic treatment should be delayed in promptly replanted teeth with open apices,[226] but infection makes pulp survival unlikely. Studies of transplanted third molars with incomplete roots show that resorption occurred in only a few cases and continuation of normal root growth is possible.[92 196]
- *Mature teeth.* If replanted within minutes, a small proportion of tooth pulps revascularise.[22 27 301 399] The apical foramen must be open, but artificial widening is not helpful.[112] Delaying root canal treatment by 20 days or more favours development of external inflammatory resorption.[226] However, a 1-week delay allows time for periodontal fibre reattachment, while the necrotic pulp is minimally infected.[22 423]
- *Vitality of the periodontal ligament.* A short period outside the mouth is of utmost importance to maintain the vitality of the periodontal ligament. Immediate replantation of an (immature) tooth (by the patient or, for example, a parent in a child) increases the probability of complete healing from 20% to 37%.[22] See also next section.

Retained canines that are transplanted to surgically created alveolar sockets often became ankylosed, presumably because of damage to the periodontal ligament.[267 318] Blood clot in the wound hinders establishment of the blood supply. Allowing the surgically created socket to heal for 14 days prior to the transplantation increases the chances of re-establishing the periodontal ligament blood supply through close contact with the newly formed richly vascularised tissue in the socket.[321] Transalveolar transplantation of canines did not lead to resorption,[56 371] probably because the blood clot was removed, but unexplainable cervical resorption occurred in 8%.[56] The rate of success in one sample of autotransplanted premolars was 92.5% after 10 or more years, even when the teeth had been subjected to orthodontic forces. Root formation continued and in teeth with (half)-open apices, two-thirds of the pulps were vital. A few teeth developed inflammatory resorption.[210] In another study of autotransplanted teeth, 10% were lost after 9–29 years: a few became ankylosed or had a crown-to-root ratio >1.[99]

Extra-alveolar time The sooner an avulsed tooth is replanted, the better.[25 28 64 229 262 402 419] The crucial factor in the success of the procedure is a periodontal ligament in optimal condition. Dry storage times are of greater importance than the total time elapsed before replantation.[226 227] The best predictor of overall resorption after avulsion is the total time of dryness, and that of replacement resorption is the extra-alveolar time.[68] If replanted within a *few to 10 minutes*, progressive resorption will not occur.[12 25 74 226 227] Andersson *et al.* reported that after some *15 minutes* of extra-alveolar time, one-third of teeth show some and one-third show progressive replacement resorption.[12] Teeth stored dry for *20 minutes* show inflammatory resorption,[226 227] but there is a report of a tooth replanted after *30 minutes* of extra-alveolar time which was not markedly resorbed 27 years later.[286] In one study, when teeth were replanted after longer times, mostly all teeth were resorbed.[29] Barrett *et al.* reported that dry-stored teeth replanted after *1 hour* resorbed within 3–7 years.[45] Teeth with completed roots stored under wet conditions for *2 hours* were more likely to survive than teeth with open apices. Teeth filled with $Ca(OH)_2$ exhibited more severe resorption than teeth treated first with $Ca(OH)_2$ and then with gutta-percha.[45] In another study, half of the teeth replanted after *7 hours* were lost within 1 year.[94]

Storage media If not replanted immediately, avulsed teeth must be stored under *wet conditions* as soon as possible: in milk, the mouth, or in a culture medium. *Dry storage* compromises the viability of the periodontal ligament.[11] [12 29 74 94] The critical dry time limit is 15 minutes[106] or even possibly 5 minutes.[25]

- Milk has a favourable pH and osmolarity.[133] While trying to find milk, the ability of the ligament cells to re-establish the periodontal attachment is best guaranteed by keeping the tooth under the tongue or in the buccal sulcus; the tooth should then be transferred to preferably chilled milk.[18 21 252 331] The periodontal cells

survive almost twice as long in chilled milk than in milk at room temperature. In teeth stored in milk, no difference was found in the susceptibility to resorption among those replanted immediately and those replanted after 3–6 hours,[61 63 272] but after a somewhat longer storage period in milk, the periodontal cells lose the ability to transform into fibroblasts. In such cases, healing occurs by repair; the tooth may survive for a period of time but is inevitably lost. Periodontal cells in the alveolar socket are also damaged and do not contribute to the regeneration process.[220] In Andreasen *et al.*'s study, after storage periods of 2–24 hours in milk, three of seven teeth were replanted succesfully.[27]

In 1993 in the UK, only 25% of avulsed teeth were reported to have been stored in saliva or milk.[273] After replantation of dry-stored teeth, periodontal ligament fibres developed within 1 month, but near the resorbed parts of the root the fibres were arranged haphazardly[57] and bone was in contact with the root.[41]

- Storage in *water* is associated with replacement resorption,[21] because of its osmolarity. Schatz *et al.* found that of teeth stored in water or a wet gauze, one-third of (mature) teeth that were replanted within 1 hour developed replacement and/or inflammatory resorption; 83% developed resorption when replanted after 3 hours.[381]
- Storage in *culture media* such as Dentosafe,[129] might be superior to storage in milk.[425] Dentists may not have such media at their disposal, but soaking a tooth that has been stored dry for a long time in Viaspan,[22 60 63 64] [262] to which can be added glucocorticosteroid (dexamethasone),[370] increases the chances of success;[344 424 425] Immediate replantation results in less replacement resorption.[424 425] Teeth stored for 96 hours in Conditioned Medium (supernatant of cultured fibroblasts) were found to heal as well as immediately replanted teeth,[197] but storage up to 96 hours in Viaspan led to better outcomes than with the use of Conditioned Medium.[220 344]

Doyle *et al.* found that the numbers of viable periodontal ligament cells did not differ between teeth dry-stored for 30 minutes and soaked 15 minutes in either milk or Hank's balanced salt solution.[107] Storage at −196 °C in 5% dimethylsulfoxide or −80 °C in a freezer does not lead to damage and the periodontal ligament regenerates.[458] This method can be used when damage to the alveolar socket or planned orthodontic treatment is associated with a delay in transplantation/replantation.[458] Teeth stored submucosally[208] or subcutaneously[458] may undergo resorption after replantation.[207] Storage in plastic foil is less desirable.[61] Emdogain, a protein complex derived from the enamel matrix, may facilitate the regeneration of the periodontal ligament, as has been reported in teeth with initial replacement resorption.[129]

Contamination Contamination of the periodontal ligament increases the risk of resorption.[106] The storage conditions are crucial to prevent contamination.[381] The tooth may have been in contact with the soil, be held in the hand, etc. A visibly contaminated tooth may be cleaned by holding under running water for 10 seconds to 1 minute,[387] but preferably is cleaned with a sterile physiological salt solution,[201] which also helps to remove any blood clots in the socket. Alternatively, a blood clot may be lightly aspirated. Socket irrigation is also possible with ozonised water, which is isotonic. The ozonised water disinfects the periodontal ligament, sparing its vitality, and enhances healing.[116] After replantation the patient should be advised to eat soft food, brush with a soft toothbrush and rinse twice a day with 0.1% chlorhexidine.[464]

Splinting The longer or the more rigidly a replanted tooth is immobilised, the greater is the probability and severity of replacement resorption.[17 22 306 317] Kinirons et al. found that after a splinting period of 11 days, only a very small proportion of teeth were resorbed.[226] The gingival fibres heal sufficiently within 7 days of splinting.[22]

Iatrogenic causes

Orthodontic forces Use of excessive forces, like in rapid maxillary expansion, has resulted in extensive replacement and cervical resorption of the anchor teeth.[187 245 246] Cervical resorption occurs most frequently as a delayed reaction to orthodontic treatment performed years before,[55 420] but its occurrence is unpredictable.[178 281] Genetic factors have a substantial influence.[170 224] At times the cause is indeterminable and other factors might be involved.[151 369]

Bleaching Bleaching of discoloured teeth with 30–35% hydrogen peroxide (H_2O_2) placed in the pulp chamber, with or without heat, is associated with cervical resorption, generally developing a few years later.[138 153 167 217 241 234 249 274 303 438] The bleach is assumed to reach the root surface via defects in the cementum, but if heated (and unheated?), it might even pass through intact cementum.[167 234 274 364 438] Although the associated trauma may be the cause of pulp necrosis and the resorption, in a number of cases there is no history of trauma.[98 192 241]

In an experimental study, powdered dentine and root cementum were more likely to dissolve in 30% H_2O_2 than in 3% H_2O_2.[365] A pulp chamber filled with 30% H_2O_2, 25% citric acid and sodium hypochlorite and then closed led to small cervical resorption defects 3 months later.[180] The low pH of 30% H_2O_2 may damage the periodontal ligament,[217] and may evoke a foreign body reaction[364] and osteoclastic activity.[290] Others attribute the resorption to the free radicals. Application of heat has been found to increase the numbers of free radicals on root surfaces with cementum defects.[100]

Internal bleaching with sodium perborate may counteract macrophage adhesion,[205] which is the first step in resorption.

Thermal stimulation Atrizadeh et al. found that thermal stimulation of the pulp led to necrosis of the periodontal ligament and replacement resorption.[36] Root canal obturation with gutta-percha using a rotary McSpadden file increased the temperature within the canal to 100°C,[126 132] and to a maximum of 50°C at the root surface,[95 132] enough for the periodontal ligament to develop inflammation.[36]

Compaction of gutta-percha with an instrument rotating at 8000 rpm has been found to raise the temperature at the root surface to 45–58°C;[165 166] a rise to 77–97°C is also reported,[291] The time period of compaction, 5 seconds versus 15 seconds, also determines the temperature rise.[48] Lipski et al. found that low-temperature thermoplasticised gutta-percha compaction techniques increased the root surface temperature by only a few degrees.[265]

The question is whether root resorption follows.[199] Saunders reported that at 20 and 40 days after thermomechanical compaction ankylosis was present in 5 of 18 teeth.[379] Root canal obturation with gutta-percha at 65–70°C led to transient external root resorption.[158]

One cause of heat production in periodontology is use of electro-surgery. Study results are conflicting, and damage to the periodontium seems possible.[395]

Endodontic medicaments Use of formaldehyde or formalin and trioxymethylene(-corticoid) can cause replacement resorption, often within 30 days.[122] Phenol applied to the periodontal ligament induced superficial cementum resorption without ankylosis.[367]

Intra-ligamentary injections Anaesthetic agents are sometimes injected with considerable pressure into the periodontal ligament. Damage caused by the needle has been implicated in cervical resorption.[315] The injection may lead to infection and damage the cementum.[375] However, the risk seems small and the damage is restricted.[34 142 432] Resorbed bone and cementum are replaced within weeks to 3 months.[73 341 343] Hypercementosis has also been reported.[343]

Anomalies of eruption

Retention and delayed eruption Retained maxillary canines show replacement resorption more frequently than retained third molars. Only a few are resorbed though, suggesting a protective role of the reduced enamel epithelium,[341] which fails occasionally. Of the teeth resorbing within bone, 80% may not communicate with the oral cavity,[406] but Azaz et al. found that the vast majority of impacted canines (14% with resorption) showed communication, or were infected, for instance, via an adjacent tooth.[39] The latter theory may also explain the pre-eruptive coronal resorption seen, in particular, in the mandibular second molar.[143 190 202 355 388 396 398 414] Once erupted, the lesions may be misdiagnosed as caries or developmental anomalies.[202] It is useful to bear in mind that these lesions are filled with necrotic tissue because eruption severs their blood supply.[190] The diagnosis should be confirmed with histological examination.[398] Oswald *et al.* reported development of external replacement resorption in 20 of 54 supplemental/supernumerary impacted anterior teeth.[231]

Cysts/tumours Impingement of tooth roots by tumours, cysts and osteosclerotic lesions may lead to external resorption.

Root resorption has been reported in association with an ameloblastoma, neurilemmoma, aggressive cemento-ossifying fibroma and myeloma.[121 159 311 410] Resorption is endemic in African 5–10-year-olds with Burkitt's lymphoma (malignant transformation of lymphocytes) and sporadic in adolescents with the condition living elsewhere.[186]

Tumours resulting in root resorption are often those that expand slowly.[141] Follicular and radicular cysts exert almost equal pressure, but do not cause identical amounts of resorption,[410] raising doubts about whether pressure is the cause in such cases.

Pressure from neighbouring teeth Ectopic or late-erupting teeth may press against and induce resorption of adjacent teeth/roots.[238 359 368] Late erupting permanent maxillary canines are associated with resorption of 7–12% of maxillary incisor roots,[118 123 233 378] even when erupting labially.[230] The mid-part of the lateral incisor root is affected, mainly at the age of 10–11 years. The disto(lingual) side of the central incisors is less frequently involved.[124] Kojima *et al.* reported submergence of a lateral incisor and extraction of central incisors due to resorption.[233]

Mesially tilted third molars in contact with second molar roots can cause resorption of the latter (Figure 7.14),[127 182 187 191 278 325 362] in about 1–7.5% of cases.[148 325 407] Second molars in close proximity to retained third molars showed surface and/or replacement and/or inflammatory resorption, but this does not occur if the adjacent third molars are fully erupted.[320] Bacteria in the pericoronal space around third molars may cause pulpitis in deeply resorbed second molars. Second mandibular premolars rarely resorb the roots of first molars before eruption.[325 416 433] In a young patient with amelogenesis imperfecta, external root resorption of the four first molars, the only occluding teeth, was thought be due to excessive masticatory forces.[430]

Males show resorption due to "pressure" twice as often as females, which is suggestive of a hormonal role. After the age of 30 years resorption may not occur.[325]

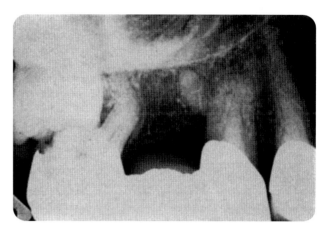

Figure 7.14 Pressure from the third molar led to the resorption of the disto-buccal root of the second molar.

Idiopathic resorption

Retained teeth with intracoronal resorption may communicate with the surrounding tissue via an occlusal fissure with thin enamel.[39 380 459] Cervical resorption of a tooth with poor-quality endodontic treatment was considered to be idiopathic; gingivitis was also present.[443] Other reported cases of idiopathic resorption, often showing multiple cervical lesions and sometimes apical lesions, were not accompanied by inflammation and dental or general health abnormalities.[54 78 101 146 193 222 223 270 304 348 449] Heredity might play a role in idiopathic resorption.[360 391]

Multiple cervical resorptive lesions may be associated with developmental aberrations such as absence of cervical cementum.[209] Others have suggested that the stimulus might be lymphokine production by lymphocytes found in dense collections near the osteoclasts.[304]

Osteoclastic activity, facilitated by prior osteoblastic activation, together with a minimal immune response in relatively young persons with little periodontitis, may be responsible for multiple lesions.[305]

Systemic diseases

A woman with nephritis and bone disease, and treated with hormones, had cervical resorption in 19 of 20 remaining teeth.[222] All the roots were resorbed in a 31-year-old who had received growth hormones for years.[393] Pankhurst *et al.* reported multiple resorptive lesions and hepatic problems in association with intravenous heroin and morphine use; hormonal abnormalities were absent.[338] Heart disease and/or intubation for anaesthesia were viewed as the cause of completely resorbed roots of the (deeply carious) maxillary first molars in a 4-year-old.[340] Multiple apical resorptive lesions were reported in a patient with hemifacial atrophy, in the affected area.[125]

Paget disease[43 87 88 401] and hyper(para)thyroidism[51 151 155 394] have been suspected, but the latter as a cause has not been confirmed.[363] Hormonal effects and systemic diseases might be co-factors.[76]

Inherited dental conditions such as amelogenesis imperfecta, dentinogenesis imperfecta, dentinal dysplasia and odontodysplasia are associated with multiple root resorption.[223]

In 179 patients with different systemic diseases, resorption appeared unrelated to the systemic condition.[193] Yet, a few diseases are associated with multiple root resorption and resorption has been seen in patients on systemic bisphosphonates.

Segmental odontomaxillary dysplasia Segmental odontomaxillary dysplasia seems indisputably related to root resorption,[232] (because of bone hyperactivity?). Atypical and irregular external resorption of deciduous molars has been reported.[35 52 337 352]

Primary hyperoxaluria (two genetic types) Primary hyperoxaluria is a rare, inherited enzymatic disorder of glyoxylate metabolism, with excessive production of oxalates. The renal tubules become blocked and kidney stones are formed. Hyperoxaluria is a feature. Haemodialysis does not remove oxalate efficiently and progressive renal dysfunction results in early death. Kidney and liver transplantation increase survival, but cannot prevent oxalate deposition.[83 173 248 446] The excessive levels of oxalate are due to hyperabsorption in the colon because of altered enterohepatic circulation.[173 248 307 446]

Chronic renal failure results in oxalosis, which is the deposition of calcium oxalate crystals in extrarenal tissues. Star-shaped oxalate crystals in the ligament cause a foreign body reaction and inflammation with generalised external root resorption,[150 354] occasionally cervical resorption, internal resorption, tooth mobility, pain and eventually tooth loss.[91 173]

Dental problems are alternatively attributed to a form of osteomalacia in association with aluminium contamination of dialysis water. Accumulation of aluminium between the osteoid and calcified matrix inhibits normal bone mineralisation.[91] Aluminium contamination seems a historic problem due to advances in dialysis.

Secondary oxalosis is common after ileojejunal bypass surgery[248] for morbid obesity.

1-hydroxyethylidene-1,1-bisphosphonate (HEBP) Administration of bisphosphonates along with application of a cold stimulus to mice caused extensive root resorption and ankylosis.[439 440] The periodontal ligament regained its normal thickness after discontinuation of HEBP, but extensive resorption developed.[439 441] Saucer-shaped lacunae, developing in areas of aseptic root resorption after application of dry ice to the crowns in rats, were seen to be repaired at day 28 with cementum. Animal teeth subjected to multiple or long periods of freezing showed more extensive external root resorption, attributed to sterile degeneration of the periodontal ligament.[110]

After HEBP administration in rats, a thick layer of atypical cementum deposited, which then rapidly resorbed under the influence of an orthodontic force.[3] In another study in rats, atypical cementum, already present after a single injection of HEBP, showed resorption 2 weeks later.[4]

Other agents ^{224}Ra and other radioactive agents used in the treatment of diseases such as bone tuberculosis have been found to induce multiple external (cervical) and internal resorption.[356]

7.5 Prevention and treatment of progressive external resorption

After trauma, early detection and diagnosis of the type of resorption requires repeat examinations, vitality tests and radiographs at 2, 3 and 6 weeks, and after 3, 12 and 24 months. The method of prevention of external root resorption is dictated by the cause.

7.5.1 Inflammatory resorption

To prevent inflammatory resorption, endodontic treatment of *mature avulsed teeth* must be performed within 2 weeks after replantation,[24 41] before the splint is removed.[22] In monkeys, intracanal application of chlorhexidine in teeth with external inflammatory resorption reduced the inflammation and might be a useful adjunct.[263]

Ledermix is the best endodontic medicament for traumatised and avulsed teeth to prevent inflammatory resorption. At the time of treatment, which is 1–2 weeks after the trauma, the periodontal ligament may not be fully healed. Ledermix is then preferred over $Ca(OH)_2$ (see Section 7.4.2).[427] The pH of $Ca(OH)_2$ suppresses the inflammation, but any effect on osteoclasts is absent or for a short time only.[22] Ledermix seems superfluous when endodontic treatment is performed correctly.

Endodontic treatment of a tooth "in the hand" may contaminate the periodontal ligament; thus replantation must be done first,[22 24] unless the tooth was dry stored for a minimum of 2 hours. External inflammatory resorption requires endodontic management,[86 92 285] but following treatment it may change into replacement resorption.[381]

Inflammatory resorption on the lateral aspect of a mandibular canine was not halted by root canal treatment, but extraction of the adjacent first premolar with a periradicular infection stopped the process.[133]

When periapical inflammation develops in replanted teeth with *incomplete roots*, the canal is temporarily filled with $Ca(OH)_2$[409] to counter the inflammation and to promote apical closure, which enables lateral condensation of gutta-percha. The positive effect of filling a root canal with Ca(OH)$_2$ is debatable.[287] The American Association of Endodontics advises Ca(OH)$_2$ temporisation for 2 weeks, and for much longer in immature teeth, but MTA[460] and the intracanal medicament alendronate are just as effective and may limit root resorption.[461]

Resorption of bone occurs at pH <6.[59] Sealing Ca(OH)$_2$ within the pulp cavity causes the pH at the cementum to become alkaline.[419] Use of Ca(OH)$_2$ plus iodoform paste in perforated roots may cause hypercementosis.[72] Under aseptic circumstances the application of Ca(OH)$_2$ or Teflon on root perforations has been found to result in ankylosis.[49] Ca(OH)$_2$ may be bactericidal, however, Peters reported that the number of colony-forming units increased within 4 weeks.[342] Shortly after the application of Ca(OH)$_2$ the formation of reparative cementum, before being stimulated, may temporarily slow down.[160]

Pohl et al. found that among extracted traumatised immature teeth, which were endodontically treated by apical resection and replanted, no resorption developed in uninfected teeth. Otherwise inflammatory resorption followed, leading to extraction after an average of 4 years.[347]

7.5.2 Replacement resorption

Excessive drying out of avulsed teeth always leads to progressive ankylosis.[22] Removal of the non-vital periodontal ligament caused complete replacement resorption within 1 month.[267] Attempts to save dry-stored teeth have included trying to increase the resistance to resorption with use of fluorides, enzymes and antibiotics after periodontal ligament removal with citric acid or sodium hypochlorite.[42 57 58 111 154 157 220 322 404 451 452] Results of these studies are conflicting.[400] After removal of the periodontal ligament, endodontic treatment may be performed before replantation.

Use of citric acid in periodontics promotes a new periodontal attachment by inhibiting the downward growth of epithelium, but extensive resorption was also seen.[257] When the epithelium did not grow downwards,[215] citric acid promoted reattachment of surgically repositioned gingiva, occasionally with the apposition of new cementum.[5 96] Application of citric acid in experimental subepithelial cavities accelerated cementogenesis: the authors proposed that the epithelial cells were unable to compete with the connective tissue cells.[316]

Replacement resorption cannot be treated, because the stimulus cannot be removed and the replacement of the root with bone-like material often occurs in a periradicular fashion.[421] Recently, Filippi et al. extracted traumatised ankylosed teeth, obturated the root canals, and replanted the teeth after applying Emdogain to the root and alveolar bone. There was no recurrence of ankylosis, unless the teeth were severely traumatised.[129] However, Emdogain did not prevent replacement resorption in dry-stored replanted teeth in rats.[462] Filippi et al. also showed that resection of the resorbed (ankylosed) part after extraction and replantation with a post extending beyond the pulp cavity prevented further ankylosis in 7 of 16 teeth.[463]

Teeth are commonly lost 3–7 years after initiation of replacement resorption.[12] The rate of progression of the process depends on first, the extent of the periodontal damage, i.e. presence of large necrotic areas rapidly results in total resorption, and second, age, i.e. a high bone turnover rate in young patients increases the rate of progression.[22] Substitution of resorbed maxillary incisors with transplanted immature mandibular premolars is the preferred treatment option in young people rather than implants because it allows further alveolar bone growth.[22 328]

When replacement resorption develops in replanted mature teeth, a gutta-percha root canal filling is preferred over Ca(OH)$_2$, because of less extensive ankylosis.[427] Delayed replantation in monkeys resulted in replacement resorption of almost all teeth, regardless of whether the canals were filled with Ca(OH)$_2$ or gutta-percha.[113]

After removal of the crown and cervical part of the root of ankylosed teeth, Malmgren et al. reported that the remaining root preserved the alveolar process, even when a major part was replaced with bone.[280] In young patients, the available space determines whether one should opt for this procedure.[444] Removal of impacted ankylosed mandibular wisdom teeth is associated with the risk of damaging the mandibular nerve.[428]

Replacement resorption of the apical part of the root may be transient. In cases where it is not transient, apical resection seems ineffective because one does not know how much the root must be removed to prevent further resorption. In many patients most of or the entire periodontal ligament is damaged. Curettage of the root surfaces also does not stop the process.[304]

Anterior teeth with root resorption to the level of the alveolar crest may remain functional for decades (Figures 7.15 and 7.16),[11 12 92 131 339 411] in particular if they are stabilised by fixing them with composite to the neighbouring

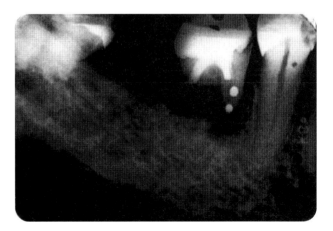

Figure 7.15 The molar with external inflammatory resorption was left in place, causing periodontal damage on the distal side of the premolar.

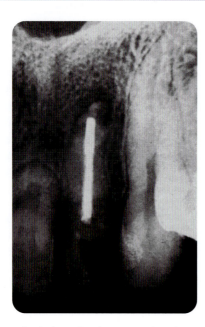

Figure 7.16 The incisor showing external replacement resorption was left in place and functioned adequately for many years.

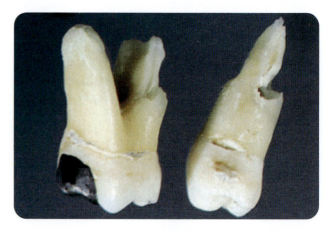

Figure 7.17 Extracted teeth exhibiting resorption defects.

teeth.[149] Advantages of leaving the tooth *in situ* are maintenance of the alveolar bone and a temporary aesthetic solution. Eventually the tooth will need to be extracted. Figure 7.17 shows resorptive defects.

7.5.3   Cervical resorption

Prevention of cervical resorption after internal bleaching with 30–35% H_2O_2 (which is now obsolete, although dentists may not be aware that cervical resorption is caused by hydrogen peroxide in higher concentrations) seems possible by sealing $Ca(OH)_2$ in the pulp chamber, which makes the pH at the root surface alkaline.[217] Closure of the dentinal tubules running from the pulp canal to the root surface with a cement to prevent diffusion of H_2O_2 to the surface,[242] interferes with bleaching of the cervical part of the crown.[137] Inclusion of sodium perborate with water is locally harmless.

Cervical resorption can be treated curatively, unless extensive or difficult to reach. The blood supply must be cut off, which may necessitate either bone removal beyond the apical boundary of the lesion[9 294 442] or orthodontic extrusion.[55] Both treatments have cosmetic disadvantages. Debridement of all the involved tissue stops the process.[46] Brief application of 90% trichloroacetic acid destroys the granulation tissue in the lesion.[176] Treatment from within the pulpal cavity[134] seems risky.

Treatment of 101 affected teeth with topical application of aqueous 90% trichloroacetic acid for 1–2 minutes caused coagulation necrosis of the resorbing tissue. Curettage was followed by restorative treatment, sometimes after endodontic therapy. The adjacent soft tissues were protected with glycerol. The approach was 100% successful in lesions that did not extend beyond a third of the root length. Treatment of deeper lesions was less successful.[179] Excessive infra-osseous cervical resorption requires extraction.[250] Moody found that curettage of the roots and restoration of the multiple cervical lesions with amalgam or glass ionomer cement could not halt the process.[304]

8

Tooth Wear and Other Signs of Ageing

8.1 Introduction

Tooth wear is the progressive loss of enamel and exposed cementum and dentine because of frictional contact between teeth and contact between teeth and the food or foreign bodies. Tooth wear is a complex process, and the rate of loss is difficult to predict;[260] teeth may wear prematurely or as part of ageing. Each contact of a tooth with its antagonists, food, etc. results in the loss of a few nanometres of the tooth surface, which over time results in a marked loss of tissue.[205] Determinants of wear include: hardness, size and shape of the food particles, the pH of the food, friction and intensity of the compressive force, the force direction, and the amount and nature of the saliva.[260]

8.2 Ageing

8.2.1 Enamel

Enamel wear increases with age and its permeability changes due to the uptake of ions from the environment. In forensic science and anthropology age is estimated of degree of wear and signs of ageing of dentine.[120 218]

8.2.2 Dentine

The mineralisation and hardness of dentine increase while tubular diameter decreases with age. Empty tubules are the result of peripheral irritation and form opaque areas called *dead tracts*. Normally, the tubules scatter light, but *sclerosis*, i.e. the deposition of minerals within the tubules lying underneath slow, destructive lesions caused by external stimuli, minimises the light refraction and makes the dentinal areas translucent.[347] The increase in translucency of the apical part of the tooth[23] is a physiological age change,[120] which ultimately can extend over two-thirds of

the root. Predentine and odontoblasts are absent underneath in these areas.[328 348] The correlation between root translucency and age varies by tooth type, from 0.55 (mandibular central incisor) to 0.83 (first molar roots).[22] A larger part of the root becomes transparent in Caucasians than in Malaysians and Chinese.[394] The length of the translucent part as a percentage of the root length is a slightly better determinant of age. The correlation was very low ($r = 0.08$) in a sample of teeth from the nineteenth century, because filiform structures (fungal, bacterial?) lying along the paths of the tubules caused a chalky root appearance.[327]

After death, the organic component, particularly in dentine, disintegrates. The enamel is then easily removed, like removing as a cap from over the opaque, chalky and brittle crown dentine. Wet earth and mummification delay disintegration.[172] Further, the enamel of teeth stored under dry conditions for a long time becomes brittle.

The intensity of the dentinal (and cemental) fluorescence under green light increases linearly with age.[176]

8.2.3 Pulp

Secondary dentine

After eruption, $0.5\,\mu m$[68] of physiological secondary dentine is formed daily, which leads to narrowing of the pulp cavity; in posterior teeth this occurs disproportionately at the floor and roof of the pulp chamber. The mean pulp length ($10-12\,mm$) in elderly people is about $7\,mm$ less than in young adults. The mesiodistal pulp width at the cervix decreases from $1.1-1.4\,mm$ to $0.2-0.3\,mm$.[233] The deposition of fibro-dentine also reduces the pulp space in maxillary and mandibular canines, but not before the age of 60 years; there is greater reduction in the size of the pulp cavities in the incisors.[269 318] The tubules bend at the junction between the primary and secondary dentine. Secondary dentine (and cementum) is also formed in retained (unerupted) teeth.[247]

Pathology of the Hard Dental Tissues, First Edition. Albert Schuurs.
© 2013 Albert Schuurs. Published 2013 by Blackwell Publishing Ltd.

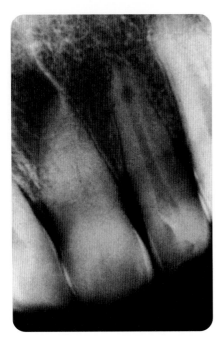

Figure 8.1 The pulp cavity of the (caries-free) central incisor is almost totally obliterated after an accident.

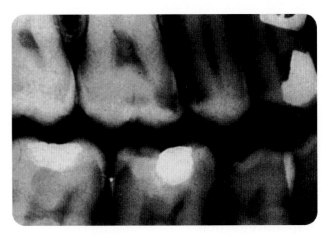

Figure 8.2 Radiograph showing a pulp stone in the pulp chamber of the maxillary first molar.

Tertiary dentine

External stimuli induce the formation of *tertiary* dentine (Chapter 5), in general with few and irregular tubules,[317] but tertiary dentine is a poor barrier to ingress of bacteria and bacterial toxins.[362]

Ivanovic *et al.* found that within 3 months, the largest amount of tertiary dentine was formed underneath a lining of calcium hydroxide, a smaller amount underneath Ledermix, and the smallest under zinc oxide eugenol. Thereafter, the daily rates of tertiary dentine production were similar.[146] Others have found no difference, after 5 and 8 weeks, in the thickness of tertiary dentine underneath calcium hydroxide and zinc oxide eugenol.[68]

Deposition of tertiary dentine leads to obliteration of the pulp cavity (Figure 8.1); in older persons tertiary dentine is laid down in response to chronic stimuli and, in young persons, to a single strong (traumatic) stimulus. Pulps that appear to be obliterated on radiographs are often vital (90% in one study).[300]

Denticles and pulp stones

Calcified structures in the pulp (Figure 8.2) are more common in older than younger persons.[132 288] Such denticles are found throughout the dentition in both anomalous (dentine dysplasia, see Chapter 3) and healthy teeth, and are attached to the pulpal walls or are free floating within the pulp. They are classified as true or false denticles and diffuse calcification of the pulp.[212 288 329 367 372]

- *True* denticles are mainly found in the pulp chamber and may occupy almost the entire pulpal space. They consist of an organic matrix and dentinal tubules.

True denticles may be present in teeth that are nonfunctional, for example due to lack of contact with an antagonist.

- *False* denticles, called *pulp stones*, are found within the pulp chamber and the root canal. They consist of concentric or lamellar layers, which probably consist of calcified, degenerated pulp tissue. Heavy masticatory forces are associated with an increase in the number of pulp stones.

- *Diffuse* calcifications[147] occur along the long axis of the radicular pulp and are associated with the pulpal blood vessels or collagen fibrils.

In an Indian study, 3% of deciduous incisors and about 25% of second molars showed diffuse calcifications.[175] About 20% of the teeth of a sample of Iraqi 13–14-year-olds and 20–40-year-old Israelis contained denticles; Israeli women were more likely to have denticles than men.[22 360] "Pulp stones" are present in all tooth types, regardless of eruptive status. Blood chemistry, such as phospholipid levels, is normal.[288 335]

8.2.4   Cementum

The apical cementum thickness triples or even quadruples (from about 150 μm) with age,[350 406] including in impacted teeth.[16 308 406] Human age is estimated using the cementum thickness in ancient and forensically recovered teeth,[350] or by a microscopic count of the number of cementum layers deposited during life,[355] which correlates highly with chronological age: Pearson's $r = 0.98$ for persons up to 55 years. For older persons, a formula is used to adjust for discrepancies.[351]

Hypercementosis

Hypercementosis is a post-developmental, anomalous increase in the deposition of cementum, mainly at the apex, within the furcation and, in case of periodontal problems, at the proximal root surfaces.

The causes are either idiopathic,[16] for instance in impacted teeth,[161 363] or local and systemic, or drug-induced.[281] Hypercementosis may delay eruption and is a secondary cause of root curvature and ankylosis.[272]

Local causes

Almost 2% of 42-years-olds showed hypercementosis in an average of 3.8 teeth, mainly the second and first premolars and first molars, in this order.[105 272] Others have found lower prevalence rates (0.1–0.3% of teeth).[161 346] Excessive eruption after extraction of an antagonist, heavy occlusal forces and forced premature functioning of transplanted and partly developed teeth are associated with hypercementosis.[231 232 346 363 391] Periodontal infection may lead to hypercementosis, either in the apical region or along the length of the root.[183 217 363] Marked hypercementosis (Figure 8.3) makes a root club-shaped.[76] The excess cementum may separate from the root during extraction.[46] The periodontal space and the lamina dura of the bone are normal on radiographs (Figures 8.4 and 8.5).[105 183]

Acromegaly

Increased secretion of growth hormone factor by the hypothalamus (mostly due to an adenoma) leads to the release of excess growth hormone by the pituitary gland.[100] The consequent increase in production of an insulin-like growth factor (IGF I) in the liver prompts skeletal growth, where the potential for growth is still present. In children there is gigantism, and in adults there is enlargement of, for instance, the terminal phalanges of the hands and feet. Swelling of the lips and submandibular glands may be the first sign.[382] The face becomes coarse.[369]

Condylar growth leads to an increase in the size of the mandible, sometimes unilaterally.[123] Lengthening of the mandibular body leads to the development of diastemata between the lower incisors and causes them to occlude anterior rather than lingual to the upper incisors (negative overjet). Pressure from the enlarged tongue contributes to development of an open bite.[61 123 234] Hypercementosis has been observed in some adult patients in one or more teeth.[105 391] Attempts to treat the open bite will be fruitless as long as the causative factor is not addressed.[61]

Osteitis deformans (Paget's disease of bone)

Osteitis deformans is a chronic bone disease in which: (1) an increased number of osteoclasts resorb bone at an increased rate; followed by (2) osteoblastic activity which leads to bone hypertrophy; and finally (3) sclerotic bone persists without an increase in turnover (rest stage).[1] Viruses, e.g. the measles virus, have been demonstrated in the osteoclasts.[56 255]

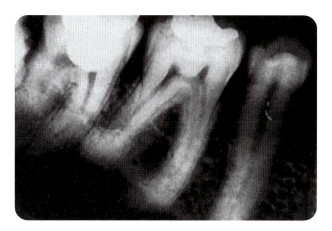

Figure 8.4 Hypercementosis in a first mandibular molar.

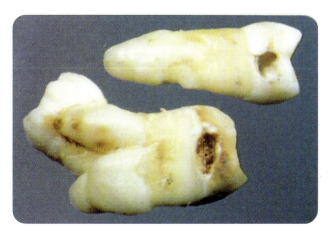

Figure 8.3 Club-shaped hypercementosis in a premolar and concrescence of two molars.

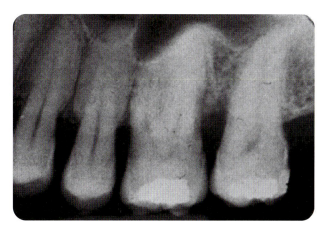

Figure 8.5 Premolars with hypercementosis, a feature also present in the other teeth in this dentition. (Courtesy of N.A. Bakx.)

Solitary lesions may remain unnoticed. In other cases, the accelerated resorption leads to soft bones that bend under weight-bearing. Later the bones become hard and their thickness increases. Secondary symptoms are caused by compression of the nerves by the hypertrophic bone (headache, deafness, blindness, facial paralysis). Sarcomas may develop.[29 52 56]

Hypertrophied facial bones give the patient the appearance of a lion, *leontiasis ossea*, which may be considered as a separate disease entity.[67] In some 20% of patients, the jaws are involved, the maxilla twice as often as the mandible. Extraction may lead to jaw fracture,[340] and in the osteolytic phase there may be prolonged bleeding, and in the osteo-sclerotic phase, a "dry socket" may result.[52 330] Pressure from the widened alveolar ridge may lead to fracture of a prosthesis or a prosthesis may cause ulcers in the mucosa. The teeth in the enlarged and broadened alveolar processes become loose and spaced, and may exfoliate spontaneously.[330] Later, sclerosis is observed around the tooth apices together with hypercementosis. The pulps are obliterated. Hypercementosis leads to ankylosis: the periodontal space and the lamina dura are absent on X-rays.[46 189]

The therapy is symptomatic: plicamycin administration prevents sarcoma and heart failure. Calcitonins are used to stabilise the calcium metabolism. Diphosphonates and sodium fluoride may prevent resorption.[52 56 340] Use of gallium nitrate is still in experimental stages.[1]

Other causes

Hypercementosis is associated with hypothyroidism, calcinosis (mineral deposits in soft tissues), arthritis, hypovitaminosis A and hypervitaminosis D, and some syndromes, such as the oculodentodigital syndrome, in which there is enamel hypoplasia and syndactyly as well as eye abnormalities with hypertelorism.[38 55 81 109] In acute rheumatism, hypercementosis appears more radiolucent on X-rays than normal cementum.[217] Autosomal dominant *cementum dysplasia*, an inherited anomaly, affects the cementum and adjacent bone. It is not clear whether the dysplasia, just like benign cementoblastoma,[162] belongs to the group of hypercementoses.[322]

Ciclosporin A, an immunosuppressive agent that prevents rejection of transplanted organs, has been shown to induce the formation of large volumes of new cementum with an irregular outline, in particular in the cervical third of the roots.[14]

8.3   Nomenclature

Physiological attrition is tooth wear caused by particles in masticated food pulp, which exert a cutting action under the masticatory forces; the term is also applied to tooth wear caused by non-functional tooth contacts.

Pathological attrition is tooth wear caused by chewing with a mutilated dentition and parafunctional movements (non-functional movements). *Abrasion* is tooth wear caused by frictional contact with foreign bodies other than food and tooth brushing. The occlusal, facial and lingual surfaces are affected.[117] In particular circumstances, tooth wear progresses rapidly, and is distinguished by the cause.[39 117 144 145 219 380]

The term "attrition" did not become popular. Tooth wear due to tobacco chewing has been classified as abrasion,[71 380] pathological attrition[320] and attrition.[329] In several countries, "abrasion" is used to refer to all kinds of tooth wear,[271 317] and even to indicate erosion,[260] and is also called *corrosive wear*[205] and *corrosion*.[117] Physiological attrition has also been called "abrasion".[407] Furthermore, other conditions have been distinguished:[116 144 180 258] *abfraction*, which is the fracturing of cervical enamel and occlusal splintering of thin enamel under physical stress; and *demastication*, which refers to mesiodistal grooves in the incisal edges and cupping on occlusal surfaces caused by contact with hard food or foreign bodies.

Many clinical cases do not fit neatly into the categories mentioned above, and are often not readily diagnosed;[17] this is also because several causes of tooth wear can act on a tooth simultaneously or at different points in time. The term "wear" covers all the categories mentioned above,[260] although the different origins of tooth wear may be of preventive importance.

8.4   Physiological and progressive tooth wear

Tooth wear is characterised by well-demarcated wear facets, which are related to the tooth contacts[186] and there is a close fit between opposing facets.

Vigorous and prolonged mastication is a characteristic solely of mammals, and their teeth undergo wear. Compensatory mechanisms and adaptations (ongoing eruption, cementum deposition) guarantee an efficient masticatory system for the lifetime.[241]

The degree of wear differs greatly between the two dentitions. A balanced physiological state is said to exist when the distance between the occlusal plane and the alveolar crest remains constant throughout life,[31 267 396] but when wear compromises functioning or survival of a tooth, the process is considered pathological.

Skeletal material excavated in Athens, near the Acropolis, is representative of almost the entire time span between the Neolithic period and the Turkish Domination, and of persons of all ages. The material showed that the occlusal plane-to-bone distance remains constant during life, in spite of tooth wear, except when the wear is pathological. In the physiological process, the length of the crown may be reduced to zero or even less than that, with root separation.[267] A Romano-British population study supports the findings. Tooth wear is compensated by movement of the teeth in occlusal direction.[396]

In contemporary humans, a small amount of tooth wear underlies the increase in the lower face height (~0.4 mm/year)[397] because of alveolar bone growth and continuing tooth eruption. The cementum becomes exposed.[241]

Deciduous dentition

Wear starts at the incisal edges of the incisors in an edge-to-edge bite (Figure 8.6). Next the occlusal molar surfaces are affected. Wear often progresses into the dentine (Figure 8.7).

In contrast with deciduous molars, the spaced deciduous anterior teeth do not come into contact with each other and are not flattened approximally. The wear is in general most severe in the maxillary arch and the anterior teeth.[387]

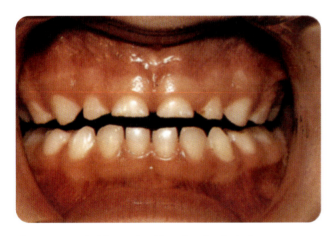

Figure 8.6 A deciduous dentition showing incisal wear.

Permanent dentition

Occlusal wear in the permanent dentition starts in the teeth that erupt first, commonly the permanent mandibular first molars. Wear facets on cusp tips increase in size, rapidly or slowly, as the case dictates. The cusps become shorter and flatter.[228] The masticated food leaves scratches on the enamel. Abrasive particles trapped in the scratches cause wear of the antagonists.[205]

Next, the incisor mamelons disappear, together with the height differences between the perikymata and imbrication lines. A normal bite is associated with labial wear facets on the incisal edges of the mandibular incisors and palatal facets on the maxillary incisors. A reversed bite causes wear on the opposite surfaces. The first mandibular incisor has one antagonist and thus shows one wear facet; the lateral incisor has two antagonists and two wear facets.

As more permanent teeth erupt, more tooth contacts are made, which slows down the tooth wear.[334] The buccal cusps of the mandibular posterior teeth and the palatal cusps of the maxillary posterior teeth, called centric cusps or stops, receive the brunt of the forces during mastication. The deeper enamel that is thereby exposed shows normal ultrastructure.[256]

Over time, tissue loss may be substantial (Figure 8.8). Differences in incisal heights are gradually levelled and cusps in the post-canine zone become flatter. The wear progresses more rapidly when the dentine is exposed. The enamel of first molars already shows in teenagers (erosive) *cupping* (*ditching*) near the mesio-buccal cusp tip. Penetration of dietary agents discolours the exposed dentine brown.[372] The incisal edges have a margin of white enamel surrounding brown discoloured secondary dentine; in the centre is the darker tertiary dentine. However, the core may be white.

Approximal wear occurs because the fibres of the periodontal ligament allows the teeth to rub to against each

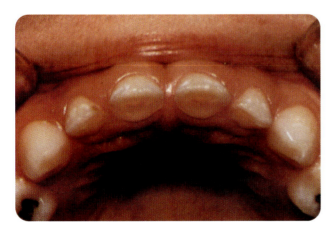

Figure 8.7 The wear has exposed the dentine of the deciduous teeth.

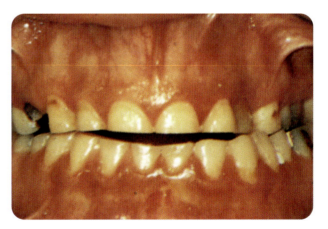

Figure 8.8 Excessive wear of the permanent anterior teeth (possibly the result of parafunction).

other during functioning, which together with the action of food flattens the approximal contact points. Mesial migration of the (pre)molars maintains the tooth contacts. The occluso-gingival width of the contacts increases from 1.5–2.5 mm to 3 mm. The bucco-lingual width of 2–3 mm broad contacts becomes 4–4.5 mm. Thereafter, wear reduces progressively because of greater resistance of the enlarged contacts.[267]

In the Lengua Indians (Paraguay) living in primitive conditions, approximal wear decreased after the eruption of the third molars.[164]

8.4.1 Measurements

The absence of stable reference points impedes quantitative measurement of occlusal wear. The upper border of the mandibular canal provides a fixed reference line that allows measuring the distance to the mandibular occlusal surfaces. There is no maxillary reference line.[241]

A number of qualitative indices are available to record occlusal wear, often using photographs or stone casts. Qualitative indices are non-linear and mean values are misleading. Broca's index (1879) for occlusal wear[372] was suggested to be arbitrary, ambiguous and subjective. The distinction between various tooth wear stages is relative:[211]

- 0 = no wear
- 1 = wear, but cusps still present
- 2 = occlusal dentine partly denuded
- 3 = only peripheral enamel present
- 4 = wear progression to or near the amelo-cementum junction.

Other scales, sometimes modified, are similar to Broca's index.[97 150 151 338] An eight-point scale, which was later modified,[104 295] used quantitative and morphological criteria.[227] Other indices assess the ratio between the denuded dentine and the total occlusal surface,[228 385] the morphology of the centric and non-centric cusps,[113] and the distance from the cusp tips to the intersection of the occlusal grooves (which, however, also undergo wear).[229]

The Tooth Wear Index (TWI) records per tooth the extent of (1) occlusal, lingual, buccal, (2) incisal and (3) cervical wear. Per age decade, "acceptable" threshold wear values have been proposed per tooth type,[338 339] but age itself neither causes the defects nor determines the effects.[42 83] Because of the difficulty in distinguishing wear from erosion, the index is applicable in both cases.

The Incisal wear Index (IwI) for children records the disappearance of the mamelons, followed by presence of smooth wear facets and finally incisal "ditching".[333] Ryge's scoring system (Table 8.1) aids treatment decision making. A score is given corresponding to the most severe wear category of 90% of the tooth ratings. Colour photographs illustrate the wear stages.[253]

Table 8.1 Rating scale (simplified) for occlusal wear[253]

Rating	Operational explanation
Satisfactory (= acceptable wear)	
R (Romeo)	Neither visible wear nor change in anatomical form
S (Sierra)	Limited (normal) wear. Limited change in morphology (enamel wear facets, small areas with exposed dentine)
M (Mike)	Considerable wear with obvious morphological change (length reduction, large dentine exposures without sensitivity) but without need for treatment
Non-acceptable wear	
T (Tango)	Considerable wear with marked morphological changes (tooth length reduction, large areas of exposed dentine that is soft and discoloured). Further damage to teeth and surrounding tissue is likely
V (Victor)	Excessive wear. Extreme morphological, aesthetic and functional changes (fracture of tooth tissues, soft dentine, pulp exposure, pain, gingival irritation). Damage to the teeth and/or surrounding tissues is *now* occurring

8.4.2 Determinants of wear

A number of partly interdependent factors determine the rate of tooth wear.

Age

Wear is age dependent,[233 250] as in ancient humans,[267] but cultural, regional (diet) and individual differences confound the determination of average tooth wear rates.[177 229 274 332] Many children, teenagers and young adults show wear, and nearly 100% of older people, often into dentine.[140 222 333] The almost equal tooth wear scores in younger and older people indicate that wear starts at an early age.[326] Incisal wear is not related to loss of the posterior teeth. Unacceptable increase in wear (TWI) has been proposed as 5% for <15-year-olds and 9% for those >65-years-old.[342] From the fifth decade onwards, wear in the canines and (pre)molars is not unrelated, probably because the canine guidance also disappears.[325]

In an Inuit study and in ancient Anglo-Saxon skulls, tooth wear was found to be an accurate predictor of age.[227 241] Wear of contemporary 10-year-old bruxists predicts wear reasonably well 20 years later,[169] but generally, age explains only 12% of the wear over the whole dentition.[298] Sollberg *et al.* found that the correlation between age and premolar wear was 0.7 and with the anterior teeth 0.2, but correlations between wear and age vary considerably,[345] due to scoring methods, differences in wear in different tooth, dietary differences (carbonated drinks),[221] salivary composition and flow, participation in craft activities, etc. Scores in a sample of young Saudi

Arabians varied depending on variables such as nail- and pen-biting, an erosive diet, use of a "miswak" (chewing stick used as a toothbrush) and bruxism. Tooth wear is more pronounced in Saudi Arabia than in Western countries, because of presence of fine airborne dust particles in the desert environment.[150 151]

Diet
Consumption of hard or uncooked foods promotes occlusal and approximal wear in both dentitions.[135 143]

The varying food of evolving hominids maintained the versatility of the omnivore.[89] Davies *et al.* found that wear in Western Greenland was less than in the more isolated Eastern Greenland, where the food requires heavy and long mastication.[72] Marked wear occurred in ancient tribes and populations due to consumption of uncooked food, methods of food preparation, and contamination of the food with sand.[31 71 94 130 135 175 176 181 184 211 228 229 303 311 385] The hunter-gatherer community had more anterior tooth wear at a younger age than the later farming settlements due to habits; the molars in both groups were equally worn. At an older age, farmers lost their posterior teeth through caries, which promoted wear of the anterior teeth, contrary to the more contemporary findings noted above.[143]

Anthropologists use the degree of tooth wear as a benchmark for age determination. For example, an individual who died at age 13–14 years will show severely worn first permanent molars due to consumption of an abrasive diet but unabraded second premolars.[31] Food availability and religious and cultural factors and habits largely determined the diet[71] and underlie marked differences in tooth wear in prehistoric humans, which precludes age determination based on tooth wear alone. The diet must be studied, based on, for example, fossilised excrements.

A medieval population (AD400–800) exhibited more occlusal wear and cupping than an age-matched contemporary group with an acidic, raw diet, while the latter showed greater wear than their contemporaries with an average diet. Buccal concavities were common in the acidic diet group (63%), infrequent in the average diet group (8%), and absent in the medieval group.[104]

Masticatory force/time
Men tend to have more tooth wear than women[91 151 326 342 345] because their masticatory muscles are more developed.[70 152 329 386] Kiliaridis *et al.* found that subjects with advanced wear had a comparatively high biting force.[165] Chewing times depend on the diet: a sample of 7000-year-old Indian dentitions showed considerable wear as a consequence of long and forceful mastication of raw vegetables and seeds.[135]

Saliva
Reduced saliva and salivary proteins, in particular lubricating mucins and proline-rich proteins, and a low buffering capacity, promote tooth wear.[91 152 345 372 374] The permanent viscoelastic salivary film on tooth surfaces reduces friction.[374] Ligation of the salivary gland ducts in rats increased tooth wear.[54] Many medicaments, especially used by older persons, cause xerostomia (Chapter 5). Otherwise, salivary glands of elderly people function well, although mucin content decreases.[381] It is not clear whether salivary lubrication is thereby substantially affected. Excessive tooth wear (enhanced by consumption of erosive beverages) has been reported in dehydration (leading to a reduced salivary flow) and in drug-induced xerostomia.[405]

Other factors causing wear
Crossbites are associated with severe wear of the deciduous molars and a Class III canine relationship is associated with wear of incisors.[387] Angle's Class II and III molar relationships are associated with deviating wear patterns.[326] The presence of some types of amelogenesis and dentinogenesis imperfecta increases the likelihood of tooth wear as fluoride may do.[210] In diabetes mellitus, the first permanent molars develop typical saucer-like wear facets occlusally.[283] Excessive wear in 100 patients was caused by "erosion" (in 35) and by "erosion-attrition" (in 25),[329] as were the teeth in a pygmy.[365] In a sample of young swimmers and cyclists using sport drinks, incisal edge tooth wear into dentine was found to be the rule than the exception.[220] (Rough) porcelain and ceramics promote tooth wear, other restoratives hardly.

Contact with quartz-filled composite restorations in antagonist teeth affects mainly incisal dentine, if exposed, of the mandibular incisors.[57 400] In *in vitro* experiments, composites with the greatest wear resistance (with quartz or zirconium silicate fillers) damaged the enamel more than other composites.[357] Gold (type III) and composite inlays are equally abrasive.[139] Porcelain is most damaging,[80 139 204 324] more so when the glaze disappears,[149] but a glazed ceramic may be worse than other polished ceramics (and gold).[407] Aluminous and bonded porcelains cause greater wear of the enamel than hydrothermal and machinable porcelain, the latter causing the least wear.[7] Rough porcelain is highly abrasive: after occlusal adjustment, the porcelain must be polished.[149] In an *in vitro* study, type III gold and a glaze caused the same amount of wear, but some brands were more damaging.[285]

8.4.3 Consequences of wear

Dental arches
Regressive periodontal changes with ageing make teeth less resistant to the horizontal component of masticatory forces. But the teeth are able to resist the forces better when wear flattens the occlusal surfaces, whereby the horizontal component of the masticatory forces is reduced. Broad approximal contacts stabilise the dental arches. Some researchers doubt the compensatory effect.

Due to wear, the occlusal surfaces of the teeth of Australian aboriginals were found to flatten and gradually inclined more buccally. The masticatory movements in the aboriginals were broader than in Europeans.[37] The idea that occlusal flattening would be desirable is based on the great amounts of wear observed in ancient skulls and in "primitively living" people.[35]

However, chewing with flat teeth requires the use of greater forces, which increases the horizontal component of the masticatory forces, but does not result in alveolar bone resorption.[111 188] A load that is too high will displace a tooth,[112] unless it is stabilised by adjacent teeth. Approximal wear increases this form of stabilisation.[296]

Anthropologists question whether wear was responsible for the edge-to-edge bite seen in so many ancient skulls. Ongoing wear decreases the anterior and post-canine lateral overjet.[295] An edge-to-edge relationship of the anterior teeth may be a consequence of occlusal wear when, due to abrasion of the upper incisors, the labial displacement of the mandibular incisors is not prevented.[31]

In the past, progressive approximal wear with mesial migration of teeth led to shortening of the dental arches, which ensured sufficient space for third molar eruption. The minor loss of approximal enamel per tooth was averaged over the dental arch around 1900 as about 1 cm during a 40-year period,[211] and in the "primitive" peoples as 1.6 cm.[31 311]

Approximal wear is associated with the diet, which has changed significantly over time.[63] Due to less approximal wear, the percentage of retained third molars increased from 12% in the prehistoric times to 35% in the medieval period and 50% in the Victorian times to 55% in modern dentitions.[328]

Tooth wear in the prehistoric period was a universal mechanism that reduced the "too large" mesio-distal tooth widths, leading to accommodation of a full complement of teeth with few instances of malocclusion.[31] With the modern diet, the teeth remain too wide mesio-distally, which often necessitates extraction therapy. However, malocclusions in present-day aboriginals with unworn teeth are the consequence of jaws that are too small instead of teeth that are too large; the increase in overjet with crowding might be explained by this point of view.[65]

Teeth may migrate when wear is extreme.[241]

Enamel

Worn and thin occlusal enamel may succumb to masticatory forces, as has been found in prehistoric Inuits.[272] Chewing on the hard abfracted enamel particles increases the occlusal tooth wear.

Dentine

To reiterate, the peritubular dentine becomes richer in minerals,[269] making the dentine harder. Sclerotic dentine and dead tracts that are present in about 50% of teeth[348] are not so much due to ageing as to tooth wear.[214]

Pulp

Tertiary dentine is found in many worn teeth,[349] but it is also deemed to be secondary dentine,[268] because tertiary dentine is said to not form in the roof of the pulp chamber. However, wear induces tertiary dentine formation like caries.[270 317 362] Wear disrupts the odontoblastic layer and bacterial endotoxins are able to penetrate the pulp via the tubules of the exposed dentine.[362]

Temporomandibular joint (TMJ)

The TMJ and masticatory apparatus must adapt to a decreased vertical occlusal dimension after wearing away of the occlusal enamel. The efficiency of the response of the masticatory apparatus depends on the load applied and the adaptive capacity of the TMJ. Slow, steady wear does not seem problematic.

Generalised steady wear reduces the depth of the articular fossa of the TMJ. More marked wear leads to an increase in fossa depth and alters the slope of the articular eminence, followed either by levelling off of the fossa depth due to later wear of anterior teeth, or a sharp decrease due to later wear of the molars.[133]

An increase in the height of the alveolar bone compensates for wear.[35 359] Nowadays, "insufficient" wear increases the height of the face. Wear might therefore be functional.[35] Luke et al. suggest that if the cusps are considered as merely representative of adaptations to chew food of specific quality, severe wear may be an anomaly.[195]

The adaptive capacity of the TMJ seems limited, so that marked wear might result in craniomandibular dysfunction;[43] but tooth wear and TMJ disturbances appear unrelated in studies on contemporary Americans and an ancient British population.[97 299 395 396] TMJs in skulls from the seventeenth century frequently show remodelling in association with extensive tooth wear and, rarely, deformative changes or osteoarthrosis.[390] Remodelling is indicative of adaptation rather than pathology. Alterations in the TMJ have been found to be associated with tooth loss.[396] Yet, severe tooth wear might cause degenerative changes in the temporomandibular disc.[167 297] Tooth wear and joint pathology have been found to be associated,[297 400] but not in young adults.[326]

Cementum

Hypercementosis may compensate for tooth wear by allowing continuous eruption.[331]

8.4.4 Prevention and treatment

Patients (vegetarians) must be made aware of severe wear that can be caused by frequent consumption of raw (acidic) food. The consequences of xerostomia require active management, eventually with artificial saliva.

Substantial tooth wear with involvement of dentine requires intervention, but not in deciduous teeth. Curative treatment, with composite restorations prevents deterioration. When the adaptive mechanisms fail,[48] severe wear is an indication for gold and/or porcelain crowns, preceded by temporary crowns to test the effect of restoring the vertical dimension of occlusion.[36] A "Dahl appliance", a splint placed on the palatal surfaces of the maxillary anterior teeth, allows eruption of the discluded posterior teeth.[302] The posterior jaw interference guide may help create sufficient space for restorations in the anterior region.[34] Very severe cases require "overdentures".

8.5 Pathological tooth wear in mutilated dentitions

Commonly, wear patterns in many patients are more or less similar. Different patterns are found in asymmetrical and mutilated dentitions, following tilting and migration of teeth into extraction spaces and overeruption of antagonists (Figures 8.9 and 8.10). Removable partial denture clasps may cause unusual tooth wear.[128]

8.5.1 Epidemiology

Mutilated dentitions are suspected to be common. Studies have found that substantial wear of the (pre)molars correlates with a small number of post-canine contacts, significant crowding, a small overjet and overbite, although presence of a Class II molar relationship in the worn

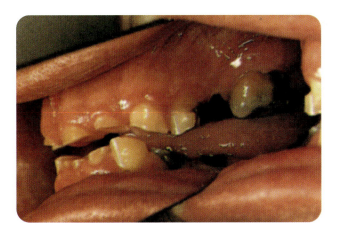

Figure 8.9 Buccal view of a mutilated dentition with excessive wear.

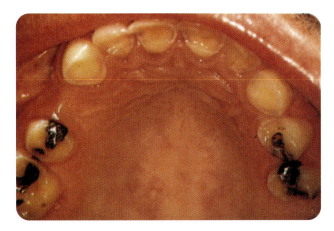

Figure 8.10 Inciso-occlusal view of the same dentition as in Figure 8.9. The palatal surfaces of the incisors are grooved due to heavy contact with the lower incisors.

dentitions was rare.[151 152] Tooth wear is promoted in dentitions with an abnormal number of teeth,[60] but some studies have found that anterior tooth wear is unrelated to the number of posterior teeth,[239] which contradicts the aforementioned paleontological findings.[134]

8.5.2 Consequences

Pulp
Studies of ancient skulls indicate that when the rate of tooth wear surpasses the rate of tertiary dentine production it leads to exposure of the pulp,[212 242 399] which may have already become necrotic due to the combination of wear, bacterial toxins, hypermobility and apical overloading.

Periodontium
Teeth that are subjected to abnormally directed masticatory forces show a wide periradicular space[64 320] and migrate to a position in the dental arch where the occlusion and articulation forces are lower.[111] If such teeth cannot migrate, they become permanently hypermobile and resorption may ensue. Traumatic occlusion and articulation do not cause periodontitis, but existing periodontitis becomes more severe.[49 110 111 188 276]

Periodontal changes include capillary thrombosis, deviations in the orientation of the collagen fibres, increased numbers of fibroblasts and osteoclasts, hyaline degeneration and necrosis. During healing vascularity increases and connective tissue is formed,[64] manifesting finally as hypermobility, a broad periradicular space,[158] resorption of alveolar bone and development of periodontal abcesses.[48 64]

Pain
Slow tooth wear is painless, because the dentine becomes sclerotic. More abrupt wear may cause pain: contact with an antagonist initially leads to a short and sharp pain, but in later stages there is a permanent, dull pain that intensifies during contact. Response of the patient to percussion and pressure applied in the direction of the overload aids the diagnosis.[362] Premature contacts and occlusal interferences in asymmetrical dentitions may have repercussions for the TMJ and the masticatory musculature,[362] but whether dysfunction develops is still being debated.[298]

Facial changes
Excessive tooth wear leads to facial changes. Crothers *et al.* found that severely worn maxillary anterior teeth were 5 mm shorter and the mandibular incisors 3.3 mm shorter than in controls. Overjet was reduced and alveolar bone growth counterbalanced the loss in vertical dimension. The lower face became shorter and the upper face longer.[69] A small angle between the mandibular and palatal planes and a small gonial angle characterise advanced tooth wear. Patients with severely worn teeth have an open bite less frequently than is found in the general population.[151 152 165]

8.5.3 Prevention and treatment

Dental arch asymmetries must be prevented or treated with orthodontics, implants, bridges, partial dentures and overdentures.[19 82] Splints may be needed (see Section 8.6). Masseter muscle activity is sensitive to occlusal instability. In a study of patients with myogenous craniomandibular disorders, non-uniform distribution of tooth contacts along the dental arches tended to disturb the symmetry of the masticatory muscles. Properly adjusted full-arch maxillary stabilisation splints immediately improved the symmetry; splints with occlusal interferences worsened the masseter muscle asymmetry (but not that of the temporal muscle).[148]

Reconstruction of the vertical dimension may be indicated.[48] Intrusion of the mandibular anterior teeth helps restore normal overjet and overbite.[69]

8.6   Bruxism and tooth clenching

Bruxism consists of non-functional mandibular movements characterised by unconscious, involuntary, non-functional articulation. Forceful occlusion of the teeth (clenching/vertical bruxism) during sleep and/or by day is considered as a type of bruxism. Many people audibly grind or silently clench the teeth. The duration, frequency, force and direction of mandibular movements, the steepness of the occlusal cusps and the quality of periodontal support determine the consequences.

8.6.1   Epidemiology

Tooth grinding is a universal phenomenon,[233] and is found not only in adults but also in younger people.[245] The reported prevalence rates in children vary from 5% to 88%.[6 98 145 174 289 305] In Grodfeld et al.'s study, more than half of 6–8-year-olds and two-thirds of 13–15-year-olds exhibited signs of bruxism,[118] which increased from adolescence into adulthood and decreased thereafter.[98] In a sample of psoriasis patients who were frequent bruxists, the decrease started at the age of 35 years.[170] A small number of patients are aware of their parafunction,[98 120 305] which creates a bias in studies using self-reports. Prevalence rates based on self-reports are between 5% and 21%.[103 246 251 289 326]

The diagnosis requires presence of clinical symptoms besides frequently repeated rhythmic muscle activities during sleep. Masticatory muscle activity without tooth contact may have led to the high prevalence rates reported. All-night electromyographic (EEG; masseter muscle) recordings and registration of rapid eye movements (REM) has revealed that half of the grinding periods occur during REM sleep.[179 290 376] Clenchers have been noted among control subjects.[290] A relationship has also been established with light sleep,[279 376] during periodic transient arousals, abruptly changing sleep levels characterised by body movements, especially early at night, with EEG alterations and increased heart rates.[201 336 401]

Rjamford studied bruxism electromyographically,[284] but masticatory muscle activity is not proof of grinding of teeth. Some 60% of the adult population show nocturnal rhythmic masticatory muscle activity, but a considerably lower proportion fulfil the criteria for the diagnosis of bruxism.[194] Instead of electromyography, polysomnography must be used.[79 193]

The clenching force and the number of grinding episodes varies between individuals.[59] Bruxists (clenchers) clench (grit) the teeth for about 10 seconds, 5–10 times/night,[60] and sometimes for 25 seconds.[352] The grinding forces exceed those used normally in the day.[60] The biting force and how long bruxists are able to bite exceed the force and time in non-bruxists,[200 262 285] with exceptions.[80 108] Dahl et al. did not find any relation between the maximum bite force and tooth wear,[70] but the bite force of those with marked tooth wear has been found to be higher than that found in the general population.[165]

8.6.2   Aetiology

The aetiology is said to be multifactorial.[356] Nadler distinguished local, systemic, psychological and occupational factors.[235] Bruxism in children and adults may be aetiologically different.[305]

Peripheral factors
Local causes include occlusal interferences.[356 361] Some authors have suggested that premature contacts can be highly irritating, and patients try to get rid of them by clenching and grinding the teeth,[84 314] which then may become habitual.

Persistent parafunctions may be deeply ingrained habits. Premature tooth contact forces the mandible in an eccentric closing position and the occlusal discrepancies may be enough to exceed an "irritation threshold". Therefore bruxism may develop, giving rise to discomfort and muscle pain, which in turn increases the tendency to bruxism. Some studies support this point of view, but others do not.[48 50 156 245 284 286 304]

Children, who may already have been rubbing their gum pads against each other as infants, may later clench and grind the teeth in an unconscious attempt to position the individual teeth such that the musculature obtains rest. Other non-validated causes in children include vesical irritability, hyperacidic urine, nervousness and local and psychological factors.[235]

Electromyographic (EMG) studies have indicated that malocclusion does not result in bruxism.[275 290 301] Human and animal studies with artificial occlusal interferences (or eliminated premature contacts) have not confirmed their role:[304] rather, bruxism has been found to reduce;[21 27] premature contacts may be so painful that tooth contact and bruxism are avoided.

Studies found that slightly "high" inlays were associated with a decrease in tooth pain threshold. After height adjustment of the inlays the symptoms disappeared[26 142] and bruxism ceased.[284] However, others have found that elimination of occlusal interferences does not reduce bruxism.[20] Even small interferences can cause spontaneous pain. Chronic overload might result in periodontal (and pulpal) damage.[12] Some studies have found a high correlation between periodontal breakdown and bruxism.[120 204]

Daytime tooth grinding and clenching are also not related to malocclusion.[287] Bruxism habits in the daytime and at night may differ,[290] perhaps because of the difference in the levels of consciousness.

Occlusal interferences are present in many dentitions, but not everyone grinds and not all bruxists have occlusal interferences,[115] which are harmful only when they act as a trigger.[261] Lobbezoo et al. found no difference between bruxists and non-bruxists on 26 occlusal variables.[193] A review concluded that bruxism must be treated both dentally and psychologically.[216] Bruxism, craniomandibular and temporomandibular dysfunction (CMD and TMD) may be correlated, but causality is still being debated.[192] [349] Causality is difficult to establish because of the multifactorial character of CMD. A deficiency in neuromuscular adaptation may play a role.[90 388]

The relationship between CMD, clenching/bruxism, and joint anomalies (ankylosis spondylitis, whereby the head is pressed ventrally on a stiff neck and the patients cannot open their mouth wide) is unclear,[392] but in studies, CMD patients have been found to grind their teeth more frequently than controls and to more often experience different types of headache, including migraine.[226]

Systemic and central factors

As mentioned above, nocturnal bruxism episodes in non-REM sleep are associated with transient arousal.[201] Kato et al. found that transient arousals, experimentally induced during sleep, were followed more frequently by rhythmic masticatory muscle activity and grinding in patients with bruxism than in controls. Spontaneous micro-arousals occur about 15 times per sleeping hour, as shown by a sudden increase in EEG and EMG activity and heart rate.[160] Bruxists show a significantly higher number of such transient arousals than controls.[201]

The term "bruxomania" has been used in the past to refer to bruxism assumedly caused by cortical brain lesions and disturbances in the medulla and pons.[209 235] Bruxomania was distinguished in the past from tooth grinding in nephritis and in cerebral diseases such as meningitis.[235] Bruxism indeed seems to be a neurological disorder, involving a disturbance in the equilibrium between the direct and indirect output pathways from the basal ganglia in the brain involved in the coordination of movements. Disturbances in central neurotransmitter pathways (e.g. dopaminergic system) may be aetiological.[193 194] Use of pharmaceutical agents, such as amphetamines, enhances bruxism,[306] as does smoking.[5 178 203] Nicotine stimulates central dopaminergic activity. Long-term use of dopamine antagonists by psychiatric patients

and excessive use of amphetamines lead to bruxism in the day, as do other medicaments. Two types of bruxism may be distinguished: idiopathic bruxism, which is suppressed by administering dopamine, and iatrogenic bruxism, which develops with long-term use of dopaminergic therapeutic agents.[193]

Gastrointestinal disturbances, chronic middle ear infection, subclinical dietary deficiencies, endocrine disturbances, inheritance, nephritis, brain damage, allergies, drugs, alcohol abuse, trauma, etc. are other factors suggested to be causative.[6 193] A low oesophageal pH after reflux, in particular in the supine position, relates to the frequency of rhythmic masticatory muscle activity, but no more than 10% of episodes include parafunctions.[223] Rett's syndrome is associated with bruxism (this progressive neurological disturbance starting before the age of 2 years in females, and includes progressive dementia, stereotypical wrenching movements of the hands and epilepsy).[9 47 263] While associations between bruxism and the abovementioned causes may be indirect, cerebral spastic palsy is a direct systemic cause.[264]

Alternately sleeping on the left and right sides is the most common postural factor associated with right and left side bruxism; the mandible is usually forced lateroprotrusively. Sleeping for a long time in one side position may lead to unilateral clenching. Sleeping in the supine position seems to be the most compromising posture, with bilateral tooth wear and a high incidence of posterior neck pain and stiffness.[63]

Occupational factors

Three groups of factors have been distinguished:[235]

- *Physical factors.* Athletes who, like aerialists and stunt men pulling automobiles with their teeth, engage in strenuous activities, show habitual tooth wear. Porters, dock-workers, etc. may clench their teeth during exertion. People who stretch and yawn a great deal may clench their teeth tightly.[235] Tractor drivers clench their teeth to avoid the disconcerting "shocks" to the mandible due to the bumpy motion of the tractor. When this becomes habitual, the consequences become more severe. Chewing gum can be looked upon as a form of bruxism because of the unconscious and rhythmic motor activity associated with it.[235]
- *Emotional factors.* Precision workers such as watchmakers and diamond cleavers whose work involves slight physical but strenuous nervous exertion may be susceptible to bruxism.
- *Occupational stress* (see Section 8.8.2).

Psychological factors

As the aforementioned causes are unable to explain bruxism consistently, psychological factors have also been studied. Some psychoanalysts regarded bruxism as an expression of anger and aggression,[356] others as an expression of, for instance, anxiety[117 140 317] or emotional disturbance[190] or the level of stress on the previous day.[171]

Chronic mental stress may result in dental parafunction if aggression alleviates the stress insufficiently,[114] but the way in which aggression becomes manifest appeared unrelated to the degree of non-functional tooth wear.[102] The importance of and the very role of stress in bruxism is still unclear, because it is "difficult to say what mental stress is the cause".[235] Mental stress during occupational activities (e.g. in pilots) may lead to bruxism or clenching.[75] Pingitore et al. found that stress and bruxism were associated only in persons with type A behaviour (competitive, impatient, putting work first), but even in this group, bruxism could not be predicted accurately.[273] Neither anticipated nor actual stress correlated at the group level with bruxism: positive correlations were established for a large minority.[271] Others have found an association between self-reported frequent bruxism and severe stress experience and the authors concluded that in patients with bruxism the history usually revealed ongoing stress in their "normal" work life.[3 4] In other studies, stress-clenchers (daytime) scored consistently higher on the factor "obsession" than non-stress bruxists (at night).[109 170] Two-thirds of a sample of longstanding bruxists reported somatic, psycho-social and sleep disorders. They considered stress as the cause.[157] The relationship between bruxism and stress may be associated with a perceived imbalance between a demand and the (in)ability to meet that demand, which has consequences for the subject that they consider to be important. The result is heightened activity of the (para)sympathetic nervous system, which may manifest in somatisation, and thus bruxism and clenching.[84]

Bruxism in children may not have significant psychological connotations,[174] but children with bruxism have been reported to have greater levels of stress and nervous symptoms such as bed-wetting, sleep disturbances,[191] high levels of aggression and somatisation.[174] Altogether, bruxism in childhood may signify psychological problems. While a psychological basis may be likely,[356] the influence of psychological factors is uncertain.[109 174] Personality and emotional disturbances may be related to nocturnal bruxism,[155 174 290 305] but neither psychological (nor dental) problems appear causative.[171] Bruxists and non-bruxists have been reported to achieve similar scores on psychological tests.[287] Yet, anxiety and depression may be more prevalent among bruxists than controls.[225]

The paradigms concerning TMD have shifted from the mechanistic and a psychophysical origin of the disorder to a biopsychosocial concept.[224] Peripheral aetiological factors are considered to play a minor role, if any, and central factors seem more relevant.[5 194] Other factors[6] seem unlikely and a relationship with bruxism has not either been convincingly elucidated or explained.

8.6.3 Consequences

Bruxism is associated with headache,[145 226] pain and stiffness of the masticatory, neck and shoulder muscles, hypertrophy of the masticatory musculature,[98 157 273 305 378] and a tired feeling in the jaw muscles when waking up, which may be tender on palpation.[284] Myofacial pain may develop[305 337 338] due to the eccentric activity of the temporalis and pterygoid muscles.[201] Treatment may resolve headaches.[146]

Bruxism may cause TMJ instability, movement impairment and pain.[262 377] The fluid in the articular disc absorbs the masticatory forces, but it is drained away under longer-term and heavier bruxing and clenching loads. Then, the fibres of the disc must absorb the load and may become damaged. However, a causal relationship between bruxism and TMJ disorders is not established. Bruxism might have an initiating role though when other factors have reduced the adaptive capacity of the TMJ and associated tissues.

Microfractures of the subchondral bone is a predisposing factor. The bone becomes sclerotic and is unable to withstand the overloading and the cartilage of the joint becomes more vulnerable to pressure. Coping mechanisms of the patient may interfere with healing. A possible predisposing biological factor concerns the oestrogenic joint receptors: more women than men report joint disorders, which are also uncommon in children.[349]

Extensive occlusal wear facets are signs of broad horizontal bruxing movements. Pronounced palatal wear of the incisors occurs mainly due to vertical parafunction. In the case of deep overbite and upright incisors, the wear is distributed over a great area of the labial surfaces of the mandibular incisors. A reduced functional space limits jaw excursions. A normal space allows ventral bruxism, which results in a wide area of contact between the opposing incisors.[27]

Epidemiological data regarding tooth damage are limited. Lyons et al. reported that during a period of 6 months, tooth wear was greater in bruxists than non-bruxists. Eccentric jaw movements resulted in excessive canine wear.[200] Substantial wear of anterior teeth depends, as stated previously, on the angle between the mandibular and maxillary incisors, etc.[173] Heavier masticatory forces may lead to fracture of or cracks in the teeth.[98] Bruxism and clenching cause surface irregularities in the enamel, which further increase the wear.[403] Cervical abfraction lesions are frequently present.[262] Bruxism results in loss of alveolar bone and hypermobile teeth at the overloaded jaw site.[49]

In sum, many people grind or clench their teeth, but not all of them show excessive wear. Figures 8.11 and 8.12 show wear in a bruxist's dentition with an edge-to-edge bite and Figure 8.13 shows wear in a dentition with a normal overjet and overbite.

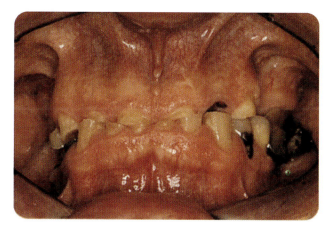

Figure 8.11 Frontal view of a dentition of a bruxist. Note the edge-to-edge anterior bite.

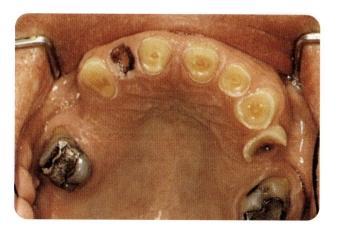

Figure 8.12 Inciso-occlusal view of the maxillary teeth of the same dentition as in Figure 8.11. The incisal edges have flattened and are surrounded by a white line, representing the enamel. Centrally, there is tertiary dentine within the less dark primary (and secondary) dentine.

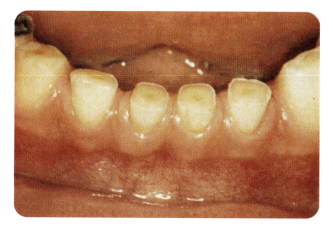

Figure 8.13 Wear of the lower incisors in a patient with a normal overbite and overjet.

8.6.4 *Prevention and treatment*

Management of bruxism should include consideration of the pathophysiological, psychological and occlusal factors. In view of the causative uncertainties[99] it is not surprising that several different therapies have been proposed for bruxism.

- *Counselling* may make patients aware that they clench or grind their teeth in the day. Bruxism at night may decline with counselling to avoid alcohol, coffee, tea, heavy meals, smoking, and watching television and exercising in the evening.[374]
- *Peripheral treatment.* Correction of occlusal interferences is always desirable. The high muscle tone in bruxists hinders ascertaining the right occlusion. The effect of elimination of premature contacts on bruxism is doubtful,[6] but favourable results have been reported.[59 388]
- *Bite plate.* A splint covering the occlusal surfaces at night may prevent the grinding movements, but it must not lead to a change in the occlusal relationship.[284] The splint is not intended to resolve CMD, but it is the standard preventive treatment for nocturnal bruxism,[373] and aims to protect the teeth from wear, reduce parafunctional activity and deprogramme the muscles. Splint therapy for some years has been found to reduce tooth wear.[55] In one study on young children, use of an acrylic resin bite plate prevented worsening of wear facets, even after the removal of the plate; in the children in the control group the wear facets became worse.[121]

Splints fabricated from a soft material[262] may reduce effects of the grinding forces on the dentition, but they have not been found to eliminate the parafunction.[185] Okeson reported that the soft splint may even promote masticatory muscle activity, which decreased with the use of a hard splint:[254] 60% of splints consistently showed signs of wear and 30% occasionally,[137] indicating persistence of bruxism. Half of bruxists in another study benefited from use of a hard splint but bruxism became worse in 25%.[58] The use of the splint might decrease EMG activity during submaximal biting, in particular of the masseter muscle.[373]

- *Medication.* Some pharmaceutical agents show promise. The sedative diazepam, which reduces muscle tone, is prescribed for only a short period because of its side effects. A dopamine precursor and a dopamine antagonist are effective, but side effects preclude their use in general practice. A β-blocker and botulinum toxin A, which block acetylcholine, may be worthwhile, but further research is required.[373]

- *Physiotherapy* is aimed at alleviating the musculoskeletal symptoms of bruxism and teaching patients to recognise and alter their behaviour.[15][379] Biofeedback[159] methods may afterwards increase bruxism,[103] and the same has been suggested for the splint method.[307]
- *Psychotherapy* consists of a diagnostic examination with psychological tests and the treatment[44][109] nowadays often consists of cognitive behaviour therapy.[368][371] The approach does not seem very effective.[109][131] Attention to somatic, psychological and social factors is recommended, in other words, a multifactorial treatment plan.[84]
- *Prosthetic-restorative treatment* aims at the restoration of functional, aesthetic and phonetic problems and pain relief, and is directed by the dental findings, the aetiological factors and patient expectations. The description here is mainly based on a literature review by Donachie *et al.*[83] Occlusal therapy with adhesive restorative techniques prevents ongoing wear and restores occlusal function.
- *Vertical bruxism*, characterised by the absence of lateral jaw movements, in which all muscles show activity,[202] affects in particular the palatal surfaces of maxillary incisors. The ongoing eruption of these teeth increases the overbite. The Dahl bite plane and use of palatal composite stops allows the posterior teeth to erupt. Alternatively, orthodontic intrusion of the anterior teeth, a lengthy process, allows local restorative treatment. An artificially pronounced cingulum prevents relapse.
- *Horizontal bruxism* affects the incisal and occlusal surfaces. The vertical dimension is preferably restored with composite because persistent bruxism requires re-restoration. Canine guidance and simple cusp–fossa contacts between the posterior antagonists reduce the large horizontal jaw movements. In severe cases, overdentures may be indicated. Partial dentures may wear rather quickly and accelerate bone resorption. Porcelain and gold-porcelain crowns might not withstand the heavy occlusal forces. Before making crowns and bridges, the neuromuscular adaptation to the restored vertical and horizontal positions is tested with a splint.

8.7   Cervical lesions caused by tooth brushing

Cervical defects, chiefly on the buccal root surfaces (Figure 8.14), are initiated and worsen by tooth brushing with a dentifrice, but a toothpaste needs to be abrasive to aid removal of plaque and stains.[309]

Tooth brushing affects all the brushed surfaces, which is in general difficult to see. Cervical lesions tend to be steep and deep on the enamel side and taper off in the apical direction. In the pulp, tertiary dentine formation is

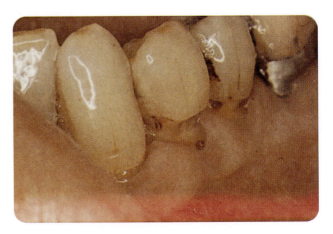

Figure 8.14 Cervical wear.

observed (Figure 8.15A). The wear may compromise the longevity of the tooth (Figure 8.15B). However, studies show that the manner of tooth brushing could not explain the form of all cervical lesions noted; abfraction grooves also exist (see Chapter 9).[45][168] Restorative materials, in particular temporary fillings and glass ionomer cement, are also abraded. A toothpaste may increase the toxicity of casting alloys, in particular under acidic conditions, such as present underneath plaque.[389] The clinical relevance of the findings is presumably small.

8.7.1   Epidemiology

Less abrasion of dentine occurs *in vivo* than is expected on the basis of *in vitro* experiments,[312] because of factors such as saliva and differences in brushing power of different people. Cervical tooth wear concerns mainly the labial/buccal dentine in the incisors, canines and premolars,[141] but the molars are not free from the defects. Lingually erupted teeth undergo less abrasion than buccally erupted teeth.[141] Cervical wear aggravates and becomes more prevalent with age, because of gingival recession. The cementum and dentine wear more than the adjoining enamel.[238][316] A low bleeding index, which indicates "good" oral hygiene, was associated with greater gingival recession and cervical root lesions in 25% of patients who brushed 2–3 times/day.[316] The dexterity of the brushers was related to the gingival recession.[215]

Donachie *et al.* found that the mean cervical TWI score was relatively low, even among older age cohorts, the maxillary canines frequently having score 2 (defect <1 mm deep). Maxillary and mandibular premolars tended to have worse levels of cervical wear than mandibular molars. The first maxillary molar had higher TWI scores after the age of 65 years.[83] Reported prevalences of cervico-buccal abrasion lesions vary from 18% to 65%; in one study, 32% of 65-year-olds showed grade 3 lesions.[141]

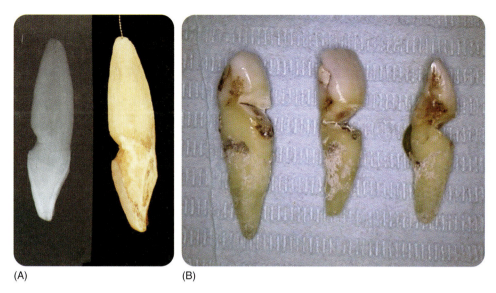

Figure 8.15 (A) Cervical wear: the radiograph shows tertiary dentine underneath the defect that has divided the pulp cavity in two. (B) Excessive cervical wear threatens the longevity of the tooth.

A relationship with age and, according to some, with sex exists.[33 127 282 310 343 344] In a Swiss study, about 20% of 26–30-year-olds and about 50% of 46–50-year-olds exhibited cervical defects more than 1 mm deep; the majority were painful.[196] In a Swedish study, 85% of 21–60-year-olds had at least one superficial cervical lesions and about 20% deep lesions; the latter occurred more frequently in older persons.[32] In a cross-sectional study of randomly selected sample of Croatians every sixth tooth and every third premolar was affected, but the authors did not make any distinction based on cause. The study showed that most lesions start at an early age and become more severe with time.[42]

The prevalence and severity of abrasive cervical defects increase with age, but extractions, cervical erosion, abfraction and caries are confounding factors.[127 398] Cervical tooth wear progresses at a rate of about 75 μm/year,[248] with large individual differences depending on the abrasiveness of the toothpaste.[313] Ultimately the pulp may become exposed.[212 248] Not much is known about the hardness of the teeth in relation to tooth wear.[229] Fluorotic enamel in rat molars has not been found to be very resistant to wear.

8.7.2 Aetiology

Wear caused by tooth brushing is a function of the abrasiveness of the toothpaste, frequency and duration of brushing, brushing power, and factors such as acids and the tooth tissue being brushed. Saxton *et al.* compared the results of clinical studies (by using dental casts obtained after taking impressions) with those obtained from *in vitro* experiments. They found that *in vivo* on average 1 μm/week of dentine at the dentino-enamel junction was lost due to abrasion, which was much less than that predicted by the laboratory experiments.[313]

Abrasive ingredients in toothpastes

Toothpastes must exert a scouring action on teeth,[101] but they must not damage the dental hard tissues.[28] As abrasives form a major component of a dentifrice[206 239] (Table 8.2), a compromise is required between the desired abrasiveness of the paste and dental damage.[236] International standards for toothpastes include abrasiveness limits in order to achieve a balance between their efficacy and the damage caused by the scouring action.

The relationship between the abrasiveness and cleaning effect of a dentifrice is not simple.[166] A higher degree of abrasiveness does not equate with better cleaning,[309] but a linear correlation may exist between *in vitro* dentine abrasiveness and clinical stain cleaning.[10] Some toothpastes contain abrasives that are harder than the enamel, but do not affect the softer dentine. The hardness, in general, slightly exceeds that of dentine and is decisively lower than that of enamel.[101] Besides the abrasive's hardness,[73] particle size,[51 77] the proportion in the toothpaste, surface properties and chemical influence of other ingredients also determine the abrasiveness of a toothpase.[353 354 356 401] For example, the foaming agent sodium lauryl sulfate (which is a mucosal irritant in xerostomia)[341] affects the abrasiveness of silicon dioxide.[291] Larger particles of this agent cause greater wear of dentine than smaller ones.[53 77] Baxter *et al.* reported that an increase in the size of calcium carbonate particles from 0.1 μm to 10 μm increased its abrasiveness; the larger particles were

Table 8.2 Toothpaste ingredients

Common basic ingredients

20–50%	Abrasives
20–40%	Water
1–2%	Binding agents (stabilisers, anti-separation components)
1–3%	Detergents (e.g. surfactant – sodium lauryl sulfate)
1–3%	Flavourings, sweeteners, colouring agents and preservatives

Therapeutic ingredients

Fluoride	Anti-caries
Sodium hexamethaphopsphate + soluble pyrophosphate[a]	Anti-stain
Pyrophosphates	Anti-tartar (plus methoxy-ethylene and maleic acid)
Zinc citrate + triclosan[b]	Anti-tartar (anti-calculus and anti-gingivitis)
Peroxide/carbamideperoxide	Tooth whitening (+ aluminium oxide or silica; Chapter 10)
Strontium chloride	Desensitising
Potassium nitrate[c]	Desensitising
Sodium citrate	Desensitising
Titanium fluoride	Desensitising (Chapter 6)
Lysozyme, lactoferrin + peroxidase	Anti-xerostomia (not proven)
Betaine (= trimethylglycine)[d]	Subjective relief of xerostomia symptoms only
NaF + 0.3% triclosan + polyvinylmethylether malic acid[e]	Anti-caries, anti-gingivitis
Sodium hexametaphosphate + SnF_2 toothpaste	Anti-erosive (Chapter 6)

[a]Experimentally superior in stain prevention compared with a highly abrasive alumina-based dentifrice. The experimental and other highly abrasive dentifrices removed stains with equal efficacy (Chapter 10).[106 107 393]
[b]Broad-spectrum antibacterial agent, reduces plaque and gingivitis.
[c]Weak evidence for efficacy.[278]
[d]The mucosal appearance remained unchanged.[341]
[e]A herbal toothpaste, which has been found to reduce the risk of gingivitis, gingival bleeding, plaque and stains.[96]
After Mandel (1998).[206]

less effective at cleaning, however.[28] Other determinants are the crystal structure, friability and surface properties of the tooth, toothpaste cleavage of the particles during brushing, and solubility of the abrasive. Presence of plaque worsens the deleterious effect.[24] Wülknitz found a moderate correlation ($r = 0.66$) between the cleaning power of 41 European toothpastes and dentine abrasion.[402]

Flour of pumice and the softer powdered chalk, which were added in the past to toothpastes, inactivate fluoride in dentifrices. The highly abrasive pumice is in any case not required; the cleaning power of less abrasive agents is sufficient.[101] Brushing 1–2 minutes twice a day with, for instance, a calcium carbonate abrasive should result in stains being left in less than 10% of each tooth surface in the majority of the patients.[73]

Newer abrasive substances include calcium pyrophosphate, insoluble sodium metaphosphate (IMP), polymethylmethacrylate and polyvinylchloride, and silica and aluminium oxides. Pyrophosphates inhibit the transformation of plaque into calculus, but are rapidly broken down by salivary enzymes. Combined with fluoride, high concentrations of pyrophosphates (and polyphosphate salts) reduce calculus build-up. Other anti-calculus products include zinc citrate with triclosan.[206] The so-called "whitening toothpastes" possess abrasive properties

similar to the conventional silica-based dentifrices.[265] IMP has low while silicon dioxide has higher abrasiveness.[86] Hydrated silica (= H_2SiO_3, silicic acid with water in form of granules) is incorporated in many dentifrices: its abrasiveness depends on the particle size and morphology. Wülknitz found that hydrated silica toothpaste was the best among toothpastes with a single abrasive agent, regardless of the kind.[402]

In Europe, aluminium oxide, IMP, and calcium carbonate and phosphate are often included in tooth pastes.[24] Other abrasives, either in or not in combination, which are incorporated less often include: aluminium trihydrate, (precipitated) calcium carbonate, sodium (bi)carbonate, dicalcium phosphate dihydrate, calcium pyrophosphate. Others such as polishing alumina are rarely included.

Acidic toothpastes promote wear. Svinnseth *et al.* found that the pH of 23 toothpastes ranged from 3.7 to 10.1.[358] Regular brushing with a gel (pH = 5.2) did not increase the risk of development of cervical lesions.[315] The dentine abrasiveness of a number of toothpastes ranges from 20 to 202,[66] as determined *in vitro* in comparison with a standard paste with calcium pyrophosphate (abrasiveness = 100) in a brushing machine.[66 236] However, clinically, subject (patients) and specimen variations exist both within and between toothpastes.[3] Some pastes are relatively very abrasive.[236 358]

Several *in vitro* methods are used to measure the abrasiveness of toothpastes: scanning electron microscopy, light (laser)-reflection, profilometry before and after brushing, radioactivity measurement of the paste slurry after brushing dentine irradiated prior to brushing, and weighing tooth tissue before and after brushing.[3 13 24 51 66 75 77 92 124 129 182 187 248 249 256 266 292 293 312] Barbakow *et al.* found that two measurement methods rank ordered the same pastes very differently; therefore and owing to flaws in both methods,[25] it was not possible to say which paste was the least abrasive.

A toothpaste for smokers contained an abrasive form of silica,[206] and another toothpaste for smokers caused more abrasion of dentine and enamel than a regular toothpaste, but *in vivo*, individual factors (plaque, dilution with saliva) will modify the abrasive action.[249] An investigation of 41 European toothpastes, of which 11 were intended for smokers, showed the abrasiveness of eight pastes exceeded that of the standard paste, but all were within the acceptable range (= 2.5 × reference value) as per the DIN (Deutsche Institut für Normung)/International Standards Organization (ISO) standard[402] revised in 1995.[141] More recently, in a Dutch study of 35 toothpastes one appeared too abrasive for enamel and three others were too abrasive for use on dentine.[78]

When a number of abrasives themselves were rank ordered according to their abrading properties, the abrasiveness of calcium pyrophosphate and insoluble sodium metaphosphate was found to be relatively mild.[239] Sodium bicarbonate (baking soda, Moh hardness 2.5) is harder than dentine (Moh 2–2.5).[187] One study found that greater amounts of silica led to greater abrasion of dentine compared with similar amounts of baking soda of similar particle size.[53]

Baking soda possesses relatively low intrinsic hardness and high solubility. In higher concentrations, it is bactericidal towards most bacteria implicated in periodontitis, but has no anti-caries activity *per se.*[240]

Tooth powders are highly abrasive. Kitchin *et al.* reported that over a period of 8 years, brushing with Dr Lyon's tooth powder will abrade about 3.5 mm of the 7 mm bucco-lingual width of the canine. Tooth brushing with water would have the same effect in 6686 years.[166] In another study, a tooth powder intended for smokers appeared highly abrasive.[358]

Tooth brushing frequency and duration

Brushing twice a day is associated with greater tooth wear lesions than brushing once a day or less.[33 310] What counts, in fact, is the number of brushing movements.[59 77]

Brushing twice a day for 3 minutes results in 10 000 strokes/tooth/year.[166] Many people do not brush that long.[85] In an *in vitro* study, smooth, polished enamel appeared to wear 0.2 μm/day with the use of 500 strokes.[337]

The site in the dental arch where one starts to brush is of importance because: (1) the paste at this site is minimally diluted by the saliva and usually abrades maximally; (2) the toothbrush filaments are stiffer to start with than later; and (3) the brushing force might also be higher

initially.[41 208 282] Dilution rapidly lowers the abrasive concentration in the toothpaste slurry to a fifth, which further lowers to a tenth as brushing proceeds.[85] However, some toothpastes become more abrasive after dilution, because ingredients such as glycerine in the undiluted paste decrease the abrasiveness more than saliva.[358] Volpe *et al.* found that over a period of 4.5 years there was no difference in cervical tooth wear in relation to use of a strongly and a less abrasive toothpaste.[384]

A higher likelihood of wear related to tooth brushing has been found in people living in urban areas compared with those living in rural areas,[215] because the authors speculated that those in urban areas may be brushing their teeth more frequently.

Brushing technique

Along with the toothpaste used, the type of movement of the toothbrush – horizontal ("scrubbing"), vertical or rotary – also affects the degree of abrasion.[282 310] Rotary and alternating horizontal and vertical brushing are more likely to cause cervical lesions.[215] Some researchers suggest the roll brushing technique is worse than horizontal,[259] but others have noted the opposite[88] because of the longer-lasting contact with the teeth.[40] The scrubbing action is abrasive on the root, but not on the enamel.[257] Bergström *et al.* found that tooth brushing frequency had greater influence than bristle stiffness and the dentifrice abrasiveness.[33] Stain removal is in general more effective with rotary than horizontal brushing movements.[88]

Brushing power

The sex-dependent[41 266] brushing power co-determines the degree of wear.[383] "Hard" brushing increases the likelihood of cervical lesions.[18] The brushing power contributed most to cervical tooth wear when a more abrasive toothpaste is used than when a less abrasive one is used.[313] Right-handed people brush the left side of their dentition better than the right, yet tooth wear lesions have sometimes been noted to develop more frequently, and of somewhat greater depth, on the left side.[1 2 196 252 310 329] No left-right difference was noted in a sample of left-handed individuals;[215] plaque scores also showed the same pattern.[1 2] Scrubbing and circular brushing in combination with brushing power contributes to cervical wear.[383]

Compared with the penholder grip, brushing with the toothpaste held in a palm grip causes more gingival damage,[244] and probably also more root abrasion.

Toothbrush

The role of the toothbrush in causing tooth wear is controversial. The (nylon filament) toothbrush itself damages the hard dental tissues minimally.[41 141 257 282 309] In an older study, the toothbrush was concluded to be the major factor in dentine abrasiveness.[313] In another study, a medium-hard toothbrush was 1.4 times more abrasive than a soft one, almost independent of the abrasiveness of the toothpaste.[77] An *in vivo* study found that without a use of toothpaste, hard toothbrushes increased the surface roughness of dentine more than medium-hard brushes, although the latter were still more abrasive than soft brushes.[237] Natural and synthetic bristles are not very dissimilar in abrasiveness, but their stiffness is a factor.[207] Since tooth brushing in practice is rarely performed without a toothpaste, few epidemiological data are available on the effect of the toothbrush alone. Remarkably, Dyer *et al.* found that with a toothpaste, toothbrushes with stiff filaments caused the least and those with soft filaments the most abrasion. The authors suggested this was due to: (1) the increased retention of toothpaste in the soft brushes because of the smaller diameter of the filaments and denser tufts, and (2) the greater flexion of the soft filaments, which increased the area of contact between the filaments and the tooth surface. However, over a lifetime, the differences in abrasion caused by filaments of different stiffness were considered to be insignificant.[87]

Powered toothbrushes with rotary-oscillation movements reduce the risk of plaque formation moderately more than manual brushes.[126] Electric brushes are less damaging to the gingiva than manual brushes because of they enforce correct movements and a lower brushing force; the toothbrush stops moving when an increased force is exerted.[119 125 243 315 371 375] The accuracy of this claim has been debated.[81 138 371]

In Africa, use of the miswak "chewing stick" leads to significant tooth wear.[163] The miswak is widely used, more so by men than women, in particular among the less educated groups. Miswak use reduces the risk of development of plaque and gingivitis and inhibits growth of *Actinomyces actinomycetemcomitans*, which is related to periodontal disease. The miswak is as effective as the toothbrush.[8]

Restorations

Momoi *et al.* found that two relatively soft light-cured resin-modified glass ionomer cements were less resistant to abrasion than glass ionomer cements. A hybrid composite and a spherical high-copper amalgam had superior qualities.[230]

In a study comparing the rate of wear of three veneering materials, two materials seemed to have acceptable rates. The ceramic and composite restorations had a rate of wear of roughly 12–14 μm/year in height and 10–12 μm³/year in volume. The respective values for the negative control poly(methylmethacrylate) were 50 μm/year and 45 μm³/year.[11]

8.7.3   Prevention and treatment

Patients with cervical lesions should use low-abrasive toothpastes and brush well but not excessively. Restora-

tive treatment is indicated when the cervical lesion is about 1 mm deep, or sooner if a lesion is compromising the fit of the clasp of a partial denture.[122] Composite restorations are associated with the risk of marginal leakage between the restoration and root dentine.[323] Although the adhesiveness of composites has improved, the risk of microleakage remains. Alternatives include compomers, glass ionomer cements and resin-modified glass ionomer cements.[197 370]

8.8   Other causes of tooth wear

8.8.1   Prophylactic pastes

Prophylactic pastes may be 20-fold more abrasive than toothpastes.[74] Professional cleaning prior to local fluoride application seems superfluous.[364] Stains may be polished selectively, if possible with a toothpaste.

The abrasiveness of prophylactic pastes also differs widely. Particle size and abrasiveness are not well related. Dentine abrades more than enamel, which influences the choice of the prophylactic paste used (Table 8.3).[213] Magnesium and aluminium silicates are not very abrasive and polish rather well.[280]

Smooth enamel abrades less than rough enamel.[187 353] Biller *et al.* found that polishing (30 seconds) with rubber cups at 2000 rpm and an abrasive prophylactic paste resulted in a cervical groove of 2–4 μm and more incisally, a groove 1 μm deep, which were related to pressure from the rim of the rubber cup.[38] Use of most prophylactic pastes roughens the surface of enamel, dentine and restorations, which necessitates polishing. However, Perlite

Table 8.3 Particle size and abrasiveness of prophylactic polishing powders[a] with regard to enamel and dentine

Powder	Particle size (μm)	Abrasiveness (rank order)[b] Enamel	Dentine
Flour of pumice, medium	38	2.68 (2)	56.6 (1)
Silicon carbide	14.3	5.56 (1)	26.3 (5)
Aluminium oxide	13.8	1.86 (5)	24.8 (6)
Flour of pumice, fine	12.8	1.00 (7)	30.6 (2)
Feldspar	12.2	1.50 (5)	28.8 (4)
Silex extra fine	7.2	2.58 (3)	30.3 (3)
Zirconium silicate	7.1	2.45 (4)	22.6 (7)
Cerium oxide	4.4	0.78 (8)	14.4 (8)

[a]In paste form, which is less abrasive than dry powder.
[b]The rank order indicates the comparative degree of abrasiveness.[213] The lower the rank order number, the more abrasive is the powder.

particles (volcanic glass) become blunt and disintegrate under load and become a (super)fine non-abrasive polishing paste.[198 199] Perlite has been recently incorporated in a "whitening" toothpaste (Chapter 10).

The presence of orthodontic brackets obstructs professional and self maintenance of oral hygiene. Professional removal of plaque is facilitated by use of air-powder abrasive devices. In one study, one apparatus abraded about 7 μm of enamel per minute and left a smooth surface and another abraded 100 μm of enamel per minute, which was why the author advised against its routine application. All the devices caused too much abrasion of dentine.[153]

8.8.2 Oral and occupational habits

Oral habits

People working in open air environments, such as those working on farms and in the fishing industry, may chew tobacco. Frequent and long-term chewing on the small and irregular silica and calcium particles in the tobacco abrades the teeth, eventually to the level of the gingiva.[43] The teeth are also stained brown. There is usually no pain due to tertiary dentine formation.

From India to Indonesia, millions of people chew betel preparations (e.g. the Indian *paan*),[404] which usually consist of an areca nut wrapped in a tobacco or sirih leaf, along with lime (erosive) and/or other ingredients.[270 294] The oral mucosa discolours red-brown (mahogany) and the teeth become red-brown to black. In Central Europe and Russia cracking open of sunflower seeds with the incisors cause triangular defects in the incisal edges.[145 277] In Jordan, the same habit involves roasted watermelon and pumpkin seeds.[93]

Pipe smoking, nail-biting[150] (40–50% of children and adolescents),[246 251] excessive use of toothpicks,[62 166] and other oral habits occasionally lead to specific loss of hard dental tissues. Biting on a pipe causes defects closely reflecting the form and diameter of the stem of the pipe. Elongated bucco-lingual, oval and unilateral tapered grooves located near the cervix in premolars and molars have been noted in the remains of ancient peoples found in particular geographical, that is temporal, regions, (the early hominins: *Homo habilis*, *Homo erectus*, *Homo heidelbergensis* and *Homo sapiens*). The shape of these interproximal grooves is consistent with the shape and positioning of toothpicks.[366]

Hlusko *et al.* experimentally created approximal half-oval grooves in premolar roots with grass-stalk "toothpicks", which are rigid, fairly inflexible and highly abrasive (silica). Use of toothpicks is a persistent human habit and toothpicks represent one of the oldest human tools.[136]

Occupational habits

Hair stylists who hold or open hairpins with their teeth, seamstresses who bite off thread with their teeth and carpenters who hold nails between their teeth often show notches/grooves in these teeth. Sandblasters, miners[95] and metalworkers frequently have excessive tooth wear owing to exposure to air-borne abrasive particles, unless precautions are taken. A dental technician, who moistened the brush used to apply porcelain powder on crowns with his lips, had severely worn anterior teeth.[30] Professional wind musicians who need to hold the reed of the wind instrument between their incisors develop tooth abrasion. Moreover, these instruments exert a lever action that may affect the longevity of the tooth being used as a support in cases with periodontal disease.

Tooth wear has also been noted in remains of ancient craftspeople who stripped animal hides with their teeth for producing ropes and other binding materials. The fibrous material was intensively chewed and repeatedly pressed or pulled across the teeth.[319 366]

9

Tooth Fractures and Traumatic Dentoalveolar Injuries

9.1 Introduction

Dental trauma is a mechanically caused tooth and/or periodontal injury.

9.2 Abuse

Physical abuse may cause oral injury.

9.2.1 Battered child syndrome[289] (non-accidental injury)[24]

Every year, 0.35–0.8% children in the USA are physically abused or neglected.[358 361] The frequency of abuse varies between countries, cultures and over the time.[8 24] At the minimum, half of those abused suffer head and facial injuries, yet two-thirds of American paediatric and even more Dutch dentists claim to have never observed abuse.[222 358 405] They profess a lack of knowledge and fear making false accusations.[405]

Scepticism is required when clinical findings in a child with facial or oral injuries are incompatible with explanations given by parents.[232] One should have a high index of suspicion in children presenting with wounds in different healing stages, several healed root fractures, a lacerated upper lip, torn maxillary frenum, oral mucosal lacerations and discoloured teeth.[159 289 360] During bouts of anger, force is often directed towards the mouth of the child in an effort to silence him or her. Unscrupulous abusers try to avoid leaving marks. Most victims are younger than 4 years, and are often babies.[397] Round burns (cigarettes), burns around the wrists (binding ropes), facial bite wounds, and pulled out hair (forcing down during sexual assaults) are obvious signs of child abuse. Skull fractures and intracranial injuries will be seen in those presenting to hospitals.[216 358]

Dentists should be suspicious in cases of children who are unable to establish communication, including eye contact, occasionally present with enticing behaviour towards the dentist,[405] and children who appear vigilant, or are in a state of frozen watchfulness or show distant or shy interaction with the parents. Long sleeves and high-necked clothes on hot days in the summer may be a cover-up for injuries.[232] Abused children may be unwanted (stepchildren) or born after an extra-marital relationship, they may have disabilities, or were born prematurely and were kept in an incubator for some time, which interferes with establishing a bond. When the child with visible injuries attends the dental office, one could consider the list of features in Table 9.1.

The dentist should consider the following questions: Were there witnesses? Have they come with the child? Have adequate steps been undertaken by the parents/caregivers? Is the perpetrator present? Most perpetrators are 20–30 years of age, emotional, impulsive and immature, and self-oriented with a tendency towards poorly controlled aggressive behaviour. Abusive parents often have a history of being abused in childhood themselves. Poverty, alcohol, drugs and matrimonial problems may play a role.[216]

9.2.2 Partner and parental abuse

Mistreatment of (fe)male partners happens frequently but is often concealed.[270] Abuse of parents by adult and teenage children is beginning to draw attention.

Fighting
Alcohol and drug intoxication is linked to assaults in which the maxillofacial region is often the target. In Britain, one-quarter of injuries are due to violence.[420]

Torture
Orofacial blows, teeth fractured with the use of forceps, oral (and facial) electrical torture cause all kinds of facial/oral injuries.[24]

Table 9.1 Features of oral injuries in child abuse[8]

Injury	
Type	Bruises, stab wounds, burns, cuts?
Site	Is the injury at a "usual" location?
Characteristics	Colour, form/shape. A common injury?
Time	Does the appearance of the injury correspond with the reported time of injury?
Cause	Does the parents' explanation correspond with the type, site and appearance of the injury?
Previous injuries	Signs of healed wounds and fractures?

Brutal removal of teeth was used as torture in the days of the Roman Empire (St Apollonia, Alexandria, AD249) and was a common medieval practice to punish, for example, heretics.[238]

The biblical saying "an eye for an eye and a tooth for a tooth" was already practised in Babylon. The Codex Hammurabi (1750BC) decreed that physicians must treat their patients with care: he who knocked out a tooth of person of equal rank must lose a tooth.

9.2.3 Dealing with cases of suspected abuse

Speak separately with the child and parent. Ask specific questions regarding the injury, but avoid angering the parent. Documented findings must be reported to appropriate agencies.

9.2.4 Brain damage

Referral for a medical consultation has priority when there is evidence of blood or other fluid leakage from the nose or ears (brain damage). The patient may show:

- Problems with walking. Can he or she turn the head in both directions without paraesthesia (cranial nerve damage)?[351]
- Lethargy, confusion. Decreased consciousness may point to increased intracranial pressure (hypertension, low pulse)[361]
- Abnormal eye position/movements, double vision, asymmetrical pupil sizes, delayed pupil reaction to a bright light. Can the patient follows a moving finger with the eyes? Can they read?
- Low blood pressure, increased pulse (shock)[52]
- Nausea/vomiting, inability to swallow
- Breathing problems
- Facial paralysis (touch with cotton wool)
- Hoarse, unclear speech/diction.[234 289]

Facial bone discontinuities, mobility and pain on application of rotational pressure on the temporomandibular joint and haematomas around the eyes are indicative of fractures.

9.3 Spontaneous cracks and fractures of the teeth

9.3.1 Spontaneous cracks (infractions, craze lines)

A *spontaneous crack* is an incomplete fracture that occurs under application of routine masticatory forces or due to parafunctions. The fractured tooth segments are not separated and the depth and direction of the infraction is not clearly known. Posterior teeth in particular, either healthy (one-third or even two-thirds) or not (carious, worn or restored) are prone to cracks when subjected to the lateral component of masticatory forces.[53 76 195 379 436] The often encountered mesiodistal infraction propagates deeper with time.[72 118] The crack is centrally located or peripherally directed and may lead to complete (cuspal) fracture of the tooth.[75]

Epidemiology
Persons over the age of 30 are predominantly affected,[75 112 119 157 195 379 400] and there are no differences between the sexes.[411] Mandibular molars in particular are prone to crack near the lingual cusps,[1 43 50 75 76 112 157 195 400 413] because the mesio-palatal cusps of the maxillary molars act like a wedge, pushing the mandibular molar cusps apart.[107 195] The oblique ridge protects the maxillary molars against cracks,[195] but a few studies have found that these teeth experience cracks more frequently than their antagonists.[322 436]

A prevalence of 80–100 cases/year in general practice is reported.[117] Per tooth the rate varies from 1% to 32%, with cracks extending into dentine.[285 323 414] After caries and periodontal disease, spontaneous cracks may be considered the third most frequent cause of tooth loss in older persons,[63 157] but this has been noted to be a "subjective impression" due to lack of sufficient evidence.[257]

Aetiology
Causes and contributing factors are: unexpectedly biting on hard objects (pips, stones), tooth wear, excessive erosion, caries, cavity preparation and endodontic treatment, and bruxism.[2 75 119] Changes in the oral temperature can lead to cracking of the enamel of the incisors[24] due to differences in the expansion coefficients of enamel and dentine.[66 104 366]

Little dentine remaining after cavity preparation increases the probability of a crack. Sharp internal line angles in a preparation promote stress concentration related to masticatory forces, which initiates and propagates cracks. Other iatrogenic causes are: non-passively fitting cast restorations that have been forced into place and excessive hydraulic forces during luting; placement of parapulpal pins close to the enamel; restorations with steep occlusal slopes that result in an increase in the horizontal component of masticatory forces; use of high condensation pressures when carrying out an amalgam restoration; and moisture contamination during condensation of a poor-quality amalgam.[261 350]

Amalgam restorations minimally restore the stiffness of a tooth. Excursive interferences make teeth twice as vulnerable to cracks, and when restored with amalgam, the odds ratio increases to 6.[330] Teeth with three-surface amalgam restorations crack more frequently than teeth with two-surface fillings.[322 413] Studies have found that over 90% of fractured posterior teeth are filled with amalgam, often a Class II or a broad Class I restoration;[114] [281] the lingual wall tends to fracture.[39] As the cavity floor is deepened and as the cusp width is reduced, cuspal deflection under loading increases considerably. The cracks are more superficial in teeth with large restorations. In healthy teeth, the crack will be deeper and closer to the pulp.[199]

Dentinal collagen, which is present specially around the pulp, makes the tooth more resilient.[231] Endodontic preparation reduces the tooth's internal coherence and increases the probability of spontaneous cracks developing in posterior teeth, even more so when the final restoration is amalgam.[158 175 413] With use of bonded amalgam, 40–60% of the tooth stiffness is recovered.[323] Dias De Souza reported that cements lack this property,[108] but teeth with amalgam restorations bonded with cement did not fracture.[265] Non-vital teeth lack the feedback mechanism that protects against extreme loading: the masticatory force may surpass the resistance of the tooth.[306 329]

Endodontic treatment leads to loss of some free water[188] making the tooth more brittle,[306] but this is disputed, as is the claimed loss of collagen cross-linking in the dentine of non-vital teeth.[202 316 317 365]

Bonded composite restorations are associated with reduced cuspal flexing. Caron *et al.* found that teeth with a three-surface composite restoration fractured under a lower occlusal loading and more severely than teeth with two boxed restorations separated by enamel.[78] Bonded three-surface composite restorations in premolars help recover the stiffness of the teeth more than bonded amalgam[435] and improve their fracture strength.[369] However, the polymerisation contraction-shrinkage of the resin deforms the cusps [275 320] and may cause enamel infractions (Figure 9.1) that extend into the thin dentine.[403] The volumetric shrinkage starts during the light-curing stage and a loss of 2–3% of the volume occurs by day 1.[126] A bonded two-surface composite restoration bends the buccal and lingual cusps by 16 μm and a three-surface restoration by 23 μm, but the cuspal tips bend by 38 (± 44) μm.[320] Comparable values have been reported by others.[403] Use of a lower intensity light and a two-step curing method with first a low and then high light exposure has been found to reduce contraction stress[103 127] without affecting the total volumetric shrinkage.[252]

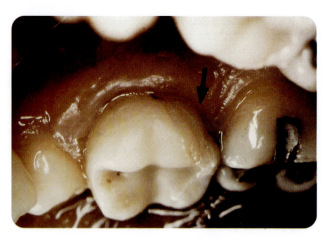

Figure 9.1 Cracks in the enamel caused by the setting contraction/shrinkage of the bonded composite restoration.

Vertical crown-root infraction

The probability that cracks extend beyond the epithelial attachment increases the more distally the tooth is situated. Crack progression into the root may split the tooth[158 175] (the risk is increased in dentinogenesis imperfecta owing to the low dentine microhardness).[24]

The shape, size and material of canal posts co-determine success or failure.[363] Tapering canal posts, large diameters and use of a large torsion force while inserting threaded posts increase the risk of longitudinal infractions and fractures. Tapered posts cause radicular cracks in the coronal third of the root while parallel posts cause cracks in the apical third,[105 324] although use of the latter may be less risky.[106] Cast metallic posts are associated with more unfavourable outcomes than glass fibre posts with diameters smaller than the root canal.[437] A post must fit passively and be seated with a low-viscosity cement, without rotation, to minimise the hydraulic pressure force.[350] Cracks post insertion may not clinically manifest for 1–2 years.[105 387] Corrosion expansion of (silver) posts causes longitudinal cracks/fractures.[4 34 96 173 253 387]

Pilo *et al.* found that premolars with different types of post showed mainly oblique radicular fractures.[324] In another study, the incisors performed equally well with different post-core systems;[192] more than 80% survived for 6 years.[193] Fibre-reinforced composite posts fail under relatively low loadings, but root fractures are less likely.[290]

Diagnosis and appearance

Diagnosing a crack (Figure 9.2) may be difficult. Cracked vital teeth are rarely (about 15%) painful,[284 413] but even then often remain undetected or are misdiagnosed as, for example, sinusitis or ear pain.[72 75 168 412] A crack in the enamel cannot cause pain, but deeper cracks open

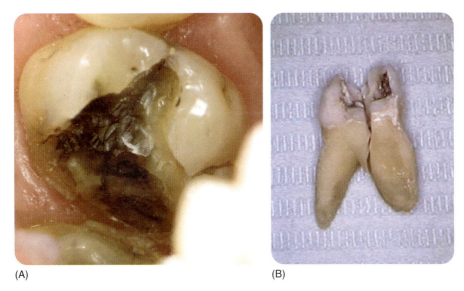

(A)   (B)

Figure 9.2 (A) Following removal of a large restoration, a dark-coloured vertical fracture line is visible (which is sometimes difficult to see, like in this figure), running from top of the figure to the bottom. (Courtesy of M. van der Zwet.) (B) After an endodontic access opening was made in the crown because of pulpitis, a crack was observed in the bottom of the pulp chamber. After extraction and cleaning, the tooth appeared to be totally split.

minutely under pressure and when they close after cessation of the pressure, the consequent movements of the fluid in the dentinal tubules can cause pain.[76][117] Pain elicited by chewing, cold (rarely hot) stimuli, sweet and acidic stimuli (micro-leakage) may represent a dentinal crack (*greenstick fracture*).[75][375] Dentine caries may develop underneath sound enamel when plaque accumulates in deep cracks.[407] Cracks extending to the pulp lead to pulpitis. Bacteria colonise subgingivally, and penetrate the cracks giving rise to small, deep periodontal defects that appear on radiographs as diffuse radiolucencies.[2][105][412]

A sharp short pain when biting on a cotton roll is indicative of a crack.[76][117] In spite of the presence of an avoidance pattern during chewing because of the sudden, sharp, lacerating pain, the patient may be unable to identify the involved tooth.[261][284][396] Percussion in the axial direction is often inconclusive. Application of lateral pressure on the pertinent cusp may be painful, but pressure applied in another direction will not cause any problem;[50] even gentle occlusal rubbing may elicit pain. The pain may become continuous,[366] but then disappear when a part of the tooth breaks away.[412]

Tooth by tooth information may be gained with the use of occlusal biting devices (Tooth Slooth or Fracfinder) or with the application of some polymerised composite on a suspected cusp.[274] Cracks are often difficult to observe, including on radiographs,[2] unless they run parallel to the X-rays.[50] The outline of a crack usually coincides with a groove or fissure. The adjoining teeth impede approximal

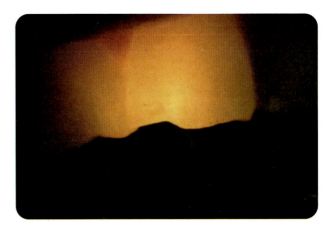

Figure 9.3 Cracks (the dark line in the right central incisor) may be difficult to see, even with transillumination.

examination.[400] Disclosing solution is not rinsed away from a crack,[218] in particular when the crack reaches into the dentine,[413] but it does not mark new cracks.[117] Transillumination (Figure 9.3; or with the Penlight), meticulous drying and directing light perpendicular to the long axis of the tooth, and use of methylene blue dye, may be helpful.[218][256][322][330] Older cracks resemble discoloured grooves, especially in the marginal ridges.[330]

Application of fluorescent oil 8 minutes after polishing shows a yellow-green line at the place of the crack with application of ultraviolet light under a surgical microscope.[260]

Prevention and treatment

Cavity preparations must be kept small and shallow, and internal line angles should not be sharp. Steep occlusal cuspal slopes must be avoided during carving of the restoration. When a crack is present, grinding of the cusps is an acceptable provisional measure;[3] despite this, however, the food bolus may load the tooth unfavourably.[157] A temporary solution to avoid crack propagation, fracture and pulpitis[256] is fitting a stainless steel band, which also helps alleviate the pain.[117]

Endodontic access preparations increase cuspal flexure,[316] which may require partial coverage crowns rather than composite restorations.[85] Older data on protection offered by composites were contradictory,[112 156 263 283 385 410] but contemporary composite systems (and bonded amalgam) seem satisfactory.[40 65 174 175 176 323 382] However, bonded amalgam restores the stiffness of the tooth to a lesser degree,[323] may debond with time,[41] and cyclic loading reduces the shear bond strength progressively.[269] All this, together with thermal cycling, nullifies the bonding advantage.[59]

The adhesive restorative approach in non-vital premolars is promising,[236] but the resistance against fractures is reduced within 3 years.[175] *In vitro* studies show that the adhesion of composite systems to dentine decreases with time[113 132 181 182 183 184] through hydrolysis and enzymatic degradation.[51 52] The longer the observation period, the higher is the noted prevalence rate of fractures.[67] The enamel bond may seal and protect the hybrid resin-dentine layer,[102] but dentinal fluid flow and diffusion of fluid compromise the bond.

Unstable polymeric hydrogels within hybrid layers leach out, and total etching alters the collagen fibrils.[183 184] Partly demineralised collagen became almost completely destroyed by proteolytic enzymes.[318] Storage in saline increased nanoleakage with hydrolysis of the bond.[250]

Long etching times,[319] and excessive drying and wetting, increase micro- and nanoleakage.[131] Water degrades the bond[38] and lowers the bond strength[169] of two-step, but not of three-step, dentine adhesives.[102]

Thermocycling reduced the shear bond strength by 38–50%, depending on the pretreatment of dentine (acid-etching, self-etching, or neodymium:yttrium aluminum garnet (Nd:YAG) laser).[203] The microtensile bond strength achieved with the use of a self-etching primer declined after 1 year from 39 MPa to 14 MPa and that of a wet bonding system reduced from 48 to 12 MPa.[235]

Treatment of an enamel crack in a healthy tooth might be delayed,[257 412] but an associated amalgam restoration must be substituted with a bonded composite, a composite onlay or a cast restoration when the crack extends into the dentine.[2 86 204] The prognosis may be unfavourable,[86 375] but in one study only about 10% of the teeth restored with bonded composite were lost[2] and in another study using bonded composite onlays, 7% were lost in 6 years.[438] In cases of pulpitis, prevention of crack propagation should be prioritised over endodontic treatment.[86]

In the past, attempts were made to melt and fuse the cracked enamel segments with laser treatment.[287] Not much is known, however, about the quality of the solidified enamel.[407]

A crack that is visible in the pulp chamber during endodontic treatment makes extraction unavoidable,[158] particularly when a pocket is present. Attempts have been made to save such teeth with crowns,[392] but bacteria still have access to the periodontium via the cracks in the enamel.

9.3.2 Spontaneous tooth fractures

A *spontaneous fracture* is the separation and loss of a tooth segment due to loading with masticatory forces or parafunctions. Tooth fractures (Figure 9.4) have the same

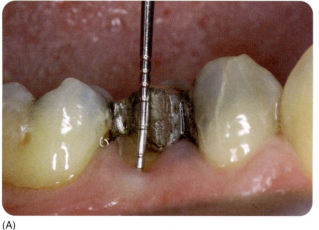
(A)

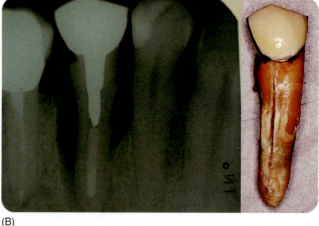
(B)

Figure 9.4 (A) Spontaneous cusp fracture; the explorer shows the depth at which the fracture line is located. (Courtesy of M. van der Zwet.) (B) Typical radiographic appearance of a vertical fracture (left panel) and the tooth after extraction (right panel). The spontaneous fracture of the root 35 years after treatment was caused by corrosion of the canal post.

causes as cracks, or a crack may propagate and become a fracture. Such fractures sometimes manifest when chewing soft food, because the fractured part of the tooth becomes incorporated in the food bolus. A cusp or a whole wall of the restoration may be lost after removal of a filling.[117] A *horizontal* fracture is often restorable.[86] A *vertical* fracture poses a serious problem and may require extraction.

Fractures may occur in healthy teeth,[247 279] but are more common in decayed or filled teeth, especially after endodontic treatment, in mainly patients younger than 50 years.[128 241] Bader *et al.* reported that of 39 potential risk factors, only the presence of a crack and the amount of dentine supporting the cusps were predictive of posterior tooth fracture. Parafunctions, biting on hard objects and factors such as endodontic treatment, steep cusps and sharp internal cavity line angles were poor predictors.[44]

Particularly affected are the posterior teeth, except the mandibular premolars.[45 82 128 241] The cusps of intact maxillary premolars deflect up to 11 μm under stress; with small two-surface cavities they deflect up to 20 μm, and with extended three-surface cavities the deflection reaches 32 μm.[200] The deflection may exceed the resilience of the tooth. The larger a cavity, the more likely it is that the tooth will fracture. A narrow isthmus offers better fracture resistance.[114 281] The rate of fracture of functional and non-functional cusps may not be different,[241] but centric stops are less prone to fracture than other cusps, especially those in the mandibular molars.[82 114] A left/right difference has been noted.[258]

One per cent of amalgam fillings are replaced due to tooth fracture.[7] The estimated fracture rate in Bader *et al.*'s study was 4.4/100 adults for posterior teeth and 5/100 for all teeth,[42] but proportionally more fractures occur. Other authors have proposed an annual rate of some 20 fractured teeth/1000 patients,[128] but a rate of 70/1000 has also been reported.[43] In the mandible, twice as many lingual than buccal cusps fracture. The opposite has been found for maxillary premolars.[44 45 391]

In 3–4% of fractures the pulps are exposed and 25% extend subgingivally.[44 45] Bader *et al.* reported that some 3% of fractured teeth had to be extracted.[45] The majority of fractures of endodontically treated premolars are located at the base of the cusps.[391] If these teeth are crowned, apical transmission of the masticatory forces increases the risk of root fracture.[355] Hansen *et al.* found that only a small proportion of endodontically treated posterior teeth restored with a two-surface amalgam fractured within 3 years versus almost 30% with three-surface amalgam restorations, half of which were extracted within 10 years. Fractures of the lingual cusp caused the most periodontal damage and these are more common in the molars.[176]

In studies, the presence of an unfilled three-surface cavity halved the fracture resistance of maxillary premolars. Amalgam and composite bonded with one-step and two-step adhesives reinforced the teeth equally; without the adhesive, both materials protected minimally.[87 207 391 419 439] The fracture resistance of maxillary premolars restored with bonded composite (inlays) has been found to differ from that of intact premolars; a bonded amalgam performed less well.[99 160 440] A ceromer functioned the best.[99]

Research shows that creep and expansion of amalgam and weakening of the coronal root due to use of Gates Glidden drills in endodontically treated teeth increases the risk of fracture;[178] even a composite bonded only to the enamel has a higher survival rate.[177] A cast-metal onlay was superior to resin composite onlays or fibre-reinforced composite and ceramics,[68] but the failure mode of the former was commonly unfavourable.[425]

In one study, restorations including the palatal cusp of maxillary premolars with a bonded composite, bonded amalgam or reinforced glass ionomer cement were subjected to axial loading. The teeth with reinforced glass ionomer cement exhibited lower resistance against fracture, but more tooth tissue was retained. Use of dentine pins did not improve the protection.[327]

9.3.3 Cervical abfraction (physical stress-induced or non-carious cervical lesion)

Cervical abfraction lesions are small V-shaped defects with sharp margins that are found mainly on the buccal enamel surface of the permanent teeth, and which may primarily be caused by occlusal forces.

The horizontal component of masticatory forces bends the crown (200–400 μm)[385] on the firmly fixed root. Repeated flexures generate alternating cervical tension and compression. The tensile stresses may disrupt the chemical bonds between the hydroxyapatite crystals. Ions and small molecules penetrate the microcracks and prevent re-establishment of the bonds. The flexures cause fatigue, tearing and abrasion of the cervical enamel,[164 166 243 244 276 313] and even more so because the interdigitation between the cervical enamel and dentine is relatively weak.[161 307] In experimental studies, the maximum principal stresses exceeded the failure stresses for enamel.[337] The more elastic dentine better withstands bending.[243]

The initial phase of development of abfraction lesions may comprise loss of cervical dentine, undermining the enamel. In a finite element study (which involves using a computer modelling technique), an artificially created discontinuity between the cervical enamel and root dentine increased the principal stress upon occlusal loading dramatically in excess of the failure stress rate for the cervical enamel.[339]

The lesions are characteristically wedge-shaped and located at sites of tensile stress concentration. Erosion, in contrast, results in more disc-shaped lesions.[243 249 307] Initially, a wave-like or corrugated pattern is seen on the cervical enamel surface.[64] Abfraction occurs predominantly on the buccal surfaces and may occur at an angle toward the mesial or distal,[243] because each point along the occlusal plane generates slightly different forces near the fulcrum.[293] Lesions also develop approximally, encircle the whole crown, resulting in breaking away of the tooth crown.[164] A shift in the fulcrum apically, for instance after occlusal wear or changes in the periodontal attachment, may lead to several stacked lesions.[64 239 243 249]

Some studies support the abfraction theory, but others do not. Studies supporting this theory are those involving (1) models in which a tooth with piezoelectric transducers is mounted and subjected to loadings, (2) photo-elastic models, in which a tooth made of birefringent plastic after loading shows areas of stress concentration under polarised light, and (3) strain gauge and (4) finite element analysis. These techniques have been criticised.[336 441]

A tooth mounted in plaster behaves differently from a tooth with a periodontal ligament.[308] Photo-elastic teeth have a lower elastic modulus than enamel.[336] In computer models, the enamel is considered to be isotropic (all prisms oriented in the same direction), but the enamel is anisotropic. In the anisotropic enamel the load flux is directed especially towards the dentine and in the isotropic model towards the rigid enamel. A more realistic enamel model altered the stress direction and decreased the maximum tensile stresses. The finite model simplifies reality, and thus may result in false conclusions.[100]

The models illustrate, however, the ability of occlusal forces to cause damage.[336] Use of the models indicates that lingual lesions should be present as often as buccal ones, but this is not supported by clinical findings.

During biting, chewing and swallowing, the lower and upper teeth come into contact, but such forces are not usually harmful. Larger forces, which develop during bruxism[194] with large horizontal jaw movements[271] or tooth clenching,[96] or are seen with premature contacts and malocclusion may cause the V-shaped cervical defects.[243 337 390] The magnitude, direction and patterns of strain developed on the cervical enamel depend highly on the loading patterns. Point loadings on the outer and inner inclines of cusps results in asymmetrical cervical strains[315] and concordantly shaped cervical lesions.[155 243] Abfraction does not occur in mobile teeth, due to the absence of a fulcrum. Kuroe et al. found that cuspal loading appeared to concentrate stresses around the cervical region below the loaded cusp, and the stresses were highest under buccal cusp loading,[239] the site where the majority of the abfractions occur. Almost all teeth with abfraction in one study showed coronal wear facets, canine disclusion was common and balancing interferences were present in one-fifth of the teeth.[277] Progression of occlusal and cervical tissue loss were strongly associated.[325]

The lesions develop chiefly in the maxillary and mandibular premolars,[121] but the commonest sites seem to be: (1) labial surfaces of the maxillary incisors, (2) buccal surfaces of the maxillary premolars and (3) the labial surfaces of the maxillary canines. Rees et al. found that peak local and peak principal stresses seemed, indeed, highest in the maxillary incisors, intermediate in the maxillary first premolars and lowest in the maxillary canines.[338] When one of two adjacent premolars is affected, abfraction seems likely. Erosion and tooth brushing may be the principal causes when both premolars show lesions. Acidic attacks accelerate the loss of cervical tissue.[165]

Bending generates a small piezoelectric charge between the dentinal regions, which may be attributed to "stress corrosion", i.e. loss of tooth material.[166] Piezoelectricity may cause enamel demineralisation or the cyclic changes can attract and repel charged erosive agents.

The lesions may be multifactorial[249 307] or multicausal[277 309] and abfraction may not be the primary cause.[255] Currently there is insufficient evidence to be absolutely certain of the cause.[441] Occlusal forces might be major contributors, but are unlikely to be entirely responsible for the defects.[262] The association of cervical abfraction lesions with occlusal forces does not necessarily support a causal relationship.[25 45] Bader et al. found that, from a number of factors investigated, forceful brushing three times/day, starting on the buccal sides, bruxism, drinking fruit juice more than once/day, and a low salivary buffering capacity were separately associated with cervical lesions. Interactions between these factors were almost nil.[46] Subgingival lesions exclude tooth brushing as a cause[64] and wedge-shaped lesions likely develop under the influence of another factor.[309]

Epidemiology

In Dawid et al.'s study, some 50% of pilots had cervical abfraction lesions versus about 10% of other air force personnel. The authors concluded that tooth clenching under stress could have be responsible. The pilots were older than the controls, but age did not seem a decisive factor.[96] However, in another study including mostly bruxists, older persons had more defects than younger people. Most patients were bruxists.[162] In a Nigerian population, one-third of cervical defects were found to be abfraction lesions, associated with occlusal wear facets.[295] Although abfraction should be more frequently present in teeth with occlusal wear than in those with occlusal erosion, this was not found to be the case in another study.[226]

Prevention and treatment

Occlusal adjustment reduces cervical stress. The tensile stresses may lead to debonding and loss of cervical restorations, for which reason microfilled composites that flex with the tooth are preferred to stiffer ones.[194 244] A thick layer of a flexible liner and mechanical retention are recommended. Abrasive/erosive lesions are preferably restored with composites resistant to wear.[244] Dentists should consider erosion in the diagnosis and treatment of non-carious cervical lesions,[226] but abfraction must be kept in mind as a primary cause.

9.4   Traumatic tooth fractures

An external force may fracture the enamel and/or crown dentine or the root. Precise registration and history taking of the injury is essential for evaluation and medicolegal and financial reasons. Information must be gained regarding general health and use of medicaments that may affect the treatment, such as presence of blood coagulation disorders, immune system deficiencies, diabetes mellitus, acute rheumatism, epilepsy, allergies and heart diseases.

Based on the aetiology, pathology, etc., several classifications of tooth fracture have been proposed.[24 142] The classification by Andreasen and Andreasen[24] has been adopted by the World Health Organization and is also followed here. The guidelines presented in this chapter for the management of traumatic dental injuries are in accordance with those of the International Association of Dental Traumatology.[442] Recent guidelines can also be found at www.dentaltrauma.guide.

Pulp survival and healing after crown fractures with and without pulp exposure depend on the developmental stage of the root and damage to the apical blood supply.[345] Traumatic forces transmitted to the periodontium may damage the periodontal tissues. Dental injuries are treated on an emergency basis, but limited evidence suggests that a treatment delay of 24 hours has no serious consequences for crown and root fractures[27] and intrusion.[443] The risk of fracture is greater in adults than in children, who are more likely to experience tooth displacement because of their more resilient alveolar bone and incomplete (thus shorter) tooth roots.[24 36 60 251]

Each case of dental trauma should have radiographs and sensibility tests for obtaining information regarding pulp cavity size, root development, root fractures and other injuries. However, immediately after trauma the pulp may not react due to transient pulp damage. Sensibility may return[88 347] after 6–10 weeks,[332 431] sometimes even after years.[11] At 3 months, some 80% of pulps of traumatised teeth will react.[444] It is worth bearing in mind that non-traumatised immature teeth may not react to sensibility testing.[139]

The pulp can become necrotic after some time.[11 332 352 431] Radiographs and sensibility testing of permanent teeth are repeated after 6 weeks, 6 months, 1 year and, for fractures, 5 years,[442] to check for resorption, periapical granuloma formation, pulp obliteration, absence of secondary dentine formation and cessation of root development. A yellow discolouration of the crown points to pulp obliteration, a grey-blue to black colour signifies a necrotic pulp, and a pink spot signifies internal crown or cervical resorption (Chapter 7). Immature teeth may also temporarily appear pink.[10 11] Most traumatised deciduous teeth are assessed clinically after 1 week, 6–8 weeks and 1 year (clinically and with radiographs at both follow-ups), and

root fractures and intrusive injuries are also assessed at 2–3 weeks and 6 months.[442]

After an injury, the patient should brush with a soft brush and rinse with 0.1% chlorhexidine.[442]

9.4.1   Crown infraction

Traumatic crown infraction is an incomplete fracture (crack) in the enamel and/or dentine caused by an external force, without separation of the segments.[24] Infraction, usually limited to the enamel,[24] occurs in about 10% of teeth affected by trauma,[332] and most commonly in the permanent maxillary anterior teeth. Infractions into dentine, in, for instance, maxillary premolars, are caused by a blow to the chin. The infraction may be difficult to see.

Treatment
The prognosis is usually favourable.[331] An infracted anterior tooth does not need treatment, unless the tooth is heavily loaded functionally, in which case grinding is indicated. The crack may be sealed with an unfilled composite to prevent staining.[24] Pulpitis develops in 0–3.5% of cases.[24 332] A part of the tooth may fracture between dental follow-ups.

Deciduous teeth
Crown infractions of deciduous teeth are rare. A grey discolouration that becomes yellow in 75% of cases[60] is indicative of pulp obliteration, and a grey-blue to black discolouration is due to pulp necrosis.[362] With respect to the sequelae of the injury, it does not matter whether dark discoloured deciduous teeth are endodontically treated or not.[445] Where pain develops, or the permanent succedaneous tooth germ is in danger or there is lack of cooperation, extraction is indicated. Traumatic injuries to the teeth in children younger than 4 years often may only slightly intrude the tooth.[24]

9.4.2   Uncomplicated crown fracture

In a traumatic, uncomplicated crown fracture due to an external force, part of the enamel breaks away and eventually a part of the dentine as well. Generally, an incisal edge, in particular of a permanent central incisor, breaks away (Figure 9.5); occasionally it is held in place by the periodontal fibres. Pain occurs when:

- The dentine is exposed. Temperature changes, sweet/acidic stimuli and touching elicit pain because the (wide) dentinal tubules are suddenly exposed
- The periodontium is injured.

Most crown fractures are uncomplicated.[24] Often the enamel alone is fractured.[220] Inspection, palpation and

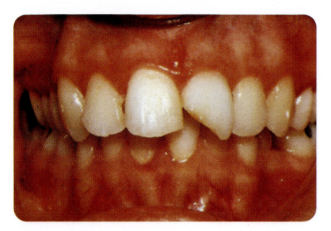

Figure 9.5 Uncomplicated fracture of the crown: both the enamel and dentine are involved.

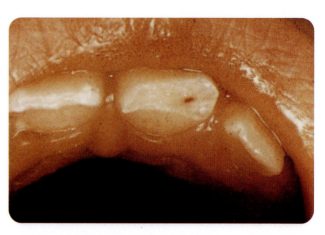

Figure 9.6 Complicated crown fracture: in addition to the enamel and dentine, the pulp is also involved.

radiographs may reveal embedded tooth fragments in the soft tissues, which if not removed can cause infection and malformation, for example of the lips. Late detection may necessitate removal via an extraoral approach[109]

Treatment and prognosis

When dentine is exposed, bacterial ingress and their toxins endanger the pulp. Provisional protection can be achieved by application of a varnish or glass ionomer cement due to lack of time (emergency appointment) or patient cooperation. Dentine that has been exposed for a few days does not have to be treated as if it was carious, as has been advised previously.[301] A pulp visible through the dentine (<0.2 mm) should be protected against the etchant by application of a layer of lining cement. The pulp is necrotic when follow-up radiographs show arrested root formation or periapical pathology. The pulp undergoes necrosis in up to 2% of uncomplicated fracture cases,[333] and in 30% of cases where the periodontium is also damaged.[332 334]

The tooth is restored with composite, but when only the enamel has fractured, just smoothening of the sharp edges may suffice. The fractured segment may be reattached with a low-viscosity composite, after pretreatment with a calcium chelator.[24 376] When carrying out indirect pulp capping, removal of a segment of the dentine is required to accommodate the capping material;[16] an internal groove prepared before bonding will be sufficient.[340] Compared with intact teeth, some studies have found that the fracture resistance of the reattached part is >90%,[123] [340] but according to others it is 10–45%.[101] Use of a chemically cured composite increases fracture resistance the most; a light-cured composite resin is second best, followed by resin cement; use of an adhesive only results in least increase in fracture resistance. A bevel also increases the fracture resistance.[101] A fragment stored dry

for more than 1 hour will discolour and be prone to fracture again, unless it is rewetted for at least 1 day.[124] Ries *et al.* found that a composite restoration functions as effectively as a reattached fragment, provided internal grooves are prepared.[340] If the treatment plan includes grinding of the incisal edge, which reduces the crown length, orthodontic extrusion may provide an acceptable cosmetic solution.[146]

Deciduous teeth

The treatment of uncomplicated fractures (about 8%)[60] may be limited to smoothening of sharp edges or application of, for instance, a glass ionomer cement on exposed dentine.[134] Prior to deciding on the treatment, the stage of root development and time to exfoliation should be assessed. Stainless steel crowns are used on posterior teeth in cases where a large part of the tooth has been lost.[24]

9.4.3 Complicated crown fracture

In a traumatic complicated crown fracture, there is loss of enamel and dentine leading to exposure of the pulp. All kind of external stimuli will cause pain. The exposed pulp (Figure 9.6) may proliferate through the exposure point if treatment is delayed. Only a small proportion of crown fractures are complicated.[220 335]

Treatment and prognosis

The treatment is dictated by the period of contamination of the exposed pulp, retention of the wound dressing, and the developmental stage of the root. The treatment options are direct pulp capping or partial vital amputation and extirpation and eventually apexification.[406] The pulp is extirpated when the root is fully developed. If not, extirpation is the least desirable option: a vital pulp is the best condition for ongoing root development.

- In teeth where the pulp has been exposed for even several hours, direct pulp capping is still warranted, because the pulp should be minimally contaminated.[92][335]
- The contamination is more severe where the trauma occurred (up to) 2 weeks ago, but partial pulpotomy is an option, because pulpal inflammation should be no more than about 2 mm deep.[92][345] Fuks *et al.* reported a high success rate after 7.5–11 years,[138] but others have had decidedly less success with pulpotomy carried out after 24 hours of the exposure.[153] Any pulpal blood clot must be removed to prevent internal resorption (Chapter 7).

Fractures accompanied by periodontal trauma have a less positive outcome, but the size of the exposure and the time interval between accident and treatment have not been found to affect outcomes.[24][92][98] Pulp obliteration (5%) and necrosis (25%) are seen after complicated crown fractures with concomitant luxation. In cases with no periodontal trauma, 99% of the pulps remained healthy.[345] In teeth with incomplete root development the chances of pulp survival are greater.[24][345]

- A necrotic pulp in an immature tooth requires extirpation and apexification with calcium hydroxide $(Ca(OH)_2)$. The $Ca(OH)_2$ should be replenished every 3 months to induce the formation of an apical barrier and thus to enable condensation of gutta-percha (Figures 9.7 and 9.8).[154][406]

- Insertion of $Ca(OH)_2$ in the first endodontic session leads to narrowing of the open apex within 9 months.[97] If the root canal is filled with $Ca(OH)_2$ in the second session it can take up to 20 months.[427]
- Addition of a disinfectant to the $Ca(OH)_2$ filling has been found to promote apical closure,[245] but is not indicated.[406]
- After apexification with $Ca(OH)_2$ the fracture resistance of the root is halved within 1 year:[29] Al-Jundi *et al.* found that one-third of teeth treated in this way fractured, the majority subsequent to a minor injury and 15% spontaneously.[6] Mineral trioxide aggregate (MTA) performs better than $Ca(OH)_{2;}$[446] but use of MTA also weakens the dentine considerably after a week of the filling.[447]

The retention possibilities determine the choice of restoration, although often this is a composite restoration or the fractured segment of the tooth crown is reattached, combined with, if necessary, a canal post.

Deciduous teeth

Depending on the expected exfoliation time and the child's cooperation, complicated fractures are treated with direct pulp capping/vital amputation[134] or extraction. Prevention of damage to the successor tooth germ after pulp necrosis requires cleaning the canal up to 3 mm of the apex, copious irrigation with sodium hypochlorite, and use of a resorbable root canal filling.

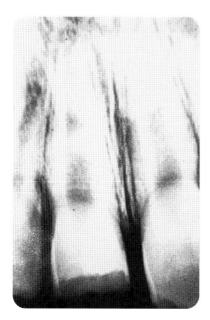

Figure 9.7 Crown fracture of an immature tooth. Because the pulp became non-vital, the root canal was filled with $Ca(OH)_2$ to encourage apexification (development of an apical dentinal bridge).

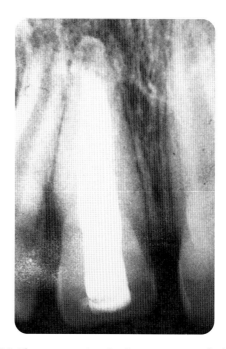

Figure 9.8 The same tooth as in Figure 9.7, 6 months later; the root canal was filled by condensation of gutta-percha up to the newly formed apical dentinal bridge.

Complications after crown fractures Development of secondary pulpal pathology is infrequent if the periodontium was not injured.[332][386] An untreated pulp exposure invariably results in pulp necrosis. Ravn reported that when exposed dentine was treated, 5% of the pulps became necrotic.[332][334] If the periodontium was injured too, the risk of complications increased with the increased severity of the insult.[335] In an intruded fractured tooth the pulp will invariably become non-vital.[24] Another complication is external root resorption, because of which traumatised permanent central incisors have been extracted.[349] If the root sheath is severely damaged but infection is absent, a bone-like tissue occasionally develops in the pulp space of permanent immature teeth.[190]

9.4.4 Crown-root fracture

A traumatic crown-root fracture is when a part of the tooth crown and root breaks off, with or without pulp exposure. The crown-root fracture often extends from the incisal edge to 2–3 mm underneath the gingival attachment, commonly with pulp exposure.[24] In maxillary premolars that are injured via a blow to the mandible, there is usually loss of the buccal cusp.[355] The gingival fibres may hold the fractured segment *in situ* (Figure 9.9), because of which the fracture may go unnoticed. However, under application of pressure, the tooth fragments will separate. The periodontium is also injured in these cases.

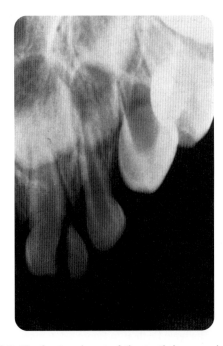

Figure 9.9 The fractured part of the tooth has remained more or less *in situ* because of its attachment to the gingiva.

Treatment and prognosis

Extraction must be considered when the required crown preparation for a restoration will damage the adjacent teeth or the fracture extends more than 3–4 mm below the gingival attachment. A fracture ending below the attachment may require gingivoplasty to ensure a periodontally acceptable restoration. When the fracture extends deep below the epithelial attachment, the crown:root ratio must be minimally 1:1 to warrant restoring the tooth. Orthodontic or surgical extrusion can be used to bring the fracture site to a supragingival level, where a ferrule of 2–3 mm can be prepared.[73][208][217][341] Absence of a ferrule lowers the fracture resistance.[458] Rapid orthodontic extrusion requires 1 month of stabilisation per mm of extrusion.[111] Surgically extruded teeth are stabilised for 3 weeks.[120] It has been proposed to "over-extrude" the tooth to allow restoration, and also to then enable intruding the tooth into its original position.[384] Gingivoplasty and extrusion result in a relatively small cervix and a tapering crown shape, which may, however, be acceptable.[208][394]

Surgical extrusion (3–7 mm) is performed with elevators and cutting of the periodontal fibres with a scalpel. The tooth is stabilised with interdental sutures. The root may be rotated, with the palatal surface facing labially. After the stabilisation period, endodontic treatment is insituted.[73]

Compensatory growth of bone and soft tissue occurs with *slow* orthodontic extrusion, which is indicated when interproximal bone is required as a substructure for maintenance of the interdental papillae or correction of a bony defect. Forced *rapid* orthodontic eruption will outpace bone growth. Extrusion at the rate of 1 mm/week is expected with a force of 25–30 g. Gingival recontouring is often needed. An endodontically treated, intruded tooth can be extruded via a metal hook cemented into the root canal.[111]

Anterior teeth

Exposed dentine with a closed pulp cavity must be protected, but which may not be possible. If the pulp is exposed, endodontic treatment is performed prior to extrusion. Gingivoplasty and/or extrusion and a post may be needed to save the tooth.[24] Treatment choices post extraction are: orthodontic treatment, a bridge or implant, or autotransplantation of a premolar into the space previously occupied by the traumatised tooth.[24]

- A large overbite is an indication for orthodontic closure of the extraction space.[414] Post-treatment complications include loss of bone and gingival retraction around the adjacent teeth.[55] When a lateral incisor is used to replaced a lost central, this leads to an asymmetry (Figure 9.10A): correction of the asymmetry with a wide crown or composite restoration (Figure 9.10B) may create periodontal problems. The shape of a canine replacing a lost lateral incisor is adjusted by cuspal grinding and composite build-up of the margins.

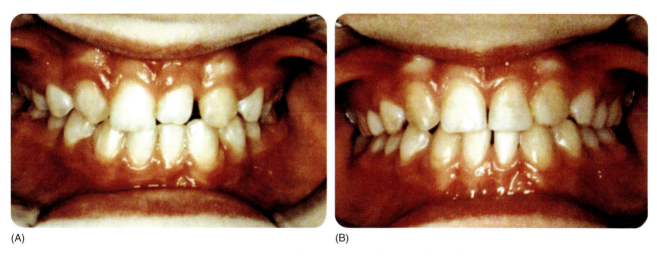

(A)   (B)

Figure 9.10 (A) Following the loss of the upper left central incisor in an accident, the lateral incisor and canine were orthodontically moved in a mesial direction to close the space. (B) The lateral incisor was then built up with a composite resin to resemble a central incisor.

- Tooth replacement with a Maryland bridge or an implant is anther option, although the latter is contraindicated in young people.
- Autotransplantation of preferably a mandibular first premolar, including Hertwig's epithelial sheath,[294] into the place of a lost maxillary central incisor seems the best solution when orthodontic extraction therapy is indicated. To prevent external root resorption, the transplant tooth should remain outside the donor site for a minimal amount of time: the recipient site must be prepared in advance. The tooth shape is adjusted with grinding and composite build-up.[62]

Posterior teeth

Crown-root fractures in posterior teeth are often uncomplicated. In most cases, crown preparation is possible, eventually after gingivoplasty and ostectomy or orthodontic extrusion. If the fracture is complicated, endodontic treatment is performed, along with apexification in the case of an immature root. In most instances the provisional restoration poses no problem. Fractured premolars in children with tooth size-arch size discrepancy are candidates for extraction.

Deciduous teeth

The fractured fragment is often held in place by the gingiva.[134] The teeth are usually extracted,[388] but can be saved when the fracture line is situated close to the cervix and a restoration/temporary crown will have sufficient retention. Root canal posts cannot be used. Apical root fragments are not removed to avoid damaging the successor tooth germ.[134]

9.4.5 *Vertical crown-root fracture*

A traumatic vertical crown-root fractures involves splitting of a tooth by an external force, over its entire length. These fractures are not clearly seen on radiographs, but later a halo-like, large radiolucency around the root, or a lateral radiolucency extending apically from the crestal bone, may be (but does not have to be) present.[448] Examination with localised computed tomography is more efficacious in the detection of longitudinal fractures, but it (modestly) increases the radiation dose.[449] In a few instances, the traumatic force splits the tooth vertically; these are mainly endodontically treated teeth. In one study, about 10% of such teeth referred for extraction were vertically fractured.[140] Another study found:[259]

- Two-thirds of the affected teeth were maxillary premolars, one-third were mandibular molars (mesial roots) and 10% were mandibular premolars.
- 57% patients had chronic symptoms and 31% had acute symptoms.
- Bone resorption was present, the majority of lesions being V-shaped and often narrow.

Roots with deeper grooves on the surfaces are especially more at risk.[225]

An inappropriate restoration, use of a canal post, thin root walls of young teeth or removal of excessive amounts of radicular dentine compromises the structural integrity of the tooth. As already stated, the dentine surrounding the pulp has more dentinal tubules and is richer in collagen than the outer dentine. Collagen is resilient and stores energy. The inner dentine deforms under loading, the outer dentine is stressed. Conservation of the inner core of dentine offers greater resiliency to the tooth. Use of a morphologically shaped root canal pin will minimise dentine removal[231] and the resistance this provides against vertical root fracture is different from that provided by root canal sealers.[36 246]

The occlusal load during mastication is three times higher on the mandibular premolars than on the canines.[372] The amount of dentine remaining in the mandibular premolars (not the mandibular canines) after endodontic treatment is related to the fracture resistance of the treated tooth.[423]

A tooth with a longitudinal fracture was endodontically treated and restored with amalgam and a post inserted within the amalgam. Two years later, there was no inflammation.[306]

9.4.6   Root fracture

A traumatic root fracture involves intra-alveolar splitting of the root, including the cementum, dentine and pulp, and is accompanied by rupture/compression of the periodontal ligament and bone involvement. Transverse fractures can occur at every level of the root. An external force can result in fracture of a small proportion of roots, especially in the permanent dentition, with periodontal damage. The coronal fragment may be luxated, but is rarely avulsed.

As the fracture plane is seldom parallel to the X-ray beam, the fracture appears ellipsoid in shape on radiographs, giving the impression of two fractures (Figures 9.11 and 9.12). Two more radiographs, taken with a posi-

tive and negative angulation, provide greater insight. A beam delivered at too steep an angle does not display the fracture.[24] Radiographs may not show a fracture until after a few days, when the coronal root fragment is displaced by blood and oedema, mechanical forces or resorption. They may also not show a fracture that is located at the labial or lingual margin of the alveolar bone.[125]

Healing

Four kinds of tissue are formed between the two intrabony root fragments.[24 25 26 30] Which kind of tissue is formed in a particular case depends on the mobility of the coronal fragment and[212] presence of infection. The position of the fragments relative to each other[15] might, however, be irrelevant[73 74 125] unless the fracture is level with or coronal to the alveolar bone crest. There may be self-limiting resorption in the fracture plane and obliteration of the pulp in the coronal fragment. The type of resorption that occurs is predictive of the kind of tissue that will be formed.[14 24]

Type 1 healing: formation of (osteo)dentine   Union of the fragments within 2–3 months by deposition of (osteo) dentine covered by cementum (Figure 9.13) occurs when: the root is immature and the fragments are close together; after rapid and optimal repositioning; adequate splinting; and when the pulp and periodontium are healthy. Untreated fractures may also heal in this way.[9 74 80 91] Union with dentine is uncommon,[125] taking place only when superficial internal resorption is present.[14]

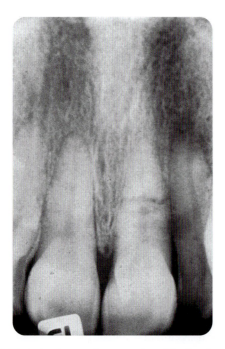

Figure 9.11 A simple root fracture: the oblique orientation of the radiograph has caused a projection on the film suggestive of a double fracture.

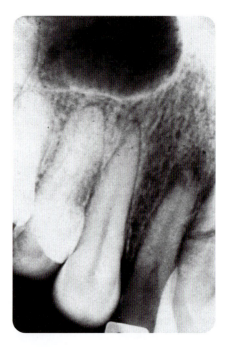

Figure 9.12 Incidentally detected simple root fracture of an upper central incisor.

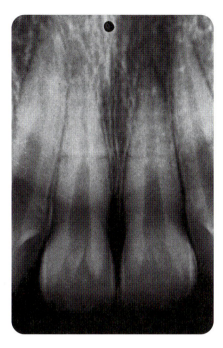

Figure 9.13 Healed fractures in the roots of both the upper central incisors after callus formation. The fracture lines are visible despite healing.

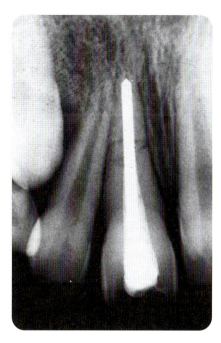

Figure 9.15 This root fracture was "immobilised" with an internal pin. It has been noted that in cases of root fracture, the pulp in the apical part of the root usually remains vital.

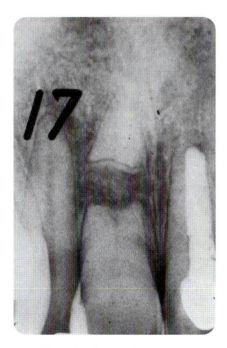

Figure 9.14 Healing of a fractured root with interposition of bone.

When the odontoblasts are traumatised or absent at the fracture line, new cells are recruited from the pulp, which transform into odontoblast-like cells. A zone of unorganised mineralised tissue is formed, upon which a highly organised dentine layer develops.[383] Radiographs often show a remnant of the fracture line after healing. The crown often becomes yellow (due to pulp obliteration). The pulp may react less strongly on sensibility tests, but will remain vital for years.

Type 2 healing: formation of connective tissue When the tooth fragments are dislocated, periodontal cells dominate the healing process. A connective tissue "bridge" is formed before the severed or stretched pulp can react. This mode of healing is also seen in teeth with restorations, marginal periodontitis,[15] and inadequately splinted teeth. The pulp cavities in the fractured fragments are often obliterated.[14] Radiographs show a radiolucent area between the fragments, with edges smoothed due to resorption. The tooth reacts on sensibility tests. Tooth mobility may be normal, but permanent interproximal splinting could be indicated.[24]

Type 3 healing: interposition of bone (and connective tissue) Inadequate repositioning of coronal fragments leads to interposition of bone.[268] The coronal part "erupts" while the apical fragment stays behind. The bony bridge is separated from the fragments by a periradicular space (Figure 9.14). Mobility of the coronal part may be normal. Sensibility tests provoke a reaction.

Type 4 healing: interposition of granulation tissue Granulation tissue (Figures 9.15 and 9.16) is formed when the

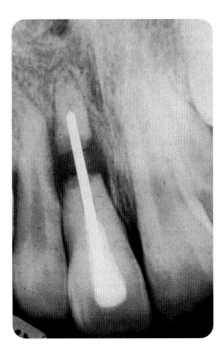

Figure 9.16 The same tooth as in Figure 9.15, 3 months later: note the interposition of granulation tissue.

pulp of the coronal fragment is infected or necrotic, or bacteria from the sulcus gain access to the fracture site. More than half, or 20–40%, of the pulps remain vital after root fracture and if the pulp becomes necrotic, this usually happens in the coronal part, [24 71 74 80 91 93 125 429] determined by the degree of extrusion of the coronal fragment.[30] A sinus tract may be present. The coronal fragment is mobile and the tooth is tender on percussion. Consecutive radiographs show broadening of the fracture line, due to resorption of the root fragments. The probability of granulation tissue formation is higher when the coronal fragment of a tooth with a closed apical foramen is somewhat extruded or laterally displaced and rigid fixation (see Section 9.8) is used.[15 24]

Interposition of hard tissue is reported to occur in 3–30% of cases of root fractures, bone and periodontal ligament interposition in 5–8%, and the periodontal ligament alone in 36–43%; pulp necrosis and inflammatory changes are reported in 20–23% of cases.[25 26 91 429] The quality of healing progressively worsens with increased separation of the fragments. Optimal repositioning of a fragment with an initial displacement <1 mm enhances the likelihood of type 1 and 2 healing, which is more desirable. Rigid splints affect healing negatively, while non-rigid splints promote healing.[24 297] Andreasen *et al.* reported that a splinting period longer than 4 weeks did not affect the kind of healing process and tissue deposited in the region of the fracture.[25 26]

Treatment and prognosis

The distance between the fracture and the gingival sulcus co-determines the treatment, which is directed towards repositioning the displaced coronal fragment and fixation with a semi-rigid splint. Immediate repositioning is easiest, as later the blood clots in the space between the fragments prevent optimal repositioning.[428] Severe periodontal disease is a contraindication for treatment.

1. A fracture *near the gingival sulcus* has a poor prognosis, because immobilisation (for up to 5 months)[442] of the coronal fragment is almost impossible, but the location of the fracture may not influence the type of healing.[91] If the fracture area becomes infected, extraction is unavoidable, but a long apical root fragment may be preserved and orthodontically/surgically extruded above the alveolar crest.[195 186 189] The remaining root must be long enough to accept a canal post. Gingival and bone reshaping may also be needed.

2. When the fracture is situated to the *middle of the root*, the tooth can be saved.
   - A dislocated coronal fragment and fractured alveolar bone are repositioned with finger pressure, first on the bone on the buccal side and then with forward pressure on the lingual surface of the tooth.[24]
   - Immobilisation. The coronal part is fixed to two neighbouring teeth with a flexible splint (composite). Cvek reported that a splinting period of <60 days to >90 days affected neither the healing frequency nor healing with hard tissue,[91] but 4 weeks of splinting is recommended.[442] The prognosis of mid-root fractures after treatment delay is rather good; Al-Jundi reported an 80% survival rate.[6]
   - If repositioning partly fails or the biting/masticatory forces applied to the tooth are quite heavy, grinding of the tooth or antagonist(s) is carried out after fixation.
     In fractured teeth with loss of the coronal fragments, Bühler removed the apical segments atraumatically and apically lengthened (4–5 mm) them with a titanium screw. After replantation, the apical fragments were immobilised for 3 weeks. Two years later, 75% of the teeth had survived.[70]
   - With a necrotic pulp, the coronal fragment is endodontically treated with $Ca(OH)_2$ or MTA. In one study, neither removal of the apical fragment nor endodontic treatment of both root fragments improved the prognosis and periodontal healing.[450]

3. A tooth with an *apical root fracture* is not splinted if it is not mobile. Repositioning, splinting and/or endodontic treatment may, however, be required.

4. *Vertical* fractures of the roots (mostly endodontically treated (pre)molars) are often seen on radiographs only years later. The root fragments are sometimes visibly separately. In other cases a V-shaped radiolu-

cency is seen at either the apex, the bifurcation or the proximal side of the root. After a longer time, the periodontal space on one of the two proximal sides widens, with sometimes extensive bone loss, which is visible as a radiolucent area or diffuse "halo" around the root.[285]

During lateral condensation if a snapping sound is heard or pain suddenly develops or blood wells up in the canal, the root is vertically fractured.[401] A force of 5 kg exerted with the spreader seems safe; a force of 7 kg is borderline safe.[254] The preparation form and type of spreader, preferably not excessively tapered, influence the tendency of the root to break because the force may deform the root.[286] Teeth with a vertical root fracture cannot be saved, unless by hemi-section of a multi-rooted tooth.[54] Bonding of the root fragments (cyanoacrylate, glass ionomer cement, composite) has been attempted, but there is a lack of reports of long-term follow-up of this approach.[285]

Deciduous teeth

Splinting of a deciduous tooth is difficult, but it may be attempted if the coronal fragment of a tooth with a complete root is not displaced. A dislocated coronal fragment is extracted.[134] The apical part is left *in situ* to avoid damage to the permanent tooth germ.

Complications after root fracture A "stretched" pulp may survive in the coronal part of the root;[429] if it is severed, revascularisation may take place along the fracture line. Pulp necrosis, often in the coronal part only, cannot be diagnosed reliably within the first year after trauma,[428] unless the patient presents with pain, a sinus tract or granulation tissue across the fracture line.[125] Complications include internal and external resorption and obliteration. Check-ups at the already mentioned time intervals (see Section 9.4) are mandatory. Table 9.2 shows the fate of pulps and teeth in a 15-year retrospective study of traumatised teeth.[343]

In general the pulp is obliterated in teeth with healed root fractures,[90] [210] unless it is necrotic.[212] Pulp necrosis

necessitates extraction when the fracture is located in the coronal third of the root. When the fracture is located more apically, a necrotic pulp in the coronal part is an indication for endodontic therapy. Root canal sealer may squeeze through the fracture line (Figure 9.17). A dislocated coronal fragment impedes access to the apical part of the root, which is then removed surgically in case of pulpitis/necrosis. The pulp in the apical part remains mostly vital, but may become obliterated.[90] [210]

Application of Ca(OH)$_2$ in the coronal fragment promotes fracture healing with dentine and cementum or with bone and connective tissue[8] and induces formation of a bridge apical to the coronal root fragment within 6–12 months, enabling condensation of gutta-percha. Ca(OH)$_2$ is placed only once,[84] unless bleeding continues, which necessitates reapplication after 1 week.

In patients with haemophilia or a deficient immune system (e.g. in leukaemia, neutropenia, acquired immune deficiency syndrome (AIDS)) extraction must be avoided. The trauma and treatment should not interfere with the diet in people with diabetes due to risk of hypoglycaemia.

9.5 Traumatic periodontal injury

Trauma associated with tooth movement may damage the periodontal tissues. Complications are pulp obliteration or necrosis, resorption and damage to the succedaneous teeth. The periodontal ligament has considerable

Table 9.2 Types of permanent teeth injury and the likely pulpal reactions[343]

	Pulpal reaction (%)			
	Survival	Obliteration	Necrosis	Extraction (%)
Complicated crown fracture	50	0	50	0
Crown-root fracture	0	0	40	60
Root fracture	0	50	0	50

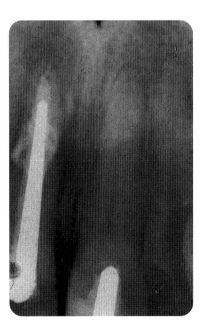

Figure 9.17 The endodontic cement has squeezed through the fracture line in the root.

potential for repair. Mechanoreceptors in the ligament enable determination of the touch threshold of teeth and to assess changes in the ligament after trauma. In cases of periodontal trauma, the touch thresholds (with von Frey hairs) are increased from a mean of around 1.3 g (range 0.5–2.5) to around 3.5 g (range 1–10). A few weeks later thresholds rapidly fall and often return to normal in 3–6 months. The more severe the periodontal damage, the higher is the initial post-traumatic threshold and the more delayed is the recovery.[151]

Sound teeth with a healthy periodontium in the line of bone fractures are left in place, unless they are an obstacle.[370 388] An alveolar bone fragment must be repositioned; splinting is done indirectly via the adjacent teeth for 4 weeks.[442]

9.5.1   Concussion

Concussion refers to traumatic periodontal injury without loosening or displacement the tooth. A minor injury makes the tooth tender on horizontal and/or vertical percussion. The percussion sound (a reliable diagnostic test of ankylosis)[451] is normal.[13] The Periotest (Chapter 7), a device that measures tooth mobility quantitatively, cannot diagnose ankylosis accurately.[452]

The damage consists of vascular rupture and bleeding from the gingival sulcus, oedema and injured periodontal fibres, followed by transient external root resorption. Radiographs do not show the damage in concussion.

Treatment
The prognosis is good, but the tooth should be kept under observation. Pain during biting and articulation can be remedied by lightly grinding the antagonist. Several periodontally injured teeth should be splinted semi-rigidly for 1 week. The patient should be advised to eat soft food for 1–2 weeks.[442]

Deciduous teeth
About one-third of deciduous teeth discolour and one-quarter of pulps are obliterated. Reported rates of pulp necrosis range from a few cases to about 20%,[60 326] but if the crown discolours, the pulp is necrotic in nearly all such cases, without radiographic and clinical signs.[198]

9.5.2   Subluxation

Subluxation is a traumatic periodontal injury with tooth mobility but without tooth displacement. Percussion and biting/chewing are painful. The percussion sound will be dull.[13] The damage consists of haemorrhages, oedema and torn periodontal fibres, followed by transient external root resorption. Radiographs do not show other abnormalities.

Treatment
Grinding of the antagonist teeth is recommended and if several teeth are involved, semi-rigid splinting should be done for 1–2 weeks.[442]

Deciduous teeth
The gingival sulcus may bleed.[134] The majority of subluxated deciduous teeth do not need treatment (80%), but they should be kept under observation. The mobility of most teeth returns to normal. Discomfort and occlusal interferences are absent.[137] Discolouration and the likelihood of pulp obliteration increase with time:[137] about 40% of the teeth discolour grey to black,[60] and one-quarter of the pulps are obliterated and 7% to half become necrotic.[60 326] The exfoliation times in 75% of subluxated deciduous teeth and the eruption of the succedaneous teeth are not affected. Radiographic, and sometimes clinical, evidence of pathology is present in almost one-third of cases. Enamel hypoplasia in the succedaneous teeth is very rare,[24 380] but there has been a report of a complicated crown fracture, a small root and periapical periodontitis.[1]

9.5.3   Luxation

Luxation is a traumatic periodontal injury, often accompanied by tooth mobility and always accompanied by displacement. Lingual and labial palpation will help determine whether the tooth sockets are fractured, which is likely when several teeth are displaced. After luxation, the pulpal blood circulation is interrupted because of the apically crushed or severed neurovascular supply. Revascularised pulps in incomplete roots may not respond to electrical and thermal pulp testing.[56] Laser Doppler flowmetry is more sensitive.[152 302]

Intrusion
Intrusion is traumatic partial or total displacement of the tooth into the jaw. Radiographs show the periradicular space to be absent and aid in determining the position of the intruded tooth. The displacement may be considerable; there is a report of a root apex protruding into the nasal cavity.[328] The percussion sound is clear, high and metallic,[7] as the tooth is wedged into the alveolar bone. Percussion is not painful because of the locked position,[24] but Strobl *et al.* reported a positive pain reaction in their sample.[395] The periodontal membrane and blood vessels are severely crushed. Compression of the blood vessels causes ischaemia, increasing the likelihood of root resorption.

Treatment of intruded permanent teeth
Intruded teeth have been repositioned and splinted. After the therapy, pulp laser Doppler flowmetry dropped to almost nil in 36 weeks in one study.[328] The more complete

is the root development and the more severe the intrusion, the higher is the probability of root resorption/ankylosis.[4][205] Three treatment modalities are available:

- *Spontaneous re-eruption*[69] warrants a wait-and-see approach,[209] and is recommended when the degree of intrusion is small.[115][312] Of 40 intruded teeth, 37 were left untreated, of which two became ankylotic,[209] but spontaneous eruption is unpredictable and is not comparable to the normal eruption process.[205][224] Permanent teeth with immature roots often re-erupt spontaneously (Figures 9.18, 9.19 and 9.20).[209][367] A slight luxating force may be required to free the tooth from its locked position.[24] Ebeleseder *et al.* reported a positive association between intrusion that was not deep and periodontal and pulpal healing.[115]
- *Immediate surgical extrusive repositioning* reduces the long spontaneous repositioning times, but may induce external resorption and bone sequestration. Minimal

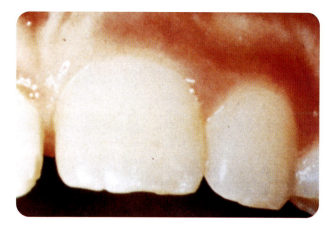

Figure 9.20 Final position of the tooth shown in Figure 9.18.

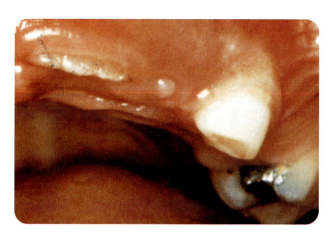

Figure 9.18 Accidental intrusion of an immature central incisor with a wide-open apical foramen.

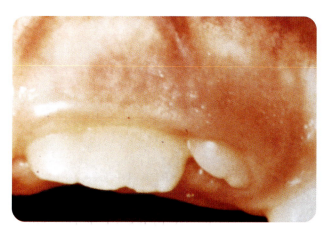

Figure 9.19 The intruded tooth in Figure 9.18 showing spontaneous re-eruption.

surgical manipulation had a positive effect on periodontal healing and more radical manipulation with forceps increased the risk of ankylosis.[115][312] Ebeleseder *et al.* found that pulps became necrotic in about 60% of surgically extruded immature teeth and about 90% of mature teeth. External inflammatory and replacement resorption developed in two-thirds to three-quarters.[115] The repositioned tooth was splinted with (wire and)composite for 3–4 weeks. A few teeth discoloured in the short term and about half were discoloured after a few years.[115] Surgical repositioning may lead to unintended extraction of the tooth.

- *Orthodontic repositioning* for 3–4 weeks might be preferred in more severe cases.[17][24][201][312] A few days before the orthodontic treatment, the tooth may be slightly loosened with forceps.[24] The traction forces exceed those used in conventional orthodontic treatment; as a severely intruded tooth does not have a functional periodontal ligament,[205] it requires stabilisation for a longer period.

There is no agreement about the best treatment method;[24][205] more teeth may be saved by surgical repositioning than by spontaneous realignment, regardless of the degree of intrusion.[229] No method significantly increases the likelihood or rate of root resorption.[4] More than half of the pulps die and external root resorption is common. A two-week delay in active repositioning increases the risk of failure.[205] The guidelines of the Royal College of Surgeons of England are shown in Table 9.3.[224]

In teeth in more advanced stages of root development, the probability of pulp necrosis is higher. Pulpitis or pulp necrosis in intruded immature permanent teeth requires endodontic attention on the day of the trauma to prevent external resorption,[24] with $Ca(OH)_2$ placed in the root canal.[273] Mature permanent teeth are treated endodontically within 3 weeks, because the pulp invariably dies:

Table 9.3 Treatment options for intrusive injuries of permanent teeth[224]

Intrusion (mm)	Treatment
<3 (mild)	Wait and watch for passive repositioning
3–6 (moderate)	Wait and watch for passive repositioning or immediate orthodontic traction
>6 (severe)	Extraction or immediate surgical repositioning (orthodontic treatment is unpredictable), or extraction followed by immediate root canal treatment, removal of damaged periodontal ligament and replantation

cases of slow spontaneous eruption may require active extrusion[24] or just excision of the gingiva.[367]

Presently, it is recommended that immature permanent teeth are allowed to erupt spontaneously. If within 3 weeks no movement is noted, rapid orthodontic extrusion should be instituted. Mature teeth may be rapidly (with orthodontics) repositioned[442 443] when the patient is older than 17 years and the intrusion is <7mm (www.dentaltrauma.guide), but forced eruption of immature teeth leads to pulp necrosis, external resorption and defective marginal bone healing.[443]

Deciduous teeth
A deciduous tooth may be intruded totally; the apex is commonly displaced labially,[134] but the succedaneous tooth germ may be damaged as it is located palatal to the deciduous root apex.[32] The likelihood of enamel hypoplasia and discolouration of the permanent teeth is highest after intrusion of the predecessor; the more severe the intrusion, the more frequent and severe are the defects.[415 416]

The literature is not explicit on whether intruded deciduous teeth should be extracted[218] or repositioned. When left alone (or with space maintenance for re-eruption),[438] complete spontaneous repositioning has been reported in 60–80%.[60 438] The incidence and types of developmental disturbance of the succedaneous teeth seem not to be related to whether intruded deciduous teeth are extracted or left to re-erupt spontaneously.[416 453]

A maxillary permanent central incisor showed a 3mm wide zone of hypoplastic enamel. The predecessor was intruded at a young age and was still present in the bone, buccal to the permanent incisor.[282]

A deciduous tooth that is intruded in the direction of the permanent successor should be extracted without using elevators, with the forceps grasping the approximal surfaces.[24] However, immediate extraction leads more frequently to developmental anomalies in the succedaneous teeth than no or delayed treatment (55% versus 44% in the literature),[407 417] The intrusion of the deciduous tooth may or may not have damage the successor,[418] but delayed acute inflammation around the re-erupting deciduous

tooth may still do so.[24] Compared with other types of luxation, intrusion may be associated with a decreased risk of pulp necrosis,[381] but an non-vital pulp in the long term may be more damaging than immediate active treatment.[407] About half of the pulps of a sample of traumatised deciduous teeth became necrotic.[60 326]

Extrusion
Traumatic extrusion is a luxation injury in which the tooth is partially displaced in a more or less axial direction, out of the socket. Extrusion is accompanied by bleeding from the ligament. Unequal incisal levels of adjacent teeth are suspicious of minor extrusive injuries. If the injury is more severe, the "elongation" of the tooth is obvious. The teeth are commonly displaced in a lingual direction and are excessively mobile in contrast with lateral luxation. Radiographs show the torn periodontal ligament as a widened periradicular space. The percussion sound is dull.[13] The blood flow in a sample of extruded permanent incisors was lower than in control teeth and remained unaltered 36 weeks after splint removal.[395]

Treatment
Extruded teeth must be repositioned as soon as possible with finger pressure and a semi-rigid splint applied. Spontaneous repositioning is unlikely. The splint, left in place for 14 days, must allow small functional movements, which promote healing.[24 297] The tooth is fixed with composite to the mesial/distal corners of the incisal edges of the adjacent teeth, and reinforced with a piece of nylon thread[35] or "soft stainless steel" (0.3mm),[297] or with a suture running from the palatal gingiva over the incisal edge and bonded with composite on the labial tooth surface.[167] If the alveolar bone is fractured, rigid splinting is required for 6–8 weeks.

A mature extruded tooth requires endodontic therapy; an immature tooth should be kept under observation and tested at the time intervals mentioned above. More than 40% of the pulps became necrotic, mostly during the first year post-injury, especially if the teeth are severely extruded. Obliteration (35%) is also related to the degree of extrusion.[242] In Robertson *et al.*'s study, the 20-year rate of survival was 84% for pulps with all kinds of periodontal damage and subsequent pulp canal obliteration;[344] in another study very few extruded roots resorbed.[242]

Deciduous teeth
Extruded deciduous teeth should be extracted or repositioned;[24] fixation is difficult, but is recommended to avoid avulsion.[134] The majority of extruded deciduous teeth discolour after some time and the pulp is obliterated.[60]

Lateral luxation
Lateral luxation is traumatic tooth displacement in a direction other than axial intrusion and extrusion. The

luxated tooth is immobile, with comminution or simple fracture(s) of the socket. The crown is frequently displaced to the lingual and the apex to the buccal side and may perforate the socket wall. When the crown is displaced to the buccal side, the apical periradicular space is enlarged, which is visible on occlusal radiographs. The intimate contact between root and bone makes the percussion sound metallic.[13] Strobl *et al.* found that the blood flow in laterally luxated permanent incisors remained low for 36 weeks after splint removal.[395] In the incisors, especially mature ones, independent of degree of luxation, studies show a similar risk of the pulp becoming necrotic or obliterated (40% risk).[17 293]

Treatment

Repositioning of the luxated tooth with the fingers, first of the apex and next of displaced bone fragments, and suturing of torn gingiva should be done as soon as possible. The tooth may be locked to such degree that repositioning may require use of forceps. Non-rigid fixation for 4 weeks is desirable; in cases with fractures of the alveolar bone, rigid splinting for 4 weeks is required. If left untreated, the luxated tooth will remain in its new position, but spontaneous realignment is possible, and may be encouraged with some orthodontic treatment.

Deciduous teeth

When the apex is laterally displaced, a luxated deciduous tooth realigns spontaneously in the absence of incisal interference; in more than half the cases, this occurs without complications,[60] but the pulp is prone to necrosis.[381] Repositioning increases the risks of necrosis[381] and damage to the succedaneous tooth. Pulp vitality testing is difficult. Grey discolouration, apical swelling, periapical radiolucency on radiographs, increased mobility and return of pain signal necrosis.[60] Owing to risk of damage to the permanent successors, deciduous teeth with a palatally displaced apex are extracted non-traumatically.[24]

Complications after (sub)luxation In mature permanent teeth, one-quarter of the pulps become necrotic after concussion and subluxation and almost all are necrosed after more severe periodontal injury.[13 110] Findings of a long-term retrospective study are presented in Table 9.4.[343]

Pulp obliteration is evidenced as a grey discolouration of the crown, within 6 weeks to 3 months[12] and sometimes after years,[11] but a yellow discolouration of the crown is more common.[343] Teeth with necrosed pulps become black in colour. Survival of the pulp depends on the diameter of the apical foramen.[19 20] The more mature the root and the more severe the (sub)luxation (Table 9.5), the greater is the risk of pulp necrosis and obliteration.[12 17 371]

In immature roots, the pulp may revascularise, but it will be obliterated.[12 18] The "obliterated" pulp may be vital,[18 152] and thus it is advisable to abstain from endodontic intervention.[343] After (sub)luxation, a vital pulp may temporarily not react to vitality tests.[24] When, after a few weeks, the pulp does react, it indicates pulpal survival or revascularisation. Check-ups at time intervals as described above are necessary. Gazelius *et al.* reported that in a sample of almost mature incisors showing no signs of blood flow at baseline, this was partially renewed after 6 weeks and fully restored after 9 months. However, after another 9 months, the pulps were obliterated.[152]

There is a risk of self-limiting resorption,[10 11] and of external inflammatory and replacement resorption especially in luxated mature teeth.[88] Approximately 70% of incisors that have been intruded by greater than half the crown length become ankylosed.[115] Palatally luxated molars (young rats) may show palatal root resorption. On the buccal side, the periodontal ligament is torn.[278]

Table 9.5 Pulpal reactions of mature and immature permanent teeth to periodontal trauma[12]

Injury	Apex	Pulpal reaction (%)	
		Necrosis (%)	Obliteration (%)
Concussion	Open	0	3
	Closed	4	6
Subluxation	Open	0	12
	Closed	15	9
Extrusion	Open	9	61
	Closed	55	20
Lateral luxation	Open	9	71
	Closed	77	11
Intrusion	Open	63	13
	Closed	100	0

Table 9.4 Types of periodontal injuries of permanent teeth and the likely pulpal reactions[343]

	Pulpal reaction (%)			
	Survival	Obliteration	Necrosis	Extraction (%)
Concussion/subluxation	67	17	13	3
Extrusion/lateral luxation	48	19	26	6
Intrusion	57	29	14	0
Crown fracture + luxation[a]	47	15	30	8

[a]More crown fractures are seen in subluxation than luxation.[88]

Some 10% of the enamel anomalies in the permanent dentition are caused by trauma to the deciduous teeth. After intrusion of the primary tooth/teeth, 50% of the successors are affected, after extrusion 33%, and after subluxation 25% are affected.[23] The main consequences are opacities, hypoplastic enamel, dilaceration, root angulation, root duplication and sequestration of the permanent tooth germ.[33 417] The tooth germ is especially sensitive to trauma during the early developmental and initial calcification stages.[402]

In deciduous teeth, most pulps show osteodentine and sometimes denticles or fibrotic tissue and signs of degeneration, but they often remain vital.[346] Other common consequences are discolouration, pulp obliteration and necrosis.[60] The grey colour seen in 50% of (sub)luxations eventually disappears.[60 211] In the long-term, however, the teeth become yellow (due to pulp obliteration) and only a few pulps become necrotic.[211] Deciduous teeth with periradicular lesions, gingival swelling and (spontaneous) pain have been treated successfully with a combination of antibacterial drugs including minocycline, without the need for endodontic treatment. The succedaneous teeth erupt without any problems.[399]

Avulsion (exarticulation)

Avulsion is a traumatic periodontal injury in which the tooth is totally displaced out of the socket. The neurovascular supply of an avulsed tooth is severed, as is the periodontal ligament. The cementum and the alveolar bone may also be damaged or fractured.

Treatment and prognosis

Consequences of late replacement (primary teeth are not replanted), dry storage of the avulsed tooth and use of particular storage media are described in Chapter 7. In sum, viable periodontal ligament cells allow reattachment of the tooth with minimal and transient inflammation. Although dry storage is associated with a very poor prognosis, Sheroan et al. replanted avulsed permanent teeth with complex dentoalveolar trauma after an extended extraoral dry time, with the long-term goal of achieving ankylosis to preserve bone in the anterior maxilla.[368] When the ankylosed tooth is infra-occluded by more than 1 mm, the crown should be removed,[442] which allows vertical apposition of the alveolar bone.[454]

When despite a wide open apex, revascularisation of the pulp fails, treatment efforts should be directed against the toxins in the pulp,[409] with closure of the apical foramen with Ca(OH)$_2$ or MTA. One prerequisite for replantation is the absence of severe periodontitis.[24]

An incisor was replanted successfully in a patient who had been treated in the past for periodontal disease but who now had good oral hygiene.[81]

Other contraindications to replantation are a comminuted socket (although some successful cases have been reported),[237] lack of space within the dentition and large carious lesions. Contamination must be removed. The extra-alveolar time period could be a decisive factor in the likelihood of contamination of the periodontal tissues.[359] In Kinirons et al.'s study, resorption occurred in 57% of replanted teeth without visible contamination, 75% of teeth with contamination that was washed clean, 87.5% of teeth which were rubbed clean, and in all the teeth (100%) with visible contamination.[228]

Any blood clots in the socket should be removed by irrigation; curettage is not recommended. If the tooth cannot be seated in its proper place with light finger pressure, either blood or a bone fragment is present within the socket. Intermitting finger pressure allows overcoming the blood barrier.[191] A blood clot could serve as a matrix for bacterial growth.[359] Interfering bone fragments are repositioned with a blunt instrument.[408] The occlusion should be checked and radiographs taken to see whether the tooth has been seated correctly.[77] The tooth is non-rigidly splinted for 7–10 days.[22 172 288] Any endodontic treatment should be performed before the removal of the splint, because the replanted tooth will still be rather mobile.[24] Cases with fractured alveolar bone require rigid splinting for 4–6 weeks.[408]

Fully developed roots

The notion that within 7 (to 14) days after replantation, root canal treatment must be performed[18 47] is based on consensus and not on research.[48] There are guidelines stating that after avulsion the root canal must be filled with Ca(OH)$_2$ between day 7 and 14 to aid healing of the periodontal ligament. Again, a week later, but not later than a fortnight, the root canal must be filled permanently.[48] When the apical foramen has a diameter less than 1 mm, the pulp is not revascularised.[233] Endodontic treatment prior to replantation has been proposed,[187] but is not advisable.

Incomplete roots

An avulsed immature tooth replanted within three-quarters of an hour may show revascularisation and root completion.

Greer reported a case with avulsion of a tooth with a wide-open apex, in which the pulp was left behind in the socket. Over time, dentine was laid down and a periodontal space formed around the tooth.[163]

The condition of Hertwig's sheath determines whether the root will be completed.[28 31] Removal of the sheath stops the root development and partial removal and concussion of the sheath results in defective development.[31] After extra-alveolar time exceeding 60 minutes the probability of revascularisation is low.[408] Complications after avulsion are external inflammatory and replacement resorption (Chapter 7) and arrested root development.[28] When ankylosis develops, the replanted tooth is, depending on the age and sex of the patient,[223] increasingly infra-occluded, with local arrest of dento-alveolar growth.[223]

In one study, infra-occlusion in boys younger than 16 years increased yearly by 0.4 mm and in girls younger than 14 years by 0.6 mm. After the pubertal growth spurt the annual increase was much smaller. When ankylosis develops after the age of 20–30 years, the increase in infraocclusion is small (0.07 mm/year), because the adjacent teeth erupt more slowly.[223]

Deciduous teeth

Avulsion of deciduous teeth is the most frequent dental injury after crown fractures and luxations.[221] An exarticulated deciduous tooth[13 442] is rarely replanted, because of the risk of mobility, abscess formation, resorption and damage to the succedaneous tooth germ.[24 433] After exarticulation of a deciduous tooth, development of half of the succedaneous teeth is disturbed.[24] Preservation of avulsed deciduous teeth has been considered challenging,[421] but despite limited evidence, it is advocated to promote the development of the maxilla and speech,[130] space maintenance and the child's self-esteem. One treatment that has been suggested is holding the crown with a pair of forceps, resecting the apex and filling the root canal with $Ca(OH)_2$. The replanted tooth is splinted for 1 week.[130] In the presence of a fistula and inflammatory resorption,[421] replantation of a deciduous tooth is contraindicated. In one study, of eight replanted deciduous incisors, four had to be extracted soon.[230] Parents who request replantation must be cautioned about the risk of pathological consequences. When an exarticulated deciduous mandibular anterior tooth is not replanted, a space maintainer is indicated.[389]

Chest radiography is recommended when an avulsed deciduous tooth cannot be found and may have been aspirated/inhaled.

Antibiotics

Prophylactic antibiotics (see also Chapter 7) are advised when bacteraemia is likely,[442] and are definitely administered to patients with heart conditions and a medium to high and risk of endocarditis after replantation.[5 240] Antibiotics may prevent inflammatory root resorption,[288 408 409] although in a study in rats they were ineffective after delayed replantation.[455] In case of dry-stored avulsed teeth and teeth with an injured periodontal ligament and infected pulp, systemic tetracycline is preferred because of its antiresorptive actions.[353 354] Soaking in doxycycline promotes the rate of revascularisation and continuation of root development.[408 426] In immature teeth kept dry for 5 minutes before replantation, pulp revascularisation occurred in 91% when coated with minocycline, 73% when soaked in doxycycline, and 33% when soaked in saline.[342]

A Tanzanian study found that antibiotics were prescribed by about two-thirds of practitioners for soft tissue injuries and by almost half for concussion.[219] Antibiotics have been stated to be useful for fractured alveolar bone, contaminated soft tissue wounds (if administrated within the first 3 hours)[24] and severely contaminated avulsed teeth.[191]

The side effects of antibiotics may present a contraindication to the use of antibiotics as far as possible, including local application.[37 406] Administration of antibiotics after root fractures was found to promote, paradoxically, healing with both hard tissue formation and pulp necrosis.[25 26] Bacteria may produce enzymes that inactivate medications or they may become less permeable to a drug or be able to excrete that drug. Their ability to mutate (and genetic transfer) may make them resistant to antibiotics.[180]

Degloving

Degloving refers to traumatic apical displacement of the gingiva, with denudation of the alveolar bone. In cases of trauma, the oral mucosa may be pushed apically so that a sheet of soft tissue, like a surgical flap, is separated from the bone. The injury is uncommon.[373]

Treatment

Where early treatment is instituted, the wound is cleaned and the sheet repositioned and sutured for 4–5 days. When the treatment is delayed, granulation tissue develops. The management then focuses on plaque control with chlorhexidine rinses. Healing is very slow and may be unsatisfactory.[373]

9.6   Epidemiology

The low annual rate of dental injuries[61 171 394] is associated with considerable between-country variation in the cumulative incidence rate over the years from 1% in young children to 35% and even up to about 50% in adolescents.[9 18 24 32 79 135 145 179 310 348 374 430] The few available data may not include traumatised teeth with healed periodontal ligaments and injured deciduous teeth because of shedding. Concussion, the most frequent injury in the (deciduous) dentition,[326] is often not recorded owing to the absence of severe symptoms. Many patients with dental injuries do not or cannot seek (or delay) treatment.[74 311]

The prevalence of facial injuries with dental trauma decreases with age: 39% in the first decade, 24% in the second, 18% in the third and 8–9% thereafter.[149] Almost half of patients presenting with facial injuries to an Austrian clinic had dental injuries, most frequently subluxation (51%) and crown fractures (38%), followed by avulsion (7%).[149] One-third of cases with dento-alveolar trauma needed treatment.[171] The epidemiological features are summarised below:

- Boys experience 1.5 to >2 times more injuries to the permanent dentition than girls, although the sex differences may be small or even absent.[143 145 220 267] This is also true for luxations, in which the subluxation type prevails.[61 89 94 135 149 170 205 292 305 321 404 434] In the deciduous dentition the difference between the sexes in the frequency of dento-alveolar trauma is small, if present,[57 424] but differences based on age categories have also reported.[264] Boys between the ages of 2 and 10 years have a greater probability of dental trauma than girls, due to more rough playing.[32] Most tooth trauma occurs at the start of a new school year.[272]

- The maxillary central incisors in particular are injured, usually from the labial aspect. With the exception of vehicular accidents, damage to one tooth is most common, but according to some research the teeth are more usually injured together.[24 80 89 122 214 296 303 331 393 404 428 434] Protruding maxillary anterior teeth with inadequate lip coverage,[267] increased overjet (>4 mm),[136 213 215] and overbite[267 404] are the most frequently traumatised.[9 49 112 136 206 220 304 310] The severity of the injury also increases with increasing overjet and in the extreme overjet group, injury to the maxillary central incisors occurs at an earlier age,[213 215 267 374] although possibly not in the deciduous dentition.[9] Because age, gender and ethnicity may confound the incisor–trauma relationship, relevant data must be adjusted.[291 374] Trauma to mandibular permanent incisors is associated with overbites that are five to six times more deep.[374]

- In serious (vehicular) accidents, luxations and bone fractures are most common.[24] Victims are, in particular, teenagers sitting next to the driver. Following car accidents, avulsion is most common[422] and occurs more commonly in the mandible than the maxilla.[305]

- In the deciduous dentition, (sub)luxations and exarticulation predominate,[24 60 61 135 218] in particular between the first and third year of life.[57] According to the literature, one-third of all deciduous dentitions are traumatised,[32 129 428] in particular periodontally.[144 272 280] In a sample of 4-year-old Mexican boys, 72% were injured.[356]

- In a sample of Norwegian 9–17-year-olds, the large majority of dental injuries occurred at school and while playing during leisure time. Sporting accidents were responsible for 8% of injuries. Mild injuries prevailed (89%).[377] Living in overcrowded households is another risk factor.[268]

9.6.1   Type of injury

Avulsion occurs in 1% to 13% of trauma cases.[94 135 331 357 434] The periodontium in children does not offer much resistance against external forces. Contact with a hard object will injure the dental hard tissues, while that with a softer object will damage the periodontal tissues.[96 296]

About half to 80% of the injuries lead to uncomplicated crown fractures and one-third to periodontal damage ranging from concussion to avulsion.[94 299 356 434] The same applies to the deciduous dentition[356] and a fracture of one type or another may be present in about 15%.[60]

Damage to the incisors is mostly limited to the enamel:[267 374] uncomplicated/complicated crown fractures (70%), cracks (4%); and root fractures (2%).[311] In the permanent dentition about 10% of the injured teeth are infracted.[332] Social deprivation (London) increases the risk of dental injuries: in such populations, Mata et al. reported that fractures of the enamel alone were left untreated more often than enamel-dentine fractures.[268]

About half of the traumatic injuries in the permanent dentition are concussions and (sub)luxations,[135 143] more so in the deciduous dentition.[57] However, uncomplicated crown fractures may constitute more than 90% of the injuries.[352] A minority of 1–2% of the injuries consist of root fractures.[58 94 434] Half of the root fractures are located in the middle third of the root, one-third are apical fractures and rest occur more cervically.[80] (Un)complicated crown fractures are most common in sportspeople, who also have a fairly high chance of multiple fractures and luxation.[357]

9.6.2   Causes

A "danger period" exists when toddlers learn to walk (due to falls) and cycle.[185 394 434] Fighting among boys, just playing around and falls are responsible for almost 70% of the injuries.[136 185] Incidents associated with horse riding, pool diving, skiing, skateboarding, etc. cause 13% of the dental injuries and vehicular accidents almost 10%.[185] Fist fighting is of less importance.[89 331 432] The probability of avulsion is, however, highest during rough and tumble playing,[141] assumedly related to sex and age. Most dental injuries occur at home; contact sports are the second most common cause in the UK,[95] but violence leading to falls due to being pushed is the major cause in some other countries.[266]

High-risk sports include contact sports such as football (UK; soccer USA) and (ice) hockey and (roller)skating (Figure 9.21) and cricket,[196 357] and combat sports such as boxing and wrestling. In medium-risk sports, such as basketball, a third of the accidents are associated with orofacial injuries.[133] Women have a higher rate of basketball-associated injuries than men, who are more accustomed to using a mouthguard. Other medium-risk sports are squash, diving and gymnastics.[24] Alpine skiing is a high-risk sport, causing multiple facial trauma, of which around 40% are accompanied by dental injuries, in particular luxation and fractures.[150] Gassner et al. reported that concomitant facial and dental injuries were in particular due to sports and play/household, and a minority are due to physical assault and vehicular accidents.[149]

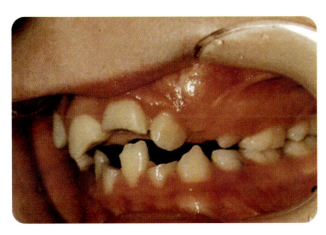

Figure 9.21 Multiple crown fractures caused by injury from a hockey stick.

9.7 Prevention

Besides learning appropriate sporting techniques and using mouth and face guards/helmets/seat belts/protective clothing, prevention of dental injuries is often impossible. Mouth/faceguards considerably decrease the risk of dental trauma, jaw (condyle) fracture,[24 83 133 147] and of brain concussion through shock absorption of blows to the chin. Mouthguards protect somewhat against the rare dental injury that may occur during setting up of general anaesthesia and orotracheal intubation.[24 300 324 378] The population at large is either uneducated about tooth protection or is insufficiently motivated to use the devices. Although 27% of an Israeli sample were aware of the existence of protective sport devices, less than 3% actually used these.[248] In the UK, girls from lower socio-economic backgrounds used mouthguards less frequently than boys and after some time the use decreased even more.[3] Requirements for a mouthguard include:[24]

- Absorption and dispersal of the energy provided by the external force.
- The device stays in place (no risk of being swallowed or inhaled) and is easily removed.
- The device does not interfere with the occlusion, mouth breathing and speech, and should be odourless and tasteless, must not irritate the soft tissues and should not provoke vomiting.
- The device is easily cleaned and disinfected.

A mouthguard designed for the maxilla should comply with the following requirements:

- It should cover the incisal edges of anterior teeth, the occlusal surfaces of the premolars and the buccal gingiva up to 3 mm from the mucobuccal fold, without interfering with movement of frenal attachments. Covering the molars gives a better distribution of the external forces, but may be uncomfortable.
- It should be 2 mm thick.
- It should cover 5–6 mm of the palatal mucosa and have a palatal thickness of 2 mm with a thin ending.
- It should be 3–4 mm thick incisally.
- The occlusal thickness must not exceed the freeway space.

Professionally made mouthguards seem more effective,[24 364] safe and comfortable (retention) than the cheaper stock and (boil-and-bite) mouth protectors.[197] The custom device is made in the dental laboratory on plaster models from individual impressions and fits well. Details about producing individual mouthguard from resilient acrylic resins are described elsewhere.[300 314] A mouth-formed type has a hard outer shell with a soft resilient liner (vinyl chloride lining with a self-curing acrylate).[24] None of the modern mouthguard materials stands out as more superior to the others, but latex is least appropriate.[456] More research is needed to determine the effectiveness of mouthguards against specific sports equipment (baseball bat, ice hockey puck), because the transmitted forces depend on the impacting objects and the material from which the mouthguard is made.[398]

The latex or plastic stock type (boxers) is available in three sizes. The poor fit requires biting on the mouthguard to keep it in place. The mouth boil-and-bite type protector is fitted by the user themselves and thus its disadvantages include a poor fit.

A mouthguard must be able to compensate for the ongoing eruption of teeth of young patients through the provision of adequate spaces within the mouthguard. Before taking impressions, any fixed orthodontic appliances are covered with a soft wax. After use, the mouthguard must be cleaned with soap and water and when dry, stored in a perforated box. Before use the device should be rinsed with water or a mild disinfectant.

9.8 Splints

Neither the necessity of splinting nor the method and period of splinting are well documented. The efficacy of long-term splinting after intra-alveolar root fractures[91] and after avulsion is doubtful.[21] More than half of untreated root fractures heal uneventfully[74] and healing with hard tissue seems to occur considerably more frequently when the tooth is *not* splinted, most likely due to the functional movements of the coronal part of the affected tooth. A fractured root with no (or slight) loosening of the coronal fragment should not to be splinted.[91] A splint:[24]

- Should stabilise the tooth in its normal position during the immobilisation period

- Should be made directly at the chairside
- Should not damage the teeth during insertion or removal
- Must not exert orthodontic or traumatic forces
- Must not promote gingivitis or caries
- Must not affect the occlusion or articulation
- Should not interfere with sensibility tests and endodontic treatment
- Should preferably be cosmetically acceptable
- Must allow some movement in case of periodontal trauma, although socket fractures require rigid splinting to protect the developing callus.

The older splinting methods include a gold or acrylic cap splint, made on a cast of an alginate impression, and orthodontic bands on the injured and adjacent teeth connected with an archwire.[91] Prior to splinting, the teeth are cleaned with 2% sodium hypochlorite.

Acceptable methods are:

1. A *non-rigid* splint made from composite resin. In the maxilla, the splint connects the incisal half or third of the labial surface of the injured tooth to the two neighbouring teeth. In the mandible, the splint is applied lingually. A gap in the dentition requires splint reinforcement with a thin orthodontic wire or a nylon thread.[24]
2. A *rigid* splint is made from composite reinforced with an orthodontic wire (diameter 0.8 mm) adapted to the contours of the tooth surfaces.[298] The wire is bonded with composite bonding material on the gingival third of the labial surfaces and connects the traumatised tooth with two teeth on either side of it.

The patient must avoid using the splinted tooth and should be shown how to clean the teeth. The composite splint is removed by cutting away the bulk of the composite with a diamond bur in the high-speed handpiece. The remaining composite is removed with a scaler or a straight chisel (held at the enamel–composite interface) and with flexible discs. The splint is left in place for as short a time period as possible. Recommended splinting periods (Table 9.6) are based on the literature,[24] [120] [218] [442] but should be tailored to individual circumstances,[116] because both the type of split and the fixation period are generally not significantly related to healing outcomes.[457]

Table 9.6 Splinting periods

Injury	Splint type	Splinting period
Replantation, root fully developed	Non-rigid	1 week[a]
Replantation, incomplete root	Non-rigid	3–4 weeks[b]
Subluxation	Non-rigid	2 weeks
Luxation:		
• Extrusion	Non-rigid	2 weeks
• Lateral luxation	Non-rigid	4 weeks
• Lateral luxation + alveolar fracture	Rigid	4 weeks
• Rapidly extrusion after intrusion	Non-rigid	3–4 weeks
Alveolar fracture	Rigid	4 weeks
Root fracture	Rigid	4 weeks[c]

[a]Mobility >1.5 mm requires a splinting period of a fortnight.[191]
[b]Splinting time of avulsed teeth >10 days relates to replacement resorption.[227]
[c]Formerly, a splinting period of 2–3 months was proposed, but a period exceeding 4 weeks does not enhance the healing pattern.[25][26]

10

Discoloration of Teeth

10.1 Introduction

Discoloration of teeth is when the colour of all or several teeth or (part of) a tooth is outside the white-yellow spectrum. The colour (=*hue*) of an object is determined by which wavelengths of white light it absorbs and reflects, for instance a red object only reflects the red wavelength and absorbs the rest. *Chroma* (=*saturation*) refers to the strength of the colour, its purity, that is, how more or less intense it is. *Brilliance* (=*value*) is the brightness of colours on a scale from black (=0) to white (=100). The amount and spectral composition of the light co-determine the hue and brilliance, for instance the differences in blue colour of the northern sky in the day or at dusk. The colour that is perceived is affected by a number of factors, including the observer.[115]

The permanent teeth are commonly white-yellow in colour, with hints of brown, pink and grey-green. The deciduous teeth are bluish white. Inheritance is responsible for inter-individual tooth colour differences.[114] Intra-individually, the colours of the different classes of teeth differ slightly, for example, the permanent maxillary canines are darker than the permanent incisors.

The enamel surface reflects most wavelengths, but the light that is transmitted through the translucent enamel scatters and is reflected by the dentine before it emerges from the tooth. The impact of the yellow-orange dentine on the perceived tooth colour is greater in the cervical region than in the centre of the crown due to differences in the enamel thickness in these areas. At the incisal edges, the thin enamel is darker, reflecting the lack of light within the mouth, more so when it is worn. Locally, different wavelengths of light may be absorbed, resulting in, for instance, brown spots (combined red, green and yellow wavelengths). Darker skin makes the teeth appear whiter: in one study, 50% of subjects with darker teeth had a fair and 17% had a dark complexion.[179] More severe discolorations are expressions of generalized or local pathological processes, which may have diagnostic implications.[367]

Colour determination

The colour of a tooth can be determined and recorded by comparing the tooth with a set of artificial teeth, for instance the Vitapan Classical or the Trubyte Bioform colour-ordered shade guide. The Vitapan shade guide has 16 shades divided into four colour groups ("hues"), each one ordered from light to dark, that is, A1–A4 (including A3.5), B1–B4, C1–C4 and D2–D4, The Trubyte Bioform colour-ordered shade guide has 24 shades When used to evaluate the effects of bleaching, the four groups are pooled and ordered from the lightest to the darkest shade, as shown in Figure 10.1. Colour photos or slides may be used to record tooth colours.[359]

The tooth colour also can be determined by photospectrometry, which measures the different colours of the whole labial surface at once. Colorimeters and high-resolution digital cameras may misread the real colours, sometimes considerably.[94] The colour measurement is presented as, for instance, the Vitapan shade guide number and as a numerical value. *Every* colour can be described with the numerical three-dimensional CIE (International Commission on Illumination) L*a*b* colour system, in which:

- L* represents the brilliance (L = 0 is perfect black, and L = 100 is perfect white)
- a* is the parameter for the green-red axis: positive values are red, negative values are green (an object cannot be red and green at the same time)
- b* represents the yellow-blue axis: positive values are yellow, negative values are blue.

Classification of tooth discoloration

Discoloration can occur during odontogenesis (*endogenous/intrinsic discoloration*) due to incorporation

Pathology of the Hard Dental Tissues, First Edition. Albert Schuurs.
© 2013 Albert Schuurs. Published 2013 by Blackwell Publishing Ltd.

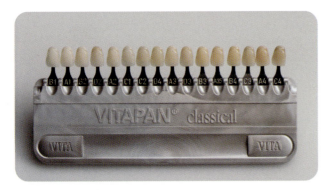

Figure 10.1 Vitapan Classical shade guide: the colours are ordered from light to dark.

Table 10.1 Classification of tooth discoloration

Type of discoloration	Description
1. Endogenous	
1.1 Developmental	Discolouring pigments are incorporated into the dental hard tissues during odontogenesis
	Examples: hypocalcification and biliary anomalies
1.2 Post-eruptive	Infiltration of discolouring pigments into dentine occurs via the pulp
	Examples: sclerotic dentine, tertiary dentine and necrotic pulp
2. Exogenous – post-eruption	
2.1 Infiltrative	Discolouring pigments infiltrate the enamel/dentine from the mouth
	Examples: agents from cavity fillings/ root canal fillings infiltrating dentine
2.2 Pseudo-discoloration	Stains on tooth surfaces
	Example: chlorhexidine stain
3. Endogenous or exogenous – post-eruption breakdown	Enamel loss leads to exposed dentine, which is eventually secondarily infiltrated exogenously
	Example: Pulp showing through after internal or cervical dentine resorption

of pigments in the developing hard tissues. Developmental hypocalcification also causes the tooth colour to change. Post-eruption, infiltration of the enamel/dentine by pigments can occur via the pulp (*endogenous*) or the mouth (*exogenous/extrinsic*).[367] Deposits of exogenous pigments on the enamel surface,[368] that is, the acquired salivary pellicle, does not discolour the tooth tissues themselves: the term *pseudo-discoloration* seems more appropriate here. Loss of enamel or dentine underlies other pseudo-discolorations. Based on such considerations, tooth discoloration can be classified as shown in Table 10.1.

Attribution to a discoloration category may be difficult. For instance, enamel that is opaque due to irradiation with high-intensity laser which causes water loss with light scattering, and brown-coloured dentine due to non-enzymatic collagen denaturation or oxidation of a dentine component.[22]

10.2 Endogenous discoloration

Often all the teeth are affected, although occasionally only a few may be discoloured. Development enamel hypocalcification (opacities) and hypoplasia and their numerous causes are described in detail in Chapter 3.

10.2.1 Endogenous developmental discoloration

Endogenous developmental tooth discoloration is due to incorporation of discolouring pigments in the dental hard tissues at the time of odontogenesis.

Amelogenesis imperfecta (pp. 79–86)
The subtypes are associated with different discolorations: brown (to black), mottled brown, (opaque-)white, yellow, glass-like, alternating white and normal coloured bands (Figure 10.2 and Table 3.4).

Biliary anomalies
In people with congenitally defective biliary ducts or biliary atresia (1:10 000 live births)[389] dark green to yellow-brown bile pigments are deposited in both dentitions.[97 149 232 316 389] Dentine formed after liver transplantation has a normal colour.[144 316]

Coeliac disease (p. 63)
Symmetrical enamel hypoplasia may be accompanied by discoloration, which is chronologically distributed per quadrant.

Molar-incisor hypocalcification (cheese molars) (pp. 53–4)
The partly brown discoloured first permanent molars may be accompanied by white and yellow opacities in the incisors.

Chemotherapy (pp. 77–8)
Discoloration of teeth, mostly likely brown colour, have been reported in children after chemotherapy.

Congenital syphilis (pp. 54–5)
The corkscrew-shaped incisors can be dirty grey in colour. The hard tissue between the multiple cusps of the first permanent molars may be brown in colour.

Congenital porphyria
Porphyrin traces are present in all people. Increased porphyrin levels lead to discoloration of all hard dental tissues. In particular, the dentine in the deciduous dentition discolours a dark yellow-brown, red-brown and

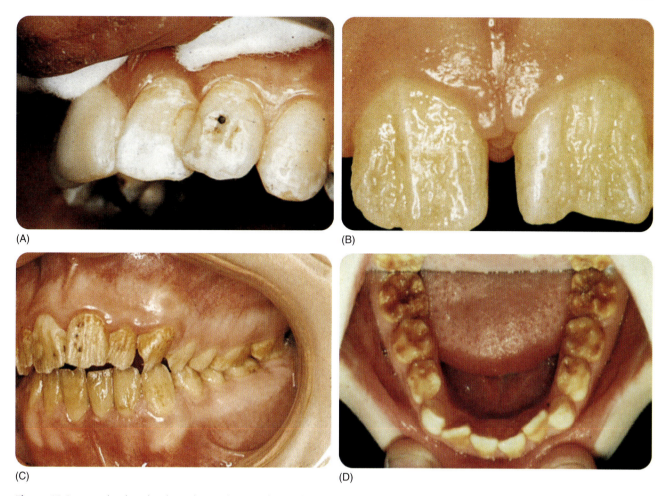

(A)

(B)

(C)

(D)

Figure 10.2 A–D Discoloration in various subtypes of hereditary amelogenesis imperfecta.

purple-brown (erythrodontia), all of which fluoresce red under ultraviolet light.[227] The enamel may be thin.

Porphyrin is needed to synthesise haemoglobin. An inherited enzyme disturbance precludes the formation of one of the precursors from which "haem" (=ferroprotoporphyrin, part of haemoglobin) is formed. There are many types of porphyrin and they occur across the whole of the animals and plant kingdoms.

The skin of patients with congenital porphyria is hypersensitive to ultraviolet (UV) light and it blisters and scars under the light in the operating theatre. The oral mucosa is vulnerable to mild trauma. The patients also have haemolytic anaemia. The porphyrin level is raised in faeces, urine (red) and calcified (dental) tissues.[98 112 231] Root resorption has been reported.[96]

The "Swedish" variant, acute intermittent porphyria, a rare condition that includes mental retardation, peripheral neuropathy and acute respiratory paralysis, is probably due to decreased levels of uroporphyrinogen-I synthase. In such patients, use of substances such as ethanol, erythromycin, corticosteroids and some anaesthetic agents (lidocaine) is life-threatening.[48]

Dentine dysplasia (DD) (pp. 86–8)
In type II DD, the crowns of the deciduous teeth show a translucent amber colour,[334] and the permanent teeth may be grey or brown.[280] In radicular type I DD yellow-brown[319] and light blue-brown discoloration of the crowns is occasionally observed.[225]

Dentinogenesis imperfecta (pp. 88–93)
The crowns in type I and II dentinogenesis imperfecta are amber and opal coloured,[319] but not all teeth are necessarily affected. Violet, red-brown, purple-brown,[123] grey-blue[305] and grey-green[123] colours have been reported and such discolorations are caused by secondary deposition of minerals in the hypocalcified dentine (Figure 10.3). Ongoing rapid dentinogenesis with pulpal obliteration intensifies the stains.[312] The enamel tends to chip away.

The grey or amber opalescent enamel in type III dentinogenesis imperfecta crumbles rapidly, exposing the shiny, amber dentine.[178]

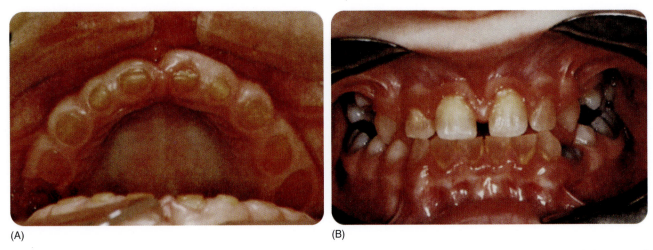

(A)   (B)

Figure 10.3 Dentinogenesis imperfecta. The anterior teeth are amber in colour (A) and the molars are somewhat blue (B). (Courtesy of Department of Oral Surgery, University of Groningen.)

Fluorosis (pp. 68–75)

Fluorotic enamel shows fine or merging white lines due to superficial porosities, which in more severe cases extend into the dentine. Very porous enamel breaks down, which causes pitting. Brown discoloration probably develops due to the post-eruption infiltration of the porosities by dietary pigments.[270] The white and brown colours (Figure 10.4) might also be due to causes other than fluorosis, which are then diagnosed as "discoloration possibly associated with excessive fluoride".[79]

Haemolytic anaemias

Haemolytic diseases of the newborn produce jaundice.

Erythroblastosis fetalis (Rh incompatibility) (pp. 56–7)

Mild neonatal jaundice is common, but jaundice can be severe in cases of rhesus incompatibility, which is diagnosed when the bilirubin concentration is 1.5 mg/100 mL in the serum. It is clinically visible at 7 mg/100 mL.[171] The liver of the neonate is unable to process the large amounts of haemoglobin degradation products: the reddish yellow bilirubin of the destroyed erythrocytes is oxidised to the yellow-green biliverdin. Incorporation of these pigments in the calcifying dentine of the deciduous teeth is responsible for the discoloration that shows through the enamel if the concentration exceeds 30 mg/100 mL,[386] which explains why not all affected children have discoloured teeth. A green (incorrectly named *chlorodontia*), yellow-green, blue, grey or brown hue is visible.[271 374] The discoloration gradually disappears.[171] Bilirubin might also be found within the enamel.[98]

Thalassaemia and sickle cell anaemia (p. 58)

The erythrocytes are broken down in these hereditary diseases and the haemoglobin is released into the blood plasma. The circulating bilirubin is incorporated in the developing dentition and leading to grey discoloration of the permanent dentition in particular.[160]

The haemoglobin molecule consists of two α- and two β-globulin chains. In thalassaemias the production of the globulin chains is reduced.[363] Sickle cell anaemia occurs in homozygotic carriers of the defective gene.

Maternal–fetal ABO incompatibility (p. 57)

Blood group incompatibility is accompanied with jaundice in the infant, but tooth discoloration has been only occasionally reported, including green (bilirubin)[102] and black and grey stains.[30 232]

Transfusion reaction haemolysis

In this condition, the teeth are discoloured grey due to haemosiderin deposition.[136]

Hypophosphataemic vitamin D-resistant rickets (pp. 63–6) and hypovitaminosis D (pp. 62–3)

In both these conditions, the (hypoplastic) enamel in affected children may be discoloured yellow and brown.

Inborn metabolism errors

Ochronosis (p. 58)

In this condition, abnormal phenylalanine degradation leads to blue-black discoloration of the permanent teeth, occasionally dark brown due to the presence of homogentisic acid.[160 191 368 377]

Primary hyperoxaluria and oxalosis (p. 188)

Hyperoxaluria is an inherited disorder of glyoxylate metabolism with renal failure. In oxalosis, oxalate crystals accumulate in extrarenal sites such as the muscles and skin,[384] pulp and dentine, and initiate a foreign body reac-

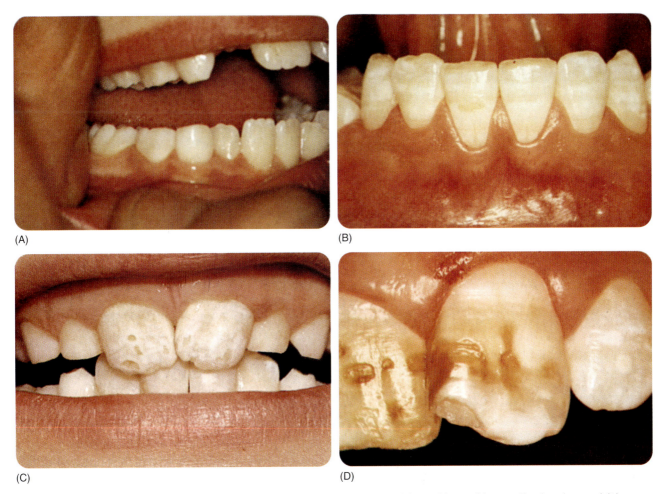

Figure 10.4 (A) Fluorotic opacities in a deciduous dentition, (B) mild fluorosis, (C) opacities and brown discoloration, and (D) severe discoloration due to fluorosis with hypoplasia.

tion in the periodontal ligament, resulting in root resorption.[254 384] Grey coloured teeth have also been reported.[137 279]

Phenylketonuria (p. 58)
Inhibition of the transformation of the amino acid phenylalanine (toxic to the brain) to tyrosine results in phenylalanine accumulation, which discolours the permanent teeth brown.

Infection and trauma in the deciduous teeth (p. 79)
Periradicular pathology of the deciduous teeth after trauma or caries may disturb the developing enamel structure of the succedaneous teeth (occasionally with deposition of cementum on the enamel), which secondarily stain brown due to infiltration of dietary chromogenic pigments.[129] White discolorations are seen in Turner teeth[46] and yellow and brown discoloration also occurs (Figure 10.5).

Low birthweight and prematurely born children (p. 59)
The enamel may show yellow-brown bands.

Orotracheal intubation (p. 57)
Children may have yellow-brown discoloured enamel on the side on which the tube was inserted.

(Pseudo)hypoparathyroidism (p. 67)
Both hypoparathyroidism and a lack of response to parathormone are accompanied by hypoplastic yellow enamel.

Regional odontodysplasia (ghost teeth, pp. 93–5)
If the teeth erupt, the (thin) enamel of the teeth is yellow to brown.

Syndromes
Enamel hypoplasia seen in many syndromes may resemble that seen in hereditary amelogenesis imperfecta. In

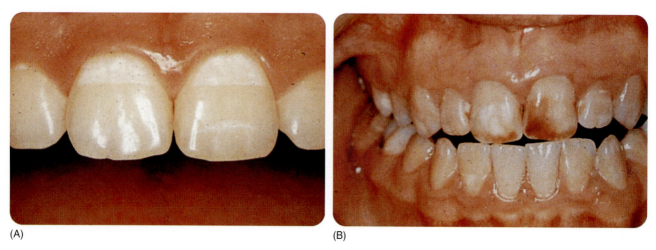

(A)   (B)

Figure 10.5 (A) These opacities developed following (mild) trauma to the deciduous predecessors. (B) Brown discoloration, following possibly more severe trauma and/or infection in the predecessors.

tuberous sclerosis, small brown pits appear on the teeth. In the Crigler–Najjar syndrome, glucuronidation of bilirubin is absent, whereby the teeth become green to brown.[98]

Tetracyclines (pp. 75–7) and ciprofloxacin

The earliest tetracyclines caused yellow discoloration of the teeth, which fluoresces under UV light. Tetracycline use in pregnancy or in children leads to discoloration of the children's teeth. Due to oxidation under daylight, the yellow colour changes to brown (purple-red dentine).[65 88] The posterior teeth, which are least exposed to light, remain yellow for longer. Use of other tetracyclines caused yellow, grey-brown, blue-grey, (brown-)yellow/ cream-white discolorations (Figure 10.6).

Three degrees of severity of tetracycline discoloration have been distinguished:

1 = yellow or grey discoloration, uniformly distributed throughout the dentition and tooth
2 = darker grey or yellow discoloration, also uniformly distributed
3 = dark-grey to blue discoloration, this is the most severe and is characterised with marked (cervical) banding.

A fourth degree has been proposed,[115] which is too dark a discoloration to attempt vital bleaching. In a sample of cystic fibrosis patients, 25% had tetracycline-discoloured teeth, mainly in the permanent dentition. About two-thirds of them had grey teeth, one-quarter had yellow teeth, and one-tenth had brown teeth.[110]

Later generations of tetracyclines are less discolouring, but the more severely discolouring earlier tetracyclines continued to be used in some countries. Severely affected dentitions are now mostly found in people older than 35

years. The new generation of tetracyclines (doxycycline (Vibramycin and Doxymycin)) only incidentally discolour the teeth and this is usually not severe. Minocycline (see Section 10.2.2) is an exception.

10.2.2   Endogenous post-eruption discoloration

Endogenous post-eruption tooth discoloration occurs due to infiltration of the dental hard tissues by chromatic agents via the pulp, with the discoloured dentine showing through the enamel. A second category of causes includes dentinal sclerosis and pulpal obliteration.

(Capillary) bleeding

Trauma to a newly erupted tooth may cause pulpal bleeding. A pinkish red colour shines through the enamel, becomes grey-blue within a few days, dark-grey after a few weeks, fading after 2–3 months once the pulp has healed and the blood products have been resorbed.[12 153]

In a sample of traumatised deciduous teeth, 15% (or less)[173] showed transitory discoloration,[41] and the rest remained grey: the pulp either became necrotic or was obliterated. The transient character of the discoloration has been questioned because all pulps in another sample of discoloured deciduous teeth showed irreversible pathological changes, including obliteration.[331] Left untreated, the majority of discoloured deciduous teeth will function until their normal exfoliation time.[283 328] Holan observed that about half of such teeth become lighter in colour. Infection was present when the teeth remained dark. In some dark teeth, root growth was arrested and in others inflammatory external root resorption developed. In the majority of the teeth that became lighter, the pulp was obliterated, which happened in only a few teeth that

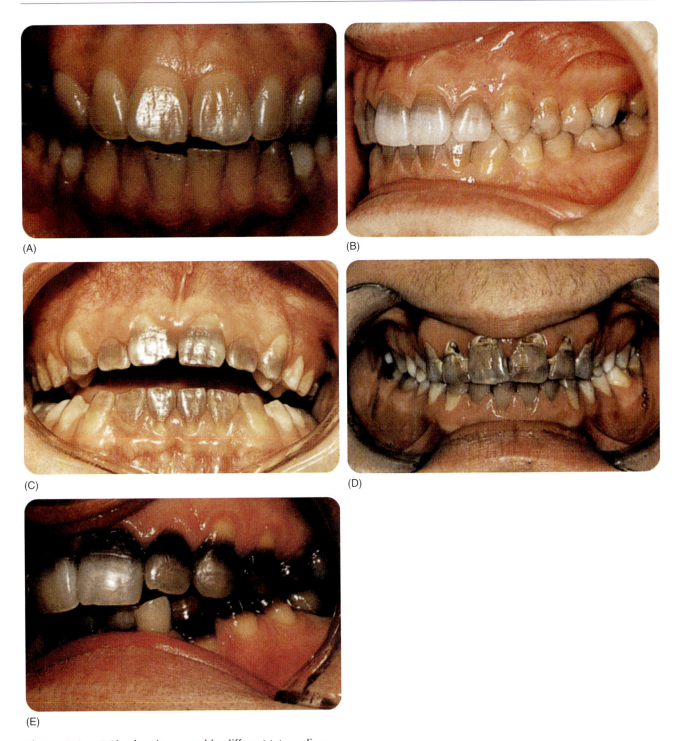

(A)

(B)

(C)

(D)

(E)

Figure 10.6 A–E Discoloration caused by different tetracyclines.

remained dark. Expansion of the dental follicle of the suc-cedaneous tooth occurred in nearly all cases, which may signify a dentigerous cyst indicating the need to remove the deciduous tooth; the permanent tooth was deflected from its position and failed to continue erupting. [173]

Drowning/suffocation

Blood accumulating passively in the head because of a head-down position after drowning and, less likely, suf-focation, leads to red discoloration of the teeth after some time ("pink teeth"): haemolytic derivates from pulpal blood penetrate the dentine. Exposure to sunlight changes the red colour to brown within a few days. In some archaeological material, such discoloration was absent.[47]

Lepromatous leprosy

Leprosy is a chronic infectious disease affecting the nerves, skeleton and skin. Leprosy is classified into different types, based on clinical, bacteriological, immunological and histopathological criteria. Depending on the innate capacity of the host to mount a cellular reaction, at least three types are recognised: a malignant lepromatous type, a benign tuberculoid type and a dimorphous (mixed) type.[304] In the lepromatous type, *Mycobacterium leprae* are abundant in the pulps and tubules, leading to discoloration of the incisors, which are reddish in about 10% to possibly one-third of the patients.[52 304] The pulps often become necrotic. Premaxillary bone recession leads to loss of the anterior teeth in all types.[288 304 333]

Necrotic pulp

A necrotic pulp causes progressive darkening of the dentine (Figure 10.7). The root is darker than the crown because the enamel partly masks the dark dentine.

- Following trauma (or application of excessive orthodontic force)[157] erythrocyte breakdown products from the ruptured pulpal blood vessels penetrate the dentinal tubules.[233] With time, the products become yellow-brown to blue-black. Iron from the erythrocytes forms a coloured compound with hydrogen sulfide. Formation of a haematoma prior to the breakdown of the erythrocytes may first give rise to light-pink discoloration. A similar discoloration develops after endodontic treatment of vital pulps when pulpal remnants are left behind.
- When the pulp became necrotic because of caries, blood will be absent. The grey-brown discoloration of the

crown in such cases is caused by degradation of proteins (Figure 10.8).[115]

Pulpal obliteration (ageing and trauma)

Ongoing dentinogenesis with age and dentine sclerosis make the crowns yellow and brown, respectively.[98 179 249 327] Solheim reported the correlation between tooth yellowing and age to be 0.85 for the maxillary incisors and 0.6 for mandibular counterparts.[327] An alternative explanation for yellowing of dentine with age is the incorporation of nitrogen and blood derivates into the tissue. Enamel, especially enamel cracks and lamellae, darkens also because of infiltration of dietary pigments (Figure 10.9).

After (sub)luxation, the pulp of deciduous teeth may be obliterated (partially or totally), causing a mild yellow discoloration.[182] Andreasen reported partial and total obliteration in 15% and 1% of teeth, respectively, after periodontal trauma.[11]

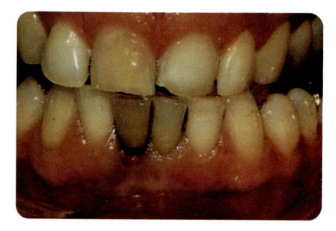

Figure 10.8 Brown discoloration (see text) in a non-vital tooth and amalgam discoloration of the first left maxillary premolar.

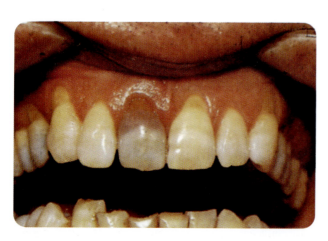

Figure 10.7 A dark non-vital tooth.

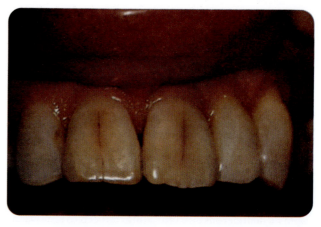

Figure 10.9 Discolouring pigments infiltrate cracks in the enamel or the enamel lamellae.

Tetracycline and other antibiotics

Tetracycline products, when these drugs are administered to adults for extended periods, are incorporated in the secondary dentine and may slightly discolour the teeth.

Minocycline

Minocycline is used to treat severe inflammatory acne and systemic infections including atypical pneumonias and sexually transmitted diseases.[354] It stains the bone and nail beds, breast milk (black colour), the lips (brown) and causes blue-black pigmentation (macules) of the tongue. Cutaneous hyperpigmentations have different colours and are divided into several types. Roots of erupted teeth become dark-green. Roots of extracted teeth exposed to the drugs during their development appear black.[55 70 264 354 379] Brown-black minocycline pigment (spherical structures) has been observed within the oral mucosa overlying the hard palate,[354] but the attached gingiva usually appears blackish-blue,[55 116] due to the dark-green alveolar bone showing through.

Minocycline is completely absorbed in the gastrointestinal tract even when administered with dairy products. Once inside the tissues, the drug is oxidised and transformed into a coloured product. There are other theories of discoloration, such as chelation of iron by haemosiderin (a degradation product of minocycline), forming a melanin-like molecule.[45 55 70 175]

Minocycline is rapidly bound by plasma proteins and collagen binds minocycline to a significant degree, so that pigmentation occurs in tissues rich in collagen: scars, bones, teeth.[45] Use of minocycline >100 mg daily leads to darkening of the crowns of already erupted teeth, to green-grey, grey, black, yellow or a striking blue-grey hue of the incisal three-quarters of the crowns, especially the middle third, fading incisally. The teeth are affected in only 3–6% of long-term users of the drug. Staining may already develop after 1 month and even 1 week of using the drug.[45 55 63 65 142 175 266 354 379]

Palliative treatment of rheumatoid arthritis and management of periodontal disease with minocycline may increase the prevalence of stained teeth in the future.[55 175 354 379]

Other antibiotics

Staining following use of antibiotics such as amoxicillin has been reported a few times,[93] but this is disputable. Ciprofloxacin, which is given intravenously to young children with *Klebsiella pneumoniae* infection, stains the teeth green.[351]

Typhus/cholera

The pink discoloration seen in some typhus and cholera victims[98] may be categorised as endogenous post-eruption discoloration.

10.3 Exogenous discoloration

10.3.1 Exogenous-infiltrative discoloration

Exogenous-infiltrative discoloration of teeth is due to post-eruption penetration of the teeth by chromogenic agents from the environment (mouth). A filling in a tooth cavity and an endodontic filling in the pulp cavity are considered as belonging to the environment of the tooth.

Amalgam and other filling materials

Radiographs sometimes show opaque areas underneath amalgam fillings.[300 362] This is because metal ions from the corroding restorations, in particular stannic ions, penetrate the demineralised dentine and to a lesser degree the enamel.[98 154 204 236 362 377] Besides stannic ions, some silver ions,[377] as well as copper and mercury ions have been observed.[236 308 330] Clinically, the tooth appears blue-black,[98] sometimes green-black, and further away from the copper-containing amalgams it is green-brown.[236] The opaque areas on the radiographs become larger with time[236] due to ongoing infiltration by corrosion products. Contact with other metals worsens the corrosion,[40 308] as well as with the non-γ-2 and copper-rich amalgams.[6 282]

Condensation may lead to pushing of amalgam components into the dentinal tubules,[315] but metal ions may be displaced by galvanic action.[236] Conventional amalgams may be less able to conduct electric currents than copper-containing amalgams.[181]

The layer of unfilled bonding agent between the enamel surface and the composite restorations may discolour brown after some time. A grey hue may develop around pins, and composite and glass ionomer cement fillings.

Diet

Infiltration of enamel by dietary pigments from foods and beverages – into the enamel lamellae, cracks, and carious and developmental opacities – and the exposed dentine cause a permanent brown discoloration of these tissues. The teeth of many older people also have accumulated brown-orange-yellow stains, leading to an unaesthetic appearance.[68]

Filling materials in the pulp cavity

Tooth discoloration of various types (Table 10.2) has been reported within days to weeks of obturating the pulp cavity with an endodontic filling material; the discoloration becomes more severe with time.[267 346 360 361]

Ions liberated by corrosion of a silver root canal post cause a grey-black discoloration.[138] Use of Durelon, Fuji glass ionomer cement, Fletcher's cement and zinc phosphate cement does not alter the tooth colour. IRM and Dycal make the teeth slightly darker.

Table 10.2 Tooth discoloration produced by various endodontic cements/pastes

Discoloration	Material
Brown-yellow	Iodoform paste
Grey (moderate discoloration)	AH26 (silver free), Duopercha
Light pink	Diaket, gutta-percha
Orange-red/yellow-brown	Grossman's cement, zinc oxide-eugenol cement, N2, Tubli Seal, Endomethasone
Pinkish (later becomes dark red)	Riebler paste
Yellow-green (moderate discoloration)	Cavit

Table 10.3 Tooth discoloration due to exposure to various industrial chemical dusts

Colour	Chemical
Black	Silver, iron, manganese
Grey	Mercury, lead
(Blue-)green	Copper, nickel, antimony
Orange	Chromic acid fumes
Bright yellow	Cadmium
Green, red, orange	Para-amino salicylic acid, copper, nickel

Industrial discoloration

Incorporation of air-borne dust particles and fumes of metallic salts causes characteristic discoloration of the teeth (Table 10.3).[89 98]

Silver nitrate and silver diamine fluoride

Silver nitrate (AgNO$_3$), which was used in the past to arrest dentine caries, resulted in an intense black discoloration.[98 368]

Below a superficial layer of the black precipitate, carious dentine is brown stained by free silver colloid. The deeper dentine and the pulp became black due to reduced silver globules. Sclerotic dentine remains stain-free,[98] and the discoloration is well defined.[236]

Nowadays, application of *silver diamine fluoride* to carious tissue causes black discoloration of the dentine. Yellow silver phosphate is formed and turns black under sunlight.[222]

10.3.2 Exogenous pseudo-discolorations: superficial stains

Exogenous superficial pseudo-discoloration is due to adherence of environmental chromogenic agents to the salivary pellicle or plaque. Most cases of "tooth discoloration" are due to the coating of the tooth surface, i.e. pigments adhering to the pellicle (and plaque). The pig-

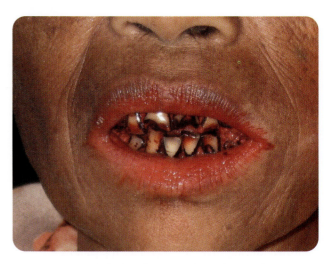

Figure 10.10 Relatively mildly discoloured teeth in a person with a betel chewing habit. (Courtesy of N.A.M. Rosema.)

ments originate from the diet, e.g. tea, coffee, wine, tobacco, etc., or are associated with cationic antiseptics and metal salts that interact with dietary chromogens and precipitate on the tooth surface.[376] Some of the staining agents also penetrate the tooth tissues.

Indices have been developed to evaluate the colour, intensity and distribution of such stains.[103] The stains have also been classified according to their origin, metallic or non-metallic,[376] but neither the mechanism nor the variable extent of the stain, or the fact that not all metals stain the teeth, have been accounted for in these classifications. To overcome these problems, Nathoo classified extrinsic stains as follows:[255]

N1 type – direct dental stain: in direct staining, the dietary chromogens are taken up by the pellicle that then shows the natural colour of the chromogen

N2 type – direct dental stain: in this type, the colour of the chromogen may also change after binding.

N3 type – indirect dental stain: indirect staining agents are initially colourless or tooth coloured, and discolour after becoming chemically altered.[255 376]

Betel chewing (p. 209)

The betel nut is derived from the orange-red nut of the *areca*, *arang*, *betel* and *pinang palms*, and is wrapped in a fresh or fermented betel leaf coated with lime and sometimes tobacco or other ingredients.[284] Betel chewing is widespread in southern Asia.[385] It stains the lips, tongue and mucosa a mahogany brown, with a red-brown to black coating on the teeth (Figure 10.10). Oxidation of polyphenols (tannins and gallotannins) accounts for the red colour. Brown to black, complex polymeric end-products precipitate on the teeth.[247] The rather thick layer has a tartar-like structure.[285] Tooth wear is common. Frequent use leads to pathological, cancerous changes in the oral mucosa.[284][313]

In Thailand, many rural people are betel chewers, but most are older.[287] In many other countries betel-chewing is also quite common. In the city of Kaohsiung in Taiwan, some 13% of men, mainly of low educational level, chew betel, although unawareness of the negative consequences has been reported.[64] Among a sample of 16–18-year-old Taiwanese adolescents, 10% reported chewing betel and 31% reported doing so in the past.[385]

Calculus
Calculus is mineralised plaque, the calcium salts being derived from the salivary film which covers the plaque.

- The yellow-white *supragingival* calculus may become brown due to stains of dietary origin, smoking and so on. This calculus, in particular, is found on tooth surfaces near the orifices of the salivary glands, especially on the lingual surfaces of the mandibular anterior teeth and the buccal surfaces of the maxillary molars. Starting just above the gingiva, the calculus extends over the tooth surface.
- The brown to black (haemoglobin-derived) discoloured *subgingival* calculus may be visible through the gingiva. Compared with supragingival deposits, it is harder, more "stone"-like,[224] more evenly distributed over the dentition and more firmly attached to irregularities in the root surface.[224]

The proportion of the population with calculus increases with age to some 80%. Dialysis patients have abundant calculus deposits due to their high salivary urea concentration. Use of some medicaments decreases the formation of calculus.[224]

Chlorhexidine and other mouthwashes
The brown-discolouring chlorhexidine (Figure 10.11) is used as an antibacterial rinse after periodontal surgery

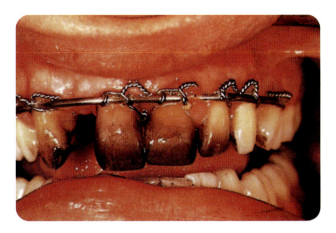

Figure 10.11 Discoloration caused by chlorhexidine.

and for caries prevention.[4] Compared with controls, greater amounts of brown staining was noted in a group using a dentifrice with 0.12% chlorhexidine. Addition of zinc to the toothpaste made the discoloration less severe,[302] as did peroxyborate.[145] Differences have been noted in the intensity of discoloration between individuals. Solheim *et al.* noted that the retention time of chlorhexidine was longer in patients with discoloured than non-discoloured dentitions;[326] the composition of the salivary pellicle of both groups was similar.[102]

Chlorhexidine probably stains the teeth because of an interaction with dietary chromogens in tea, coffee, red wine[6] and polyphenolic compounds. Thus, chlorhexidine may bind dietary chromogens to the tooth surface,[376] but the discoloration could also be due to sulfide (which is, however, still under discussion[376]), because chlorhexidine denatures proteins (in the pellicle) coupled to dietary iron.[104][372]

Sodium lauryl sulfate (foam-forming) in toothpastes inactivates chlorhexidine. An experimental toothpaste with no sodium lauryl sulfate was effective against plaque, but was not considered fit for use because of discoloration with long-term use.[180] The staining produced was independent of the abrasiveness of the toothpaste.[199] Stannous fluoride might prevent staining[100] by a redox reaction, like oxidising agents (1% peroxy-monosulfate).[109] Oxidising agents remove established stains[100] and can be used prophylactically in combination with chlorhexidine.

- *Benzethonium chloride*, a quaternary ammonium salt added to toothpaste, discolours the plaque brown.[101] Eriksen *et al.* found that addition of a weak chelator did not alter the tendency to discolour.[101] Another mouthwash contains copper ions as an anti-caries and anti-plaque agent.[7] Compared with chlorhexidine, a mouthwash with copper sulfate was less effective and caused green staining.[370]
- A *potassium permanganate* mouthwash induces violet to black staining.[157][368]
- *Cetylpyridinium chloride*, a toxic quaternary ammonium compound, is present in several mouthwashes and toothpastes, and stains the teeth brown like *benzalkonium chloride*.

Chromogenic bacteria
In a sample of 11–12-year-old children, Sutcliffe found several extrinsic tooth stains: brown (20%), green (10%), black (2%) and orange (2%) stains.[337] A yellow stain has also been observed in children.[216] Of a sample of 5–14 year Mexican children more than 10% had (undefined) extrinsic stains.[314]

- *(Brown) black stain.* In a sample of caries-free children[344] with a normal oral hygiene[337] a brown to anthracite-black line or band was observed, especially the anterior teeth.[216] The "mesenteric line" is a line of plaque formed by coalescence of brown or black spots along the cervical margin, which often follows the contour of the gingiva[98] but is separated from the gingiva by a small unstained zone. The prevalence varies from some 5% to 20%, especially in younger children.[195 198 337] The plaque is characterised by Gram-positive rods (commonly about 35% but up to 90% has been reported); several *Actinomyces* species dominate. Streptococci average 5% of the flora.[323] The characteristic plaque is very stable,[323] and tends to calcify.[344] The black pigment consists of an insoluble ferric salt,[286] formed from hydrogen sulfide produced by bacteria and dietary iron, and also contains calcium, silicon, magnesium, lead, manganese, phosphorous, silver and sodium.[318] Brown stains are more easily removed than black stains, and both tend to recur.[98] Kinirons *et al.* found that patients with *cystic fibrosis* showed black stains (besides tetracycline discoloration) more frequently than controls (some of whom also had tetracycline discoloration).[195]

• *Green stain.* A grey- to brown-green, thick, tenacious stains may be present (Figure 10.12) on mainly the buccal surfaces of (deciduous) teeth,[337] and are seen twice as often in boys than girls.[216] The pigment is possibly formed from bacterial hydrogen sulfide and blood traces.[318] The oral hygiene of the affected individuals is usually poor.[337] These stains contains many chemical elements (aluminium, barium, nickel, boron, copper, titanium, strontium and potassium) in addition to those in the brown stain.[318] Underneath the stain, the enamel is rough and demineralised,[98] but this is not always reported.[216] Among the associated micro-organisms are *Bacillus pyocyaneus*, which creates a typical garlic odour; and fungi, such as *Aspergillus* and *Penicillium glaucum*.[98] The fungi need light to grow and the stain is therefore often restricted to the anterior teeth.

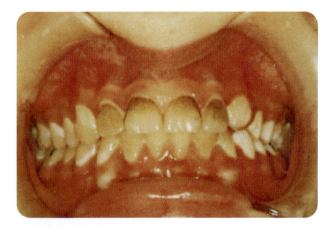

Figure 10.12 Green discoloration due to chromogenic bacteria.

• *Orange stain.* A more rare stain is an orange to bright red stain on the middle and gingival third of the buccal and lingual surfaces of all teeth.[216] Several micro-organisms have been identified, but not much is known about them.[309] Children with this stain have poor oral hygiene.[337] The stain is easily removed, but will recur.[368]

Associated with the stain are *Bacillus prodigius, Bacillus Rouge de Kiel, Bacillus mesentericus ruber, Bacillus roseus, Sarcina rosea* and *Micrococcus roseus*.[98] *Serratia marcescens* and *Flavobacterium lutescens* have also been found.[157]

However, conclusive evidence for discoloration by the action of chromogenic bacteria is still lacking.[376]

Khat chewing

Habitual chewing of khat leaves (a psychostimulant that has amphetamine-like substances) in the southern Arabian peninsula and East Africa leads to a yellowish-brown dental stain.[157]

Iron solutions and other medicaments

Iron ions have an affinity for the hard dental tissues. Iron solutions, prescribed for iron deficiency, some anaemias and gastric irritation, produce a black discoloration,[98 368] acting in combination with the salivary pellicle or by penetration into the enamel. Medicaments containing manganese oxide and potassium chlorate also stain the teeth.[368] Sulfa drugs, such as sulfaethidole, cause black and green staining, assumedly because of icterus.[136 232] Bismuth-containing drugs cause a yellow discoloration.

One composite bonding agent contains iron chloride. Fe^{3+} ions are released under the influence of the etchant and $Fe(OH)_3$ is formed. Both Fe^{3+} and $Fe(OH)_3$ react with sulfide and form the yellow-green Fe_2S_3 and black FeS;[332] whether local stains develop has not been reported.

Plaque

Around 75% of plaque consists of a variety of bacteria ($>10^8/mm^3$) that are attached supra- and subgingivally to the salivary pellicle. When the plaque is thick enough, its white colour is clearly visible (Figure 10.13).

Calcium bridges link the pellicle glycoproteins to the enamel. The bacteria adhere to the salivary pellicle through mechanisms that involve combination of free energy and electrostatic and hydrophobic forces.[255]

Ageing pellicle may become brown, by denaturation through acids and detergents and the Maillard reaction, i.e. an initially colour-free material becomes brown with time, for example a slice of an apple. The Maillard reaction (non-enzymatic browning) is based upon a reaction between sugars and amino acids. Furthermore, redox reactions also occur.[255] The plaque may become discoloured by the action of many agents, for instance antibacterial agents.

Stannous fluoride

Local application of SnF_2 (8%) often causes light-brown to gold-yellow tooth stains,[186][378] consisting of stannic sulfide,[99] also visible on radiographs.[260]

The stain contains tin and sulfur, probably tin sulfide that oxidises. The sulfur may originate from the salivary pellicle proteins, which denatured at the low pH of SnF_2.[100] In an *in vitro* study, denatured proteins did not form a salt with tin chloride.[6] In view of the complexity of the chemical process involved in the production of a metal sulfide, it has been questioned whether such processes occur in the mouth.[376]

Some 30 years ago a toothpaste with stannous fluoride was taken off the market, for reasons including discoloration and instability. More recently, stabilised SnF_2 toothpastes have been reintroduced.[373]

Swimming (p. 161)

The teeth of swimmers, who exercise more than 6 hours/week in disinfected swimming pools with pH >7, show

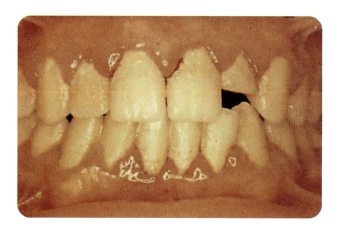

Figure 10.13 Plaque deposits are clearly visible in this figure.

brown discoloration. Tooth brushing neither prevents nor is able to remove the stain.

Tannins in wine and tea

Both red and white wines and (black) tea contain tannins (polyphenols) that may cause a black discoloration of teeth. In one case reported, daily swirling of 1.5 L white wine (pH 3.2, 21.5 mg tannin/L) was associated with tooth erosion and denudation of the dentine, which was stained an intensive black (Figure 10.14). The stain contained tannin.[310] In another study, a brown discoloration was observed. Wines discolour the teeth even more when chlorhexidine is used.[262]

The phenols attach by way of an ion-binding mechanism directly to the enamel.[255] Tannins are divided into derivates of flavonols and hydrolysable tannins, which are esters of sugars.[310] Tannin and chlorhexidine denature the pellicle proteins: iron and stannous sulfides may be formed,[102][346] but it is not clear where the required amounts of iron (low concentration in saliva) and stannum originate from.[6] Bleeding gums might be a source of iron. Coloured dietary precipitates are another likely source, specially in patients using antiseptic mouthwashes. An *in vitro* study showed that precipitation of wine and tea occurred with chlorhexidine.[6] *In vivo* studies have reported brown tooth stains after rinsing with chlorhexidine and tea, and a rinse of an iron tonic with tea led to a grey to black stain. Rinsing with chlorhexidine alone, or tea or iron tonic alone did not cause tooth discoloration.[5]

Temporary discoloration due to dietary causes

Several temporary discolorations are caused by various foodstuffs such as berries, pepper, saffron and liquorice.[98]

Tetracyclines (pp. 75–7)

Large yellow tetracycline crystals bind to the pellicle proteins.[369] Bjorvatn found that immersion in an aqueous

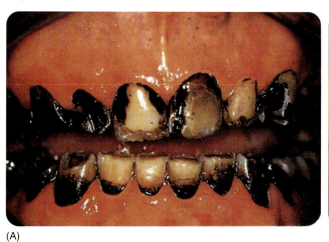
(A)

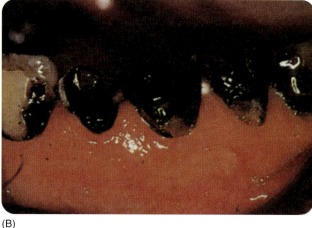
(B)

Figure 10.14 A,B The denuded dentine (due to erosion) in this patient was discoloured black by tannins in *white* wine. The patient consumed (after swirling) 1.5 L of an acidic wine daily.

solution of tetracycline (tablets) etched the enamel, to which the tetracycline crystals then attached firmly.[38] Minocycline stained the teeth black. The minocycline concentration in the gingival crevicular fluid is much higher than in the serum: minocycline attaches to the pellicle's glycoproteins, etches the enamel, and is oxidised, with the degraded aromatic ring forming the insoluble black quinone ("extrinsic" theory).[45 55 70 175]

Tobacco, marihuana

Smoking and chewing tobacco give rise to a brown-black coal tar coating, in particular on the lingual tooth surfaces. Tar products dissolve in the saliva and decrease the pH, thereby facilitating penetration into the fissures, grooves, enamel defects, lamellae, cracks and denuded dentine.[89 368] Marijuana smoking causes a cervical dark-brown to black discoloration.[111]

Traditional staining of the teeth

Black teeth were considered fashionable in the past in Japan.[114] Women in Southeast Asia still stain their teeth black,[157] and tooth mutilation with secondary staining used to be a rather common tribal tradition in African countries.

Ashes from burned bark, the juice of the Euphorbiaceae plant and iron-containing soil was used for blackening the teeth. In some tribes, the enamel was etched with lemon and black paint, ginger and mango was used to stain the teeth. Iron with herbal mixes were used by Japanese women and later the samurai: the "honourable" tooth black appeared to protect the teeth against carious demineralisation.[157]

10.4   Discoloration due to breakdown

Endogenous and exogenous breakdown of dental hard tissues results in pseudo-discolorations.

Amalgam/other filling materials

Dental silver amalgam restorations and white filling materials tend to be reflected.

Caries

The initial caries lesion is chalky white because the increased pore volume reduces the translucency of the enamel. On drying the lesion, the fluid in the pores is replaced by air, which reduces the refractive index. (The refractive index of enamel is 1.62, that of water is 1.33 and that of air is 1.0.[376]) The white spot then becomes brown, as chromogenic dietary pigments penetrate into the pores.[193]

Discoloured carious dentine, if not directly visible, may be visible (white/grey/brown) through the enamel, for instance approximal caries may be observed from the occlusal or buccal aspect. A brown zone occurs ahead of bacterial progress within demineralised dentine.[122] The colour of exposed carious dentine depends on the state of activity in the lesion, the more active the lesion, the lighter (white, yellow) is the colour; arrested lesions appear dark brown.

The brown colour of dentine is attributed to Maillard pigmentation[197] or melanin or, alternatively, pigments such as lipofuchsin and bile acids.[376]

Exposed dentine

As the enamel becomes thinner due to tooth wear or erosion, its colour becomes darker because the more yellow-orange dentine shines through more easily. Incisally the darkness of the oral cavity interior shows through.

Dentine is exposed by wear, erosion, in hereditary amelogenesis imperfecta and dentinogenesis imperfecta, and in traumatic tooth fractures and due to gingival recession, when the softer cementum is brushed away and so on. The dentine is less mineralised than the enamel and its surface is interrupted by the many orifices of the dentinal tubules, so that dietary pigments are more easily taken up, causing a brown stain.

External cervical and apical and internal resorption (Chapter 7)

Cervical and internal resorption of crown dentine create the "pink spot" when the process reaches the enamel and the red granulation-like tissue shows through (Figure 10.15). Most pink spots represent cervical resorption.[353]

A grey colour of luxated teeth, which may or may not disappear with time, is associated with temporary apical bone resorption,[11] or with external (apical) root resorption of a vital tooth that responds to pulp sensitivity tests.[71]

10.5   Prevention

10.5.1   Patient

Use of an adequately abrasive toothpaste, abstaining from smoking, the combination chlorhexidine wine/tea, and avoidance of the consumption of tooth-staining beverages, such as black tea, will prevent infiltrative staining and pseudo-discolorations. The African meswak (a chewing stick) is an effective alternative because of its abrasive silica content and calcium phosphate salts.[158] Workers exposed to industrial dusts should wear a mask.[157]

Anti-calculus dentifrices

These contain (see also Chapter 8, Table 8.2) pyrophosphate salts with copolymers or antibacterial zinc compounds (in particular zinc citrate) and reduce the formation of calculus by 30% and more.[72] The inhibitors include sodium metidronate (a diphosphonate), a copoly-

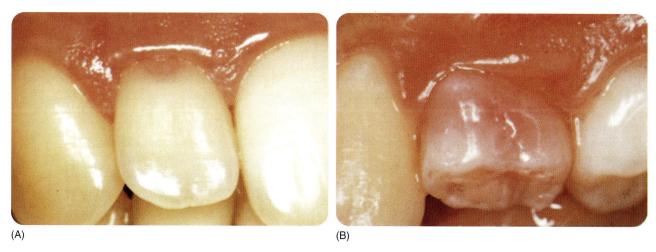

(A)   (B)

Figure 10.15 (A) A pink spot due to cervical resorption and (B) a red deciduous crown due to internal resorption that occurred shortly before shedding.

mer of polyvinylmethylether with malic acid.[224] Subgingival calculus formation is not inhibited.

Chewing gum

Yankell *et al.* reported a sustained reduction in chlorhexidine staining with chewing gum containing baking soda five times/day for 20 minutes;[386] the reduction in staining was also greater than with a placebo.[329] Biesbrock *et al.* found that sodium hexametaphosphate in gum prevented stain formation and facilitated stain removal and showed reasonable results when added to dentifrices.[34]

Whitening toothpastes

The term "whitening toothpaste" suggests a change in the tooth colour, but most of these toothpastes simply clean the tooth surfaces. Their stain removal ability depends on their content: the abrasives, the detergents, the chelating agents and calcium phosphate absorbents, and proteolytic enzymes. Some toothpastes contain oxygenating agents with the aim of changing the intrinsic tooth colour (see Section 10.6.3).

Toothpastes with surface-active ingredients (poly- and pyrophosphates) are effective stain removers. Sodium pyrophosphate may, however, cause tooth sensitivity. Use of dentifrices with tripolyphosphate reduces the amount of calcium available for the formation of calculus. Other toothpastes contain papain, a proteolytic enzyme that breaks down the salivary pellicle. *In vitro* studies have demonstrated that toothpaste brands are not equally effective, but all are better than brushing only with water.[274 341]

Interestingly, Kleber *et al.* showed that 30 minutes brushing in the laboratory with dentifrices containing the mild abrasive sodium bicarbonate (baking soda) altered the intrinsic hue of teeth more effectively than a dentifrice with silica and a dentifrice containing dicalcium phosphate.[196]

Bacterial affinity for enamel pre-brushed with two whitening toothpastes was greater than for enamel brushed with a regular toothpaste,[335] causing a rougher surface.

The chemical stain removal properties of 28 "whitening" toothpastes, a fluoride toothpaste, two oxidising mouthrinses (positive controls) and water were investigated by way of shaking externally stained acrylic specimens in standard test slurries. The cleaning ability of the products varied greatly. Two dentifrices outperformed all of the others and achieved 100% stain removal within 5 minutes.[317] The toothpastes abraded both enamel and dentine differently, in the order of a few micrometres.[357] Most of the 28 toothpastes affected the stain minimally.[317] Brushing with ineffective toothpastes may increase the severity of stains in the oral environment, due to calcification of organic stains.

Some toothpastes contain chelating agents (sodium citrate, citric acid). Their erosive action may remove the superficial (discoloured) layer from the tooth surface. Other newer anti-calculus and stain-inhibiting toothpastes have a dual action, i.e. stain prevention as well as stain removal, and are as protective as a sodium fluoride-containing toothpaste against caries. They also inhibit calculus formation as efficiently as a conventional calculus-control toothpaste.[269] One such multicare "whitening" dentifrice contains polypyrophosphate (=sodium hexametaphosphate) and stain-controlling ingredients.[132 380]

To induce the formation of stains, volunteers in one study rinsed three times daily with tea and once with chlorhexidine for a period of 3 weeks. Next, they brushed with the "whitening" toothpaste, which reduced the stains significantly more than with use of a regular dentifrice.[132] The whitening, calcium-control toothpaste performed at least comparably with a more abrasive dentifrice.[131] Pretreatment of powdered hydroxyapatite with another toothpaste containing sodium hexametaphosphate resulted in better desorbtion of tea components compared with a number of other dentifrices.[24]

Allen et al. reported that another toothpaste with a highly cleaning silica base,[9] a soluble pyrophosphate and sodium hexametaphosphate prevented and removed tea and chlorhexidine stains.

In other studies, thanks to the greater cleaning action of silica in one paste relative to the other, the extent of the stained area and the stain intensity following the use of the pastes was significantly different.[21 321] Allen et al. found that some whitening toothpastes were superior to the negative control paste.[9]

The two dentifrices described above do not contain bleaching agents. They remove and prevent (to some degree) extrinsic discolorations, due to their abrasive, enzyme (papain), phosphates and fat solvent content. Inhibition of external staining and stain removal by way of chemicals added to other dentifrices has also been investigated. A "whitening" dentifrice promoted rather than reduced stain formation, in spite of containing the surfactant sodium lauryl sulfate, which is known to reduce staining. Addition of polyvinylpyrrolidone (PVP) and/or sodium tripolyphosphate in a toothpaste has been shown to reduce the staining effect of rinsing with chlorhexidine/tea.[67 274]

In a study involving rinsing with either a slurry of a whitening toothpaste or a slurry of an experimental toothpaste containing PVP and sodium tripolyphosphate, or water, the experimental paste was superior to water, which in turn was superior to the whitening toothpaste that promoted the chlorhexidine/tea stain. It is not clear whether PVP or the sodium tripolyphosphate was effective.[67] Another similar rinsing study with a PVP toothpaste found that water and the "whitening" toothpaste were equally ineffective.[274]

The prophylactic abrasive perlite has been incorporated into one toothpaste. Perlite is a glassy silicate of volcanic origin, chemically inert and of neutral pH. The mildly abrasive and lightly polishing perlite possesses excellent stain removal qualities and does not scratch the tooth surface. Compared with standard silica-containing toothpastes, the perlite paste appeared superior for stain prevention and removal, while being equally abrasive.[185 186 237] Some whitening toothpastes contain a metal (titanium) oxide, which leaves behind a thin white layer that quickly disappears.

Electric powered toothbrushes

The brushing time with a manual toothbrush is on average 15 seconds per quadrant.[364] To compensate for short brushing times, an inefficient dentifrice or a rather persistent stain, one may brush for a longer period, which increases the number of brushing movements. The latter is more easily achieved with electric toothbrushes, especially the rotary-oscillating types.[306 307 366] Many studies have found that these are more effective than a manual toothbrush,[188 253 281 290 343 364 365] although some studies have not.[29] Research also shows that they do not cause more damage to the teeth and gingivae than manual toothbrushes.[146]

Differences exist between the cleaning ability of electric brushes, including the approximal surfaces.[23 303 364] In 2004, a Dutch judge ruled that the claims of marketing the best electric toothbrush could not be substantiated by the manufacturers.

Persulfate

After rinsing with chlorhexidine, a second rinse with 1% persulfate (Caroat[R]) might prevent tooth discoloration.[105]

Eriksen et al. found that use of peroxymonosulfate stabilised with a succinic acid/sodium hydroxide buffer (pH 5) led to a decrease in staining in dentitions severely stained with chlorhexidine from 50% to 5%. Those with heavily stained teeth consumed thrice as much tea (and smoked) than the individuals without staining. The experimental solution did not affect the action of chlorhexidine. The toxicity and other disadvantages of the solution were said to need further research,[105] but no follow-up publications could be found.

In another study, use of oxidising mouthrinses (sodium perborate-monohydrate) for 1 minute before rinsing with chlorhexidine (0.12%) for a fortnight reduced the proportion of stained tooth surfaces from 48% to 28%. Increased plaque inhibition and milder gingivitis was observed. The patients did not brush their teeth during the experimental period.[146] Oxidising mouthrinses remove external stains (tea + chlorhexidine) quite well.[317]

Other patient factors

Pulp necrosis due to caries may be prevented by timely dental visits. Trauma prevention is described in Chapter 9.

10.5.2   Dentist

Professional tooth cleaning, adequately and timely performed endodontic treatment, choice of adequate (endodontic) filling materials and so on, may prevent tooth discoloration. With a few exceptions, discolorations associated with a developmental cause cannot be prevented. One exception is fluorosis prevention by use of a correct fluoride regimen and if needed, the defluoridation of water. Another example is minocycline discoloration in young adults, which might be prevented by high doses of vitamin C, because this antioxidant blocks the pigment formation (a quinone ring),[44 55] but the dose of vitamin C required to achieve this needs further research.[63]

10.6   Treatment

In a sample of people asked to self-assess the colour of their teeth, many reported that the colour of their teeth was not normal and about 5% thought that their teeth

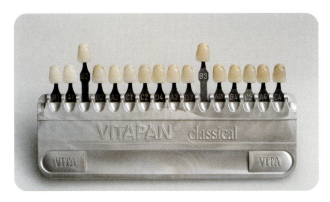

Figure 10.16 After bleaching, the tooth colour may change from, for instance, Vitapan C3 to C2, which is an improvement of seven shades.

were severely discoloured.[10] Joiner reported that a around one-third of a US and UK sample were dissatisfied with their tooth colour. Younger subjects in particular desired whiter teeth.[183] Exogenous pseudo-discolorations can be treated with prophylaxis. Superficially discoloured enamel may be removed. Intrinsic discolorations can be bleached by the dentist or the patient,[66 115 143 168 311] although some stains are quite resistant and cannot be removed completely.[168]

The tooth colour must be assessed at baseline and after bleaching. If, for example, the tooth colour prior to bleaching equals Vitapan shade tab C3 (rank order number 14) and after bleaching C2 (number 7), the tooth became seven shades lighter (Figure 10.16). Bleaching effects as measured with electronic devices such as spectrophotometers may be presented as Vita shades or altered values for b* and a* and L*. From the baseline values b_1, a_1 and L_1 and the values after bleaching, b_2, a_2 and L_2, the colour change ΔE is calculated using the equation:[53 130 183]

$$\Delta E = [L^*_1 - L^*_2) + (a^*_1 - a^*_2)(b^*_1 - b^*_2)]^{1/2}$$

If $\Delta E = 1$, half of the observers will not notice a colour change. Values of ΔE between 2 and 4 indicate small colour differences and $\Delta E > 4$ a clear difference.

Prior to bleaching, an appropriate bleaching method is selected, based on the diagnosis of the discoloration, but often several methods or combinations of methods can be used.

10.6.1 Polishing

Exogenous pseudo-discolorations may be removed with polishing. Pits, fissures, cracks, and so on will remain stained. A polishing cup with for instance the relatively very abrasive flour of pumice may leave grooves in the enamel surface that are 1–4 μm deep.[37]

10.6.2 Abrasion

The tooth colour improves when superficial stained enamel is removed. Brown fluorotic stains and Turner enamel stains often reside in the outer enamel and may be removed with fine diamond burs followed by polishing. Often less than one-tenth of a millimetre of enamel has to be removed; deeper reaching stains may be bleached afterwards. White fluorotic blemishes, opacities, decalcifications, and snow-capped lesions (Chapter 3) may be abraded, but bleaching the surrounding enamel masks the white colour.

Micro-abrasive(-erosive) technique
Alternatively, PREMA Compound (hydrochloric acid blended with fine silicon carbide particles) is rubbed over the discoloured areas with a latex applicator tip. Variations in the method exist: 18% phosphoric acid (rubber dam should be applied first) mixed with pumice is rubbed over the stain with a prophylactic cup, for 30–60 seconds, using a low-speed handpiece, and repeated 5–10 times. The enamel is rinsed clean for colour assessment between the applications.[76 77 78 79 80 81 276] To save time, one may start with a fine-grit diamond bur.

Finally, neutral 1% sodium fluoride gel is applied for 4 minutes, which is proven to make the surface caries-resistant. The results are good (Figure 10.17), unless the discolorations are deep. In a case of brown hypomature-tive hereditary amelogenesis imperfecta treated with this method, the tooth surfaces were healthy looking and shiny 4 years later.[15] The treatment, which needs to be performed just once, is stopped when:

- The wet enamel attains the desired colour
- The discoloured enamel surface becomes concave
- Dentine is exposed.

If the stains persist, one may bleach (or restore) the teeth.

10.6.3 External bleaching

Bleaching agents
Many bleaching agents exist, but because of side effects few are used in the clinical situation.

- *Hydrogen peroxide* (H_2O_2) is available as 25–45% gel (polyethylene glycol or propylene glycol) for professional use and in lower concentrations for at-home use. In higher concentration, the pH of H_2O_2 is about 4. Therefore manufacturers add sodium hydroxide (NaOH) or phosphates to the gels. H_2O_2 generates within 0–60 minutes, unstable reactive radicals (H·, O·, OH·, HO$_2$) and ions (OH$^-$, OOH$^-$).[143 239] The most powerful radical, perhydroxyl (·OH$_2$), exists in the free

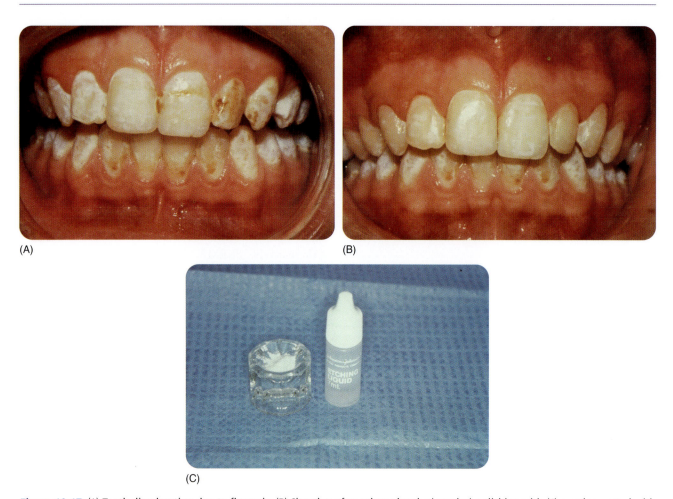

Figure 10.17 (A) Tooth discoloration due to fluorosis. (B) Situation after micro-abrasive(-erosive) polishing with (C) pumice wetted with phosphoric acid.

form in an alkaline environment, which is another reason to raise the pH. The radicals reach the dentine (and pulp) via enamel. They oxidise (break down) and thereby discolour pigmented carbon rings, cyclic conjugated chemicals and unsaturated double bonds of organic molecules, and reduce metallic oxides (e.g. Fe_2O_3 becomes colourless FeO).[143]

- *Carbamide peroxide* (CP) consists of urea + hydrogen peroxide ($H_2NCONH_2.H_2O_2$) in an unstable gel (glycerine, polyacrylic acid carbopol and carboxypolymethylene, pH 5–7.5). When CP comes in contact with saliva, about one-third vol% becomes free H_2O_2; this reaction occurs rapidly the first 2 hours and gradually slows down. Ten per cent CP is equivalent to about 3.5% H_2O_2 and 6.5% urea, which is broken down into ammonia and carbon dioxide. Carbopol adheres to the teeth and slows down the delivery of the active oxygen because the gel slowly dissolves in the saliva. Concentrations of 10–22% CP are available for use at home (in the USA 10% is approved) and for in-office bleaching concentrations of about 35% are available.

- *Sodium perborate* (*trihydrate*), $2 \times [NaBO_2(OH_2)]4H_2O$ powder ≈ about 10% H_2O_2, is used mainly for internal bleaching and acts slowly, but is long acting. Once it is wetted with water, the pH becomes alkaline.
- *Hydrocarbonoxoborate* is meant for at-home use. A recently marketed gel is non-peroxide in-office *chlordioxide* (CLO_2; pH 3–5), which is nowadays used as an ingredient in a whitening toothpaste.

It should be noted that from 1 November 2012, a new European directive (2011/84/EU; http://eur-lex.europa.eu/LexUriServ/LexUriServ.do?uri=OJ:L:2011:283:0036:0038:EN:PDF) will come into effect. This directive clearly indicates the concentrations of bleaching agents, which will be permissible for use from that date onwards both in the dental office and at home by patients in Europe and UK (e.g. H_2O_2 and carbamide peroxide maximum strength 6% and 16%, respectively). Therefore dentists practising in the Europe and the UK should refer to this directive when reading this section of the book and providing treatment or advice for home treatment for their patients.

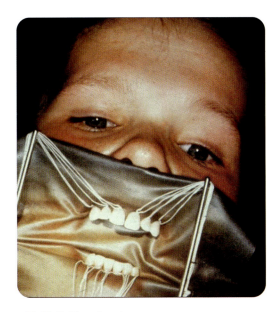

Figure 10.18 Rubber dam in use.

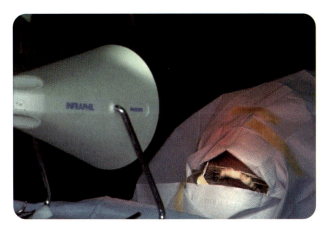

Figure 10.19 Patient protection during treatment involving heating 30% H_2O_2 with an Infraphil lamp.

Bleaching agents also include: sodium fluoride (anti-demineralisation), potassium nitrate (analgesic), iron (catalyst), amorphous calcium phosphate (against pain) or casein phosphopeptide – amorphous calcium phosphate (which attaches to the pellicle and plaque and releases on an acidic challenge, calcium and phosphate ions that counteracts demineralisation and promotes remineralisation), water (against drying out the enamel) and activators (in-office bleaches). Other chemicals promote penetration of the at-home bleach and better-controlled activation.

Power-bleaching

Prior to in-office bleaching with lamps and highly concentrated H_2O_2 and CP gels, the gingiva is protected by application of rubber dam (Figure 10.18) or paint-on dam. The bleach is mixed with an activator before use, and the gel bleaches the teeth after application. However, light from a lamp promotes the dissociation of the bleach and shortens the treatment time. Some brands require the use of brand-specific lamps, others will react to common curing lights (such as halogen light and LEDs), formerly a red light (Figure 10.19). The benefit of using lamps continues to be doubtful;[39][311] in some studies, the use of lamps improved (somewhat) the bleaching results,[226][263][336] but the efficacy of using a lamp depends on the brand of the bleach employed.[226]

With the CO_2 laser, addition of colorant to the bleaching gel is not necessary. The argon laser emits blue light that acts on a photochemically sensitive gel and has been found to be effective; remarkably 35% carbamide peroxide in one brand appeared more efficacious than 37% carbamide peroxide in another brand.[59] A few authors are

not in favour of the laser-bleach technique, but the argon laser performs well.[311]

Nowadays, sodium perborate is also used in external bleaching, as is a gel that contains chlorine dioxide (ClO_2) and is activated with an LED lamp or plasma arc lamp. (ClO_2 is slower to activate but remains active longer than H_2O_2, but it may be mixed with 35% H_2O_2 for optimal action.) The gel is commonly applied several times per session (about three-quarters of an hour) and is briefly activated with light from the lamp every so often.

De Silva Gotardi reported that patients with baseline colours C2 to B4 were satisfied after three to four visits. The teeth became two to four Vita shades lighter per visit.[92] Others have also reported that more than one visit is needed to get an optimal result.[142][202] Another, comparative studies have established improvements ranging from 2 to 4 shades with different bleaches and lamps;[226] but improvements of 6–9[124][263] and 10–15 shades have also been reported.[159][336] Drying out of the teeth makes them temporarily lighter (whiter), which is why the change in colour should be evaluated 1 week after the treatment.

Enamel stains and discoloured dentine can be treated with power-bleaching (Figure 10.20), but people with more or less normal tooth colour also desire whiter teeth. The patient should be informed about the possibility of pain, which usually lasts for 1 day and occasionally for a few days. Prior to the treatment, the patient may take analgesics; local anaesthesia should not be used.[147][259] Some observations about power-bleaching are warranted.

- Power-bleaching of vital teeth with a large pulp cavity or denuded dentine (but the latter is highly questionable) or with leakage along restorations is contraindicated.
- Because 30–35% H_2O_2 burns the gingiva (and skin), a rubber dam should be used, although the pain is

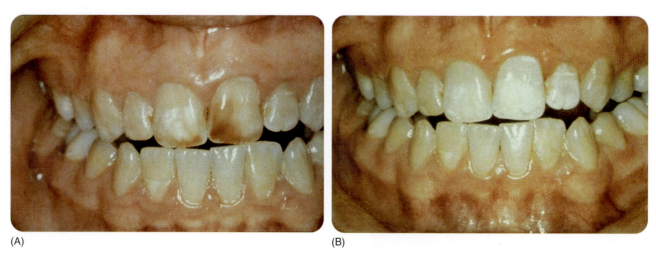

(A)   (B)

Figure 10.20 (A) Before and (B) after power bleaching.

temporary. Adequate steps should be taken to protect the eyes, skin and clothes of both the patient and the dental team.

- A moderate tetracycline stain requires up to six treatment sessions whereas a light stain requires three (or fewer) sessions. Yellow and brown tetracycline discolorations respond better than those with banding. Tetracycline released from the skeleton into the blood circulation may cause a relapse.
- Fluoride must be applied after bleaching.
- Because the enamel is more porous after bleaching with an acidic bleach, discolouring agents (such as tea, wine, coal tar) are best avoided for some weeks.
- An alternative to power-bleaching is slower at-home bleaching.

Bleaching in the waiting room
Patients can be treated without a lamp in the waiting room, with 35% CP applied in a custom tray prior to (or in lieu of) at-home bleaching or to restore previously bleached tooth colour following relapse. The tray (Figure 10.21) is made from soft ethylvinylacetate using a stone cast.[164] The surfaces to be bleached are blocked out on the cast with light-cured resin before the tray is vacuum formed. The scalloped tray extends to the gingival margin, or alternatively extends 2–3 mm onto the gingival to assure maximum retention.[166]

The bleach is warmed under hot water and the reservoirs in the tray are refilled every 30–45 minutes. The total time required is up to 120 minutes, if necessary followed by at-home bleaching. Severe discolorations are preferably treated with power-bleaching, but at-home bleaching under supervision seems at the least equally effective, certainly in case of tetracycline discoloration, if these have not already been internally bleached.

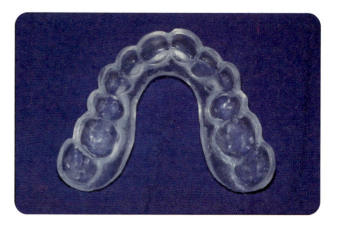

Figure 10.21 Custom-made disposable bleaching tray.

External at-home bleaching, supervised by the dentist
Custom tray-based systems
At home, the patient can fill the reservoirs in a custom tray using a syringe with 10% CP gel (or higher concentration). The system is called "nightguard" because the tray was intended for use while sleeping (about 8 hours), but it is often used while the patient is awake; a refill within three to four hours may be beneficial, because then the salivary flow is greater than at night. In one study, remnants of the active ingredient of a CP gel were collected from the tray and teeth after intervals ranging from 15 seconds to 10 hours. After 15 seconds, 87% of the gel was recovered, after 2 hours more than 50% was recovered, and after 10 hours 10% was recovered, but the amount recovered each time varied considerably by brand.[238] Some gels contain ingredients that promote penetration of the gel into the tooth and control its activ-

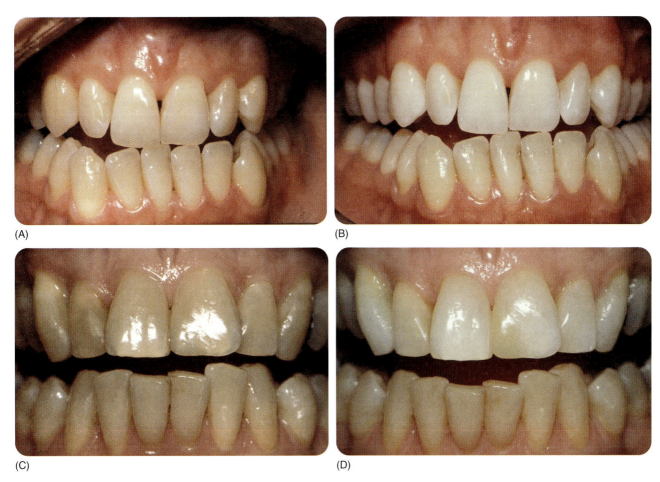

Figure 10.22 (A,B) Teeth before and after bleaching. (C,D) Another patient before and after bleaching; note the unchanged colour of the composite restoration in the left maxillary central incisor.

ity.[229] The pH of the gels ranges from about 5.5 to 7 or more.

The patients are asked to visit the office every week. Generally the results are acceptable (Figure 10.22A,B) after 2–4 weeks. Within a few days the enamel may become splotchy and unevenly white, presumably due to local differences in the enamel structure; such colour differences gradually disappear. [110] The most pronounced effect is seen the first 2 weeks. In Fasarano's study, after 6 weeks, 97% of fluorosis and 100% of discolorations related to ageing,[248] were effectively treated.[110] Nicotine staining is more tenacious.[161 240]

Tetracycline stains require bleaching longer times, depending on the location and colour of the stain. Light tetracycline discolorations confined to the incisal three-quarters and discoloration without banding respond quicker than other tetracycline stains, as has been discussed above. In one study, an improvement was seen in 75% of tetracycline discolorations.[165] Matis found that after 6 months at-home bleaching of tetracycline discoloration, 91% of the patients were satisfied.[240] In another

group of patients the most tenacious discoloration required 1213 treatment hours, but in other patients less time was needed.[163] In such situations one may consider the more rapid internal bleaching technique,[2] but this will require "unnecessary" endodontic treatment first.

Niederman found that neither the time (overnight versus <4 hours/day) nor the treatment duration had a significant effect, but the brand of the bleach did have a significant effect (on the average, an overall lightening effect of 5.9 shades): mean changes in shade guide units by brand varied between 11.4 and 3.6 shades. Some brands act slower than others.[261] Browning found about 5 shades improvement with low-sensitivity whiteners.[51]

Yellow spots left after micro-abrasive removal of brown fluorotic stains have been treated with professional external and supervised at-home bleaching.[77 85 164 194 244] Good results have been reported in cases of dentinogenesis imperfecta.[82]

External stains must not be bleached. Caries and leaking restorations should be treated prior to bleaching. Enamel with cracks and denuded dentine are not bleached (and pain is not more frequent in such cases) and neither are teeth with a large pulp cavities as mentioned above. Composite and porcelain restorations cannot be bleached (Figure 10.22C,D) and may need to be replaced 1–2 weeks after bleaching of teeth with such restorations (see Section 10.6.6).

Whitening strips

Whitening strips are flexible, polyethylene strips coated with 10–13% H_2O_2, and are prescribed for at-home use under supervision. They are indicated for difficult discolorations like tetracycline stains. The strip is applied to the labial surfaces of the anterior teeth by aligning the straight edge with the gingiva and folding the other back over the incisal edges (Figure 10.23). The strips are left *in situ* for 30 minutes and are applied twice a day for 2–3 weeks. If the teeth become sensitive, the strips may be used once a day or the treatment may have to be stopped.

Many reports about whitening strips are to be found in several supplements of the *Compendium for Continuing Education in Dentistry* (years 2000, 2001, 2003), sponsored by the manufacturer. Some researchers involved in the investigations of the strips have had competing interests, for instance Gerlach,[129–135] but all articles were peer-reviewed. Generally teeth became two Vita shades lighter,[133] but in one publication, a mean change of 5.5 shades was reported, with a quarter of the sample showing an average of 8 shades.[135] The strips gave an improvement of 6.6 shades of tetracycline discoloration within 2 months.[203] Patients with yellow teeth, in particular younger patients, benefit most from using these strips.

Over-the-counter products

Over-the-counter bleaching systems have been subjected to few clinical trials, with the exception of whitening strips and paint-on gels. These trials are often performed

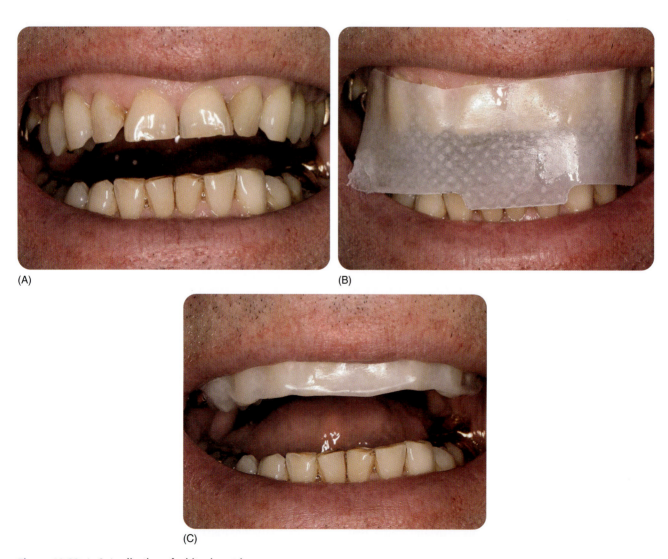

(A)

(B)

(C)

Figure 10.23 A–C Application of whitening strips.

by paid researchers and published in dental journal supplements sponsored by the manufacturers.

In the European Union (EU), products with concentrations >0.1% H_2O_2 belong to the category of medical devices and thus may not be sold to the public, which will not be changed in the near future. In the USA, over-the-counter bleaching products may contain up to 6% H_2O_2. Disadvantages of commercial products include, first, the type of discoloration is not diagnosed, and second, people may bleach the teeth for too long.

Acid/rinse/toothpaste

The so-called three-step bleaching systems had been particularly popular in the USA. The typical procedure was as follows: the labial enamel was "conditioned" with acetic acid or citric acid (pH 2.6–3.8) for 15 seconds; dabbed with cotton wool soaked with a 3–6% H_2O_2 solution or gel for 1–2 minutes; and finally the teeth were brushed with a titanium dioxide toothpaste, which left behind a temporary white pigment on the tooth. The procedure resulted in loss of dentine and cementum after 8 weeks comparable with that lost after 6 months of tooth brushing. A loss of even 50% of the enamel was reported.[371] In *in vitro* experiments, the enamel was more severely affected after immersion for 1 hour in a commercial product than in a supervised agent. After 15 hours of soaking in some products, the enamel became more porous with an altered surface.[36] The American Dental Association has advised against the use of these products. Long-term use might also damage the pulp.

Commercial trays

Presently, some commercial tray-based bleaching systems are available, containing peroxides in different concentrations, flavouring agents, desensitising agents and other modifications. For instance, a 10% CP gel can be used in a stock tray ("boil-and-bite" tray), sometimes with a pre-bleaching toothpaste (sodium fluoride whitening paste) and a post-bleaching rinse. The trays fit poorly, may leak and irritate the gingivae mechanically, and may exert "orthodontic" forces.

Whitening strips and wraps

Over-the-counter whitening strips with about 5% H_2O_2 are available for non-pathological discolorations. Their advantages over the custom-tray systems are: shorter contact time, ease of use and no need for tray fabrication. The strips allow bleaching to be done while carrying out daily activities. The Whitening Strip System consists of a dual-action whitening/anti-calculus toothpaste. The newer whitening *wraps* contain 8% H_2O_2 and resemble the strips to a degree. According to Matis, the wraps used for 30 minutes, 7 days long, lightened the wraps the teeth 10 shades and the strips 7.7 shades.[241]

Paint-on-gel (CP or H_2O_2)

Over-the-counter gels in jars are also available, containing 18% CP or 5.9% and 8.7% H_2O_2. The colourless gel is painted on the teeth with a brush, like nail polish on nails, and allowed to dry for 30 seconds. The gel adheres quite well to the teeth and dissolves slowly. It can be used for both intrinsic and extrinsic stains. Some research has shown that after treatment twice a day for 2 weeks, teeth can become almost four shades lighter,[126] similar to the effect of using 18% CP in trays,[256] but Cronin reported that the product has little effect (1 shade change versus 2.6 shades change with whitestrips).[83] Because the painting brush is reused and stored in the jar with the gel, there is a risk of microbial contamination and breakdown of the gel. A supplement of the *Journal of Dentistry* (2004) sponsored by Unilever dealt with an improved "format" of the paint-on gel, which is supplied as disposable cotton bud applicators. In one study, compared with a silica-sodium fluoride toothpaste, the paint-on procedure led to a significantly greater change in the mean Vita shade score.[187] One new product in this category is the "on the go" whitening pen.

Whitening toothpastes

Some toothpastes include oxygenating agents, often in low concentration; there is one toothpaste with 18% CP. They may prevent and remove pseudo-discolorations, but significant bleaching seems unlikely.[256] A 0.4 shade improvement after 6 months has been reported,[256] assumedly because of the short contact time with the teeth. Prolonged daily use is not recommended.

Comparison of some bleaching procedures

Gerlach found that 6% H_2O_2 gel in a tray had a poorer whitening effect than whitening strips and caused pain more frequently (22% versus 13%, respectively).[134] A 16% CP equivalent bleached more effectively within 21 days than 6.5 and 7.5% H_2O_2 strips, with less (mostly mild) toothache and gingival irritation. The tooth contact times of the systems are different.[220 229] Kugel reported that whitening strips performed better than a tray system with 10% CP and required 14 versus 28 bleaching hours. In another study, whitening strips used for 2 months for moderate to severe tetracycline staining improved the appearance of the teeth by 6.6 shade units and a custom-tray with 19% CP 4.1 shades.[203] Other studies have shown comparable results and the strips outperformed some over-the-counter systems.[129 130] Whitening strips performed better than wraps,[241] and a 6% whitestrip had better results than a 18% carbamide paint-on gel.[83] Also, 10% H_2O_2 whitestrips had similar effects to 10% carbamide peroxide used in trays.[155] Table 10.4 shows a comparison of three bleach systems and Table 10.5 shows the relationship between bleaching times and the colour change produced. Auschill found that in order to make

Table 10.4 Time required to lighten canines by six Vita shades[196]

Commercial product	Bleaching agent	Length of session	Total hours required Mean (SD)
Opalescence	30% H_2O_2/lamp	15 minutes	0.8 (0.1)
Whitening strips	6% H_2O_2 gel	30 minutes, twice a day	18.0 (3.2)
Opalescence	10% CP/at-home	8 hours/night	50.7 (16.4)

Table 10.5 Colour change (ΔE) of the enamel and underlying dentine after several bleaching sessions with different bleaching methods[381]

Commercial product	Bleaching agent	Time (hours)	Effect (ΔE) Enamel	Dentine
Opalescence	10% CP	80	6.8	13.2
Opalescence	15% CP	40	5.6	12.4
Opalescence Quick	35% CP	2	8.3	13.5
Opalescence Extra Boost	35% H_2O_2	2	7.2	12.2
Rapid White	$NaClO_2$	3	2.2	3.0
Whitening strips	6% H_2O_2	10	2.3	2.4

teeth 6 shades lighter, power-bleaching with a 30% H_2O_2 gel required 0.8 hours, 5,3 % H_2O_2 whitestrips 16 hours and a 10% carbamide peroxide at-home gel 50.7 hours.[20] However, in a split-mouth study, bleaching at-home for 14 days with a 10% carbamide peroxide performed better than power-bleaching twice.[392] Wiegand established that a 35% carbamide peroxide and a 35% H_2O_2 gel performed equally well (within 2 hours) and that lower concentration gels required much more time (80 and 40 hours with 10% and 15% carbamide peroxide, respectively,) and 6% H_2O_2 whitestrips required 10 hours.[381]

10.6.4 Internal bleaching

Since external bleaching of stained dentine is followed by relapse, it has been suggested that discoloured dentine must be directly de-stained.[16] In the 1960s, sodium perborate powder wetted with water was enclosed in the pulp chamber for several days ("walking bleach"). Compared with external bleaching, the method required less chairside time,[119] was more effective, and had good initial[16 113 174 177] and longer-lasting results.[13] Internal bleaching is the method of choice when endodontic treatment of a discoloured tooth has been performed or is necessary.[1 2] To avoid the use of veneers, the "walking bleach" method might be used for severe tetracycline stains in teeth that otherwise do not need endodontics.

The procedure is as follows. The pulp chamber is opened and, after checking the endodontic filling, and any pulpal remnants and coloured material such as the endo-

dontic cement are removed using a bur. Discoloured dentine is left *in situ*. The root canal filling is removed to 2–3 mm past the cemento-enamel junction; if the filling is not removed to this level, the cervical part of the crown will not be bleached due to the orientation of the S-shaped tubules (Figure 10.24). When a denuded root has to be bleached, more of the canal filling is removed. To prevent leakage in apical direction, exposed gutta-percha is sealed with a layer of, for instance, a (resin-modified) glass ionomer cement. When due to gingival recession de-staining of the root is required, the root canal filling is removed up to 3 mm beyond the gingival level. It does not appear necessary, as was previously thought, to etch the internal dentine with phosphoric acid and clean with dehydrating alcohol.[58 138 152 176]

Wetted sodium perborate (toxic to reproduction) is enclosed in the pulp chamber. The temporary filling should provide an adequate seal (without any risk of leakage). After 3–4 days the sodium perborate paste is refreshed. The procedure is repeated until the tooth is somewhat whiter in colour than the neighbouring teeth, because of a possible colour relapse. Wetting of sodium perborate with H_2O_2 has been proposed, but the low pH introduces the risk of cervical resorption, but 3% gives good results.[296]

H_2O_2 (30%) has been shown to de-stain more effectively than sodium perborate.[234] Other commercial agents include Enzymatic Cleaner (amylase, trypsin and lipase), HiClean (composition unknown), Liquid Iron Chelator and Desferal (also an iron chelator). In studies these products reduced blood staining inefficiently, with the latter two even increasing the intensity of the stain.[234]

Tetracycline-stained teeth attained a more natural gloss and colour after insertion of sodium perborate with 10% CP in the final treatment session.[8] Recently, Teixeira inserted 37% CP instead of sodium perborate into the pulp cavity on a weekly basis; a satisfactory tooth colour was obtained after 4 weeks,[342] but the advantage of this approach is not clear.

The "walking bleach" method is more efficient and effective in younger than older people, because of greater diffusion through the wider dentinal tubules in younger people.[56 113] The results and prognosis of internal bleaching with sodium perborate are quite good: in 10% the results were not acceptable, in about 25% they were acceptable and in 65% the treatment was deemed a success.[174] Waterhouse also found an initial success rate of 60%.[375] Internal bleaching of dark yellow teeth required more sessions and bleached less successfully than grey teeth.[1] Corrosion products of amalgam restorations in the dentine cannot be bleached.

Internal-external bleaching

In this method, the patients applies CP in a tray to the labial surfaces and on the palatal side in the open pulp

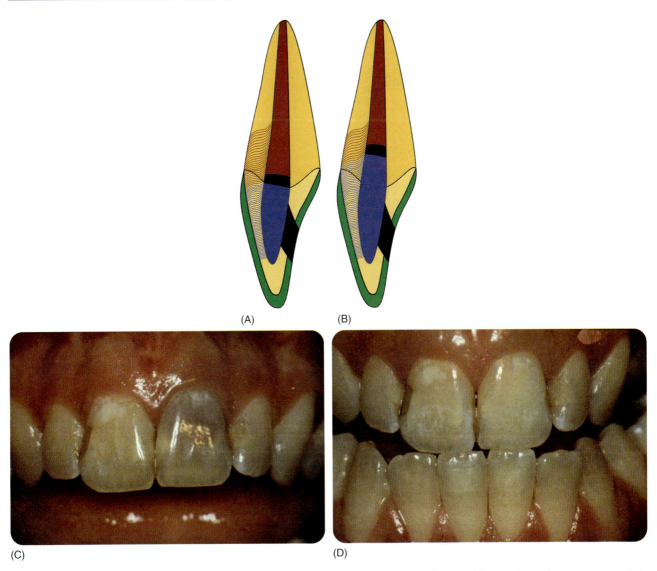

(A)   (B)

(C)   (D)

Figure 10.24 (A) The root canal filling (red) has not been sufficiently removed to allow the bleaching product (blue) to penetrate into those dentinal tubules running from the root canal to the cervical crown. (B) Correct amount of root canal filling removed, allowing the cervical enamel to be bleached. A non-vital tooth before (C) and after (D) internal bleaching ("walking bleach"). This method can be used to bleach tenacious tetracycline discolorations such as those shown in Figure 10.6E.

chamber. During the day, the patient should seal the palatal opening with a cotton pellet. Alternatively, the patient is asked to fill the pulp chamber with CP using a syringe and to change the solution every 2 hours. Next, the patient inserts a custom-made splint to retain the bleach; between the bleach sessions a cotton pledget is inserted to prevent ingress of debris. Mild/moderate discolorations commonly require five to eight applications.[221] However, a pulp chamber left open for several days introduces the risk of leakage along the root canal filling.

10.6.5   Colour relapse

With the *micro-abrasive(-erosive) technique* all stained tissue is removed, making relapse unlikely.

The colour change after *at-home bleaching* may remain stable for 6 months to 3 years or more,[82 128 165 212 238 261 298 324 382] even 25 years.[164 168] The efficacy of the method is 98%, unless the teeth had tetracycline stains, although extended treatment times often lighten these teeth.[211] In one study, after 90 months, 60% of patients who had bleached tetracycline discolorations at home reported an incomplete relapse, but only few requested re-treatment.[214] A slight darkening of tetracycline stained teeth was seen 54 months after treatment with 10% carbamide peroxide during 6 months in 2 of 10 patients.[210] Relapse of staining has also been reported after 22 weeks in one-third of the patients.[214] In some cases, considerable relapse was seen within 1 week, even as much as a return of the original colour; thereafter the colour remained stable.[298]

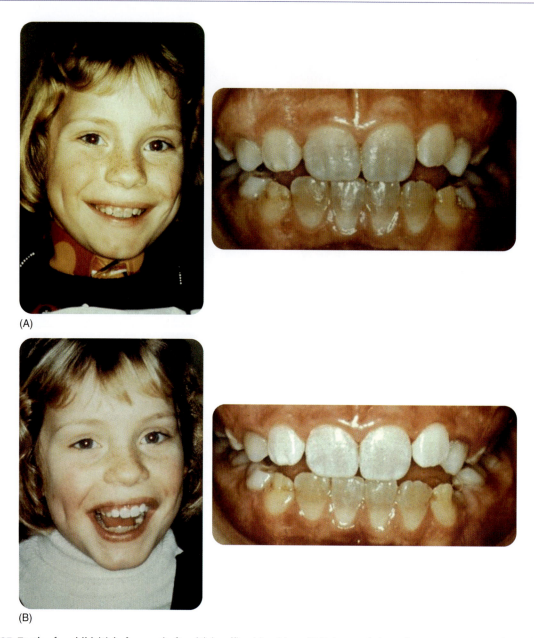

Figure 10.25 Teeth of a child (A) before and after (B) in-office bleaching. (C) Relapse of the colour some 20 years later. (D,E) Colour relapse in an internally bleached tooth. (E) The white spot is due to the cement shining through the enamel. All the local dentine was removed because the opening was made incorrectly.

Two-thirds of the patients were still satisfied with the tooth colour after 3 years and some 40% after 7 years.[211] Of a small sample treated with 10% CP, 60% reported no obvious relapse after 7 years, but the rest were re-treated.[214] Another study reported colour stability of 43% after 9–12 years.[168] Colour relapse has also been reported after H_2O_2 bleaching (Figure 10.25A–C) and internal bleaching (Figure 10.25D,E).

Haywood *et al.* found that 1–3 years after *power-bleaching*, the procedure had to be repeated.[164] Following

relapse within the first week after bleaching,[298] the color remained stable.[128] Zekonius found after 6 weeks a decrease of about 3 ΔE units.[392] Wiegand established that ΔE 1 year after bleaching fell from 13 to 12, the value of ΔL^* became almost equal to the base value, but according to Δb^* the teeth were still less yellow.[392]

Use of the *walking bleach method* improved discolorations caused by endodontic sealers, but relapse has been observed after 6 months.[375] In Feiglin's study, 1 year after walking bleach with H_2O_2 (heated/unheated) and sodium

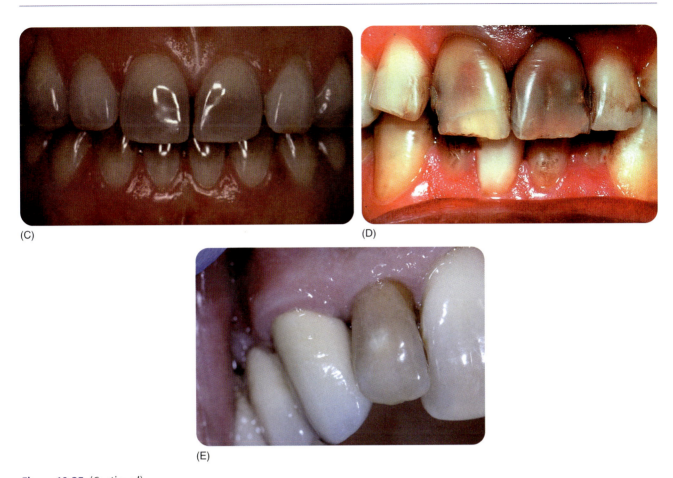

(C)

(D)

(E)

Figure 10.25 (*Continued*)

perborate, about half of the teeth become darker, and this proportion rose after 2 and 6 years; yet the patients were still satisfied.[113] A combination of the walking bleach with power-bleaching has also been found to be successful.[172] In other study, teeth that became 14 shades lighter, were still 13 shades lighter two years later,[91] but Wiegand found that ΔE fell from 16 to 10 within 1 year.[382] Four of 20 tetracycline-discoloured teeth had to be re-treated within 5–15 years.[3] Retreatment was needed for 10% of another sample within 1–2 years and 40% within 8 years.[121] In a sample of internally bleached teeth, on the one hand, 20% showed an unacceptable relapse within a period of 3 years,[174] but on the other hand, after 5–15 years the success rate was still 90%.[130 139] Re-treatment every 2 years may be required.[110] Leakage around fillings, which allows ingress of bacteria and staining agents, underlies failure of treatment. The more difficult a tooth is to bleach, the more likely is a colour relapse,[177] but opinions in this regard differ.[16] However, 6 years after bleaching of tetracycline staining, good results were reported by Aldecoa.[8] When the teeth become darker again, the whitening procedure may be repeated; this usually requires less time than the first treatment. Within

1–5 years after internal bleaching, in 50–65% of one sample, the colour was not considered satisfactory any more,[121] but others have reported similar success rates after 8 years' follow-up.[8 16]

10.6.6   Side effects

Enamel

The bleaching products may alter the physical properties and chemical composition, and affect the organic[190] and inorganic components of the enamel, but reports are conflicting, even when the same bleaches have been studied. The severity of the alterations depends on the concentration of the bleaching agent, the pH, treatment times and the product brand. Changes in enamel microhardness and roughness (erosion) caused by, in general, low concentrations of carbamide peroxide and hydrogen peroxide are absent or minimal, superficial and invisible to the naked eye.[35 36 39 54 59 69 74 106 108 162 187 189 190 212 213 223 230 243 248 252 265 275 278 291 322 388] Carbopol seems to have a role here.[31] Joiner concluded after reviewing the literature that neither the morphology, the subsurface microhardness or the chemical composition, nor the ultrastructure of the enamel was altered by bleaching.[184] However, somewhat more serious consequences have also been reported,[97 291 292] such as a decrease in the subsurface microhardness and strength (MPA) of the enamel with consequently an increase in wear,[90] but Cadenaro did not observe an increased roughness of the enamel after application of 38% hydrogen peroxide or 35% carbamide peroxide.[54] In contrast, use of acidic hydrogen peroxide bleaches (pH often between 4 and 5) and acidic 10% carbamide peroxide considerably decrease the enamel microhardness, both on the surface and in the deeper layers, lower its fracture resistance, and lead to development of deep pores and erosion, and may also alter the enamel chemical composition.[17 18 19 62 90 215 217 242 301] Therefore, patients must be advised against consuming wine and tea and using chlorhexidine for a period of 1–2 weeks, due to the higher risk of re-coloration. It is worth remembering that most experiments are performed in the laboratory, often using artificial saliva and bovine teeth, and the changes *in vivo* will be less profound because of the positive action of saliva. Generally speaking, H_2O_2 seems to affect the microhardness more than CP, but carbopol causes demineralisation;[32] among others, Da Silva reported a decrease in the tensile strength due to all bleaching products.[90] A paint-on gel (8.75% with phosphoric acid) was found to lower the microhardness by some 25%.[215] Urea may degrade the organic matrix.[190] Exaggerated bleaching (and high concentrated H_2O_2) makes the enamel unnaturally white and lustreless.

Dentine

Bleaches, both carbamide peroxide and hydrogen peroxide up to 35%, applied to the enamel may affect the organic due to urea[190 293 391] and inorganic components[39 62 257 243] of dentine, but again study results with respect to the microhardness and fracture resistance of dentine are not in agreement.[31 61 223 340] The microhardness of the dentine may decrease slightly, which is most probably clinically irrelevant.[242 243] A bleach applied on the tooth surface with pH 3.7 decreased the microhardness of the enamel as well as of dentine; five other bleaches with either H_2O_2 or CP of different concentration did not.[18] Effects on cementum have been little studied, but it is reported to become pitted and thinner.[107 294]

Cervical resorption

The risk of cervical resorption, which develops some years after internal bleaching, is non-existent,[228] unless H_2O_2 in concentrations higher than a few per cent is used.[121 148 156 169 170 200 205 206 251 352] The resorption seems related to the presence of free radicals on the root surface. Is has been stated the resorption develops because of a foreign body reaction[87 245] or because in contrast with sodium perborate H_2O_2 promotes the adherence of macrophages.[14 228]

Pulp

An increase in pulpal temperature during power-bleaching, ranging from 7 °C to 13 °C, may cause pain and endanger the pulp. The dental hard tissues transfer heat moderately. An excessive high temperature causes aspiration of the odontoblasts into the dentinal tubules and their destruction, and induces tertiary dentine formation and pulpal inflammation.[115] In an animal experiment a pulpal temperature rise of 16.5 °C damaged the pulps irreversibly.[390] In humans, a rise of 7–13 °C had no effect.[26] Some lamps (halogen, plasma, infrared, CO_2 laser) may increase the intrapulpal temperature by 18–39°C.[25 226] The activity of pulpal enzymes can be reduced by the rise in temperature.[42 43 141 186 278] However, lamps are used for too short a time to cause such damaging effects.

Free radicals appeared to cause damage in cell cultures,[151 355] and therefore H_2O_2 and CP may, in principle, cause infection in the pulp and may affect pulpal enzymes, but the amounts that seep into the pulp are small, in particular from a paint-on gel.[184] The higher the amount of carbopol in CP bleaches, the greater is the amount of peroxide (up to 2.5 µg) found in the pulp,[16 43 73 218 345] but free radicals are normally present in the body.

Bleaching at home frequently evokes toothache. Widely diverging prevalences are reported, from 10% to 78%, a few days after starting the bleach procedure or between bleaching sessions.[49 50 51 125 140 150 163 164 165 166 201 209 212 229 240 250 263 272 287 324 340] The transient pain is in most cases moderate, but some people abstain from further treatment. Toothache may depend on the percentage of CP or H_2O_2 in the product being used and its brand, the concentration of the bleach and the carbopol concentration, the frequency and duration of the gel application, and the number of times the gel is reapplied. For example, 17% carbamide peroxide caused more pain than 10%.[201] Teeth already sensitive prior to bleaching are a risk factor for pain.[209] Children may experience severe toothache, because of their dentine is still thin. The amount of active oxygen reaching the pulp may be a factor determining the risk for toothache. A product with a lower concentration of CP gel (5%) with potassium nitrate has been marketed, but tooth sensitivity has still also been reported. Pain depends to a degree, on the presence of potassium nitrate (KNO_3).[50 51] Movement of the fluid in the dentinal tubules of denuded dentine causes pain (Chapter 6). However, such a mechanosensitive process does not occur after the bleach is applied to the enamel. Markowitz hypothesized that oxidising substances may activate the intradental nerves via a chemosensitive ion channel (TRPA1). TRAP1 has indeed been observed in the pulpal nerves.[235]

Gingival (and skin) irritation and throat sensitivity

Several studies have shown that various brands of CP do not damage ("burn") the gingiva,[155 392] although others have reported damage,[209] as with whitening strips.[155] Gin-

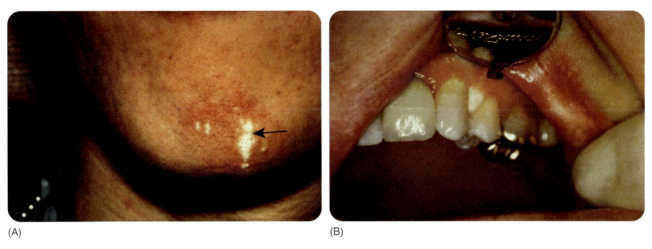

Figure 10.26 Caustic effect of a bleaching gel (A) spilling on the skin and (B) leaking through an incorrectly placed rubber dam.

gival pain may occur without clinical symptoms,[209] but paper-white gingival stains signals gingival damage and is associated with pain. A beneficial effect is claimed on gingivitis and plaque scores.[77 126 212 218 277] However, in a meta-analysis no significant differences were found in the plaque index and gingivitis scores between the bleached and control groups.[261] Although bleaches are reported not to damage the gingiva,[128] erythema and oedema do occasionally occur,[324] but these signs are short-lasting, as is the pain. More serious damage involves vacuolisation and formation of vesicles, and ultimately gingival destruction.[352] Thus power-bleaching requires use of rubber dam (although even then leakage between the dam and the teeth may lead to pain)[392] and bleaching in the waiting room (35% CP) requires careful removal of excess bleach material (Figure 10.26). Throat and tongue sensitivity has been reported,[50 51 164] but is less likely than tooth and gingival sensitivity.

Composites
The attachment of a new composite restoration to a tooth that has been bleached will be temporarily decreased,[27 33 84 90 117 127 164 250 268 320 325 347 348 349 350] due to peroxide that remains behind with the use of carbamide peroxide or H_2O_2, but not with sodium perborate.[317] This is why following bleaching, restoration with composite needs to be postponed by about 7–14 days, tending towards 14 days if the restoration involves the dentine,[27 33 350 358] after which the peroxide is no longer present,[27 90 117 320] unless katalase is applied.[90 268] Several investigators have reported discontinuous contact between the bonding agent and the tooth, with no penetration (tags) of the bonding agent.[250 348 350] Some, however, blame structural changes in the dental tissues instead,[189 268] and yet again others have denied a decrease in attachement.[75 258 352] Reports on increased microleakage around composite restorations

after at-home bleaching[28] are conflicting and are based on *in vitro* experiments.

Existing composite (and compomer) restorations might become whiter[77] due to changes occurring within the resin matrix. Moreover, their surface and that of glass ionomer and porcelain restorations may become softer and rough,[57 208 356 387] although some researchers did not (almost) find this[57 207 231 252 273 299 339 356 387]

Amalgam
An existing grey hue around amalgam restorations has been observed to change to green after extensive bleaching of tetracycline-stained teeth with 10% CP.[167] The pH of the bleaching and bleaching time (brand dependent), increase the amount of mercury released from the fillings, from a few micrograms to >100 µg after a bleaching time of hours, more so from newer restorations than older ones.[57 95 167 289 295 297 305 338] This finding is, however, not unanimous.[159]

Systemic effects
Bleaching agents leaking out of custom trays are swallowed, which could have an impact on health. Caution may be required in elderly people and children.[118] In animal experiments and in tissue cultures, large doses appear to be toxic,[60 86 120 149 218 383] but the amounts swallowed by patients is (much) too low for systemic toxic effects to occur.[86 219] Free radicals, the hydroxyl oxygen radical in particular, has been associated with carcinogenesis, genotoxicity, cytotoxicity, etc. However, it should be stressed that hydrogen peroxide is a normal metabolite in humans,[352] which breaks down into water and oxygen, and that the body is well equipped with extracellular and intracellular metabolic defence mechanisms, such as the enzymes catalase, peroxidase and selenium-dependent glutathione peroxidases.[192]

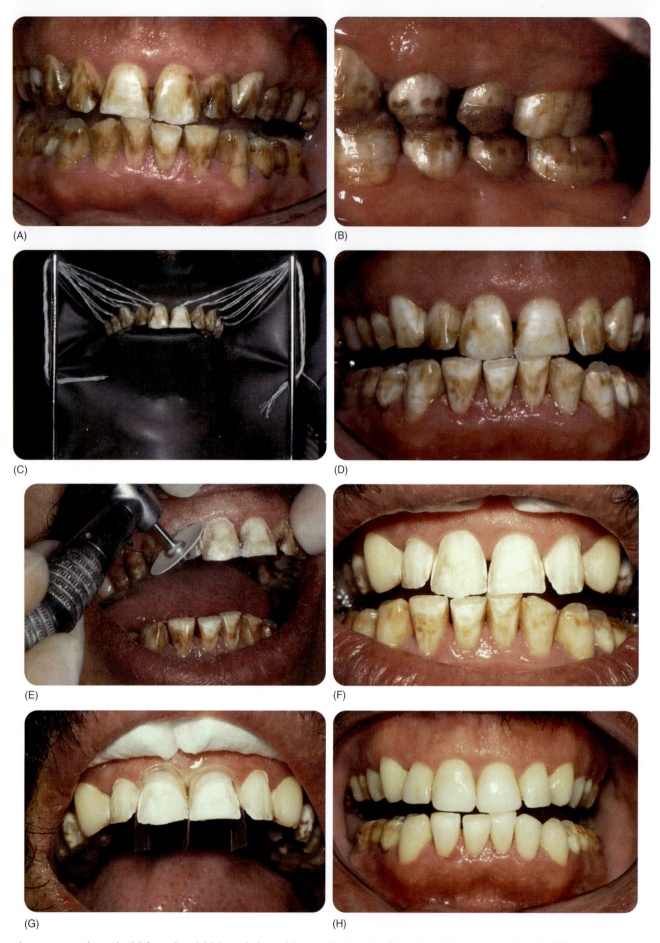

Figure 10.27 Fluorosis: (A) frontal and (B) lateral views. (C) Correctly placed rubber dam. (D) The teeth after in-office bleaching with 30% H$_2$O$_2$. The result is not satisfactory because of the severity of the fluorotic lesions. The lateral incisor showed the most improvement. The same teeth after grinding (E) with an abrasive disc (an alternative is a diamond-coated disc). (F) Further grinding led to removal of too much enamel. (G) Tooth preparations for veneer restorations with Vivadent contour strips in place. (H) The veneers *in situ*.

Table 10.6 Recommended bleaching treatments for various types of tooth discoloration

Type of discoloration	Polishing or micro-abrasive[a]	External bleaching[b]	Internal bleaching	Curative treatment
1. Developmental				
Fluorosis				
Brown	X	X		
Opacities	X	x (go through splotchy stage)		
Pits, brown	(x)	?		x (local)[c]
Tetracyclines		x	x	(x)
Amelogenesis imperfecta		?		x (crowns)
Turner teeth	(x)	x		x (local)[c]
Dentinogenesis imperfecta		x		(x)
Odontodysplasia				x (extraction)
2.1 Infiltrative endogenous				
Non-vital pulp			x[d]	
Capillary pulp bleeding	Wait and watch approach: may disappear spontaneously			
Pulp obliteration				
Vital/ageing		x		(x)
Non-vital			x[d]	(x)
2.2 Infiltrative exogenous				
Iatrogenic				
Endodontic fillings		(x)	x	
Amalgam/metal salts				x (replacement)
Local brown	X	x	x	x
Industrial	X	x	x	x
3.1 Exogenous pseudo-discoloration				
Plaque	X			
Calculus	X			
Tar (smoking)	X	(x)		
Tin fluoride	X			
Chlorhexidine	X			
Tea/wine	X	(x)		
Chromogenic bacteria				
Brown(black)	X			
Green	X			x (local)
Orange	X			
Iron solution/medicaments	X	(x)		
3.2 Breakdown pseudo-discoloration				
Resorption				
Internal				Endodontics
External (cervical)				x (local)
Shining through restoration				x (local)
Shining through caries				x (local)

[a]With acid added to the abrasive agent (such as flour of pumice).
[b]Either in-office with 30% H_2O_2 (alternative Quik Start Bleaching gel and other 35% carbamide containing bleaches) or (waiting room) or supervised at-home bleaching (e.g. Opalescence Quick and Rembrandt X-tra-Comfort).
[c]Composite or veneer restorations, crowns.
[d]Or the combination of internal and at-home bleaching.
x, additional treatment; ?, doubtful result.

Some 90 mg of the bleaching agent is applied in tray-based methods.[219] Depending on the viscosity of the agent and the shape of the tray, some bleach will leak and be swallowed. But 90 mg is a small amount in view of the doses that appear to be seriously toxic in rats.[192] The dif-ference between a toxicologically suspected dose and the actual swallowed amount of a CP bleach used at home is reported to be equivalent to a factor of 100 or more.[219] The initial concerns about safety (general health) have dissipated but are nowadays again reason for concern.

10.6.7   *Restoration*

When bleaching is unsatisfactory or contraindicated (Figure 10.27), tooth-coloured restorations are the last treatment option. If hypoplasia is also present, restorations may be the preferable treatment. Composite or porcelain (veneers) may be used to treat discoloured labial surfaces; this option is indicated in cases of exogenous breakdown (psuedo-discoloration) or when large labial restorations are already present. It is advisable to bleach the labial surfaces before restoration with a porcelain veneer, otherwise an opaque veneer will be required to mask the discoloration, resulting in a lifeless appearance of the tooth. A translucent veneer has better aesthetics. An incisal edge-to-edge occlusion is a contraindication to veneer placement as is bruxism. Nightguard bleaching may be possible in patients with existing veneers.[168]

Table 10.6 shows the preferred treatment modalities for a number of discolorations.

11

Congenital Syndromes with Dental Anomalies

11.1 Introduction

A *syndrome* is currently defined as the presence of multiple congenital developmental malformations, deformations and/or dysplasias, occurring in varying combinations with or without mental abnormalities, as a result of genetic aberrations or the effect of a teratogenic agent.

Congenital anomalies can be distinguished into:

- *Malformations*: morphological defects due to intrinsic disturbances of development
- *Disruptive defects*: developmental malformation due to an extrinsic cause
- *Deformations*: when abnormal mechanical or functional forces, such as lack of fetal movement, affect morphology, frequently in late fetal life (some disruptions cause secondary deformations)
- *Dysplasias*: morphological defects due to abnormal cell organization or function in a specific tissue.[55 114]

A "true" syndrome is due to a single etiological cause leading disturbances with primary effects in several tissues. In "false syndromes" several anomalies are present and they are caused by more than one etiological factor.[51] Use of the term "syndrome" is incorrect in anomalies such as "crack(ed) tooth syndrome" and "Riga–Fedes syndrome".[176] A "sequence" is a primary structural abnormality, which through secondary and tertiary consequences results in a pattern or combination of developmental defects. Syndromes and sequences are named after their first and/or most important reporter or the main affected body part(s) or are referred to by the number (and part) of the chromosome responsible for the defects.[51 52]

11.1.1 Causes of syndromes

- In many syndromes, the cause is a single mutated gene. Thousands of such monogenetic syndromes exist, and new ones are described every week. Mutations in several genes are associated with craniofacial and dental aberrations.[328] Spontaneous mutations, which may become inheritable, occur, for instance, in more than half of tuberous sclerosis patients.[106]
- Other syndromes are caused by abnormalities in chromosome number. The germ cell or the female gamete may contain a pair instead of one chromosome; after fertilisation, three chromosomes instead of two will be present in the somatic cells. When only a part of a chromosome pair splits, the fertilised egg has two chromosomes plus that part. A (micro-) part of a chromosome may be absent: after fertilisation, the chromosome pair will be incomplete.
- Embryonic malformation may also occur due to the effects of *exogenous teratogenic agents*. Examples are: alcohol abuse, antenatal infections (congenital syphilis), metabolic disturbances and use of teratogenic medications such as thalidomide. The dosage, vulnerability of the mother/fetus, time of exposure and interactions between different agents determine the severity of the disturbances.[106] Alcohol abuse by the expectant mother is estimated to affect 2:1000 newborns in the USA and the risk increases when alcohol is used together with tobacco.[299]
- Syndromes also result from a combination of genetic and exogenous causes (e.g. clefts).[114]

11.1.2 Causes of sequences

The diagnostic determinants of the most frequent sequence, the Pierre Robin sequence (1:2000–30000 births, Europe, ~9:100000 births) develop in the 10th–12th week *in utero*. Pathognomonic features are: mandibular micrognathia, cleft palate and glossoptosis (falling back of the tongue leading to airway obstruction). The causes of this sequence include:[6 52 106 302]

- Owing to insufficient amniotic fluid, the fetal mandible is pressed against the sternum leading to deformation.

Pathology of the Hard Dental Tissues, First Edition. Albert Schuurs.
© 2013 Albert Schuurs. Published 2013 by Blackwell Publishing Ltd.

The tongue is located between the unfused palatal processes and prevents their fusion.

- Inadequate mandibular movements due to neurogenic hypotonia.
- Syndromes, including isolated cleft palate.
- Teratogenic agents.
- Collagen disturbances.

Severe airway obstruction and prolonged hypoxia further lead to cor pulmonale, brain damage, feeding problems, (lethal) apnoea,[161] etc. Procedures such as intubation are used to bring the mandible forwards and to prevent glossoptosis. An orthodontic appliance that stimulates the vomiting reflex may help teach the patient to avoid responding to the reflex, by holding the mandible in a forward position.[272]

11.1.3   Genotype and phenotype

In a number of syndromes, early ossification of the cranial sutures inhibits the growth of the skull ("craniosynostosis" with sometimes high intracranial pressure) due to mutation of a fibroblast growth factor receptor.[7 56 121] There are a limited number of clinical manifestations of abnormal development. Thus, craniosynostosis, dwarf stature, polydactyly (too many fingers), microcephaly (small head) and micrognathia, to name a few, are not syndrome-specific, and are pathogenetically heterogeneous.[52 121] In contrast, a mutated gene may lead to markedly varied phenotypes.[99]

11.1.4   Diagnosis

The overall pattern of anomalies, the mode of inheritance and the molecular basis (if known), all help in reaching a diagnosis, but the clinical diagnosis of a syndrome with non-specific and variable symptoms may be very difficult. Syndromes with a known aetiology are distinguished by the frequency and in what combination certain characteristic anomalies occur.

Immediately after birth, the head and neck may be deformed because of intra-uterine constriction, but this corrects spontaneously within a few days. If it does not, further examination must be carried out to check whether the deformation represents a true malformation. An example of late spontaneous disappearance is dolichocephaly (long-headedness) in prematurely born children. The heavy head and weak neck muscles force the child to lie on either the right or left side; the head becomes long and narrow because the soft and thin bones deform. After about 3 months, the dolichocephalic pattern disappears because the child increasingly moves his or her head. Dolichocephaly persists, however, in full-term children with premature closure of the side sutures in the skull.[130]

Many variations exist in the size and form of facial features such as the forehead, face, ears, distance between the eyes, nose and nostrils, lips and mouth (palate, uvula), etc., which can be measured and compared with normal values,[101] but often one has to rely on subjective assessments.[54] A single minor craniofacial deviation is in general no more than a family characteristic. Three minor deviations are associated with a major defect in more than half of the children;[245] these deviations may be statistically uncommon in the population overall, yet may be part of normal familial morphological variants.[51] However, a combination of minor facial anomalies may result in a specific appearance, such as in trisomy 21 and through their recognition lead to the diagnosis.[54]

The history, including pregnancy and birth history, contact with teratogenic and mutagenic agents, presence of dysmorphological features in other identically affected family members and a careful clinical examination may point to a diagnostic hypothesis. Additional genetic and molecular tests may confirm the diagnosis, which is a prerequisite for determining the prognosis, therapy (if possible) and need for genetic counselling.[114] The general dental practitioner will encounter common syndromes such as clefts and trisomy 21, but it may be rare to see other uncommon ones. Thus the dentist must have some knowledge of the common syndromes for making appropriate referrals and arranging consultation and collaboration with geneticists and paediatricians/physicians.

11.1.5   Dental anomalies

Either higher or lower frequency of occurrence of a dental anomaly in patients with a syndrome compared with the general population makes it likely that the dental anomaly is associated with the syndrome.[51] Hyperdontia, double teeth, taurodontism, enamel hypoplasia, etc. are sometimes reported to occur as a part of a rare syndrome,[118 139 275] but their presence may simply be coincidental (see Chapter 2 for detailed description of deviations of tooth number and shape). Isolated dental anomalies, such as hypodontia, may be micro-manifestations of a syndrome. For example, the combination of 10 agenetic maxillary posterior teeth, partial absence of the alveolar process and otitis media[227] may or may not represent an as-yet unknown syndrome, but a deaf-mute patient with 14 congenitally missing teeth does not,[240] because oligodontia may occur in some deaf-mute persons.

11.1.6   Nomenclature

The following terms are frequently used in relation to syndromic features.

- *Brachy*: short, such as brachycephaly (short head) and brachydactyly (short fingers).

- *Chondros*: cartilage (dyschondroplasia, achondroplasia = disturbed development of the cartilage).
- *Dyshidrosis*: disturbed function or absence of the sweat glands. Anhidrosis, hypohidrosis- and hyperhidrosis refer to, respectively, the absence, under- and over-production of sweat.
- *Dysostosis*: disturbed bone development, in particular disturbed ossification.
- *Frontal bossing*: prominent, pronounced forehead (brow).
- *Hypertelorism*: larger than normal distance, often pertaining to the eyes.
- *Hypogenitalism*: underdeveloped function/under-development of the gonads.
- *Onychodysplasia*: abnormal nails.
- *-ploid*: a suffix indicating number of chromosomes. Haploid means 23 chromosomes, as normally present in the gametes. Diploid refers to the 23 chromosome pairs in the somatic cells. Aneuploidy indicates both fewer and more chromosomes than the haploid number.
- *Poly*: presence of extra elements in a body part: polydactyly (more than five fingers).
- *Strabismus*: cross-eyed.
- *Syn*: together, syndactyly (fused fingers or toes), craniosynostosis (early ossification of the sutures of the skull, sometimes one or more).
- *Trichodysplasia*: abnormal hair.

11.1.7 Classification

Of the monogenetic syndromes, more than 1000 manifest in the orofacial region. Most chromosomal syndromes have orofacial effects as do many syndromes with a multifactorial cause.[275] Included here are only those monogenetic syndromes that include dental anomalies, unless they are very rare (arbitrarily considered as an prevalence rate of about 1 or <1:100 000, with one or two exceptions).

Extensive, well-documented descriptions of syndromes may be found in several textbooks,[100 268 275 276] in particular in the lavishly illustrated, encyclopaedic *Syndromes of the Head and Neck* by Gorlin *et al.*[106] The web-based "OMIM database" developed by McKusick *et al.* contains exhaustive descriptions of syndromes, grouped by the mode of inheritance and then alphabetically within the groups.[211] Each syndrome has a six-digit identification number, unless allelic variants are known (when it has 10 digits). Other classifications also exist.[53] In this chapter, McKusick's classification is partly followed. Autosomal dominant (AD) syndromes are described in Section 11.2, which also includes the autosomal recessive (AR) and X-linked syndromes with identical names. Section 11.3 describes the AR syndromes, Section 11.4 the X-linked syndromes, and Section 11.5 the syndromes due to chromosomal abnormalities. Prevalence figures for Europe are based

upon the "Prevalence of rare diseases: a bibliographic survey, September 2006" (last updated 2011; Orphanet Reports Series, http://www.orpha.net/orphacom/cahiers/docs/GB/Prevalence_of_rare_diseases_by_decreasing_prevalence_or_cases.pdf). For a few syndromes, only the number of cases is given.

11.2 Autosomal dominant syndromes

100800. Achondroplasia, chromosome 4
Prevalence: 1:16 000–32 000.[106]

Bone growth impairment causes short-limb dwarfism (120–130 cm) with a normal torso. Striking features are an enlarged head (hydrocephalus internus), frontal bossing, depressed nasal bridge, midfacial dysplasia, mandibular protrusion, short neck, lordosis (abnormally curved spine), joint hypermobility but limitation of elbow extension, and trident (three pronged) hands.[106 211]

Anomalies in the teeth are seldom described.[38] Besides taurodontism the incisor crowns may converge towards the incisal edge, with prominent mamelons suggestive of fusion with supernumerary or supplemental teeth.

101200. Acrocephalosyndactyly type I, (Apert's (Crouzon's) syndrome)
Prevalence: 1:65 000–100 000 births.[55 106]

This syndrome, which is one of the syndromes featuring craniosynostosis, is often due to a fresh mutation. Many affected babies die in the neonatal period.[137] The premature fusion of skull sutures prevents the growth-related anterior displacement of the cranial base, orbits and maxilla. Late closure of the fontanelles underlies "acrocephaly" (tower skull) and "acrobrachycephaly" (short skull).

Facial characteristics include a steep and high forehead, hypertelorism and exophthalmia (bulging eyes), underdeveloped midface with a beaked nose and mandibular prognathism, abnormally shaped ears with hearing problems, symmetrical syndactyly and often mental retardation, but rarely an IQ = 35 has been reported.[106 211] The high-arched palate is narrow, with lateral bony swellings, and sometimes present a cleft,[244] ending in a bifid uvula.[211] Other dental anomalies that have been reported are malocclusions (crowding), hypodontia,[249 322] hyperdontia,[106] delayed eruption,[268 278 323] root resorption and transposition of teeth.[323]

Craniofacial measurements in Apert's and Crouzon's syndromes (see 101 200) deviate from the normal ranges, in general more so in Apert's than Crouzon's.[156] After infancy, the differences become less exaggerated.[158]

113650. Branchio-oto-renal dysplasia (Bor's syndrome), chromosome 8
Prevalence: 1:40 000.[221]

There are fistulas or cysts in the lower neck, ear malformations, hearing loss and renal anomalies.[106 211 221] Oral findings include an arched cleft palate, bifid uvula and retrognathia,[106 211] generalised microdontia (rare in the permanent dentition) and malformed premolars.[221]

118400. Cherubism (familial benign giant cell tumour of the jaw), chromosome 4

Prevalence: about 200 patients, twice more likely in males than females.

In this non-familial, inherited syndrome there is painless fibrous cyst-like dysplasia (central giant cell granuloma with failure of osteoclastogenesis).[355] This results in overdevelopment of the jaws, starting at age 3–4 years and sometimes earlier, leading to an "angelic" round face with broad cheeks and hypertelorism.[211]

The deciduous teeth exfoliate early. Displacement of permanent tooth germs may lead to ectopic impaction[301] and resorption. Oligodontia is also reported. After puberty, there is partial remission of cherubism. Surgical reconstruction should be delayed until the end of puberty,[107 318] and ranges from tooth removal to correction of the shape of buccal bone, removal of giant cell tumour and autotransplantation of teeth to normal bone areas.[301] The grade of severity of cherubism is related to the number of agenetic or impacted molars.[301]

Cherubism may be present in Noonan's syndrome (Section 11.5) and also occur in combination with fibromatoses.[106]

Orofacial clefts
119530. Orofacial cleft 1, chromosome 6

602966. Orofacial cleft 2, (AD?), chromosome 2

600757. Orofacial cleft 3, (AD?), chromosome 19
See also: 119300 and 119540
Prevalence: varies by country.

In the Netherlands, about 2.9:1000 children are born every year with orofacial clefts. Boys are affected more often than girls,[44 84 290] and 0.4:1000 have a cleft palate (see also 119540).[291] In Sweden, the incidence is double that in France and California, when patients from Asian ethnic backgrounds are excluded.[237] All kinds of clefts are present in 0.2–3.6:1000 of newborns worldwide (although racial variation is there: Indians > Mongoloid > Caucasian > African).[84 106] The relationship with race suggests an association with the facial or palatal width. More severe defects are generally noted in boys, although not in all races.[106] Orofacial clefts should be distinguished from the isolated clefts of the palate and from the cleft of the lip and palate.

Cleft lip and/or palate present in 200–250 syndromes.[106] [211] In about 15% of cases, orofacial clefts occur in combination with other anomalies, such as the Van der Woude syndrome (119300) and chromosomal syndromes such as the trisomies.[141 237 291] Isolated clefts occur in 75–80% of cases, 10–15% are familial and about 15% occur as parts of a syndrome. If one parent and one child have a cleft, there is a 17% probability that a subsequent child will be affected.[211] Neither higher maternal age nor higher birth order or paternal age is associated with the risk of isolated clefts.[297] Environmental influences, including maternal drug and alcohol intake and smoking, are of importance.

In a sample of monozygotic twins, in about a third of cases, both twins exhibited orofacial clefts and a palatal cleft was present in one-quarter of both twins.[121] Most dizygotic twins in another sample were discordant.[205] A gene on the short arm of chromosome 6 has been implicated in clefts, but (modifying) effects of genes on chromosomes 4, 17 and 19 are also possible.[121] Orofacial cleft 2 is linked to chromosome 2.[211] In regards to race and environment, different transcription factors (such as transforming growth factors) regulating skull development are possibly involved, but which ones are is not known.[165]

Facial and cranial clefts are caused by non-fusion of embryonic parts (from the 7th embryonic week). The clefts are classified from 0 to 14.[275] Cranial clefts above the eye are numbered 8–14 and facial clefts occurring under the eyes 0–7 (from the nose to the ear). Clefts of the lip, alveolar bone and palate are included in general in clefts 1, 2 and 3.

The severity of cleft lip, unilateral or bilateral, varies from a small notch in the lip to an actual cleft involving the alveolus and premaxilla. The palatal cleft manifests as a shallow groove in the midline of the hard palate or a full cleft through the bone. Unlike other clefts, palatal clefts are more prevalent in females than males and more frequently on the left than the right side. Two years after birth, development (weight) lags behind in children with cleft palates, and is attributed to feeding problems, airway infections and surgery.[84 138] The child's ability to learn to speak is hampered.

"Micro-clefts" in the middle of the lower lip are present in a small proportion of children with orofacial clefts and the Pierre Robin sequence.[225]

Solitary hypodontia is common in orofacial clefts;[112] 70–80% prevalence is reported.[44] The findings related to hypodontia may be summarised as follows:

- Hypodontia is most frequent in the maxilla.[228] The maxillary lateral incisor is most frequently agenetic, also when there is only a cleft lip (Figure 11.1).
- Hypodontia in the deciduous dentition is more often associated with non-alveolar clefts than in controls.[63] The permanent lateral incisor in the cleft region is agenetic considerably more often than the deciduous incisor; when the latter is absent, its successor will be agenetic.[296] Van der Wal reported that the lateral incisor was absent in half of one sample of patients with facial clefts and was malformed in one-quarter of the

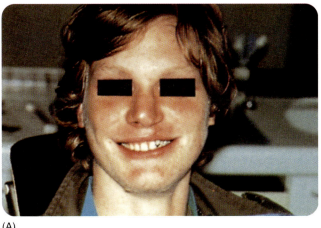

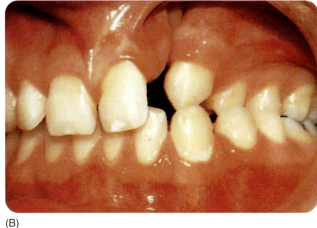

(A)   (B)

Figure 11.1 Patients with clefts of the lip (A) and palate (B).

patients.[292] The profile shows a retrusive upper lip/jaw.[175]

- The more severe the cleft, the more severe is the hypodontia,[116 228] including the parts of the dental arches beyond the cleft region.[6 228]
- The upper central incisor is agenetic in small proportion of patients.[296] The second maxillary and mandibular premolars are frequently agenetic in similar proportions[312] (18% of the patients), and this is more on the left than the right side, where the clefts are more common.[258]
- The second molars are missing in about 4% (3% of contralateral teeth develop late).[116]
- Hypodontia is present to the same degree in familial and sporadic clefts.[44]
- The development of the dentition is delayed.[116 270]

The deciduous teeth are relatively small, yet crowding is almost the rule.[63] The permanent teeth have normal measurements.[215] Tooth development and eruption are delayed in particular in cases with hypodontia and worsens with age.[224 228] The morphology of, in particular, the upper lateral incisor is affected;[296] T-shaped incisors have been reported.[113 155] The enamel of the central incisor is more often hypoplastic than that of the lateral incisor,[296] as found in 20–45% of one series of cases,[109] perhaps as a consequence of surgery,[3] although this also occurs in non-surgical patients. Enamel opacities (of which many are carious white spots) are present in 95% of 5–17-year-olds with clefts.[109] Caries develops 3.5 times more often than in controls and is not restricted to the teeth near the cleft.[31] Intranasal teeth have been reported a few times, attributed to the presence of clefts and surgery.[147] Small morphological tooth deviations have been described in the region outside the cleft.[35] Lip and palate clefts are regularly accompanied by hyperdontia, also in combination with hypodontia and natal and neonatal teeth,[5 44 63 126 155 197 207 229 236 296 309] outside the cleft region.

In about 20% of cleft cases, there are extra lateral incisors and fewer extra central incisors in both dentitions.[296] In about 25% of the deciduous and about 10% of the permanent dentitions supplemental lateral incisors are present,[5] on average about 0.3 extra teeth/dentition,[44 155] in particular when the lip is involved in an alveolar cleft.[308]

Early removal of (impacted) extra teeth in the cleft results in unfavourable loss of bone; the tooth must be removed during secondary bone plastic surgery, at the age of 7–12 years.[92]

Other syndromes with clefts
119300. Van der Woude syndrome, chromosome 1

607613. Van der Woude syndrome 2, chromosome 1
Prevalence: 1:35000–100000.[106]

The "lower lip sinus syndrome" is attributed to absence of a part of chromosome 1 (or 2). The majority shows symmetrical pits and/or sinuses (pits connected to small salivary glands) in the lower lip. The penetrance is high and the expressivity is variable.[42] Sometimes slight bulges are present and less often a cleft lip and/or palate and/or uvula, frequently with hypodontia.[211 231]

119540. Cleft palate, chromosome 2

303400. Cleft palate with ankyloglossia, X-linked
Prevalence: 0.4:1000.[106]

Non-familial cleft palates seem related to environmental factors (maternal age).[211] Clefts of only the palate are more common in females.[5] (Submucosal) palatal clefts occur in association with other anomalies more often than orofacial clefts.[106] Half of 139 patients with cleft palates had multiple anomalies, and 34, in particular, had

Stickler's syndrome: a flat midface, joint problems, hearing loss and myopia (short-sightedness).[141] Additional problems, e.g. the Pierre Robin sequence (261800) and the Van der Woude syndrome (119300), were present in more than half of another sample of 50 cleft palate patients.[291] Associations with Apert's (101200) and the de Lange (122470) syndromes are also reported.[143]

Agenetic maxillary lateral incisors (more frequently absent in the Pierre Robin sequence)[6] and enamel hypoplasia of the central incisors are associated dental anomalies. Anterior tooth agenesis is less frequent than in patients with orofacial clefts, but has been noted to occur more often than in controls.[5]

Ranta et al. found that children with hypodontia had similar proportions of 1–11 agenetic teeth as children with cleft palates, but in the latter a larger number of maxillary teeth were absent. More teeth were symmetrically agenetic in the maxilla of children without a cleft and in the mandible of children with a cleft.[230]

In about 15% of patients, a submucous cleft palate is associated with isolated dental agenesis, mainly the mandibular second premolars followed by the maxillary lateral incisors and second premolars. Heliovaara et al. reported peg-shaped lateral incisors in 10%, transposition (Mx.C.P$_1$) in 4% and supernumerary teeth in 3% of their sample of cleft palate patients.[120]

In cleft palate patients, odontogenesis is delayed, and more so when there is associated hypodontia.[226]

119600. Cleidocranial dysplasia (formerly dysostosis cleidocranialis), chromosome 6
Prevalence: 1:1 000 000.[256]

The syndrome is caused by mesodermal dysfunction due to anomalous actions of osteoclasts, resulting in multiple bone anomalies. About a third are due to spontaneous mutation.[106] The cranial sutures are wide open, and some of them and the frontal fontanelles do not ossify (requiring autologous bone transplantation). The features include brachycephaly, frontal bossing, hypertelorism, depressed nose bridge, hypoplastic zygomas and maxillae, hypoplastic frontal and paranasal sinuses and a small midface. The patients have drooping, narrow shoulders and a long neck, with short stature. The clavicles may be (partially) absent, which allows the affected individual to bring the shoulders close together (Figure 11.2).[34 106 211]

The jaw bones may show coarse trabeculation and the alveolar crestal bone may be very dense.[181] The underdeveloped maxilla makes the mandible appear more prominent.[8 115] There is a high palatal vault[101] and occasionally a cleft, which may or may not be submucous. The permanent dentition may have a few to more than 30 extra teeth,[8 13 24 47 137 324] mainly in the mandibular premolar region,[144] which develop after the age of 12 years,[181] and in the premaxilla.[12 88 137] These teeth may develop from remnants of the dental lamina.[157] The permanent teeth mature late, which is more evident when accompanied by hyperdontia.[256] One sample of siblings showed discordance in the location and numbers of extra teeth.[325] Rarely, a tooth from the normal series is agenetic.[24 65]

The eruption of the permanent teeth is delayed (Figure 11.3) or fails[65] (partially in some incisors),[24] except for the permanent

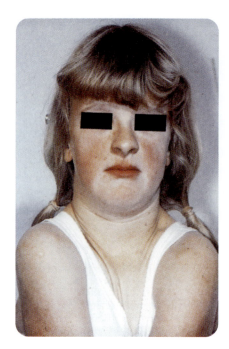

Figure 11.2 Cleidocranial dysplasia: the shoulders can be brought much closer together than in normal individuals.

first molars. The deciduous teeth resorb late and persist into adulthood.[8 9 144 245 256 311] Cellular cementum is absent and acellular cementum is grossly lacking on the impacted teeth.[254] A number of teeth, in particular the first molars,[137] erupt in spite of the absence of cellular cementum.[258 267] The eruption delay seems to be caused by the reduced resorption of bone and roots of the deciduous teeth.[106 157 244] The roots of the unerupted teeth are (almost) completely developed, though they may be curved,[144] long or short, with a sharply pointed apex or malformed otherwise.[181] The crowns are often small.

Correction of the underdeveloped midface is achieved with surgery.[89] Surgical intervention enables the eruption of impacted teeth, with formation of cementum,[122] but in some patients orthodontic traction is desirable.[65] Stepwise early removal of the extra and persisting deciduous teeth, along with the overlying bone, is followed by spontaneous eruption of the normal teeth.[137] Other authors state that the bone must be saved as much as possible: the permanent successor is extruded through an opening in the bone after extraction of the deciduous tooth.[24]

Presence of different mutations was established in two patients belonging to the same family and in another patient from a different family.[99 315] The mutations concern the gene *CBFA1*. In an experimental study, homozygous mice did not develop a skeletal system and heterozygous mice had cleidocranial dysplasia without the dental anomalies.[315]

122470. Cornelia de Lange syndrome (Brachmann–de Lange syndrome; typus degenerativus amstelodamensis), chromosome 3
Prevalence: 0.6:100 000 (Denmark),[137] 1:16 744 (Taipei) and 1:10 000 births (USA).[106]

Most cases are isolated.[211] The syndrome, characterised by a delay in growth and development, has a mild, classical expres-

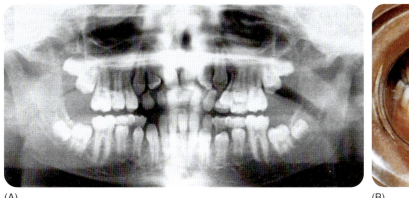
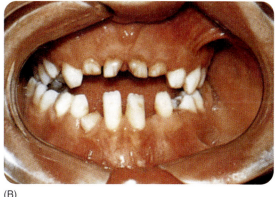

(A)   (B)

Figure 11.3 (A,B) The dentition of a patient with cleidocranial dysplasia; this case does not demonstrate hyperdontia.

sion. The patients have low birthweight, short stature and micro-brachycephaly. The characteristic facial features are: hirsutism (with hair growth extending down to the neck and covering the forehead), approximating eyebrows above a depressed nose bridge and long eyelashes, anteverted nostrils with a long philtrum and an upward tilt of the nose tip, and maxillary prognathism with a thin upper lip and drooping oral commissures. The eyes show several anomalies. The characteristic facies does not develop until the age of 2 years in the mild phenotype and is present at birth in the classical type. The low-set ears may be small and curly hair may be present, for instance, on the back. The extremities in particular are also malformed, with oligodactyly and syndactyly of the second and third toes. Other abnormalities concern the gastrointestinal and genitourinary tract, such as hypospadias (ectopic external urethral orifice), hypoplastic kidneys and cardiovascular defects. Severe to borderline mental retardation exists.[211]

As regards the dentition, patients may show deciduous double teeth,[72] delayed eruption, hypodontia and microdontia[326 75] with spaced teeth.[211] Gastric reflux causes dental erosion.[326]

123500. Crouzon's (or morbus) syndrome, chromosome 10
Prevalence: 1:25 000.[106]

A third of craniofacial dysostosis/pseudo-Crouzon's syndrome cases[211 256] are caused by fresh mutations. The growing skull is displaced downwards under pressure from the growing brain in one or another direction, depending on which sutures close early.[235] The face is often broadest at the level of the eyebrows.[206] Abnormalities in the vicinity of the eyes are the most frequent,[153] and hearing deficits are also frequent,[106 262] including hypertelorism and exophthalmia; blindness is not uncommon. The midface, including the maxillary arch, is hypoplastic (Figure 11.4). The nose may be beak shaped, above a short upper lip.[211] Early surgery[90] is done to reopen the sutures; screws are inserted to provide traction that promotes growth of the skull in the desired directions. The hands (and feet) exhibit syndactyly, brachydactyly and other defects.[7 262]

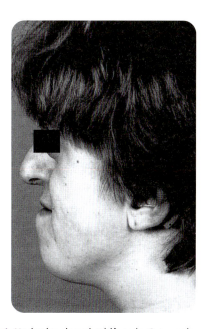

Figure 11.4 Underdeveloped midface in Crouzon's syndrome.

The short maxilla has a high palate, with lateral bony swellings. The associated malocclusions include crowding, open bite, cross bites, and a Class III molar relationship. Other dental anomalies that have been reported are hypodontia and small crowns,[208] shovel-shaped incisors[106] and impacted teeth.

129200–129550. The ectodermal dysplasias
Prevalence: (all types): 7:10 000.

The ectodermal dysplasias are a heterogeneous group of congenital disorders in which structures of ectodermal origin exhibit dystrophy; however, non-ectodermal tissues may also be affected.[164] The main characteristic features concern the hair, teeth, nails and sweat glands:[217]

- Hypotrichosis: sparse, thin and sometimes dry hair
- Oligodontia
- Onychodysplasia (dystrophic nails)
- Dyshidrosis: affected sweat glands may be anhidrotic, hypohidrotic (in 80%) or hidrotic.

Salivary production is also reduced. Perspiration is possible to a degree in those with hypohidrosis; anhidrotic patients are in fact hypohidrotic. Consequences include pyrexia of unknown origin in children and excessive rise in body temperature in hot weather (which can cause brain damage that is sometimes fatal) and even after mild exercise. In a group of patients with various forms of ectodermal dysplasia, the number of aplastic teeth ranged from 2 to 26; all the third molars were missing. The teeth least affected were the maxillary central incisors and the mandibular canines, (which were, however, most affected by malformation) and the mandibular first molars.[327]

Two of the four characteristic features must be present in order to diagnose ectodermal dysplasia; the validity of the diagnosis increases when the triad of hypohidrosis, hypotrichosis and oligodontia is present. Moreover, patients often have:

- Asteatosis (reduced production by the sebaceous glands)
- A thin, smooth skin
- Full lips.

Other features include a small face, depressed nose bridge (saddle nose) with frontal bossing, absence of or more than two nipples, aplastic or hypoplastic mammary glands, patchy distribution of body hair, mental retardation[106 288] and lacrimal gland hypoplasia. In the Christ–Siemens–Touraine syndrome (the most common form; see below) patients have short stature[211] and cranial abnormalities (smaller face because of frontal bossing). Clefts, syndactyly, polydactyly[241] and other features, such as deafness, absent dermal ridges or immunodeficiency with osteoporosis may also be present.[211] The (oral) mucosa may be affected,[98] and xerostomia may be present.[260]

Pinheiro et al. in 1981 described 18 types of ectodermal dysplasia, each of which included at least two characteristic features.[217]

Later, other forms were described, for instance odonto-onycho-dermal dysplasia (with features such as hidrotic palmoplantar hyperkeratosis, persisting deciduous teeth, severe hypodontia, dystrophic nails, erythema of cheeks/nose)[81 183 186] and a variant with metal retardation and marked oligodontia of the permanent dentititon.[187] More than 150 ectodermal dysplasias have been recognised.[164]

Presently, more than 200 types[363] are classified according to all possible combinations of the four main features. When only two of the four principal defects are present, with or without other malformations, the syndrome belongs to group A. If only one of the four principal characteristics is present with at least one other ectoder-

mal defect, the syndrome belongs to group B. Eleven subgroups are distinguished, based on the combinations of the presence of the principal characteristics, for instance defects of hair and teeth, hair and nails, hair and sweat glands, teeth and nails, teeth and sweat glands, and so on,[216] but the classification is said to be arbitrary and based on criteria that do not take into account biological considerations such as the pathogenesis and genetic background.[196 216]

The mode of inheritance differs in the different "types", but for some the cause is unknown.[216] The X-linked forms are phenotypically indistinguishable from the autosomal recessive disorders.[193] Carrier females show mild expressions of the mutated gene and male carriers usually have pronounced symptoms. The hypohidrotic form is the most frequently seen form and is often X-linked.[30 106 164 288] The anhidrotic form is sometimes autosomal recessive but closely resembles the X-linked recessive type.[19] The syndrome does not have a predilection for females, as was previously thought.[164]

305100. Ectodermal dysplasia 1, X-linked

This is the Christ–Siemens–Touraine syndrome, and patients are said to have both anhidrosis and hypohidrosis.[164]

The responsible gene (EDA) codes for a small protein (ectodysplasin A), which may be a tumour necrosis factor-related ligand.[196 264] Furthermore, another protein has been isolated and characterized, called edar.[193] Ectodysplasin binds to edar to form a unique ligand–receptor pair that regulates the embryologic morphogenesis.[196]

The clinical identification of heterozygous females is difficult because of the variability in the severity of the signs caused by X-chromosome inactivation. However, they show increased agenesis of permanent teeth compared with normative data, while affected males have multiple missing teeth, mostly in the mandible.[356]

Besides hypotrichosis with mild abnormalities of the sweat glands and breasts in heterozygous females and fine silky hair (and alopecia), patients may show short stature, saddle nose, high and broad cheekbones, a pointed chin, protuberant lips, lacrimal gland hypoplasia, corneal dystrophy and mental retardation.[211 280] Pigmented skin lesions might progress to melanomas.[328]

The maxilla is retruded with relative mandibular protrusion.[363] Reported dental features are microdontia, conical and tapered crown shapes, hypodontia, also in the deciduous dentition,[329] and anodontia,[246] enamel hypoplasia and delayed eruption.[280] The roots may be short and conical in shape.[356] The first deciduous tooth, often a conical canine, appears at 1.5 years of age or later. Early dental treatment, often done to prevent teasing and bullying, consists of recontouring the conical teeth with composite resin or removable dentures. The number of tooth germs present should be established early on with radiographic examination.[28]

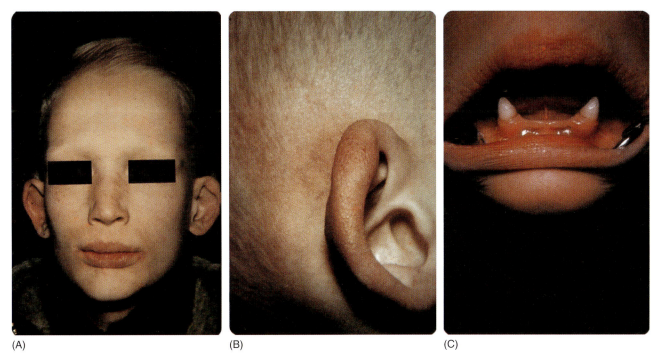

(A)   (B)   (C)

Figure 11.5 (A) Face, (B) ear and hair, and (C) conical teeth in a boy with ectodermal dysplasia. (Courtesy of W.A.M. van der Kwast.)

129490. Ectodermal dysplasia 3 (anhidrotic), chromosome 2
Prevalence: 1 : 10 000–100 000.[30 280]

In a sample of about 1500 patients, one patient had this type of ectodermal dysplasia.[241] The patients show variable degrees of hypohidrosis and mild hypotrichosis. Mild hypodontia may exist, but in ectodermal dysplasia oligodontia is common, sometimes also in other family members and carriers.[19 30 164 180 214 260 288] Anodontia and the presence of just one premolar are also reported.[279] When more teeth are present, they often have a conical crown, enlarged pulp cavities and exhibit rhizomicry and disturbances in eruption.[19 134] The maxillary central incisors and the first permanent molars are the least frequently absent. There are indications that the dominant and recessive modes of inheritance differ in regards to which teeth will be agenetic,[287] but if this is true, it cannot be used to distinguish the mode of inheritance. (Hypohidrotic) ectodermal dysplasia is associated with oligodontia and taurodontism.[192 273]

The conical crowns may be restored with composite[98] or crowns; crown and bridge restorations[2] may be used if the oligodontia is not very severe. Partial dentures fitted in young children with few teeth help overcome problems with speech development and eating, and prevent cosmetic, craniomandibular joint and psychological problems, but bone support for the prosthesis is minimal. The tongue (that previously had more space) poses a problem, just like the decreased salivary flow.[14 30 321] In a prospective study without bone grafting, mandibular endosteal implants were placed anterior to the mental foramen and maxillary implants mesial to the first molars, and overdentures provided to subjects judged to be mature. The patients were aged 8–68 years. In growing children, implants are usually not indicated. Of the implants placed, 91% in the mandible and 76% in the maxilla survived. The 24-month survival rate was lowest in patients under 11 years.[110]

Figures 11.5, 11.6 and 11.7 show ectodermal dysplasia patients with characteristic facies and other features.

To illustrate the variety of presentations of ectodermal dysplasia the rare ectrodactyly-ectodermal dysplasia-clefting syndrome (129900, over 100 reported patients).[106] is briefly described. The hands resemble the claws of a lobster (pincers) and the feet are sometimes malformed (cleft). Cleft lip and palate, oligodontia or anodontia,[101] [241] taurodontism, double teeth, enamel dysplasia and xerostomia are reported.[211]

189500. "Tooth and nail" syndrome (dysplasia; Witkop's syndrome), chromosome 4
Prevalence: 1–2 : 10 000.[211]

In this simplest form of ectodermal dysplasia the sweat glands and scalp hair are affected.[211] The spoon-shaped, hypoplastic, longitudinally ridged and pitted nails, in particular those of the toes,[307] improve with age.[211] The syndrome often draws attention only when the permanent teeth fail to erupt. The teeth may be small, sharp and conical. The permanent mandibular incisors and second molars and maxillary canines are frequently agenetic,[97][131][307][337] but all permanent teeth may be absent. The reduced vertical dimension is manifested as a pouting lower lip.[307] The dermatoglyphs show abnormalities.[338] The syndrome is particularly seen in Canadian Mennonites of Dutch origin.

The peculiar dermatoglyphic patterns are also observed in family members, and in amelogenesis imperfecta[13] and hypodontia.[11] The epidermal skin characteristics develop in the third to sixth months *in utero*. Development of the dermatoglyphs of the feet lags behind by 2–3 weeks.[13]

308300. Incontinentia pigmenti type II ("classical incontinentia pigmenti")

Prevalence: 1:40 000,[171] 95% females.

The Bloch–Sulzberger syndrome, a dermatosis, belongs to the tricho-odonto-onychal subgroup of the ectodermal dysplasias, but mesodermal anomalies also exist.[171] Many cases are not familial.[349] The skin is pigmented with "*café au lait* spots", sometimes associated with a variety of other malformations (eyes, teeth, skeleton, heart, etc.). The trunk and limbs show erythema (rash), linear vesicles and pustules that develop in the newborn period (stage 1).[170] After a few months (stage 2) there is development of skin papules (purulent), verrucous lesions (warty keratotic papules and plaques) and hyperkeratosis of the distal limbs and scalp. Stage 3 starts at age 1 year and consists of slowly fading brown or blue-grey hyperpigmentation (tattoos) on primarily the trunk. In stage 4, the skin of especially the legs of adults is pale (hypopigmentation), atrophic (lower limbs), usually fading with time, but scarring. The stages may overlap and not all are seen in every patient.[171][211][300] Features include skeletal disturbances (short stature, microcephaly, syndactyly), eye defects in 30% (retinal bleeding, myopia, strabismus, blue sclerae, blindness) and neurological problems (seizures, mental retardation, spastic paralysis).[300] The nails (ridged, dystrophic, pitted) and hair (alopecia, frizzy coarse hair, thin sparse hair) are involved.[211] The patients may have learning disabilities. Females may have nipple and breast hypoplasia or aplasia or even supernumerary nipples. The

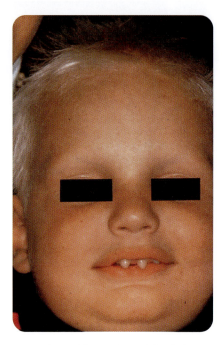

Figure 11.6 A patient with ectodermal dysplasia.

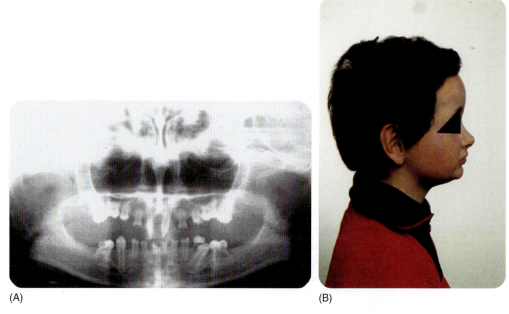

(A)   (B)

Figure 11.7 (A) Oligodont dentition and (B) facial profile of a girl with ectodermal dysplasia.

syndrome in males is often lethal *in utero*. Surviving males, and there are many of them,[350] are equally affected as females.[106 171 211]

Orofacial features include cleft lip and palate,[300] severe hypodontia or oligodontia (40%) in the deciduous and permanent dentitions, with persisting deciduous teeth.[87] [106 133 217 233] Extra cusps occur mainly in posterior teeth.[170] [171 203] The eruption of the malformed (dysplastic), conical teeth (30%) is delayed,[106 171 223 233 242] but the developmental stages of the teeth in a young child were nearly normal.[133] Mandibular molars of the deciduous dentition may show taurodontism[75 170] and the anterior teeth may show elongated crowns and shortened roots.[351]

130000–130090. Ehlers–Danlos types I–IV, VII–VIII, X, chromosomes 2, 7, 9, 17

225310. Ehlers–Danlos syndrome with platelet dysfunction due to fibronectin abnormalities, type 10, chromosome 11

225400–225410. Ehlers–Danlos syndrome, types VI–VII, AR, chromosomes 1, 5

305200. Ehlers–Danlos syndrome, type V, X-linked
Prevalence: Types I and II, 1 : 10 000–20 000.[106]

In this heterogeneous series of syndrome types (type IX is now called occipital horn syndrome)[106 211] the connective tissue is affected. Depending on the type, the skin is very elastic. For instance, in type I the skin can be stretched considerably after which it springs back into it is original position (hyperextensibility). Periodontal destruction is reported in several types.[330] The atrophic skin is fragile (showing the characteristic "cigarette paper" scars after tearing), prone to bruising and may not retain sutures following surgery and cutaneous bleeding is common. The joints are hypermobile. In the rare and malignant type IV, the skin is translucent, there is joint hyperlaxity,[330] and spontaneous rupture of the bowel and arteries (which makes the patient prone to haemorrhage, which may also happen after block anaesthesia) is associated with sudden death; however, presence of these features depends on complete penetrance. Cardiac (mitral) valve problems are present in some types.[92]

About half of type I patients can touch their nose with their tongue.[104] Excessive bleeding after extraction[269] (which has been questioned)[204] may apply to some types only. Intraosseous fibrous lesions of the jaws and other bones may represent a manifestation of tuberous sclerosis.[64] Small and irregularly positioned teeth are reported in types I and VI.[211] Type IV seems to be associated with early tooth loss. Orthodontic treatment takes the usual amount of time or the tooth movement may be faster, but the oral mucosa is very vulnerable to ulcerations and the risk of rapid relapse requires long-term use of retainers.[142 190 204]

The dentine may be dysplastic and patients are diagnosed as having dentinogenesis imperfecta;[16] the condition may also resemble radicular dentine dysplasia.[268 312] In type I, the dentition is normal appearing, and in type VII C multiple permanent tooth agenesis and dysplastic dentine are seen.[331]

In a 13-year-old patient with subtype VIIC (dermatosparaxis), opalescent teeth, root dysplasia and pulp obliteration were reported, but the features were not consistent with a full dentinogenesis imperfecta diagnosis. A female proband in addition had hypodontia and microdont lateral incisors.[70]

The (pre)molars show elongated occlusal cusps and deep fissures,[142 204] characteristic pulp stones (in some types) and malformed roots, sometimes rhizomicry.[204 268] Often, the presence of small (pinhole) enamel pits in mentally retarded children have led to an early diagnosis.[126] In one sample of patients, 100% had pits versus 75% of their relatives and 72% of controls. The number of pits was significantly greater in the patients, but this cannot be used as a screening feature.[86] Some type III patients show hyperdontia,[185] and micrognathia is also reported. Severe and generalised periodontal problems characterise type VIII.[93]

Epidermolysis bullosa
Prevalence: at least 1 : 17 000.

In epidermolysis bullosa there is increased skin and mucosal fragility with involvement of the mucosa of the mouth, oropharynx and oesophagus, and the nails (absent, dystrophic) and teeth. The anomalies are due to the absence or alteration of a glycoprotein in the basal membrane, which leads to deficiencies in the connections between the cell layers. Minor trauma produces blisters.

Tooth brushing may cause formation of bullae,[210] usually in all types. In the past, extractions were considered unavoidable,[123] but curative treatment is possible using certain types of general anaesthesia (local anaesthesia provokes formation of bullae), and application of 1% hydrocortisone cream on the mucosa,[313] and erythromycin prevention.[162] Intubation for general anaesthesia causes oral blistering and bulla formation in the larynx and pharynx with airway obstruction. Oral surgery must be avoided, if possible, for the associated iatrogenic trauma may cause severe problems.[194] Prostheses are mostly contraindicated,[314] in particular in the junctional types. Problems in especially the recessive subtypes include restricted mouth opening due to contractures and ankyloglossia.[210]

131760–132000. Epidermolysis bullosa, chromosomes 3, 7, 12

226440–226700. Epidermolysis bullosa, AR, chromosomes 1, 3, 10, 17, 18
Epidermolysis bullosa has 27 types, with mainly inherited skin anomalies.[106 210] The skin and sometimes the mucosa

are fragile. Following trauma, vesicles or bullae develop, which can progress to form painful ulcers. In some types, eating hard foods lead to formation of palatal blood blisters, which rapidly ulcerate. In the absence of bullae, the same phenomenon is seen on sites external to the oral cavity, the pathogenesis of which is unknown.[62] Rough clothing material and a higher room temperature may provoke the formation of bullae or they may arise spontaneously. Scarring depends on the anatomical level (deep or more superficial) at which the separation of the skin (that forms the bullae) takes place, and which this is used to establish the type present (Table 11.1). There are three types:[184]

- *Type I, the suprabasal* simplex type, (prevalence 2.5:100 000 in Europe). Blisters develop through cleavage of the basal epidermal cell layer, in some types only on the hand and foot, which heal without scarring within 2–10 days. In contrast with adults, children develop painful oral blisters and wounds. Dental anomalies are rare, but the mucosa is vulnerable.
- The *junctional transbasal type II* (with atrophic skin), (prevalence 0.06:100 000 in Europe). This type has a poor prognosis: half of the affected children die within 2 years. Cleavage takes place in the lamina lucida.
- The *sub-basal dystrophic type III* (prevalence 0.27:100 000 in Europe). This often heals with scars and contractures (pseudo-syndactyly may develop).

Based on the mode of inheritance and patient typing (with diagnostic tools such as immunohistochemistry and immunofluorescence), the subdivision is established.[106] The *autosomal dominant simplex* types (in which sometimes only the hands and/or feet are affected versus the generalised defects that are present at or shortly after birth) may not show scarring, unless there is secondary infection.[97][211] The oral mucosa is (almost) free of defects.[102] The enamel is affected in the Dowling–Meara type.[106]

In all the *junctional* types (226450–226700) except dystrophica neurotrophica (226440), 30–40% of patients have generalised thin or pitted enamel.[314] The dentino–enamel junction is flat in the deciduous dentition and the dentine is locally unmineralised.[10] The cementum is abnormal. Severe forms of epidermolysis bullosa lead to extensive caries, which is not associated with a reduced salivary flow.[314]

Presence of enamel hypoplasia in a young child with epidermolysis bullosa simplex led to re-evaluation of the diagnosis, which was consequently changed to junctional epidermolysis.[29]

In some *autosomal recessive junctional* types, healing occurs without scarring, but in more severe cases, crippling contractures develop (mitten-like deformities of the hands, microstomia).[261] Bullae are not present in all types. Hallopeu–Siemens (226600) is a serious and destructive

form, starting either at birth or in young children, with oral mucosal bullae.

Mental development may not progress.[79][313] Pitted enamel and more severe enamel hypoplasia are commonly associated with the dystrophic recessive types. The dominant dystrophic form has rough enamel, appearing "globular" on radiographs,[280] delayed eruption with many retained teeth[103] taurodontism,[280][313] hyperdontia or anodontia,[166] and poorly mineralised hypercementosis.[268] Removable prosthetic appliances are not indicated,[79] and even if extractions are the only treatment option, dentures cannot be made when the mouth is poorly accessible.[313] Oral hygiene may be impaired owing to mucosal sensitivity. Dental treatment often requires general anaesthesia, in particular in the dystrophic recessive forms.[261]

Bullae in an "infantile" form of junctional epidermolysis bullosa (226730) do not heal, but the syndrome is commonly fatal at an early age because of secondary infection and dehydration.[37]

Only the dentine formed before birth is normally calcified,[10][37] but this does not imply a specifically altered structure of the later forming dentine.[96] The cellular cementum is hypoplastic and hypocalcified.[122] Ameloblasts function normally until the first layer of dentine is formed; after this there is development of metaplasia.[96]

In a simplex form (601001), blisters are seen on the plantar, dorsal and lateral surfaces of the feet.[211]

149000. Angio-osteo-hypertrophy syndrome
Prevalence: >1000 patients (Europe).

The Klippel–Trénaunay–Weber syndrome/angio-osteo-hypertrophy syndrome is characterised by large cutaneous haemangiomas (varicose veins, port-wine marks) with locally hypertrophied bones, often in one leg or arm, or the toes are elongated.[106][211] The hands may show macrodactyly, syndactyly, polydactyly and oligodactyly. Additionally, seizures and mental retardation have been reported.[211]

Where facial haemangiomas exist, the jaw is hypertrophic and the rapidly formed teeth erupt early.[198][211]

154400. Mandibulofacial dysostosis 1, Nager type, chromosome 9
Prevalence: 1:10 000 born alive.

The syndrome, alternatively called acrofacial dysostosis or Treacher Collins type, affects the structures derived from the first and second branchial arches and is characterised by hypoplastic supraorbital rims and zygomas in a small face, down-slanting of the lower eye lids and recessive chin, which makes the nose seem large.[106][211] The ears may be malformed, sometimes rudimentary (like in trisomy 18)[320] and the patients have conductive deafness. The hair may slant towards the cheeks. The radius and thumbs may be lacking and finger and toe syndactyly, or missing toes, has also been reported. Other features include unilateral renal agenesis, urticaria pigmentosa and

Table 11.1 Features (simplified) of epidermolysis bullosa[106 162 211 252]

Number/(sub)type	Period of development	Hand	Foot	Face	Elsewhere	Mouth (mucosa)	Teeth	Nails
I: SIMPLEX (intra-epidermal blisters)								
A. Non-scarring, AD								
131760. Herpetiformis, Dowling–Meara	1st month	Yes	Yes	Yes	Yes	No	Some	Yes
131800. Weber–Cockayne	1–3rd decade	Yes	Yes	No	No	No	No	No
131900. Koebner type	0–0.5 years	Yes	Yes	Moderate involvement	Yes	Some	No	No
131950. Ogna	?	Yes	Yes	No	Rarely	No	No	Yes
131960. Mottled pigmentation	Childhood	Yes	Yes	No	Yes	No	No	Yes
132000. Dystrophy with localised absence of skin, Bart's	At birth	Yes	Yes	No	Yes	No	No	Yes
B Atrophic scarring, AR								
226670. Simplex and muscular dystrophy	At birth	Yes	Yes	Yes	Yes	Yes	No	Yes
II: JUNCTIONAL (blistering, atrophic skin)								
Non-scarring, AR								
226440. Localisata[a]	at birth	no	yes	no	yes	no	yes	yes
226600. Inversa dystrophica	Neonatal period	No	No	No	Yes	Rarely	Yes	Yes
226500. Dystrophica neurotrophica (progressiva)	5–8 years	Yes	Yes	No	Yes	Yes	No	No
226650. Generalisata benign	At birth	Yes	Yes	No	Yes	Yes	Yes	Yes
226700. Letalis (generalisata gravis), Herlitz[b]	Neonatal	Yes infants	Yes infants	Yes	Yes	Yes	Yes	Yes
III: DERMAL (dermolytic, blistering, dystrophic skin)								
A. Scarring, AD								
Cockayne–Touraine	0–5 year(s)	Yes	Yes	No	Yes	Rarely	No	Yes
131750. Dystrophica albupapuloid, Pasini	Neonatal period and infancy	Yes	Yes	Yes	Yes	Yes	No	Yes
131850. Pretibial, Kuske–Portugal	11–24 years	No	No	No	Yes	No	No	Yes
B. Scarring, AR								
226450. Dystrophica inversa	Neonatal period	No	No	No	Yes	Yes	Yes	No
226600. Hallopeau–Siemens								
Localised	Neonatal period and infancy	Yes	Yes	Yes	Yes	Yes	Moderate involvement	Moderate involvement
Generalized	Neonatal period and infancy	Yes	Yes[c]	Yes	Yes[c]	Yes[c]	Mild	Yes
Mutilans	Neonatal period and infancy	Yes[c]	Yes[c]	Yes	Yes[d]	Yes[d]	Mild	Moderate involvement
IV. ACQUIRED (dystrophic skin)								
Acquisata	Adulthood	Yes	Yes	No	Yes	Mild	No	Yes

[a]With mental retardation.
[b]Often lethal within months after birth.
[c]Signifies severe symptoms.
[d]Signifies very severe ones.
AD, autosomal dominant; AR, autosomal recessive.

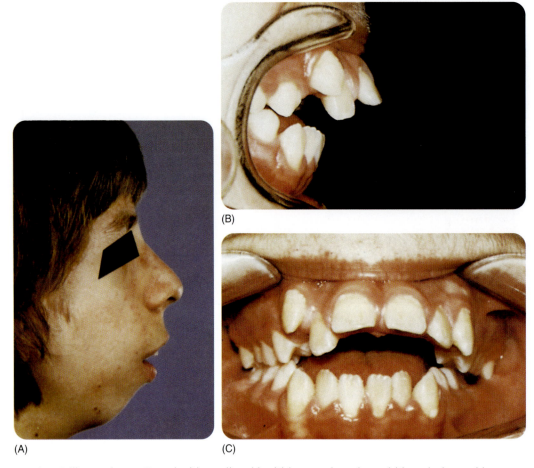

Figure 11.8 Treacher Collins syndrome. Note the (A) receding chin, (B) increased overjet and (C) marked open bite.

hydrocephalus.[211] Some 60% of cases are due to new mutations.[106]

The palate may have a cleft or be partially absent (soft palate). Hypoplasia or absence of the parotid gland is reported.[106] A micrognathic mandible (hypoplastic rami and condylar processes) and eruption disturbances with crowding and anterior open bite (Figure 11.8) are also reported.[211] Restricted opening of the mouth is rarely reported.[91] Dental treatment consists mainly of distraction (elongation) of the lower jaw,[152] which may, however, affect the development of the molars and change their position.[332] Hypodontia and enamel hypoplasia exist.

154700. Marfan's syndrome (type I), chromosome 15
Prevalence: 1.5–10:10 000 births.[137]

Abnormalities of the connective tissue (mutated fibrillin-1 gene)[211] results in skeletal abnormalities (tall stature, dolichocephaly, long narrow face, premature arthritis, spine abnormalities, joint hypermobility and contractures, slender, tall stature and long extremities, fingers, feet and toes). There are also eye abnormalities (myopia, subluxation of the lens, iris hypoplasia, early glaucoma, etc.) and cardiovascular problems (aorta aneu-

rysms, increased risk of endocarditis).[194] The ligaments are weak (e.g. flat feet).[106][211]

The prevalence of temporomandibular joint dysfunction (pain, clicking) in this syndrome is about 50% and of temporomandibular joint subluxation is about 25%.[21] The high-arched palate sometimes has a cleft. The elongated but narrow teeth are crowded in around 30%.[106][211] Mandibular and maxillary retrognathia and an extreme overjet are reported.[306] In both dentitions the roots may be either very short or curved with normal length, the pulp chambers may be either reduced in height or mildly taurodont.[69] Occasionally severe periodontitis is seen, related to the presence of malocclusion and anomalies of the elastic ligament fibres.[333]

164200. Oculo-dento-osseous dysplasia, chromosome 6[36]

257850. Oculo-dento-osseous dysplasia, AR
Prevalence: about 250 cases (Europe).

Syndrome 164200 is known as oculo-dento-digital dysplasia,[78][250][316] which refers to dysplasia of the eyes, teeth, fingers and toes. It belongs to the ectodermal hair-tooth-nail (tricho-odonto-onychal) subgroup and resembles the Hallerman–Streiff syndrome (234100). The small face has a narrow nasal bridge,

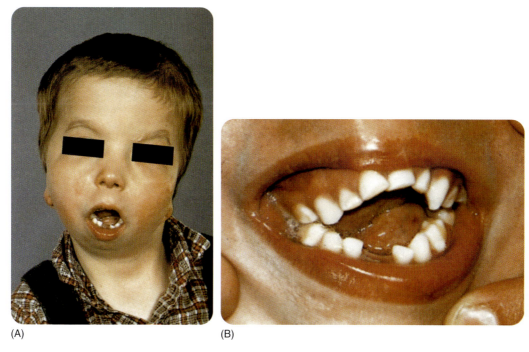

(A)   (B)

Figure 11.9 Goldenhar's syndrome: (A) asymmetrical face and (B) malocclusion with hypodontia and open bite.

hypoplastic nose alae and small anteverted nostrils. The small deep-set eyes show hypertelorism and iris anomalies (microcornea, glaucoma and cataracts). Other features are hearing loss, hypotrichotic hair, syndactyly with missing or hypoplastic middle phalanx of the fifth (and fourth?) finger and toe, which are bent,[106 211] and neurological (that is, mental retardation) and skeletal abnormalities (hip dislocation, broad tubular bones).[211] Half of the cases are non-familial in origin.[106] In some families, the neurological symptoms and dysmorphic features appear to increase in successive generations.[36] The palatal vault is high and sometimes has a cleft, as does the lip. Generalised microdontia and oligodontia are observed. The hypoplastic enamel resembles amelogenesis imperfecta.[36 68 211] The recessive form shows eye and hand abnormalities, but lacks most of the characteristics of the dominantly inherited syndrome.[211]

164210. Oculo-auriculo-vertebral spectrum, chromosome 14
Prevalence: 1:3000–6000?

Due to the complexity of the syndrome the term "spectrum" has been proposed.[106 211] It had also been given other names such as hemifacial microsomia.[128] Growth of the eyes, ears and the mandible is mostly unilaterally affected. In the variant Goldenhar's syndrome the vertebrae are involved. Chromosome anomalies that are associated with "Goldenhar's" belong to trisomies 7, 9 and 18, one or two extra X-chromosomes and absence of a part of chromosomes 5, 6 and 18.[106]

The wide range of anomalies, which also vary in severity, have prompted researchers to develop classification

systems to aid treatment planning, including orthodontic treatment planning.[304] The pathognomonic feature is hemifacial microsomia (underdevelopment of half of the face, maxilla). The face is markedly asymmetrical (in 20%) or to a lesser degree (in 65%),[106] which sometimes becomes apparent a few years after birth, with hypoplasia of the facial muscles. Other anomalies concern the eye/eyelid (microphthalmia, anophthalmia), the external ears, which may be absent (sometimes an accessory lobe is present in front of the ear and there is conductive hearing loss) or displaced, and the vertebrae (such as fusion). The zygomatic arches may be hypoplastic (Figure 11.9A). Other problems concern the lungs (hypoplasia), kidneys (renal agenesis, cysts), heart (e.g. septal defects), brain (most cranial nerves may be involved, mental retardation, hydrocephalus), etc.[128 211]

The cleft palate has a high vault and the mandibular ramus is hypoplastic.[101] Lateral facial clefts may occur,[106] including a cleft lip.[211] There is a tendency towards hypodontia on the affected side,[82 305] in particular of the mandibular premolars.[304] Other dental anomalies include severe malocclusion, open bite (Figure 11.9B), delayed eruption,[25] and enamel opacities in the central and lateral incisors.[304] The mesio-distal width of molars is reduced bilaterally; the more distally located the tooth, the smaller is the width. The latter finding suggests that both halves of the face are involved in microsomia.[255] A solitary median maxillary central incisor has been reported.[334] The parotid gland may be agenetic.[211]

1662001–166220. Osteogenesis imperfecta, types I, II and IV, chromosomes 17 and 7

259420. Osteogenesis imperfecta, type III, AR, chromosomes 17 and 7 (see also Chapter 3)
Birth prevalence: all types 1 : 20 000,[55] type III – possibly 25% of patients.

This connective (collagen) tissue disorder (Chapter 3) is characterised by (multiple) bone fractures due to mild to severe bone fragility, which sometimes results in disability.

- Type I patients have blue sclerae and progressive hearing loss. Although the teeth are stated to be normal,[211] 50% may have abnormal dentine. Three subtypes are distinguished: IA with normal teeth, IB with opalescent teeth and IC with dentinogenesis imperfecta.
- Type II is a perinatal form that is lethal.
- Type III patients have blue sclerae, the colour fading slowly with age, and either normal or opalescent teeth. The limbs deform progressively in childhood and the spine deforms during late childhood and adolescence. Laxity of the ligaments is described. Death (due to pulmonary hypertension and heart failure) is not uncommon in the first decades of life, but generally not in infancy. The triangular face shows frontal bossing and micrognathia. Severe generalised osteoporosis with multiple fractures is present already *in utero*.[106 211] Dentinogenesis imperfecta manifests more prominently in the deciduous than the permanent teeth.
- Type IV patients have normal white sclerae and osteoporotic bones that do not fracture. (Osteoporosis is not a unique feature of osteogenesis imperfecta and may be present in elderly people and in cases of diseases such as thalassaemia).[220] Mutations of the type I collagen genes underlie the multiple bone abnormalities, such as wormian bones, abducted hips, a large anterior fontanelle and scoliosis, depending on the type.[211]

Besides opalescent teeth or dentinogenesis imperfecta, the eruption of permanent teeth may be considerably accelerated, but delayed eruption is also reported.[234] Dens invaginatus (10%) and agenesis of permanent teeth (18%) are reported in osteogenesis imperfecta although the types associated were not specified.[167]

166750. Otodental dysplasia (or syndrome)
High-frequency sounds are not heard by affected patients, sometimes at a young age; later the hearing loss involves lower frequencies. Iris abnormalities may be present.[163] The diagnostic features of the teeth in both dentitions are: macrodontia (a product of fusion?), bulbous canines with labial enamel hypoplasia; taurodont, globe-shaped posterior teeth (globodontia, with fused cusps, most evident in the deciduous dentition); bifurcated pulp chambers; agenetic premolars (also microdontia); hyperdontia; delayed eruption; canines with short and curved roots; peg-shaped teeth; pulp calcifications and denticles; and double teeth (fusion?).[45 108 187 211 253 293 310 312 357]

175100. Gardner's syndrome (familial adenomatous polyposis), chromosome 5
Prevalence: 1 : 1400–12 000.[73 106]

Characteristic features are multiple intestinal polyps, in particular in the colon and rectum, which often develop in the pubertal period and are usually detected in the third decade of life. Left untreated, they become malignant at about the age of 40. Carcinomas may also develop elsewhere, for instance thyroid and bone sarcomas and malignant ovarian tumours.[106 211] Lipomas, fibromas, epidermoid cysts of the skin and osteomas of the facial bones make the face asymmetrical. Oral osteomas are present in more than 70%,[308] in particular in the mandible, and manifest as exostoses and diffuse sclerosis, which may be the initial clinical finding.[358] The skin and oral mucosa may be pigmented.

The teeth may show hypercementosis and failure of eruption.[254 317] Some 35% of the patients show impactions, 10–20% have hyperdontia and 10% have (large) odontomes.[106 211 269 335 358] The number of extra teeth in hyperdontia may be indicative of the severity of other symptoms.[80] About 75% of the patients have other tooth anomalies, including fused roots, agenetic teeth,[43] and persisting deciduous teeth. The dental manifestations should alert the dentist, who might be the first to detect the presence of the syndrome.[73]

176270. Prader–(Labhart)–Willi syndrome, chromosome 15
Prevalence: 1 : 25 000.[15]

This postnatal obesity syndrome is caused in 50–90% by the absence of a small part of chromosome 15 (deletion of paternal copies of some genes on the proximal long arm or maternal disomy 15,[211] or translocation of chromosomes 13 and 15).[243] There are several characteristic features.[106 211] Neonates often experience asphyxia with a weak or squeaky cry and feeding problems due to severe muscle hypotonia and hypo-reflexia, which, however, improve gradually. After the first year of life, patients may become overweight. Life-threatening obesity starts to develop at 3–5 years and becomes worse during adolescence. The patients feel excessively hungry, but weight gain also occurs on a normal diet. Diabetes mellitus develops. Males show hypogonadism, small penis, and cryptorchidism (non-descent of testes in the scrotum) and females have hypoplastic labia. The syndactylic hands and feet are small. Additional features are: osteoporosis with reduced bone mass and scoliosis, and a relative short stature. Patients have often a low IQ, are ill-tempered, stubborn with sudden aggression and neurological problems (e.g. seizures, poor motor coordination). The iris and hair are lighter coloured (blond) than in other family members and skin depigmentation (sun sensitivity) often occurs.[23 211]

Oral features are a triangular mouth, micrognathia and microdontia, high palatal vault, delayed eruption of both dentitions, enamel hypoplasia (in possibly about 40%, although absent in a group of 15 patients),[359] hypodontia, hyperdontia, mucous saliva or xerostomia and caries.[15 23 243 336]

191100–191191 and 605284. Tuberous sclerosis 2, 3 4, and 1, chromosomes 16, 12(?), 11, 9, respectively

Prevalence: 1: about 6000–10 000,[125 202] or 1:50 000–150 000[239] (8.8:100 000 in Europe).

The complex of neurocutaneous syndromes used to be known as epiloia,[105] and Bourneville–Pringle syndrome.[59] The majority were said to be caused by spontaneous mutations, but this may be based upon an incorrect diagnosis: milder forms may not have been recognised.[169 202] A generalised description of the complex is presented here, but the clinical expressions vary widely.

Epilepsy, mental retardation, skin lesions and hamartomas (benign tumour-like nodules) are the main features. Pigmented (*café au lait*) and depigmented skin with white macules at birth resembles the leaves of the mountain ash tree (sebaceous adenoma originating from the sebaceous glands).[239] Red-pigmented skin or skin coloured more or less symmetrically (butterfly-form) angiofibromas (0.1–1.0 cm, sometimes large plaques) are found in 50–90% of the adults. Heart, brain and viscera show multiple hamartomas. The nails may be discoloured, but the main feature is the presence of many peri- and subungual fibromas. Cardiac rhabdomyoma is associated with tuberous sclerosis (Figure 11.10) and many patients have renal lesions. Half of the patients are mentally retarded and epileptic seizures, both grand and petit mal, are common from the second year of age.[106 125 211]

Although some patients survive to old age,[282] 75% die before the age of 30.[239] Treatment (with phenytoin) of epilepsy results in gingival hyperplasia, which is not related to the typical mucosal anomalies,[173] i.e. fibromatous swellings covered with normal mucosa in 10–50% of the patients,[105 106 169] sometimes only on the tongue or gingiva.[66] The palate may be arched and macroglossia may exist.[169] The alveolar processes may be enlarged due to hyperostosis.[127] Tooth eruption may be delayed. In some reports, the buccal and lingual enamel in almost 100% of cases shows small pits, but others have found much lower proportions.[106 211] The pits, sometimes the size of a pin point, can be observed with disclosing solution and on radiographs.[202] The enamel defects (and mucosal anomalies) may be the first signs and an increased number of the striae of Retzius are seen around the pits.[59] Many relatives of patients (and other controls) also show enamel pits, but in smaller numbers. The pits are not a useful screening feature,[86] but as said above, they may alert the dentist. A few patients have impacted teeth. Dental treatment with general anaesthesia may be complicated by pulmonary fibrous degeneration, which is associated with dyspnoea and even spontaneous pneumothorax.[59]

192430. Velocardiofacial syndrome (Sphrintzen VCF syndrome; chromosome 22q11 deletion syndrome), chromosome 22

Prevalence: 1:2000–5000 live births.

The syndrome consists of cleft palate (occasionally just a submucous cleft), multiple heart and arterial anomalies, microcephaly and a characteristic long facies with small optic discs, a square-shaped nasal root, and a prominent tubular nose with hypoplastic alae and a bulbous tip that may be bifid; velopharyngeal insufficiency (pertaining to the soft palate and pharynx; nasal speech) is also present. Other features are learning disability with delayed language development and poor social interaction. The

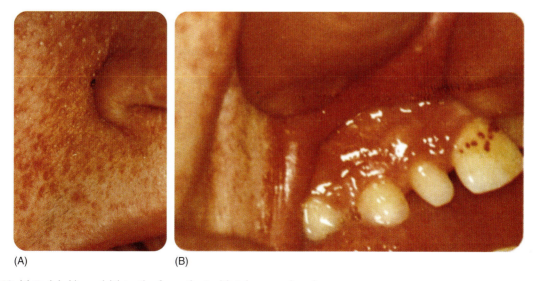

(A)   (B)

Figure 11.10 (A) Facial skin and (B) teeth of a patient with tuberous sclerosis.

hands are slender.[26][106][211] Thymus aplasia or hypoplasia leads to decrease in the number of T cells. Hypocalcaemia (due to hypoparathyroidism) occurs,[151][360] possibly in all patients and most have cardiac defects.[360]

There is a small mouth with incompetent (open) lips and cleft palate,[211] mandibular retrognathia and micrognathia (Pierre Robin sequence) with malocclusion.[26][106][211] Enamel hypoplasia,[26] often symmetrical and chronological, and hypomineralisation have been reported, but are not necessarily associated with the condition. Hypodontia, peg-shaped and "narrow" teeth, delayed tooth development and eruption times are common, as is a Class II molar relationship.[151] Presence of a solitary median central incisor (due to fusion of the right and left central incisors) is reported.[334]

194050. Williams–Beuren syndrome, chromosome 7
Prevalence: 1 : 10 000.[211]

Most cases are isolated. The characteristics are so varied, either with aortic stenosis or infantile hypocalcaemia, that two syndromes have been suspected. A number of cardiovascular defects are always present. The patients are short, the circumference of the head is small but in some patients it is increased. The midface is flat and the cheeks are full (Elvin face). The nose bridge is depressed, the nares are anteverted and the philtrum is long. The lips are thick and often wide open, and the mandible may be hypoplastic. Growth, which is initially slow with coordination problems, soon catches up; the friendly patients easily make social contacts. IQ on the average is <60. The nails are also hypoplastic.[124][211]

The teeth are agenetic or there is microdontia with generalised thin enamel.[106][211] The dentine of deciduous teeth is locally dysplastic (due to hypocalcaemia in adolescents and young people).[195] Crossbites, sometimes bilateral, are often seen in the molar region.[106]

11.3 Autosomal recessive syndromes

216400, 216411. Cockayne syndrome type I (or type A), chromosome 5

133540. Cockayne syndrome type II (or type B), AD, chromosome 10
Prevalence: 200 cases (Europe) in 2006.

Among the many signs and symptoms are dwarfism (starting in the second year), microcephaly, prematurely aged appearance, loss of subcutaneous fat, mental retardation due to impaired neurological development, loss of hearing and sight, disproportionately long limbs and flexion contractures of the joints. The thin nose is prominent and scalp hair is fine. Cryptorchidism, micropenis and small breasts are other manifestations.[106][211] The dry, anhidrotic skin becomes photosensitive to ultraviolet light (due to the inability to restore RNA synthesis)[211] and becomes scarred and pigmented in older patients.[106] The patients do not necessarily show symptoms at a young age (type I) and may

reach early adulthood,[32] but only few survive further. Type II is more severe than type I: death from pneumonia may occur at age 6–7 years.

The deciduous dentition erupts late. Some patients have oligodontia of the permanent dentition, in others some teeth are missing. The roots of teeth with hypoplastic enamel,[339] may be short and conical and the maxillary central incisors may be wide. The risk of caries is increased.[106][248][361]

225500. Ellis–van Creveld syndrome, chromosome 4
Prevalence: 7 : 1 000 000 births,[106] 0.9 : 100 000 in Europe.

Half of the patients with "short-limb dwarfism" with chondroectodermal dysplasia are to be found in an inbred isolate, the Old Order Amish of Pennsylvania, USA. In this form of ectodermal abnormality, the mesodermal cartilage is involved. The patients show dwarfism (Figure 11.11A), in particular of the distal parts of the extremities, short ribs, polydactyly (six fingers) and syndactyly, thin and wrinkled nails (Figure 11.11B), thin and sparse hair, a narrow thorax and heart defects (50–60%).[106][211] Hypospadias and cryptorchidism are reported and occasionally mental retardation.[211]

The middle of the short upper lip has a notch and is connected to the oral mucosa (partial harelip, lip-tie). Many other lip- and cheek ties exist.[119] The teeth are dysplastic (Figure 11.11C), and other dental features include conical shaped incisors, which may have several mamelons and a well-developed cingulum[244] or a talon.[119] Deciduous double teeth are reported and the deciduous (mandibular) incisors and canines may be absent, but hyperdontia and oligodontia have also been reported.[106][119][340] Further, 25% of patients have neonatal or natal teeth,[244] which may exfoliate early.[211] The enamel may be hypoplastic,[217][341] and eruption is delayed.[211]

234100. Hallermann–Streiff syndrome
Prevalence: about 150 patients,[106] all sporadic cases.[211]

Characteristics include small stature, brachycephaly and microcephaly, small eyes, blue sclerae, strabismus and cataracts, hypotrichosis and atrophic skin (nose, scalp sutural areas). Frontal and parietal bossing, a thin nose and underdevelopment of the mandible cause a "bird face" appearance. Other reported features include syndactyly, spina bifida and scoliosis, hypogenitalism and cryptorchidism, tonic-clonic seizures and sometimes mental retardation.[106][211]

Dental anomalies are present in 50–80% of the patients.[61][174] The mandible is hypoplastic with short rami and the condyles may be absent. The underdeveloped maxilla[61] has a high-arched palate.[265] Malocclusion, open bite and crowding,[61] hypodontia, oligodontia and anodontia have been reported.[71][265] Supernumerary teeth and persisting natal and neonatal teeth with rhizomicry may be present,[209][211][244] but hyperdontia may not occur.[1] Eruption may be delayed.[278] The report of a double tooth and a canine with two crowns[71] might have been a coincidence. The enamel may be hypoplastic. The anatomical features hinder anaesthesia via intubation through the mouth and nose.[68]

240300. Hypoadrenocorticism with hyperparathyroidism and moniliasis (AR and AD), chromosome 21
Prevalence: at least 70 patients have been described.[168]

The syndrome, presently named autoimmune polyendocrine syndrome, type I, is characterised by the presence of a minimum

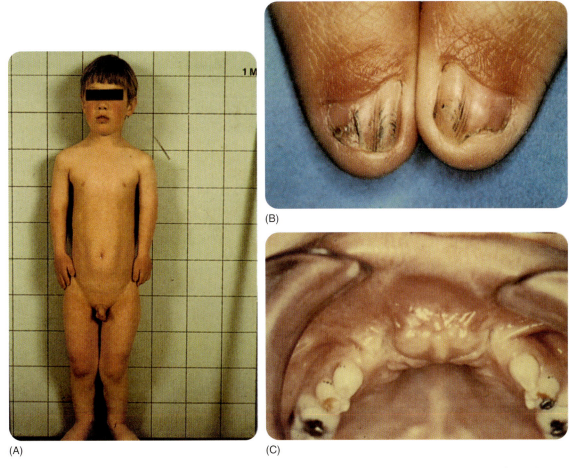

Figure 11.11 Ellis–van Creveld syndrome: (A) dwarf stature, (B) dystrophic nails and (C) dental agenesis and malformations.

of two of three major features: Addison's disease (that is, adrenal insufficiency), hypoparathyroidism and chronic mucocutaneous candidiasis. Three subtypes are recognised. In type I (endocrine candidiasis syndrome), two of the three clinical symptoms mentioned above present. It has its onset in childhood and the parathyroid cortex function is compromised (idiopathic atrophy). Hepatitis, pernicious anaemia and hypogonadism are common. Chronic oral and nail candidiasis is the third major symptom. Acquired hypothyroidism is rare and is preceded by tetany because of decreased serum calcium and increased phosphorous levels.[106 211] Type II (269200) is not associated with dental anomalies. In type III, Addison's disease is absent, but autoimmune thyroid disease and other autoimmune disorders are present.[106] The lethal disorder results in progressive weakness, malabsorption of food, diabetes mellitus, anorexia, and pigmentation of the skin and oral mucosa.[211] Tissues of ectodermal origin are affected (alopecia, nails). The enamel is chalky white and hypoplastic, either completely or in alternating bands,[201] and is insensitive to treatment with calcium and vitamin D.[303] The dental anomalies may precede (and occur independent of)[168] the hypocalcaemia.[106] The roots (of premolars) are short while the pulp chambers are large. The eruption of the teeth is sometimes delayed. Hypodontia is observed.[106]

241500, 241510. Infantile hypophosphatasia, chromosome 1

146300. Adulthood hypophosphatasia, AD, chromosome 1
Prevalence: 1 : 100 000.[94]

The syndrome is principally manifest as defectively mineralised bones and teeth. Clinical manifestations vary between affected kindred, but are relatively consistent within each kindred. The recessive mode of inheritance has the most severe symptoms.[129] Several forms are distinguished, dependent on the age of development.[342] Serum alkaline phosphatase is 7–10 times lower than normal.[179] If the syndrome starts *in utero* or early life (241500), the features include severe skeletal abnormalities (craniosynostosis and others), hypercalcaemia and early death. Many of the children who have the second type (241510) are initially normal, but gradually develop malaise, eating problems, anorexia, dehydration, constipation and irritability.[106] Rachitis-like bone disorders may be present.[219]

A characteristic feature, sometimes the only one, called *odonto-hypophosphatasia*, consists of very premature exfoliation of one or some deciduous (anterior) teeth, a consequence of absence of (normal) cementum and loss of alveolar bone.[40 178 219] Space must be maintained for the permanent teeth.[46] The pulp cavities are large. Hypoplastic enamel,[39] shell teeth[178] and premature resorption may occur. Delayed eruption of deciduous teeth is reported, as is rampant caries,[172] but premature exfoliation of fully rooted deciduous teeth seems characteristic.[342] Cortisone and a diet rich in phosphates seem somewhat promising treatments.[39]

252100. Orofaciodigital syndrome, type OFD II

Prevalence: 1:300 000,[106] 1.2:100 000 (Europe).

311200. Orofaciodigital syndrome, type OFD I, X-linked dominant

Prevalence: 1:50 000[106] or 1:250 000,[148] in cleft lip and/ or palate patients 15:1000.[148]

At least nine OFD types are distinguished,[148] which some common, moderate defects in the face, digits and intraorally.[106] Some of them are described in just one family.[106] OFD II or Mohr's syndrome patients are deaf, have short stature and possess broad hands with polydactyly, syndactyly and brachydactyly. The face shows hypertelorism, zygomatic arch hypoplasia, a low nasal bridge and a broad, sometimes bifid nasal tip. Some of the other features are hydrocephaly and scoliosis.[106 211] Contrary to OFD I, the skin and hair are normal.[211] The upper lip has a central cleft and the lobulated tongue shows a midline cleft or nodules. The mandible may be hypoplastic. Many hypertrophied frena are present, though less than in OFD I.[106] The mandibular central incisors are either normal or agenetic, but hyperdontia is also observed and more incidentally, microdontia, taurodontism and talons.[100]

OFD I (or Papillon–Léage–Psaume) mostly presents in females, and affects the face, mouth and hands/feet. The penetrance of the syndrome in males is either very incomplete or the syndrome is lethal in utero. The mandibular rami, zygomatic arches and the nostrils are not fully developed. The face shows frontal bossing and hypertelorism and there is hypersecretion from the sebaceous glands. The broad hands show syndactyly with unilateral polysyndactyly or brachydactyly. The second to fifth toes and fingers are hypoplastic. The dry scalp is covered with sparse, dry, rough and brittle hair (local alopecia).[106 111 148] About 30–50% of the patients have an IQ of 70–90, with brain malformation, seizures and hydrocephalus. Hamartomas in the hypothalamus are associated with precocious puberty. The short upper lip may show a pseudo-cleft in the midline and there may also be a cleft in the palate. A lateral cleft may divide the upper jaw in three segments: one anterior part containing the incisors and canines and two post-canine segments. The tongue may show several clefts (of the rim) resulting in a lobulated or a bifid tongue and hamartomas.[106] Besides agenesis of the maxillary lateral incisors[100] or mandibular incisors and eventually the canines,[78 111] hyperdontia and malocclusion have been reported.[101 148 259] A double tooth was reported once[148] and may not be part of the syndrome. Multiple hyperplastic frena connect the lip and cheeks with the jaws[78] and may cause ankyloglossia.[106]

252800–253220. Mucopolysaccharidoses (Table 11.2), chromosomes 4, 5, 7, 12, 14, 16, 17

309900. Mucopolysaccharidosis, X-linked

Mutations in genes lead to deficient lysosomal enzymes that split the glycosaminoglycans, formerly called

Table 11.2 Mucopolysaccharidoses (MPS)

Number/MPS type	Period of development	Enzyme deficiency	IQ	Skeletal
252800 I-H (Hurler)[a,b]	0–2 years	α-L-iduronidase	±	++++
252900 III-A (Sanfilippo)[b]	4–6 years	Heparan sulfate N-sulfamidase	–	+
252920 III-B (Sanfilippo)[b]		α-N-acetyl-glucosaminidase	–	+
252930 III-C (Sanfilippo)[b]		Acetyl CoA: α-glucosaminide-N-acetyltransferase	–	+
252940 II-D (Sanfilippo)[b]		α-N-acetylgalactosamine-6-sulfatase	–	+
253000 IV-A (Morquio)[c]	1–2 years	N-acetylgalactosamine-6-sulfate sulfatase	+	++++
253010 IV-B (Morquio)[c]		β-Galactosidase	+	++++
252300 IV-C (Morquio) (252800 V = Type I-S [Scheie], see text)		β-N-acetylhexoaminidase B		
253200 VI (Maroteaux -Lamy)[d]	2–6 years	N-acetylgalactosamine-4-sulfatase	+	+++
253220 VII (Sly)[e]		β-glucuronidase	±	+++

[a]Excessive urinary excretion of dermatan sulfate.
[b]Excessive urinary excretion of heparan sulfate.
[c]Excessive urinary excretion of keratan sulfate.
[d]Excessive urinary excretion of GAGs (glycosaminoglycans).
[e]Excessive urinary excretion of acid mucopolysaccharides.
+, normal; ±, reduced; –, considerably reduced. Greater number of + signs indicates more severe skeletal aberrations.[106 146 266]

mucopolysaccharides. The syndrome concerns dermatan sulfate, heparan sulfate and keratan sulfate. The family of the metabolic disorders is still known as "mucopolysaccharidoses". Rare types are not covered here. Glycosaminoglycans, which are not or are insufficiently degraded, are to a large degree stored intracellularly, and the urinary excretion of the three sulfates increases. Common findings (except in Morquio's syndrome) in the clinically differing phenotypes are skeletal malformations ("dysostosis multiplex"), such as short stature (not a feature of Scheie's syndrome), stiff joints, stiffening of the thorax and in some types mental retardation. The severity of the features differs by type. Other disturbances are cardiovascular abnormalities, again differing by type, eye problems (corneal clouding), abnormal hair and hepatosplenomegaly. The face often becomes coarse.

Ad 252800. Type I: MPS I-H (The letter "H" refers to Hurler)
Prevalence: 1:100000.[160]

Scheie's syndrome is less severe than Hurler's syndrome and the Hurler–Scheie syndrome is an intermediate type.[106 146] The full picture in Hurler's syndrome develops during the second year of life[106] and the syndrome is lethal,[95] usually before age 10. Deficient α-L-iduronidase activity precludes the intralysosomal degradation of the glycosaminoglycans sulfates that contain α-L-iduronidin. Therefore non-degraded or partially degraded mucopolysaccharides accumulate and interfere with the functioning of affected cells. Hurler patients are severely mentally retarded and have skeletal malformations (such as an enlarged skull, gargoyle-like face, claw-like hands); the abdomen is protruded due to hepatic and splenic enlargement, the cornea shows clouding and the skin becomes dry, pale and coarse. Death occurs because of lethal blockage of the coronary arteries and pneumonia. Bone marrow transplantation is effective, but many patients do not have matching relatives and use of material from unrelated donors is associated with an increased risk of morbidity. Infusion of the missing enzyme may result in clinical and biochemical improvement.[281]

Oral features are: macroglossia; a high-arched palate; short mandibular rami and spaced, hypoplastic peg-shaped teeth with retarded eruption; narrow, irregular dentinal tubules with a decreased protein content; irregularly arranged enamel prisms; and microgaps at the dentino–enamel junction.[343] Dentigerous cysts occur bilaterally,[344] and also in other mucopolysaccharidoses (Maroteaux–Lamy).[345]

Ad 252900–252940.
Clinically the four types do not differ much, but biochemically they are well distinguished. **Sanfilippo's types IIIA–IIID** patients show severe mental and neurological degeneration with relatively mild mucopsolysaccharidosis features. The degradation of heparan sulfate requires activity of four different enzymes (Table 11.2). Failing activity of each one results in one of the four subtypes and consequently there is lysomal accumulation of heparan sulfate. Type IIIA is more severe than types IIIB and IIIC and has an earlier onset. The relatively mild features resemble those of Hurler's syndrome (type I). The mildly coarse facial appearance of patients with normal stature is dull and the abundant (scalp) hair is coarse. Hearing loss occurs. Joint stiffness

and hepatosplenomegaly are also mild and the corneas are clear. Dysostosis multiplex (dense calvaria and, in IIIA, thickened ribs, egg-shape vertebrae) develops slowly.[106 211] The main clinical feature is a progressive mental deterioration.[298]

The tongue does not protrude. Dental abscesses may develop. There has been one report of pulp obliteration, which have may been coincidental.[106] Patients may also have microdontia, delayed formation and eruption of the teeth[278] and bruxism.[298]

Ad 253000. MPS IV-A, Morquio's syndrome
Prevalence: 1:40000.[149]

The specific enzyme deficiency (Table 11.2) due to which keratan sulfate is not degraded enables a genotypical diagnosis. Some of the general features, which have three grades of severity, include dwarfism (short trunk), a short neck, progressively flattening vertebrae with consequent neurological symptoms, flexed knees, long limbs, flat feet, osteoporosis, a flaring rib cage with marked kyphosis, weak musculature and hyperflexible joints. The IQ is normal. Patients do not die before middle age. The corneas slowly opacify and progressive deafness starts in adolescence.

The mouth is broad, the maxilla prominent and the nose short. The teeth may be widely spaced, either due to the large jaws or, more likely,[149] because of thin, hard enamel that breaks away. The very porous enamel makes the crowns appear dull white, grey or yellow. Pitting and concave or vertical indentations of the buccal and occlusal enamel have been reported.[238] Typically, the cusps of the molars are small and sharp/pointed[254] (Figure 11.12), but they become flattened because the enamel flakes off.[17 149 254] The anterior teeth are spaced and flared.[346] The severity of the dental anomalies is not related to the severity of the biochemical and other clinical findings.[149]

Ad 253010. MPS IVB, Morquio's syndrome (or Morquio's disease)
Prevalence: 0.4:100 000 (Europe).

In general a milder or moderately severe (different alleles)[106] phenotype than IVA is present. The two types

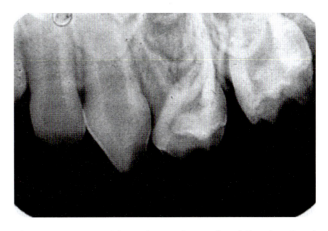

Figure 11.12 Morquio's syndrome: the small and sharply pointed molar cusps are typical of this syndrome.

may be distinguished by the quality of enamel: hypoplastic enamel in IVA and normal enamel in IVB.[149 238]

Ad 252300. A (possible) third subtype of **Morquio's syndrome, IV-C,** is caused by another deficient enzyme (Table 11.2) that is involved in the degradation of keratan sulfate.[106] However, keratosulfate is not excreted in the urine.[211] To our knowledge, no dental anomalies have been reported.

265800. Pyknodysostosis, autosomal recessive, chromosome 1
Prevalence: >100 patients.[20]

Pyknodysostosis (**pycnodysostosis**) consists of sclerosing osteochondrodysplasia. The diagnosis requires the combination of osteopetrosis (on radiographs there is increasing bone density, but the numbers of osteoclasts, which lack a major resorbing protease, is normal) and dwarfism (height <1.50 m due to shortness of the extremities). Features are cranial dysplasia (persisting fontanelles, open cranial sutures), obtuse mandibular angle and dysplastic or short terminal phalanges (brachydactyly).[57 140] Additional findings are clavicular dysplasia, hypermobile joints, thin and hypoplastic nails with grooves on stubby fingers, a tendency to fractures, a deformed head (that is, frontal bulging), small face and blue sclerae (in bulging eyes). The French painter Toulouse–Lautrec may have had pyknodysostosis.[106 132 211]

The eruption of the permanent dentition is delayed and premature eruption of the deciduous dentition has been reported.[57 200 268 347] During the eruption of permanent teeth in the small jaws, the deciduous teeth persist due to delayed root resorption,[140] resulting in delayed eruption and two rows of teeth.[278] Unerupted maxillary teeth have been observed in the floor of the hypoplastic maxillary sinus and may protrude in the antrum.[348] In older patients, the palate is high and narrow with a deep groove. The teeth are severely crowded and there is a high risk of caries.[57 132 140 294] A deep carious lesion leads to pulpal death, which in turn causes infection in the apical bone, which may develop further into osteomyelitis. Periodontitis is another cause of osteomyelitis.[294 229] The patients frequently have an open bite.[57 140] Sometimes the teeth are agenetic, and others have reported enamel hypoplasia[200 254] and hypercementosis.[200]

268400. Rothmund–Thomson syndrome, chromosome 8
Prevalence: 70% of the 130 reported cases are in females.[106]

The syndrome belongs to the tricho-odonto-onychal subgroup of the ectodermal dysplasias. Skin lesions develop first (3–6 months) on the cheeks and ears, which become red and swollen. Developing later is a poikilodermatous (mottled) appearance due to local atrophy, (de)pigmentation and telangiectasia on the buttocks, hands, forearms and legs. Other features are alopecia and early grey hair, frontal bossing, juvenile cataracts and microphthalmia. Hypersensitivity to sunlight (blistering in 33%), warty keratosis and squamous and basal cell carcinoma may be related, but osteosarcoma and fibrosarcoma, which have also been reported, are likely not to be related. The voice is high-pitched and there is hypospadias/hypogonadism in 25%. A bird-face appearance has been noted. Occasional cases of dwarfism, diabetes mellitus and mental retardation are reported.[106 211] The

slender arms may lack the radius, ulna and thumbs.[106] The dentition shows microdontia, absence of secondary occlusal grooves and enamel ridges,[312] short conical roots,[35] taurodontism,[154] oligodontia combined with hyperdontia, sometimes anodontia,[217] and delayed eruption.[35 217 278]

11.4   X-linked syndromes

305400. Facio(digito)genital dysplasia (Aarskog(–Scott) syndrome)
Prevalence: about 200 cases (Europe).

Patients have a slightly short stature, but not at birth. Males have a "saddle-bag" bifid scrotum and cryptorchidism, but are able to reproduce after delayed puberty. The face is round with low-set ears and a broad forehead, hypertelorism, strabismus, drooping upper eyelids and anteverted nostrils under a broad nasal bridge. The short neck may be webbed. The hands show brachydactyly (the terminal phalanges may be missing), soft tissue webbing between the fingers and hyperextensible finger joints. Both mental retardation and normal intelligence have been reported. Females show less severe features than males.[106 211]

A cleft of the lip and palate may occur. Other dental findings are enamel hypoplasia and hypocalcification, hypodontia, rhizomicry and delayed eruption.[106 268] Due to hypoplasia of the maxilla, the mandible shows relative prognathism. Crowding, malocclusion, persisting deciduous teeth and taurodontism have been reported.[67]

305600. Focal dermal hypoplasia syndrome (Goltz–Gorlin syndrome)
Prevalence: 90% females,[106] 200–300 cases in Europe.

The ectodermal and mesodermal tissues are affected. Female reproductive ability is reduced. Homozygotic males die *in utero.*[182] The first sign is the substitution of connective tissue of the thin skin by fat nodules or large fat herniations. Papillomas are present on the atrophic and linearly hyperpigmented or hypopigmented skin, and there is urticaria as well as desquamation and angiofibromatous nodules (anus, lips). The extremities are short and the face and trunk are asymmetrical (scoliosis of the spine). The brittle hair is locally thin. A number of eye aberrations exist and the ears are deformed. The nails are dysplastic, spooned, grooved or absent. Other reported anomalies are: hand defects, such as syndactyly and polydactyly, missing fingers and palmar and plantar hyperhidrosis or hypohidrosis. Often the patient has more than two nipples. Mild mental retardation, hydrocephalus and hearing loss are also seen.[22 106 211] Oral features are a cleft tongue, lip and palate, underdeveloped mandible and microdont teeth that are peg-shaped with enamel pits;[182 312] high pulp horns have also been noted. The incisal edges are grooved and hyperdontia is reported,[312] but hypodontia and anodontia may be more common,[41 182 254] as are delayed odontogenesis and eruption,[182 268] and taurodontism.[182] Gingival hypertrophy and gingival/mucosal arborescent papillomas are reported.[23] Deciduous double teeth and mulberry molars have also been reported,[289] and root resorption is suggested to be part of the syndrome.[23]

11.5 Chromosomal syndromes

These syndromes were previously classified as "chromosomal",[211] but presently they are grouped under either autosomal or X-linked and Y-linked syndromes. Because more than one gene is involved, they are dealt with separately in this book.

190685. Down's syndrome, trisomy 21 included, X-linked (chromosomal)

Prevalence: 1:600–1000 live births.[74 251]

Down's syndrome (mongolism and trisomy G) is caused by meiotic non-disjunction, resulting in three copies of chromosome 21 (trisomy 21) in the somatic cells. In a small proportion, the condition is inherited. The older the mother, the higher is the risk of the syndrome, but the majority of the children are born to mothers younger than 35 years. The age of the father (>55 years) has a role in non-disjunction during spermatogenesis.[232] Some women (2–3%) show mosaics: cells with 46 chromosomes and others with 47 chromosomes. The extra chromosome 21 may be partially present (partial trisomy 21).[211]

Not all patients have a low IQ (25–70, small brain with a reduced number of cortical convolutions). Features include generalised growth retardation with short extremities, congenital heart defects, duodenal and/or pyloric stenosis, risk of leukaemia, immunological disorders, small penis and scrotum, cryptorchidism, and hyperflexible joints. There is brachycephaly with small ears. The skull base and midface are underdeveloped at birth and although growth occurs thereafter, development still lags behind.[85 106 211] The characteristic facies is flat with a rounded profile (upslanting palpebral fissures, epicanthal folds, convergent strabismus, nystagmus, broad nose with flat nose bridge). The life span, in spite of medical advancements, is usually 16–40 years. An estimated 75–90% die *in utero*.[58]

Common intraoral features are a narrow palate, small jaws with broad, incompetent, cracked lips and a relatively large protruding tongue that can be grooved (lingua plicata).[77 106] Both the irregular, macrodont deciduous and the microdont permanent dentition erupt late in an unusual sequence,[18 106 213 271] but not in patients with a mosaic pattern.[199] Other reported features are hypocalcification and hypoplasia (related to diseases in youth[74] due to immunodeficiency),[106] conical teeth, hypodontia (in 27–50%, but also as low as in 13% is reported) in the incisor and premolar region,[33 102 212 352] in particular of the mandibular central incisors,[3 74] the permanent canine[33] and maxillary lateral incisors.[3] Third molar agenesis, which occurs more often in the maxilla than in the mandible, is more frequent than in the general population,[159] and could be as high as about 75%.[257] Anodontia (20%) is proven to occur,[352] and hyperdontia[48] might be coinci-

dental. Shovel-shaped incisors are also seen,[251] and taurodontism (50–66%),[3 135 352] mainly meso-taurodontism, is observed more frequently in females (33%) than males (23%). The second molars are more often affected (53%) than the first (40%) and third molars (7%).[223] Two-thirds of cases have Angle's Class III malocclusion.[33] The teeth (including roots) are small and the molars show morphological reduction, with absence of Carabelli's cusps,[222] but the reverse is true in the deciduous dentition.[284] The second deciduous and permanent first molars have a reduced mesio-distal crown width, thin enamel and dentine, with large pulp width (due to reduced proliferation and functioning of the ameloblasts and odontoblasts).[319] Asymmetries in the deciduous and permanent dentition may point to the influence of environmental factors.[283] Maxillary canine/first premolar transposition was found in 15% of 34 patients.[257]

The eruption is delayed, and the tooth morphology simpler than in siblings. Periodontitis is frequent (90%),[106] already at a young age, due to which many younger patients become edentulous.[74 191 234] Compared with age-matched children with mental retardation, Down's syndrome patients appear to have deep pockets and an early onset of severely destructive periodontal disease, which seemingly depends on alterations in their immunological response.[49] Preventive management seems ineffective.[353]

The serum interleukin-2 receptor level is much higher in Down's patients with periodontitis than in controls. Interleukin acts as an immunological messenger and triggers cellular immune response, but if the interleukin binds to free receptors in the serum, the specific receptor function found on the cell surfaces is blocked.[60]

There is severe tooth wear, associated with bruxism and reflux of gastric juices and vomiting.[27] In relation to the pH of stimulated saliva, studies are contradictory.

A lower salivary flow rate and a lower salivary potassium and a higher sodium concentration have been established. The anti-caries activity of the enzymes amylase and peroxidase is reduced in the syndrome.[263]

Klinefelter's syndrome and variants, X-linked and Y-linked (chromosomal)

Prevalence: about 2:1000 boys.

Males may possess one extra X chromosome, 47,XXY, and exhibit female characteristics. Occasionally patients have more than two X-chromosomes, 48,XXXY and 49,XXXXY, which is the most severe syndrome (prevalence: 1:85000–100000 male births).[117] Other aneuploidy variants are 48,XXYY and 46XY/47,XXY (mosaicism).[106] Postpubertally, males lack testosterone and show eunuchoid growth, hypogonadism (normal penis, but small testes, azoospermia), gynaecomastia (breast formation), elevated levels of urinary gonadotropins, varicosities and leg ulcerations, coarse face with hypertelorism and upslanting palpebral fissures. The extremities may be long. Patients often have low IQ and, generally, the greater the number of X chromosomes, the more severe are the features.

Taurodontism of the deciduous and permanent molars, hypodontia (that is, of the premolars), delayed permanent tooth development, shovel-shaped incisors and mandibular prognathia are reported.[117] The crowns of the permanent teeth are larger in size, due to the increased enamel thickness and long roots, which are due to the stimulatory effects of the Y chromosome.[364]

278850. XX male syndrome[211]
Prevalence: 1:25 000.[106]

Maleness is inherited predominantly. However, females with a normal sex chromosome constitution may show masculinisation, possibly due to reciprocal X–Y interchange at paternal meiosis.[211] The phenotype of 46,XX males is that of 47,XXY, but they are not as tall and the disproportion between limbs and trunk is absent.[106] Males with extra X-chromosomes have taurodontism,[50 145 247 277] as do 47,XXX and 48,XXXX females; moreover, hypodontia occurs in 49,XXXXX.[106] Males have taurodontism only when they possess two extra X-chromosomes,[83] but (hypo)taurodontism in the second and third molars has been observed in a third of men with one additional X-chromosome,[50 295] which lead to the diagnosis of the syndrome.[50] The degree of taurodontism is possibly determined by the number of additional X-chromosomes,[274] and certainly its prevalence (in a statistical sense).[106] One additional X-chromosome is associated with larger than normal permanent teeth and shovel-shaped incisors.[145 285] Patients frequently have open bite, crossbites and mesial occlusion as a consequence of mandibular prognathism.[160]

Some males possess one extra Y-chromosome (for instance 47,XYY). They have macrodont teeth and shovel-shaped incisors.[106] The increased tooth size has been suggested to be a direct genetic effect. Both the X- and Y-chromosomes have dental growth promoting gene(s), but the Y-chromosome gene(s) may be more effective than the X-chromosome gene(s).[4]

45,X females (Turner's syndrome)
Prevalence: 1:2500 births.

Females may lack one X-chromosome or miss a part of one of the X-chromosomes (i.e. a transversal split), whereas, again, others have mosaicism (45,X/46,XX or 45X/47,XXX or 45X/46,XY, respectively).[106 211] About 60% of patients with pterygia (a webbed neck and for instance webbed popliteal spaces (back of the knees)) have one X-chromosome.

Until 12–14 years the bone age is normal, after which the growth spurt fails to occur, causing short stature. Gonadal dysgenesis in sterile patients is characteristic.[106] The maxilla and mandible are retrognathic due to underdevelopment of the skull base.[135 136] Skeletal abnormalities include radial deviation of the forearm, short metacarpals and metatarsals, chest deformity and osteoporosis. The nails are hypoplastic and the webbed neck is short and broad. The skin shows pigmented nevi and lymphoedema of the hand and feet. Sight abnormalities (often strabismus) and auditory problems are common. The risk of cardiovascular defects (prevalence 15–50%) depends on the karyotype present.[106]

The dental development of permanent teeth is 1 year ahead,[188] but their eruption is ahead by only a few months.[150 189] The numerical aberration in the X-chromosome likely affects the amount and quality of secretion of amelogenin.[354] Consequently, the size of the deciduous molars and the mesio-distal and sometimes the bucco-lingual width of the permanent teeth is smaller than normal, the enamel being thin,[150 177 189 286] with, for instance, morphologically deviating disto-lingual cusps of first permanent molars.[150 177] About a third have two-rooted mandibular premolars.[362]

In 45,X/46,XX mosaics an asymmetry in the occlusal morphology of the first permanent molars is possibly due to different cell lines being regulated by discrete genes.[218] The maxillary incisors are often not mirrored. Although a number of aberrations involve morphological reduction, the opposite has also been noted, such as large, conical premolars.[189]

Females with dysmorphic Noonan's syndrome (163950, chromosome 12) have a normal chromosomal constitution, yet show many features of Turner's syndrome, such as short stature, broad or webbed neck, chest deformity, hypertelorism, mild mental deficiency, congenital heart disease and a triangular face, which is why this was previously considered to be pseudo-Turner's syndrome. Males are affected too, with the condition then called male Turner's syndrome. The prevalence is 1:1000–2500 among females.[76] Other features are possibly due to cherubism.[76] The dental anomalies are as described above.[189]

References

Introduction and Chapter 1: Anomalies of Number

1. AASHEIM B, ÖGAARD B. Hypodontia in 9-year-old Norwegians related to need of orthodontic treatment. Scand J Dent Res 1993; 101: 257–60.
2. ABRAMOVITCH K et al. Bulky maxillary central incisor. Gen Dent 1989; 37: 421–3.
3. ACS G et al. Bilateral double primary molars: case report. Pediatr Dent 1992; 14: 115–16.
4. ACTON CHC. Multiple supernumerary teeth and possible implications. Aust Dent J 1987; 32: 48–9.
5. ADLER P, ADLER-HRADECKY C. Die Agenesie des Weisheitszahnes. Dtsch Zahnärztl Z 1963; 18: 1361–9.
6. AGUILO L, GANDIA JL. Late development of maxillary supernumerary tooth: a case report. J Clin Pediatr Dent 1997; 22: 41–4.
7. AGUILO L et al. Primary triple teeth: histological and CT morphological study of two case reports. J Clin Pediatr Dent 2001; 26: 87–92.
8. ALALUUSUA S et al. Natal and neonatal teeth in relation to environmental toxicants. Pediatr Res 2002; 52: 652–5.
9. ALALUUSUA S et al. Developmental dental aberrations after the dioxin accident in Seveso. Environm Health Perspect 2004; 112: 1313–18.
10. AL-EMRAN S. Prevalence of hypodontia and developmental malformation of permanent teeth in Saudi-Arabian schoolchildren. Br J Orthod 1990; 17: 115–18.
11. ALEXANDER SA et al. Deciduous tooth anomalies and partial anodontia. Oral Surg 1985; 60: 230.
12. ALEXANDER-ABT J. Apparent hypodontia. Am J Orthod Dentofac Orthop 1999; 116: 321–3.
13. ALLWRIGHT WC. Natal and neonatal teeth. Study among Chinese in Hong Kong. Br Dent J 1958; 105: 163–72.
14. ALMEIDA CM, GOMIDE MR. Prevalence of natal/neonatal teeth in cleft lip and palate children. Craniofacial J 1996; 33: 297–9.
15. ALMEIDA JD et al. Supernumerary mesiodentes with familial character. Quint Int 1995; 26: 343–5.
16. ALPASLAN G et al. Disturbances in oral and dental structures in patients with pediatric lymphoma after chemotherapy. Oral Surg Oral Med Oral Pathol Oral Radiol Endod 1999; 87: 317–21.
17. ALVAREZ I, CREATH CJ. Radiographic considerations for supernumerary tooth extraction: report of case. ASDC J Dent Child 1995; 62: 141–4.
18. ALVAREZ MP et al. Natal molars in Pfeiffer syndrome type 3: a case report. J Clin Pediatr Dent 1993; 18: 21–4.
19. ALVESALO L, PORTIN P. The inheritance pattern of missing, peg–shaped, and strongly mesio–distally reduced upper lateral incisors. Acta Odont Scand 1969; 27: 563–75.
20. ANDERSON RA. Natal and neonatal teeth: histologic investigation of two black females. ASDC J Dent Child 1982; 49: 300–3.
21. ANDREASEN JO et al. The effect of traumatic injuries to primary teeth on their permanent successors. I. A clinical and histologic study of 117 injured permanent teeth. Scand J Dent Res 1971; 79: 219–83.
22. ANEGUNDI RT et al. Natal and neonatal teeth: a report of four cases. J Indian Soc Pedod Prev Dent 2002; 20: 86–92.
23. ANNEROTH G et al. Clinical, histological and microradiographic study of natal, neonatal and pre–erupted teeth. Scand J Dent Res 1978; 86: 58–66.
24. ARCHER WH, FOX LS. Choroiditis caused by a palatally impacted unerupted maxillary rudimentary supernumerary cuspid. Oral Surg 1952; 5: 861–3.
25. ARTE S et al. Gene defect in hypodontia: exclusion of EGF, EGFR, and FGF–3 as candidate genes. J Dent Res 1996; 75: 1346–52.
26. ARYA BS, SAVARA BS. Familial partial anodontia: report of a case. ASDC J Dent Child 1974; 41: 47–54.
27. ARYANPOUR S et al. Endodontic and periodontal treatment of a geminated mandibular first premolar. Int Endod J 2002; 35: 209–14.
28. ATASU M, AKYUZ S. Congenital hypodontia: a pedigree and dermatoglyphic study. J Clin Pediatr Dent 1995; 19: 215–24.
29. ATASU M, ERYILMAZ A. Synodontia between maxillary central incisor and a supernumerary incisor teeth: a dental,

genetic and dermatoglyphic study. J Clin Pediatr Dent 1996; 20: 247–51.

30. ATKINS CO, MOURINO AP. Management of a supernumerary tooth fused to a permanent maxillary central incisor. Oral Surg 1986; 61: 146–8.

31. BÄCKMAN B, WAHLIN YB. Variations in number and morphology of permanent teeth in 7-year-old Swedish children. Int J Paediatr Dent 2001; 11: 11–17.

32. BADGER GR. Pulpectomy treatment for fused deciduous teeth: a case report. J Endod 1980; 6: 752–3.

33. BAILIT HL. Dental variation among populations: an anthropologic view. Dent Clin North Am 1975; 19: 125–39.

34. BANKS HV. Incidence of the third molar development. Angle Orthodont 1934; 4: 223–33.

35. BARAC-FURTINOVIC V. Double teeth in primary dentition and findings of permanent successors. Acta Stomatol Croat 1991; 25: 39–43.

36. BARTLEMAN PC. Supernumerary teeth. Dent Cosmos 1932; 74: 1028.

37. BAUM BJ, COHEN MM. Studies on agenesis in the permanent dentition. Am J Phys Anthropol 1971; 35: 125–8.

38. BAUM BJ, COHEN M. Patterns of size reduction in hypodontia. J Dent Res 1971; 50: 779.

39. BECKER A et al. Interdisciplinary treatment of multiple unerupted supernumerary teeth. Am J Orthod 1982; 81: 417–22.

40. BEDI R, MOODY GH. A primary double molar tooth in a child with Russell-Silver syndrome. Br Dent J 1991; 171: 284–6.

41. BEERE D et al. Mirror image supplemental primary teeth in twins: case report and review. Pediatr Dent 1990; 12: 390–2.

42. BECKTOR KB et al. Segmental odontomaxillary dysplasia: clinical, radiological and histological aspects of four cases. Oral Dis 2002; 8: 106–10.

43. BEDI R, YAN SW. The prevalence and clinical management of natal teeth – a study in Hong Kong. J Paediatr Dent 1990; 6: 85–90.

44. BELTES P, HUANG G. Endodontic treatment of an unusual mandibular second molar. Endod Dent Traumatol 1997; 13: 96–8.

45. BEN-BASSAT Y, BRIN I. Skeletodental pattern in patients with multiple congenitally missing teeth. Am J Orthod Dentofac Orthop 2003; 124: 521–5.

46. BERENDSEN WJH, WAKKERMAN HL. Continued growth of the dentinal papillae after extraction of neonatal teeth: report of a case. ASDC J Dent Child 1988; 55: 139–41.

47. BERGSTRÖM K. An orthopantomographic study of hypodontia, supernumeraries and other anomalies in school children between the ages of 8–9 years. Swed Dent J 1977; 1: 145–57.

48. BETTS A, CAMILLERI E. A review of 47 cases of unerupted maxillary incisors. Int J Paediatr Dent 1999; 9: 285–92.

49. BEYER-OLSEN EMS et al. Double formation of teeth. Dentomaxillofac Radiol 1986; 15: 99–105.

50. BIER SJ. Fusion. N Y State Dent J 1958; 24: 246–7.

51. BIGEARD L et al. Clinical and ultrastructural study of the natal tooth: enamel and dentin assessments. ASDC J Dent Child 1996; 63: 23–31.

52. BIGGERSTAFF RH. Heritability of the Carabelli cusp in twins. J Dent Res 1973; 52: 40–4.

53. BJERKLIN K, BENNETT J. The long-term survival of lower second primary molars in subjects with agenesis of the premolars. Eur J Orthod 2000; 22: 245–55.

54. BJUGGREN G. Premature eruption in the primary dentition – a clinical and radiological study. Swed Dent J 1973; 66: 343–55.

55. BLAINEY JR, HILL IN. Congenitally missing teeth. J Am Dent Assoc 1967; 74: 298–9.

56. BLANEY TD et al. Endodontic management of a fused tooth: a case report. J Endod 1982; 8: 227–30.

57. BLANK BS et al. A fused central incisor. Periodontal considerations in comprehensive treatment. J Periodont 1985; 56: 21–4.

58. BODENHAM RS. The treatment and prognosis of unerupted maxillary incisors associated with the presence of supernumerary teeth. Br Dent J 1967; 123: 173–7.

59. BODENHOFF J, GORLIN RJ. Natal and neonatal teeth; folklore and fact. Pediatr 1963; 32: 1087–93.

60. BODIN I et al. Hyperodontia. Dentomaxillofac Radiol 1978; 7: 15–17.

61. BOLAÑOS MV et al. Radiographic evaluation of third molar development in Spanish children and young people. Forensic Sci Int 2003; 133: 212–19.

62. BOLK L. Welcher Gebissreihe gehören die Molaren an? Zeitschr Morphol Anthropol 1914; 17: 83–118.

63. BORAN TL et al. Overdentures as treatment for severe hypodontia. Gen Dent 1988; 36: 472–4.

64. BORUCHOV MJ, GREEN LJ. Hypodontia in human twins and families. Am J Orthod 1971; 60: 165–74.

65. BOS H. Een opmerkelijk geval van dubbeltandformatie. Ned Tijdschr Tandheelkd 1968; 75: 537–41.

66. BOTAZZO AC et al. Natal teeth: case report. J Clin Pediatr Dent 1996; 20: 325–7.

67. BOTTOMLEY WK. Fused supernumerary tooth. Oral Surg oral Med Oral Pathol 1987; 64: 13.

68. BOWDEN DEJ. Post-permanent dentition in the premolar region. Br Dent J 1971; 131: 113–16.

69. BOYD JD, MILES AEW. Erupted tooth in a cyclop foetus. Br Dent J 1951; 91: 173–81.

70. BOYNE J. Gemination – report of two cases. J Am Dent Assoc 1955; 50: 194.

71. BOYNE PJ. Supernumerary maxillary incisors. Oral Surg 1954; 7: 901–5.

72. BRABANT H. Comparison of the characteristics and anomalies of the deciduous and the permanent dentition. J Dent Res 1967; 46 (suppl 5): 897–902.

73. BREDY E et al. Häufigkeit der Zahnunterzahl bei Anlage und Nichtanlage von Weisheitszähnen. Dtsch Zahn–Mund– Kieferheilkd 1991; 79: 357–63.

74. BRICKER SL, MARTIN R. Bilateral gemination of maxillary permanent central incisors. Oral Surg 1987; 63: 120.

75. BRIN I et al. The unerupted maxillary central incisor: review of its etiology and treatment. ASDC J Dent Child 1982; 49: 352–6.

76. BROADWAY SE, BROADWAY RT. Some cases of composite odontomes. Br Dent J 1953; 94: 87–93.

77. BRONNER-FRASER M et al. Analysis of neural crest cell lineage and migration. J Craniofac Genet Dev Biol 1991; 11: 214–22.

78. BROOK AH. The prevalence of dental anomalies in 11–14 year old children: a comparison of the continuous and discontinuous residents of a natural fluoride area. Proc Brit Paedod Soc 1974; 4: 7–12.

79. BROOK AH. A unifying aetiological explanation for anomalies of human tooth number and size. Arch Oral Biol 1984; 29: 373–8.

80. BROOK AH, EKANAYAKE NO. The etiology of oligodontia: a family history. ASDC J Dent Child 1980; 47: 32–5.

81. BROOK AH, WINTER GB. Double teeth. A retrospective study of "geminated" and "fused" teeth in children. Br Dent J 1970; 129: 123–30.

82. BROOK AH, WINTER GB. Dental anomalies in association with achondroplasia. Br Dent J 1970; 129: 519–20.

83. BROWN WB. Fusion of mandibular anterior teeth. Oral Surg 1968; 25: 708–9.

84. BRUCE KW. The effect of irradiation on the developing dental system of the Syrian hamster. Oral Surg 1950; 3: 1468–77.

85. BRUCE KW, STAFNE EC. The effect of irradiation on the dental system as demonstrated by the roentgenogram. J Am Dent Assoc 1950; 41: 684–9.

86. BRUNSVOLD MA. A geminated tooth with adjacent cyst. J Endod 1984; 10: 381–3.

87. BRUSZT P. Zwillingsbildung der obere mittleren Milchschneidezähne bei zwei Brüdern. Schizodontie oder Synodontie. Zahnärztl Welt Zahnärzt Rundschau Zahnärztl Ref 1978; 87: 498–9.

88. BUCHANAN S, JENKINS CR. Riga-Fedes syndrome: natal or neonatal teeth associated with tongue ulceration. Case report. Aust Dent J 1997; 42: 225–7.

89. BUENVIAJE TM, RAPP R. Dental anomalies in children: a clinical and radiographic survey. ASDC J Dent Child 1984; 51: 42–6.

90. BURGERSDIJK R, TAN HL. Oral symptoms of the Wolf syndrome: report of case. ASDC J Dent Child 1978; 45: 488–9.

91. BURLEY MA, REYNOLDS CA. Gemination of three anterior teeth. Br Dent J 1965; 118: 169–70.

92. BURZYNSKI NJ, ESCOBAR VH. Classification and genetics of numeric anomalies of dentition. Birth Defects Orig Artic Ser 1983; 19: 95–106.

93. BUTLER PM. The ontogeny of mammalian heterodonty. J Biol Buccale 1978; 6: 217–27.

94. BYRD ED. Incidence of supernumerary and congenitally missing teeth. ASDC J Dent Child 1943; 10: 84–6.

95. CACEDA JH et al. Unilateral fusion of primary molars with the presence of a succedaneous supernumerary tooth: case report. Pediatr Dent 1994; 16: 53–5.

96. CALDO-TEIXEIRA AS, PUPPIN-RONTANI RM. Management of severe partial hypodontia: case report. J Clin Pediatr Dent 2003; 27: 133–6.

97. ÇALISKAN MK. Traumatic gemination – triple tooth. Survey of the literature and report of a case. Endod Dent Traumatol 1992; 8: 130–3.

98. CAMM JH, WOOD AJ. Gemination, fusion, and supernumerary tooth in the primary dentition: report of case. ASDC J Dent Child 1989; 56: 60–1.

99. CARTON A, REES RT. Mirror image dental anomalies in identical twins. Br Dent J 1997; 162: 193–4.

100. CARVALHO JC et al. Malocclusion, dental injuries and dental anomalies in the primary dentition of Belgian children. Int J Paediatr Dent 1998; 8: 137–41.

101. CASSETTA M et al. Hyperdontia: an epidemiological survey. J Dent Res 2001; 80: 1295.

102. CASSIA A et al. Five mandibular incisors: an autosomal recessive trait? Br dent J 2004; 197: 307–9.

103. CASTALDI CR et al. Incidence of congenital anomalies in permanent teeth of a group of Canadian children aged 6–9. J Can Dent Assoc 1966; 32: 154–9.

104. CHADWICK SM, KILPATRICK NM. Late development of supernumerary teeth: a report of two cases. Int J Paediatr Dent 1993; 3: 205–10.

105. CHAPMAN KW. Fused supernumerary tooth. Oral Surg 1984; 58: 119.

106. CHATE RAC. Supernumerary molars. Oral Surg 1978; 45: 857–9.

107. CHAUDRY SI et al. Dental twinning. Br Dent J 1997; 182: 185–8.

108. CHAWLA HS, TEWARI A. Problems of gemination, fusion, twinning and supernumerary teeth. J Indian Dent Assoc 1975; 47: 348–54.

109. CHEN RJ, WANG CC. Gemination of a maxillary premolar. Oral Surg Oral Med Oral Pathol 1990; 69: 656.

110. CHOSACK A et al. Hypodontia: a polygenic trait–a family study among Israeli Jews. J Dent Res 1975; 54: 16–19.

111. CHOW MH. Natal and neonatal teeth. J Am Dent Assoc 1980; 100: 215–16.

112. CLAYTON JM. Congenital dental anomalies occurring in 3,557 children. ASDC J Dent Child 1956; 23: 206–8.

113. CLEM WH, NATKIN E. Treatment of the fused tooth. Oral Surg 1966; 21: 365–70.

114. COBURNE MT. The genetic control of early odontogenesis. Br J Orthod 1999; 26: 21–8.

115. COCHRANE SM et al. Late developing supernumerary teeth in the mandible. Br J Orthod 1997; 24: 293–6.

116. COHEN MM. Chromosomal disorders. Dent Clin North Am 1975; 19 (1): 87–111.

117. COUPLAND MA. Apparent hypodontia. Br Dent J 1982; 152: 388.

118. COZZA P et al. Early diagnosis and treatment of supplemental mandibular teeth: report of case. ASDC J Dent Child 2002; 69: 180–3.

119. CROLL TP et al. Fusion and gemination in one dental arch: report of a case. ASDC J Dent Child 1981; 48: 297–9.

120. CUNAT JJ, COLLORD J. Late developing premolars: report of two cases. J Am Dent Assoc 1973; 87: 1835.

121. CUNHA RF et al. Natal and neonatal teeth: review of the literature. Pediatr Dent 2001; 23: 158–62.

122. CURZON JA, CURZON MEJ. Congenital dental anomalies in a group of British Columbia children. J Can Dent Assoc 1967; 33: 554–8.

123. DANFORTH RA et al. Segmental odontomaxiallry dysplasia. Report of eight cases and comparison with

hemimaxillofacial dysplasia. Oral Surg Oral Med Oral Pathol 1990; 70: 81–5.

124. DARWISH S *et al.* Natal teeth, bifid tongue and deaf mutism. J Oral Med 1987; 42: 49–56.

125. DAS P *et al.* Novel missense mutations and a 288-bp exonic insertion in PAX9 in families with autosomal dominant hypodontia. Am J Med Genet A 2000; 118: 35–42.

126. DAS P *et al.* Haploinsufficiency of PAX9 is associated with autosomal dominant hypodontia. Hum Genet 2002; 110: 371–6.

127. DA SILVA FILHO OG *et al.* Delayed formation of a lower second premolar. J Clin Pediatr Dent 2004; 28: 299–301.

128. DAVID HT *et al.* Nonendodontic coronal resection of fused and geminated vital teeth. Oral Surg Oral Med Oral Pathol Oral Radiol Endodont 1997; 83: 501–5.

129. DAVIES PL. Agenesis of teeth of the permanent dentition: a frequency study in Sydney schoolchildren. Aust Dent J 1968; 13: 146–50.

130. DAVIS GB, TIDEMAN H. Completely fused third and fourth molars. Oral Surg 1978; 45: 981.

131. DAVIS PJ. Hypodontia and hyperdontia of permanent teeth in Hong Kong schoolchildren. Community Dent Oral Epidemiol 1987; 15: 218–20.

132. DAVIS PJ. Findings from 1163 panelipse radiographs of 12-year-old children living in Hong Kong. Community Dent Health 1988; 5: 243–9.

133. DAUGAARD-JENSEN J *et al.* Comparison of the pattern of agenesis in the primary and permanent dentitions in a population characterized by agenesis in the primary dentition. Int J Paediatr Dent 1997; 7: 143–8.

134. DAUGAARD-JENSEN J *et al.* Pattern of agenesis in the primary dentition: a radiographic study of 193 cases. Int J Paediatr Dent 1997; 7: 3–7.

135. DE BOER JG. Een mandibulaire mesiodens. Ned Tijdschr Tandheelkd 1968; 75: 258–62.

136. DE BOER JG. Odontologische spelingen der natuur. Ned Tijdschr Tandheelkd 1974; 81: 334–6.

137. DE BOER M. Aspecten van de gebitsontwikkeling bij kinderen tussen vijf en tien jaar. Verslag van een longitudinaal onderzoek bij 422 kinderen. Thesis, University of Utrecht, 1970.

138. DE BOER M. Een patiënt met agenesie van de blijvende laterale bovensnijtanden. Ned Tijdschr Tandheelkd 1987; 94: 2–4.

139. DE BOER M, KOOI SK. Dentes natales. Ned Tijdschr Tandheelkd 1998; 105: 326–8.

140. DECHAUME M. Anomalies dentaires congénitales. Précis de Stomatologie. Paris: Masson et Cie., 1966, pp. 208–9.

141. DE HAAS JM. Syndroom van Cornelia de Lange. Ned Tijdschr Tandheelkd 1972; 79: 246–7.

142. DE OLIVEIRA MATTOS-GRANER R *et al.* Anomalies of tooth form and number in the permanent dentition. ASDC J Dent Child 1997; 64: 298–302.

143. DE JONGE THE. Beschouwingen over de synodontie. Ned Tijdschr Tandheelkd 1955; 62: 828–34.

144. DE JONGE THE. Dubbeltandformatie bij de onderkaakspraemolares van 's mensen gebit [een additionele mededeling]. Ned Tijdschr Tandheelkd 1963; 70: 765–73.

145. DE JONGE THE. Verschmelzung und Verwachsung im Bereich der Molares des menslichen Gebisses. Dtsch Zahnärtl Zeitschr 1965; 20: 922–5.

146. DE JONGE THE. De mandibulaire mesiodens. Ned Tijdschr Tandheelkd 1965; 72: 95–101.

147. DELANY GM, GOLDBLATT LI. Fused teeth: a multidisciplinary approach to treatment. J Am Dent Assoc 1981; 103: 732–4.

148. DELBEM AC *et al.* Natal teeth: case report. L Clin Pediatr Dent 1996; 20: 325–7.

149. DE LAPERSONNE F. Supernumerary teeth. Dent Cosmos 1921; 63: 660.

150. DE MUYNCK S *et al.* A novel MSXI mutation in hypodontia. Am J Med Genet 2004; 127A: 401–3.

151. DERMAUT LR *et al.* Prevalence of tooth agenesis correlated with jaw relationship and dental crowding. Am J Orthod Dentofac Orthop 1986; 90: 204–10.

152. DE SIQUEIRA VCF *et al.* Dental fusion and dens evaginatus in the permanent dentition: literature review and clinical case report with conservative treatment. ASDC J Dent Child 2004; 71: 69–72.

153. DETOMASI DC *et al.* Cherubism: report of a nonfamilial case. J Am Dent Assoc 1985; 111: 455–7.

154. DIBIASE DD. The management of mid-line supernumeraries. J Int Assoc Dent Child 1971; 2: 21–6.

155. DICK HM, HONORÉ LH. Dental structures in benign ovarian cystic teratomas (dermoid cysts). Oral Surg 1985; 60: 299–307.

156. DICK HM, SIMPSON WJ. Dental changes in osteopetrosis. Oral Surg 1972; 34: 408–16.

157. DI FELICE R, LOMBARDI T. Fusion of permanent mandibular molars associated with periodontitis: a case report. Periodont Clin Invest 1993; 15: 17–18.

158. DIXON GH, STEWART RE. Genetic aspects of anomalous tooth development. In: STEWART RE, PRESCOTT GH (eds) Oral facial genetics. St Louis, MO: CV Mosby, 1976.

159. DOLDER E. Zahn-Unterzahl. Schweiz Monatsschr Zahnheilkd 1936; 46: 663–701.

160. DOLDER E. Deficient dentition. Statistical survey. Dent Rec 1937; 57: 142–3.

161. DOLINE S *et al.* The effect of radiotherapy in the treatment of retinoblastoma upon the developing dentition. J Pediatr Ophthalmol Strabismus 1980; 17: 109–13.

162. DRAKE DL. Segmental odontomaxillary dysplasia: an unusual orthodontic challenge. Am J Orthod Dentofac Orthop 2003; 123: 84–6.

163. DUNCAN K, CRAWFORD PJM. Transposition and fusion in the primary dentition: report of case. ASDC J Dent Child 1996; 63: 365–7.

164. DUNCAN WK, HELPIN ML. Bilateral fusion and gemination: a literature analysis and case report. Oral Surg 1987; 64: 82–7.

165. DUTHIE N. Partial anodontia. A prosthetic solution. Br Dent J 1981; 150: 46.

166. EAGLAND MC. Congenital absence of the second permanent molar. Br Dent J 1970; 128: 247–8.

167. ECKERT SE, WOLLAN PC. Retrospective review of 1170 endosseous implants placed in partially edentulous jaws. J Prosthet Dent 1998; 79: 415–21.

168. EDWARDS TSF. Supplemental teeth. A review and case report. Dent Pract 1966; 16: 291–2.

169. EGERMARK-ERIKSSON I, LIND V. Congenital numerical variation in the permanent dentition. Odontol Revy 1971; 22: 309–15.

170. EIDELMAN E et al. Hypodontia: prevalence amongst Jewish population: prevalence amongst Jewish populations of different origin. Am J Phys Anthropol 1973; 39: 129–33.

171. ELLISDON PS, MARSHALL KF. Connation of maxillary incisors. Br Dent J 1970; 129: 16–21.

172. ENDO T et al. Association of advanced hypodontia and craniofacial morphology in Japanese orthodontic patients. Odontology 2004; 92: 48–53.

173. ERDEM GB et al. Primary incisor triplication defect. ASDC J Dent Child 2001; 68: 322–5.

174. ERSIN NK et al. Mesiodens in primary, mixed and permanent dentition: a clinical and radiographic study. J Clin Pediatr Dent 2004; 28: 295–8.

175. FARIAS M, VARGERIK K. Dental development in hemifacial microsomia I. Eruption and agenesis. Pediatr Dent 1988; 10: 140–3.

176. FAVALLI O et al. Bilateral twinning: report of case. ASDC J Dent Child 1998; 65: 268–71.

177. FERGUSON JW. An unusual lateral incisor. Br J Orthod 1984; 11: 163–6.

178. FERGUSON NC et al. An investigation of the occurrence of diastemata and supernumerary teeth. J Am Dent Assoc 1973; 87: 1409–10.

179. FINK HD. Posterior fusion. Oral Surg 1976; 42: 852.

180. FISCHER-BRANDIES H. Probleme bei der Kieferorthopädisch-prosthetischen Behandlung bei Patienten mit Zahnunterzahl. Dtsch Zahnaerztl Z 1985; 40: 137–40.

181. FLEISCHER-PETERS A, QUAST U. Klinisch-röntgenologische Untersuchungen über Art und Häufigkeit von Zahnanomalien. Dtsch Zahnärzteblatt 1970; 24: 255–60.

182. FLINCK A et al. Oral findings in a group op newborn Swedish children. Int J Paediatr Dent 1994; 4: 67–73.

183. FOLEY J. Surgical removal of supernumerary teeth and the fate of incisor eruption. Eur J Paediatr Dent 2004; 5: 35–40.

184. FOLIO J et al. Clinical management of multiple maxillary anterior supernumerary teeth: report of a case. ASDC J Dent Child 1985; 52: 370–3.

185. FOSTER TD, TAYLOR GS. Characteristics of supernumerary teeth in the upper central incisor region. Dent Pract 1969; 20 (Sept): 8–12.

186. FRAZIER-BOWERS SA et al. A novel mutation in human PAX9 causes molar oligodontia. J Dent Res 2002; 81: 129–33.

187. FRAZIER-BOWERS SA et al. Mutational analysis of families with molar agenesis. Connect Tissue Res 2002; 43: 296–300.

188. FRIEDMAN S et al. Endodontic therapy of a fused permanent maxillary lateral incisor. J Endod 1984; 10: 449–51.

189. FRIEDMAN S et al. Endodontic management of molars with developmental anomalies. Int Endodont J 1986; 19: 267–76.

190. FROHBERG U. Bilaterale Gemination zentraler Incisivi im Oberkiefer. Dtsch Zahn- Mund-Kieferheilkd 1991; 79: 451–4.

191. FUJITA H. Median incisor fusion. Oral Surg 1984; 57: 578–9.

192. FUKUTA Y et al. Supernumerary teeth with eumorphism in the lower incisor region: report of five cases and a review of the literature. J Oral Sci 1999; 41: 199–202.

193. FULSTOW ED. The congenital absence of an upper central incisor. Br Dent J 1968; 124: 186–8.

194. GADBOIS RE. The mesiodens in the Alaskan Eskimo. ASDC J Dent Child 1969; 36: 187–8.

195. GAGE JP et al. Abnormal amino acid analyses obtained from osteogenesis imperfecta dentin. J Dent Res 1988; 67: 1097–102.

196. GALASSI MS et al. Natal maxillary primary molars: case report. J Clin Pediatr Dent 2004; 29: 41–4.

197. GARDINER JH. Erupted teeth in the newborn. Proc R Soc Med 1961; 54: 504–6.

198. GARN SM, LEWIS AB. Effect of agenesis on the crown-size profile pattern. J Dent Res 1969; 48(II): 1314.

199. GARN SM, LEWIS AB. The gradient and the pattern of crown-size reduction in simple hypodontia. Angle Orthod 1970; 40: 51–8.

200. GARN SM et al. Third molar polymorphism and the timing of tooth formation. Nature 1961; 192: 989.

201. GARN SM et al. Third molar agenesis and reduction in the number of other teeth. J Dent Res 1962; 41: 717.

202. GARVEY MT et al. Supernumerary teeth – An overview of classification, diagnosis and management. J Can Dent Assoc 1999; 65: 612–16.

203. GAZIT E, LIEBERMAN MA. Macrodontia of maxillary central incisors: case reports. Quint Int 1991; 22: 883–7.

204. GELFAND G. Fused mandibular molars. Oral Surg 1977; 44: 968.

205. GELLIN ME. The distribution of anomalies of primary anterior teeth and their effect on the permanent successors. Dent Clin North Am 1984; 28: 69–80.

206. GIBSON ACL. Concomitant hypo-hyperodontia. Br J Orthod 1979; 6: 101–5.

207. GIBSON N. A late developing mandibular premolar supernumerary tooth. Aust Dent J 2001; 46: 51–2.

208. GIMNES HT. Congenital absence of teeth in Oslo school children. Dent Abstr 1964; 9: 237.

209. GISSEN BN. Supernumerary and impacted teeth. Dent Cosmos 1935; 77: 203.

210. GLENN FB. A consecutive six-year study of the prevalence of congenitally missing teeth in private pedodontic practice of two geographically separated areas. ASDC J Dent Child 1964; 3: 264–70.

211. GOHO C. Neonatal sublingual traumatic ulceration (Riga-Fedes diseases): reports of cases. ASDC J Dent Child 1996; 63: 362–4.

212. GOLDBERG JM et al. Endodontic therapy involving fused mandibular second and third molars. J Endod 1985; 11: 346–7.

213. GOLDENBERG M et al. Clinical radiographic, and genetic evaluation of a novel form of autosomal-dominant oligodontia. J Dent Res 2000; 79: 1469–75.

214. GOLDMAN HM, BLOOM J. A collective review of dental anomalies and diseases. Oral Surg 1949 2: 880–905.

215. GOLDMAN JJ, NEWTON NJ. Supernumerary tooth bud in the maxillary antrum. Oral Surg 1949; 2: 993–4.

216. GORLIN RJ *et al*. Syndromes of head and neck. New York, NY: Oxford University Press, 1990.

217. GORLIN RJ, MESKIN LH. Severe irradiation during odontogenesis. Oral Surg 1963; 16: 35–8.

218. GRABER LW. Congenital absence of teeth: a review with emphasis on inheritance patterns. J Am Dent Assoc 1978; 96: 266–75.

219. GRAHNÉN H. Hypodontia in the permanent dentition. Odontol Revy 1956; 7 (3): 1–100.

220. GRAHNÉN H, GRANATH LE. Numerical variations in primary dentition and their correlation with the permanent dentition. Odontol Revy 1961; 12: 348–57.

221. GRAUBARD SA. Fusion of a lower second and third molar and macrodontia of a lower first molar. Oral Surg 1977; 44: 817.

222. GRAVELY JF, JOHNSON DB. Variation in the expression of hypodontia in monozygotic twins. Dent Pract 1971; 21: 212–20.

223. GREGG TA. Surgical division and pulpotomy of a double incisor tooth. Br Dent J 1985; 159: 254–5.

224. GRIFFIN GJ. Case report: a possible variant of otodental syndrome. J Paediatr Dent 1995; 1: 27–9.

225. GRIMANIS GA *et al*. A survey on supernumerary molars. Quint Int 1991; 22: 989–95.

226. GROSSMAN KE. Endodontics involving an unusual case of fusion. J Endod 1981; 7: 40–1.

227. GROVER PS *et al*. Panographic survey of US army recruits: analysis of health status. Military Med 1982; 147: 1059–62.

228. GROVER PS, LORTON L. The incidence of unerupted permanent teeth and related clinical cases. Oral Surg 1985; 59: 420–5.

229. GROVER PS, LORTON L. Gemination and twinning in the permanent dentition. Oral Surg 1985; 59: 313–18.

230. GYSEL C. Diagnose en frequentie der agenesie van de eerste molaar. Ned Tijdschr Tandheelkd 1965; 72: 597–604.

231. HAAVIKKO K. Hypodontia of permanent teeth. An ortho-pantomographic study. Suom Hammaslääk Toim 1971; 67: 219–25.

232. HAGMAN FT. Fused primary teeth: a documented familial report of case. ASDC J Dent Child 1985; 52: 459–60.

233. HAGMAN FT. Anomalies of form and number, fused primary teeth, a correlation of the dentitions. ASDC J Dent Child 1988; 55: 359–61.

234. HAIDAR Z, SHALHOUB SY. The incidence of impacted wisdom teeth in a Saudi community. Br J Oral Maxillofac Surg 1986; 15: 569–71.

235. HALL RK. Congenitally missing teeth – a diagnostic feature in many syndromes of the head and neck. J Int Assoc Dent Child 1983; 14: 69–75.

236. HALL RK *et al*. Solitary median maxillary central incisor, short stature, choanal atresia/midnasal stenosis (SMMCI) syndrome. Oral Surg Oral Med Oral Pathol Oral Radiol Endodont 1997; 84: 651–62.

237. HALS E. Natal and neonatal teeth. Oral Surg 1957; 10: 509–21.

238. HAMASHA AAH, AL-KHATEEB T. Prevalence of fused and geminated teeth in Jordanian adults. Quint Int 2004; 35: 556–9.

239. HANRATTY WJ. Odontectomy of seven impacted supernumerary bicuspids. J Am Dent Assoc 1960; 61: 80–2.

240. HANSEN LS, ENGLISH JA. Histologic changes in the incisor teeth of rats serially sacrificed after receiving 1,500 R of 200 KV. X-ray irradiation. J Dent Res 1967; 36: 417–31.

241. HANSEN L, KJAER I. A premaxilla with a supernumerary tooth indicating a developmental region with a variety of dental abnormalities: a report of nine cases. Acta Odontol Scand 2004; 62: 30–6.

242. HARRIS WE. Endodontic treatment of a fused mesiodens: report of case. J Am Dent Assoc 1971; 83: 643–6.

243. HARRISON M *et al*. Solitary maxillary central incisor as a new finding in CHARGE association: a report of two cases. Int J Paediatr Dent 1997; 7: 185–9.

244. HARTNEY PC. Unusual dentitions. Dent Radiogr Photogr 1981; 54: 16–17.

245. HARVEY CE. Veterinary dentistry. Philadelphia, PA: W.B. Saunders, 1985, p. 79.

246. HASHIM HA. Orthodontic treatment of fused and gemi-nated central incisors: a case report. J Contemp Dent Pract 2004; 5 (1): 1–6.

247. HASIAKOS PS *et al*. Treatment of an unusual case of fusion. ASDC J Dent Child 1986; 53: 205–9.

248. HASSAN FS, AL-SARRAJ FR. Fusion of primary teeth: a case report. Quint Int 1989; 20: 149–52.

249. HASUND A, BANG G. Morphologic characteristics of the Alaskan Eskimo dentition: IV. Cusp number and groove patterns of mandibular molars. Am J Phys Anthropol 1985; 67: 65–9.

250. HATTAB FN *et al*. Impaction status of third molars in Jordanian students. Oral Surg Oral Med Oral Pathol Oral Radiol Endod 1995; 79: 24–9.

251. HATTAB FN *et al*. Supernumerary teeth: report of three cases and review of the literature. ASDC J Dent Child 1994; 61: 382–93.

252. HAYES PA. Hamartomas, eruption cyst, natal tooth and Epstein pearls in a newborn. ASDC J Dent Child 2000; 67: 365–8.

253. HEGDE SV, MUNSHI AK. Late development of supernu-merary teeth in the premolar region: a case report. Quint Int 1996; 27: 479–81.

254. HELING B. A two-rooted central incisor. Oral Surg 1977; 43: 649.

255. HELLMAN M. Our third molar teeth; their eruption, pres-ence, and absence. Dent Cosmos 1936; 78: 750–62.

256. HEMMIG SB. Third and fourth molar fusion. Oral Surg 1979; 48: 572.

257. HENNIS I *et al*. Supernumerary teeth in the anterior section of the maxilla with special attention to dentoid structures (I). Quint Int 1984; 15: 731–40.

258. HERBST E, APFFELSTAEDT M. Atlas und Grundriss der Misbildungen der Kiefer und Zähne. München: J.F. Leh-manns Verlag, 1928, pp. 261–71.

259. HERNÁNDEZ-GUISADO JM *et al*. Dental gemination: report of case. Med Oral 2002; 7: 234–6.

260. HIMMELHOCH DA. Separation of fused primary incisors: report of case. ASDC J Dent Child 1988; 55: 294–7.

261. HITCHIN AD. A primary double molar tooth in a child with Russell-Silver Syndrome. Br Dent J 1992; 172: 46.

262. HITCHIN AD, MORRIS I. Geminated odontome-connation of the incisors in the dog – Its etiology and ontogeny. J Dent Res 1966; 45: 575–83.

263. HOBKIRK JA, BROOK AH. The management of patients with severe hypodontia. J Oral Rehabil 1980; 7: 289–98.

264. HOFFMANN C. Partielle Anodontie – Eine Fallbeschreibung. Quintessenz 1992; 43 947–55.

265. HÖGSTRÖM Å, ANDERSSON L. Complications related to surgical removal of anterior supernumerary teeth. ASDC J Dent Child 1987; 54: 341–3.

266. HOLCOMB JQ, PITTS DL. Endodontic treatment of an anomalous mandibular molar. J Endod 1985; 11: 87–9.

267. Holländer K. Klinisch -röntgenologische Untersuchung von drei Geschwistern mit Doppelbildungen von Milchfrontzähnen. Dtsch Zahnärztl Zeitschr 1980; 35: 831–4.

268. HOROWITZ JM. Aplasia and malocclusion: a survey and appraisal. Am J Orthod 1966; 52: 440–53.

269. HOLM AK, ARVIDSON S. Oral health in preschool Swedish children. 1. Three-year-old-children. Odontol Revy 1974; 25: 81–98.

270. HOLM AK, LUNDBERG L. Hypodontia of both primary and permanent central upper incisor. Description of a case. Odontol Revy 1972; 23: 429–35.

271. HOOLEY JR. The infant's mouth. J Am Dent Assoc 1967; 75: 95–103.

272. HOWARD RD. The unerupted incisor. A study of the postoperative eruptive history of incisors delayed in their eruption by supernumerary teeth. Dent Pract 1967; 17: 332–41.

273. HOU GL, TSAI CC. Fusion of maxillary third and supernumerary fourth molars. Aust Dent J 1989; 34: 219–22.

274. HOSOMI T *et al*. A Maxillary central incisor having two root canals geminated with a supernumerary tooth. J Endod 1989; 15: 161–3.

275. HUANG WS *et al*. Mesiodens in the primary dentition stage: a radiographic study. ASDC J Dent Child 1992; 59: 186–9.

276. HUGOSON A, KUGELBERG CF. The prevalence of third molars in a Swish population. An epidemiologic study. Community Dent Health 1988; 5: 121–38.

277. HÜLSMANN M *et al*. Hemisection and vital treatment of a fused tooth – literature review and case report. Endod Dent Traumatol 1997; 13: 253–8.

278. HUMERFELT D *et al*. Hyperodontia in children below four years of age: a radiographic study. ASDC J Dent Child 1985; 52: 121–4.

279. HUNSTADBRATEN K. Hypodontia in the permanent dentition. ASDC J Dent Child 1973; 40: 115–17.

280. HUNT NP. Hypodontia – problems of permanent space closure. Br J Orthod 1985; 12: 149–52.

281. HURLEN B, HUMERFELT D. Prevalence of premaxillary supernumerary teeth in Norwegian children: a radiographic study. Dentomaxillofac Radiol 1984; 13: 109–15.

282. HURLEN B, HUMERFELT D. Hyperdontia in 14th–18th century Norwegian populations: a radiographic study on skulls. Dentomaxillofac Radiol 1984; 13: 135–9.

283. HURLEN B, HUMERFELT D. Characteristics of premaxillary hyperodontia. A radiographic study. Acta Odontol Scand 1985; 43: 75–81.

284. ILTIS H. Inheritance of missing incisors. J Heredity 1948; 39: 363–6.

285. INTERNATIONAL HUMAN GENOME SEQUENCING CONSORTIUM. Finishing the euchromatic sequence of the human genome. Nature 2004; 431: 931–45.

286. ISMAEL SS. Supplemental maxillary deciduous canines. Br J Orthod 1987; 14: 251–2.

287. ITKIN AB, BARR GS. Comprehensive management of the double tooth: report of case. J Am Dent Assoc 1975; 90: 1269–72.

288. IVY RH. A case of non-eruption of entire permanent denture. Dent Cosmos 1933; 75: 689–90.

289. JÄRVINEN S. Congenitally missing first permanent molars: unusual course of development. ASDC J Dent Child 1984; 51: 374–5.

290. JÄRVINEN S, LETHINEN L. Supernumerary and congenitally missing primary teeth in Finnish children. Acta Odontol Scand 1981; 39: 83–6.

291. JÄRVINEN S *et al*. Epidemiologic study of joined primary teeth in Finnish children. Community Dent Oral Epidemiol 1980; 8: 201–2.

292. JENNINGS JK. Multiple supernumerary impacted mandibular bicuspids. J Am Dent Assoc 1957; 55: 877–8.

293. JIMÉNEZ-RUBIO A *et al*. A case of combined dental development abnormalities. Endod Dent Traumatol 1998; 14: 99–102.

294. JOHANNSDOTTIR B *et al*. Prevalence of malocclusion in 6-year-old Icelandic children. Acta Odontol Scand 1997; 55: 398–402.

295. JOONDEPH DR, McNEILL RW. Congenitally absent second premolars: an interceptive approach. Am J Orthod 1971; 59: 50–66.

296. JORGENSON RJ. Clinician's view of hypodontia. J Am Dent Assoc 1980; 101: 283–6.

297. JUMLONGRAS D et al. A novel missense mutation in the paired domain of PAX9 causes non-sdyndromic oligodontia. Hum Genet 2004; 114: 242–9.

298. KAFFE I *et al*. Fusion of permanent molars. Quint Int 1982; 13: 1237–9.

299. KAJII TS *et al*. Agenesis of third molar germs depends on sagittal maxillary dimensions in orthodontic patients in Japan. Angle Orthod 2004; 74: 337–42.

300. KALER LC. The incidence of mesiodens in children of Hispanic descent. J Pedodont 1986; 10: 164–8.

301. KAMANSKI FW. Gemination. Oral Surg 1978; 46: 331.

302. KANTOR ML *et al*. Duplication of the premolar dentition. Oral Surg Oral Med Oral Pathol 1988; 66: 62–4.

303. KARAÇAY S *et al*. Multidisciplinary treatment of "twinned" permanent teeth: two case reports. ASDC J Dent Child 2004; 71: 80–6.

304. KATES GA *et al*. Natal and neonatal teeth: a clinical study. J Am Dent Assoc 1984; 109: 441–3.

305. KATZ RW. An analysis of compound and complex odontomas. ASDC J Dent Child 1989; 56: 445–9.

306. KAUGARS GE *et al.* Odontomas. Oral Surg Oral Med
Oral Pathol 1989; 67: 172–6.

307. KAYALIBAY H *et al.* The treatment of a fusion between
the maxillary central incisor and supernumerary tooth:
report of case. J Clin Pediatr Dent 1996; 20: 237–40.

308. KEENE HJ. The relationship between third molar agenesis
and the morphologic variability of the molar teeth. Angle
Orthod 1965; 35: 289–98.

309. KEIL A, SPETH-ESCHENBRENNER J. Über Zahnanomalien bei 3400 Patienten nach Röntgenstaten. Dtsch Zahn
Mund Kieferheilkd 1963; 40: 360–76.

310. KELLY JR. Gemination, fusion, or both? Oral Surg 1978;
45: 655–6.

311. KERLEY MA, KOLLAR EJ. Supernumerary tooth formation in mouse molar transplants. J Dent Res 1977; 56:
1344.

312. KILLIAN CM, CROLL TP. Dental twinning anomalies:
the nomenclature enigma. Quint Int 1990; 21: 571–6.

313. KIM SG, LEE SH. Mesiodens: a clinical and radiographic
study. ASDC J Dent Child 2003; 70: 58–60.

314. KIMOTO S *et al.* Hypoplasia of primary and permanent
teeth following osteitis and the implications of delayed
diagnosis of a neonatal maxillary primary molar. Int J
Paediatr Dent 2003; 13: 35–40.

315. KINDELAN JD *et al.* Hypodontia: genotype or environment? A case report of monozygotic twins, Br J Orthod
1998; 25: 175–8.

316. KINIRONS MJ. Unerupted premaxillary supernumerary
teeth. A study of their occurrence in males and females. Br
Dent J 1982; 153: 110.

317. KINIRONS MJ. Candidal invasion of dentine complicating hypodontia. Br Dent J 1983; 154: 400–1.

318. KING NM *et al.* Multiple supernumerary premolars: their
occurrence in three patients. Aust Dent J 1993; 38:
11–16.

319. KIRVESKARI P *et al.* Crown size and hypodontia in the
permanent dentition of modern Skolt Lapps. Am J Phys
Anthropol 1978; 48: 107–12.

320. KJAER I *et al.* Aetiological aspects of mandibular tooth
agenesis – focusing on the role of nerve, oral mucosa, and
supporting tissues. Eur J Orthod 1994; 16: 371–5.

321. KLIMEK J *et al.* Rasterelektronenmikroskopische Untersuchungen und klinische Beobachtungen bei Dentes
connati. Dtsch Zahnaerztl Z 1982; 37: 685–91.

322. KLOEPPEL W. Zwillingszähne. Fortschr Kieferorthop
1956; 17: 249–51.

323. KNAPP JF, McMAHON JI. Treatment of triple tooth:
report of a case. J Am Dent Assoc 1984; 109: 725–7.

324. KNUDSEN PA. Congenital malformations of upper incisors in exencephalic mouse embryos, induced by hypervi-
taminose A. II. Morphology of fused upper incisors. Acta
Odontol Scand 1965; 23: 391–409.

325. KNUDSEN PA. Malformations of upper incisors in mouse
embryos with exencephaly, induced by trypan blue. Acta
Odontol Scand 1966; 24: 647–75.

326. KNYCHALSKA-KARWAN Z *et al.* The mesiodens teeth
under an electron scanning microscope and X-ray micro-
analyser. J Int Assoc Dent Child 1984; 15: 7–13.

327. KOBIELAK A *et al.* The novel polymorphic variants within
paired box of the PAX9 gene are associated with selective
tooth agenesis. Folia Histochem Cytobiol 2001; 39:
111–12.

328. KOCH H *et al.* Indications for surgical removal of supernumerary teeth in the premaxilla. Int J Oral Maxillofac
Surg 1986; 15: 273–81.

329. KODACERELI I *et al.* Late-forming supernumeraries in
the premolar regions. J Clin Orthod 1994; 38: 143–4.

330. KOOI SK. Aspecten van het tijdelijke gebit. Thesis, University of Utrecht, 1982.

331. KOKTEN G *et al.* Supernumerary fourth and fifth molars:
a report of two cases. J Contemp Dent Pract 2003; 4 (4):
67–76.

332. KOPP WK. A hereditary congenitally missing maxillary
central incisor. Oral Surg 1967; 24: 367.

333. KORENHOF CAW. Fylogenie van het gebit. In: VAN DE
VELDE JP (ed.) De ontwikkeling van het tand-kaakstelsel.
Ontogenie en fylogenie. Alphen aan den Rijn: Samsom
Stafleu, 1987, pp.198–286.

334. KOTSOMITIS N, FREER TJ. Inherited dental anomalies
and abnormalities. ASDC J Dent Child 1997; 64: 405–8.

335. KOZAKIEWICZ M, PERCZYNSKA-PARTYKA W,
KOBOS J. Cherubism – clinical picture and treatment.
Oral Dis 2001; 7: 123–30.

336. KRAYER JW. A supernumerary tooth located at the facial
of a mandibular lateral incisor: a case report. J Periodont
1989; 60: 410–12.

337. KRYSINSKI Z. The three-digit system of designating
supernumerary teeth. Quint Int 1986; 17: 127–8.

338. KUROL J. Early treatment of tooth-eruption disturbances.
Am J Orthod Dentofac Orthop 2002; 121: 588–91.

339. LAATIKAINEN T, RANTA R. Hypodontia in twins discordant or concordant for cleft lip and/or palate. Scand J
Dent Res 1994; 102: 88–91.

340. LAINE T, HAUSEN H. Cross-sectional study of orthodontic treatment and missing of permanent teeth in two birth
cohorts of Finnish students according to sex. Community
Dent Oral Epidemiol 1982; 10: 209–13.

341. LAMMI L et al. Mutations in AXIN2 cause familial tooth
agenesis and predispose to colorectal cancer. Am J Hum
Genet 2004; 74: 1043–50.

342. LAMMI L *et al.* A missense mutation on PAX9 in a family
with distinct phenotype of oligodontia. Eur J Hum Genet
2003; 11: 866–71.

343. LANGOWSKA-ADAMCZYK H, KARMANSKA B.
Similar locations of impacted and supernumerary teeth in
monozygotic twins: a report of two cases. Am J Orthod
Dentofac Orthop 2001; 119: 67–70.

344. LAPEER GL. Congenitally missing maxillary first permanent molars: a case report. J Can Dent Assoc 1990; 56:
535–6

345. LAUWERYNS I *et al.* Mirror image in aplasia of a premolar in a monochorial twin: case report and review. J Clin
Pediatr Dent 1992; 17: 41–4.

346. LAVELLE CLB *et al.* Cusp pattern, tooth size and third
molar agenesis in the human mandibular dentition. Arch
Oral Biol 1970; 15: 227–37.

347. LAW L *et al.* Endodontic treatment of mandibular molars
with concrescence. J Endod 1994; 20: 562–4.

348. LAWS TF. Triple mesiodentes. J Am Dent Assoc 1979; 99: 483.

349. LE BOT P, SALMON D. Congenital defects of the upper lateral incisors (ULI): condition and measurements of other teeth, measurements of the superior arch, head and face. Am J Phys Anthropol 1977; 46: 231–44.

350. LEE VAHLSING H et al. Cyclophosphamide – induced abnormalities in the incisors of the rat. J Dent Res 1977; 56: 809–16.

351. LEONARDI R, BARBATO E. A late-developing supernumerary premolar. J Clin Orthod 2004; 38: 331–2.

352. LERVIK T, COWLEY GC. Observations of dental disease and anomalies in 9- to 11-year-old Norwegian children. Acta Odontol Scand 1983; 41: 45–51.

353. LESLIE JC. Multiple supernumerary teeth. Oral Surg 1984; 57: 463.

354. LEVESQUE GY et al. Sexual dimorphism in the development, emergence, and agenesis of the mandibular third molar. J Dent Res 1981; 60: 1735–41.

355. LEVITAS TC. Gemination, fusion, twinning and concrescence. ASDC J Dent Child 1965; 32: 93–100.

356. LIBFELD H et al. Endodontic therapy of bilaterally geminated permanent maxillary central incisors. J Endod 1986; 12: 214–16.

357. LIDRAL AC, REISING BC. The role of MSX1 in human tooth agenesis. J Dent Res 2000; 81: 274–8.

358. LINDERSTRÖM A et al. Is tooth agenesis related to brainstem anomalies in myelomeningocele patients with Chiari II malformations? Acta Odontol Scand 2002; 60: 337–40.

359. LINDQVIST B. Extraction of deciduous second molars in hypodontia. Eur J Orthod 1980; 2: 173–81.

360. LINN EK. Concrescence: a case report. Gen Dent 1998; 46: 338–9.

361. LIU JF. Characteristics of premaxillary supernumerary teeth: a survey of 112 cases. ASDC J Dent Child 1995; 62: 262–5.

362. LOCHT S. Panoramic radiographic examination of 704 Danish children aged 9–10 years. Community Dent Oral Epidemiol 1980; 8: 375–80.

363. LORBER CG. Zur Klinik connataler und neonataler Zähne. Dtsch Zahnaerztl Z 1969; 24: 255–62.

364. LOWELL RJ, SOLOMON AL. Fused teeth. J Am Dent Assoc 1964; 68: 162.

365. LUDWIG FJ. The mandibular second premolars: morphologic variation and inheritance. J Dent Res 1957; 36: 263–73.

366. LUTEN JR. The prevalence of supernumerary teeth in primary and mixed dentitions. ASDC J Dent Child 1967; 34: 346–53.

367. LYON MF. Sex chromatin and gene action in the mammalian X–chromosome. Am J Hum Genet 1962; 14: 135–48.

368. MACDONALD-JANKOWSKI DS. Odontomas in a Chinese population. Dentomaxillofac Radiol 1996; 25: 186–92.

369. MADER CL. Fusion of teeth. J Am Dent Assoc 1979; 98: 62–4.

370. MADER CL. Concrescence of teeth: a potential treatment hazard. Gen Dent 1984; 32: 52–5.

371. MAGNÚSSON Te. Prevalence of hypodontia and malformations of permanent teeth in Iceland. Community Dent Oral Epidemiol 1977; 5: 173–8.

372. MAGNÚSSON Te. Hypodontia, hyperodontia, and double formation of primary teeth in Iceland. Acta Odontol Scand 1984; 42: 137–9.

373. MAIN DMG. Tooth identity in ovarian teratomas. Br Dent J 1970; 129: 328–32.

374. MAKLIN M et al. A study of oligodontia in a sample of New Orleans Children. ASDC J Dent Child 1979; 46: 478–82.

375. MAMOPOULOU A et al. Agenesis of mandibular second premolars. Spontaneous space closure after extraction therapy: a 4-year follow-up. Eur J Orthod 1996; 18: 589–600.

376. MANDEVILLE LC. Congenital absence of permanent maxillary lateral incisor teeth: a preliminary investigation. Ann Eugen 1950; 15: 1–10.

377. MARÉCHAUX SC. The treatment of fusion of a maxillary central incisor and a supernumerary: report of a case. ASDC J Dent Child 1984; 51: 196–9.

378. MARÉCHAUX SC. The single maxillary central primary incisor. ASDC J Dent Child 1986; 53: 124–6.

379. MARYA CM, KUMAR BR. Familial occurrence of mesiodentes with unusual findings: case reports. Quint Int 1998; 29: 49–51.

380. MASATOMI Y et al. Unusual multiple natal teeth. Pediatr Dent 1991; 13: 170–2.

381. MASON C et al. A retrospective study of unerupted maxillary incisors associated with supernumerary teeth. Br J Oral Maxillofac Surg 2000; 38: 62–5.

382. MASON C et al. Multiple supernumeraries: the importance of clinical and radiographic follow-up. Dentomaxillofac Radiol 1996; 25: 109–13.

383. MASSLER M, SAVARA BS. Natal and neonatal teeth. A review of twenty-four cases reported in the literature. J Pediatr 1950; 36: 349–59.

384. MATTHEEUWS N et al. Has hypodontia increased in Caucasians during the 20th century? A meta-analysis. Eur J Orthod 2004; 26: 99–103.

385. MAIBAUM WW. Fusion or confusion? Oral Surg Oral Med Oral Pathol 1990; 69: 656–7.

386. MAYHALL JT. Natal and neonatal teeth among the Tlinget Indians. J Dent Res 1967; 46: 748–9.

387. McGINNIS JP et al. Mandibular third molar development after mantle radiation in long–term survivors of childhood Hodgkin's disease. Oral Surg 1987; 63: 630–3.

388. McKIBBEN DR, BREARLY LJ. Radiographic determination of the prevalence of selected dental anomalies in children. ASDC J Dent Child 1971; 38: 390–8.

389. McNAMARA CM et al. The management of premolar supernumeraries in three orthodontic cases. J Clin Pediatr Dent 1977; 22: 15–18.

390. MEADORS LW, JONES HL. Fused primary incisors with succedaneous supernumerary in the area of a cleft lip: case report. Pediatr Dent 1992; 14: 397–9.

391. MEHLMAN ES. Management of a totally fused central and lateral incisor with internal resorption perforating the lateral aspect of the root. J Endod 1978; 4: 189–91.

392. MELHADO RM *et al*. Bilateral gemination. Oral Surg 1984; 54: 605.

393. MEMMOTT JE, SULLIVAN RE. A very delayed developing premolar: clinical report. Pediatr Dent 1985; 7: 137–9.

394. MENCZER LF. Anomalies of the primary dentition. ASDC J Dent Child 1955; 22: 57–62.

395. MERCURI LG, O'NEILL R. Multiple impacted and supernumerary teeth in sisters. Oral Surg 1980; 50: 293.

396. MERCEDES GALLAS M, GARCIA A. Retention of permanent incisors by mesiodens: a family affair. Br Dent J 2000; 188: 63–4.

397. MEWS JRC. Skeletodental patterns associated with missing teeth. Am J Orthod Dentofac Orthop 2004; 125 (3): 20.

398. MILANO M *et al*. Bilateral fusion of the mandibular primary incisors. Report of case. ASDC J Dent Child 1999; 66: 280–2.

399. MILLAZZO A, ALEXANDER SA. Fusion, gemination, oligodontia and taurodontism. J Pedodont 1982; 6: 194–9.

400. MILES AEW. Malformations of the teeth. Proc R Soc Med 1954; 47: 817–26.

401. MINA M, KOLLAR EJ. The induction of odontogenesis in non–dental mesenchyme combined with early murine mandibular arch epithelium. Arch Oral Biol 1987; 32: 123–7.

402. MITCHELL L, BENNETT TG. Supernumerary teeth causing delayed eruption – A retrospective study. Br J Orthod 1992; 19: 41–6.

403. MÖLLER P *et al*. Variable expression of familial hypodontia in monozygotic triplets. Scand J Dent Res 1981; 89: 16–18.

404. MOODY E, MONTGOMERY B. Hereditary tendencies in tooth formation. J Am Dent Assoc 1934; 21: 1774–6.

405. MOORE KH. A case report of bilateral double teeth. Br J Orthod 1984; 11: 40–1.

406. MORGAN GA *et al*. Recurring mandibular supplemental premolars. Oral Surg 1970; 30: 501–4.

407. MORRIS DO. Fusion of mandibular third and supernumerary fourth molars. Dent Update 1992; 19: 177–8.

408. MOSQUEDA-TAYLOR A *et al*. Odontogenic tumors in Mexico. A collaborative retrospective study of 349 cases. Oral Surg Oral Med Oral Pathol Oral Radiol Endod 1997; 84: 672–5.

409. MOSTOWSKA A *et al*. Novel mutation in the paired box sequence of PAX9 gene in a sporadic form of oligodontia. Eur J Oral Sci 2003; 111: 272–6.

410. MULLER TP *et al*. A survey of congenitally missing permanent teeth. J Am Dent Assoc 1970; 81: 101–17.

411. MUNRO D. Gemination in the deciduous dentition. Br Dent J 1958; 108: 238–40.

412. NANDA RS. Agenesis of the third molar in man. Am J Orthod 1954; 40: 698–706.

413. NAZIF MM *et al*. Impacted supernumerary teeth: a survey of 50 cases. J Am Dent Assoc 1983; 106: 201–4.

414. NEAL JJD, BOWDEN DEJ. The diagnostic value of panoramic radiographs in children aged nine to ten years. Br J Orthod 1988; 15: 193–7.

415. NEWMAN GV, NEWMAN RA. Report of four familial cases with congenitally missing mandibular incisors. Am J Orthod Dentofac Orthop 1998; 114: 195–207.

416. NIEMINEN P *et al*. A graphical www-database on gene expression in tooth. Eur J Oral Sci 1998; 106 (suppl 1): 7–11.

417. NIEMINEN P *et al*. Identification of a nonsense mutation in the PAX9 gene in molar oligodontia. Eur J Hum Genet 2001; 9: 743–6.

418. NIK-HUSSEIN NN. Bilateral symmetrical fusion of primary and permanent mandibular lateral incisors and canines. J Pedodont 1989; 13: 378–83.

419. NIK-HUSSEIN NN. Natal and neonatal teeth. J Pedodont 1990; 14: 110–2.

420. NIK-HUSSEIN NN, Salcedo AH. Double teeth with hypodontia in identical twins. ASDC J Dent Child 1987; 44: 179–81.

421. NISWANDER JD, SUJAKU C. Congenital anomalies of teeth in Japanese children. Am J Phys Anthropol 1963; 21: 569–74.

422. NOMURA R *et al*. Genetic mapping of the absence of third molars in EL mice to chromosome 3. J Dent Res 2003; 82: 786–90.

423. NORDGARDEN H *et al*. Oligodontia is associated with extra–oral ectodermal symptoms and low salivary flow rates. Oral Dis 2001; 7: 226–32.

424. NORDQUIST GG, McNEILL RW. Orthodontic vs. restorative treatment of the congenitally absent lateral incisor – long-term periodontal and occlusal evaluation. J Periodont 1975; 46: 139–43.

425. O CARROLL MK. Fusion and gemination in alternate dentitions. Oral Surg Oral Med Oral Pathol 1990; 57: 655.

426. ODELL EW, HUGHES FJ. The possible association between localized juvenile periodontitis and supernumerary teeth. J Periodont 1995; 66: 449–51.

427. OLSEN CB *et al*. Management of fused supernumerary teeth in children using guided tissue regeneration: long-term follow up of 2 cases. Pediatr Dent 2002; 24: 566–71.

428. ONLINE MENDELIAN INHERITANCE IN MAN (OMIM™). McKusick-Nathans Institute for Genetic Medicine, John Hopkins University (Baltimore, MD) and National Center for Biotechnology Information, National Library of Medicine (Bethesda, MD), 2000. Available at: www.ncbi.nlm.nih.gov/omim/.

429. OOÉ T. On the development of position of the tooth germs in the human deciduous front teeth. Okajimas Folia Anat Japon 1956; 28: 317–40.

430. O'REILLY PMR. A structural and ultrastructural study of a fused tooth. J Endod 1989; 15: 442–6.

431. OSTLER MS, KOKICH VG. Alveolar ridge changes in patients congenitally missing mandibular second premolars. J Prosthet Dent 1994; 71: 144–9.

432. OWENS BM *et al*. Dental odontomas: a retrospective study of 104 cases. J Clin Pediatr Dent 1997; 21: 261–4.

433. PACKOTA GV *et al*. Radiographic features of segmental odontomaxillary dysplasia: study of 12 cases. Oral Surg Oral Med Oral Pathol Oral Radiol Endod 1996; 82: 577–84.

434. PANDERS AK *et al*. Het odontoom. Klinische en röntgenologische aspecten. Ned Tijdschr Tandheelkd 1988; 95: 131–4.

435. PARKER PR, VANN WF. Solitary maxillary central incisor: clinical report. Pediatr Dent 1985; 7: 134–6.

436. PARKS CR. Fusion and gemination. Oral Surg 1970; 29: 394.

437. PASSARGE B, BOSMAN H. Fusion of lateral incisors as autosomal dominant trait. Birth Defects Original Article Series 1971; VII: 194–5.

438. PATEL JR. Gemination. Oral Surg Oral Med Oral Pathol 1984; 57: 232.

439. PECK S *et al*. Prevalence of tooth agenesis and peg–shaped maxillary lateral incisor associated with palatally displaced canine (PDC) anomaly. Am J Orthod Dentofac Orthop 1996; 110: 441–3.

440. PECK S *et al*. Concomitant occurrence of canine malposition and tooth agenesis: evidence of orofacial genetic fields. Am J Orthod Dentofac Orthop 2002; 122: 657–60.

441. PELTOLA JS *et al*. Radiographic findings in the teeth and jaws of 14– to 17–year–old Estonian schoolchildren in Tartu and Tallin. Acta Odontol Scand 1997; 55: 31–5.

442. PERETZ B, BREZNIAK N. Fusion of primary mandibular teeth: report of case. ASDC J Dent Child 1992; 59: 366–8.

443. PEYRANO A, ZMENER O. Endodontic management of mandibular lateral incisor fused with supernumerary tooth. Endod Dent Traumatol 1995; 11: 196–8.

444. PINDBORG JJ. Pathology of the dental hard tissues. Copenhagen: Munksgaard, 1970.

445. PLAETSCHKE J. Okklusionanomalien in Milchgebiss. Dtsch Zahn- Mund- Kieferhleilkd 1938; 5: 435–51.

446. POLDER BJ *et al*. A meta-analysis of the prevalence of dental agenesis of permanent teeth. Community Dent Oral Epidemiol 2004; 32: 217–26.

447. PORTEL MB *et al*. Unusual case of multiple natal teeth. J Clin Pediatr Dent 2004; 29: 37–40.

448. POTTER RHY. The genetics of tooth size. In: STEWART RE, PRESCOTT GH (eds) Oral facial genetics. St Louis, MO: CV Mosby, 1976.

449. POWELL RE. Fusion of maxillary lateral incisor and supernumerary tooth. Oral Surg 1981; 51: 331.

450. PÖYRY M, RANTA R. Anomalies in the deciduous dentition outside the cleft region in children with oral clefts. Proc Finn Dent Soc 1985; 81: 91–7.

451. POYTON HG *et al*. Median incisor fusion. Oral Surg 1969; 28: 76–8.

452. POYTON GH *et al*. Recurring supernumerary mandibular premolars. Report of a case of postmature development. Oral Surg 1960; 13: 964–6.

453. PRABHAKAR AR *et al*. Duplication and dilaceration of a crown with hypercementosis of the root following trauma: a case report. Quint Int 1998; 29: 655–7.

454. PRABHU NT, MUNSHI AK. Surgical management of a labially placed permanent maxillary central incisor after supernumerary tooth extraction: report of a case. J Clin Pediatr Dent 1997; 21: 201–4.

455. PRAHL-ANDERSEN B. Gebitsontwikkelingen bij agenesieën. Ned Tijdschr Tandheelkd 1984; 91: 515–18.

456. PRICE C, HOGGINS GS. A category of supernumerary premolar teeth. Br Dent J 1969; 126: 224–8.

457. PRIMOSCH RE. Anterior supernumerary teeth-assessment and surgical intervention in children. Pediatr Dent 1981; 3: 204–15.

458. PROGREL H. Case of bilateral gemination of deciduous incisors with congenital absence of permanent successors. Dent Pract Dent Rec 1956; VII: 13–14.

459. PRUSACK N *et al*. Segmental odontomaxillary dysplasia. A case report and review of the literature. Oral Surg Oral Med Oral Pathol Oral Radiol Endod 2000; 90: 483–8.

460. PUNJABI AP. Oral rehabilitation in two siblings with anhidrotic ectodermal dysplasia – prosthetic considerations. J Indian Dent Assoc 1983; 55: 119–23.

461. PUY L *et al*. Double teeth: case reports. J Clin Pediatr Dent 1991; 15: 120–4.

462. RADLANSKI RJ *et al*. The origin of tooth number of the human deciduous dentition: a hypothesis. Med Hypotheses 1988; 25: 139–40.

463. RAJAB LD, HAMDAN MAM. Supernumerary teeth: review of the literature and a survey of 152 cases. Int J Paediatr Dent 2002; 12: 244–54.

464. RANTA R. Premature mineralization of permanent canines associated with aplasia of their primary predecessors: report of four cases. ASDC J Dent Child 1983; 50: 274–7.

465. RANTA R. Numeric anomalies of teeth in concomitant hypodontia and hyperodontia. J Craniofac Genet 1988; 8: 245–51.

466. RANTA R, TULENSALO T. Symmetry and combinations of hypodontia in non-cleft and cleft palate children. Scand J Dent Res 1988; 96: 1–8.

467. RANTA R, YLIPAAVALNIEMI P. Developmental course of supernumerary premolars in childhood: report of two cases. ASDC J Dent Child 1981; 48: 385–8.

468. RASMUSSEN P. Severe hypodontia: diversities in manifestations. J Clin Pediatr Dent 1999; 23: 179–88.

469. RAVN JJ. Aplasia, supernumerary teeth and fused teeth in the primary dentition. An epidemiologic study. Scand J Dent Res 1971; 79: 1–6.

470. RAZAK IA, NIK-HUSSEIN NN. A retrospective study of double teeth in the primary dentition. Ann Acad Med Singapore 1986; 15: 393–6.

471. REAGAN SE, DAO TM. Oral rehabilitation of a patient with congenital partial anodontia using a rotational path removable partial denture: report of case. Quint Int 1995; 26: 181–5.

472. REEH ES, ElDEEB M. Root canal morphology of fused mandibular canine and lateral incisor. J Endod 1989; 15: 33–5.

473. REITMAN AA. Gemination: a case report of bilateral geminated incisors. N Y State Dent J 1976; 42: 605–7.

474. RICHARDSON M. Late third molar genesis: its significance in orthodontic treatment. Angle Orthod 1980; 50: 121–8.

475. RIESENBERGER RE, KILLIAN CM. Triplication and twinning in one dental arch: report of case. Quint Int 1990; 21: 621–3.

476. RINGQVIST M, THILANDER B. The frequency of hypodontia in an orthodontic material. Sven Tandlak Tidskr 1969; 62: 535–41.

477. RIPAMONTI U, THACKERAY J. A supernumerary tooth in a 1.7 million-year-old Australopithecus robustus from Swartkrans, South Africa. Eur J Oral Sci 1999; 107: 317–21.

478. RIZUTTI N, SCOTTI S. A case of hyperodontia with twenty-two supernumeraries: is surgical-orthodontic treatment. Am J Orthod Dentofac Orthop 1997; 111: 471–80.

479. ROBERT JC. Supernumerary teeth. Oral Surg 1968; 25: 577–8.

480. ROBERTS MW. Multiple familial dental anomalies: report of case. ASDC J Dent Child 1973; 40: 482–3.

481. ROBERTS MW et al. Two natal maxillary molars. Oral Surg Oral Med Oral Pathol 1992; 73: 543–5.

482. ROBERTSSON S, MOLIN B. The congenitally missing upper lateral incisor. A retrospective study of orthodontic space closure versus restorative treatment. Eur J Orthod 2000; 22: 697–710.

483. ROCK WP. A case of bilateral supplemental maxillary central incisors. Int J Paediatr Dent 1991; 1: 155–8.

484. ROLAND STILL WH. A short study of supernumerary teeth in Southern Nigeria. Br Dent J 1945: 79: 215–17.

485. RØLLING S. Hypodontia of permanent teeth in Danish schoolchildren. Scand J Dent Res 1980; 88: 365–9.

486. ROME WJ. Endodontic therapy involving an unusual case of gemination. J Endod 1984; 10: 546–8.

487. ROMITO LM. Concrescence: report of a rare case. Oral Surg Oral Med Oral Pathol Oral Radiol Endod 2004; 97: 325–7.

488. ROSE JS. A survey of congenitally missing teeth, excluding third molars, in 6000 orthodontic patients. Dent Pract 1966; 17: 107–14.

489. ROSENBERG GERTZMAN GB. Genetics – a tool for the dentist. Report of a case of inherited oligodontia. Clin Prev Dent 1982; 4: 19–21.

490. ROTH PM et al. Congenitally missing lateral incisor treatment. J Clin Orthod 1985; 19: 258–62.

491. ROTH P, HIRSCHFELDER U. Zahnunterzahl bei Anlage aller vier Weisheitszähne. Dtsch Zahnärztl Z 1990; 45: 267–9.

492. ROTSTEIN I et al. Endodontic therapy for a fused mandibular molar. Endod Dent Traumatol 1997; 13: 149–51.

493. RUBENSTEIN LK et al. Development of supernumerary premolars in an orthodontic population. Oral Surg Oral Med Oral Pathol 1991; 71: 392–5.

494. RUBIN MM et al. A comparison of identical twins in relation to three dental anomalies: multiple supernumerary teeth, juvenile periodontosis, and zero caries incidence. Oral Surg 1981; 52: 391–4.

495. RUFFALO RC et al. A comparative study of three radiographic surveys in preschool children. ASDC J Dent Child 1983; 50: 422–4.

496. RUHLMAN DC, NEELY AR. Multiple impacted and erupted supernumerary teeth. Report of a case. Oral Surg 1964; 17: 199–203.

497. RUNE B, SARNÄS KV. Tooth size and tooth formation in children with advanced hypodontia. Angle Orthod 1974; 44: 316–21.

498. RUNNER MN. New evidence for monozygotic twins in the mouse: twinning initiated in the late blastocyst can account for mirror image asymmetries. Anat Rec 1984; 209: 399–406.

499. RUPRECHT A et al. Double teeth: the incidence of gemination and fusion. J Pedod 1985; 9: 332–7.

500. RUPRECHT A et al. The incidence of taurodontism in dental patients. Oral Surg 1987; 63: 743–7.

501. RUPRECHT A et al. The incidence of dental invagination. J Pedodont 1986; 10: 265–72.

502. RUPRECHT A, CRAM R. Gemination of the mandibular right lateral incisor. Oral Surg 1984; 57: 693.

503. RUPRECHT A, ROSS AS. Gemination of a mandibular third molar. Oral Surg 1985; 58: 432.

504. RUSHMA M. Natal and neonatal teeth: a clinical and histological study. J Clin Pediatr Dent 1991; 15: 251–3.

505. RUSHTON MA. Effects of radium on the dentition. Am J Orthod Oral Surg 1947; 33: 828–30.

506. SAAD AY. Regressive changes of the dental pulp complex in retained primary molars with congenitally missing successor teeth. J Clin Pediatr Dent 1997: 22 (1): 63–7.

507. SAITO T. A genetic study on the degenerative anomalies of deciduous teeth. Jap J Hum Genet 1959; 4: 27–31.

508. SALEM G. Prevalence of selected dental anomalies in Saudi Children from Gizan region. Community Dent Oral Epidemiol 1989; 17: 162–3.

509. SÀNDOR GKB et al. Genetic mutations in certain head and neck conditions of interest to the dentist. J Can Dent Assoc 2001; 67: 549–60.

510. SANTORO FP, WESLEY RK. Clinical evaluation of two patients with a single maxillary central incisor. ASDC J Dent Child 1983; 50: 379–81.

511. SAPOKA AAM, DEMIRJIAN A. Dental development of the French Canadian child. J Can Dent Assoc 1971; 37: 100–4.

512. SARNAT H et al. Developmental dental anomalies in chrondoectodermal dysplasia (Ellis-van Creveld syndrome). ASDC J Dent Child 1980; 47: 28–31.

513. SASS T. Zahnüberzahl im oberen Eckzahnbereich als seltene Anomalie und Ursache einer Retention. Dtsch Zahnaerztl Z 1986; 41: 711–13.

514. SAWYER M et al. Endodontic therapy in an unusual case of fusion. J Endod 1980; 6: 796–8.

515. SCANLAN PJ, HODGES SJ. Supernumerary premolar teeth in siblings. Br J Orthod 1997; 24: 297–300.

516. SCAREL RM et al. Absence of mutations in the homeodomain of the MSX1 gene in patients with hypodontia. Am J Med Genet 2000; 92: 346–9.

517. SCHALK-VAN DER WEIDE Y. Oligodontia. A clinical, radiographic and genetic evaluation. Thesis, University of Nijmegen, 1992.

518. SCHALK-VAN DER WEIDE Y et al. Symptomatology of patients with oligodontia. J Oral Rehabil 1994; 21: 247–61.

519. SCHEINER MA, SAMPSON WJ. Supernumerary teeth: a review of the literature and four case reports. Aust Dent J 1997; 42: 160–5.

520. SCHMIDT RE. Fusion. Oral Surg 1965; 19: 478.

521. SCHNEIDER PE. Eineiïge Zwillinge vom Spiegelbild – Typ mit geminierten (verdoppelten) Schneidezähnen: ein Fallbericht. Quintessenz 1986; 9: 1547–9.

522. SCHUFFENHAUER S et al. De novo deletion (14) (q11.2q13) including PAX9: clinical and molecular findings. J Med Genet 1999; 36: 233–6.

523. SCHULZE C. Developmental abnormalities of the teeth and jaws. In: GORLIN RJ, GOLDMAN HM (eds) Thoma's oral pathology. St Louis, MO: CV Mosby, 1970.

524. SCHULZE C. Anomalien und Missbildungen der menschlichen Zähne. Berlin: Quintessenz Verlags–GmbH, 1987.

525. SCHUURS AHB. Spelingen der natuur. Ned Tijdschr Tandheelkd 1984; 91: 315–18.

526. SCHUURS AHB, VAN LOVEREN C. Double teeth: review of the literature. ASDC J Dent Child 2000; 57: 313–25.

527. SCHWARTZ JH. Supernumerary teeth in anthropoid primates and models of tooth development. Arch Oral Biol 1984; 29: 833–42.

528. SCHWEITZER G. Seltene Zahnmissbildungen. Dtsch Zahnärztl Wochenschr 1932; 35: 511–19.

529. SCOTT R, TURNER CG. The anthropology of modern human teeth. Dental morphology in recent human populations. Cambridge: Cambridge University Press, 1997.

530. SEDANO HO, GORLIN RJ. Familial occurrence of mesiodens. Oral Surg 1969; 27: 360–2.

531. SEDANO HO, SAUK JJ, Gorlin RJ. Oral manifestations of inherited disorders. Woburn: Butterworth (Publishers) Inc, 1977.

532. SEJRSEN B et al. Agenesis of permanent incisors in a mediaeval maxilla and mandible: aetiological aspects. Eur J Oral Sci 1995; 103: 65–9.

533. SERRANO JV. Bilateral fusion of teeth. Oral Surg 1972; 34: 348–9.

534. SHAFER WG et al. A textbook of oral pathology. Philadelphia, PA: W.B. Saunders, 1983.

535. SHAH RM, BOYD MA. The relationship between presence and absence of third molars hypodontia of other teeth. J Dent Res 1979; 58: 544.

536. SHAH RM, PAULS V. Supernumerary premolars: report of two cases. J Can Dent Assoc 1978; 44: 114–15.

537. SHAPIRA Y, KUFTINEC MM. Multiple supernumerary teeth. Report of cases. Am J Dent 1989; 2: 28–30.

538. SHARMA A. A rare non-syndrome case of concomitant multiple supernumerary teeth and partial anodontia. J Clin Pediatr Dent 2001; 25: 167–9.

539. SHTEYER A. Fusion of a third mandibular molar with a distomolar. Oral Surg 1976; 42: 410.

540. SIGAL MJ et al. Bilateral mandibular hamartomas and familial natal teeth. Oral Surg Oral Med Oral Pathol 1988; 65: 731–5.

541. SILVERMAN NE, ACKERMAN JL. Oligodontia: a study of its prevalence and variation in 4032 children. ASDC J Dent Child 1979; 46: 470–7.

542. SILVESTRI AR. The unresolved problem of the third molar. J Am Dent Assoc 2003; 134: 450–5.

543. SLAVKIN HC, BAVETTA LA. Odontogenic epithelial – mesenchymal interactions in vitro. J Dent Res 1968; 47: 779–85.

544. SLAVKIN HC. Entering the era molecular dentistry. J Am Dent Assoc 1999; 130: 413–17.

545. SLETTEN DW et al. Retained deciduous mandibular molars in adults: a radiographic study of long–term changes. Am J Orthod Dentofac Orthop 2003; 124: 625–30.

546. SMALL BW. Esthetic management of congenitally missing lateral incisors with single–tooth implants: a case report. Quint Int 1996; 27: 585–90.

547. SMITH GA. "Double teeth". Br Dent J 1980; 148: 163–4.

548. SNAWDER KD. Considerations in dental treatment of children with ectodermal dysplasia. J Am Dent Assoc 1976; 93: 1177–9.

549. SO LSY. Unusual supernumerary teeth. Angle Orthod 1990; 60: 289–92.

550. SOFAER JA et al. Developmental interaction, size and agenesis among permanent maxillary incisors. Human Biol 1971; 43: 36–45.

551. SOLARES R, ROMERO MI. Supernumerary premolars: a literature review. Pediatr Dent 2004; 26: 450–8.

552. SOMMERMATER JI, HEMMERLE J. Dents natale et post–natale: leur email. Rev Mens Suisse Odontostomatol 1994; 104: 11–19.

553. SONI NN et al. Polarized light and microradiographic study of natal teeth. ASDC J Dent Child 1967; 34: 433–8.

554. SONNABEND E. Zur Unterzahl der Zähne insbesondere der 3.Molaren. Dtsch Zahn- Mund-Kieferheilkd 1966; 46; 34–43.

555. SOUTHAM JC. Retained dentine papillae in the newborn. A clinical and histopathological study. Br Dent J 1968; 125: 534–8.

556. SOUTHAM JC. The structure of natal and neonatal teeth. Dent Pract 1968; 18: 423–7.

557. SPATAFORE CM. Endodontic treatment of fused teeth. J Endod 1992; 18: 628–31.

558. SPEISER AM, BIKOFSKY VM. Premolars with double occlusal surfaces. J Am Dent Assoc 1981; 103: 600–1.

559. SPERBER GH. Anodontia. Two cases of different etiology. Oral Surg 1963; 16: 73–82.

560. SPERBER GH et al. Mirror–image dental fusion and discordance in monozygotic twins. Am J Medic Genet 1994; 51: 41–5.

561. SPYROPOULOS ND et al. Simultaneous presence of partial anodontia and supernumerary teeth. Oral Surg 1979; 48: 53–6.

562. STABHOLZ A, FRIEDMAN S.Endodontic therapy of an unusual maxillary permanent first molar. J Endod 1983; 9: 293–5.

563. STAFNE EC. Supernumerary upper central incisors. Dent Cosmos 1931; 73: 976–80.

564. STAFNE EC. Supernumerary teeth. Dent Cosmos 1932; 74: 653–9.

565. STAFNE EC, BOWING HH. The teeth and their supporting structures in patients treated by irradiation. Am J Orthod Oral Surg 1947; 33: 567–81.

566. STAMATIOU J, SYMONS AL. Agenesis of the permanent lateral incisors: distribution, number and sites. J Clin Pediatr Dent 1991; 15: 244–6.

567. STEEN WHA. De oligodontiepatiënt: indicatie en behandeling. Ned Tijdschr Tandheelkd 1986; 93: 2–5.

568. STELLZIG A et al. Mesiodentes: incidence, morphology, etiology. J Orofac Orthop 1997; 58: 144–53.

569. STERMER BEYER-OLSEN EM et al. Changing positions of supernumerary teeth in the premaxilla: a radiographic study. ASDC J Dent Child 1985; 53: 428–30.

570. STEVENSON W. Supernumerary canines. Report of an unusual case. Br Dent J 1965: 118: 257–8.

571. STILLWELL KD, COKE JM. Bilateral fusion of the maxillary central incisors to supernumerary teeth: report of case. J Am Dent Assoc 1986; 112: 62–4.

572. STIMSON JM et al. Features of oligodontia in three generations. J Clin Pediatr Dent 1997; 21: 269–76.

573. STOCKDALE CR. An unusual case of gemination. Oral Surg Oral Med Oral Pathol 1969; 27: 59.

574. STRITZEL F et al. Agenesis of the second premolar in males and females: distribution, number and sites affected. J Clin Pediatr Dent 1990; 15: 39–41.

575. SUAREZ BK, SPENCE MA. The genetics of hypodontia. J Dent Res 1974; 53: 781–5.

576. SURMONT PA et al. A complete fusion in the primary human dentition: a histological approach. ASDC J Dent Child 1988; 55: 362–7.

577. SVEDMYR B. Genealogy and consequences of congenitally missing second premolars. J Int Assoc Dent Child 1983; 14: 77–82.

578. SVIRSKY JA. Bilateral gemination. Oral Surg 1979; 47: 300.

579. SWAN RH. Odontomas. A review, case presentation and periodontal considerations in treatment. J Periodont 1987; 58: 856–60.

580. SYMONS AL et al. Anomalies associated with hypodontia of the permanent lateral incisor and second premolar. J Clin Pediatr Dent 1993; 17: 109–11.

581. SZENTHE S. Das gemeinsame Vorkommen des Zusammenmenwachsens des untere Milcheckzahnes mit dem laterale Schneidezahn und der Aplasie des bleibenden lateralen Schneidezahnses. Fortschr Kieferorthop 1958; 19: 244–50.

582. TAGGER M. Tooth gemination treated by endodontic therapy. J Endod 1975; 1: 181–4.

583. TAL H. Familial hypodontia in the permanent dentition: a case report. J Dent 1981; 9: 260–4.

584. TALOUMIS LJ, NISHIMURA RS. Treatment of an unusual instance of fusion with a talon cusp. Gen Dent 1989; 37: 208–10.

585. TANAKA S et al. A rare case of bilateral supernumerary teeth in the mandibular incisors. Br Dent J 1998; 185: 386–8.

586. TANNENBAUM KA, ALLING EE. Anomalous tooth development. Case reports of gemination and twinning. Oral Surg 1963; 16: 883–7.

587. TASA GL, LUKACS JR. The prevalence and expression of primary double teeth in western India. ASDC J Dent Child 2001; 68: 196–200.

588. TAVAJOHI-KERMANI H et al. Tooth agenesis and craniofacial morphology in an orthodontic population. Am J Orthod Dentofac Orthop 2002; 122: 39–47.

589. TAY WM. Natal canine and molar in an infant. Report of case. Oral Surg Oral Med Oral Pathol 1970; 28: 598–602.

590. TAY F et al. Unerupted maxillary anterior supernumerary teeth: report of 204 cases. ASDC J Dent Child 1984; 51: 289–94.

591. Thesleff I. Genetic basis of tooth development and dental defects. Acta Odontol Scand 2000; 58: 191–4.

592. THESLEFF L, ÅBERG T. Tooth morphogenesis and the differentiation of ameloblasts. In: CIBA FOUNDATION (ed) Dental enamel. Chichester: John Wiley & Sons, 1997.

593. THESLEFF I et al. Epithelial-mesenchymal interactions in tooth morphogenesis: the roles of extracellular matrix, growth factors, and cell surface receptors. J Craniofac Genet Dev Biol 1991; 11: 229–37.

594. THILANDER B, MYRBERG N. The prevalence of malocclusion in Swedish schoolchildren. Scand J Dent Res 1973; 81: 12–20.

595. THOMPSON GW, POPOVICH F. Probability of congenitally missing teeth: results in 1,191 children in the Burlington Growth Centre in Toronto. Community Dent Oral Epidemiol 1974; 2: 26–32.

596. THOMPSON GW et al. Third molar agenesis in the Burlington Growth Centre in Toronto. Community Dent Oral Epidemiol 1974; 2: 187–92.

597. TINN CA. Excess, deficiency and gemination in the deciduous and permanent dentitions of school children. Br Dent J 1940; 68: 236–38.

598. TO EWH. A study of natal teeth in Hong Kong Chinese. Int J Paediatr Dent 1991; 2: 73–6.

599. TOMIZAWA M et al. Bilateral maxillary fused primary incisors accompanied by succedaneous supernumerary teeth: report of a case. Int J Paediatr Dent 2002; 12: 223–7.

600. TOPPER DC et al. A dental and facial anomaly not previously reported with VACTERL association: report of case. ASDC J Dent Child 1990; 57: 216–19.

601. TORETTI EF et al. Odontomas: an analysis of 167 cases. J Pedodont 1983; 8: 282–4.

602. TÓTH A, CSÉMI L. Zwillingszähne im Milchgebiss. Dtsch Zahnärztl Zeitschr 1967; 22: 546–54.

603. TOWNSEND GC, MARTIN NG. Fitting genetic models to Carabelli trait data in south Australian twins. J Dent Res 1992; 71: 403–9.

604. TOWNSEND G, RICHARDS L. Twins and twinning, dentists and dentistry. Aust Dent J 1990; 35: 317–27.

605. TRUBMAN A, SILBERMAN SL. Triple teeth: case reports of combined fusion and gemination. ASDC J Dent Child 1988; 55: 298–9.

606. TSESIS I et al. Endodontic treatment of developmental anomalies in posterior teeth: treatment of geminated/fused teeth – report of two cases. Int Endod J 2003; 36: 372–9.

607. TUCKER AS et al. The activation level of the TNF family receptor, Edar, determines cusp number and tooth number during tooth development. Dev Biol 2004; 268: 185–94.

608. TURNBULL NR, LAI NN. Eruption of a permanent mandibular canine in a 5-year-old boy. Int J paediatr Dent 2003; 13: 117–20.

609. ULRICH K. Sommersprossen und Dysplasien der Augenbrauen als Indikatoren für genetisch bedingte Störungen der Zahn– und Gebissentwicklung. Stomatol DDR 1990; 40: 64–6.

610. TSUBONE H *et al*. Clinico-pathological aspects of a residual natal tooth: a case report. J Oral Pathol Med 2002; 31: 239–41.

611. TSURUMACHI T, KUNO T. Endodontic and orthodontic treatment of a cross-bite fused maxillary lateral incisor. Int Endod J 2003; 36: 135–42.

612. UCOCK M. Fusion involving both maxillary central incisors. Oral Surg 1984; 58: 238–9.

613. ÜNER O *et al*. Delayed calcification and congenitally missing teeth. Aust dent J 1994; 39: 167–71.

614. URELES SD, NEEDLEMAN HL. Focal dermal hypoplasia syndrome (Goltz syndrome): the first dental case report. Pediatr Dent 1986; 8: 239–44.

615. UZAMIS M *et al*. Clinical and ultrastructural study of natal and neonatal teeth. J Clin Peiatr Dent 1999; 23: 173–7.

616. VALIATHAN A, PRASHANTH VK. Cherubism: presentation of a case. Angle Orthod 1997; 67: 237–8.

617. VAN DER WAAL *et al*. Pathologie van de mondholte. Houten: Bohn Stafleu Van Loghum, 1996.

618. VAN LIMBORGH J, GRIFFIOEN FMM. Storingen in de tandkiemontwikkeling. Ned Tijdschr Tandheelkd 1983; 90: 180–5.

619. VASTARDIS H. The genetics of human tooth agenesis: new discoveries for understanding dental anomalies. Am J Orthod Dentofac Orthop 2000; 117: 650–6.

620. VEGH T. Gemination and fusion. Oral Surg 1975; 40: 816–17.

621. VELASCO LFL *et al*. Esthetic and functional treatment of a fused permanent tooth: a case report. Quint Int 1997; 28: 677–80.

622. VELEZ I *et al*. Segmental odontomaxillary dysplasia. Report of two cases and review of the literature. Todays FDA 2002; 14: 20–1.

623. VENO H *et al*. Dental anomalies in the midline. Oral Surg Oral Med Oral Pathol 1988; 65: 638–9.

624. VERMEEREN JIJF. Zes incisives superiores. Ned Tijdschr Tandheelkd 1970; 77: 107–8.

625. VIEIRA AR. Oral clefts and syndromic forms of tooth agenesis as models for genetics of isolated tooth agenesis. J Dent Res 2003; 82: 162–5.

626. VIEIRA AR *et al*. MSX1, PAX9 and TGFA contribute to tooth agenesis in humans. J Dent Res 2004; 83: 723–7.

627. VISSER JB. Over hypodontie, oligodontie en de behandeling van de daaruit voortvloeiende gebitsdeficiënties. I en II. Ned Tijdschr Tandheelkd 1981; 88: 52–6, 90–5 [and thesis].

628. VISSER JB. Speciële pathologie van het menselijk gebit. Leiden: Staleu & Tholen BB, 1974.

629. VOLK A. Über die Häufigkeit des Vorkommens von fehlenden Zahnanlagen. Schweiz Monatschr Zahnheilkd 1963; 73: 320–34.

630. VRIJMAN A. Agenesieën: implanteren of verplaatsen? Tandartspraktijk 2003; September: 29–31.

631. VRIJMAN A. Agenesieën (3). Niet–aangelegde tweede premolaren in de onderkaak. Tandartspraktijk 2004; January: 2–7.

632. WABEKE KB, PRAHL-ANDERSEN B. Oligodontie: etiologie, frequentie, verschijningsvormen, preprosthetische orthodontie. Ned Tijdschr Tandheelkd 1986; 93: 9–13

633. WATSON JD *et al*. Molecular biology of the gene. Menlo Park, CA: Benjamin/Cummings Publishing Company, 1987.

634. WEBER FN. Supernumerary teeth. Dent Clin North Am 1964; July: 509–17.

635. WEISS JK. The double tooth. J Clin Orthop 1980; XIV: 780–7.

636. WEISZ AS, DOHAN LM. Dens in dente. Oral Surg Oral Med Oral Pathol 1988; 65: 264.

637. WELSCH MJ, STEIN SL. A syndrome of hemimaxillary enlargement, asymmetry of the face, tooth abnormalities, and skin findings. Pediatr Dermatology 2004; 21: 448–51.

638. WERTHER R, ROTHENBERG F. Anodontia. A review of its etiology with presentation of a case. Am J Orthod 1939; 25: 61–81.

639. WESLEY RK *et al*. Solitary maxillary incisor and normal stature. Oral Surg Oral Med Oral Pathol 1978; 46: 837–42.

640. WHITTINGTON BR, DURWARD CS. Survey of anomalies in primary teeth and their correlation with the permanent dentition. N Z Dent J 1996; 94: 4–8.

641. WILLIAMS DW. The early eruption of a supernumerary tooth (mesiodens). Br Dent J 1976; 140: 209–10.

642. WILLIAMS P. An unusual case of hyperodontia. Br Dent J 1998; 184: 371–2.

643. WILLIAMS P *et al*. The use of osseointegrated implants in orthodontic patients: I. Implants and their use in children. Dent Update 2004; 31: 287–90.

644. WINSTANLEY RB. Prosthodontic treatment of patients with hypodontia. J Prosthet Dent 1984; 52: 687–91.

645. WINTER GB. Local pathological conditions influencing the development of the upper labial segment. Dent Pract Dent Rec 1966; 17: 153–61.

646. WINTER GB. Hereditary and idiopathic anomalies of tooth number, structure and form. Dent Clin North Am 1969; 13: 355–73.

647. WINTER GB. The association of ocular defects with the otodental syndrome. J Int Assoc Dent 1983; 14: 83–7.

648. WISTH PJ *et al*. Frequency of hypodontia in relation to tooth size and dental arch width. Acta Odontol Scand 1974; 32: 201–6.

649. WITKOP CJ. Genetics and dentistry. Eugen Quart 1958; 5: 15–21.

650. WONG M. Treatment considerations in a geminated maxillary lateral incisor. J Endod 1991; 17: 179–81.

651. YAMZAKI H *et al*. Mesiodens in the primary dentition: a case report. Pediatr Dent J 1997; 7: 109–13.

652. YANUKOGLU F, KARTAL N. Endodontic treatment of a fused maxillary lateral incisor. J Endod 1998; 24: 57–9.

653. YODA T *et al*. Multiple macrodonts with odontoma in a mother and son – a variant of Ekman-Westborg-Julin syndrome. Report of a case. Oral Surg Oral Med Oral Pathol Oral Radiol Endodont 1998; 85: 301–3.

654. YONEZU T *et al*. Prevalence of congenital dental anomalies of the deciduous dentition in Japanese children. Bull Tokyo Dent Coll 1997; 38: 27–32.

655. YUEN SWH *et al*. Double primary teeth and their relationship with the permanent successors: a radiographic study of 376 cases. Pediatr Dent 1987; 9: 42–8.

656. YÜKSEL S, ÜÇEM T. The effect of tooth agenesis on dentofacial structures. Eur J Orthod 1997; 19: 71–8.

657. YUSOF WZ. Non-syndrome multiple supernumerary teeth: literature review. J Can Dent Assoc 1990; 56: 147–9.

658. ZACHARIADES N, SKOURA-KAFOUSSIA C. Geminated lower third molar. Report of an uncommon case. J Oral Med 1985; 40: 208.

659. ZAJICEK G, MICHAELI Y. On the potential of the adult rat incisor odontogenic organ to differentiate into two intact teeth. J Biol Buccale 1978; 6: 339–42.

660. ZHU J, KING D. Natal and neonatal teeth. ASDC J Dent Child 1995; 62: 123–8.

661. ZHU J et al. Supernumerary and congenitally absent teeth: a literature review. J Clin Pediatr Dent 1996; 20: 87–95.

662. ZILBERMAN Y et al. Assessment of 100 children in Jerusalem with supernumerary teeth in the premaxillary region. ASDC J Dent Child 1992; 59: 44–7.

663. ZVOLANEK JW, SPOTTS TM. Supernumerary mandibular premolars: report of case. J Am Dent Assoc 1985; 110: 721–3.

664. NORDGARDEN H et al. Reported prevalence of congenitally missing teeth in two Norwegian counties. Community Dent Health 2002; 19: 258–61.

665. ALBASHAIREH ZS et al. The prevalence and pattern of hypodontia of the permanent teeth and crown size and shape deformity affecting upper lateral incisors in a sample of Jordanian dental patients. Community Dental Health 2006; 23: 239–43.

666. ITH-HANSEN K, KJAER I. Persistence of deciduous molars in subjects with agenesis of the second premolars. Eur J Orthod 2000; 22: 239–43.

667. ORHAN AS et al. Familial occurrence of nonsyndromal multiple supernumerary teeth. Angle Orthod 2006; 76: 891–7.

668. BATRA P et al. Non-syndromic multiple supernumenrary teeth transmitted as an autosomal dominant trait. J Oral Pathol Med 2005; 34: 621–5.

669. KUROL J. Impacted and ankylosed teeth: Why and when to intervene. Am J Orthod Dentofac Orthop 2006; 129 (suppl 1): S86–S90.

670. LIU MH, HUANG WH. Oral abnormalities in Taiwanese newborns. ASDC J Dent Child 2004; 71: 118–20.

671. CHEN S et al. Altered gene expression in human cleidocranial dysplasia pulpal cells. Arch Oral Biol 2005; 50: 227–36.

672. HALL RK. Solitary median maxillary central incisor (SMMCI) syndrome. Orohanet J Rare Dis 2006; 1: 12.

Chapter 2: Deviations in Tooth Morphology and Size

1. AAS IHM. Variability of a dental morphological trait. Acta Odontol Scand 1983; 41: 257–63.

2. AASENDEN R et al. Effects of fluoride Supplementation form birth on human deciduous and permanent teeth. Arch Oral Biol 1974; 19: 321–6.

3. ABBOTT PV. Labial and palatal "talon' cusps" on the same tooth. Oral Surg Oral Med Oral Pathol Oral Radiol Endod 1998; 85: 726–30.

4. ACKERMAN JL et al. Taurodont, pyramidal and fused molar roots associated with other anomalies in a kindred. Am J Phys Anthropol 1973; 38: 681–94.

5. ACS G et al. Shovel incisors, three rooted molars, talon cusp, and supernumerary tooth in one patient. Pediatr Dent J 1992; 14: 263–4.

6. AL-EMRAN S. Prevalence of hypodontia and developmental malformation of permanent teeth in Saudi-Arabian schoolchildren. Br J Orthod 1990; 17: 115–18.

7. ALBUM MM. Taurodontia in deciduous first molars. J Am Dent Assoc 1958; 56: 562.

8. AL-KHATEEB T et al. The incidence of taurodontism in permanent molars in Saudi Arabian dental patients. Pediatr Dent J 1997; 7: 69–72.

9. ALLWRIGHT WC. Odontomes of the axial core type as a cause of osteomyelitis of the mandible. Br Dent J 1958; 105: 363–5.

10. ALT KW. Radicula appendiciformis an einem lateralen Oberkieferschneidezahn. Quintessenz 1990; 10: 105–8.

11. ALTINBULAK H et al. Multiple dens invaginatus. Oral Surg Oral Med Oral Pathol 1993; 76: 620–2.

12. ALVESALO L, PORTIN P. The inheritance pattern of missing, peg–shaped, and strongly mesio-distally reduced upper lateral incisors. Acta Odont Scand 1969; 27: 563–75.

13. ALVESALO L et al. 47,XXY males: sex chromosomes and tooth size. Am J Hum Genet 1980; 32: 955–9.

14. ALVESALO L et al. The cusp of carabelli. Acta Odontol Scand 1975; 33: 191–7.

15. AMOS ER. Incidence of the small dens in dente. J Am Dent Assoc 1955; 51: 31–3.

16. ANDEREGG CR et al. Treatment of the palato-gingival groove with guided tissue regeneration. J Periodontol 1993; 64: 72–4.

17. ANDREASEN JO, RAVN JJ. The effect of traumatic injuries to primary teeth on their permanent successors. II. A clinical and radiographic follow-up study of 213 teeth. Scand J Dent Res 1971; 79: 284–94.

18. ANDREASEN JO et al. The effect of traumatic injuries to primary teeth on their permanent successors. Scand J Dent Res 1971; 79: 219–83.

19. ANTONIADES K et al. Congenital hemifacial hyperplasia. Br J Oral Maxillofac Surg 1988; 26: 344–8.

20. APAJALAHTI S et al. Short root anomaly in families and its association with other dental anomalies. Eur J Oral Sci 1999; 107: 97–101.

21. ARYS A et al. Les perles d'émail des dents de lait. J Biol Buccale 1987; 15: 249–55.

22. ASKENAS BG et al. Cervical enamel projection with gingival fenestration in a maxillary central incisor. Quint Int 1992; 23: 103–7.

23. ATASU M et al. Generalized microdontia and associated anomalies: a clinical, genetic, radiological and dermatoglyphic study. J Clin Pediatr Dent 1996; 20: 161–72.

24. ATKINSON SR. The permanent maxillary lateral incisor. Am J Orthod 1943; 29: 685–98.

25. AXELSSON G et al. Crown size of permanent teeth in Icelanders. Acta Odontol Scand 1983; 41: 181–6.
26. AXELSSON G et al. Cusp number and groove pattern of lower molars in Icelanders. Acta Odontol Scand 1981; 39: 361–6.
27. BÄCKMAN B, WAHLIN YB. Variations in number and morphology of permanent teeth in 7-year-old Swedish children. Int J Paediatr Dent 2001; 11: 11–17.
28. BAILEY SE. A closer look at Neanderthal postcanine dental morphology: the mandibular dentition. Anat Rec 2002; 269: 148–56.
29. BAILIT HL. Dental variation among populations: an anthropologic view. Dent Clin North Am 1975; 19: 125–39.
30. BANNER H. Bilateral dens in dente in mandibular premolars. Oral Surg Oral Med Oral Pathol 1978; 45: 827–8.
31. BARKHORAR RA. Maxillary canine with two roots. J Endod 1985; 11: 224–7.
32. BARTON DH et al. Oral-facial characteristics of circumscribed scleroderma. J Clin Pediatr Dent 1993; 17: 239–42.
33. BAZOPOULOU-KYRKANIDOU E et al. Microdontia, hypodontia, short bulbous roots and rootcanals with strabismus, short stature, and borderline mentality. Oral Surg Oral Med Oral Pathol 1992; 74: 93–5.
34. BEDI R et al. Dens evaginatus in the Hong Kong Chinese population. Endod Dent Traumatol 1988; 4: 104–7.
35. BELL RA et al. Complex congenital hemihypertrophy. J Pedod 1984; 8: 300–13.
36. BELTES P. Endodontic treatment in three cases of dens invaginatus. J Endod 1997; 23: 399–402.
37. BENJAMIN MR et al. Multiple macrodontic multituberculism. Am J Med Genet 2003; 120A: 283–5.
38. BERNABÉ E et al. Tooth-width ratio discrepancies in a sample of Peruvian adolescents. Am J Orthod Dentofac Orthop 2004; 125: 361–5.
39. BERNICK SM. Taurodontia. Oral Surg 1970; 29: 549.
40. BEYNON AD. Developing dens invaginatus (dens in dente). Br Dent J 1982; 153: 255–60.
41. BHATT AP et al. Radicular variety of double dens invaginatus. Oral Surg 1975; 39: 284–7.
42. BIGGERSTAFF RH. Heritability of the Carabelli cusp in twins. J Dent Res 1973; 52: 40–4.
43. BISSADA NF et al. Incidence of cervical enamel projections and its relationship to furcation involvement in Egyptian skulls. J Periodont 1973; 44: 583–5.
44. BØHN A. Dens in dente. Acta Odontol Scand 1948; 8: 53–80.
45. BOLANOS OR et al. A unique approach to the treatment of a tooth with dens invaginatus. J Endod 1988; 14: 315–17.
46. BORGES SOARES A et al. Bilateral talon cusp. Quint Int 2001; 32: 283–6.
47. BOSSHARDT DD et al. Immunocytochemical characterization of ectopic enamel deposits and cementicles in human teeth. Eur J Oral Sci 2003; 111: 51–9.
48. BOTTOMLEY WK. Fused supernumerary tooth. Oral Surg 1987; 64: 132.
49. BOVÉDA C et al. Root canal treatment of an invaginated maxillary lateral incisor with a C-shaped canal. Quint Int 1999; 30: 707–11.
50. BRABANT H. Comparison of the characteristics and anomalies of the deciduous and the permanent dentition. J Dent Res 1967; 46 (suppl 5): 897–902.
51. BRABANT R et al. Beitrag zur Kenntnis der "dens in dente" benannten Zahnanomalie. Stoma 1955; 9: 12–27.
52. BRAMANTE CM et al. Dens invaginatus in mandibular first premolar. Oral Surg Oral Med Oral Pathol 1993; 76: 389.
53. BRKIC H et al. The treatment options of dens invaginatus complications in children. ASDC J Dent Child 2003; 70: 77–81.
54. BROOK AH. A unifying aetiological explanation for anomalies of human tooth number and size. Arch Oral Biol 1984; 29: 373–8.
55. BRUCE KW. The effect of irradiation on the developing dental system of the Syrian hamster. Oral Surg 1950; 3: 1468–77.
56. BRUCE KW, STAFNE EC. The effect of irradiation on the dental system as demonstrated by the roentgenogram. J Am Dent Assoc 1950; 41: 684–9.
57. BRYANT RH et al. Four birooted primary canines. ASDC J Dent Child 1982; 49: 441–2.
58. BURKE FJT et al. The effect of irradiation on developing teeth. Oral Surg 1979; 47: 11–13.
59. BURTON DJ et al. Multiple bilateral dens in dente as a factor in the etiology of multiple periapical lesions. Oral Surg 1980; 49: 496–9.
60. CABO-VALLE M et al. Maxillary central incisor with two root canals. J Oral Rehabil 2001; 28: 797–8.
61. CABRERIZO MERINO MC et al. Dental anomalies caused by oncological treatment. J Clin Pediatr Dent 1998; 22: 261–4.
62. CARBONELL VM. The tubercle of carabelli in the Kish dentition, Mesopotamia, 3000 BC. J Dent Res 1960; 39: 124–8.
63. CARL W et al. Effects of radiation on the developing dentition and supporting bone. J Am Dent Assoc 1980; 101: 646–8.
64. CARLSEN O et al. Radix entomolaris: identification and morphology. Scand J Dent Res 1990; 98: 363–73.
65. CARLSEN O et al. Radix paramolaris in permanent mandibular molars: identification and morphology. Scand J Dent Res 1991; 99: 189–95.
66. CARLSEN O et al. Radix paramolaris and radix distomolaris in Danish permanent maxillary molars. Acta Odontol Scand 1999; 57: 283–9.
67. CARLSEN O et al. Radix mesiolingualis and radix distolingualis in a collection of permanent maxillary molars. Acta Odontol Scand 2000; 58: 229–36.
68. CARTER AC et al. Canine substitution. Am J Orthod Dentofac Orthop 1997; 112: 316–19.
69. CARVALHO JC et al. Malocclusion, dental injuries and dental anomalies in the primary dentition of Belgian children. Int J Paediatr Dent 1998; 8: 137–41.
70. CASAMASSIMO PS et al. An unusual triad: microdontia, taurodontia, and dens invaginatus. Oral Surg 1978; 45: 107–12.
71. CAVANHA AO. Enamel pearls. Oral Surg 1965; 19: 373–82.

72. CECÍLIA MS *et al*. The palato-gingival groove. A cause of failure in root canal treatment. Oral Surg Oral Med Oral Pathol Oral Radiol Endod 1998; 85: 94–8.

73. CHADWICK SM *et al*. Dilaceration of a permanent mandibular incisor. Br J Orthod 1995; 22: 279–81.

74. CHASE RH. Unusual macrodontia. Gen Dent 1994; 42: 216.

75. CHEN RJ. Conservative management of dens evaginatus. J Endod 1984; 10: 253–7.

76. CHEN RJ *et al*. Talon cusp in primary dentition. Oral Surg 1986; 62: 69–72.

77. CHOHAYEB AA. Dilacerations of permanent upper lateral incisors: frequency, direction, and endodontic treatment implications. Oral Surg Oral Med Oral Pathol 1983; 55: 519–20.

78. CHU FCS *et al*. Fractured dens evaginatus and unusual periapical radiolucency. Dent Traumatol 2002; 18: 339–41.

79. COHEN DA. Shortened roots in the maxilla and mandible. Oral Surg Oral Med Oral Pathol 1991; 71: 252.

80. CONGLETON J *et al*. Amelogenesis imperfecta with taurodontism. Oral Surg 1979; 48: 540–4.

81. CONKLIN WW. Bilateral dens invaginatus in the mandibular incisor region. Oral Surg Oral Med Oral Pathol 1978; 45: 905–8.

82. CONSTANT DA *et al*. A review of taurodontism with new data on indigenous southern African populations. Arch Oral Biol 2004; 46: 1021–29.

83. CORRUCCINI RS *et al*. Developmental correlates of crown component asymmetry and occlusal discrepancy. Am J Phys Anthropol 1981; 55: 21–31.

84. CRAWFORD JL. Concomitant taurodontism and amelogenesis imperfecta in the American Caucasian. ASDC J Dent Child 1970; 37: 171–5.

85. CREAVEN J. Dens invaginatus-type malformation without pulpal involvement. J Endod 1975; 1: 79–80.

86. CROFT LK. Periodontal abscess from enamel pearl. Oral Surg 1971; 32: 154.

87. CUDZINOWSKI L. Dens in dente. ASDC J Dent Child 1982; 49: 139–41.

88. CURZON MEJ *et al*. Evaginated odontomes in the Keewatin Eskimo. Br Dent J 1970; 129: 324–8.

89. CURZON MEJ *et al*. Three-rooted mandibular molars in the Keewatin Eskimo. J Can Dent Assoc 1971; 37: 71–2.

90. CURZON MEJ. Three-rooted mandibular permanent molars in English Caucasians. J Dent Res 1973; 52: 181.

91. DAHLBERG AA. The paramolar tubercle (Bolk). Am J Phys Anthropol 1945; 3: 97–103.

92. DAHLLÖF G *et al*. Disturbances in dental development after total body irradiation in bone marrow transplant recipients. Oral Surg Oral Med Oral Pathol 1988; 65: 41–4.

93. DANFORTH RA *et al*. Segmental odontomaxiallry dysplasia. Report of eight cases and comparison with hemimaxillofacial dysplasia. Oral Surg Oral Med Oral Pathol 1990; 70: 81–5.

94. DANKNER E *et al*. Dens evaginatus of anterior teeth. Literature review and radiographic survey of 15,000 teeth. Oral Surg Oral Med Oral Pathol Oral Radiol Endod 1996; 81: 472–6.

95. DARWAZEH AM *et al*. Prevalence of taurodontism in Jordanian dental patients. Dentomaxillofac Radiol 1998; 27: 163–5.

96. DARWAZEH AM *et al*. Radiographic evidence of enamel pearls in Jordanian dental patients. Oral Surg Oral Med Oral Pathol Oral Radiol Endod 2000; 89: 255–8.

97. DAVIS PJ. Findings from 1163 panelipse radiographs of 12-year-old children living in Hong Kong. Community Dent Health 1988; 5: 243–9.

98. DAVIS PJ *et al*. The presentation of talon cusp: diagnosis, clinical features, associations and possible aetiology. Br Dent J 1985; 159: 84–8.

99. DEBALL S *et al*. Homozygous beta thalassemia in an African-American pediatric patient. J Clin Pediatr Dent 1997; 21: 315–19.

100. DE BOER JG. Dens in dente. Ned Tijdschr Tandheelkd 1962; 69: 707–14.

101. DE BOER JG. Endodontische anatomie. Ned Tijdschr Tandheelkd 1966; 73: 268–87.

102. DE BOER JG. Drukanomalieën. Ned Tijdschr Tandheelkd 1972; 79: 97–100.

103. DE BOER JG. Glazuurparels. Ned Tijdschr Tandheelkd 1974; 81: 422–5.

104. DE BOER JG. Een merkwaardig element. Ned Tijdschr Tandheelkd 1975; 82: 167–8.

105. DE JONGE COHEN THE. Ein neuer Beitrag zur Morphogenese des "Dens in dente". Vierteljahrschr Zahnheilkd 1925; 41: 125–30.

106. DE JONGE-COHEN THE. Drukanomalieën. Bijdrage tot de pathologische anatomie van 's menschen gebit. Ned Tijdschr Tandheelkd 1928; 35: 636–44.

107. DE JONGE THE. Anatomie der Zähne. Zahn-Mund-Kieferheilkd 1954; Band I Lig. 5: 169–232.

108. DE LA PARRA C. Een eerste onderpraemolaar met drie wortels. Ned Tijdschr Tandheelkd 1953; 60: 287–9.

109. DE MAN K. Abnormal root development, probably due to erythema multiforme (Stevens-Johnson syndrome). Int J Oral Surg 1979; 8: 381–5.

110. DE SMIT A *et al*. An histological investigation of invaginated human incisors. J Biol Buccale 1984; 12: 201–9.

111. DE SOUSA SMG *et al*. Dens invaginatus: treatment choices. Endod Dent Traumatol 1998; 14: 152–8.

112. DE SOUSA SMG *et al*. Unusual case of bilateral talon cusp associated with dens invaginatus. Int Endod J 1999; 32: 494–8.

113. DE SOUZA-\-FREITAS JA *et al*. Anatomic variations of lower first permanent molar roots in two ethnic groups. Oral Surg 1971; 31: 274–8.

114. DIXON GH *et al*. Genetic aspects of anomalous tooth development. In: STEWART RE *et al*. Oral facial genetics. St Louis, MO: CV Mosby, 1976.

115. DE SIQUEIRA VCF *et al*. Dental fusion and dens evaginatus in the permanent dentition: literature review and clinical case report with conservative treatment. ASDC J Dent Child 2004; 71: 69–72.

116. DRAKE DL. Segmental odontomaxillary dysplasia: an unusual orthodontic challenge. Am J Orthod Dentofac Orthop 2003; 123: 84–6.

117. DUCKMANTON PM. Maxillary permanent central incisor with abnormal crown size and dens invaginatus. Endod Dent Traumatol 1995; 11: 150–2.

118. DUGMORE CR. Bilateral macrodontia of mandibular second premolars. Int J Pediatr Dent 2001; 11: 69–73.

119. DURR DP *et al*. Clinical significance of taurodontism. J Am Dent Assoc 1980; 100: 378–81.

120. DURY DC *et al*. Dental root agenesis secondary to irradiation therapy in a case of rhabdomyosarcoma of the middle ear. Oral Surg 1984; 57: 595–99.

121. ECHAVE-KRUTWIG MDE *et al*. Impacted incisors with dilacerated roots. J Clin Orthod 2002; 36: 641–5.

122. EDEN EK *et al*. Dens invaginatus in a primary molar. ASDC J Dent Child 2002; 69: 49–53.

123. EISENBUD L *et al*. Oral presentations in non-Hodgkin's lymphoma. Part III. Oral Surg 1985; 59: 44–51.

124. EKMAN-WESTBORG B *et al*. Multiple anomalies in dental morphology: macrodontia, multituberculism, central cusps, and pulp invaginations. Oral Surg 1974; 38: 217–22.

125. Elvery MW *et al*. Radiographic study of the Broadbeach Aboriginal dentition. Am J Phys Anthropol 1998; 107: 211–19.

126. FABRA-CAMPOS H. Failure of endodontic treatment due to a palatal gingival groove in a maxillary lateral incisor with talon cusp and two root canals. J Endod 1990; 16: 342–5.

127. FAHID A *et al*. Maxillary second molar with three buccal roots. J Endod 1988; 14: 181–3.

128. FALOMO OO. The cusp of Carabelli: frequency, distribution, size and clinical significance in Nigeria. West African J Med 2002; 21: 322–4.

129. FARIAS M *et al*. Tooth size and morphology in hemifacial microsomia. Int J Paediatr Dent 1998; 8: 197–201.

130. FISCHER H. Die "prismatischen" Molaren van Krapina/Kroatien im Lichte rezenter Funde. Dtsch Zahnaerztl Z 1961; 16: 8–15.

131. FISCHER-BRANDIES H *et al*. Odontometrische Studie über die Abhängigkeit von Zahn- und Körpergrösse. Fortschr Kieferorthop 1988; 49: 96–107.

132. FLEISCHER-PETERS A, QUAST U. Klinisch-röntgenologische Untersuchungen über Art und Häufigkeit von Zahnanomalien. Dtsch Zahnärzteblatt 1970; 24: 255–60.

133. FOLWACZNY M *et al*. Impaired dentofacial development after radiotherapy of a non-Hodgkin lymphoma. ASDC J Dent Child 2000; 67: 428–30.

134. FONG CD *et al*. Sequential expression of an amelin gene in mesenchymal and epithelial cells during odontogenesis in rats. Eur J Oral Sci 1998; 106: 324–30.

135. FRAYER DW. Metric dental changes in the European upper paleolithic and mesolithic. Am J Phys Anthropol 1977; 46: 109–20.

136. FRONER IC *et al*. Complex treatment of dens invaginatus type III in maxillary lateral incisor. Endod Dent Traumatol 1999; 15: 88–90.

137. FUJIKI Y *et al*. Clinical and radiographic observation of dens invaginatus. Dentomaxillofac Radiol (Proc) 1974; 3: 343.

138. FUKS AB *et al*. Multiple taurodontism associated with osteoporosis. J Pedod 1982; 7: 68–74.

139. FUKUTA Y *et al*. A central tubercle on the lingual surface of the upper lateral incisor. J Nipon Univ Sch Dent 1997; 39: 86–8.

140. GARDNER DG *et al*. Talon cusps: a dental anomaly in the Rubinstein-Taybi syndrome. Oral Surg 1979; 47: 519–21.

141. GARN SM, LEWIS AB. Effect of agenesis on the crown-size profile pattern. J Dent Res 1969; 48 (II): 1314.

142. GARN SM *et al*. Genetic independence of Carabelli's trait from tooth size or crown morphology. Arch Oral Biol 1966; 11: 745–7.

143. GARN SM *et al*. Sex difference in tooth size. J Dent Res 1964; 43: 306.

144. GARN SM *et al*. Relationship between buccolingual and mesiodistal tooth diameters. J Dent Res 1968; 47: 495.

145. GAZIT E *et al*. Macrodontia of maxillary central incisors. Quint Int 1991; 22: 883–7.

146. GAYNOR WN. Dens evaginatus – how does it present and how should it be managed? N Z Dent J 2002; 98: 104–7.

147. GEDIK R *et al*. Multiple taurodontism. ASDC J Dent Child 2000; 67: 216–17.

148. GEIST JR. Dens evaginatus. Oral Surg Oral Med Oral Pathol 1989; 67: 628–31.

149. GENC A *et al*. Taurodontism in association with supernumerary teeth. J Clin Pediatr Dent 1999; 23: 151–4.

150. GEURTSEN W *et al*. Palatinal-gingivale Furchung und Wurzelüberzahl bei Oberkieferschneidezähnen. Dtsch Zahnaerztl Z 1986; 41: 667–71.

151. GIBSON ACL. Continued root development after traumatic avulsion of partly-formed permanent incisor. Br Dent J 1969; 126: 356–6.

152. GIBSON AC. Bilateral macrodontism of mandibular third molars with impaction of second molars. Oral Surg Oral Med Oral Pathol 1970; 29: 717–18.

153. GIRSCH WJ, McCLAMMY TV. Microscopic removal of dens invaginatus. J Endod 2002; 28: 336–9.

154. GOLDMAN HM. Oral pathology. A collective review and atlas of dental anomalies and diseases. Oral Surg 1949; 2: 880–905.

155. GOLDSTEIN AR. Enamel pearls as contributing factors in periodontal breakdown. J Am Dent Assoc 1979; 99: 210–11.

156. GOLDSTEIN E, GOTTLIEB MA. Taurodontism: familial tendencies demonstrated in eleven of fourteen. Oral Surg 1973; 36: 131–44.

157. GOLDSTEIN E *et al*. Mohr syndrome of oral-facial-digital II. J Am Dent Assoc 1974; 89: 377–82.

158. GÖLLNER L. Über Schmelztropfen. Dtsch Monatschr Zahnheilkd 1928; 46: 225–40.

159. GONÇALVES A *et al*. Dens invaginatus type III. Int Endod J 2002; 35: 873–9.

160. GOODMAN HO. Genetic parameters of dentofacial development. J Dent Res 1965; 44 (suppl 1): 174–84.

161. GOODMAN JR *et al*. Dental problems associated with hypophosphataemic vitamin D resistant rickets. Int J Pediatr Dent 1998; 8: 19–28.

162. GOODMAN NJ *et al*. Dens in dente in a mandibular canine. Oral Surg Oral Med Oral Pathol 1976; 41: 267.

163. GOOSE DH *et al*. Size and morphology of children's teeth in North Wales. In: KURTÉN B (ed.) Teeth: form, function, and evolution. New York, NY: Columbia University Press, 1982.

164. GOOSE DH *et al*. The mode of inheritance of Carabelli's trait. Hum Biol 1971; 43: 64–9.

165. GORLIN RJ *et al*. Syndromes of head and neck. New York, NY: Oxford University Press, 2001.

166. GORLIN RJ *et al*. Severe irradiation during odontogenesis. Oral Surg 1963; 16: 35–8.

167. GOTOH T *et al*. Clinical and radiographic study of dens invaginatus. Oral Surg 1979; 48: 88–91.

168. GOUND TG *et al*. Nonsurgical management of a dilacerated maxillary lateral incisor with type III dens invaginatus. J Endod 2004; 30: 448–51.

169. GRAHNÉN H *et al*. Palatal invaginations ("dens in dente") of the second maxillary permanent incisors. Odontol Revy 1958; 9: 163–6.

170. GRAHNÉN H *et al*. Dens invaginatus. I. A clinical, roentgenological and genetical study of permanent upper lateral incisors. Odontol Revy 1959; 10: 115–37.

171. GREWE JM *et al*. Cervical enamel projections: prevalence, location, and extent; with associated periodontal implications. J Periodont 1965; 36: 460–5.

172. GRULICH F *et al*. Häufigkeiten und Lokalisation von Schmelzparaplasien an mehrwurzeligen menschlichen Zähnen. Dtsch Zahnärztl Z 1993; 48: 247–9.

173. GÜNGÖR HC *et al*. Pulpal tissue in bilateral talon cusps of primary central incisors. Oral Surg Oral Med Oral Pathol Oral Radiol Endod 2000; 89: 231–5.

174. GUSTAFSON G *et al*. Dens in dente. Br Dent J 1950; 88: 83–8, 111–22, 144–6.

175. HAGARTY TJ *et al*. Stellate central incisors. Oral Surg 1984; 54: 112.

176. HALLETT GEM. The incidence, nature, and clinical significance of palatal invaginations in the maxillary incisor teeth. Proc R Soc Med 1953; 46: 491–9.

177. HAMAMOTO Y *et al*. Production of amelogenin by enamel epithelium of Hertwig's root sheath. Oral Surg Oral Med Oral Pathol Oral Radiol Endod 1996; 81: 703–9.

178. HAMASHA AA *et al*. Prevalence of dens invaginatus in Jordanian adults. Int Endod J 2004; 37: 307–10.

179. HAMASHA AA *et al*. Prevalence of dilacerations in Jordanian adults. Int Endod J 2002; 35: 910–12.

180. HAMNER JE III *et al*. Taurodontism. Oral Surg 1964; 18: 409–18.

181. HARTUP GR. Dens invaginatus type III in a mandibular premolar. Gen Dent 1997; 45: 584–7.

182. HARZER W. A hypothetical model of genetic control of tooth-crown growth in man. Arch Oral Biol 1987; 32: 159–62.

183. HATA S *et al*. The dentofacial manifestations of XXXXY syndrome. Int J Paediatr Dent 2001; 11: 138–42.

184. HATTAB F *et al*. Talon cusp – Clinical significance and management. Quint Int 1995; 26: 115–20.

185. HATTAB F *et al*. Talon cusp in permanent dentition associated with other dental anomalies. ASDC J Dent Child 1996; 63: 368–76.

186. HATTAB FN *et al*. Oral manifestations of Ellis–van Creveld syndrome. J Clin Pediatr Dent 1998; 22: 159–65.

187. HATTAB FN, HAZZA'A AM. An unusual case of talon cusp on geminated tooth. J Can Dent Assoc 2001; 67: 263–6.

188. HAYES PA. Hamartomas, eruption cyst, natal tooth and Epstein pearls in a newborn. ASDC J Dent Child 2000; 67: 365–8.

189. HAYWARD JR. Cuspid gigantism. Oral Surg 1980; 49: 500–1.

190. HELD M *et al*. Multiple localized root agenesis. ASDC J Dent Child 1985; 52: 45–7.

191. HELPIN ML *et al*. Complications following radiation therapy to the head. Oral Surg 1986; 55: 209–12.

192. HICKS MJ. Dens invaginatus with partial coronal agenesis. Oral Surg Oral Med Oral Pathol 1990; 70: 240–1.

193. HICKS MJ *et al*. Dens invaginatus with partial coronal agenesis. ASDC J Dent Child 1985; 52: 217–19.

194. HOLAN G. Dens invaginatus in a primary canine. Int J Paediatr Dent 1998; 8: 61–4.

195. HOLT RD *et al*. Taurodontism: a criterion for diagnosis and its prevalence in mandibular first permanent molars in a sample of 1115 British schoolchildren. J Int Ass Dent Child 1979; 10: 41–47.

196. HOLTON WL *et al*. Prevalence and distribution of attached cementicles on human root surfaces. J Periodontol 1986; 57: 321–4.

197. HOOIJER DA *et al*. Numerous radicular enamel pearls in a premolar of a wild sheep. Oral Surg 1975; 39: 637–40.

198. HOU GL *et al*. Cervical enamel projection and intermediate bifurcational ridge correlated with molar furcation involvements. J Periodontol 1997; 68: 687–93.

199. HOU GL *et al*. Relationship between periodontal furcation involvement and molar cervical enamel projections. J Periodontol 1987; 58: 715–21.

200. HOU GL *et al*. The morphology of root fusion in Chinese adults. (I). Grades, types, location and distribution. J Clin Periodontol 1994; 21: 260–4.

201. HOU GL *et al*. Relationship between molar root fusion and localized periodontitis. J Periodontol 1997; 68: 313–19.

202. HOVLAND EJ *et al*. Nonrecognition and subsequent endodontic treatment of dens invaginatus. J Endod 1977; 3: 360–2.

203. HRDLICKA A. Shovel-shaped teeth. Am J Phys Anthropol 1920; 3: 429–65.

204. HSU JW *et al*. Ethnic dental analysis of shovel and Carabelli's traits in a Chinese population. Aust Dent J 1999; 44: 40–5.

205. HÜLSMANN M. Der Dens invaginatus-ätiologie, Inzidenz und klinische Besonderheiten. Schweiz Monatschr Zahnmed 1995; 105: 765–76.

206. HÜLSMANN M. Dens invaginatus: aetiology, classification, relevance, diagnosis, and treatment considerations. Int Endod J 1997; 30: 79–90.

207. IKEDA H *et al*. Importance of clinical examination and diagnosis. Oral Surg Oral Med Oral Pathol Oral Radiol Endod 1995; 79: 88–91.

208. IRELAND EJ *et al*. Short roots, taurodontia and multiple dens invaginatus. J Pedod 1987; 11: 164–75.

209. IWASAKI H *et al*. Morphological investigation of deciduous teeth in Shanghai, China – Carabelli's tubercle and protostylid. Pediatr Dent J 2001; 11: 5–9.

210. JAYAWARDENA CK *et al*. On the origin of intrinsic acellular extrinsic fiber cementum: studies on growing cementum pearls of normal and biphosphonate-affected guinea pig molars. Eur J Oral Sci 2002; 110: 261–9.

211. JASPERS MT. Taurodontism in the Down syndrome. Oral Surgery 1981; 51: 632–6.

212. JENG JH, LU KH *et al*. Treatment of an osseous lesion associated with a severe palato-radicular groove. J Periodontol 1992; 63: 708–12.

213. JIMÉNEZ-RUBIO A *et al*. Multiple dens invaginatus affecting maxillary lateral incisors and a supernumerary tooth. Endod Dent Traumatol 1997; 13: 196–8.

214. JOHO JP *et al*. Microdontia: a specific tooth anomaly. ASDC J Dent Child 1979; 46: 483–6.

215. JONAS I, SCHIENLE R. Veränderungen der Zahnmorphologie unter dem Einfluss von fluoridierten Trinkwasser. Schweiz Monatschr Zahnmed 1984; 94: 399–408.

216. JØRGENSEN KD. The deciduous dentition. Acta Odontol Scand 1956; 4 (suppl 20): 72–140.

217. JORGENSON RJ. The conditions manifesting taurodontism. Am J Med Genet 1982; 11: 435–42.

218. JORGENSON RJ *et al*. The prevalence of taurodontism in a select population. J Craniofac Genet Develop Biol 1982; 2: 125–35.

219. JOSHI MR. Carabelli's trait on maxillary second deciduous molars and first permanent molars in Hindus. Arch Oral Biol 1975; 20: 699–700.

220. JOWHARJI N *et al*. An unusual case of dental anomaly: a "facial" talon cusp. ASDC J Dent Child 1992; 59: 156–8.

221. JU Y. Dens evaginatus – A difficult diagnostic problem? J Clin Pediatr Dent 1991; 15: 247–8.

222. KABBAN M *et al*. Tooth size and morphology in twins. Int J Padiatr Dent 2001; 11: 333–9.

223. KANNAPAN JG *et al*. A study of dental morphological variation. Tubercle of Carabelli. Indian J Dent Res 2001; 12: 145–9.

224. KANNAN SK *et al*. Dens in dente (dens invaginatus). Indian J Dent Res 2003; 14: 125–9.

225. KARACA I *et al*. Multiple bilateral dens in dente involving all the premolars. Aust Dent J 1992; 37: 449–51.

226. KASTE SC *et al*. Dental abnormalities in children treated for neuroblastoma. Med Pediatr Oncol 1998; 30 (1): 22–7.

227. KAWATA T, TANNE K. Early detection of dens evaginatus appearing on premolars and clinical management: histological study. J Clin Pediatr Dent 2002; 26: 199–201.

228. KAUFMAN AY *et al*. Developmental anomaly of permanent teeth related to traumatic injury. Endod Dent Traumatol 1990; 6: 183–8.

229. KEELER C. Taurodont molars and shovel incisors in Klinefelter's syndrome. J Heredity 1973; 64: 234–7.

230. KEENE HJ. The relationship between Carabelli's trait and the size, number and morphology of the maxillary molars. Arch Oral Biol 1968; 13: 1023–5.

231. KEREBEL B *et al*. Les perles d' émail: étude histopathologique. J Biol Buccale 1986; 14: 239–48.

232. KEREBEL B *et al*. Dentinogenesis imperfecta with dens in dente. Oral Surg 1983; 55: 279–85.

233. KHABBAZ MG *et al*. Dens invaginatus in a mandibular lateral incisor. Int Endod J 1995; 28: 303–5.

234. KHANNA JN *et al*. Hemifacial hypertrophy. Int J Oral Maxillofac Surg 1989; 18: 294–7.

235. KHARAT DU *et al*. Shovel-shaped incisors and associated invagination in some Asian and African populations. J Dent 1990; 18: 216–20.

236. KIESER JA *et al*. On the non-existence of compensatory tooth size interaction in a contemporary human population. J Dent Res 1986; 65: 1105–7.

237. KILPATRICK NM *et al*. Dilaceration of a primary tooth. Int J Paediatr Dent 1991; 1: 151–3.

238. KNEŽEVIC G. Dens invaginatus with ameloblastoma. Oral Surg Oral Med Oral Pathol 1980; 49: 274.

239. KOGON SL. The prevalence, location and conformation of palato-radicular grooves in maxillary incisors. J Periodontol 1986; 57: 231–4.

240. KOH ET *et al*. Prophylactic treatment of dens evaginatus using mineral trioxide aggregate. J Endod 2001; 27: 540–2.

241. KOLAKOWSKI D *et al*. A Differential environmental effect on human anterior tooth size. Am J Phys Anthropol 1981; 54: 377–81.

242. KORENHOF CAW. Morphogenetical aspects of the human upper molar. Thesis, University of Utrecht, 1960.

243. KOSINSKI RW *et al*. Localized deficient root development associated with taurodontism. Pediatr Dent 1999; 21: 213–15.

244. KOVACS I. Contribution to the ontogenetic morphology of roots on human teeth. J Dent Res 1967; 46 (suppl 5): 865–74.

245. KRAMER IRH. The pathology of pulp death in non-carious maxillary in incisors with minor palatal invaginations. Proc R Soc Med 1953; 46: 503–6.

246. KRAUS BS. Carabelli's anomaly of the maxillary molar teeth. Observations on Mexicans and Papago Indians and an interpretation of the inheritance. Am J Hum Genet 1951; 3: 348–55.

247. KREUTZ RW *et al*. "Pseudo fracture" of mandibular first molar. Oral Surg Oral Med Oral Pathol 1987; 64: 774–5.

248. KUPIETZKY A *et al*. Enamel pearls in the primary dentition. ASDC J Dent Child 1993; 60: 63–6.

249. KUSTALOGLU OA. Paramolar structures of the upper dentition. J Dent Res 1962; 41: 75–83.

250. LAATIKAINEN T *et al*. Taurodontism in twins with cleft lip and/or palate. Eur J Oral Sci 1996; 104: 82–6.

251. LARA VS *et al*. Macroscopic and microscopic analysis of palato-gingival groove. J Endod 2000; 26: 345–50.

252. LAU TC. Odontomes of the axial core type. Br Dent J 1955; 99: 219–25.

253. LAVELLE CLB. Angle-Saxon and modern British teeth. J Dent Res 1968; 47: 811–15.

254. LE BOT P, SALMON D. Congenital defects of the upper lateral incisors (ULI): condition and measurements of other teeth, measurements of the superior arch, head and face. Am J Phys Anthropol 1977; 46: 231–44.

255. LEE GTR *et al.* The inheritance of dental traits in a Chinese population in the United Kingdom. J Med Genet 1972; 9: 336–9.

256. LE HUCHE R. Füllungen, Inlays-Onlays und Kronen als Funktion der Form des Zahnes. Berlin: Quintessenz, 1971.

257. LEIB AM *et al.* Furcation involvements correlated with enamel projections from the cementoenamel junction. J Periodontol 1967; 38: 330–4.

258. LEONARD M. Diminished root formation. Oral Surg 1972; 34: 205–8.

259. LERVIK T *et al.* Observations of dental disease and anomalies in 9- to 11-year-old Norwegian children. Acta Odontol Scand 1983; 41: 45–51.

260. LEWIS R *et al.* Palatal invaginations in incisors and the presence of cusps of Carabelli. J Pedod 1984; 8: 285–92.

261. LIN L *et al.* Bilateral dilaceration. J Endod 1982; 8: 85–7.

262. LLAMAS R *et al.* Taurodontism in premolars. Oral Surg Oral Med Oral Pathol 1993; 75: 501–5.

263. LIBFELD H *et al.* Incidence of four-rooted maxillary second molars: literature review and radiographic survey of 1200 teeth. J Endod 1989; 15: 129–31.

264. LIN YTJ. Treatment of an impacted dilacerated maxillary central incisor. Am J Orthod Dentofac Orthop 1999; 115: 406–9.

265. LIND V. Short root anomaly. Scand J Dent Res 1972; 80: 85–93.

266. LINDNER C *et al.* A complex treatment of dens invaginatus. Endod Dent Traumatol 1995; 11: 153–5

267. LINDSTEN R *et al.* Dental arch space and permanent tooth size in the mixed dentition of a skeletal sample from the 14th to the 19th centuries and 3 contemporary samples. Am J Orthod Dentofac Orthop 2002; 122: 48–58.

268. LIU JF *et al.* Talon cusp affecting the primary maxillary central incisors in two sets of female twins. Pediatr Dent 1995; 17: 362–4.

269. LOH FC. Paramolar with bifid crown. Oral Surg Oral Med Oral Pathol 1993; 76: 257–8.

270. LOH HS. Incidence and features of three-rooted permanent mandibular molars. Aust Dent J 1990; 35: 434–7.

271. LOMÇALI G *et al.* Talon cusp. Quint Int 1994; 25: 431–3.

272. LORENA SC *et al.* Multiple dental anomalies in the maxillary incisor region. J Oral Sci 2003; 45: 47–50.

273. LOVIUS BBJ *et al.* The effect of fluoridation of water on tooth morphology. Br Dent J 1969; 127: 322–4.

274. LOWE PL. Dilaceration caused by direct penetrating injury. Br Dent J 1985; 159: 373–4.

275. LUNT Da. "Molarization" of the mandibular second premolars. J Dent 1976; 4: 83–6.

276. LYSELL L. Taurodontism. Odontol Revy 1962; 13: 158–74.

277. LYSELL L. Taurodontism in both dentitions. Odontol Revy 1965; 16: 359–62.

278. LYSELL G *et al.* A unique case of dilaceration. Odontol Revy 1969; 20: 43–6.

279. LYSSEL L *et al.* Mesiodistal tooth size in the deciduous and permanent dentitions. Eur J Orthod 1982; 4: 113–22.

280. MaCDONALD-JANKOWSKI DS *et al.* Taurodontism in a young adult Chinese population. Dentomaxillofac Radiol 1993; 22: 140–4.

281. MACHTEI EE *et al.* The relationship between cervical enamel projection and class II furcation defects in humans. Quint Int 1997; 28: 315–20.

282. MADEIRA MC *et al.* Prevalence of taurodontism in premolars. Oral Surg 1986; 61: 158–62.

283. MADER CL. Talon cusp. J Am Dent Assoc 1981; 103: 244–6.

284. MADER CL *et al.* Primary talon cusp. ASDC J Dent Child 1985; 52: 223–6.

285. MADER CL *et al.* Incomplete dens in dente in a fused tooth. Oral Surg 1982; 53: 439.

286. MAVRODISZ K *et al.* Prevalence of talon cusp in patients aged 7–18. Fogorv Sz 2003; 96: 257–9.

287. MANABE Y *et al.* Non-metric tooth crown traits of the Thai, AKA and YAO tribes of Northern Thailand. Arch Oral Biol 1997; 42: 283–91.

288. MANGANI F *et al.* Endodontic treatment of a "very particular" maxillary central inicisor. J Endod 1994; 20: 560–1.

289. MANN RW *et al.* Anomalous morphologic formation of deciduous and permanent teeth in 1 5-year-old 15Th century child: a variant of the Ekman-Westborg-Julin syndrome. Oral Surg Oral Med Oral Pathol 1990; 70: 90–4.

290. MANSON-HING LR. Taurodontism. Oral Surg 1963; 16: 305.

291. MARCUSHAMER M *et al.* Microdontic teeth succedaneous to natal teeth. Pediatr Dent 1992; 14: 400–1.

292. MARKLUND M *et al.* The relationship between mandibular morphology and apical root curvature in man. Arch Oral Biol 1988; 33: 391–4.

293. MASTERS DH *et al.* Projection of cervical enamel into molar furcations. J Periodontol 1964; 35: 49–53.

294. MATSUOKA T *et al.* Crown dilacerations of a first premolar caused by extraction of its deciduous predecessor. Endod Dent Traumatol 2000; 16: 91–4.

295. MATTISON GD *et al.* Lateral root dilaceration: a multidisciplinary approach to treatment. Endod Dent Traumatol 1987; 3: 135–40.

296. McCULLOCH KJ *et al.* Dens invaginatus from orthodontic perspective. Am J Orthod Dentofac Orthop 1997; 112: 670–5.

297. McCULLOCH KJ *et al.* Dens evaginatus. J Can Dent Assoc 1998; 64: 104–13.

298. McGINNIS JP *et al.* Tooth root growth impairment after mantle radiation in long-term survivors of Hodgkin's disease. J Am Dent Assoc 1985; 111: 584–8.

299. McKAIG SJ *et al.* Dens invaginatus on the labial surface of a central incisor Dent Update 2001; 28: 210–12.

300. McKEE JK. A genetic model of dental reduction through the probable mutation effect. Am J Phys Anthropol 1984; 65: 231–41.

301. McNAMARA CM *et al.* Root abnormalities, talon cusps, dens invaginati with reduced alveolar bone levels. Int J Paediatr Dent 1998; 8: 41–5.

302. MEHROTRA KK *et al.* Microdontic maxillary lateral incisor. J Clin Pediatr Dent 1992; 16: 119–20.

303. MELLOR JK *et al.* Talon cusp: a clinically significant anomaly. Oral Surg 1970; 29: 225–8.

304. MENA CA. Taurodontism. Oral Surg 1971; 32: 812–23.

305. MEON R. Talon cusp in primary dentition. Singapore Dent J 1990; 15: 32–4.

306. MEON R. Talon cusp in two siblings. N Z Dent J 1990; 86: 42–4.

307. RUSHMA, MEON. See reference 389.

308. MEREDITH HV *et al.* Frequency, size, and bilateralism of Carabelli's tubercle. J Dent Res 1954; 33: 435–40.

309. MERRILL RG. Occlusal anomalous tubercles on premolars of Alaskan Eskimos and Indians. Oral Surg 1964; 17: 484–96.

310. METRO PS. Taurodontism: a dental rarity in modern man. Oral Surg 1965; 20: 236–7.

311. MIDDLETON SHAW JC. Taurodont teeth in South African races. J Anat 1928; 62: 476–99.

312. MILAZZO A *et al.* Fusion, gemination, oligodontia and taurodontism. J Pedod 1982; 6(winter): 194–9.

313. MILLER WA. Pulp calcifications in a taurodont tooth. Br Dent J 1969; 126: 456–8.

314. MINICUCCI EM *et al.* Dental abnormalities in children after chemotherapy treatment for acute lymphoid leukaemia. Leukemia Research 2003; 27: 45–50.

315. MIYOSHI S *et al.* Bifurcated root canals and crown diameter. J Dent Res 1977; 56: 1425.

316. MJÖR IA. The structure of taurodont teeth. ASDC J Dent Child 1972; 39: 459–63.

317. MOORREES CFA *et al.* Mesiodistal crown diameters of the deciduous and permanent teeth in individuals. J Dent Res 1957; 36: 39–47.

318. MOREAU JL *et al.* Etudes du taurodontisme au Sénégal. Rev Mens Suisse Odonto-Stomatol 1985; 95: 515–21.

319. MORFIS AS. Chemical analysis of a dens invaginatus by S.E.M. microanalyses. J Clin Pediatr Dent 1992; 17: 79–82.

320. MOSKOW BS. Some observations on radicular enamel. J Periodontol 1971; 42: 92–6.

321. MOSKOW BS *et al.* Studies on root enamel. (2) Enamel pearls. A review of their morphology, localization, nomenclature, occurrence, classification, histogenesis and incidence. J Clin Periodontol 1990; 17: 275–81.

322. MOULE AJ *et al.* Unusual root formation in a premolar with dens evaginatus. Aust Dent J 1987; 32: 354–6.

323. MÜLLER-LESSMANN V *et al.* Rudimentäre Wurzelbildung und ausbleibender Zahndurchbruch im bleibenden Gebiss. Dtsch Zahnärztl Zeitschr 2002; 57: 124–6.

324. MUPPARAPU M *et al.* A rare presentation of dens invaginatus in a mandibular lateral incisor occurring concurrently with bilateral maxillary dens invaginatus. Aust Dent J 2004; 49: 90–3.

325. MYERS CL. Treatment of a talon-cusp incisor. ASDC J Dent Child 1980; 47: 119–21.

326. NAKAGAWA T *et al.* Ekman-Westborg-Julin syndrome. Int J Oral Maxillofac Surg 1997; 26: 49–50.

327. NAMDAR F *et al.* Macrodontia in association with a contrasting character microdontia. J Clin Pediatr Dent 1999; 23: 271–4.

328. NASHASHIBI IA. Orthodontic movement of a palatally displaced, dilacerated, unerupted maxillary central incisor. J Pedod 1986; 11: 83–90.

329. NATKIN E *et al.* A case of talon cusp associated with other odontogenic abnormalities. J Endod 1983; 9: 491–5.

330. NAZIF MM *et al.* Dens invaginatus in a geminated central incisor. Pediatr Dent 1990; 12: 250–2.

331. NEAL JJD, BOWDEN DEJ. The diagnostic value of panoramic radiographs in children aged nine to ten years. Br J Orthod 1988; 15: 193–7.

332. NGUYEN AM *et al.* Pyramidal molar roots and canine-like dental morphologic features in multiple family members. Oral Surg Oral Med Oral Pathol Oral Radiol Endod 1996; 82: 411–16.

333. NOIKURA T *et al.* Double dens in dente with a central cusp and multituberculism in bilateral maxillary supernumerary central incisors. Oral Surg Oral Med Oral Pathol Oral Radiol Endod 1996; 82: 466–9.

334. NUNN JH *et al.* Dental caries and dental anomalies in children treated by chemotherapy for malignant disease: a study in the north of England. Int J Paediatr Dent 1991; 1: 131–5.

335. OGDEN GR. The significance of taurodontism in dental surgery. Dent Update 1988; 15: 32–4.

336. OGDEN GR. Taurodontism in dermatologic disease. Int J Dermatol 1988; 27A: 360–4.

337. OMNELL K *et al.* Dens invaginatus. II. A microradiographical, histological and micro X-ray diffraction study. Acta Odontol Scand 1960; 18: 304–30.

338. OEHLERS FAC. Dens invaginatus (dilated composite odontome). I. Variations of the invagination process, associated anterior crown forms. Oral Surg 1957; 10: 1204–18 and 1302–16.

339. OEHLERS FAC. The radicular variety of dens invaginatus. Oral Surg 1958; 11: 1251–60.

340. OGINNI A *et al.* Talon cusp. Pediatr Dent J 2001: 11: 85–8.

341. OHISHI K *et al.* Examination of the roots of paramolar tubercles with computed tomography. Oral Surg Oral Med Oral Pathol 1999; 88: 479–83.

342. OIDA S *et al.* Amelogenin gene expression in porcine odontoblasts. J Dent Res 2002; 81: 103–8.

343. OLMEZ S *et al.* Dens invaginatus of a mandibular central incisor: surgical endodontic treatment. J Clin Pediatr Dent 1995; 20: 53–6.

344. Online Mendelian Inheritance in Man (OMIM™). McKusick-Nathans Institute for Genetic Medicine, John Hopkins University (Baltimore, MD) and National Center for Biotechnology Information, National Library of Medicine (Bethesda, MD), 2006. Available at: www.ncbi.nlm.nih.gov/omim/.

345. ONYEASO CO *et al.* Need for preventive and interceptive orthodontic treatment in 3–5-year-old Nigerian children in two major cities. Afr J Med Med Sci 2002; 31: 115–18.

346. OOSHIMA T *et al.* The prevalence of developmental anomalies of teeth and their association with tooth size in the primary and permanent dentitions of 1650 Japanese children. Int J Paediatr Dent 1996; 6: 87–94.

347. ORUP HI JR *et al*. Prenatal anticonvulsant drug exposure: teratogenic effect on the dentition. J Craniofac Genet Dev Biol 1998; 18: 129–37.

348. PACKOTA GV *et al*. Radiographic features of segmental odontomaxillary dysplasia: study of 12 cases. Oral Surg Oral Med Oral Pathol Oral Radiol Endod 1996; 82: 577–84.

349. PAJARI U *et al*. Effect of anti-neoplastic therapy on dental maturity and tooth development. J Pedod 1988; 12: 266–74.

350. PALMER ME. Case reports of evaginated odontomes in Caucasians. Oral Surg 1973; 35: 772–9.

351. PARKER JL *et al*. Hypoplastic-hypomaturation amelogenesis imperfecta with taurodontism. ASDC J Dent Child 1975; 42: 379–83.

352. PARNELL AG *et al*. Frequency of palatal invagination in permanent maxillary anterior teeth. ASDC J Dent Child 1978; 45: 392–5.

353. PAULSON RB *et al*. Double-rooted maxillary primary canines. ASDC J Dent Child 1985; 52: 195–8.

354. PAYNE M *et al*. A radicular dens invaginatus. Br Dent J 1990; 169: 94–5.

355. PEARLMAN J *et al*. An evaginated odontoma in an American negro. J Am Dent Assoc 1977; 95: 570–2.

356. PÉCORA JD *et al*. Study of the incidence of radicular grooves in maxillary incisors. Braz Dent J 1992; 3: 11–16.

357. PERZIGIAN AJ. Allometric analysis of dental variation in a human population. Am J Phys Anthropol 1981; 54: 341–5.

358. PETERSSON A. A case of dentinal dysplasia and/or calcification of the dentinal papilla. Oral Surg 1972; 33: 1014–17.

359. PIATELLI A *et al*. Dens invaginatus: a histological study of undemineralized material. Endod Dent Traumatol 1993; 9: 191–5.

360. PIETROVSKI J *et al*. Tooth dwarfism and root underdevelopment following irradiation. Oral Surg 1966; 22: 95–9.

361. PINDBORG JJ. Pathology of the dental hard tissues. Copenhagen: Munksgaard, 1970.

362. PITTS DL *et al*. Talon cusp management: orthodontic-endodontic considerations. ASDC J Dent Child 1983; 50: 364–8.

363. POLLOCK RA *et al*. Congenital hemifacial hyperplasia. Cleft Palate J 1985; 22: 173–84.

364. POTTER RHY. The genetics in tooth size. In: STEWART R, PRESCOTT G (eds) Oral facial genetics. St Louis, MO: CV Mosby, 1976.

365. POYTON HG. Dens in dente. Dent Radiogr Photogr 1966; 39: 27–33.

366. POYTON HG *et al*. Thalassemia. Changes visible in radiographs used in dentistry. Oral Surg 1968; 25: 564–76.

367. POYTON HG *et al*. Three evaginated odontomes. J Can Dent Assoc 1965; 31: 439–42.

368. PRIMACK JE. Individual bilateral megadontism. J Am Dent Assoc 1967; 75: 655–7.

369. PRUSACK N *et al*. Segmental odontomaxillary dysplasia. A case report and review of the literature. Oral Surg Oral Med Oral Pathol Oral Radiol Endod 2000; 90: 483–8.

370. RADNZIC D. Dental crowding and its relationship to mesiodistal crown diameters and arch dimensions. Am J Orthod Dentofac Orthop 1988; 94: 50–6.

371. REGATTIERI LR *et al*. Taurodontism. Oral Surg 1972; 34: 691.

372. REICHART PA *et al*. Three-rooted permanent mandibular first molars in the Thai. Community Dent Oral Epidemiol 1981; 9: 191–2.

373. REICHART P *et al*. Morphologic findings in dens evaginatus. Int J Oral Surg 1982; 11: 59–63.

374. REICHART P *et al*. Dens evaginatus in the Thai. An evaluation of fifty-one cases. Oral Surg 1975; 39: 615–21.

375. RIDDEL K *et al*. Dens invaginatus: a retrospective study of prophylactic invagination treatment. Int J Paediatr Dent 2001; 11: 92–7.

376. RISNES S. The prevalence and distribution of cervical enamel projections reaching into the bifurcation on human molars. Scand J Dent Res 1974; 82: 413–19.

377. RISNES S. Ectopic tooth enamel. A SEM study of the structure of enamel in enamel pearls. Adv Dent Res 1989; 3: 258–64.

378. RITZAU M *et al*. The Ekman-Westborg-Julin syndrome. Oral Surg Oarl Med Oral Pathol Oral Radiol Endod 1997; 84: 293–6.

379. ROBBINS IM *et al*. Multiple morphologic dental anomalies. Oral Surg 1964; 17: 683–90.

380. ROSS IF *et al*. Root fusion in molars: incidence and sex linkage. J Periodontol 1981; 52: 663–7.

381. ROLAND NM. Periapical lesions associated with dens in dente. Oral Surg 1979; 48: 190.

382. ROOTKIN-GRAY VFAI *et al*. Macrodontia of a mandibular second premolar. ASDC J Dent Child 2001; 68: 347–9.

383. ROTSTEIN I *et al*. Clinical considerations in the treatment of dens invaginatus. Endod Dent Traumatol 1987; 3: 249–54.

384. RUFFALO RC *et al*. A comparative study of three radiographic surveys in preschool children. ASDC J Dent Child 1983; 50: 422–4.

385. RUPRECHT A *et al*. The incidence of taurodontism in dental patients. Oral Surg 1987; 63: 743–7.

386. RUPRECHT A *et al*. The incidence of dental invagination. J Pedodont 1986; 10: 265–72.

387. RUPRECHT A *et al*. The clinical significance of dental invagination. J Pedod 1987; 11: 176–81.

388. RUPRECHT A *et al*. Macrodontia of the mandibular left first premolar. Oral Surg 1979; 48: 573.

389. RUSMAH, M. Talon cusp in Malaysia. Aust Dent J 1991; 36: 11–14.

390. RUSHTON MA. Effects of radium on the dentition. Am J Orthod Oral Surg 1947; 33: 828–30.

391. RUSHTON MA. Unilateral hyperplasia of the jaws in the young. Int Dent J 1951; 2: 41–67.

392. RUSHTON MA. Invaginated teeth (dens in dente): contents of the invagination. Oral Surg 1958; 11: 1378–87.

393. SABALA CL *et al*. Bilateral root or root canal aberrations in a dental school population. J Endod 1994; 20: 38–42.

394. SALAMA FS *et al*. Talon cusp: a review and two case reports on supernumerary primary and permanent teeth. ASDC J Dent Child 1990; 57: 147–9.

395. SALEM G. Prevalence of selected dental anomalies in Saudi Children from Gizan region. Community Dent Oral Epidemiol 1989; 17: 162–3.

396. SARR M et al. Taurodontism and pyramidal tooth at the level of the molars. Prevalence in the Senegalese population 15 to 19 years of age. Odontostomatol Trop 2000; 23: 31–4.

397. SAUK JJ et al. Taurodontism, diminished root formation, and microcephalic dwarfism. Oral Surg 1973; 36: 231–5.

398. SCHALK-VAN DER WEIDE Y. Oligodontia. A clinical, radiographic and genetic evaluation. Thesis, University of Nijmegen, 1992.

399. SCHALK-VAN DER WEIDE Y et al. Taurodontism and length of teeth in patients with oligodontia. J Oral Rehabil 1993; 20: 401–12.

400. SCHROEDER HE. Pathobiologie oraler Strukturen. Basel: Karger, 1983.

401. SCHULZE C. Developmental abnormalities of the teeth and jaws. In: GORLIN RJ, GOLDMAN HM (eds) Thoma's oral pathology. St Louis, MO: CV Mosby, 1970.

402. SCHULZE C. Anomalien und Missbildungen der menschlichen Zähne. Berlin: Quintessenz Verlags–GmbH, 1987.

403. SCIULLI PW et al. Canine size: an aid in sexing prehistoric Amerindians. J Dent Res 1977; 56: 1424.

404. SEDANO HO et al. Clinical orodental abnormalities in Mexican children. Oral Surg Oral Med Oral Pathol 1989; 68: 300–11.

405. SEGURA JJ et al. A. Talon cusp affecting permanent maxillary lateral incisors in 2 family members. Oral Surg Oral Pathol Oral Med Oral Radiol Endod 1999; 88: 90–2.

406. SEGURA-EGEA JJ et al. Dens evaginatus of anterior teeth (talon cusp). Quint Int 2003; 34: 272–7.

407. SEGURA-EGEA JJ et al. Talon cusp causing occlusal trauma and acute periodontitis. Dent Traumatol 2003; 19: 55–9.

408. SEOW WK et al. Association of taurodontism with hypodontia: a controlled study. Pediatr Dent 1989; 11: 214–19.

409. SEOW WK et al. A controlled study of the morphometric changes in the primary dentition of pre-term, very-low-birthweight children. J Dent Res 2000; 79: 63–9.

410. SERMAN NJ et al. The radiographic incidence of multiple roots and canals in human mandibular premolars. Int Endod J 1992; 25: 234–7.

411. SERT S et al. Taurodontism in six molars. J Endod 2004; 30: 601–2.

412. SHAFER WG et al. A textbook of oral pathology. Philadelphia, PA: WB Saunders, 1983.

413. SHAPIRA Y et al. Multiple-rooted mandibular second premolars. J Endod 1982; 8: 231–2.

414. SHARMA K et al. Genetic basis of dental occlusal variations in Northwest Indian twins. Europ J Orthod 1986; 8: 91–7.

415. SHARMA K et al. Genetic variance in dental dimensions of Punjabi twins. J Dent Res 1985; 64: 1389–91.

416. SHAW L. Short root anomaly in a patient with severe short-limbed dwarfism. Int J Paediatr Dent 1995; 5: 249–52.

417. SHAW L et al. Size and development of the dentition in endocrine deficiency. J Pedod 1989; 13: 155–60.

418. SHEY Z et al. Clinical management of an unusual case of dens evaginatus in a maxillary central incisor. J Am Dent Assoc 1983; 106: 346–8.

419. SHIELDS ED et al. Odontometric variation among American black, European, and Mongoloid populations. J Craniofac Genet 1990; 10: 7–18.

420. SHIFMAN A et al. Prevalence of taurodontism found in radiographic dental examination of 1,200 young adult Israeli patients. Community Dent Oral Epidemiol 1978; 6: 200–3.

421. SIM TPC. Management of dens invaginatus: evaluation of two prophylactic treatment methods. Endod Dent Traumatol 1996; 12: 137–40.

422. SKINNER MA et al. The role of enamel pearls in localized severe periodontitis. Quint Int 1989; 20: 181–3.

423. SMITH DMH et al. Root dilaceration of maxillary incisors. Br Dent J 1981; 150: 125–7.

424. SMITH S et al. An unusual oral complication of herpes zoster infection. Oral Surg 1984; 57: 388–9.

425. SOAMES JV et al. A radicular dens invaginatus. Br Dent J 1982; 152: 308–9.

426. SOFAER JA et al. A developmental basis for differential tooth reduction during hominid evolution. Evolution 1971; 25: 509–17.

427. SOFAER JA et al. Developmental interaction, size and agenesis among permanent maxillary incisors. Hum Biol 1971; 43: 36–45.

428. SOMOGYI-CSIZMAZIA W et al. Three-rooted mandibular first permanent molars in Alberta Indian children. J Can Dent Assoc 1971; 37: 105–6.

429. SPERBER GH et al. Study of the number of roots and canals in Senegalese first permanent mandibular molars. Int Endod J 1998; 31: 117–22.

430. STECKER S et al. Dens evaginatus: a diagnostic and treatment challenge. J Am Dent Assoc 2002; 133: 190–3.

431. STEELE-PERKINS G et al. Essential role for NFI-C/CTF transcription-replication factor in tooth root development. Mol Cell Biol 2003; 23: 1075–84.

432. STEELMAN R. Incidence of an accessory distal root on mandibular first permanent molars in Hispanic children. ASDC J Dent Child 1986; 53: 122–3.

433. STEINBERG AG et al. Hereditary generalized microdontia. J Dent Res 1961; 40: 58–62.

434. STENVIK A et al. Taurodontism and concomitant hypodontia in siblings. Oral Surg 1972; 33: 841–5.

435. STEWART DJ. Dilacerated unerupted maxillary central incisors. Br Dent J 1978; 145: 229–33.

436. STEWART RE. Taurodontism in X-chromosome aneuploid syndromes. Clin Genet 1974; 6: 341–4.

437. STEWART RE et al. Dens evaginatus (tuberculated cusps): genetic and treatment considerations. Oral Surg 1978; 46: 831–6.

438. SUCHINA JA et al. Dens invaginatus of a maxillary lateral incisor: endodontic treatment. Oral Surg Oral Med Oral Pathol 1989; 68: 467–71.

439. SUNDE OE et al. Dental changes in a patient with hypoparathyroidism. Br Dent J 1961; 111: 112–17.

440. SUTALO J *et al.* Häufigkeit von Schmelzformationen an Wurzeln bleibender Zähne. Schweiz Monatschr Zahnmed 1989; 99: 174–80.

441. SUZUKI M *et al.* Shovel-shaped incisors among the living Polynesians. Am J Phys Anthropol 1964; 22: 65–72.

442. SWAN RH *et al.* Cervical enamel projections as an etiologic factor in furcation involvement. J Am Dent Assoc 1976; 93: 342–5.

443. SYKARAS SN. A two-rooted maxillary lateral incisor. Oral Surg 1972; 34: 349.

444. SYKARAS SN. Occlusal anomalous tubercle on premolars of a Greek girl. Oral Surg 1974; 38: 88–91.

445. TAGGER M. Nonsurgical endodontic therapy of tooth invagination. Oral Surg 1977; 43: 124–9.

446. TAKEDA Y *et al.* Failure of root development of human permanent teeth following irradiation. Int J Oral Maxillofac Surg 1987; 16: 376–82.

447. TAKINAMI S *et al.* Radiation-induced hypoplasia of the teeth and mandible. Oral Surg Oral Med Oral Pathol 1994; 78: 382–4.

448. TALOUMIS LJ, NISHIMURA RS. Treatment of an unusual instance of fusion with a talon cusp. Gen Dent 1989; 37: 208–10.

449. TAN JL *et al.* Dens invaginatus: three clinical presentations of dens invaginatus in children. ASDC J Dent Child 1994; 61: 330–3.

450. TARJÁN I *et al.* Endodontic treatment of immature tooth with dens invaginatus. Int J Paediatr Dent 1999; 9: 53–6.

451. TAYLOR GN *et al.* Extraradicular communicating dens invaginatus. Oral Surg 1977; 44: 931–8.

452. TAYLOR RMS. Aberrant maxillary third molars. Morphology and developmental relations. In: KURTÉN B (ed.) Teeth: form function, evolution. New York, NY: Columbia University Press, 1982.

453. TENNANT RD. Taurodontism. Dent Dig 1966; 72: 355–7.

454. THEWS ME *et al.* Aberrations in palatal root and root canal morphology of two maxillary first molars. J Endod 1979; 5: 94–6.

455. THODEN VAN VELZEN SK *et al.* Endodontologie. Alphen aan den Rijn: Stafleu & Tholen BV 1995.

456. THODEN VAN VELZEN SK *et al.* Een zeldzame combinatie van dens invaginatus en mesiodens. Ned Tijdschr Tandheelkd 1973; 80: 244–6.

457. THOMAS CJ *et al.* The Carabelli trait in the mixed deciduous and permanent dentitions of five south African populations. Arch Oral Biol 1986; 31: 145–7.

458. THOMAS JG. A study of dens in dente. Oral Surg 1974; 38: 653–5.

459. THORNBURN DN *et al.* Familial ogee roots, tooth mobility, oligodontia, and microdontia. Oral Surg Oral Med Oral Pathol 1992; 74: 576–81.

460. TOURE B *et al.* Prevalence du taurodontism au niveau molaire chez les Senegalais melanoderme age de 15 a 19 ans. Odonto Stomatol Trop 2000, 89: 36–9.

461. TOWNSEND G *et al.* Tooth size in 47,XYY males: evidence for a direct effect of the Y chromosome on growth. Aust Dent J 1985; 30: 268–72.

462. TOWNSEND GC *et al.* Heritability of permanent tooth size. Am J Phys Anthropol 1978; 49: 497–504.

463. TOWNSEND GC *et al.* Family studies of tooth size factors in the permanent dentition. Am J Phys Anthropol 1979; 50: 183–90.

464. TOWNSEND GC *et al.* Fitting genetic models to Carabelli trait data in south Australian twins. J Dent Res 1992; 71: 403–9.

465. TSAI SJJ *et al.* A catalogue of anomalies and traits of the permanent dentition of southern Chinese. J Clin Pediatr Dent 1998; 22: 185–94.

466. TSATSAS B *et al.* Cervical enamel projections in the molar teeth. J Periodontol 1973; 44: 312–14.

467. TSE CSM *et al.* Endodontic treatment of a canine with a talon cusp. Endod Dent Traumatol 1988; 4: 235–7.

468. TSESIS I *et al.* Taurodontism: an endodontic challenge. J Endod 2003; 29: 353–5.

469. TSURUMACHI T *et al.* Non-surgical root canal treatment of dens invaginatus type 2 in maxillary lateral incisor. Int Endod J 2002; 35: 310–14.

470. TSUTSUMI T *et al.* Labial talon cusp in a child with incontinentia pigmenti achromians. Pediatr Dent 1991; 13: 236–7.

471. TÜRKER M *et al.* Early pulpal involvement in an unusual case of dens in dente. Aust Dent J 1993; 38: 439–41.

472. TURNER CG II. Three-rooted mandibular first permanent molars and the question of American Indian origins. Am J Phys Anthropol 1971; 34: 229–41.

473. TÜZÜM MS *et al.* Multiple bilateral dens invaginatus and an impacted cuspid in the maxillary region. Aust Dent J 1990; 35: 128–9.

474. UBIOS AM *et al.* Mandibular growth and tooth eruption after localized X-radiation. J Oral Maxillofac Surg 1992; 50: 153–6.

475. UFOMATA D. Microdontia of a mandibular second premolar. Oral Surg Oral Med Oral Pathol 1988; 65: 637–8.

476. ULMANSKY M *et al.* Double dens in dente in a single tooth. Oral Surg 1964; 17: 92–7.

477. UNEOKA M. Pyramidal molars. Oral Surg 1985; 59: 433.

478. VARRELA J. Root morphology of mandibular premolars in human 45,X females. Arch Oral Biol 1990; 35: 109–12.

479. VARRELA J. Effect of 45,X/46,XX mosaicism on root morphology of mandibular premolars. J Dent Res 1992; 71: 1604–6.

480. VERTUCCI FJ *et al.* Root canal morphology of the maxillary first premolar. J Am Dent Assoc 1979; 99: 194–8.

481. VIRE DE. Two-rooted maxillary lateral incisor. Oral Surg 1985; 59: 321.

482. VISSER JB. Beitrag zur Kenntnis der menschlichen Zahnwurzelformen. Thesis, University Zürich, 1948.

483. VON ARX T. Developmental disturbances of permanent teeth following trauma to the primary dentition. Aust Dent J 1993; 38: 1–10.

484. VON ARX T. Milchzahnintrusionen und Odontogenese der bleibende Zähne. Schweiz Monatschr Zahnmed 1995; 105: 11–17.

485. WALKER RT. Root form and canal anatomy of mandibular second molars in a southern Chinese population. J Endod 1988; 14: 325–9.

486. WALKER RT *et al.* The palato-gingival groove and pulpitis. Int Endod J 1983; 16: 33–4.
487. WALKER RT *et al.* Three-rooted lower first permanent molars in Hong Kong Chinese. Br Dent J 1985; 159: 298–9.
488. WANG JC *et al.* Cervical projection and bifurcational ridge correlating with furcation involvement. J Dent Res 1996; 75: 212.
489. WARREN EM *et al.* The relationship between crown size and the incidence of bifid root canals in mandibular incisor teeth. Oral Surg 1981; 52: 425–9.
490. WEISZ AS. Dens in dente. Oral Surg Oral Med Oral Pathol 1988; 65: 264.
491. WEYMAN J. The effect of irradiation on developing teeth. Oral Surg 1968; 25: 623–9.
492. WINKLER MP *et al.* Multirooted anomalies in the primary dentition of native Americans. J Am Dent Assoc 1997; 128: 1009–11.
493. WINTER GB. Hereditary and idiopathic anomalies of tooth number, structure and form. Dent Clin North Am 1969; 13 (2): 355–73.
494. WITHERS JA *et al.* The relationship between palato-gingival grooves to periodontal disease. J Periodontol 1981; 52: 41–4.
495. WITKOP CJ. Manifestations of genetic diseases in the human pulp. Oral Surg 1971; 32: 278–316.
496. WITKOP CJ. Hereditary defects of dentin. Dent Clin North Am 1975; 19 (1): 25–45.
497. WITKOP CJ *et al.* Teeth with short, thin, dilacerated roots in patients with short stature: a dominantly inherited trait. Oral Surg 1982; 54: 553–9.
498. WOELFEL JB. Dental anatomy: its correlation with Dental Health Service. Philadelphia, PA: Lea & Febiger, 1984.
499. WONG MT *et al.* Management of dens in dente. Gen Dent 1992; 40: 300–3.
500. WORLD HEALTH ORGANIZATION. Fluorides and human health. Geneva: World Health Organization, 1970.
501. YAMAOKA M *et al.* Relationship between third molar development and root angulation. J Oral Rehabil 2001; 28: 198–205.
502. YANG ZP *et al.* The root and root canal anatomy of maxillary molars in a Chinese population. Endod Dent Traumatol 1988; 4: 215–18.
503. YEH SC *et al.* Dens invaginatus in the maxillary lateral incisor: treatment of 3 cases. Oral Surg Oral Med Oral Pathol Oral Radiol Endod 1999; 87: 628–31.
504. YIP WK. The prevalence of dens evaginatus. Oral Surg 1974; 38: 80–7.
505. YODA T *et al.* Multiple macrodonts with odontoma in a mother and son – a variant of Ekman-Westborg-Julin syndrome. Report of a case. Oral Surg Oral Med Oral Pathol Oral Radiol Endod 1998; 85: 301–3.
506. ZEE KY *et al.* Prevalence of cervical enamel projection and its correlation with furcation involvement in Eskimos dry skulls. Swed Dent J 2003; 27: 43–8.
507. ZEE KY *et al.* Cervical enamel projections in Chinese first permanent molars. Aust Dent J 1991; 36: 356–60.
508. ZHU JF *et al.* Talon cusp with associated adjacent supernumerary tooth. Gen Dent 1997; 45: 178–81.
509. ZILLICH RM *et al.* Maxillary lateral incisor with two roots and dens formation. J Endod 1983; 9: 143–4.
510. JAFARZADEH H *et al.* Dilaceration. J Endod 2007; 33: 1025–30.
511. MALCIC A *et al.* Prevalence of root dilacerations in adult Patients in Croatia. Oral Surg Oral Med Oraql Pathol Oral Radiol Endod 2006; 102: 104–9.
512. KAZUO E *et al.* Rare associations of dens invaginatus and Mesiodens. Oral Surg Oral Med Oral Pathol Oral Radiol Endod 2007; 104: e41–4.
513. SCHWARTZ SA *et al.* Combined endodontic-periodontal treatment of a palatal groove. J Endod 2006; 32: 573–8.
514. EZODDINI AF *et al.* Prevalence of dental developmental anomalies. Community Dent Health 2007; 24: 140–4.
515. HARILA-KAERA V *et al.* Permanent tooth crown dimensions in prematurely born children. Early Hum Dev 2001; 62: 131–47.
516. ALTUG-ATAC AT *et al.* Prevalence and distribution of dental anomalies in orthodontic patients. Am J Orthod Dentofac Orthop 2007; 131: 510–14.
517. HAZZA'A AM *et al.* Radiographic features of the jaws and teeth in thalassaemia major. Dentomaxillofac Radiol 2006; 35: 283–8.
518. LEVITAN ME *et al.* Dens evaginatus. J Endod 2006; 32: 1–9.
519. CHO SY *et al.* Concomitant developmental an anomalies in Chinese children with dens evaginatus. Int J Paediatr Dent 2006; 16: 247–51.
520. MAVRODISZ K *et al.* Prevalence of accessory tooth cusps in a contemporary and ancestral Hungarian population. Eur J Orthod 2007; 29: 166–9.
521. Lopes NN *et al.* Dental abnormalities in children submitted to antineoplastic therapy. ASDC J Dent Child 2006; 73: 140–5.

Chapter 3: Developmental Structural Anomalies of Enamel and Dentine

1. AASENDEN R *et al.* Effects of fluoride supplementation from birth on human deciduous and permanent teeth. Arch Oral Biol 1974; 19: 321–6.
2. AASENDEN R *et al.* Effects of fluoride supplementation from birth on dental caries and fluorosis in teenaged children. Arch Oral Biol 1978; 23: 111–15.
3. ABE K *et al.* The occurrence of interglobular dentin in incisors of hypophosphatemic mice fed a high-calcium and high-phosphate diet. J Dent Res 1992; 71: 478–83.
4. ABE K *et al.* Structural deformities of deciduous teeth in patients with hypophosphatemic vitamin D-resistent rickets. Oral Surg Oral Pathol Oral Med 1988; 65: 191–8.
5. ABRAMS AM *et al.* Odontodysplasia. ASDC J Dent Child 1966; 33: 353–62.
6. ACIL Y *et al.* Detection of mature collagen in human dental enamel. Calcif Tissue Int 2004; 76 (2): 121–6.
7. ADVIESCOLLEGE PREVENTIE MOND and TANDZIEKTEN. Consequenties toename gebruik fluoride. Ned Tijdschr Mondhyg 1981; 5: 9–11.

8. AGUIRRE JM *et al*. Dental enamel defects in celiac patients. Oral Surg Oral Med Oral Pathol Radiol Endod 1997; 84: 646–50.

9. AINE L. Coeliac-type permanent-tooth enamel defects. Ann Med 1996; 28: 9–12.

10. AINE L *et al*. Enamel defects in primary and permanent teeth of children born prematurely. J Oral Pathol Med 2000; 29: 403–9.

11. AINE L *et al*. Dental enamel defects in celiac disease. J Oral Pathol Med 1990; 19: 241–5.

12. AKPATA ES *et al*. Dental fluorosis in 12–15-year-old rural children exposed to fluorides from well drinking water in the Hail region of Saudi Arabia. Community Dent Oral Epidemiol 1997; 25: 324–7.

13. ALALUUSUA S *et al*. Developmental dental aberrations after the dioxin accident in Seveso. Environ Health Perspect 2004; 112: 1313–18.

14. ALALUUSUA S *et al*. Developing teeth as biomarker of dioxin exposure. Lancet 1999; 353: 206.

15. ALALUUSUA S *et al*. Developmental dental defects associated with long breast feeding. Eur J Oral Sci 1996; 104: 493–7.

16. ALDRED MJ. Unusual dentinal changes in dentinogenesis imperfecta associated with osteogenesis imperfecta. Oral Surg Oral Med Oral Pathol 1992; 73: 461–4.

17. ALDRED MJ *et al*. Variable expression in amelogenesis imperfecta with taurodontia. J Oral Pathol 1988; 17: 327–33.

18. ALDRED MJ *et al*. Genetic heterogeneity in X-linked amelogenesis imperfecta. Genomics 1992; 567–73.

19. ALDRED MJ *et al*. Amelogenesis imperfecta – towards a new classification. Oral Dis 1995; 1: 2–5.

20. ALDRED MJ *et al*. Clinical and radiographic features of a family with autosomal dominant amleogenesis imperfecta with taurodontism. Oral Dis 2002; 8: 62–8.

21. ALDRED MJ *et al*. Amelogenesis imperfecta: a classification and catalogue for the 21ar century. Oral Dis 2003; 9: 19–23.

22. AL-ALOUSI W *et al*. Enamel mottling in a fluoride and in a non-fluoride community. Br Dent J 1975; 138: 9–15 and 56–60.

23. ALEXANDER SA. The treatment of hypocalcified amelogenesis imperfecta in a young adolescent. J Pedod 1984; 9: 95–100.

24. ALEXANDER WN. Composite dysplasia of a single tooth as a result of electric burn damage. J Am Dent Ass 1964; 69: 589–91.

25. ALEXANDER WN *et al*. Odontodysplasia. Oral Surg 1966; 22: 814–20.

26. ALLEY TR *et al*. Hereditary opalescent dentine. Oral Surg 1953; 6: 328–34.

27. ALLMARK C *et al*. A community study of fluoride tablets for school children in Portsmouth. Br Dent J 1982; 153: 426–30.

28. ALmquist AL. Aplasia of the crown of the tooth: hereditary hypoplasia of the enamel. J Am Dent Assoc 1944; 31.

29. AL-SHAWI A. Experience in the treatment of missile injuries of the maxillofacial region in Iraq. Br J Oral Maxillofac Surg 1986; 24: 244–50.

30. ANATOLIOTAKI M *et al*. Congenital rickets due to maternal vitamin D deficiency in a sunny island of Greece. Acta Paediatr 2003; 92: 389–91.

31. ANDERSEN L *et al*. Parathyroid glands, calcium, and vitamin D in experimental fluorosis in pigs. Calcif Tissue Int 1986; 38: 222–6.

32. ANDREASEN JO *et al*. Textbook and color atlas of traumatic injuries to the teeth. Copenhagen: Munksgaard, 1994.

33. ANDREASEN JO *et al*. The effect of traumatic injuries to the primary teeth on their permanent successors – II. Scand J Dent Res 1971; 79: 283–94.

34. ANDREASEN JO *et al*. Traumatic injuries to the teeth. Copenhagen, Munksgaard, 1981.

35. ANDREASEN JO *et al*. The effect of traumatic injuries to primary teeth on their permanent successors. I. Scand J Dent Res 1971; 79: 219–83.

36. ANDREASEN JO *et al*. Enamel changes in permanent teeth after trauma to their primary predecessors. Scand J Dent Res 1973; 81: 203–9.

37. ANGELILLO IF *et al*. Prevalence of dental caries and enamel defects in children living in areas with different water fluoride concentrations. Community Dent Health 1990; 7: 229–36.

38. ANGELILLO IF *et al*. Caries and fluorosis prevalence in communities with different concentrations of fluoride in the water. Caries Res 1999; 33: 114–22.

39. ANGELOS GM *et al*. Oral complications associated with neonatal oral tracheal intubation: a critical review. Pediatr Dent 1989; 11: 133–9.

40. ANGMAR-MÅNSSON B *et al*. Plasma fluoride and enamel fluorosis. Calcif Tissue Res 1976; 22: 77–84.

41. ANGMAR-MÅNSSON B *et al*. Single fluoride doses and enamel fluorosis in the rat. Caries Res 1985; 19: 145–52.

42. ANONYMUS. Overzicht tandpasta's. NVM Tijdschrift 1995; 19: 84–93.

43. ANSARI G *et al*. Dentinal dysplasia type I. ASDC J Dent Child 1997; 64: 429–34.

44. ANTALOVSKÁ Z *et al*. Disturbances of dentine mineralization following oral administration of tetracycline. Oral Surg 1966; 22: 803–10.

45. AOBA T *et al*. Dental fluorosis: chemistry and biology. Crit Rev Oral Biol Med 2002; 13: 155–70.

46. APONTE-MERCED L *et al*. Pre-eruptive protein-energy malnutrition and acid solubility of rat molar enamel surfaces. Arch Oral Biol 1980; 25: 701–5.

47. APPLEBAUM E *et al*. Discoloration of the teeth in patients with cystic fibrosis of the pancreas. Oral Surg 1964; 17: 366–7.

48. ARCHARD HO. The dental defects of vitamin D-resistant rickets. Birth Defects Orig Artic Ser 1971; 7: 196–9.

49. ARCHARD HO *et al*. Hereditary hypophosphatemia (vitamin D-resistant rickets) presenting primary dental manifestations. Oral Surg 1966; 22: 184–93.

50. ARKLE PW. Prevalence of enamel opacities and hypoplasia in the permanent teeth of schoolchildren. J Dent Res 1962; 41: 511–12.

51. ARMSTRONG C *et al*. Histopathology of the teeth in segmental odontomaxillary dysplasia: new findings. J Oral Pathol Med 2004; 33: 246–8.

52. ARMSTRONG WD *et al.* Placental transfer of fluoride and calcium. Am J Obstet Gynec 1970; 107: 432–4.

53. ARQUITT CK *et al.* Cystic fibrosis transmembrane regulator gene (CFTR) is associated with abnormal enamel formation. J Dent Res 2002; 81: 492–6.

54. AST DB *et al.* Newburgh–Kingston caries-fluoride study XIV. Combined clinical and roentgenographic dental findings after 10 years of fluoride experience. J Am Dent Assoc 1956; 52: 314–25.

55. ATASU M *et al.* Hypocalcification type amelogenesis imperfecta in permanent dentition in association with heavily worn primary teeth, gingival hyperplasia, hypodontia and impacted teeth. J Clin Pediatr Dent 1999; 23: 117–21.

56. ATASU M *et al.* Enamel hypoplasia and essential staining of teeth from erythroblastosis fetalis. J Clin Pediatr Dent 1998; 22: 249–52.

57. AWADIA AK *et al.* An attempt to explain why Tanzanian children drinking water containing 0.2 or 3.6 mg fluoride per liter exhibit a similar level of dental fluorosis. Clin Oral Invest 2000; 4: 238–44.

58. AXRUP K *et al.* Children with thalidomide embryopathy: odontological observations and aspects. Acta Odontol Scand 1966; 24: 3–21.

59. BACKER DIRKS O. Fluoriden voor tandheelkundig gebruik. Geneesmiddelenbulletin 1982; 16 (14): 61–6 and 10.

60. BACKER DIRKS O *et al.* Dental and medical aspects in high fluoride area. Caries Res 1976; 10: 135.

61. BACKER DIRKS O *et al.* Total and free ionic fluoride in human and cow's milk as determined by gas-liquid chromatography and the fluoride electrode. Caries Res 1974; 8: 181–6.

62. BACKER DIRKS O. Fluoride. In: HOUWINK B (ed.) Preventieve tandheelkunde. Alphen aan den Rijn: Samson Stafleu, 1984.

63. BÄCKMAN B. Amelogenesis imperfecta. Scand J Dent Res 1988; 96: 505–16.

64. BÄCKMAN B. Inherited enamel defects. In: CIBA FOUNDATION (ed.) Dental enamel. Chichester: John Wiley & Sons, 1997.

65. BÄCKMAN B *et al.* Mineral distribution in the enamel of teeth with amelogenesis imperfecta as determined by quantitative microradiography. J Dent Res 1994; 102: 193–7.

66. BÄCKMAN B *et al.* Microradiographic study of amelogenesis imperfecta. Scand J Dent Res 1989; 97: 316–29.

67. BÄCKMAN B *et al.* Amelogenesis imperfecta. J Oral Pathol Med 1989; 18: 140–5.

68. BÄCKMAN B *et al.* Amelogenesis imperfecta: prevalence and incidence in a northern Swedish county. Community Dent Oral Epidemiol 1986; 14: 43–7.

69. BÄCKMAN B *et al.* The absence of correlations between a clinical classification and ultrastructural findings in amelogenesis imperfecta. Acta Odontol Scand 1993: 51: 79–89.

70. BADGER GR. Incidence of enamel hypoplasia in primary canines. ASDC J Dent Child 1985; 52: 57–8.

71. BAELUM V *et al.* Posteruptive tooth age and severity of dental fluorosis in Kenya. Scand J Dent Res 1986; 94: 405–10.

72. BAKA'EEN G *et al.* Dentinal dysplasia type I. ASDC J Dent Child 1985; 52: 128–9.

73. BAKER KL. Tetracycline-induced tooth changes. Part 5. Med J Aust 1975; 2: 301–4.

74. BALL SP *et al.* Linkage between dentinogenesis imperfecta and Gc. Ann Hum Genet 1982; 46: 35–40.

75. BARDSEN A. "Risk periods" associated with the development of dental fluorosis in maxillary permanent central incisors: a meta-analysis. Acta Odontol Scand 1999; 57: 247–56.

76. BARNHART WE *et al.* Dentifrice usage and ingestion among four age groups. J Dent Res 1974; 53: 1317–22.

77. BARTA JE *et al.* ABO blood group incompatibility and primary tooth discoloration. Pediatr Dent 1989; 11: 316–18.

78. BASU K *et al.* A new look on neonatal jaundice. J Indian Med 2002; 100: 556–60, 574.

79. BATTAGEL JM *et al.* Dentinogenesis imperfecta: an interdisciplinary approach. Brit Dent J 1988; 165: 329–331.

80. BAUER W. Zur Entstehung der rachitischen Schmelzhypoplasien. Vierteljschr Zahnheilkd 1929; 45: 62–79.

81. BAUMANN MA. Neue morphologische Erkenntnisse zur Dentinogenesis imperfecta typ II. Dtsch Zahnärztl Z 1992; 47: 377–380.

82. BAUME LJ *et al.* The effect of thyroid hormone on dental and paradental structures. Parodontologie 1952; 6: 87–106.

83. BAUME LJ *et al.* Hormonal control of tooth eruption – II. J Dent Res 1954; 33: 91–103.

84. BAWDEN JW *et al.* The effects of parathyroid hormone, calcitonin, and vitamin D metabolites on calcium transport in the secretory rat enamel organ. J Dent Res 1983; 62: 952–5.

85. BAWDEN JW *et al.* Fluoride uptake in hard tissues of fetal Guinea pigs in response to various dose regimens. Arch Oral Biol 1992; 37: 929–33.

86. BAXTER PT *et al.* Prolonged use of doxycycline in patients with small asymptomatic abdominal aortic aneurysms. J Vasc Surg 2002; 36: 1–12.

87. BAXTER PM. Toothpaste ingestion during toothbrushing by school children. Br Dent J 1980; 148: 125–8.

88. BAYLESS JM *et al.* Diagnosis and treatment of acute fluoride toxicity. J Am Dent Assoc 1985; 110: 209–11.

89. BECK DJ. The epidemiology of dental caries. In: COHEN B *et al.* (eds) Scientific foundations of dentistry. London: William Heinemann Medical Books, 1976.

90. BECKS H. Histologic study of tooth structure in osteogenesis imperfecta. Dent Cosmos 1931; 73: 437–54.

91. BECKTOR KB *et al.* Segmental odontomaxillary dysplasia. Oral Dis 2002; 8: 106–10.

92. BEENTJES VE *et al.* Factoren die een rol kunnen spelen bij het ontstaan van kaasmolaren. Ned Tijdschr Tandheelkd 2002; 109: 387–90.

93. BELTRAN ED *et al.* Fluoride in toothpastes for children: suggestion for a change. Pediatr Dent 1988; 10: 185–8.

94. BENUSIS KP *et al.* Enamel hypoplasia in children with galactosemia associated with periods of poor control. ASDC J Dent Child 1978; 45: 73–5.

95. BEN-BASSAT Y *et al.* Effect of trauma to the primary incisors on permanent successors in different developmental stages. Pediatr Dent 1985; 7: 37–40.

96. BEN-BASSAT Y *et al.* Effects of trauma to he primary incisors on their permanent successors: multidisciplinary treatment. ASDC J Dent Child 1989; 56: 112–16.

97. BERGMAN G *et al.* Studies on mineralized dental tissues – VIII. Histologic and microradiographic investigation of hereditary opalescent dentine. Acta Odontol Scand 1956; 14: 103–17.

98. BERGMAN G *et al.* Unilateral dental malformation. Oral Surg 1963; 16: 48–60.

99. BERNARD WV. Roentgenographic and histologic differentiation of dentinogenesis imperfecta and dentinal dysplasia. J Dent Res 1960; 39: 674–5.

100. BERNSTEIN ML *et al.* Oral lesion in a patient with calcinosis and arthritis. J Oral Pathol 1985; 14: 8–14.

101. BEVELANDER G, *et al.* The effect of the administration of tetracycline on the development of teeth. J Dent Res 1961; 40: 1020–24.

102. BHATT M *et al.* Developmental enamel defects in primary teeth in children with cerebral palsy, mental retardation, or hearing defects: a review. Adv Dent Res 1989; 3: 132–42.

103. BHATT M *et al.* Lack of stability in enamel defects in primary teeth of children with cerebral palsy or mental retardation. Pediatr Dent 1989; 11: 118–20.

104. BIERI JG. The role of vitamin E in clinical medicine. ASDC J Dent Child 1984; 51: 133–6.

105. BIREK C. Herpesvirus-induced diseases. Cal Dent Assoc J 2000; 28: 911–17.

106. BISCHOFF JI *et al.* Relationship between fluoride concentration in enamel, DMFT index and degree of fluorosis in a community in an area with a high level of fluoride. J Dent Res 1976; 55: 37–42.

107. BIXLER D. Heritable disorders affecting dentin. In: STEWART RE *et al.* (eds) Oral facial genetics. St Louis, MO: CV Mosby, 1976.

108. BIXLER D. Developmental abnormalities of dentin. In: STEWART RE *et al.* (eds) Pediatric dentistry. St Louis, MO: CV Mosby, 1982, pp. 117–29.

109. BIXLER D *et al.* Dentinogenesis imperfecta. J Dent Res 1969; 48: 1196–9.

110. BJORVATN K. Antibiotic compounds and enamel demineralization. Acta Odontol Scand 1982; 40: 341–52.

111. BJORVATN K. In vitro study by fluorescence microscopy and microradiography of tetracycline-tooth interaction. Scand J Dent Res 1983; 91: 417–24.

112. BJORVATN K *et al.* The effect of penicillin – and tetracycline – containing medicaments on the microhardness of human dental enamel. Acta Odontol Scand 1982; 40: 299–305.

113. BLACHARSH C. Dental aspects of patients with cystic fibrosis: a preliminary clinical study. J Am Dent Assoc 1977; 95: 106–10.

114. BLINKHORN AS. Influence of social norms on toothbrushing behavior of children. Community Dent Oral Epidemiol 1978; 6: 222–6.

115. BOHATY BS *et al.* The prevalence of fluorosis-like lesions associated with topical and systemic fluoride usage in an area of optimal water fluoridation. Pediatr Dent 1989; 11: 125–8.

116. BONUCCI E *et al.* Morphological studies of hypomineralized enamel of rat pups on calcium-deficient diet, and of its changes after return to normal diet. Anat Rec 1996; 239: 379–95.

117. BOSSENS M. Antibiotics and pregnancy. Rev Med Brux 2001; 22: A206–3.

118. BOUYSSOU M *et al.* Sur une nouvelle dysembryoplasie systématisée: les "dents fantomes" (ghost teeth). Acta Odontologiques 1966; 75: 307–26.

119. BOUVIER D *et al.* Rehabilitation of young patients with amelogenesis imperfecta. ASDC J Dent Child 1996; 63: 443–7.

120. BOUVIER D *et al.* Amelogenesis imperfecta – a prosthetic rehabilitation. J Prosthet Dent 1999; 82: 130–1.

121. BOYDE A. Enamel structure and cavity margins. Oper Dent 1976; 1: 13–28.

122. BRADLAW RV. The dental stigmata of prenatal syphilis. Oral Surg 1953; 6 (I): 147–58.

123. BRAS J *et al.* Radiographic interpretation of the mandibular angular cortex: a diagnostic tool in metabolic bone loss. Part II. Oral Surg 1982; 53: 647–50.

124. BREARLY LJ *et al.* Characteristics and caries experience of tetracycline-affected dentitions. J Dent Res 1973; 52: 508–16.

125. BREARLY LJ *et al.* Tetracycline-induced tooth changes: part I. Med J Aust 1968; 653–8.

126. BREEN GH. Prophylactic dental treatment for a patient with vitamin D-resistant rickets. ASDC J Dent Child 1986; 53: 38–43.

127. BRENNEISE CV *et al.* Dentin dysplasia, type II. Oral Surg Oral Med Oral Pathol Oral Radiol Endod 1999; 87: 752–5.

128. BRENNEISE CV *et al.* Clinical, radiographic, and histological manifestations of dentin dysplasia, type I. J Am Dent Assoc 1989; 119: 721–3.

129. BRIN I *et al.* Trauma to the primary incisors and its effect on the permanent successors. Pediatr Dent 1984; 6: 78–82.

130. BRITISH DENTAL ASSOCIATION. Fluoride supplement dosage. Br Dent J 1997; 182: 6–7.

131. BRONCKERS ALJJ *et al.* Histological and biochemical studies of vitamin C requirements of hamster molars during development in vitro. J Biol Buccale 1982; 10: 263–9.

132. BROOK AH. Dentine dysplasia. Shields type I. ASDC J Dent Child 1984; 51: 52.

133. BROOKES SJ *et al.* Biochemistry and molecular biology of amelogenin proteins of developing dental enamel. Arch Oral Biol 1995; 40: 1–14.

134. BROOKRESON KR *et al.* Dentinal dysplasia. J Am Dent Assoc 1968; 77: 608–11.

135. BROWN EM *et al.* Calcium-receptor-regulated parathyroid and renal function. Bone 1997; 20: 303–9.

136. BRUDEVOLD F *et al*. Dental fluorosis as related to the concentration of fluoride in teeth and bone. J Am Dent Assoc 1978; 96: 459–63.

137. BURKES EJ *et al*. Dentin dysplasia II. J Endod 1979; 5: 277–81.

138. BURSTONE MS. The ground substance of abnormal dentin, secondary dentin, and pulp calcification. J Dent Res 1953; 32: 269–79.

139. BURZYNSKI NJ *et al*. Autosomal dominant smooth hypoplastic amelogenesis imperfecta. Oral Surg 1973; 36: 818–23.

140. BUTLER WT. Dentin extracellular matrix and dentinogenesis. Oper Dent 1992; 5 (suppl): 18–23.

141. BUTLER W *et al*. Describing the severity of mottling in a community. Community Dent Oral Epidemiol 1985; 13: 277–80.

142. BUZALAF MAR DAMANTE CA *et al*. Risk of fluorosis associated with infant formulas prepared with bottled water. J Dent Child 2004; 71: 110–13.

143. CABRAL LAG *et al*. Regional odontodysplasia. Quint Int 1994; 25: 141–5.

144. CABRERIZO MERINO MC *et al*. Dental anomalies caused by oncological treatment. J Clin Pediatr Dent 1998; 22: 261–264.

145. CALE AE *et al*. Pigmentation of the jawbones and teeth secondary to minocycline hydrochloride therapy. J Periodontol 1988; 59: 112–14.

146. CANADIAN DENTAL ASSOCIATION. Fluoride supplementation. J Can Dent Assoc 2000; 66: 363.

147. CARPENTER TO *et al*. 24,25 dihydroxyvitamin D supplementation corrects hyperparathyroidism and improves skeletal abnormalities in X-linked hypophosphatemic rickets. J Clin Endocrinol Metab 1996; 81: 2381–8.

148. CARTWRIGHT AR *et al*. Craniofacial features associated with amelogenesis imperfecta. J Craniofac Gent Dev Biol 1999; 19: 148–56.

149. CEHRELI ZC *et al*. Dentinogenesis imperfecta: influence of an overdenture on gingival tissues and tooth mobility. J Clin Pediatr Dent 1996; 20: 277–80.

150. CHALLACOMBE SJ. Does fluoridation harm immune function? Community Dent Health 1996; 13 (suppl 2): 69–71.

151. CHANDRA S *et al*. Community oral health assessment in a fluorotic belt. J Indian Dent Assoc 1981; 53: 21–2.

152. CHANDRA S *et al*. Determination of optimal fluoride concentration in drinking water in an area in India with dental fluorosis. Community Dent Oral Epidemiol 1980; 8: 92–6.

153. CHAUDRY AP *et al*. Odontogenesis imperfecta. Oral Surg 1961; 14: 1099–103.

154. CHAUSSAIN-MILLER C *et al*. Dental abnormalities in patients with familial hypophosphatemic vitamin D-resistant rickets. J Pediatr 2003; 142: 324–31.

155. CHEEK CC *et al*. Dental and oral discolorations associated with minocycline and other teatracycline analogs. J Esthet Dent 1999; 11: 43–8.

156. CHELLAPAH NK *et al*. Enamel defects in a fluoridated South-East Asian community. Aust Dent J 1990; 35: 530–5.

157. CHIANG Y-T. A neurohistological study on the effect of hypervitaminosis A on the development of tooth germ. J Kyushu Dent Soc 1986; 40: 31–48.

158. CHOSACK A *et al*. Amelogenesis imperfecta among Israeli Jews and the description of a new type of local hypoplastic autosomal recessive amelogenesis imperfecta. Oral Surg 1979; 47: 148–56.

159. CIARLONE AE *et al*. The quantitative binding of tetracycline to dentin. J Endod 1988; 14: 494–6.

160. CIARLONE AE *et al*. Further characterization of tetracycline's quantitative binding to dentin. J Endod 1989; 15: 335–8.

161. CIOLA B *et al*. Radiographic manifestations of an unusual combination type I and type II dentin dysplasia. Oral Surg Oral Med Oral Pathol 1978; 45: 317–22.

162. CLARK DB. Dental findings in patients with chronic renal failure. J Can Dent Assoc 1987; 53: 781–5.

163. CLARK DB *et al*. Dentin in chronic renal failure. J Oral Pathol 1988; 17: 60–9.

164. CLARK DC. Trends in prevalence of dental fluorosis in North America. Community Dent Oral Epidemiol 1994; 22: 148–52.

165. CLARKSON J. Review of terminology, classifications, and indices of developmental defects of enamel. Adv Dent Res 1989; 3: 104–9.

166. CLARKSON JJ *et al*. Prevalence of enamel defects/fluorosis in fluoridated and non-fluoridated areas in Ireland. Community Dent Oral Epidemiol 1992; 20: 196–9.

167. CLEARY MA *et al*. Oral health implications in children with inborn errors of intermediary metabolism. Int J Paediatr Dent 1997; 7: 133–41.

168. CLEREBURGH A. Enamel mottling in 15-year-old children in Barnsley area, England. Community Dent Oral Epiodemiol 1979; 7 (6): 349–52.

169. CLERGEAU-GUERITHAULT S *et al*. Dentinogenesis imperfecta type III with enamel and cementum defects. Oral Surg 1985; 59: 505–10.

170. COCHRAN JA *et al*. A comparison of the prevalence of fluorosis in 8–year-old children from seven European study sites using a standardized methodology. Community Dent Oral Epidemiol 2004; 32 (suppl 1): 28–33.

171. COCHRAN JA *et al*. Development of a standardized method for comparing fluoride ingested from toothpaste by 1.5–3.5-year-old children in seven European countries. Part I: field work. Community Dent Oral Epidemiol 2004; 32 (suppl 1): 39–46.

172. COCHRAN JA *et al*. Development of a standardized method for comparing fluoride ingested from toothpaste by 1.5–3.5-year-old children in seven European countries. Part 2. Community Dent Oral Epidemiol 2004; 32 (suppl 1): 47–53.

173. COCKINGS JM *et al*. Minocycline and oral pigmentation. Aust Dent J 1998; 43: 14–16.

174. COHEN S *et al*. Origin, diagnosis, and treatment of the dental manifestations of vitamin D-resistant rickets. J Am Dent Assoc 1976; 92: 120–9.

175. COKE JM *et al*. Dentinal dysplasia, type I. Oral Surg 1979; 48: 262–8.

176. COLE B *et al*. Malformation in the primary and permanent dentitions following trauma prior to tooth eruption. Endod Dent Traumatol 1999; 15: 294–6.

177. COLLINS MA *et al*. Dental anomalies associated with amelogenesis imperfecta. Oral Surg Oral Med Oral Pathol Oral Radiol Endod 1999; 88: 358–64.

178. COMMISSION ON ORAL HEALTH, RESEARCH AND EPIDEMIOLOGY. An epidemiological index of developmental defects of dental enamel (DDE Index). Int Dent J 1982; 32: 159–67.

179. COMMISSION ON ORAL HEALTH, RESEARCH & EPIDEMIOLOGY. A review of the developmental defects of enamel index (DDE index). Int Dent J 1992; 42: 411–26.

180. CONGLETON J *et al*. Amelogenesis imperfecta with taurodontism. Oral Surg 1979; 48: 540–4.

181. CONLEY H *et al*. Clinical and histological findings of the dentition in a hypopituitary patient. ASDC J Dent Child 1990; 57: 376–9.

182. CONNE PH *et al*. Les effets d'une hypovitaminose et d'une avitaminose A de plus en plus prolongées sur l'incisive du rat blanc. Schweiz Monatschr Zahnheilkd 1969; 79: 667–84.

183. COOK CD *et al*. Health and differential survival in prehistoric populations: prenatal dental defects. Am J Phys Anthropol 1979; 51: 649–64.

184. COOK-MOZAFFARI P. Cancer and fluoridation. Community Dent Health 1996; 13 (suppl 2): 56–62.

185. CORRÊA RODRIGUES MH *et al*. Fingernails and toenails as biomarkers of subchronic exposure to fluoride from dentifrice in 2- to 3+year-old children. Caries Res 2004; 38: 109–14.

186. COUMOULOS H. Observations on the appearance of dental enamel in an endemic fluorosis area, with particular reference to deciduous teeth. Br Dent J 1949; 86; 172–6.

187. COURSON F *et al*. Regional odontodysplasia: expression of matrix metalloproteinases and their natural inhibitors. Oral Surg Oral Med Oral Pathol Oral Radiol Endod 2003; 95: 60–6.

188. COVE DH *et al*. Fetal hyperthyroidism: experience of treatment in four siblings. Lancet 1985; I: 430–2.

189. CRALL MG *et al*. Genetic marker study of dentinogenesis imperfecta. Proc Finn Den Soc 1992; 88 (suppl 1): 285–93.

190. CRAWFORD JL. Concomitant taurodontism and amelogenesis imperfecta in the American Caucasian. ASDC J Dent Child 1970; 37: 171–5.

191. CRAWFORD PJM *et al*. Regional odontodysplasia. J Oral Pathol Med 1989; 18: 251–63.

192. CRAWFORD PJM *et al*. Amelogenesis imperfecta: autosomal dominant hypomaturation-hypoplasia type with taurodontism. Br Dent J 1988; 164: 71–3.

193. CRAWFORD PJM *et al*. X-linked amelogenesis imperfecta. Oral Surg Oral Med Oral Pathol 1992; 73: 449–55.

194. CROLL TP *et al*. The dentifrice deception revisited. Quint Int 1992; 23: 77–8.

195. CURZON MEJ *et al*. Enamel mottling in a high strontium area of the U.S.A. Community Dent Oral Epidemiol 1977; 5: 243–7.

196. CUTRESS TW *et al*. Fluoride content of the enamel and dentine of human premolars prior to and following the introduction of fluoridation in New Zealand. Caries Res 1996; 30: 204–12.

197. DAHLLÖF G *et al*. Enamel disturbances in congenital hypopituitarism. ASDC J Dent Child 1983; 50: 451–4.

198. DAHLLÖF G *et al*. Concomitant regional odontodysplasia and hydrocephalus. Oral Surg 1987; 63: 354–7.

199. DAHLLÖF G *et al*. Histologic changes in dental morphology induced by high dose chemotherapy and total body irradiation. Oral Surg Oral Med Oral Pathol 1994; 77: 56–60.

200. DAMM DD *et al*. Focal delayed eruption. Gen Dent 2001; 49: 356, 428.

201. DANFORTH RA *et al*. Segmental odontomaxillary dysplasia. Oral Surg Oral Med Oral Pathol 1990; 70: 81–5

202. DARENDELILER A *et al*. Hereditary dentinogenesis imperfecta: a treatment program using an overdenture. ASDC J Dent Child 1992; 59: 273–6.

203. DARLING AI. Some observations on amelogenesis imperfecta and calcification of the dental enamel. Proc R Soc Med 1956; 49: 759–65.

204. DAVIS H *et al*. National trends in the mortality of children with sickle cell disease, 1968 through 1992. Am J Public Health 1997; 87: 1317–22.

205. DEAN DH *et al*. Osteogenesis imperfecta congenita: dental features of a rare disease. J Oral Med 1984; 39: 119–22.

206. DEAN HT. Classification of mottled enamel diagnosis. J Am Dent Assoc 1934; 21: 1421–6.

207. DEAN JA *et al*. Dentin dysplasia, type II linkage to chromosome 4q. J Craniofac Genet Dev Biol 1997; 17: 172–7.

208. DE BOER JG. Hutchinson-tanden. Ned Tijdschr Tandheelkd 1971; 78: 308–9.

209. DE COSTER PJ. Harde tandweefsels en bindweefselstoornissen. In: DE BAAT C *et al*. (eds) Het tandheelkundig jaar 2005. Houten: Bohn Stafleu van Loghum, 2004.

210. DE KLOET HJ *et al*. In vivo remineralization and fluoride uptake after brushing with two concentrations of fluoride in dentifrices. Caries Res 1986; 65 (12): 1410–14.

211. DE LA TRANCHADE IN *et al*. Amelogenesis imperfecta and nephrocalcinosis: a new case of this rare syndrome. J Clin Pediatr Dent 2003; 27: 171–6.

212. DE LIEFDE B *et al*. Prevalence of developmental defects of enamel and dental caries in New Zealand children receiving differing fluoride supplementation. Community Dent Oral Epidemiol 1985; 13: 164–7.

213. DE LIEFDE B. Longitudinal survey of enamel defects in a cohort of New Zealand children. Community Dent Oral Epidemiol 1988; 16: 218–21.

214. DENBESTEN PK *et al*. Enamel proteases in secretory and maturation enamel of rats ingesting 0 and 100 ppm fluoride in drinking water. Adv Dent Res 1989; 3: 199–202.

215. DENT CE *et al*. Hereditary pseudo-vitamin D deficiency rickets. J Bone Joint Surg 1968; 50: 708–19.

216. DESALVO MS *et al*. Segmental odontomaxillary dysplasia (hemimaxillofacial dysplasia). Pediatr Dent 1996; 18: 154–6.

217. DESORT KD. Amelogenesis imperfecta: the genetics, classification, and treatment. J Prosthet Dent 1983; 49: 786–92.

218. DEUTSCH D et al. Changes in amino acid composition and protein distribution during development of human deciduous enamel. Growth 1987; 51: 324–54.

219. DEUTSCH D et al. Changes in mineral distribution and concentration during enamel development in the deciduous human maxillary and mandibular teeth. Growth 1987; 51: 334–41.

220. DIETRICH G et al. Molar incisor hypomineralisation in a group of children and adolescents living in Dresden (Germany). Eur J Pediatr Dent 2003; 4: 133–7.

221. DINNERMAN M. Vitamin A deficiency in unerupted teeth of infants. Oral Surg 1951; 4: 1024–38.

222. DOLINE S et al. The effect of radiotherapy in the treatment of retinoblastoma upon the developing dentition. J Pediatr Ophthalmol Strabismus 1980; 17: 109–13.

223. DONLY KJ et al. Oral electrical burns. Gen Dent 1988; 36: 103–7.

224. DOOLAND MB et al. A photographic study of enamel defects among South Australian school children. Aust Dent J 1989; 34: 470–3.

225. DOUKOUDAKIS S et al. Morphologic characteristics of dentin at the dentinoenamel junction as viewed by scanning electron microscopy. J Esthet Dent 1997; 9: 94–9.

226. DOWELL TB. The use of toothpaste in infancy. Br Dent J 1981; 150: 247–9.

227. DOWELL TB et al. Fluoride supplements – age related dosages. Br Dent J 1981; 150: 273–5.

228. DRAKE DL. Segmental odontomaxillary dysplasia: an unusual orthodontic challenge. Am J Orthod Dentofac Orthop 2003; 123: 84–6..

229. DRISCOLL WS et al. A discussion of optimal dosage for dietary fluoride supplementation. Council on dental therapeutics. J Am Dent Assoc 1978; 96: 1050–3.

230. DRISCOLL WS et al. Prevalence of dental caries and dental fluorosis in areas with negligible, optimal, and above-optimal fluoride concentrations in drinking water. J Am Dent Assoc 1986; 113: 29–33.

231. DRUMMOND BK et al. Urinary excretion of fluoride following ingestion of MFP toothpastes by infants aged two to six years. J Dent Res 1985; 64: 1145–8.

232. DRUMMOND BK et al. Estimation of fluoride absorption from swallowed fluoride toothpastes. Caries Res 1990; 24: 211–15.

233. DUCKWORTH SC et al. The ingestion of fluoride in tea. Br Dent J 1978; 145: 368–70.

234. DUMMER PMH et al. Prevalence of enamel developmental defects in a group of 11- and 12-year-old children in South Wales. Community Dent Oral Epidemiol 1986; 14: 119–22.

235. DUMMER PMH et al. Distribution of tooth enamel by tooth type in 11- and 12-year-old children in South Wales. Community Dent Oral Epidemiol 1986; 14: 341–4.

236. DUNCAN WK et al. Labial hypoplasia of primary canines in black head starts children. ASDC J Dent Child 1988; 55: 423–6.

237. DUURSMA SA et al. Fluoride bij de behandeling van patiënten met osteoporose. Ned Tijdschr Geneeskd 1986; 130: 1467–72.

238. DWORSKY ME et al. Occupational risk for primary cytomegalovirus infection among pediatric health-care workers. N Engl J Med 1983; 309: 950–3.

239. DYM H et al. Dentinal dysplasia, type I. ASDC J Dent Child 1982; 49: 437–9.

240. EGGER RJ et al. Vitaminestatus van bevolkingsgroepen. Voeding 1985; 46: 31–5.

241. EKSTRAND J et al. Pharmacokinetics of fluoride gels in children and adults. Caries Res 1981; 15: 213–20.

242. EKSTRAND J et al. Distribution of fluoride to human breast milk following intake of high doses of fluoride. Caries Res 1984; 18: 93–5.

243. ELIDRISSY ATH et al. Vitamin D deficiency in mothers of rachitic infants. Calcif Tissue Int 1984; 36: 266–8.

244. ELIOT MM et al. A study of the teeth of a group of school children previously examined for rickets. Am J Dis Child 1934; 48: 713–29.

245. ELLINGSEN JE et al. Plasma fluoride levels in man following intake of Sn2 in solution or toothpaste. J Dent Res 1985; 64: 1250–2.

246. EL-LABBAN NG et al. Permanent teeth in hypophosphatasia. J Oral Pathol Med 1991; 20: 352–60.

247. ELLWOOD RP et al. A photographic study of developmental defects of enamel in Brazilian school children. Int Dent J 1996; 46: 69–75.

248. ELLWOOD RP et al. The demographic and social variation in the prevalence of dental enamel opacities in North Wales. Community Dent Health 1994; 11: 192–6.

249. ELLWOOD RP et al. Dental enamel opacities in three groups with varying levels of fluoride in their drinking water. Caries Res 1995; 29: 137–42.

250. ELLWOOD RP et al. A comparison of information recorded using the thylstrup fejerskov index, tooth surface index of fluorosis and developmental defects of enamel index. Int Dent J 1994; 44: 628–36.

251. ELZAY RP et al. Dentinal dysplasia. Oral Surg 1967; 23: 338–42.

252. ENGSTRÖM C. Odontoblast metabolism in rats deficient in vitamin D and calcium – IV. Lysosomal and energy metabolic enzymes. J Oral Pathol 1980; 9: 246–54.

253. ENGSTRÖM C et al. Odontoblast metabolism in rats deficient in vitamin D and calcium – III. J Oral Pathol 1978; 7: 227–35.

254. ENGSTRÖM C et al. Odontoblast metabolism in rats deficient in vitamin D and calcium – II. J Oral Pathol 1977; 6: 367–72.

255. ENGSTRÖM C et al. Odontoblast metabolism in rats deficient in vitamin D and calcium – I. J Oral Pathol 1977; 6: 359–66.

256. ENWONWU CO. Influence of socioeconomic conditions on dental development in Nigerian children. Arch Oral Biol 1973; 18: 95–107.

257. ERICSSON Y. Effect of infant diets with widely different fluoride contents on the fluoride concentrations of deciduous teeth. Caries Res 1973; 7: 56–62.

258. ERICSSON Y. Report on the safety of drinking water fluoridation. Caries Res 1974; 8 (suppl): 16–27.

259. ERICSSON Y *et al*. Wide variations of fluoride supply in infants and their effect. Caries Res 1971; 5: 78–88.

260. ERPENSTEIN H *et al*. Schmelzhypoplasie und offener Biss als autosomal dominant vererbtes Merkmalspaar. Dtsch Zahnaerztl Z 1968; 23: 405–14.

261. ESCOBAR VH *et al*. A clinical, genetic, and ultrastructural study of snow-capped teeth: amelogenesis imperfecta, hypomaturation type. Oral Surg 1981; 52: 607–14.

262. EVANS DJ. A study of developmental defects in enamel in 10-year-old high social class children residing in a non-fluoridated area. Community Dent Health 1991; 8: 31–8.

263. EVANS RW. Dental fluorosis following downward adjustment of fluoride in drinking water. J Public Health Dent 1991; 51: 91–8.

264. EVANS RW. An epidemiological assessment of the chronological distribution of dental fluorosis in human maxillary central incisors. J Dent Res 1993; 72: 883–90.

265. EVANS RW *et al*. Refining the estimate of the critical period during which the human maxillary incisors are moist susceptible to fluorosis. J Public Health Dent 1995; 55: 438–49.

266. EVANS RW *et al*. Dental fluorosis following downward adjustment of fluoride in drinking water. J Public Health Dent 1991; 51: 91–8.

267. EVANS RW *et al*. An epidemiologic estimate of the critical period during which human maxillary central incisors are most susceptible to fluorosis. J Public Health Dent 1991; 51: 251–9.

268. FADAVIA S *et al*. The oral effects of orotracheal intubation in prematurely born preschoolers. ASDC J Dent Child 1992; 59: 420–4.

269. FALLER RV *et al*. The comparative anticaries efficacy of Crest toothpaste relative to some marketed Chinese toothpastes. Int Dent J 1997; 47: 313–20.

270. FANIBUNDA KB *et al*. Odontodysplasia, gingival manifestations, and accompanying abnormalities. Oral Surg Oral Med Oral Pathol Oral Radiol Endod 1996; 81: 84–8.

271. FARMER ED *et al*. Stone's oral and dental diseases. Edinburgh: E & S Livingstone Ltd., 1966.

272. FAYLE SA. Molar Incisor Hypomineralisation: restorative management. Eur J Paediatr Dent 2003; 4: 121–6.

273. FEARNE JM *et al*. Enamel defects in the primary dentition of children born less than 2000 g. Br Dent J 1990; 168: 433–7.

274. FEARNE JM *et al*. Regional odontodysplasia: a clinical and histological evaluation. J Int Ass Dent Child 1986; 17: 21–5.

275. FEJERSKOV O *et al*. Combined effect of systemic and topical fluoride treatments on human deciduous teeth. Caries Res 1987; 21: 452–9.

276. FEJERSKOV O *et al*. Clinical and structural features and possible pathogenic mechanisms of dental fluorosis. Scand J Dent Res 1977; 85: 510–34.

277. FERGUSON HW *et al*. The effect of vitamin D on the dentine of the incisor teeth and on the alveolar bone of young rats maintained on diets deficient in calcium or phosphorus. Arch Oral Biol 1964; 9: 447–60.

278. FERGUSON JW *et al*. Regional odontodysplasia. Aust Dent J 1980; 25: 148–51.

279. FESKANICH D *et al*. Vitamin A intake and hip fractures among postmenopausal women. J Am Med Assoc 2002; 287: 102–4.

280. FIEDLER MA *et al*. Review of chemicals and medication. AORN J 1998; 67: 404–5.

281. FILIPI A. Dentindysplasie Type I – oralchirurgische behandlungsmöglichkeiten periapikaler veränderungen. Quintessenz 1996; 47: 597–605.

282. FINKELMAN RD *et al*. Vitamin D and skeletal tissues. J Oral Pathol 1985; 14: 191–215.

283. FIUMARA NJ *et al*. Manifestations of late congenital syphilis. Arch Derm 1970; 102: 78–83.

284. FLEMING HS *et al*. Changes in the teeth and jaws of neonatal Webster mice after administration of NaF and CaF2 to the female parent during gestation. J Dent Res 1954; 33: 780–8.

285. FOKKER A. Peutertandpasta De stand van zaken. Ned Tandartsenbl 1999; 54 (3): 88–91.

286. FOMON SJ *et al*. Fluoride intake and prevalence of dental fluorosis: trends in fluoride intake with special attention to infants. J Public Health Dent 2000; 60 (3): 131–9.

287. FORREST JR. Mottled enamel. Br Dent J 1965; 119: 316–19.

288. FORSMAN B. Dental fluorosis and caries in high-fluoride districts in Sweden. Community Dent Oral Epidemiol 1974; 2: 132–48.

289. FORSMAN K *et al*. Localization of a gene for autosomal dominant amelogenesis imperfecta (ADAI) to chromosome 4q. Hum Mol Genet 1994; 3: 1621–5.

290. FRANQUIN JC *et al*. Effets d'une carence maternelle en vitamine A sur les structures cranio-dentaires du rat. J Biol Buccale 1981; 9: 163–81.

291. FRASER D *et al*. Pathogenesis of hereditary vitamin-D-dependent rickets. N Engl J Med 1973; 289: 817–22.

292. FRASER D *et al*. The etiology of enamel hypoplasia in children – a unifying concept. J Int Assoc Dent Child 1982; 13: 1–11.

293. FRASER D *et al*. Familial forms of vitamin D-resistant rickets revisited. X-linked hypophosphatemia and autosomal recessive vitamin D dependency. Am J Clin Nutr 1976; 29: 1315–29.

294. FRENSILLI JA *et al*. Dental changes of idiopathic hypoparathyreoidism. J Oral Surg 1971; 29: 727–31.

295. FUNAKOSHI Y *et al*. Dental observations of low birth weight infants. Pediatr Dent 1981; 3: 21–5.

296. FUNATSU T *et al*. Morphological characteristics of maxillary deciduous molars in extremely-low and very-low birth-weight infants. Pediatr Dent J 2000; 10: 103–10.

297. GAGE JP. Dentinogenesis imperfecta. Aust Dent J 1985; 30: 285–90.

298. GAGE JP *et al*. Abnormal amino acid analyses obtained from osteogenesis imperfecta dentin. J Dent Res 1988; 67: 1097–102.

299. GALEONE RJ *et al*. Odontodysplasia. Oral Surg 1970; 29: 879–80.

300. GARDNER DE *et al*. Hereditary hypophosphatemia. ASDC J Dent Child 1969; 36: 199–200, 211–12 and 216.

301. GARDNER DG. The dentinal changes in regional odontodysplasia. Oral Surg 1974; 38: 887–97.

302. GARDNER DG et al. A classification of dysplastic forms of dentin. J Oral Pathol 1979; 8: 28–46.

303. GARDNER DG et al. Regional odontodysplasia. Oral Surg 1973; 35: 351–65.

304. GARFUNKEL AA et al. Familial hypoparathyroidism, candidiasis and mental retardation. J Oral Med 1979; 34: 13–17.

305. GAVALDÁ C. Dysplasia odontomaxilar segmentaria. Med Oral 2004; 9: 181.

306. GAWENIS LR et al. Mineral content of calcified tissues in cystic fibrosis mice. Biol Trace Element Res 2001; 83: 69–81.

307. GEDALIA I. Distribution in placenta and foetus. In: World Health Organization. Fluorides and human health. Geneva: World Health Organization, 1970.

308. GEDALIA I et al. Effect of prenatal and postnatal fluoride on the human deciduous dentition. Adv Dent Res 1989; 3: 168–76.

309. GERLACH RF et al. Regional odontodysplasia. Oral Surg Oral Med Oral Pathol Oral Radiol Endod 1998; 85: 308–13.

310. GIAMBRO NJ et al. Characterization of fluorosed human enamel by color reflectance, ultrastructure, and elemental composition. Caries Res 1995; 29: 251–7.

311. GIASANTI JS. A kindred showing hypocalcified amelogenesis imperfecta. J Am Dent Assoc 1973; 86: 675–8.

312. GIANSANTI JS et al. Dentin dysplasia, type II, or dentin dysplasia, coronal type. Oral Surg 1974; 38: 911–17.

313. GIBBARD PD. The management of children and adolescents suffering from amelogenesis imperfecta and dentinogenesis imperfecta. J Oral Rehabil 1974; 1: 55–66.

314. GIBBARD PD et al. Odontodysplasia. Br Dent J 1973; 135: 525–32.

315. GIBSON WM et al. Observation of children's teeth as a diagnostic aid: 2. developmental difficulties reflected in enamel and pigment changes. J Can Dent Assoc 1964; 30: 93–101.

316. GIGLIOTTI R et al. Familial vitamin D-refractory rickets. J Am Dent Assoc 1971; 82: 383–7.

317. GIRO GM. Enamel hypoplasia in human teeth: an examination of its causes. J Am Dent Assoc 1947; 34: 310–17.

318. GITTLEMAN IF et al. Diabetes mellitus or the prediabetic state in the mother and the neonate. AMA J Dis Child 1959; 98: 342–9.

319. GRUBB BR et al. Pathophysiology of gene-targeted mouse models for cystic fibrosis. Physiol Rev 1999; 79: 193–214.

320. GIUNTA JL. Dental changes in hypervitaminosis D. Oral Surg Oral Med Oral Pathol Oral Radiol Endod 1998; 85; 410–13.

321. GLENN FB. Immunity conveyed by sodium-fluoride supplement during pregnancy: part II. ASDC J Dent Child 1979: 46: 17–24.

322. GLENN FG et al. Prenatal fluoride for growth and development: part X. ASDC J Dent Child 1997; 64: 317–21.

323. GLORIEUX FH et al. Type V osteogenesis imperfecta. J Bone Miner Res 2000; 15: 1650–8.

324. GODFREY JL. A histological study of dentin formation in osteogenesis imperfecta congenita. J Oral Pathol 1973; 2: 95–111.

325. GOMES MP et al. Regional odontodysplasia. ASDC J Dent Child 1999; 66: 203–7.

326. GOODMAN AH. Factors affecting the distribution of enamel hypoplasias within the human permanent dentition. Am J Phys Anthropol 1985; 68: 479–93.

327. GOODMAN AH. Dental enamel hypoplasias in prehistoric populations. Adv Dent Res 1989; 3: 265–71.

328. GOODMAN JR et al. Dental problems associated with hypophosphataemic vitamin D resistant rickets. Int J Pediatr Dent 1998; 8: 19–28..

329. GÖTZ W. Der Morbus haemolyticus neonatorum und seine Auswirkung, insbesondere auf Farbe und Struktur der Milchzähne. Dtsch Stomatol 1961; 11: 1–7.

330. GORLIN RJ et al. Syndromes of head and neck. New York, NY: Oxford University Press, 1976, Chapter 2.

331. GORLIN RJ et al. Syndromes of the head and neck. Oxford: Oxford University Press, 1990.

332. GOTJAMANOS T et al. Abnormally high fluoride levels in commercial preparations of 40% silver fluoride solution: contraindications for use in children. Aust Dent J 1998; 43: 422–7.

333. GOULD AR et al. Pericoronal features of regional odontodysplasia. J Oral Med 1984; 39: 236–42.

334. GOWARD PE. Mottling on deciduous incisor teeth. Br Dent J 1982; 153: 367–9.

335. GRANATH L et al. Diagnosis of mild enamel fluorosis in permanent maxillary incisors using two scoring systems. Community Dent Oral Epidemiol 1985; 13: 273–6.

336. GRAHNÉN H. Maternal rubella and dental defects. Odontol Revy 1958; 9: 181–92.

337. GRAHNÉN H et al. Maternal diabetes and changes in the hard tissues of primary teeth – I. Odontol Revy 1967; 18: 157–62.

338. GRAHNÉN H et al. Enamel defects in the deciduous dentition of prematurely born children. Odontol Revy 1958; 9: 193–204.

339. GRAHNÉN H et al. Maternal diabetes and changes in the hard tissues of primary teeth – II. Caries Res 1968; 2: 333–7.

340. GRAHNÉN H et al. The effects of rickets and spasmophilia on the permanent dentition. Odontol Revy 1954; 5: 7–26.

341. GRAHNÉN H et al. Neonatal asphyxia and mineralisation defects of the primary teeth. Caries Res 1969; 3: 301–7.

342. GRAHNÉN H et al. Mineralization defects of primary teeth in children born pre-term. Scand J Dent Res 1974; 82: 396–400.

343. GRIMER PT. An atypical form of hereditary opalescent dentine. Br Dent J 1956; 100: 275–8.

344. GROBLER SR et al. Dental fluorosis and caries experience in relation to three different drinking water fluoride levels in South Africa. Int J Paediatr Dent 2001; 11: 372–9.

345. GROBLER SR et al. Relationship between enamel fluoride levels, degree of fluorosis and caries experience in communities with a nearly optimal and a high fluoride level in the drinking water. Caries Res 1986; 20: 284–8.

346. GROENEVELD A. Longitudinal study of prevalence of enamel lesions in a fluoridated and non-fluoridated area. Community Dent Oral Epidemiol 1985; 13: 159–63.

347. GRUNDY MC. Developmental anomalies of tooth formation – II. Dent Update 1980; 7: 345–51.

348. GUGGENHEIMER J et al. Dental manifestations of the rubella syndrome. Oral Surg 1971; 32: 30–7.

349. GULLIKSON JS. Tooth morphology in rubella symdrome children. ASDC J Dent Child 1975; 42: 479–82.

350. GUZMAN R et al. Odontodysplasia in a pediatric patient. Pediatr Dent 1990; 12: 45–8.

351. GYSEL C. Een Turnersnijtand. Ned Tijdschr Tandheelkd 1968; 75: 859–61.

352. GYSEL C. Turnerpremolaren: diagnose, frequentie en classificatie. Ned Tijdschr Tandheelkd 1969; 76: 531–41.

353. HAGER TS et al. Complete prosthodontic rehabilitation of a patient with Graves' disease. Gen Dent 1997; 45: 482–4.

354. HAIKEL Y et al. Dental caries and fluorosis in children from high and low fluoride areas of Morocco. ASDC J Dent Child 1989; 56: 378–81.

355. HALL RK. Gross tooth hypocalcification in vitamin D-resistant rickets. Aust Dent J 1959; 4: 329–30.

356. HALL RK. The prevalence of developmental defects of tooth enamel (DDE) in a pediatric hospital department of dentistry population – I. Adv Dent Res 1989; 3: 114–19.

357. HALLETT KB et al. Oral health of children with congenital cardiac diseases. Pediatr Dent 1992; 14: 224–30.

358. HAMDAN M et al. The prevalence of enamel mottling on incisor teeth in optimal and low fluoride communities in England. Community Dent Health 1991; 8: 111–19.

359. HANKEY GT et al. Odontodysplasia in the deciduous dentition. Dent Pract 1968; 19: 93–5.

360. HARCOURT JK et al. In vivo incorporation of tetracycline in the teeth of man. Arch Oral Biol 1962; 7: 431–7.

361. HARGREAVES JA et al. Hypocalcification and hypoplasia in primary teeth of preschool children from different ethnic groups in South Africa. Adv Dent Res 1989; 3: 110–13.

362. HARGREAVES JA et al. Hypocalcification and hypoplasia in primary teeth of children from different ethnic groups in South Africa assessed with a new index. Adv Dent Res 1989; 3: 126–31.

363. HARGREAVES JA et al. A gravimetric study of the ingestion of toothpaste by children. Caries Res 1972; 6: 237–43.

364. HARLEY KE et al. Dental anomalies – Are adhesive castings the solution? Br Dent J 1993; 174: 15–22.

365. HARRIS R et al. Dental sequelae in deciduous dentition in vitamin D resistant rickets. Aust Dent J 1960; 5: 200–3.

366. HARRIS SS et al. In vivo and in vitro study of the effects of vitamin A deficiency on rat third molar development. J Dent Res 1986; 65: 1445–8.

367. HART PS et al. Amelogenesis imperfecta phenotype-genotype correlations with two amelogenin gene mutations. Arch Oral Biol 2002; 47: 261–5.

368. HART PS et al. A nomenclature for X-linked amelogenesis imperfecta. Arch Oral Biol 2002 47: 255–60.

369. HATTAB FN et al. Caries risk in patients with thalassaemia major. Int Dent J 2001; 51: 35–8.

370. HATTAB FN et al. Dietary sources of fluoride for infants and children in Hong Kong. Pediatr Dent 1988; 10: 13–18.

371. HEERES GJ et al. Routinematige gelapplicaties met behulp van confectielepels bij kinderen. Ned Tijdschr Tandheelkd 1984; 91: 158–63.

372. HEIER HE et al. Maternal blood group O a risk factor of neonatal hyperbilirubinemia requiring treatment. Tidsskr Nor Laegeforen 1996; 116: 34–6.

373. HEIFETZ SB et al. Prevalence of dental caries and dental fluorosis in areas with optimal and above-optimal water-fluorideconcentrations. J Am Dent Assoc 1988; 116: 490–5.

374. HITCHIN AD. Unerupted deciduous (?) teeth in youth aged 15 1/2. Br Dent J 1934; 56: 631–3.

375. HEILMAN JR et al. Fluoride concentrations of infant foods. J Am Dent Assoc 1997; 128: 857–63.

376. HEIMLER A et al. An unusual presentation of opalescent dentin and Brandywine isolate hereditary opalescent dentin in an Ashkenazic Jewish family. Oral Surg 1985; 59: 608–15.

377. HELLER KE et al. Water consumption in the United States in 1994–96 and implications for water fluoridation policy. J Public Health Dent 1999; 59 (1): 3–11.

378. HELLWIG E et al. Caries prevalence and dental fluorosis in German children in areas with different concentrations of fluoride in drinking water supplies. Caries Res 1985; 19: 278–83.

379. HELLSTRÖM I et al. Urinary fluoride excretion in small children following short-term fluoride supply with tablets or domestic salt. Scand J Dent Res 1976; 84: 187–99.

380. HEMRIKA-WAGNER AM et al. Ultrastructural changes in developing hamster molars during vitamin C deficiency in vitro. J Biol Buccale 1982; 10: 163–73.

381. HERBERT FL. Hereditary hypophosphatemia rickets: an important awareness for dentists. ASDC J Dent Child 1986; 53: 223–6.

382. HERMAN NG et al. Odontodysplasia. ASDC J Dent Child 1977; 44: 52–54.

383. HERRMANN M. Veränderung der Zahnfarbe und -struktur bei Morbus haemolyticus neonatorum. Zahnaerztl Welt 1965; 66: 595–602.

384. HERMUS RJJ et al. Vitaminevoorziening door de voeding in Nederland. Voeding 1985; 46: 19–25.

385. HEROLD RC. Fine structure of tooth dentine in human dentinogenesis imperfecta. Arch Oral Biol 1972; 17: 1009–13.

386. HEROLD RCB et al. Abnormal tooth tissue in human odontodysplasia. Oral Surg 1970; 42: 357–65.

387. HIETALA E-L et al. Mineral content of different areas of human dentin in hypophosphataemic vitamin D-resistant rickets. J Biol Buccale 1991; 19: 129–34.

388. HIETALA E-L et al. The effect of ovariectomy on dentin formation and caries in adult rats. Acta Odontol Scand 1992; 50: 337–43.

389. HILLIER S *et al*. Water fluoridation and osteoporotic fracture. Community Dent Health 1996; 13 (suppl 2): 63–8.

390. HILLMANN G *et al*. Pathohistology of undercalcified primary teeth in vitamin D-resistant rickets. Oral Surg Oral Med Oral Pathol Oral Radiol Endod 1996; 82: 218–24.

391. HILSON S *et al*. Dental defects of congenital syphilis. Am J Phys Anthropol 1998; 107: 25–40.

392. HINRICHS EH. Dental changes in juvenile hypothyroidism. ASDC J Dent Child 1966; 33: 167–73.

393. HINTZ CS *et al*. Odontodysplasia. Oral Surg 1972; 34: 744–50.

394. HODGE H *et al*. Hereditary opalescent dentin. III. Histological, chemical and physical studies. J Dent Res 1940; 19: 521–36.

395. HOFF M *et al*. Dentinedysplasie type II. Ned Tijdschr Tandheelkd 1986; 93: 45–8.

396. HOLLOWAY PJ *et al*. The prevalence, causes and cosmetic importance of dental fluorosis in the United Kingdom. Community Dent Health 1997; 14: 148–55.

397. HOLM A-K *et al*. Enamel mineralization disturbances in 12-year-old children with known early exposure to fluorides. Community Dent Oral Epidemiol 1982; 10: 335–9.

398. HOLROYD I *et al*. Amelogenesis imperfecta in triplets. Br Dent J 1995; 178: 465–8.

399. HOLT RD *et al*. Development in fluoride toothpastes. Community Dent Health 1997; 14: 4–10.

400. HONG L *et al*. Primary tooth fluorosis and amoxillin use during infancy. J Public Health Dent 2004; 64: 38–44.

401. HOROWITZ HS. Indexes for measuring dental fluorosis. J Public Health Dent 1986; 46: 179–83.

402. HOROWITZ HS. Fluoride and enamel defects. Adv Dent Res 1989; 3: 143–6.

403. HOROWITZ HS *et al*. A new method for assessing the prevalence of dental fluorosis – the tooth surface index of fluorosis. J Am Dent Assoc 1984; 109: 37–41.

404. HOTZ PR. Zahnbildungsstörungen. Schweiz Monatsschr Zahnmed 1991; 101: 45–53.

405. HOUWINK B. Het gebruik van fluoridepreparaten. Ned Tijdschr Tandheelkd 1981; 88: 366–7.

406. HÜBERS B *et al*. Zahngesundheitszustand 12–14 jähriger in zwei fluorendemischen Gebieten Nordbayerns. Dtsch Zahnaerztl Z 1980; 35: 265–7.

407. HUMMEL H *et al*. Der Einfluss eines embryonalen Mg-Mangels auf die odontogenese bei Wistar-Ratten. Zahn Mund Kiefer Heilkd 1985; 73: 18–24.

408. HUMPHREYS ER *et al*. Age related and 224Ra-induced abnormalities in the teeth of male mice. Arch Oral Biol 1985; 30: 55–64.

409. HUNTER IP *et al*. Developmental abnormalities of the dentine and pulp associated with tumoral calcinosis. Br Dent J 1973; 135: 446–8.

410. HURMERINTA K *et al*. In vitro inhibition of mouse odontoblast differentiation by vitamin A. Arch Oral Biol 1980; 25: 385–93.

411. HURSEY RJ *et al*. Dentinogenesis imperfecta in a racial isolate with multiple hereditary effects. Oral Surg 1956; 9: 641–58.

412. HUTH KC *et al*. Diagnostic features and pedodontic-orthodontic management in dentinogenesis imperfecta type II. Int J Paediatr Dent 2002; 12: 316–21.

413. HUTTON CE. Intradental lesions and their reversal in a patient being treated for end-stage renal disease. Oral Surg 1985; 60: 258–61.

414. IBRAHIM YE *et al*. Caries and dental fluorosis in a 0.25 and a 2.5 ppm fluoride area in the Sudan. Int J Paediatr Dent 1997; 7: 161–6.

415. INFANTE PF *et al*. An epidemiologic study of linear enamel hypoplasia of deciduous anterior teeth in Guatemalan children. Arch Oral Biol 1974; 19: 1055–61.

416. INTERNATIONAL WORKING GROUP ON CONSTITUTIONAL DISEASES OF BONE. International nomenclature and classification of the osteochondrodysplasias (1997). Am J Med Genet 1998; 79: 376–82.

417. ISHII T *et al*. The severity of dental fluorosis in children exposed to water with a high fluoride content for various periods of time. J Dent Res 1991; 70: 952–6.

418. ISMAIL AI. Fluoride supplements. Community Dent Oral Epidemiol 1994; 22: 164–72.

419. ISMAIL AI *et al*. The risk of fluorosis in students exposed to a higher than optimal concentration of fluoride in well water. Public Health Dent 1996; 56: 22–7.

420. IVANCIE GP. Dentinogenesis imperfecta. Oral Surg 1954; 7: 984–92.

421. IVOREN KRUIS/NIGZ. Katern fluoride advies. Woerden: Ivoren Kruis/NIGZ, 1989.

422. JACKSON D. A clinical study of non-endemic mottling of enamel. Arch Oral Biol 1961; 5: 212–23.

423. JAFFE EC *et al*. Dental findings in chronic renal failure. Br Dent J 1986; 160: 18–20.

424. JAGELS AE *et al*. Oral health of patients with cystic fibrosis and their siblings. J Dent Res 1976; 55: 991–6.

425. JACZUK Z *et al*. The enamel spots in children drinking fluoridated water. J Int Assoc Dent Child 1984; 15: 65–70.

426. JÄLEVIK B *et al*. Enamel hypomineralisation of permanent first molars: a morphological study and survey of possible aetiological factors. Int J Pediatr Dent 2000; 10: 278–89.

427. JÄLEVIK B *et al*. Etiologic factors influencing the prevalence of demarcated opacities in permanent first molars in a group of Swedish children. Eur J Oral Sci 2001; 109: 230–4.

428. JäLEVIK B. Enamel hypomineralization in permanent first molars. A clinical, histo-morphological and biochemical study. Swed Dent J Suppl 2001; (149): 1–86.

429. JANSEN TLTA *et al*. Epidemiologie van coeliakie in Nederland. Ned Tijdschr Geneeskd 1994; 138: 2544–8.

430. JASMIN JR *et al*. A scanning electron microscopic study of dentin dysplasia type II in primary dentition. Oral Surg 1984; 58: 57–63.

431. JENSEN BL *et al*. Osteogenesis imperfecta: clinical, cephalometric, and biochemical investigations of OI types I, III, and IV. J Craniofac Genet Dev Biol 1997; 17: 121–32.

432. JENSEN SB *et al*. Nature and frequency of dental changes in idiopathic hypoparathyroidism and pseudohypoparathyroidism. Scand J Dent Res 1981; 89: 26–37.

433. JOHNSEN D *et al*. Distribution of enamel defects and the association with respiratory distress in very low birth-weight children. J Dent Res 1984; 63: 59–64.

434. JOHNSON J *et al*. The fluoride content of infant formulas available in 1985. Pediatr Dent 1987; 9: 33–7.

435. JOHNSON RH *et al*. The effects of tetracyclines on teeth and bone. J Dent Res 1966; 45: 86–93.

436. JOSELL SD *et al*. Extraoral management for electrical burns of the mouth. ASDC J Dent Child 1984; 51: 47–52.

437. JOWSEY J *et al*. Effect of combined therapy with sodium fluoride, vitamin D and calcium in osteoporosis. Am J Med 1972; 53: 43–9.

438. JUDES H *et al*. The histological examination of primary enamel as a possible tool in developmental disturbances. J Pedod 1985; 10: 68–75.

439. KAHN MA *et al*. Regional odontodysplasia. Oral Surg Oral Med Oral Pathol 1991; 72: 462–7.

440. KALK WWI *et al*. Dentin dysplasia type I. Five cases within one family. Oral Surg Oral Med Oral Pathol Oral Radiol Endod 1998; 86: 175–8.

441. KALSBEEK H *et al*. Use of fluoride tablets and effect on prevalence of dental caries and dental fluorosis. Community Dent Oral Epidemiol 1992; 20: 241–5.

442. KALSBEEK H *et al*. Fluoridetabletten en glazuurfluorose. Ned Tijdschr Tandheelkd 1990; 97: 269–73.

443. KAMANN WK *et al*. Der turner-zahn. Endodontie 1997; 3: 241–9.

444. KAMEN S *et al*. Genetic aspects of shell teeth. ASDC J Dent Child 1980; 47: 187–189.

445. KANTAPUTRA PN. Dentinogenesis imperfecta-associated syndromes. Am J Med Genet 2001; 104: 75–8.

446. KELLERHOFF N-M *et al*. Die "Molaren–inzisiven-hypomineralisation". Schweiz Monatschr Zahnmed 2004; 114: 243–9.

447. KELLEY JE *et al*. Epidermal nevus syndrome. Oral Surg 1972; 34: 774–80.

448. KEREBEL B *et al*. The inorganic phase in dentinogenesis imperfecta. J Dent Res 1981; 60: 1655–60.

449. KEREBEL B *et al*. Enamel in odontodysplasia. Oral Surg 1981; 52: 404–10.

450. KEREBEL B *et al.*. Dentinogenesis imperfecta with dens in dente. Oral Surg 1983; 55: 279–85.

451. KEREM E *et al*. Prediction of mortality in patient with cystic fibrosis. N Engl J Med 1992; 326: 1187–91.

452. KERR AR, SHIP JA. Management strategies for HIV-associated aphthous stoamtitis. Am J Clin Dermatol 2003; 4: 669–80.

453. KETLEY CE *et al*. Urinary fluoride excretion by pre-school children in six European countries. Community Dent Oral Epidemiol 2004; 32 (suppl 1): 62–68.

454. KIERDORF H *et al*. Disturbed enamel formation in wild boras (*Sus scrofa* L.) from fluoride polluted areas in central Europe. Anat Rec 2000; 259: 12–24.

455. KIGUEL E. Alkaline phosphatase activity in developing molars of vitamin-D-deficient rats – II. J Dent Res 1966; 45 (II): 1816.

456. KIKUCHI K *et al*. Vitamin D-dependent rickets type II. ASDC J Dent Child 1988; 55: 465–8.

457. KIM J-W *et al*. Amelogenin p.MIT and p.W4S muatations underlying hypoplastic X–linked amelogenesis imperfecta. J Dent Res 2004; 83: 378–83.

458. KIMURA T *et al*. Fluoride intake from food and drink in Japanese children aged 1–6 years. Caries Res 2001; 35: 47–9.

459. KINDELAN J *et al*. Orthodontic and orthognathic management of a patient with osteogenesis imperfecta and dentinogenesis imperfecta. J Orthod 2003; 30: 291–6.

460. KINDELAN SA *et al*. Detection of a novel mutation in X-linked amelogenesis imperfecta. J Dent Res 2000; 79: 1978–82.

461. KING NM *et al*. Developmental defects of enamel: a study of 12-year-olds in Hong Kong. J Am Dent Assoc 1986; 112: 835–9.

462. KING NM. Developmental defects of enamel in Chinese girls and boys in Hong Kong. Adv Dent Res 1989; 3: 120–5.

463. KINIRONS MJ. Shell teeth affecting a child patient. ASDC J Dent Child 1984; 51: 441–3.

464. KINIRONS MJ. Dental health of children with cystic fibrosis: an interim report. J Pediatr Dent 1985; 1: 3–7.

465. KINIRONS MJ. Dental health of patients suffering from cystic fibrosis in Northern Ireland. Community Dent Health 1989; 6: 113–20.

466. KINIRONS MJ *et al*. The chronology of dentinal defects related to medical findings in hypoparathyroidism. J Dent 1985; 13: 346–9.

467. KINIRONS MJ *et al*. Regional odontodysplasia. Br Dent J 1988; 165: 136–9.

468. KITAHARA Y *et al*. Disturbed tooth development in parathyroid hormone-related protein (PTHrP)-gene knockout mice. Boner 2002; 30: 48–56.

469. KOBLIN I *et al*. Beitrag zur Odontodysplasie. Dtsch Zahnaerztl Z 1969; 24: 219–655.

470. KOCH G. Prevalence of enamel mineralisation disturbances in an area with 1–1.2 ppm F in drinking water. Eur J Paediatr Dent 2003; 4: 127–8.

471. KOCH G *et al*. Epidemiologic study of idiopathic enamel hypomineralization in permanent teeth of Swedish children. Community Dent Oral Epidemiol 1987; 15: 279–85.

472. KOCH G *et al*. Effect of 200 and 1000 ppm fluoride dentifrice on caries. Swed Dent J 1982; 6: 233–8.

473. KOPPANG HS *et al*. Dental features in congenital renal tubular acidosis of proximal type. Scand J Dent Res 1984; 92: 489–95.

474. KOPPE JG *et al*. Placental transport of dioxins from mother to fetus – II. Dev Pharmacol Ther 1992; 18: 9–13.

475. KORCHAGINA VV *et al*. Dental enamel hypoplasia in children with combined congenital and hereditary defects in the development of the CNS and the locomotor system (Infantile cerebral palsy, spinal cord hernias and myopathies). Stomatologiia 1997; 76: 60–4.

476. KOTSANOS N. Prevalence of tetracycline deposits in premolar teeth extracted for orthodontic purposes. Br Dent J 1982; 152: 91–2.

477. KRAUS BS. Calcification of the human deciduous teeth. J Am Dent Assoc 1959; 59: 1128–36.

478. KRESHOVER SJ *et al*. A study of prenatal influences on tooth development in humans. J Am Dent Assoc 1958; 56: 230–48.

479. KROMER B *et al*. Spätfolgen im Zahn- und Mundhöhlenbereich nach antineoplastischer Chemotherapie im Kindesalter. Deutsch Zahnärtzl Zeitschr 2002; 57: 87–95.

480. KRÖNCKE A. Schmelzflecken unter den bedingungen fluoridreicher und fluoridarmer trinkwässer. Dtsch Zahnärztl Z 1979; 34: 714.

481. KRUGER BJ. The effect of different levels of fluoride on the ultra structure of ameloblasts in the rat. Arch Oral Biol 1970; 15: 109–14.

482. KUTSCHER AH *et al*. Discoloration of the teeth induced by tetracycline. J Am Med Assoc 1963; 184: 586–7.

483. KUMAR JV *et al*. Low birth weight and dental fluorosis. J Public Health Dent 2000; 60 (3): 167–71.

484. LAGERSTRÖM M *et al*. A deletion in the amelogenin Gene (AMG) causes X-linked amelogenesis imperfecta (AIH1). Genomics 1991; 10: 971–5.

485. LAGERSTRÖM-FERMÉR M *et al*. Molecular basis and consequences of a deletion in the amelogenin gene, analyzed by capture PCR. Genomics 1993; 17: 89–92.

486. LAMB DJ. The treatment of amelogenesis imperfecta. J Prosthet Dent 1976; 36: 286–91.

487. LAMBERG M *et al*. Symptoms experienced during periods of actual and supposed water fluoridation. Community Dent Oral Epidemiol 1997; 25: 291–5.

488. LAMBROU DB *et al*. In vitro studies of the phenomenon of tetracycline incorporation into enamel. J Dent Res 1977; 56: 1527–32.

489. LANDES CA *et al*. Aspects of oral syphilis. Quint Int 2004; 35: 723–7.

490. LARIK MLMJ *et al*. Regionale odontodysplasie. Ned Tijdschr Tandheelkd 1978; 85: 238–41.

491. LARSEN MJ *et al*. Prevalence of dental fluorosis after fluoride-gel treatments in a low-fluoride area. J Dent Res 1985; 64: 1076–79.

492. LARSEN MJ *et al*. Dental fluorosis among participants in a non-supervised fluoride tablet program. Community Dent Oral Epidemiol 1989; 17: 204–6.

493. LARSEN MJ *et al*. Development of dental fluorosis according to age at start of fluoride administration. Caries Res 1985; 19: 519–27.

494. LARSEN MJ *et al*. Dental fluorosis in the primary and the permanent dentition in fluoridated areas with consumption of either powdered milk or natural cow's milk. J Dent Res 1988; 67: 822–5.

495. LARSON RH *et al*. Effect of tetracycline on the transmission of dental caries in rats. J Dent Res 1961; 40: 264–7.

496. LARSON RH *et al*. Effect of dehydroacetic acid and tetracycline on caries activity and its transmission in the rat. J Dent Res 1963; 42: 95–102.

497. LATIFAH R *et al*. Fluoride levels in mother's milk. J Pedod 1989; 13: 149–54.

498. LATIFAH R *et al*. Fluoride levels in infant formulas. J Pedod 1989; 13: 323–7.

499. LAU EC *et al*. Human and mouse gene loci on the sex chromosomes. Genomics 1989; 4: 162–8.

500. LECOMPTE EJ. Clinical application of topical fluoride products. J Dent Res 1987; 66: 1066–71.

501. LECOMPTE EJ *et al*. Pharmacokinetics of fluoride from APF gel and fluoride tablets in children. J Dent Res 1982; 61: 469–72.

502. LENCH NJ *et al*. DNA diagnosis of X-linked amelogenesis imperfecta (AIH1). J Oral Pathol Med 1997; 26: 135–7.

503. LEONARD M *et al*. Odontodysplasia. J Dent 1972; 1: 43–5.

504. LEVERETT J. Prevalence of dental fluorosis in fluoridated and non-fluoridated communities. J Public Health Dent 1986; 46 (4): 184–7.

505. LEVIN LS *et al*. Scanning electron microscopy of teeth in dominant osteogenesis imperfecta: support for genetic heterogeneity. Am J Med Genet 1980; 5: 189–99.

506. LEVIN LS *et al*. Classification of osteogenesis imperfecta by dental characteristics. Lancet 1978; I: 332–3.

507. LEVINE RS *et al*. A photographically recorded assessment of enamel hypoplasia in fluoridated and non-fluoridated areas in England. Br Dent J 1989; 166: 249–52.

508. LEVINE RS *et al*. Neonatal enamel hypoplasia in association with symptomatic neonatal hypocalcaemia. Br Dent J 1974; 137: 429–33.

509. LEVITON A *et al*. Children with hypoplastic enamel defects of primary incisors are not at increased risk of learning-problem syndromes. ASDC J Dent Child 1994; 61: 35–8.

510. LEVY FM *et al*. Nails as biomarkers of fluoride in children of fluoridated communities. J Dent Child 2004; 71: 121–5.

511. LEVY SM. A review of fluoride intake from fluoride dentifrice. ASDC J Dent Child 1993; 60: 115–24.

512. LEVY SM *et al*. Total fluoride intake and implications for dietary fluoride supplementation. J Public Health Dent 1999; 59: 211–23.

513. LEVY SM *et al*. Primary tooth fluorosis and fluoride intake during the first year of life. Community Dent Oral Epidemiol 2002; 30: 286–95.

514. LEWIS DB *et al*. Water fluoridation: current effectiveness and dental fluorosis. Community Dent Oral Epidemiol 1994; 22: 153–8.

515. LEWIS DB *et al*. Recommendations regarding total daily fluoride intake for Canadians. J Can Dent Assoc 1994; 60: 1050–60.

516. LEWIS HA *et al*. Fluorosis and dental caries in schoolchildren from rural areas with about 9 and 1 ppm F in the water supplies. Community Dent Oral Epidemiol 1992; 20: 53–4.

517. LI R, LI W *et al*. Alternative splicing of amelogenin mRNA from rat incisor ameloblasts. J Dent Res 1995; 74: 1880–5.

518. LI Y *et al*. Prevalence and distribution of developmental enamel defects in primary dentition of Chinese children 3–5 years old. Community Dent Oral Epidemiol 1995; 23: 72–9.

519. LIMEBACK H. Enamel formation and the effects of fluoride. Community Dent Oral Epidemiol 1994; 22: 144–7.

520. LIMEBACK H *et al*. The effects of hypocalcemia/ hypophosphatemia on porcine bone and dental hard tissues in

an inherited form of Type 1 pseudo-vitamin D deficiency rickets. J Dent Res 1992; 71: 346–52.

521. LINDAU BM *et al.* Morphology of dental enamel and dentine-enamel junction in osteogenesis imperfecta. Int J Paediatr Dent 1999; 9: 13–21.

522. LINDAU B *et al.* Discrimination of morphological findings in dentine from osteogenesis imperfecta patients using combinations of polarized light microscopy, microradiography and scanning electron microscopy. Int J Paediatr Dent 1999; 9: 253–61.

523. LISTGARTEN MA. A mineralized cuticular structure with connective tissue characteristics on the crowns of human unerupted teeth in amelogenesis imperfecta. Arch Oral Biol 1967; 12: 877–9.

524. LO ECM *et al.* Relationship between the presence of demarcated opacities and hypoplasia in permanent teeth and caries in their primary predecessors. Caries Res 2003; 37: 456–61.

525. LO GL *et al.* Prevalence of dental fluorosis in children in Singapore. Community Dent Oral Epidemiol 1996; 24: 25–7.

526. LOGAN J *et al.* Dentinal dysplasia. Oral Surg 1962; 15: 317–33.

527. LOZUPONE E *et al.* Morphometric analysis of the deposition and mineralisation of enamel and dentine from rat incisor during the recovery phase following a low-calcium regimen. Arch Oral Biol 1994; 39: 409–16.

528. LOWE O *et al.* Generalized odontodysplasia. J Pedod 1985; 9: 232–3.

529. LUDER HU *et al.* Mild dental findings associated with severe osteogeneis imnperfecta due to a point mutation in the (2(I) collagen gene demonstrate different expression of the genetic defect in bone and teeth. J Craniofac Genet Dev Biol 1996; 16: 156–63.

530. LUFFINGHAM JK *et al.* Dentinal dysplasia. Br Dent J 1986; 160: 281–3.

531. LUKACS JR *et al.* Epidemiology of enamel hypoplasia in deciduous teeth. J Hum Biol 2001; 13: 788–807.

532. LUKINMAA P-L *et al.* A novel type of developmental dentin defect. J Craniofac Genet Dev Biol 1996; 16: 218–27.

533. LUKINMAA P-L *et al.* Dental findings in osteogenesis imperfecta: I. J Craniofac Genet Dev Biol 1987; 7: 115–25.

534. LUKINMAA P-L *et al.* ED-A region-containing isoform of cellular fibronectin is present in dentin matrix in dentinogenesis imperfecta associated with osteogenesis imperfecta. J Dent Res 1994; 73: 1187–96.

535. LUNDSTRÖM R *et al.* Dental development in children following maternal rubella. Acta Pediatr 1962; 51: 155–60.

536. LUNIN M *et al.* The etiology of regional odontodysplasia. J Dent Res 1976; 55 (II): 189.

537. LUSTMANN J *et al.* Odontodysplasia. Oral Surg 1975; 39: 781–93.

538. LUZZI V *et al.* Case report: clinical management of hypoplastic amelogenesis imperfecta. Eur J Paediatr Dent 2003; 4: 149–54.

539. LYGAIDAKIS NA *et al.* Evaluation of composite restorations in hypomineralised permanent molars. Eur J Paediatr Dent 2003; 4: 143–8.

540. LYKOGEORGOS T *et al.* Unusual manifestations in X-linked amelogenesis imperfecta. Int J Paediatr Dent 2003; 13: 356–61.

541. MaCDONALD-JANKOWSKI DS. Multiple dental developmental anomalies. Dentomaxillofac Radiol 1991; 20: 166–8.

542. MacDOUGALL M. Dental structural diseases mapping to human chromosome 4q21. Connect Tissue Res 2003; 44 (suppl 1): 285–91.

543. MacDOUGALL M *et al.* Genetic linkage of dentinogenesis imperfecta type III locus to chromosome 4q. J Dent Res 1999; 78: 1277–82.

544. MacDOUGALL M *et al.* MEPE/OF45, a new bone/dentin matrix protein and candidate gene for dentin diseases mapping to chromosome 4q21. Connect Tissue Res 2002; 43: 320–30.

545. MacDOUGALL M *et al.* Dentin phosphoprotein gene locus is not associated with dentinogenesis imperfecta types II and III. Am J Hum Genet 1992; 50: 190–4.

546. MAGLIOLA L *et al.* Vitamin D metabolites do not alter parathyroid hormone secretion acutely. Bone Miner 1986; 1: 495–505.

547. MAHONEY EK *et al.* Mechanical properties across hypomineralizes/hypoplastic enamel of first permanent molar teeth. Eur J Oral Sci 2004; 112: 497–502.

548. MAHONEY EK *et al.* Opalescent dentine in two affected siblings. N Z Dent J 2001; 97: 15–18.

549. MÄKI M *et al.* Dental enamel defects in first-degree relatives of coeliac disease patients. Lancet 1991; 337: 763–4.

550. MÄKITIE O *et al.* Early treatment improves growth and biochemical and radiographic outcome in X-linked hypophosphatemic rickets. J Clin Endocrinol Metab 2003; 88: 3591–7.

551. MÄKITIE O *et al.* Prolonged high-dose phosphate treatment: a risk factor for tertiary hyperparathyroidism in X–linked hypophosphatemic rickets. Clin Endocrinol 2003; 58: 163–8.

552. MALCOLM A *et al.* Bone resorption and serum levels of vitamin D metabolites in the hypophosphataemic rat. Aust Dent J 1997; 42: 118–20.

553. MALMGREN B *et al.* Dentinogenesis imperfecta in a six- generation family. Swed Dent J 1988; 12: 73–84.

554. MALMGREN B *et al.* Dental aberrations in children and adolescents with osteogenesis imperfecta. Acta Odontol Scand 2002; 60: 65–71.

555. MALMGREN B *et al.* Assessment of dysplastic dentin in osteogenesis imperfecta and dentinogenesis imperfecta. Acta Odontol Scand 2003; 61: 72–80.

556. MAMELE N *et al.* Risk-benefit ratio of sodium fluoride treatment in primary vertebral osteoporosis. Lancet 1988; 2: 361–5.

557. MANJI F *et al.* Dental fluorosis in an area of Kenya with 2 ppm fluoride in the drinking water. J Dent Res 1986; 65: 659–62.

558. MANN J *et al.* Fluorosis and caries prevalence in a community drinking above-optimal fluoridated water. Community Dent Oral Epidemiol 1987; 15: 293–5.

559. MARIANI P *et al.* Coeliac disease, enamel defects and HLA typing. Acta Paediatr 1994; 83: 1272–5.

560. MARIÑO R *et al*. Prevalence of fluorosis in children aged 6–9 years-old who participated in a milk fluoridation programme in Codegua, Chile. Community Dent Health 2003; 20: 143–8.

561. MARKS SC *et al*. Dental and cephalometric findings in vitamin D resistant rickets. ASDC J Dent Child 1965; 32: 259–65.

562. MARS M *et al*. Dentinogenesis imperfecta. Br Dent J 1976; 140: 206–9.

563. MARSLAND EA *et al*. Intrinsic staining of teeth following icterus gravis. Br Dent J 1953; 94: 305–10.

564. MARSHALL JA. Dental hypoplasia. J Am Dent Assoc 1936; 23: 2074–81.

565. MARTIN JK *et al*. A study of the clinical history, tooth enamel and dermal patterns in 175 cases of cerebral palsy. Guy's Hospital Rep 1960; 109: 139–46.

566. MARTINEZ A *et al*. Prevalence of developmental defects in mentally retarded children. ASDC J Dent Child 2002; 69: 151–5.

567. MARQUES AC *et al*. Regional dysplasia. Br Dent J 1999; 186: 522–4.

568. MASCARENHAS AK *et al*. Fluorosis risk from early exposure to fluoride toothpaste. Community Dent Oral Epidemiol 1998; 26: 241–8.

569. MATTHEWS SJ *et al*. Thalidomide. Clin Ther 2003; 342–95.

570. MAUPOMÉ G *et al*. Socio-demographic features and fluoride technologies contributing to higher fluorosis scores in permanent teeth of Canadian children. Caries Res 2003; 37: 327–34.

571. McCALL DR *et al*. Fluoride ingestion following APF gel application. Br Dent J 1983; 155: 333–6.

572. McCORMICK J *et al*. Injury to the teeth of succession by abscess of the temporary teeth. ASDC J Dent Child 1967; 34: 501–4.

573. McFARLANE MW *et al*. Dentinal dysplasia. J Oral Surg 1974; 32: 867–9.

574. MACFAYDEN EE *et al*. Fluoride content of some bottled spring waters. Br Dent J 1982; 153: 423–4.

575. McDONNELL M *et al*. Hydrops fetalis due to ABO incompatibility. Arch Dis Child Neonatal Ed 1998; 78: F220–1.

576. McINNES PM *et al*. Comparison of dental fluorosis and caries in primary teeth of pre-school children living in arid high and low fluoride villages. Community Dent Oral Epidemiol 1982; 10; 182–6.

577. McKNIGHT-HANES MC *et al*. Fluoride content of infant formulas: soy-based formulas as a potential factor in dental fluorosis. Pediatr Dent 1988; 10: 189–94.

578. McLARTY EL *et al*. X-linked hypomaturation type of amelogenesis imperfecta exhibiting lyonization in affected females. Oral Surg 1973; 36: 678–85.

579. McLURE FJ. Ingestion of fluoride and dental caries. Quantitative relations based on food and water requirements of children 1–12-years-old. Am J Dis Child 1943; 66: 262–9.

580. McMILLAN RS *et al*. Relation of human abnormalities of structure and function to abnormalities of the dentition. I. Relation of hypoplasia of enamel to cerebral and ocular disorders. J Am Dent Assoc 1961; 63: 38–48.

581. McMILLAN RS *et al*. Relation of human abnormalities of structure and function to abnormalities of the dentition. III. Relation of enamel hypoplasia to epilepsy and to diagnoses associated with Rh factor. J Am Dent Assoc 1961; 63: 497–502.

582. McNALLY M *et al*. The ethics of water fluoridation. J Can Dent Assoc 2000; 66: 592–3.

583. McWHORTER AG *et al*. Prevalence of dental abscess in a population of children with vitamin D-resistant rickets. Paediatr Dent 1991; 13: 91–6.

584. MEIJER VAN PUTTEN B. Coeliakie bij volwassenen, veel ernstiger dan buikpijn. Synaps 2003; 46: 10–11.

585. MELAMED Y *et al*. Conservative multidisciplinary treatment approach in an unusual odontodysplasia. ASDC J Dent Child 1994; 61: 119–24.

586. MELLANBY M. The effect of diet on the structure of teeth. The inter-relationship between the calcium and other food factors. Br Dent J 1923; 44: 1031–49.

587. MELLANBY M. The structure of dental tissues with special reference to some stages in the development of normal and hypoplastic enamel. Br Dent J 1937; 63: 557–68.

588. MELLANDER M *et al*. Mineralization defects in deciduous teeth of low birthweight infants. Acta Pediatr Scand 1982; 71: 727–33.

589. MELLBERG JR *et al*. Fluoride in preventive dentistry. Chicago, IL: Quintessence Publishing, 1983.

590. MELLO HS. The mechanism of tetracycline staining in primary and permanent teeth. ASDC J Dent Child 1967; 34: 478–87.

591. MELNICK M *et al*. Dentin dysplasia, type II. Oral Surg 1977; 44: 592–99.

592. MELNICK M *et al*. Dentin dysplasia type I. Oral Surg 1980; 50: 335–9.

593. MENEZES DM. Opacities and hypoplasia in the enamel of Burmese children from a low fluoride area. J Dent 1975; 4: 71–2.

594. MESKIN LH. Much ado about nothing. J Am Dent Assoc 1997; 128: 1347–8.

595. MESSER HH *et al*. Influence of fluoride intake on reproduction in mice. J Nutr 1973; 103: 1319–26.

596. MIERS DR *et al*. Dentinal dysplasia, type I. ASDC J Dent Child 1990; 57: 299–302.

597. MILES DA *et al*. Hemimaxillofacial dysplasia: a newly recognized disorder of facial asymmetry, hypertrichosis of the facial skin, and hypoplastic teeth in two patients. Oral Surg Oral Med Oral Pathol 1987; 64: 445–8.

598. MILLER J. Tetracyclines and yellow teeth. Lancet 1962; I: 861–2.

599. MILLER J. Tetracycline in teeth and bone. Lancet 1962; I: 1072.

600. MILLER J *et al*. Neonatal enamel hypoplasia associated with haemolytic disease and with prematurity. Br Dent J 1959; 106: 93–104.

601. MILLER WA *et al*. Odontodysplasia. Br Dent J 1968; 125 (I): 56–9.

602. MILLER WA *et al*. Dentinogenesis imperfecta traceable through five generations of a part American Indian family. Oral Surg 1973; 35: 180–6.

603. MILSOM KM *et al.* Enamel defects in the deciduous dentition as a potential predictor of defects in the permanent dentition of 8- and 9-year-old children in fluoridated Cheshire, England. J Dent Res 1996; 75: 1015–18.

604. MINICUCCI EM *et al.* Dental abnormalities in children after chemotherapy treatment for acute lymphoid leukaemia. Leukemia Res 2003; 27: 45–50.

605. MOBLEY JA *et al.* Risk factors for congenital syphilis in infants of women with syphilis in South Carolina. Am J Public Health 1998; 88: 597–602.

606. MOCK D *et al.* Familial amelodentinal dysplasia. Oral Surg 1986; 61: 485–91.

607. MOLINARI JA *et al.* Herpes viruses, manifestations and transmission. J Can Dent Assoc 1989; 55: 24–31.

608. MÖLLER IJ *et al.* The prevalence of dental fluorosis in the people of Uganda. Arch Oral Biol 1970; 15: 213–25.

609. MONSOUR FNT *et al.* Aberrations involving the enamel epithelium in transplanted developing teeth. J Oral Maxillofac Surg 1983; 41: 377–84.

610. MOORE RS *et al.* A classification of medically handicapping conditions and the health risks they present in the dental care of children – I. J Paediatr Dent 1989; 5: 73–83.

611. MOORE RS *et al.* A classification of medically handicapping conditions and the health risks they present in the dental care of children – Part II. J Paediatr Dent 1990; 6: 1–14.

612. MORFIS AS. Enamel hypoplasia of a maxillary central incisor. Endod Dent Traumatol 1989; 5: 204–6.

613. MORGANTINI J *et al.* Traumatism dentaires chez l'enfant en âge préscolaire et répercussions sur les dents permanentes. Rev Mens Suisse Odonto-stomatol 1986; 96: 37–40.

614. MORTON ME. Excessive bleeding after surgery in osteogenesis imperfecta. Br J Oral Maxillofac Surg 1987; 25: 507–11.

615. MUNRO ND *et al.* Temporal relations between maternal rubella and congenital defects. Lancet 1987; II: 201–4.

616. MURPHY DJ *et al.* Case-control study of antenatal and intrapartum risk factors for cerebral palsy in very preterm singleton babies. Lancet 1995; 346: 1499–54.

617. MURRAY JJ. Appropriate use of fluorides for human health. Geneva: World Health Organization, 1986.

618. MURRAY JJ *et al.* Fluorides in caries prevention. Bristol: Wright, PSG, 1982.

619. MURRAY JJ *et al.* Classification and prevalence of enamel opacities in the human deciduous and permanent dentitions. Arch Oral Biol 1979; 24: 7–13.

620. MYERS HM. Dose-response relationship between water fluoride levels and the category of questionable dental fluorosis. Community Dent Oral Epidemiol 1983; 11: 109–12.

621. NAGAI I *et al.* Early influence of polyoma virus on transplanted tooth germs. J Dent Res 1963; 42: 1131–9.

622. NAKATA M *et al.* Interadicular dentin dysplasia associated with amelogenesis imperfecta. Oral Surg 1985; 60: 182–7.

623. NALBANDIAN J. The microscopic pattern of tetracycline fluorescence in the cementum of human teeth. J Biol Buccale 1978; 6: 27–41.

624. NANCI A *et al.* Morphological and immunocytochemical analyses on the effects of diet-induced hypocalcemia on enamel maturation in the rat incisor. J Histochem Cytochem 2000; 48: 1043–58.

625. NARANG A *et al.* Oral health and related factors in cystic fibrosis and other chronic respiratory disorders. Arch Dis Child 2003; 88: 702–7.

626. NAVIA JM. Nutrition in dental development and disease. Hum Nutr 1979; 1: 333–62.

627. NAVIA JM *et al.* Organ culture study of effect of vitamin-A-deficiency on rat third molar development. Arch Oral Biol 1984; 29: 911–20.

628. NEEDLEMAN HL *et al.* Macroscopic enamel defects of primary anterior teeth. Pediatr Dent 1991; 13: 208–16.

629. NELSON JF *et al.* Dental changes in familial idiopathic hypothyroidism. J Oral Med 1978; 33: 115–19.

630. NEUPERT EA *et al.* Regional odontodysplasia presenting as a soft tissue swelling. Oral Surg Oral Med Oral Pathol 1989; 67: 193–6.

631. NEVITT GA *et al.* Occurrence of nonfluoride opacities and nonfluoride hypoplasias in 588 children ages 9 to 14 years. J Am Dent Assoc 1963; 66: 65–9.

632. NEWBRUN E. Fluorides and dental caries. Springfield, IL: Charles C. Thomas, 1978.

633. NG'ANG'A PM *et al.* Prevalence and severity of dental fluorosis in primary schoolchildren in Nairobi, Kenya. Community Dent Oral Epidemiol 1993; 21: 15–18.

634. NIEGEL S. Die Odontodysplasie. Kasuistik einer asymmetrischen Hypoplasie der Zähne beider Dentitionen im linken Oberkieferquadranten. Dtsch Zahnaerztl Z 1972; 27: 434–9.

635. NIKIFORUK G *et al.* Etiology of enamel hypoplasia and interglobular dentin: the roles of hypocalcemia and hypophosphatemia. Metab Bone Dis Rel Res 1979; 2: 17–23.

636. NORDLUND AL *et al.* Fluoride-induced cystic changes in the enamel organ of the rat molar. J Oral Pathol 1986; 15: 87–92.

637. NORÉN JG. Enamel structure in deciduous teeth from low-birth-weight infants. Acta Odontol Scand 1983; 41: 355–62.

638. NORÉN JG. Microscopic study of enamel defects in deciduous teeth of infants of diabetic mothers. Acta Odontol Scand 1984; 42: 153–6.

639. NORÉN JG *et al.* Congenital hypothyroidism and changes in the enamel of deciduous teeth. Acta Pediatr Scand 1983; 72: 485–9.

640. NORÉN JG *et al.* Mineralization disturbances in the deciduous teeth of children with so called minimal brain dysfunction. Swed Dent J 1987; 11: 37–43.

641. NORÉN J *et al.* Maternal diabetes and changes in the hard tissues of primary teeth. III. Acta Odontol Scand 1978; 36: 127–35.

642. NUTRITIONAL REVIEW. Protein deficiency and tooth and salivary gland development. Nutr Rev 1974: 32:24–27.

643. NUNN JH *et al.* Distribution of developmental defects of enamel on ten tooth surfaces in children aged 12 years living in areas receiving different water fluoride levels in Sri Lanka and England. Community Dent Health 1993; 10: 259–68.

644. NUNN JH *et al*. The prevalence of developmental defects of enamel in 15–16-year-old children residing in three districts (natural fluoride, adjusted fluoride, low fluoride) in the North East of England. Community Dent Health 1992; 9: 235–47.

645. NUNN JH *et al*. Prevalence of developmental defects of enamel in areas with differing water fluoride levels and socio-economic groups in Sri Lanka and England. Int Dent J 1994; 44: 165–73.

646. O CARROLL MK *et al*. Dentin dysplasia type I. Oral Surg Oral Med Oral Pathol 1994; 78: 375–81.

647. O CARROLL MK *et al*. Dentin dysplasia: review of the literature and a proposed subclassification based on radiographic findings. Oral Surg Oral Pathol Oral Med 1991; 72: 119–25.

648. OCHI M *et al*. TEM study of enamel hypoplasia in offspring of diabetic rats experimentally-induced by streptozotocin. Pediatr Dent J 1997; 7: 81–95.

649. O'CONNELL AC *et al*. Evaluation of oral problems in an osteogenesis imperfecta population. Oral Surg Oral Med Oral Pathol Oral Radiol Endod 1999; 87: 189–96.

650. O'CARROLL MK *et al*. Dentin dysplasia: review of the literature and a proposed subclassification based on radiographic findings. Oral Surg Oral Med Oral Pathol 1991; 72: 119–25.

651. OERTEL JE *et al*. Parathyroid glands. In: ANDERSON WAD (ed.) Pathology. Volume 2. St Louis, MO: CV Mosby, 1971.

652. OGŬZ A *et al*. Long-term effects of chemotherapy on orodental structures in children with non-Hodgkin's lymphoma. Eur J Oral Sci 2004; 112: 8–11.

653. OLIVER WJ *et al*. Hypoplastic enamel associated with the nephrotic syndrome. Pediatr 1963; 32: 399–405.

654. OLSSON B. Dental caries and fluorosis in Arussi province, Ethiopia. Community Dent Oral Epidemiol 1978; 6: 338–43.

655. O'MULLANE DM *et al*. A three-year clinical trial of a combination of trimetaphosphate and sodium fluoride in silica toothpastes. J Dent Res 1997; 76: 1776–81.

656. O'MULLANE DM *et al*. Fluoride ingestion from toothpaste: conclusions of European Union-funded multicentre project. Community Dent Oral Epidemiol 2004, 32 (suppl 1): 74–6.

657. O'NEIL DW *et al*. Regional odontodysplasia. ASDC J Dent Child 1990; 57: 459–61.

658. ONLINE MENDELIAN INHERITANCE IN MAN (OMIM™). McKusick-Nathans Institute for Genetic Medicine, John Hopkins University (Baltimore, MD) and National Center for Biotechnology Information, National Library of Medicine (Bethesda, MD). Available at: www.ncbi.nlm.nih.gov/omim/.

659. ONORATO IM *et al*. Epidemiology of cytomegaloviral infections: recommendations for prevention and control. Rev Infect Dis 1985; 7: 479–97.

660. OOË T *et al*. The development of the human interradicular dentine as revealed by tetracycline-labelling. Arch Oral Biol 1984; 29: 257–62.

661. OOË T *et al*. Differential termination times of enamel formation on human deciduous anterior-tooth surfaces revealed by tetracycline labelling. Arch Oral Biol 1985; 30: 409–14.

662. OOYA K *et al*. Autosomal recessive rough hypoplastic amelogenesis imperfecta. Oral Surg Oral Med Oral Pathol 1988; 65: 449–58.

663. OPINYA GN *et al*. Fluorosis of deciduous teeth and permanent molars in rural Kenyan community. Acta Odontol Scand 1991; 49: 197–202.

664. ORUP HI *et al*. Craniofacial skeletal deviations following in utero exposure to the anticonvulsant phenytoin: monotherapy and polytherapy. Orthod Craniofac Res 2003; 6: 2–19.

665. OSUJI OO *et al*. A review of differential diagnosis of dental fluorosis and non-fluoride enamel defects. J Can Dent Assoc 1988; 54: 743–7.

666. OWEN LN. Fluorescence of tetracyclines in bone tumors, normal bone and teeth. Nature 1961; 190: 500–2.

667. OWEN LN. The effects of administering tetracyclines to young dogs with particular reference to localization of the drugs in the teeth. Arch Oral Biol 1963; 8: 715–27.

668. OZBEK M *et al*. Effects of pregnancy on the microhardness of rat incisor dentine and enamel. Arch Oral Biol 2004; 49: 607–12.

669. ÖZER L *et al*. Regional odontodysplasia. J Clin Pediatr Dent 2004; 29: 45–8.

670. ÖZKAN S *et al*. Dental manifestations of familial hypophosphatemic vitamin–D–resistant rickets. ASDC J Dent Child 1984; 51: 448–50.

671. OZOLEK JA *et al*. Prevalence and lack of clinical significance of blood group incompatibility in mothers with blood type A or B. J Pediatr 1994; 125: 87–91.

672. PACKOTA GV *et al*. Radiographic features of segmental odontomaxillary dysplasia: study of 12 cases. Oral Surg Oral Med Oral Pathol Oral Radiol Endod 1996; 82: 577–84.

673. PAJARI U *et al*. Prevalence and location of enamel opacities in children after anti-neoplastic therapy. Community Dent Oral Epidemiol 1998; 16: 222–6.

674. PANDIS N *et al*. Regional odontodysplasia, a case associated with asymmetric maxillary and mandibular development. Oral Surg Oral Med Oral Pathol 1991; 72: 492–6.

675. PAPAGERAKIS P *et al*. Differential epithelial and mesenchymal regulation of tooth-specific matrix proteins expression by 1,25-dihydroxivitamin D3 in vivo. Connect Tissue Res 2002; 43: 372–5.

676. PARKER JL *et al*. Hypoplastic-hypomaturation amelogenesis imperfecta with taurodontism. ASDC J Dent Child 1975; 42: 379–83.

677. PARTANEN AM *et al*. Epidermal growth factor receptor as a mediator of developmental toxicity of dioxin in mouse embryonic teeth. Lab Invest 1998; 78: 1473–81.

678. PENDRYS DG. Dental fluorosis in perspective. J Am Dent Assoc 1991; 122: 63–6.

679. PENNA KJ *et al*. Prevention of microstomia following facial burns. Br J Oral Maxillofac Surg 1998; 36: 146–7.

680. PEREIRA AC *et al*. Dental caries and fluorosis prevalence study in a nonfluoridated Barzilian community: trend

analysis and toothpaste association. ASDC J Dent Child 2000; 67: 132–5.

681. PEREIRA CM *et al.* Dental alterations associated with X-linked hypophosphatemic rickets. J Endod 2004; 30: 241–5.

682. PERL T *et al.* Radicular (type I) dentin dysplasia. Oral Surg 1977; 43: 746–53.

683. PERSSON M *et al.* Facial morphology and open bite deformity in amelogenesis imperfecta. Acta Odontol Scand 1982; 40: 135–44.

684. PETERSEN K *et al.* Recent findings in classification of osteogenesis imperfecta by means of existing dental symptoms. ASDC J Dent Child 1998; 65: 305–9.

685. PETERSSON A. A case of dentinal dysplasia and/or calcification of the dentinal papilla. Oral Surg 1972; 33: 1014–17.

686. PETERSSON LG. Fluorine gradients in outermost surface enamel after various forms of topical application of fluorides in vivo. Odontol Revy 1976; 27: 25–50.

687. PETRONE JA *et al.* Dentin dysplasia type I. J Am Dent Assoc 1981; 103: 891–3.

688. PETTIETTE MT *et al.* Dentinogenesis imperfecta: endodontic implications. Oral Surg Oral Med Oral Pathol Oral Radiol Endod 1998; 86: 733–7.

689. PETTIFOR JM *et al.* Endemic skeletal fluorosis in children: hypocalcemia and the presence of renal resistance to parathyroid hormone. Bone Miner 1989; 7: 275–88.

690. PEUCKMANN V *et al.* Neue Indikation für Thalidomid in der Schmerztherapie. Schmerz 2003; 17: 204–10.

691. PIMLOT JFL *et al.* Enamel defects in prematurely born, low-weight infants. Pediatr Dent 1985; 7: 218–23.

692. PINDBORG JJ. Pathology of the dental hard tissues. Copenhagen: Munksgaard, 1970.

693. PINDBORG JJ. Aetiology of developmental enamel defects not related to fluorosis. Int Dent J 1982; 32: 123–34.

694. PINKHAM JR *et al.* Odontodysplasia. Oral Surg 1973; 36: 841–50.

695. PINTO A *et al.* Management of patients with thyroid disease. J Am Dent Assoc 2002; 133: 849–58.

696. PISANTI S *et al.* Familial hypoparathyreoidism with candidasis and mental retardation. Oral Surg 1977; 44: 374–83.

697. POLEY A *et al.* Untersuchungen zu den Spätfolgen der Kiefer-osteomyelitis im Kindesalter. Dtsch Zahnaerztl Z 1967; 22: 647.

698. POLIAK SC *et al.* Minocycline-associated discoloration in young adults. J Am Med Assoc 1985; 254: 2930–2.

699. PORTEOUS JR *et al.* Tetracyclines and yellow teeth. Lancet 1962; I: 861.

700. PRICE JA *et al.* Identification of a mutation in DLX3 associated with tricho-dento-osseous (TDO) syndrome. Hum Mol Genet 1998; 7: 563–9.

701. PRIME SS *et al.* Effect of prolonged iron deficiency on enamel pigmentation and tooth structure in rat incisors. Arch Oral Biol 1984; 29: 905–9.

702. PRIMOSCH RE. Tetracycline discoloration, enamel defects, and dental caries in patients with cystic fibrosis. Oral Surg 1980; 50: 301–8.

703. PRUSACK N *et al.* Segmental odontomaxillary dysplasia. A case report and review of the literature. Oral Surg Oral Med Oral Pathol Oral Radiol Endod 2000; 90: 483–8.

704. PUNYASINGH JT *et al.* Effects of vitamin A deficiency on rat incisor formation. J Oarl Pathol 1984; 13: 40–51.

705. PURVIS RJ *et al.* Enamel hypoplasia of the teeth associated with neonatal tetany: a manifestation of maternal vitamin-D deficiency. Lancet 1973; II: 811–14.

706. PUTKONEN T. Dental changes in congenital syphilis. Acta Derm Venereol 1962; 42: 44–62.

707. REISEL JH. Klinische osteoporose en parodontopathie. Ned Tijdschr Tandheelkd 1971; 78: 132–5.

708. RABER-DURLACHER JE *et al.* Renale osteodystrofie. II. Ned Tijdschr Geneeskd 1983; 127: 1578–84.

709. RAJPAR MH *et al.* Mutation of the signal peptide region of the bicistronic gene *DSPP* affects translocation to the endoplasmic reticulum and results in defective dentine biomineralization. Hum Mol Genet 2002; 11: 2559–65.

710. RAKOCZ M *et al.* Management of the primary dentition in vitamin D-resistant rickets. Oral Surg Oral Med Oral Pathol 1982; 54: 166–71.

711. RAEZ AG. Unilateral regional odontodysplasia with ipsilateral mandibular malformation. Oral Surg Oral Med Oral Pathol 1990; 69: 720–2.

712. RAMP WK *et al.* Interrelationships of vitamin D, bone metabolism and blood calcium concentration in the chick. Bone Miner 1989; 5: 117–28.

713. RAMSEY AC *et al.* Fluoride intakes and caries increments in relation to tea consumption by British children. Caries Res 1975; 9: 312.

714. RANGGÅRD L *et al.* Effect of hypocalcemic state on enamel formation in rat maxillary incisors. Scand J Dent Res 1994; 102: 249–53.

715. RANGGÅRD L *et al.* Clinical and histologic appearance in enamel of primary teeth from children with neonatal hypocalcemia induced by blood exchange transfusion. Acta Odontol Scand 1995; 30: 123–8.

716. RANKOW H *et al.* Dentin dysplasia. J Endod 1984; 10: 384–6.

717. RANTA H *et al.* Dentin dysplasia Type II: absence of type III collagen in dentin. J Oral Pathol Med 1990; 19: 160–5.

718. RANTA H *et al.* Heritable dentin defects. Am J Med Genet 1993; 45: 193–200.

719. RAO SR *et al.* Pulpal dysplasia. Oral Surg 1970; 30: 682–9.

720. RASMUSSEN ST. Fracture properties of human teeth in proximity to the dentinoenamel junction. J Dent Res 1984; 63: 1279–83.

721. RASMUSSON CG *et al.* Celiac disease and mineralisation disturbances of permanent teeth. Int J Paediatr Dent 2001; 11: 179–83.

722. RATTNER LJ *et al.* Occurrence of enamel hypoplasia in children with congenital allergies. Oral Surg 1962; 41: 646–9.

723. READE PC *et al.* Regional dysplasia. Aust Dent J 1974; 19: 152–61.

724. REBICH T *et al.* The St. Regis environmental health issue: assessment of dental defects. J Am Dent Assoc 1983; 106: 630–3.

725. REBICH T *et al*. Dental caries and tetracycline-stained dentition in an American Indian population. J Dent Res 1985; 64: 462–4.

726. REED MW. Clinical evaluation of three concentrations of sodium fluoride in dentifrices. J Am Dent Assoc 1973; 87: 1401–3.

727. REEVER JS *et al*. Unilateral maxillary odontodysplasia. ASDC J Dent Child 1971; 38: 23–8.

728. RENK A. Dentinogenesis imperfecta. Quintessenz 1990; 41: 441–452.

729. RICHARDS A *et al*. Enamel fluoride in relation to severity of human dental fluorosis. Adv Dent Res 1989; 3: 147–53.

730. RICHARDS A *et al*. Pharmacokinetics of chronic fluoride ingestion in growing pigs. J Dent Res 1985; 64: 425–30.

731. RICHARDS A *et al*. Fluoride concentrations in unerupted fluorotic human enamel. Caries Res 1992; 26: 328–32.

732. RICHARDS LF *et al*. Determining optimum fluoride levels for community water supplies in relation to temperature. J Am Dent Assoc 1967; 74: 389–97.

733. RICHARDS LF *et al*. Nonfluoride enamel hypoplasia in varying fluoride-temperature zones. J Am Dent Assoc 1967; 75: 1412–18.

734. RICHARDSON AS *et al*. Anomalous dysplasia of dentine. J Can Dent Assoc 1970; 36: 189–91.

735. RIORDAN PJ. Dental fluorosis, dental caries and fluoride exposure among 7-year-olds. Caries Res 1993; 27: 71–7.

736. RIORDAN PJ. Dental fluorosis decline after changes to supplement and toothpaste regimens. Community Dent Oral Epidemiol 2002; 30: 233–40.

737. RIPA LW. Topical fluorides: a discussion of risks and benefits. J Dent Res 1987; 66: 1079–83.

738. RISNES S. Rationale for consistency in the use of enamel surface terms: perikymata and imbrications. Scand J Dent Res 1984; 92: 1–5.

739. RITCHIE GM. Dental manifestations of pseudohypoparathyroidism. Arch Dis Child 1965; 40: 565–72.

740. ROBERTS E *et al*. Hereditary opalescent dentine (dentinogenesis imperfecta). Am J Orthod 1939; 25: 267–76.

741. ROBINSON PB *et al*. The effects of diphenylhydantoin and vitamin D deficiency on developing teeth in the rat. Arch Oral Biol 1978; 23: 137–43.

742. ROSENBLUM FN. Odontodysplasia. ASDC J Dent Child 1971; 38: 327–30.

743. ROSENZWEIG KA *et al*. Enamel hypoplasia and dental caries in the primary dentition of prematuri. Br Dent J 1962; 113: 279–80.

744. ROTHMAN DL. Pediatric orofacial injuries. J Cal Dent Assoc 1996; 24 (3): 37–42.

745. ROTHMAN KJ *et al*. Teratogenecity of high vitamin A intake. N Engl J Med 1995; 333: 1369–73.

746. ROTHSCHILD BM *et al*. First European exposure to syphilis: the Dominican Republic at the time of Columbian contact. Clin Infect Dis 2000; 31: 936–41.

747. ROZIER RG *et al*. Dental fluorosis in children exposed to multiple sources of fluoride: implications for school fluoridation programs. Public Health Rep 1981; 96: 542–6.

748. RUBINGER D *et al*. 24,25(OH)$_2$D$_3$ affects the calcemic effects of 1,25 (OH)$_2$D$_3$ by mechanisms independent of intestinal calcium absorption. Bone Miner 1991; 5: 219–26.

749. RUBINOFF AB *et al*. Vitamin C and oral health. J Can Dent Assoc 1989; 55: 705–7.

750. RUGG-GUNN AJ *et al*. Effect of fluoride level in drinking water, nutritional status, and socio-economic status on the prevalence of developmental defects of dental enamel in permanent teeth in Saudi 14 year old boys. Caries Res 1997; 31: 259–67.

751. RUGG-GUNN AJ *et al*. Malnutrition and developmental defects of enamel in 2- to 6-year-old Saudi boys. Caries Res 1998; 32: 181–92.

752. RUGG-GUNN AJ *et al*. The water intake of 405 Northumbrian adolescents aged 12–14 years. Br Dent J 1987; 162: 335–40.

753. RUIKEN HMHM *et al*. Het gebruik van fluoridepreparaten. Ned Tijdschr Tandheelkd 1981; 88: 165–77.

754. RULE JT *et al*. The relationship between ankylosed primary molars and multiple enamel defects. ASDC J Dent Child 1972; 39: 29–35.

755. RUPRECHT A *et al*. The incidence of hypoplasia in the dental office. J Can Dent Assoc 1984; 50: 900–2.

756. RUSHTON MA. A new form of dentinal dysplasia: shell teeth. Oral Surg 1954; 7: 543–9.

757. RUSHTON MA. Anomalies of human dentine. Ann R Coll Surg Engl 1955; 16: 94–117.

758. RUSHTON MA. Some less common bone lesions affecting the jaws. Oral Surg 1956; 9: 284–304.

759. RUSHTON MA. Odontodysplasia: "ghost teeth". Br Dent J 1965; 119: 109–13.

760. RUSSELL AL. The differential diagnosis of fluoride and non-fluoride enamel opacities. J Public Health Dent 1961; 21: 143–6.

761. SABAH E *et al*. Odontodysplasia. J Clin Pediatr Dent 1992; 16: 115–18.

762. SADEGHI EM *et al*. Regional odontodysplasia: clinical, pathologic, and therapeutic considerations. J Am Dent Assoc 1981; 102: 336–9.

763. SAKAKURA Y *et al*. In vitro effects of calcitonin and/or parathyroid hormone on odontogenesis of mouse embryonic molars. J Dent Res 1989; 68: 1279–84.

764. SALIDO EC *et al*. The human enamel protein gene amelogenin is expressed from both the X and the Y chromosomes. Hum Genet 1992; 50: 303–26.

765. SANGER RC. Endocrine disorders. In: STEWART RE *et al*. (eds) Pediatric dentistry. St Louis, MO: CV Mosby, 1982, pp. 210–16.

766. SAPIR S *et al*. Dentinogenesis imperfecta: an early treatment strategy. Pediatr Dent 2001; 23: 232–7.

767. SARICI ÜS *et al*. An early (sixth- hour) serum bilirubin measurement is useful in predicting the development of significant hyperbilirubinemia and severe ABO hemolytic disease in a selective high-risk population of newborns with ABO incompatibility. Pediatrics 2002; 109: 53–64.

768. SAUK JJ *et al*. Immunohistochemical localization of type III collagen in the dentin of patients with osteogenesis imperfecta and hereditary opalescent dentin. J Oral Pathol 1980; 9: 210–20.

769. SAUK JJ et al. An electron optic analysis and explanation for the etiology of dentinal dysplasia. Oral Surg 1972; 33: 763–71.

770. SAWYER DR et al. Malnutrition and the oral health of children in Ogbomosho, Nigeria. ASDC J Dent Child 1985; 53: 141–5.

771. SAYEGH F et al. Sites of tetracycline deposition in rat dentin. J Dent Res 1967; 46: 1474.

772. SCHIENBEIN H. Über einige Fälle erblicher Dentinogenesis imperfecta. Dtsch Zahnärzteblatt 1971; 25: 164–80.

773. SCHIMMELPFENNIG CB et al. Enamel and dentin aplasia. Oral Surg 1953; 6: 1444–9.

774. SCHOUR I. The neonatal line in the enamel and dentin of the human deciduous teeth and first permanent molar. J Am Dent Assoc 1936; 23: 1946–55.

775. SCHMEISER R et al. Gibt es einen Zusammenhang zwischen dem Auftreten von Schmelzflecken und unterschiedlichen Fluoridierungsmassnahmen? Dtsch Zahnärztl Z 1996; 51: 751–5.

776. SCHMIDT CW et al. Fluoridgehalt in Milchzähnen von Kindern mit und ohne chronische Fluorexposition. Stomatol DDR 1987; 37: 599–602.

777. SCHRAITLE R et al. Zahngesundheit und Ernährung. München: Carl Hanser Verlag, 1987.

778. SCHREURS WHP et al. De invloed van farmaca en additieven op de vitaminestatus. Voeding 1985; 46: 26–31.

779. SCHROEDER HE. Pathobiologie oraler Strukturen. Basel: Karger, 1983.

780. SCHRIJVER J. Vitaminestatus bij ziektebeelden. Voeding 1985; 46: 41–5.

781. SCHÜBEL F. Über eine dysplastische form einer dentinogenesis imperfecta. Dtsch Zahnaerztl Z 1969; 10: 887–94.

782. SCHULTE A et al. Fluoridekonzentration in deutschen Mineralwässern. Dtsch Zahnärztl Z 1992; 51: 763–7.

783. SCHULZE C. Developmental abnormalities of the teeth and jaws. In: GORLIN RJ, GOLDMAN HM (eds) Thoma's oral pathology. St Louis, MO: CV Mosby, 1970.

784. SCHUURS AHB. Wel of niet te veel fluoride? Ned Tijdschr Tandheelkd 1983; 90: 489–500.

785. SCHUURS AHB et al. Niet alle kindertandpasta's geschikt voor peuters. Ned Tijdschr Tandheelkd 1990; 97: 530–1.

786. SCHWACHMAN H et al. The tetracyclines. Pediatr Clin North Am 1956; 3: 295–303.

787. SCHWACHMAN H et al. Mucoviscidosis: an evaluation of continuous and prolonged antibiotic therapy. Am J Dis Child 1954; 88: 380–2.

788. SCHWARTZ S et al. Oral findings in patients with autosomal dominant hypophosphataemic bone disease and X-linked hypophosphataemia: further evidence that they are different diseases. Oral Surg Oral Med Oral Pathol 1988; 66: 310–14.

789. SCHWARTZ S et al. Oral findings in osteogenesis imperfecta. Oral Surg 1984; 57: 161–7.

790. SCOLA SM et al. Dentinal dysplasia type I. A subclassification. Br J Orthod 1987; 14: 175–9.

791. SEEDORF H et al. Amelogenesis imperfecta in a new animal model – a mutation in chromosome 5 (human 4q21). J Dent Res 2004; 83: 608–12.

792. SEGRETO VA et al. A current study of mottled enamel in Texas. J Am Dent Assoc 1984; 108: 56–9.

793. SEOW WK. X-linked hypophosphataemic vitamin D-resistant rickets. Aust Dent J 1984; 29: 371–7.

794. SEOW WK. Enamel hypoplasia in the primary dentition. ASDC J Dent Child 1991; 58: 441–52.

795. SEOW WK. A study of the development of the permanent dentition in very low birthweight children. Pediatr Dent 1996; 18: 379–84.

796. SEOW WK. Effects of preterm birth on oral growth and development. Aust Dent J 1997; 42: 85–91.

797. SEOW WK. Clinical diagnosis of enamel defects. Int Dent J 1997; 47: 173–82.

798. SEOW WK. Taurodontism of the mandibular first permanent molar distinguishes between the tricho-dento-osseous (TDO) syndrome and amelogenesis imperfecta. Clin Genet 1993; 43: 240–6.

799. SEOW WK. Diagnosis and management of unusual dental abscesses in children. Aust Dent J 2003; 48: 156–68.

800. SEOW WK et al. The effects of acid-etching on enamel from different clinical variants of amelogenesis imperfecta: a SEM study. Pediatr Dent 1998; 20: 37–42.

801. SEOW WK et al. Dental defects in the deciduous dentition of premature infants with low birth weight and neonatal rickets. Pediatr Dent 1984; 6: 88–92.

802. SEOW WK et al. Increased prevalence of developmental dental defects in low birth-weight, prematurely born children: a controlled study. Pediatr Dent 1987; 9: 221–5.

803. SEOW WK et al. Mineral deficiency in the pathogenesis of enamel hypoplasia in prematurely born, very low birthweight children. Pediatr Dent 1989: 11: 297–301.

804. SEOW WK et al. Enamel hypoplasia in prematurely-born children. J Pedod 1990; 14: 235–9.

805. SEOW WK et al. Oral changes associated with end-stage liver disease and liver transplantation: implications for dental management. ASDC J Dent Child 1991; 58: 474–80.

806. SEOW WK et al. The spectrum of dental manifestations in vitamin D-resistent rickets. Pediatr Dent 1986; 8: 245–50.

807. SEOW WK et al. Micromorphologic features of dentin in vitamin D-resistant rickets. Pediatr Dent 1989; 11: 203–8.

808. SEYMEN F et al. Amelogenesis imperfecta. J Clin Pediatr Dent 2002; 26: 327–36.

809. SHAFER WG et al. A textbook of oral pathology. Philadelphia, PA: WB Saunders, 1983.

810. SHELLING DH et al. Relation of rickets and vitamin D to the incidence of dental caries, enamel hypoplasia and malocclusion in children. J Am Dent Assoc 1936; 23: 840–6.

811. SHIELDS ED et al. A proposed classification for heritable human dentine defects with a description of a new entity. Arch Oral Biol 1973; 18: 543–53.

812. SHINODA H. Effects of long-term administration of fluoride on physico-chemical properties of the rat incisor enamel. Calcif Tissue Res 1975; 18: 91–100.

813. SHROFF DV et al. Evaluation of aggressive pulp therapy in a population of vitamin D-resistant rickets patients. Pediatr Dent 2002; 24: 347–9.

814. SHUSTERMAN S *et al*. The prevalence of enamel defects in childhood nephrotic syndrome. ASDC J Dent Child 1969; 36: 435–40.

815. SIBLEY LC *et al*. Odontogenic dysplasia. Oral Surg 1962; 15: 1370–3.

816. SILVA M. Fluoride content of infant formulae in Australia. Aust Dent J 1996; 41: 37–42.

817. SILVA-SOUSA YTC *et al*. Enamel hypoplasia in a litter of rats with alloxan-induced diabetes mellitus. Braz Dent J 2003; 14: 87–93.

818. SJÖGREN S *et al*. 14C Vitamin A in developing rat teeth and bone. Acta Odontol Scand 1977; 35: 311–16.

819. SLAVKIN HC. Diabetes, clinical dentistry and changing paradigmas. J Am Dent Assoc 1997; 128: 638–44.

820. SLAVKIN HC. Entering the era molecular dentistry. J Am Dent Assoc 1999; 130: 413–17.

821. SLOOTWEG PJ *et al*. Regional odontodysplasia in epidermal nevus syndrome. J Oral Pathol 1985; 14: 256–62.

822. SMALL BW *et al*. Enamel opacities. J Dent 1978; 6: 33–42.

823. SMITH CE. Cellular and chemical events during enamel maturation. Crit Rev Oral Biol Med 1998; 9: 128–61.

824. SMITH CE *et al*. Developmental changes in the pH of enamel fluid and its effects on matrix-resident proteinases. Adv Dent Res 1996; 10: 159–69.

825. SMITH CE *et al*. Degradation and loss of matrix proteins from developing enamel. Anat Rec 1989; 224: 292–316.

826. SMITH DMH *et al*. Gastro-enteritis, coeliac disease and enamel hypoplasia. Br Dent J 1979; 147: 91–5.

827. SMITH G. Fluoridation – are the dangers resolved? New Sci 1983; 5 May: 286–7.

828. SOFAER JA. Single genetic disorders. In: JONES JH *et al*. (eds) Oral manifestations of inherited disorders. London: WB Saunders, 1980.

829. SOGNNAES RF *et al*. Nature and effect of tetracycline uptake in dental hard tissues. J Dent Res 1964; 43 (suppl): 753.

830. SOHN W *et al*. Fluid consumption related to climate among children in the United States. J Public Health Dent 2001; 16 (2): 99–106.

831. SONI NN. Microradiographic study of dental tissues in sickle-cell anaemia. Arch Oral Biol 1966; 11: 561–4.

832. SONI NN *et al*. Polarized light and micro-radiographic study of dental tissues in dentinogenesis imperfecta. J Dent Res 1967; 46: 434–41.

833. SORELL L *et al*. One-step immunochromatographic assay for screening of coeliac disease. Lancet 2002; 395 (3910): 945–6.

834. SPEIRS RL. Correlations between the concentrations of fluoride and some other constituents in tea infusions and their possible dental caries-preventive effect. Arch Oral Biol 1983; 28: 471–5.

835. SPEIRS RL. The relationship between fluoride concentrations in serum and in mineralised tissues in the rat. Arch Oral Biol 1986; 31: 373–81.

836. SPERBER GH. Enamel hypoplasia. Oral Surg 1967; 24: 50–1.

837. SREENATH T *et al*. Dentin sialophosphoprotein knockout mouse teeth display widened predentin zone and develop defective dentin mineralization similar to human dentinogenesis imperfecta Type II. J Biol Chem 2003; 278: 24874–80.

838. STAFNE EC *et al*. Calcifications of the dentinal papilla that may cause anomalies of the roots of teeth. Oral Surg 1961; 14: 683–6.

839. STANNARD J *et al*. Fluoride content of some bottled waters and recommendations for fluoride supplementation. J Pedod 1990; 14: 103–7.

840. STEIDLER NE *et al*. Dentinal dysplasia. Br J Oral Maxillofac Surg 1984; 22: 274–86.

841. STEIN G. Enamel damage of systemic origin in premature birth and diseases of early infancy. Am J Orthod Oral Surg 1947; 2: 831–41.

842. STEINER M *et al*. Vorkommen von schmelzopazitäten an schneidezähnen bei schulkindern einer gemeinde des kantons Zürich. Schweiz Monatsschr Zahnmed 1984; 94: 1150–5.

843. STEINER M *et al*. Epidemiologie von schmelzopazitäten im zusammenhang mit der salzfluoridierung. Dtsch Zahnrztl Z 1995; 50: 717–20.

844. STEINMAN HR *et al*. Bilateral mandibular regional odontodysplasia with vascular nevus. Pediatr Dent 1991; 13: 303–6.

845. STEPHEN KW *et al*. A 4-year double-blind fluoridated school milk study in a vitamin-D deficient area. Br Dent J 1981; 151: 287–92.

846. STEPHEN KL *et al*. Dental management of severe dentinogenesis imperfecta in a mild form of osteogenesis imperfecta. J Clin Pediatr Dent 2002; 26: 131–6.

847. STEPHEN KW *et al*. Five-year double-blind fluoridated milk study in Scotland. Community Dent Oral Epidemiol 1984; 12: 223–9.

848. STERN D *et al*. Individual variation in enamel structure of human mandibular first premolars. Am J Phys Anthropol 1985; 68: 201–13.

849. STEWART DJ. Tetracyclines: their prevalence in childrens' teeth. Br Dent J 1968; 124: 318–20.

850. STEWART DJ. Prevalence of tetracyclines in childrens' teeth – study II. Br Med J 1973; 3: 320–2.

851. STIMMLER L *et al*. Enamel hypoplasia of the teeth associated with neonatal tetany. Lancet 1973; II: 1085–6.

852. STOOKEY GK. Review of fluorosis of self-applied topical fluorides: dentifrices, mouthrinses and gels. Community Dent Oral Epidemiol 1994; 22: 181–6.

853. STORIE DQ *et al*. Management of amelogenesis imperfecta by periodontal and prosthetic therapy. J Prosthet Dent 1970; 24: 608–15.

854. SUCKLING GW *et al*. The prevalence of developmental defects of enamel in 696 nine-year-old New Zealand children participating in a health and development study. Community Dental Health 1985; 2: 303–13.

855. SUCKLING G *et al*. The macroscopic appearance and associated histological changes in the enamel organ of hypoplastic lesions of sheep incisor teeth resulting from induced parasitism. Arch Oral Biol 1986; 31: 427–39.

856. SUCKLING GW *et al*. Etiological factors influencing prevalence of developmental defects of dental enamel in 9-year-old New Zealand children participating in a health and development study. J Dent Res 1987; 66: 1466–9.

857. SUCKLING GW *et al*. Macroscopic and scanning electron microscopic appearance and hardness values of developmental defects in human permanent tooth enamel. Adv Dent Res 1989; 3: 219–33.

858. SUCKLING GW *et al*. Developmental defects of enamel in a group of New Zealand children. Community Dent Oral Epidemiol 1984; 12: 177–84.

859. SUCKLING GW *et al*. Macroscopic appearance, microhardness and microradiographic characteristics of experimentally produced fluorotic lesions in sheep enamel. Caries Res 1982; 16: 227–34.

860. SUCKLING G *et al*. Histological, macroscopic and microhardness observations of fluoride-induced changes in the enamel organ and enamel of sheep incisor teeth. Arch Oral Biol 1984; 29: 165–77.

861. SUGURJÓNS H *et al*. Parental perception of lfluorosis among 8-year-old children living in three communities in Iceland, Ireland and England. Community Dent Oral Epidemiol 2004; 32 (suppl 1): 34–8.

862. SUHER T *et al*. Localized arrested tooth development. Oral Surg 1953; 6: 1305–14.

863. SUI W *et al*. Altered pH regulation during enamel development in the cystic fibrosis mouse incisor. J Dent Res 2002; 82: 388–92.

864. SULLIVAN W *et al*. A prospective trial of phosphate and 1,25-dihydroxyvitamin D3 therapy in symptomatic adults with X-linked hypophosphatemic rickets. J Clin Endocrin Metab 1992; 75: 879–85.

865. SUNDE OE *et al*. Dental changes in a patient with hypoparathyreoidism. Br Dent J 1961; 111: 112–17.

866. SUNDELL S. Hereditary amelogenesis imperfecta: I. Swed Dent J 1986; 10: 151–63.

867. SUNDELL S *et al*. Hereditary amelogenesis imperfecta. I. Swed Dent J 1985; 9: 157–69.

868. SUNDELL S *et al*. Hereditary aspects and classification of hereditary amelogenesis imperfecta. Community Dent Oral Epidemiol 1986; 14: 211–16.

869. SUNDERLAND EP *et al*. The teeth in osteogenesis and dentinogenesis imperfecta. Br Dent J 1980; 149: 287–9.

870. SUNDERLAND EP *et al*. A histological study of the chronology of initial mineralization in the human deciduous teeth. Arch Oral Biol 1987; 32: 167–74.

871. SWALLOW JN *et al*. Side-effects to antibiotics in cystic fibrosis: dental changes in relation to antibiotic administration. Arch Dis Child 1967; 42: 311–18.

872. SWAN E. Dietary fluoride supplement protocol for the new millennium. J Can Dent Assoc 2000; 66: 362.

873. SWEENEY EA *et al*. Factors associated with linear hypoplasia of human deciduous incisors. J Dent Res 1969; 48: 1275–9.

874. SWEENEY EA *et al*. Linear hypoplasia of deciduous incisor teeth in malnourished children. Am J Clin Nutr 1971; 24: 29–31.

875. SZPUNAR SM *et al*. Trends in the prevalence of dental fluorosis in the United States. J Public Health Dent 1987; 47 (2): 71–9.

876. SZPUNAR SM *et al*. Dental caries, fluorosis, and fluoride exposure in Michigan schoolchildren. J Dent Res 1988; 67: 802–6.

877. TABARI ED *et al*. Dental fluorosis in permanent incisor teeth in relation to water fluoridation, social deprivation and toothpaste use in infancy. Br Dent J 2000; 189: 216–20.

878. TAKAGI Y *et al*. Immunochemical and biochemical characteristics in hypocalcified amelogenesis imperfecta. Oral Surg Oral Med Oral Pathol Oral Radiol Endod 1998; 85: 424–30.

879. TAKAGI Y *et al*. Dentinogenesis imperfecta: evidence of qualitative alteration in the organic dentin matrix. J Oral Pathol 1980; 9: 201–9.

880. TAKAGI Y *et al*. Histological distribution of phosphophoryn in normal and pathological human dentins. J Oral Pathol 1986; 15: 463–7.

881. TAKAGI Y *et al*. A probable common disturbance in the early stage of odontoblast differentiation in dentinogenesis imperfecta type I and II. J Oral Pathol 1988; 17: 208–212.

882. TANIGUCHI K *et al*. The effect of mechanical trauma on the tooth germ of rat molars at various developmental stages. Endod Dent Traumatol 1999; 15: 17–25.

883. TAPIAS-LEDESMA MA *et al*. Factors associated with first molar enamel defects. J Dent Child 2003; 70: 215–20.

884. TAYLOR AN *et al*. Rat intestinal vitamin D-dependent calcium-binding protein: immunocytochemical localization in incisor ameloblasts. J Dent Res 1984; 63: 94–7.

885. TEBO HG. Case report of congenital hypoplasia and hypocalcification of the enamel. Oral Surg 1950; 3: 1275–8.

886. TERVONEN SA *et al*. Regional odontodysplasia. Clin Oral Investig 2004; 8: 45–51.

887. TIDWELL E *et al*. Dentinal dysplasia. J Endod 1979; 5: 372–6.

888. TIEDER M *et al*. Hereditary hypophophatemic rickets with hypercalcuria. N Engl J Med 1985; 312: 611–17.

889. MAN UA. Hereditary hypophosphatemic rickets with hypercalciuria. N Engl J Med 1985; 312: 611–17.

890. THYAGARAJAN T *et al*. Reduced expression of dentin sialophosphoprotein is associated with dysplastic dentin in mice overexpressing transforming growth-factor–β1 in teeth. J Biol Chem 2001; 276: 11016–20.

891. THOTAKURA SR *et al*. The non-collagenous dentin matrix proteins are involved in Dentinogenesis Imperfecta Type II (DGI-II). J dent Res 2000; 79: 835–9.

892. THYLSTRUP A. Distribution of dental fluorosis in the primary dentition. Community Dent Oral Epidemiol 1978; 6: 329–37.

893. THYLSTRUP A. Posteruptive developments of isolated and confluent pits in fluorosed enamel in a 6-year-old girl. Scand J Dent Res 1983; 91: 243–6.

894. THYLSTRUP A *et al*. The influence of traumatic intrusion of primary teeth on their permanent successors in monkeys. A macroscopic, polarized light and scanning electron microscopic study. J Oral Pathol 1977; 6: 296–306.

895. THYLSTRUP A *et al*. Clinical appearance of dental fluorosis in permanent teeth in relation to histologic changes. Community Dent Oral Epidemiol 1978; 6: 315–28.

896. THYLSTRUP A, FEJERSKOV O. A scanning electron microscopic and micro-radiographic study of pits in fluorosed human enamel. Scand J Dent Res 1979; 87: 105–14.

897. THYLSTRUP A et al. Enamel changes and dental caries in 7-year-old children given fluoride tablets from shortly after birth. Caries Res 1979; 13: 265–76.

898. TOTO PD. Osteogenesis imperfecta tarda with dentinogenesis imperfecta. Oral Surg 1953; 6: 772–4.

899. TOUMBA KJ et al. The fluoride content of bottled drinking waters. Br Dent J 1994; 176: 266–8.

900. TRACY WE et al. Analysis of dentine pathogenesis in vitamin D-resistant rickets. Oral Surg 1971; 32: 38–44.

901. TREASURE ET et al. The York review – A systematic review of public water fluoridation: a commentary. Br Dent J 2002; 192: 495–7.

902. TSANG RC et al. Hypocalcemia in infants of diabetic mothers. J Pediatr 1972; 80: 384–95.

903. TURNER SD et al. Impact of imported beverages on fluoridated and nonfluoridated communities. Gen Dent 1998; 46: 190–3.

904. TYNAN JJ et al. Cystic fibrosis and oral health. J Can Dent Assoc 1984; 50: 833–5.

905. ULVESTAD H et al. Discoloration of permanent front teeth in 3,157 Norwegian children due to tetracyclines and other factors. Scand J Dent Res 1978; 86: 147–52.

906. UNDERWOOD P et al. High levels of childhood rickets in rural North Yemen. Soc Sci Med 1987; 24: 37–41.

907. USHA KK et al. Detection of high risk pregnancies with relation to ABO haemolytic disease of newborn. Indian J Pediatr 1998; 65: 863–5.

908. VADER LW et al. Specificity of tissue transglutaminase explains cereal toxicity in celiac disease. J Exp Med 2002; 195: 643–9.

909. VAIKUNTAM J et al. Regional odontodysplasia. J Clin Pediatr Dent 1996; 21: 35–40.

910. VAN AMERONGEN WE. Kaasmolaren. In: VAN DER KWAST et al. (eds) Tandheelkundig Jaar. Houten: Bohn Stafleu Van Loghum, 1995.

911. VAN AMERONGEN WE et al. Cheese molars: a pilot study of the etiology of hypocalcifications in first permanent molars. ASDC J Dent Child 1995; 4: 266–9.

912. VAN DER WAL et al. Regional odontodysplasia. Int J Oral Maxillofac Surg 1993; 22: 356–8.

913. VAN LOVEREN C. Fluoride. In: VAN LOVEREN C et al. (eds) Preventieve tandheelkunde. Houten: Bohn Stafleu Van Loghum, 1996.

914. VAN LOVEREN C et al. Fluoride ingestion from toothpaste: fluoride recovered from the toothbrush, the expectorate and the after-brush rinses. Community Dent Oral Epidemiol 2004; 32 (suppl 1): 54–61.

915. VAN NIEUWENHUIZEN J-P et al. Caries dentaires, fluorures urinaires et opacités de l'émail. Rev Mens Suisse Odontostomatol 1992; 102: 279–85.

916. VAN PALENSTEIN HELDERMAN WH. Kwaliteitscontrole van tandpasta in Nederland. Ned Tandartsenbl 2004; 59 (4): 20–2.

917. VAN WAES H et al. Erscheinungsformen der Odontodysplasie (I). Quintessenz 1992; 43: 957–64.

918. VELDHUIS AAH. Amelogenesis imperfecta. Ned Tijdschr Tandheelkd 1980; 87: 64–8.

919. VIA WF Jr et al. Relationships of cerebral disorder to faults in dental enamel. Am J Dis Child 1957; 94: 137–42.

920. VIA WF Jr et al. Relationship of enamel hypoplasia to abnormal events of gestation and birth. J Am Dent Assoc 1959; 59: 702–7.

921. VIA WF Jr et al. The effect of hypoxia upon developing enamel. J Dent Res 1959; 38: 651.

922. VIEIRA AR et al. Dentinal dysplasia type I. ASDC J Dent Child 1998; 65: 141–4.

923. VILLA AE et al. Estimation of optimal concentration of fluoride in drinking water under conditions prevailing in Chile. Community Dent Oral Epidemiol 1998; 26: 249–55.

924. VISSER WJ et al. Veranderingen aan gebitslementen bij vier kinderen met primaire vitamine D-refractaire rachitis. Ned Tijdschr Tandheelkd 1965; 72: 757–77.

925. VISSER WJ et al. Glazuurhypoplasieën en pigmentaties van glazuur en dentine waargenomen bij melkelementen van twee jonge kinderen. Ned Tijdschr Tandheelkd 1963; 70: 3–17.

926. VLACHOU A et al. Fluoride concentrations of infant food and drinks in the United Kingdom. Caries Res 1992; 26: 29–32.

927. VOGEL RI et al. Tetracycline-induced extrinsic discoloration of the dentition. Oral Surg 1977; 44: 50–3.

928. VON ARX T. Traumatologie im Milchgebiss (II). Schweiz Monatsschr Zahnmed 1991; 101: 57–69.

929. VON ARX T. Developmental disturbances of permanent teeth following trauma to the primary dentition. Aust Dent J 1993; 38: 1–10.

930. VON ARX T. Odontodysplasie. Schweiz Monatschr Zahnmed 1992; 102: 723–6.

931. VON ARX T. Autotransplantation for treatment of regional odontodysplasia. Oral Surg Oral Med Oral Pathol Oral Radiol Endod 1998; 85: 304–7.

932. VON HAAM E. Venereal diseases and spirochetal infections In: ANDERSON WAD (ed.) Pathology. Volume 1. St Louis, MO: CV Mosby, 1971.

933. VON SCHWANEWEDE M et al. Amelogenesis imperfecta hereditaria. Stomatol DDR 1983; 33: 619–25.

934. WALDMAN HB. Low birth-weight and the relationship to developmental problems. ASDC J Dent Child 1996; 63: 354–7.

935. WALDMAN HB et al. Low birthweight babies grow older, but there could be many problems. ASDC J Dent Child 2001; 68: 356–9.

936. WALLMAN IS et al. Prematurity, tetracycline, and oxytetracycline in tooth development. Lancet 1962; II: 720–1.

937. WALKER JD et al. Phenylketonuria and dentistry. ASDC J Dent Child 1982; 49: 280–4.

938. WALLMAN IS et al. Teeth pigmented by tetracycline. Lancet 1962; I: 827–9.

939. WALTER GW. Dentinogenesis imperfecta. J Am Dent Assoc 1956; 53: 455–7.

940. WALTER JB et al. Principles of pathology for dental students. Edinburgh: Churchill Livingstone, 1974.

941. WALTIMO J *et al.* Transmission electron microscopic appearance of dentin matrix in type II dentin dysplasia. Scand J Dent Res 1991; 99: 349–56.

942. WALTON JL *et al.* Dental caries and fluorosis in breast-fed and bottle-fed children. Caries Res 1981; 15: 124–37.

943. WALTON JL *et al.* Odontodysplasia. Oral Surg 1978; 46: 676–84.

944. WANG NJ *et al.* Risk factors associated with fluorosis in a non-fluoridated population in Norway. Community Dent Oral Epidemiol 1997; 25: 396–401.

945. WARNAKULASURIYA KAAS. Prevalence of selected developmental dental anomalies in children in Sri Lanka. ASDC J Dent Child 1989; 56: 137–9.

946. WARNAKULASURIYA KAAS *et al.* Determining optimal levels of fluoride in drinking water for hot, dry climates. Community Dent Oral Epidemiol 1992; 20: 364–7.

947. WARREN DP *et al.* Topical fluorides: efficacy, administration, and safety. Gen Dent 1997; 45: 134–42.

948. WARREN DP *et al.* Fluorosis of the primary dentition: what does it mean for permanent teeth? J Am Dent Assoc 1999; 130: 347–56.

949. WARREN JJ *et al.* Current and future role of fluoride in nutrition. Dent Clin North Am 2003; 47: 225–43.

950. WARREN KL *et al.* A review of fluoride dentifrice related to dental fluorosis. Pediatr Dent 1999; 21: 265–71.

951. WARREN DP *et al.* Prevalence of dental fluorosis in the primary dentition. J Public Health Dent 2001; 61: 87–91.

952. WATANABE K *et al.* Bilirubin pigmentation of human teeth caused by hyperbilirubinemia. J Oral Pathol 1999; 28: 128–30.

953. WEATHERELL JA *et al.* Changes in the fluoride concentration of the labial enamel surface with age. Caries Res 1972; 6: 312–24.

954. WEEKS KJ. Enamel mottling in a non-fluoride community since the advent of fluoride toothpastes. Br Dent J 1990; 169: 258–60.

955. WEEKS KJ *et al.* Enamel defects in 4- to 5-year-old children in fluoridated and non-fluoridated parts of Cheshire, UK. Caries Res 1993; 27: 317–20.

956. WEERHEIJM KL. Molar Incisor Hypomineralisation (MIH). Eur J Paediatr Dent 2003; 4: 115–20.

957. WEERHEIJM KL *et al.* Judgement criteria for molar incisor hypomineralisation (MIH) in epidemiologic studies. Eur J Paediatr Dent 2003; 4: 110–13.

958. WEERHEIJM KL *et al.* Prevalence of cheese molars in eleven-year-old Dutch children. ASDC J Dent Child 2001; 68: 259–262.

959. WEERHEIJM KL *et al.* Molar-incisor hypomineralisation. Caries Res 2001; 35: 390–1.

960. WEI SHY *et al.* Fluoride supplements for infants and preschool children. J Prev Dent 1977; 4 (3): 28–32.

961. WEINBERGER SJ. Bottled drinking waters: are the fluoride concentrations shown on the labels accurate? Int J Pediatr Dent 1991; 1: 143–6.

962. WEINMANN JP *et al.* Hereditary disturbances of enamel formation and calcification. J Am Dent Assoc 1945; 32: 397–418.

963. WEISSKOPF N *et al.* Idiopathische oder fluoridbedingte Schmelzflecken? Schweiz Monatschr Zahnheilkd 1972; 82: 47–56.

964. WELSCH MJ, STEIN SL. A syndrome of hemimaxillary enlargement, asymmetry of the face, tooth abnormalities, and skin findings. Pediatr Dermatol 2004; 21: 448–51.

965. WENZEL A *et al.* Dental fluorosis and localized enamel opacities in fluoride and nonfluoride Danish communities. Caries Res 1982; 16: 340–8.

966. WENZEL A *et al.* The relationship between water-borne fluoride, dental fluorosis and skeletal development in 11–15 year old Tanzanian girls. Arch Oral Biol 1982; 27: 1007–11.

967. WERLER MM *et al.* Teratogenicity of high vitamin A intake. Lancet 1995; 334: 1195.

968. WESTERGAARD J. Structural changes induced by tetracycline in secretory ameloblasts in young rats. Scand J Dent Res 1980; 88: 481–95.

969. WESTOVER KM *et al.* The relationship of breastfeeding to oral development and dental concerns. ASDC J Dent Child 1989; 56: 140–3.

970. WETZEL WE. Dentinogenesis imperfecta – Ergebnis mangelnder Differenzierungsfähigkeit des mesenchymalen Zahnbildungsgewebes. Dtsch Zahnärztl Z 1978; 33: 411–14.

971. WEYERS H. Zur Entstehung der grünen Zähne (Chlorodontie) bei Kindern mit Ikterus gravis. Kinderärztliche Praxis 1956; 24: 199–203.

972. WEYMAN J. The clinical appearances of tetracycline staining of the teeth. Br Dent J 1965; 118: 289–91.

973. WEYMAN J. Caries incidence in teeth with tetracycline incorporation. J Dent Res 1966; 45: 1817.

974. WELSCH MJ, STEIN SL. A syndrome of hemimaxillary enlargement, asymmetry of the face, tooth abnormalities, and skin findings. Pediatr Dermatol 2004; 21: 448–51.

975. WHELTON H *et al.* Dental caries and enamel fluorosis among the fluoridated and non-fluoridated populations in the Republic of Ireland in 2002. Community Dent Health 2004; 21: 37–44.

976. WHELTON H *et al.* A review of fluorosis in the European Union: prevalence, risk factors and aesthetic issues. Community Dent Oral Epidemiol 2004; 32 (suppl 1): 9–18.

977. WHITFORD GM. Acute and chronic fluoride toxicity. J Dent Res 1992; 71: 1249–54.

978. WHITFORD GM. Fluoride toxicology and health effects. In: FEJERSKOV O *et al.* (eds) Fluoride in dentistry. Copenhagen: Munksgaard, 1996.

979. WHITFORD GM *et al.* Fluorosis-like effects of acidosis, but not NH_4^+, on rat incisor enamel. Caries Res 1995; 29: 20–5.

980. WHITTAKER DK *et al.* Scanning electron microscopy of the neonatal line in human enamel. Arch Oral Biol 1978; 23: 45–50.

981. WIHR NL. Abnormal dentition in vitamin D resistant rickets. ASDC J Dent Child 1970; 37: 222–4.

982. WILSON RMH *et al.* Enamel mottling and infectious exanthemata in a rural community. J Dent 1978; 6: 161–5.

983. WILSON GW *et al.* Hereditary hypoplasia of the dentin. J Am Dent Assoc 1929; 16: 866–86.

984. WIDENHEIM J. A time-related study of intake pattern of fluoride tablets among Swedish preschoolchildren and parental attitudes. Community Dent Oral Epidemiol 1982; 10: 296–300.

985. WILLIAMS JK et al. Hypomineralised first permanent molars and the orthodontist. Eur J Paediatr Dent 2003; 4: 129–32.

986. WIKTORSSON AM et al. Prevalence of fluorosis and other enamel defects related to caries among adults in communities with optimal and low water fluoride concentrations. Community Dent Health 1994; 11: 75–8.

987. WILFART G et al. Entwicklungsbedingte Schmelzveränderungen bei Kindern mit unterschiedlicher Fluoridsupplementierung. Dtsch Zahnärztl Z 1994; 49: 879–83.

988. WILLIAMS SA et al. Odontodysplasia associated with orbital colomboma. Br Dent J 1988; 164: 390–3.

989. WILSON PHR et al. Case report: restorative options in regional odontodysplasia. Eur J Prosthet Rest Dent 2002; 10: 5–8.

990. WILSON PR et al. Mineralization levels in pre- and postnatal human deciduous molar enamel. J Paediatr Dent 1990; 6: 35–9.

991. WINTER GB. Amelogenesis imperfecta with enamel opacities and taurodontism: an alternative diagnosis for "idiopathic dental fluorosis". Br Dent J 1996; 181: 167–72.

992. WINTER GB et al. Enamel hypoplasia and anomalies of the enamel. Dent Clin North Am 1975; 19 (1): 3–24.

993. WINTER GB et al. Hereditary amelogenesis imperfecta. A rare autosomal dominant type. Br Dent J 1969; 127: 157–64.

994. WISOTZKY J. Effect of tetracycline on the phosphorescence of teeth. J Dent Res 1972; 51: 7–11.

995. WITKOP CJ JR. Genetics diseases of the oral cavity. In: TIECKE RW. Oral pathology. New York, NY: McGraw-Hill, 1965.

996. WITKOP CJ JR. Inborn errors of metabolism with particular reference to pseudohypoparathyroidism. J Dent Res 1966; 45: 568–74.

997. WITKOP CJ JR. Partial expression of sex-linked recessive amelogenesis imperfecta in females compatible with the Lyon hypothesis. Oral Surg 1967; 23: 174–82.

998. WITKOP CJ. Manifestations of genetic diseases in the human pulp. Oral Surg 1971; 32: 278–316.

999. WITKOP CJ. Hereditary defects of dentin. Dent Clin North Am 1975; 19 (1): 25–45.

1000. WITKOP CJ JR. Amelogenesis imperfecta, dentinogenesis imperfecta and dentin dysplasia revisited. J Oral Pathol 1989; 17: 547–53.

1001. WITKOP CJ JR. et al. Autosomal recessive pigmented hypomaturation amelogenesis imperfecta. Oral Surg 1973; 36: 367–82.

1002. WITKOP CJ JR et al. Heritable defects of enamel. In: STEWART RE et al. (eds) Oral facial genetics. St Louis, MO: CV Mosby, 1976.

1003. WOEHRLEN AE. Regional odontodysplasia. Gen Dent 1990; 38: 52–3.

1004. WÖLTGENS JHM et al. Fluoridegebruik. Gevlekt glazuur bij kinderen. Ned Tijdschr Tandheelkd 1989; 96: 29–33.

1005. WORLD HEALTH ORGANIZATION. Fluorine and fluorides. Environmental Health Criteria 36. Geneva: World Health Organization, 1984.

1006. WORLD HEALTH ORGANIZATION. Fluoride and oral health. Technical report 846. Geneva: World Health Organization, 1994.

1007. WORLD HEALTH ORGANIZATION. Oral health surveys, 5th edn. Geneva: World Health Organization, 1997.

1008. WRIGHT JT et al. Alteration of enamel proteins in hypomaturation amelogenesis imperfecta. J Dent Res 1989; 68: 1328–30.

1009. WRIGHT JT et al. Protein characterization of fluorosed human enamel. J Dent Res 1996; 75: 1936–41.

1010. WRIGHT JT et al. The ultrastructure of the dental tissues in dentinogenesis imperfecta. Arch Oral Biol 1985; 30: 201–6.

1011. WRIGHT JT et al. Enamel mineral composition of normal and cystic fibrosis transgenic mice. Adv Dent Res 1996; 10: 270–4.

1012. WRIGHT JT et al. The enamel proteins in human amelogenesis imperfecta. Arch Oral Biol 1997; 42: 149–59.

1013. WRIGHT JT et al. Abnormal enamel development in a cystic fibrosis transgenic mouse model. J Dent Res 1996; 75: 966–73.

1014. WRIGHT JT et al. Analysis of the tricho-dento-osseous syndrome genotype and phenotype. Am J Med Genet 1997; 72: 197–204.

1015. WRIGHT JT et al. Enamel ultrastructure in pigmented hypomaturation amelogenesis imperfecta. J Oral Pathol Med 1992; 21: 390–4.

1016. WRIGHT JT et al. Characterization of the enamel ultrastructure and mineral content in hypoplastic amelogenesis imperfecta. Oral Surg Oral Med Oral Pathol 1991; 72: 594–601.

1017. WYSOLMERSKI JJ et al. Absence of functional type 1 parathyroidhormone (PTH)/PTH-related protein receptors in humans is associated with abnormal breast development and tooth impaction. J Clin Endocrinol Metab 2001; 86: 1788–94.

1018. YAMAMOTO M et al. Human PTH(1-34) infusion test in differential diagnosis of various types of hypoparathyroidism: an attempt to establish a standard clinical test. Bone Miner 1989; 6: 199–12.

1019. YAMAZAKI H et al. A case of hypophosphatemic vitamin D-resistant rickets in which spontaneous dental abscesses were the first evidence. Jap J Pedod 1985; 23: 204–14.

1020. YASUFUKU Y et al. Dental management of familial hypophosphatemic vitamin D-resistant ricktes. ASDC J Dent Child 1983; 50: 300–4.

1021. YOUNG AB et al. Is cytomegalovirus a serious hazard to female hospital staff. Lancet 1983; 8346: 975–6.

1022. YOUNG W et al. Syndromes with salivary dysfunction predisposes to tooth wear. Oral Surg Oral Med Oral Pathol Oral Radiol Endod 2001; 92: 38–48.

1023. ZAGDWON AM et al. A prospective clinical trial comparing preformed metal crowns and cast restorations for defective first permanent molars. Eur J Paediatr Dent 2003; 4: 138–42.

1024. ZAIA AA *et al*. Oral changes associated with biliary atresia and liver transplantation. J Clin Pediatr Dent 1993; 18: 39–42.

1025. ZAMBRANO M *et al*. Oral and dental manifestations of vitamin D-dependent –rickets type I Oral Surg Oral Med Oral Pathol Oral Radiol Endod 2003; 95: 705–9.

1026. ZEGARELLI EV *et al*. Odontodysplasia. Oral Surg 1963; 16: 187–93.

1027. ZEGARELLI EV *et al*. Discoloration of the teeth in a 24-year-old patient with cystic fibrosis of the pancreas not primarily associated with tetracycline therapy. Oral Surg 1967; 24: 62–4.

1028. ZEGARELLI EV *et al*. Coloration of teeth in patients with cystic fibrosis of the pancreas. Part II. Oral Surg 1962; 15: 929–33.

1029. ZHANG X *et al*. *DSPP* mutation in dentinogenesis imperfecta Shields type II. Nat Genet 2001; 27: 151–2.

1030. ZHAO LB *et al*. Effect of a high fluoride water supply on children's intelligence. Fluoride 1996; 29: 190–2.

1031. ZIMMERMAN ER. Fluoride and nonfluoride enamel opacities. Public Health Rep 1954; 69: 1115–20.

1032. HUNTER L *et al*. Is amelogenesis imperfecta an indication for renal examination? Int J Paediatr Dent 2007; 17: 62–5.

1033. WILLIAM V *et al*. Molar incisor hypomineralization. Pediatr Dent 2006; 28: 224–32.

1034. ALALUUSUA S *et al*. Developmental dental toxicity of dioxin and related compounds. Int Dent J 2006; 56: 323–31.

1035. OGDEN AR *et al*. Gross enamel hypoplasia in molars from subadults in 16th–18th century London graveyard. Am J Phys Anthropol 2007; 133: 957–66.

1036. BOSSÚ M *et al*. Enamel hypoplasia in coeliac children: a potential marker of early diagnosis. Eur J Paediatr Dent 2007; 8: 31–7.

1037. BARONCELLI GI *et al*. Prevalence and pathogenesis of dental and periodontal lesions in children with X-linked hypophosphatemic rickets. Eur J Paediatr Dent 2006; 7: 61–6.

1038. DE ALMEIDA BD *et al*. Fluoride ingestion from toothpaste and diet in 1- to 3-year-old Brazilian children. Community Dent Oral Epidemiol 2007; 35: 53–63.

1039. ITTHAGARUN A *et al*. Effects of different amounts of a low fluoride toothpaste on primary enamel lesion progression. Eur Arch Paediatr Dent 2007; 8: 69–73.

1040. DO LG *et al*. Risk-benefit balance in the use of fluoride among young children. J Dent Res 2007; 86: 723–8.

1041. SENNHENN-KIRCHNER S *et al*. Traumatic injuries to the primary dentition and effects on the permanent successors. Dent Traumatol 2006; 22: 237–41.

1042. PAVLIC A *et al*. Severely hypoplastic amelogenesis imperfecta with taurodontism. Int J Paediatr Dent 2007; 17: 259–66.

1043. MENDOZA G *et al*. A new locus for autosomal dominant amelogenesis imperfecta on chromosome 8q24.3. Hum Genet 2006; 120: 653–62.

1044. KORBMACHER HM *et al*. Progressive preeruptive crown resorption in autosomal recessive generalized hypoplastic amelogenesis imperfecta. Oral Surg Oral Med Pral Pathol Oral Radiol Endod 2007; 104: 540–4.

1045. HU JC-C *et al*. Enamel formation and amleogenesis imperfecta. Cells Tissues Organs 2007; 186: 78–85.

1046. SPINI TH *et al*. Progressive development in regional odontodysplasia. Oral Surg Oral Med Oral Pathol Oral Radiolo Endod 2007; 104: e40–e5.

1047. MAUPOMÉ G. *et al*. Patterns of dental caries following cesstion of water fluoridation. Community Dent Oral Epidemiol 2001; 29: 37–47.

Chapter 4: Deviations in Timing and Site of Eruption

1. ADLER P. Effect of some environmental factors on sequence of permanent tooth eruption. J Dent Res 1963; 42: 605–16.

2. ADLER P *et al*. Influence of age and duration on dental development in diabetic children. J Dent Res 1973; 52: 535–7.

3. AGARWAK KN *et al*. Deciduous dentition and enamel defects. Indian Pediatr 2003; 40: 124–9.

4. AGNOSTOPOULOU S. Ectopic third molar. Oral Surg Oral Med Oral Pathol 1991; 71: 522–3.

5. AHLQWIST M *et al*. Prevalence of impacted teeth and associated pathology in middle-aged and older Swedish women. Community Dent Oral Epidemiol 1991; 19: 116–19.

6. AITASALO K *et al*. An orthopantomographic study of prevalence of impacted teeth. Int J Oral Surg 1972; 1: 117–20.

7. ALAEJOS-ALGARRA C *et al*. Transmigration of mandibular canines. Quint Int 1998; 29: 395–8.

8. ALBERS DD. Ankylosis of teeth in the developing dentition. Quint Int 1986; 17: 303–8.

9. ALDRED MJ *et al*. Precocious tooth eruption and loss in Letterer-Siwe disease. Br Dent J 1988; 165: 367–70.

10. ALLEN WA. Bilateral transposition of teeth in two brothers. Br Dent J 1967; 123: 439–40.

11. AL-SAHHAR WF *et al*. Erupted odontoma. Oral Surg 1985; 59: 225–6.

12. ALT KW. Mesiodens in der Nasenhöle bei einer frühmittelalterlichen Bestattung. Quintessenz 1988; 39: 1075–80.

13. AL-WAHEIDI EMH. Transmigration of unerupted mandibular canines. Quint Int 1996; 27: 27–31.

14. AMIR E, DUPERON DF. Unerupted second primary molar. ASDC J Dent Child 1982; 49: 365–8.

15. ANDREASEN JO *et al*. Traumatic injuries to the teeth. Copenhagen, Munksgaard, 1981

16. ANDREASEN JO *et al*. Oral health care: more than caries and periodontal disease. Int Dent J 1986; 36: 207–14.

17. AREN G *et al*. Inverted impaction of primary incisors. ASDC J Dent Child 2002; 69: 275–6, 234.

18. ATWAN S *et al*. Infraocclusion of lower primary molar with other familial dental anomalies. ASDC J Dent Child 1998; 65: 272–5.

19. AVCU N *et al*. Severe hypodontia and asymptomatic bilaterally ectopic impacted teeth in the coronoid processes. Quint Int 2004; 35: 582–3.

20. AYDIN U *et al*. Transmigration of impacted canines. Dentomaxillofac Radiol 2003; 32: 198–200.

21. BAAB DA *et al*. Caries and periodontitis associated with an unerupted third molar. Oral Surg 1984; 58: 428–30.

22. BAAB DA *et al*. Studies of a family manifesting premature exfoliation of deciduous teeth. J Periodont 1985; 56: 403–9.

23. BACETTI T. Interceptive approach to tooth eruption abnormalities. J Clin Pediatr Dent 1995; 19 (4): 297–300.

24. BACKSTRÖM MC *et al*. Maturation of primary and permanent teeth in preterm infants. Arch Dis Child Fetal Neonatal Ed 2000; 83: F104–8.

25. BALAN N. Tooth in the sigmoid notch. Oral Surg Oral Med Oral Pathol 1992; 73: 767.

26. BARSLEY RE *et al*. Impacted mandibular cuspid and lateral incisor. J Oral Med 1984; 39: 165–8.

27. BAUME LJ *et al*. Hormonal control of tooth eruption – II. J Dent Res 1954; 33: 91–103.

28. BECKER A *et al*. Submergence of a deciduous tooth: its ramifications on the dentition and treatment of the resulting malocclusion. Am J Orthod 1982; 81: 240–4.

29. BECKER A. Early treatment for impacted maxillary incisors. Am J Orthod Dentofac Orthop 2002; 121: 586–7.

30. BECKER A *et al*. The incidence of anomalous maxillary lateral incisors in relation to palatally-displaced cuspids. Angle Orthod 1981; 51: 24–9.

31. BECKTOR KB *et al*. Segmental odontomaxillary dysplasia: clinical, radiological and histological aspects of four cases. Oral Dis 2002; 8: 106–10.

32. BEERTSEN W. Wat de tand aan ons bindt. Amsterdam: "Inaugural lecture" University of Amsterdam, 1992.

33. BEERTSEN W *et al*. Microtubules in periodontal ligament cells in relation to tooth eruption and collagen degradation. J Periodont Res 1984; 19: 489–500.

34. BELL RA *et al*. Complex congenital hemihypertrophy. J Pedod 1984; 8: 300–13.

35. BEN-BASSAT Y *et al*. Occlusal disturbances resulting from neglected submerged primary molars. ASDC J Dent Child 1991; 58: 129–33.

36. BENENATI FW. Submergence of a previously restored maxillary first molar associated with mesial tilting of an adjacent tooth. Oral Surg Oral Med Oral Pathol 1992; 74: 534.

37. BERGE TI. Third molars in Norwegian general dental practice. Acta Odontol Scand 1992; 50: 17–24.

38. BIANCHI SD. Primary impaction of primary teeth. J Clin Pediatr Dent 1991; 15: 165–8.

39. BIEDERMAN W. The incidence and etiology of tooth ankylosis. Am J Orthod 1956; 42: 921–6.

40. BIEDERMAN W. Etiology and treatment of tooth ankylosis. Am J Orthod 1962; 48: 670–84.

41. BIEDERMAN W. The ankylosed tooth. Dent Clin North Am 1964; 8: 439–508.

42. BIGEARD L *et al*. Retard dentaire et microdontie chez l'enfant atteint de déficit en hormone somatotrope. J Biol Buccale 1991; 19: 291–6.

43. BIMSTEIN E. Mandibular second permanent molars impacted by the third molars. ASDC J Dent Child 1984; 51: 148–9.

44. BIMSTEIN E *et al*. Idiopathic, late, slow, and irregular dental development. ASDC J Dent Child 1984; 51: 302–4.

45. BIMSTEIN E *et al*. Root surface characteristics of primary teeth from children with prepubertal periodontitis. J Periodontol 1998; 69: 337–47.

46. BISHARA SE. Impacted maxillary canines. Am J Orthod Dentofac Orthop 1992; 101: 159–71.

47. BJERKLIN K *et al*. Ectopic eruption of the maxillary first permanent molars: etiologic factors. Am J Orthod 1983; 84: 147–55.

48. BJERKLIN K *et al*. Ectopic eruption of maxillary first permanent molars and association with other tooth and developmental disturbances. Eur J Orthod 1992; 14: 369–75.

49. BJERKLIN K, BENNETT J. The long-term survival of lower second primary molars in subjects with agenesis of the premolars. Eur J Orthod 2000; 22: 245–55.

50. BLACK SL *et al*. An unusual case of tooth migration. Oral Surg Oral Med Oral Pathol 1973; 36: 607–8.

51. BLAIR FM. Secondary retention of multiple permanent teeth. Br Dent J 1997; 182: 69–70.

52. BLOMLÖF L *et al*. Occurrence and appearance of cementum hypoplasias in localized and generalized juvenile periodontitis. Acta Odontol Scand 1986; 44: 313–20.

53. BOBO M *et al*. Self-induced displacement of a maxillary molar into the lateral pharyngeal space. Int J Oral Maxillofac Surg 1998; 27: 38–9.

54. BOCCHIEERI A *et al*. Correction of a bilateral maxillary canine – first premolar transposition in the late mixed dentition. Am J Orthod Dentofac Orthop 2002; 121: 20–8.

55. BODNER L *et al*. Impacted primary incisor. J Dent Child 1987; 54: 363–4.

56. BOHÃTKA L *et al*. Parameters of the mixed dentition in diabetic children. J Dent Res 1973; 52: 131–5.

57. BOLAÑOS MV *et al*. Approaches to chronological age assessment based upon dental calcification. Forens Sci Int 2000; 110: 97–106.

58. BORAZ RA. Hypophosphatasia. J Pedod 1988 13: 44–52.

59. BOYCZUK MP *et al*. Identifying a deciduous dentigerous cyst. J Am Dent Assoc 1995; 126: 832.

60. BRADY J. Familial primary failure of eruption of permanent teeth. Br J Orthod 1990; 17: 109–13.

61. BREARLY LJ *et al*. Ankylosis of primary molar teeth – I. ASDC J Dent Child 1973; 40: 54–63.

62. BRIN I *et al*. Position of the maxillary permanent canine in relation to anomalous or missing lateral incisors. Eur J Orthod 1986; 8: 12–16.

63. BRIN I *et al*. Eruption of rootless teeth in congenital renal disease. Oral Surg 1985; 60: 61–4.

64. BROWNBILL JW *et al*. Ectopic eruption of transposed mandibular permanent lateral incisors beneath primary first molars. Aust Dent J 1994; 39: 1–3.

65. BRUCE KW, STAFNE EC. The effect of irradiation on the dental system as demonstrated by the roentgenogram. J Am Dent Assoc 1950; 41: 684–9.

66. BRUCKNER RJ *et al*. Hypophosphatasia with premature shedding of teeth and aplasia of cementum. Oral Surg 1962; 15: 1351–69.

67. BUNTING RW. Report of the examination of the mouths of 1500 schoolchildren in the public schools of Ann Arbor, Michigan. Dent Cosmos 1909; 51: 310–22.

68. BURNETT S. Prevalence of maxillary canine – first premolar transposition in a composite African sample. Angle Orthod 1999; 69: 187–9.

69. BURTON DJ et al. Serratia infection in a patient with bilateral subcondylar impacted third molar and associated dentigerous cysts. J Oral Surg 1980; 38: 135–8.

70. BUX P et al. Ectopic third molar associated with a dentigerous cyst in the subcondylar region. J Oral Maxillofac Surg 1994; 52: 630–2.

71. CAHILL DR et al. Tooth eruption: evidence for the central role of the dental follicle. J Oral Pathol 1980; 9: 189–200.

72. CAHILL DR et al. A review and comparison of tooth eruption systems used in experimentation. In: DAVIDOVITCH Z (ed.) Biological mechanisms of tooth eruption and root resorption. Birmingham: EBSCO Media, 1988.

73. CAMM JH et al. Premature eruption of the premolars. ASDC J Dent Child 1990; 57: 128–33.

74. CARELS C. Infrapositie, ankylose, externe wortelresorptie en tandverplaatsing. Ned Tijdschr Tandheelkd 1996; 103: 63–4.

75. CARR GE et al. Ectopic eruption of the first permanent maxillary molar in cleft lip and cleft palate children. ASDC J Dent Child 1965; 32: 179–88.

76. CARVER DD et al. Intranasal teeth. Oral Surg Oral Med Oral Pathol 1990; 70: 804–5.

77. CATALANOTTO FA et al. The effects of medroxyprogesterone on dentofacial development in males with idiopathic isosexual precocity. Angle Orthod 1978; 48: 106–13.

78. CHATTOPADHYAY A et al. Transposition of teeth and genetic etiology. Angle Orthod 1996; 66: 147–52.

79. CHAUSHU S et al. Maxillary incisor impaction and its relationship to canine displacement. Am J Othod Dentofac Orthop 2003; 124: 144–50.

80. CHEYNE VD et al. Impaction of permanent first molar with resorption and space loss in region of deciduous second molar. J Am Dent Assoc 1947; 35: 774–87.

81. CHEW MT et al. Orthodontic – surgical management of an impacted dilacerated maxillary central incisor. Pediatr Dent 2004; 26: 341–4.

82. CHIAPASCO M et al. Side effects and complications associated with third molars surgery. Oral Surg Oral Med Oral Pathol 1993; 76: 412–20.

83. CHILES DG et al. The third molar question. J Am Dent Assoc 1987; 115: 575–6.

84. CHONGRUK C. Asymptomatic ectopic impacted mandibular third molar. Oral Surg Oral Med Oral Pathol 1991; 71: 520.

85. CHU FCS et al. Prevalence of impacted teeth and associated pathologies. Hong Kong Med J 2003; 9: 158–63.

86. CLARK DB. Dental findings in patients with chronic renal failure. J Can Dent Assoc 1987; 10: 781–5

87. COBOURN MT et al. Analysis of the morbidity of submerged deciduous molars: the use of imaging techniques. Oral Surg Oral Med Oral Pathol Oral Radiol Endod 2002; 93: 98–102.

88. COHEN M et al. Dental development in pituitary dwarfism. J Dent Res 1948; 27: 445–57.

89. COSTELLO JP et al. Transmigration of permanent mandibular canines. Br Dent J 1996; 181: 212–13.

90. COUTINHO S et al. Relationships between mandibular canine calcification stages and skeletal maturity. Am J Orthod Dentofac Orthop 1993; 104: 262–8.

91. CUNHA RF et al. Systemic and local teething disturbances: prevalence in a clinic for infants. ASDC J Dent Child 2004; 71: 24–6.

92. CURRAN JB et al. Bilateral transposition of maxillary canines. Oral Surg 1973; 36: 905–6.

93. CZECHOLINSKI KA et al. Frühzeitiger Milchzahnverlust. Fortschr Kieferorthop 1994; 55: 54–60.

94. DACHI SF et al. A survey of 3,874 routine full-mouth radiographs. II. A study of impacted teeth. Oral Surg 1961; 14: 1165–9.

95. DAMM DD et al. Focal delayed eruption. Gen Dent 2001; 49: 356, 428.

96. DARLING AI et al. Submerged human deciduous molars and ankylosis. Arch Oral Biol 1973; 18: 1021–40.

97. DA SILVA FILHO OM et al. Ectopic eruption of maxillary first permanent molars in children with cleft lip. Angle Orthod 1996; 66: 373–80.

98. DA SILVA FILHO, OM et al. Ectopic eruption of a mandibular lateral incisor. J Clin Pediatr Dent 1997; 21: 177–85.

99. DARWISH SM et al. Impacted primary mandibular central incisors. J Clin Pediatr Dent 2002; 26: 347–50.

100. DAVIS PJ et al. The accuracy and precision of the "Demirjian system" when used for age determination in Chinese children. Swed Dent J 1994; 18: 113–16.

101. DAYAN D et al. Reimpaction of a first permanent maxillary molar due to an obscure idiopathic etiology. Clin Prev Dent 1983; 5 (2): 22–4.

102. DE BOER JG. Transpositie van gebitselementen. Ned Tijdschr Tandheelkd 1963; 70: 671–80.

103. DE BOER JG. Een zeldzaam geval van transpositie. Ned Tijdschr Tandheelkd 1971; 78: 402.

104. DE BOER M. Early loss of primary molars. Nederlandse Vereniging voor Orthodontische Studie; Studieweek 1980: 113–32.

105. DE BOER MPJ et al. Complications after mandibular third molar extraction. Quint Int 1995; 26: 779–84.

106. DE LAPERSONNE F. Supernumerary teeth. Dent Cosmos 1921; 63: 660.

107. DE-LA-ROSA-GAY C et al. Infraocclusion of primary molars. ASDC J Dent Child 1998; 65: 47–51.

108. DEMIRJIAN A et al. Interrelationships among measures of somatic, skeletal, dental, and sexual maturity. Am J Orthod 1985; 88: 433–8.

109. DEMIRJIAN A et al. New systems for dental maturity based on seven and four teeth. Ann Hum Biol 1976; 3: 411–21.

110. DEMIRJIAN A et al. A new system of dental age assessment. Hum Biol 1973; 45: 211–27.

111. DEMIRJIAN A et al. Sexual differences in dental development and prediction of emergence. J Dent Res 1980; 59: 1110–21.

112. DESALVO MS *et al.* Segmental odontomaxillary dysplasia (hemimaxillofacial dysplasia). Pediatr Dent 1996; 18: 154–6.

113. DE VISSCHER JG *et al.* Complex odontoma in the maxilla sinus. In J Oral Surg 1982; 11: 276–80.

114. DEWHURST SN *et al.* Infraocclusion of primary molars in monozygotic twins. Int J Paediatr Dent 1997; 7: 25–30.

115. DINER H *et al.* Dental diagnostic problems of potential genetic significance. In: SALINAS CF *et al.* (eds) Dentistry in the interdisciplinary treatment of genetic diseases. New York, NY: Alan R. Liss Inc., 1980.

116. DIXON DA. Observations on submerging deciduous molars. Dent Pract 1963; 13: 303–15.

117. DOUGLASS J *et al.* The etiology, prevalence, and sequelae of infraclusion of primary molars. ASDC J Dent Child 1991; 58: 481–3.

118. DRAKE DL. Segmental odontomaxillary dysplasia: an unusual orthodontic challenge. Am J Orthod Dentofac Orthop 2003; 123: 84–6.

119. DUBAI M *et al.* Frequency of transposition and its treatment at the department Pedodondotic and Orthodontics of Semmelweis University in the last five years. Fogorv Sz 2003; 96: 21–4.

120. DUNCAN K *et al.* Transposition and fusion in the primary dentition. ASDC J Dent Child 1996; 63: 365–7.

121. EID RMR *et al.* Assessment of dental maturity of Brazilian children age 6 to 14 years using Demirjian's method. Int J Paediatr Dent 2002; 12: 423–8.

122. EISENBUD L *et al.* The importance of panographic and dental evaluation for lesions of the antrum. Lanryngoscope 1976; 86: 1004–7.

123. EKIM SL *et al.* A treatment decision-making model for infraoccluded primary molars. Int J Paediatr Dent 2001; 11: 340–6.

124. ELANGO S *et al.* Ectopic tooth in the roof of the sinus. Ear Nose Throat J 1991; 70: 365–6.

125. ELIASSON S *et al.* Pathological changes related to long-term impaction of third molars. Int J Oral Maxillofac Surg 1989; 18: 210–12.

126. EL-LABBAN NG *et al.* Permanent teeth in hypophosphatasia. J Oral Pathol Med 1991; 20: 352–60.

127. ENWONWU CO. Influence of socio–economic conditions on dental development in Nigerian children. Arch Oral Biol 1973; 18: 95–107.

128. ERICSON S *et al.* Radiographic assessment of maxillary canine eruption in children with clinical signs of eruption disturbance. Eur J Orthod 1986; 8: 133–40.

129. ERICSON S *et al.* Longitudinal study and analysis of clinical supervision of maxillary canine eruption. Community Dent Oral Epidemiol 1986; 14: 172–6.

130. ERICSON S *et al.* Radiographic examination of ectopically erupting maxillary canines. Am J Orthod Dentofac Orthop 1987; 91: 483–92.

131. EVANS R. Incidence of lower second permanent molar impaction. Br J Orthod 1988; 15: 199–203.

132. FANNING EA. Effect of extraction of deciduous molars on the formation and eruption of their successors. Angle Orthod 1963; 32: 44–53.

133. FARIAS M, VARGERIK K. Dental development in hemifacial microsomia I. Eruption and agenesis. Pediatr Dent 1988; 10: 140–3.

134. FERGUSON JW *et al.* Eruption of palatal canines following surgical exposure. Br J Orthod 1997; 24: 203–7.

135. FERGUSON NC *et al.* An investigation of the occurrence of diastemata and supernumerary teeth. J Am Dent Assoc 1973; 87: 1409–10.

136. FILIPSON R. A new method for assessment of dental maturity using the individual curve of number of erupted permanent teeth. Ann Hum Biol 1975; 2: 13–24.

137. FLEISCHER-PETERS A. Die Bedeutung der zähne für die altersschätzung von findelkindern. Dtsch Zahnärztl Z 1987; 42: 712–18.

138. FRENCH D *et al.* Papillon-Lefèvre syndrome associated early onset periodontitis: a review and case study. J Can Dent Assoc 1995; 61: 432–8.

139. FRENSILLI JA *et al.* Dental changes of idiopathic hypoparathyroidism. J Oral Surg 1971; 29: 727–31.

140. FORSBERG C-M. Tooth size, spacing, and crowding in elation to eruption or impaction of third molars. Am J Orthod Dentofac Orthop 1988; 94: 57–62.

141. FROHNE J. Das idiopathische Prämolarendiastema – zum aussergewöhnlichen Distal-, Rotations- und Angulationspotential unterer Fünfer. Quintessenz 1997; 48: 1221–36.

142. GADGIL RM. Impacted mandibular anterior teeth. Oral Surg 1986; 61: 106.

143. GAETHOFS M *et al.* Delayed dental age in boys with constitutionally delayed puberty. Eur J Orthod 1999; 21: 711–15.

144. GALEA H *et al.* The dental caries and periodontal disease experience of patients with early onset insulin dependent diabetes. Int Dent J 1986; 36: 219–24.

145. GARCIA R *et al.* The eruption of third molars in adults. Oral Surg Oral Med Oral Pathol 1989; 68: 9–13.

146. GARFUNKEL AA *et al.* Familial hypoparathyroidism, candidiasis and mental retardation. J Oral Med 1979; 34: 13–17.

147. GARN SM, LEWIS AB. The gradient and the pattern of crown-size reduction in simple hypodontia. Angle Orthod 1970; 40: 51–8.

148. GARN SM *et al.* Endocrine factors in dental development. J Dent Res 1965; 44: 243–58.

149. GEHM S *et al.* Management of ectopic eruption of permanent molars. Compend Contin Educ 1997; 18: 561–9.

150. GHOLSTON LR *et al.* Bilateral transposition of maxillary canines and lateral incisors. ASDC J Dent Child 1984; 51: 58–63.

151. GHOSE LJ *et al.* Eruption time of permanent teeth in Iraqi school children. Arch Oral Biol 1981; 25: 13–15.

152. GOLDMAN JJ, NEWTON NJ. Supernumerary tooth bud in the maxillary antrum. Oral Surg 1949; 2: 993–4.

153. GÖYENÇ Y *et al.* Unusual ectopic eruption of maxillary canines. J Clin Orthod 1995; XXIX: 580–2.

154. GREENBERG SN *et al.* Ectopic movement of an unerupted mandibular canine. J Am Dent Assoc 1976; 93: 125–8.

155. GRON AM. Prediction of tooth emergence. J Dent Res 1962; 41: 573–85.

156. GROPER JN. A simplified treatment for correcting an ectopically erupting maxillary first permanent molar. ASDC J Dent Child 1985; 52: 374–6.

157. GROVER PS *et al*. The incidence of unerupted permanent teeth and related clinical cases. Oral Surg 1985; 59: 420–5..

158. GUNGOR HC *et al*. Ectopic eruption of maxillary first permanent molars. J Clin Paediatr Dent 1998; 22: 211–16.

159. GUPTA YK *et al*. Intranasal tooth as a complication of cleft lip and alveolus in a four year old child. Int J Paediatr Dent 2001; 11: 221–4.

160. HÄGG U *et al*. Timing of tooth emergence. Swed Dent J 1986; 10: 195–206.

161. HAIDAR Z, SHALHOUB SY. The incidence of impacted wisdom teeth in a Saudi community. Br J Oral Maxillofac Surg 1986; 15: 569–71.

162. HAINLINE-RAEZ AG *et al*. Abnormal odontogenesis. ASDC J Dent Child 1985; 52: 130–3.

163. HAISHIMA K *et al*. Compound odontomes associated with impacted maxillary primary central incisors. Int J Paediatr Dent 1994; 4: 251–6.

164. HARALABAKIS NB *et al*. Premature or delayed exfoliation of deciduous teeth and root formation. Angle Orthod 1994; 64: 151–7.

165. HARILA-KAERA V *et al*. The eruption of permanent incisors and first molars in prematurely born children. Eur J Orthod 2003; 25: 293–9.

166. HARNDT E. Klinische Bemerkungen zum Zahndurchbruch. In: HARNDT E *et al*. (eds) Zahn-, Mund- und Kieferheilkunde im Kindesalter. Berlin: Verlag, 1967.

167. HARTMANN C. A treatment for ectopically erupted first permanent molars. ASDC J Dent Child 1984; 51: 363–6.

168. HARTSFIELD JK JR. Premature exfoliation of teeth in children and adolescents. Adv Pediatr 1994; 41: 453–70.

169. HARZER W *et al*. Längsschnittuntersuchung zur ersten Wechselgebissphase an 250 Dresdner Schulkindern. Stomatol DDR 1984; 34: 544–8.

170. HARZER W *et al*. Zur Dentition permanenter Zähne-Längsschnittuntersuchungen an 250 Schulkindern zwischen dem 7. und 15. Lebensjahr. Zahn- Mund- Kieferheilkd 1987; 75: 779–85.

171. HASSANALI J *et al*. Removal of deciduous canine tooth buds in Kenyan rural Maasai. East Africa Med J 1995; 72: 205–6.

172. HATTAB FN *et al*. Impaction status of third molars in Jordanian students. Oral Surg Oral Med Oral Pathol Oral Radiol Endod 1995; 79: 24–9.

173. HATTAB FN. Positional changes and eruption of impacted mandibular third molars in young adults. Oral Surg Oral Med Oral Pathol Oral Radiol Endod 1997; 84: 604–8.

174. HATTAB FN *et al*. Papillon-Lefèvre syndrome. J Periodontol 1995; 66: 413–20.

175. HAUK MJ *et al*. Delayed tooth eruption: association with severity of HIV infection. Pediatr Dent 2001; 23: 260–2.

176. HAYWARD JR. Cuspid gigantism. Oral Surg 1980; 49: 500–1.

177. HELM S. Relationship between dental and skeletal maturation in Danish schoolchildren. Sand J Dent Res 1990; 98: 313–17.

178. HELM S *et al*. Prevalence of crowding in the permanent dentition after early loss of deciduous molars or canines. Nederlandse Vereniging voor Orthodontische Studie; Studieweek 1975: 161–6.

179. HELPIN ML *et al*. Ankylosis in monozygotic twins. ASDC J Dent Child 1986; 53: 135–9.

180. HELPIN ML *et al*. Complications following radiation therapy to the head. Oral Surg 1986; 55: 209–12.

181. HENDERSON HZ. Ankylosis of primary molars. ASDC J Dent Child 1979; 46: 117–22.

182. HINRICHS EH. Dental changes in juvenile hypothyroidism. ASDC J Dent Child 1966; 33: 167–73.

183. HIRSCH A *et al*. Use of orthodontic treatment as an aid to third molar extraction. J Periodontol 2003; 74: 887–92.

184. HISLOP WS *et al*. Treatment of unerupted impacted mandibular second premolars by surgical exposure and orthodontic traction. J Pediatr Dent 1988; 4: 103–7.

185. HÖFFDING J *et al*. Emergence of permanent teeth and onset of dental stages in Japanese children. Community Dent Oral Epidemiol 1984; 12: 55–8.

186. HOLTGRAVE EA *et al*. Acceleration in dental development. Eur J Oral Orthod 1997; 19: 703–10.

187. HU JC-C *et al*. Characterization of a family with dominant hypophosphatasia. Eur J Oral Sci 2000; 108: 189–94.

188. HUGOSON A *et al*. Chapter 1.

189. HURME VO. Ranges of normalcy in the eruption of permanent teeth. ASDC J Dent Child 1949; 16: 11–15.

190. IDA-YONEMOCHI H *et al*. No developmental failure of cultured tooth germs from osteopetrotic (op/op) mice. J Oral Pathol Med 2002; 31: 374–8.

191. IDA-YONEMOCHI H *et al*. Disturbed tooth eruption in osteopetrotic (op/op) mice. J Oral Pathol Med 2002; 31: 361–73.

192. JARJOURA K *et al*. Maxillary canine impactions. Compend Contin Educ 2002; 23: 23–36.

193. HURLEN B, HUMERFELT D. Characteristics of premaxillary hyperodontia. A radiographic study. Acta Odontol Scand 1985; 43: 75–81.

194. INFANTE PF *et al*. Relation of chronology of deciduous tooth emergence to height, weight and head circumference in children. Arch Oral Biol 1973; 18: 1411–17.

195. ISERI H *et al*. Continued eruption of maxillary incisors and first molars in girls from 9 to 25 years, studied by the implant method. Eur J Orthod 1996; 18: 245–56.

196. IVY RH. A case of non-eruption of entire permanent denture. Dent Cosmos 1933; 75: 689–90.

197. JACOBS SG. The impacted maxillary canine. Aust Dent J 1996; 41: 310–6.

198. JAVID B. Transmigration of impacted mandibular cuspids. Int J Oral Surg 1985; 14: 547–9.

199. JÄRVINEN S. Mandibular incisor-cuspid transposition: a survey. J Pedodont 1982; 6: 159–63.

200. JENSEN SB *et al*. Nature and frequency of dental changes in idiopathic hypoparathyroidism and pseudohypoparathyroidism. Scand J Dent Res 1981; 89: 26–37.

201. JOSHI MR. Transmigrant mandibular canines. Angle Orthod 2001; 71: 12–22.

202. JOSHI MR *et al*. Transmigration of mandibular canines. Quint Int 1994; 25: 291–4.

203. KAIHARA Y *et al*. A case of odontoma that caused delayed eruption of mandibular first permanent molar. Pediatr Dent J 2000; 10: 129–32.

204. KALK WWI *et al*. Dentin dysplasia type I. Five cases within one family. Oral Surg Oral Med Oral Pathol Oral Radiol Endod 1998; 86: 175–8.
205. KELLER EE *et al*. Dental and skeletal development in various endocrine and metabolic diseases. J Am Dent Assoc 1970; 81: 415–19.
206. KEROS J *et al*. Heterotopia of the mandibular third molar. Quint Int 1997; 28: 753–4.
207. KERR WJS. The effect of premature loss of deciduous canines and molars on the eruption of their successors. Eur J Oral Orthod 1980; 2: 123–8.
208. KHARBANDA OP *et al*. Extreme transmigration of mandibular cuspid. J Clin Pediatr Dent 1994; 18: 307–8.
209. KHOURI SA. Periodontal adaptation following extensive extrusion and rotation of a horizontally impacted maxillary central incisor. J Periodontol 1986; 57: 251–6.
210. KIESER JA *et al*. Delayed tooth formation in children exposed to tobacco smoke. J Clin Pediatr Dent 1996; 20: 97–100.
211. KIMMEL NA *et al*. Ectopic eruption of maxillary first permanent molars in different areas of the United States. ASDC J Dent Child 1982; 49: 294–9.
212. KING NM *et al*. An intranasal tooth in a patient with a cleft lip and palate. J Am Dent Assoc 1987; 114: 475–8.
213. KIZAWA K *et al*. A case of the impacted mandibular first molar with malformation of the roots. Jap J Pedod 1985; 23: 232.
214. KJELLBERG H *et al*. Craniofacial morphology, dental occlusion, tooth eruption, and dental maturity in boys with short stature with or without growth hormone deficiency. Eur J Oral Sci 2000; 108: 359–67.
215. KOOI SK. Aspecten van het tijdelijke gebit. Thesis, University of Utrecht, 1982.
216. KOPPANG HS *et al*. Dental features in congenital renal tubular acidosis of proximal type. Scand J Dent Res 1984; 92: 489–95.
217. KOSOWICZ J *et al*. Abnormalities of tooth development in pituitary dwarfism. Oral Surg 1977; 44: 853–63.
218. KOSTOPOULOU O *et al*. Agreement between practitioners concerning removal of asymptomatic third molars. Community Dent Health 1997; 14: 129–32.
219. KOYOUMDJISKI-KAYE E *et al*. Submerging primary molars in Israeli rural children. Community Dent Oral Epidemiol 1982; 10: 204–8.
220. KRACKE RR. Delayed tooth eruption versus impaction. ASDC J Dent Child 1975; 42: 371–4.
221. KRAKOWIAK FJ. Ankylosed primary molars. ASDC J Dent Child 1978; 45: 288–92.
222. KRAMER RM *et al*. The incidence of impacted teeth. Oral Surg 1970A; 29: 237–41.
223. KRENNMAIR G *et al*. Imaging of unerupted and displaced teeth by cross–sectional CT scans. Int J Oral Maxillofac Surg 1995; 24: 413–16.
224. KRISTERSON L *et al*. Autotransplantation and replantation of tooth germs in monkeys. Effect of damage to the dental follicle and position of transplant in the alveolus. Int J Oral Surg 1984; 13: 324–33.
225. KRUGER E *et al*. Third molar outcomes from age 8 to 26. Oral Surg Oral Med Oral Pathol Oral Radiol Endod 2001; 92: 150–5.
226. KUBA Y *et al*. Inverted impaction of second premolars. J Clin Pediatr Dent 1995; 19: 205–9.
227. KUIPER L *et al*. Unilaterale neusobstructie ten gevolge van een dentogene cyste. Ned Tijdschr Tandheelkd 1986; 93: 50–1.
228. KUROL J. Infraocclusion of primary molars: an epidemiologic and familial study. Community Dent Oral Epidemiol 1981; 9: 94–102.
229. KUROL J. Early treatment of tooth-eruption disturbances. Am J Orthod Dentofac Orthop 2002; 121: 588–91.
230. KUROL J *et al*. Ectopic eruption of maxillary first permanent molars: familial tendencies. ASDC J Dent Child 1982; 49: 35–8.
231. KUROL J *et al*. Ectopic eruption of maxillary first permanent molars: a review. ASDC J Dent Child 1986; 53: 209–14.
232. KUROL J *et al*. The effect of extraction of infraoccluded deciduous molars: a longitudinal study. Am J Orthod 1985; 87: 46–55.
233. KUROL J *et al*. Infraoclusion of primary molars. Scand J Dent Res 1984; 92: 564–76.
234. KUROL J *et al*. Infraocclusion of primary molars and the effect on occlusal development. Eur J Orthod 1984; 6: 277–93.
235. KUROL J *et al*. Infraocclusion of primary molars with aplasia of the permanent successor. Angle Orthod 1984; 54: 283–94.
236. KWAN CHEN Y *et al*. Bilateral complete rotation of maxillary lateral incisors with dens invaginatus. Oral Surg Oral Med Oral Pathol 1992; 74: 532.
237. LAMB KA *et al*. Measurement of space loss resulting from tooth ankylosis. ASDC J Dent Child 1968; 35: 483–6.
238. LAMBERT M *et al*. Unusual impaction of a primary lateral incisor. ASDC J Dent Child 1994; 61: 146–8.
239. LAUTERSTEIN AM *et al*. Effect of deciduous mandibular pulpotomy on the eruption of succedaneous premolar. J Dent Res 1962; 41: 1367–72.
240. LEE CF *et al*. The daily rhythm of tooth eruption. Am J Orthod Dentofac Orthop 1995; 107: 38–47.
241. LEE-CHAN S *et al*. Mixed dentition analysis for Asian-Americans. Am J Orthod Dentofac Orthop 1998; 113: 293–9.
242. LEIVESLEY WD. Minimizing the problem of impacted and ectopic canines. ASDC J Dent Child 1984; 51: 367–70.
243. LEPE X *et al*. Absence of adult dental anomalies in familial hypophosphatasia. J Periodont Res 1997; 32: 375–80.
244. LEROY R *et al*. Impact of caries experience in the deciduous molars on the emergence of the successors. Eur J Oral Sci 2003; 111: 106–10.
245. LEVESQUE GY *et al*. Sexual dimorphism in the development, emergence, and agenesis of the mandibular third molar. J Dent Res 1981; 60: 1735–41.
246. LIN C-C *et al*. Ectopic soft-tissue mesiodens. J Oral Med 1986; 41: 124–5 and 133.
247. LIN YT. Treatment of an impacted dilacerated maxillary central incisor. Am J Orthod Dentofac Orthop 1999; 116: 15A–16A.
248. LINDSKOG S *et al*. Effect of a high dose of fluoride on resorbing osteoclasts in vivo. Scand J Dent Res 1989; 97: 483–7.

249. LIVERSIDGE HM. Dental maturation of 18th and 19th century British children using Demirjian's method. Int J Paediatr Dent 1999; 9: 111–15.

250. LIVERSIDGE HM et al. Dental maturation in British children: are Demirjian's standards applicable? Int J Paediatr Dent 1999; 9: 263–9.

251. LO RT et al. Studies in the etiology and prevention of malocclusion. Am J Orthod 1953; 39: 460–7.

252. LOEVY HT et al. Tooth eruption and craniofacial development in congenital hypothyroidism. J Am Dent Assoc 1987; 115: 429–31.

253. LOEVY HT. The effect of primary tooth extraction on the eruption of succedaneous premolars. J Am Dent Assoc 1989; 118: 715–18.

254. LOH HS. Migration of unerupted mandibular premolars. Br Dent J 1988; 164: 324–5.

255. LÓPEZ NJ et al. Histological differences between teeth with adult periodontitis and prepubertal periodontitis. J Periodontol 1990; 61: 87–94.

256. LÖHR E et al. Zur Variation der reihenfolge des seitenzahn wechsels. Zahn Mund Kieferheilkd 1985; 73: 442–7.

257. LUNDGREN T et al. Retrospective study of children with hypophophatasia with reference to dental changes. Scand J Dent Res 1991; 99: 357–64.

258. LUNDSTRÖM R et al. Dental development in children following maternal rubella. Acta Pediatr 1962; 51: 155–60.

259. LUTEN JR. The prevalence of supernumerary teeth in primary and mixed dentitions. ASDC J Dent Child 1967; 34: 346–53.

260. LYSSEL L et al. Relations between the times of eruption of primary and permanent teeth. Acta Odontol Scand 1969; 27: 271–81.

261. LYTLE JJ. Etiology and indications for the management of impacted teeth. Oral Maxillofac Surg Clin North Am 1993; 5: 63–75.

262. MACFARLANE JD et al. Dental aspects of hypophosphatasia. Oral Surg Oral Med Oral Pathol 1989; 67: 521–6.

263. MADER C et al. Transposition of teeth. J Am Dent Assoc 1979; 98: 412–13.

264. MAGNUSSON TE. Emergence of permanent teeth and onset of dental stages in the population of Iceland. Community Dent Oral Epidemiol 1976; 4: 30–7.

265. MAHANEY MC. Delayed dental development and pulmonary disease severity in children with cystic fibrosis. Arch Oral Biol 1986; 31: 363–7.

266. MAHESHWARI PK et al. Ectopic eruption of deciduous cuspid. J Indian Dent Assoc 1983; 54: 79–80.

267. MALTHA IC. The process of tooth eruption in beagle dogs. Thesis, University of Nijmegen, 1982.

268. MANCINI G et al. Primary tooth ankylosis: report of case with histological analysis. ASDC J Dent Child 1995; 62: 215–19.

269. MAPPES MS et al. An example of regional variation in the tempos of tooth mineralization and hand-wrist ossification. Am J Orthod Dentofac Orthop 1992; 101: 145–51.

270. MARÉCHAUX SC. The problems of treatment of early ankylosis. ASDC J Dent Child 1986; 53: 63–6.

271. MARKS SC et al. Tooth eruption. In: DAVIDOVITCH Z (ed.) Biological mechanisms of tooth eruption and root resorption. Birmingham: EBSCO Media, 1988.

272. MARTIN MD et al. Spontaneous exfoliation of the teeth following severe elemental mercury poisoning. Oral Surg Oral Med Oral Pathol Oral Radiol Endod 1997; 84: 495–501.

273. MATSSON L et al. Caries frequency in children with controlled diabetes. Scand J Dent Res 1975; 83: 327–32.

274. McCARTHY MF. Sports and mouth protection. Gen Dent 1990; 38: 343–6.

275. McCONNELL TL et al. Maxillary canine impaction in patients with transverse maxillary deficiency. ASDC J Dent Child 1996; 63: 190–5.

276. McDONALD F, YAP WL. The surgical exposure and application of direct traction of unerupted teeth. Am J Orthod 1986; 89: 331–40.

277. McGREGOR AJ. The impacted lower wisdom tooth. Oxford: Oxford University Press, 1985.

278. McKENNA JD et al. Localization of maxillary third molar immobilized within an infected maxillary sinus. J Am Dent Assoc 1984; 108: 208–9.

279. McKIBBEN DR, BREARLY LJ. Radiographic determination of the prevalence of selected dental anomalies in children. ASDC J Dent Child 1971; 38: 390–8.

280. McMULLAN RE et al. Investigation of premolar rotation in a group of 15–year–old Norwegian children. Eur J Orthod 1990; 12: 311–15.

281. McNAMARA CM et al. Premature dental eruption. ASDC J Dent Child 1999; 66: 70–2.

282. MEDEIROS PJ et al. Treatment of an ankylosed central incisor by single–tooth dento–osseous osteotomy. Am J Orthod Dentofac Orthop 1997; 112: 496–501.

283. MEIJER BA et al. Eenzijdige neusbloedingen als gevolg van een nasaal doorgebroken gebitselement. Ned Tijdschr Tandheelkd 2003; 110: 362–4.

284. MELCHER AH et al. The physiology of tooth eruption. In: The biology of occlusal development. Craniofacial Growth Series Monograph 7. Ann Arbor, MI: University of Michigan, 1977; 1–23.

285. MEYLE J et al. Influences of systemic diseases on periodontitis in children and adolescents. Periodontol 2000 2001; 26: 92–112.

286. MOLLAOGLU N et al. Patterns of third molar impaction in a group of volunteers in Turkey. Clin Oral Invest 2002; 6: 109–13.

287. MORGANTINI J et al. Traumatism dentaires chez l'enfant en âge préscolaire et répercussions sur les dents permanentes. Rev Mens Suisse Odonto-stomatol 1986; 96: 37–40.

288. MOORREES CFA et al. Age variation of formation stages for ten permanent teeth. J Dent Res 1963; 42: 1490–502.

289. MORI S et al. Inverted tooth eruption. Oral Surg 1979; 47: 389–90.

290. MÖRNSTAD H et al. Age estimation with aid of tooth development. Scand J Dent Res 1994; 102: 137–43.

291. MORRIS CR et al. Panoramic radiographic survey: a study of embedded third molars. J Oral Surg 1971; 29: 122–5.

292. MUELLER CT et al. Prevalence of ankylosis of primary molars in different regions of the United States. ASDC J Dent Child 1983; 50: 213–18.

293. MUELLER-LESSMANN V *et al.* Orofacial findings in the Klippel-Trénaunay syndrome. Int J paediatr Dent 2001; 11: 225–9.

294. MULLALLY BH *et al.* Ankylosis: an orthodontic problem with a restorative solution. Br Dent J 1995; 179: 426–30.

295. MUPPARAPU M. Patterns of intra-osseous transmigration and ectopic eruption of mandibular canines. Dentomaxillofac Radiol 2002; 31: 355–60.

296. MYLLARNIEMI S *et al.* Dental maturity in hypopituitarism, and dental response to substitution treatment. Scand J Dent Res 1978; 86: 307–12.

297. NANDA RS. Eruption of human teeth. Am J Orthod 1960; 46: 363–78.

298. NASTRI AL *et al.* The nasal tooth. Aust Dent J 1996; 41: 176–7.

299. NAZIF MM *et al.* The effects of primary molar ankylosis on root resorption and the development of permanent successors. ASDC J Dent Child 1986; 53: 115–18.

300. NEAL JJD, BOWDEN DEJ. The diagnostic value of panoramic radiographs in children aged nine to ten years. Br J Orthod 1988; 15: 193–7.

301. NEMCOVSKY CE *et al.* Effect of non-erupted 3rd molars on distal roots and supporting structures of approximal teeth. J Clin Periodontol 1996; 23: 810–15.

302. NEWMAN HN. Attrition, eruption, and the periodontium. J Dent Res 1999; 78: 730–4.

303. NIK-NORIAH, NIK-HUSSEIN. Early eruption and advanced root development of the permanent cuspids in a six-year-old boy. J Clin Pediatr Dent 1992; 16: 112–14.

304. NITZAN DW *et al.* Pericoronitis: a reappraisal of its clinical and microbiologic aspects. J Oral Maxillofac Surg 1985; 43: 510–16.

305. NORDENRAM Å. Impacted maxillary canines – A study of surgical treated patients over 20 years of age. Swed Dent J 1987; 11: 153–8.

306. NORTHWAY WM. The not-so-harmless maxillary primary first molar extraction. J Am Dent Assoc 2000; 131: 1711–20.

307. NORTHWAY WM *et al.* Effects of premature loss of deciduous molars. Angle Orthod 1984; 54: 295–329.

308. NYKÄNEN R *et al.* Validity of the Demirjian method for dental age estimation when applied to Norwegian children. Acta Odontol Scand 1998; 56: 238–44.

309. NYSTRÖM M *et al.* The period between exfoliation of primary teeth and the emergence of permanent successors. Eur J Orthod 1989; 11: 47–51.

310. NYSTRÖM M *et al.* Dental maturity in Finnish children, estimated from the development of seven permanent mandibular teeth. Acta Odontol Scand 1986; 44: 193–8.

311. NYSTRÖM M *et al.* Emergence of permanent teeth and dental age in a series of Finns. Acta Odontol Scand 2001; 59: 49–56.

312. O'CARROLL MK. Transmigration of the mandibular right canine with development of odontoma in its place. Oral Surg 1984; 57: 349.

313. O'CONNELL AC *et al.* Evaluation of oral problems in an osteogenesis imperfecta population. Oral Surg Oral Med Oral Pathol Oral Radiol Endod 1999; 87: 189–96.

314. O'CONNELL AC *et al.* Delayed eruption of permanent teeth in hyperimmunoglobulinemia E recurrent infection syndrome. Oral Surg Oral Med Oral Pathol Oral Radiol Endod 2000; 89: 117–85.

315. ODUSANYA SA *et al.* Third molar eruption among rural Nigerians. Oral Surg Oral Med Oral Pathol 1991; 71: 151–4.

316. OGISI FO *et al.* Ectopic nasal dentition associated with squamous cell carcinoma of palate in a 12-year-old boy. Br J Oral Maxillofac Surg 1988; 26: 58–61.

317. O'GRADY JF *et al.* Odontomes in an Australian population. Aust Dent J 1987; 32: 196–9.

318. OIKARINEN V *et al.* Similarly impacted second and third maxillary and mandibular molars in a pair of monozygotic twins. Dentomaxillofac Radiol 1990; 19: 133–4.

319. OLSSON A *et al.* Hypophosphatasia affecting the permanent dentition. J Oral Pathol Med 1996; 25: 343–7.

320. O'MEARA WF. Effect of primary molar extraction on gingival emergence of succedaneous tooth. J Dent Res 1966; 45: 1174–83.

321. OTSUKA Y *et al.* A review of clinical features in 13 cases of impacted primary teeth. Int J Paediatr Dent 2001; 11: 57–63.

322. OTUYEMI OD *et al.* Eruption times of third molars in young rural Nigerians. Int Dent J 1997; 47: 266–70.

323. OUNSTED M *et al.* A longitudinal study of tooth emergence and somatic growth in 697 children from birth to three years. Arch Oral Biol 1987; 11: 787–91.

324. PACKOTA GV *et al.* Radiographic features of segmental odontomaxillary dysplasia: study of 12 cases. Oral Surg Oral Med Oral Pathol Oral Radiol Endod 1996; 82: 577–84.

325. PAGE RC *et al.* Prepubertal periodontitis. I. Definition of a clinical disease entity. J Periodontol 1983; 54: 257–71.

326. PAGE RC *et al.* A new look at the etiology and the pathogenesis of early–onset periodontitis. J Periodontol 1985; 56: 748–50.

327. PAHKALA R *et al.* Eruption pattern of permanent teeth in a rural community in northeastern Finland. Acta Odontol Scand 1991; 49: 431–9.

328. PARNER ET *et al.* A longitudinal study of time trends in the eruption of permanent teeth in Danish children. Arch Oral Biol 2001; 46: 425–31.

329. PATEL JR. Transposition and microdontia. Oral Surg Oral Med Oral Pathol 1993; 73: 129.

330. PAYNE GS. Bilateral transposition of maxillary canines and premolars. Am J Orthod 1969; 56: 45–52.

331. PEARSON MH *et al.* Management of palatally impacted canines. Eur J Orthod 1997; 19: 511–15.

332. PECK S. On the phenomenon of intraosseous migration of nonerupting teeth. Am J Orthod Dentofac Orthop 1998; 113: 515–17.

333. PECK S *et al.* Classification of maxillary tooth transpositions. Am J Orthod Dentofac Orthop 1995; 107: 505–17.

334. PECK S *et al.* Maxillary canine-first premolar transposition, associated dental anomalies and genetic basis. Angle Orthod 1993; 63: 99–110.

335. PECK S *et al.* Concomitant occurrence of canine malposition and tooth agenesis: evidence of orofacial genetic fields. Am J Orthod Dentofac Orthop 2002; 122: 657–60.

336. PECK S *et al*. Prevalence of tooth agenesis and peg–shaped maxillary lateral incisor associated with palatally displaced canine (PDC) anomaly. Am J Orthod Dentofac Orthop 1996; 110: 441–3.

337. PEDLAR J. Crown of a tooth in the lateral pharyngeal space. Br Dent J 1986; 161: 335–6.

338. PELSMAEKERS B *et al*. The genetic contribution to dental maturation. J Dent Res 1997; 76: 1337–40.

339. PERKINS T *et al*. Improvement of dental development in osteopetrotic mice by maternal vitamin D3 sulfate administration. J Craniofac Genet 1988; 8: 83–93.

340. PHILIPPART C *et al*. Histopathology of the interactions between alveolar bone and impacted dental germs in osteopetrotic op/op rats. Oral Pathol 1989; 18: 157–62.

341. PHILIPSEN HP *et al*. Odontogenic lesions in opercula of permanent molars delayed eruption. J Oral Pathol Med 1992; 21: 38–41.

342. PICKETT AB *et al*. Oral findings in Trisomy 8 mosaicism. Pediatr Dent 1980; 2: 48–52.

343. PIERCE AM *et al*. IgE in postsecretory ameloblasts suggesting a hypersensitivity reaction at tooth eruption. ASDC J Dent Child 1986; 53: 23–6.

344. PIRINEN S *et al*. Palatal displacement of canine is genetic and related to congenital absence of teeth. J Dent Res 1996; 75: 1742–6.

345. PINDBORG JJ. Pathology of the dental hard tissues. Copenhagen: Munksgaard, 1970.

346. PINTO A *et al*. Management of patients with thyroid disease. J Am Dent Assoc 2002; 133: 849–58.

347. PISANTI S *et al*. Familial hypoparathyreoidism with candidasis and mental retardation. Oral Surg 1977; 44: 374–83.

348. PLATZER KM. Mandibular incisor-canine transposition. J Am Dent Assoc 1968; 76: 778–84.

349. PLUNKETT DJ *et al*. A study of transposed canines in a sample of orthodontic patients. Br J Orthodont 1998; 25: 203–8.

350. POPE JE *et al*. The dental status of cerebral palsied children. Pediatr Dent 1991; 13: 156–62.

351. POSEN AL. The effect of premature loss of deciduous molars on premolar eruption. Angle Orthod 1965; 35: 249–52.

352. POULSOM K. The ages of eruption of permanent teeth of children from sub-Sahara Africa. J Pediatr Dent 1988; 4: 85–8.

353. POWER SM *et al*. An investigation into the response of palatally displaced canines to the removal of deciduous canines and an assessment of factors contributing to favourable eruption. Br J Orthod 1993; 20: 215–23.

354. PRAHL-ANDERSEN B. Geretineerde hoektanden. Ned Tijdschr Tandheelkd 1974; 81: 209–15.

355. PRAHL-ANDERSEN B. Biologisches Alter bei Kindern mit Spaltbildungen. Stomatol DDR 1979; 29: 816–22.

356. PRAHL-ANDERSEN B. Gebitsontwikkeling bij agenesieën. Ned Tijdschr Tandheelkd 1984; 91: 515–18.

357. PRAHL-ANDERSEN B *et al*. Enige gevolgen van vroegtijdig verlies van tweede melkmolaren in de onderkaak. Ned Tijdschr Tandheelkd 1979; 86: 89–99.

358. PRAHL-ANDERSEN B *et al*. A mixed-longitudinal interdisciplinary study of growth and development. New York, NY: Academic Press, 1979, p. 13.

359. PRATCHYAPRUIT WO *et al*. Papillon-Lefèvre syndrome. J Dermatol 2002; 29: 329–35.

360. PROFFIT WR *et al*. Primary failure of eruption: a possible cause of posterior open-bite. Am J Orthod 1981; 80: 173–90.

361. PROGREL MA. The surgical uprighting of mandibular second molars. Am J Orthod Dentofac Orthop 1995; 108: 180–3.

362. PROVE SA *et al*. Physiological root resorption of primary molars. J Clin Pediatr Dent 1992; 16: 202–6.

363. PULVER F. The etiology and prevalence of ectopic eruption of the maxillary first permanent molar. ASDC J Dent Child 1968; 35: 138–46.

364. PUNWUTIKORN J *et al*. Symptoms of unerupted mandibular third molars. Oral Surg Oral Med Oral Pathol Oral Radiol Endod 1999; 87: 305–10.

365. PYTLIK W. Primary failure of eruption. Int Dent J 1991; 41: 274–8.

366. QUEK SL *et al*. Pattern of third molar impaction in a Singapore Chinese population. Int J Oral Maxillofac Surg 2003; 32: 548–52.

367. QUINTERO E *et al*. Primary molars in severe infraocclusion. Eur J Paediatr Dent 2003; 2: 78–83.

368. RAGHOEBAR GM *et al*. Secundaire retentie van melkmolaren. Ned Tijdschr Tandheelkd 1988; 95: 389–92.

369. RAGHOEBAR GM *et al*. Secundaire retentie van blijvende molaren – II. Therapie. Ned Tijdschr Tandheelkd 1992; 99: 485–8.

370. RAGHOEBAR GM *et al*. Secondary retention of permanent molars. J Dent 1992; 20: 277–82.

371. RAGHOEBAR GM *et al*. Secondary retention in the primary dentition. ASDC J Dent Child 1991; 58: 17–22.

372. RAGHOEBAR GM *et al*. Secondary retention as a possible cause of impaction of permanent molars in the same dentition. Quint Int 1991; 22: 807–10.

373. RAJASUO A *et al*. Comparison of clinical status of third molars in young men in 1949 and in 1990. Oral Surg Oral Med Oral Pathol 1993; 76: 694–8.

374. RAMOS-GOMEZ FJ *et al*. Oral manifestations and dental status in paediatric HIV infection. Int J Paediatr Dent 2000; 10: 3–11.

375. RANALLI DN *et al*. Comparative analysis of ectopic eruption of maxillary permanent first molars in children with clefts. ASDC J Dent Child 1986; 53: 433–5.

376. RANTA R. A comparative study of tooth formation in the permanent dentition of Finnish children with cleft lip and palate. Suom Hammaslaak Toin 1972; 68: 58–66.

377. RANTA R. Impacted maxillary second permanent molars. ASDC J Dent Child 1985; 52: 48–51.

378. RANTA R. Tooth germ transposition. ASDC J Dent Child 1989; 56: 366–70.

379. RASMUSSEN P *et al*. Inherited retarded eruption. ASDC J Dent Child 1983; 50: 268–73.

380. RASMUSSEN P *et al*. Inherited primary failure of eruption in the primary dentition. ASDC J Dent Child 1997; 64: 43–7.

381. REILLY S *et al*. Tooth eruption in failure-to-thrive infants. ASDC J Dent Child 1992; 59: 350–2.

382. REVENTLID M *et al*. Intra- and interexaminer variations in four dental methods for age estimation of children. Swed Dent J 1996, 20: 133–9.

383. RICHARDSON ER *et al*. Longitudinal study of three views of mandibular third molar eruption in males. Am J Orthod 1984; 86: 119–29.

384. RICHARDSON ME *et al*. Lower third molar development subsequent to second molar extraction. Am J Orthod Dentofac Orthop 1993; 104: 566–74.

385. RISINGER RK *et al*. The rhythms of human premolar eruption. J Am Dent Assoc 1996; 127: 1515–21.

386. RITCHIE GM. Dental manifestations of pseudohypoparathyroidism. Arch Dis Child 1965; 40: 565–72.

387. ROBERTS MW. Multiple familial dental anomalies. ASDC J Dent Child 1973; 40: 58–9.

388. ROBERTS MW *et al*. Dental development in precocious puberty. J Dent Res 1985; 64: 1084–6.

389. RÖNNERMAN A. Early loss of primary molars relation to space conditions, dental development, facial morphology and the need for orthodontic treatment. Thesis, Göteburg, 1977.

390. ROTHBERG MS *et al*. Intranasal presentation of an intruded deciduous incisor. Oral Surg Oral Med Oral Pathol 1991; 72: 263.

391. ROUSSET M-M *et al*. Emergence of permanent teeth: secular trends and variance in a modern sample. ASDC J Dent Child 2003; 70: 208–14.

392. RUNE B, SARNÄS KV. Tooth size and tooth formation in children with advanced hypodontia. Angle Orthod 1974; 44: 316–21.

393. RUPRECHT A *et al*. The incidence of transposition of teeth in dental patients. J Pedod 1985; 9: 244–9.

394. RUPRECHT A *et al*. Transposition of teeth. J Can Dent Assoc 1984; 50: 308–9.

395. SAGNE S *et al*. Transalveolar transplantation of maxillary canines. A critical evaluation of a clinical procedure. Acta Odontol Scand 1997; 55: 1–8.

396. SAĞLAM AMS *et al*. The relationship between dental and skeletal maturity. J Orofac Orthop/Fortschr Kieferorthop 2002; 63: 454–62.

397. SASS T. Retention oberer Eckzähne durch zusammengesetzte Odontome. Dtsch Zahnärztl Z 1986; 41: 708–10.

398. SAUK JJ. Genetic disorders involving tooth eruption anomalies. In: DAVIDOVITCH Z (ed.) Biological mechanisms of tooth eruption and root resorption. Birmingham: EBSCO Media, 1988.

399. SAWYER DR *et al*. Malnutrition and the oral health of children in Ogbomosho, Nigeria. ASDC J Dent Child 1985; 52: 141–5.

400. SCHEUTZEL P *et al*. Zahn- und Kieferveränderungen bei chronischer Nierinsuffizienz im Kindesalter. Dtsch Zahnärztl Z 1989; 44: 115–18.

401. SCHOEN PJ *et al*. Nabezwaren en complicaties na verwijdering van de derde molaar in de onderkaak. Ned Tijdschr Tandheelkd 1998; 105: 170–3.

402. SEGURA JJ *et al*. Maxillary canine transpositions in two brothers and one sister. ASDC J Dent Child 2002; 69: 54–8.

403. SENGUPTA A *et al*. The effects of dental wear on third molar eruption and on the curve of Spee in human archaeological dentitions. Arch Oral Biol 1999; 44: 925–34.

404. SEOW WK. A study of the development of the permanent dentition in very low birthweight children. Pediatr Dent 1996; 18: 379–84.

405. SEOW WK. Effects of preterm birth on oral growth and development. Aust Dent J 1997; 42: 85–91.

406. SEOW WK *et al*. Dental eruption in low birth-weight prematurely born children. Pediatr Dent 1988; 10: 39–42.

407. SEWERIN I *et al*. A radiographic four-year follow-up study of asymptomatic mandibular third molars in young adults. Int Dent J 1990; 40: 24–30.

408. SHAFER WG *et al*. A textbook of oral pathology. Philadelphia, PA: WB Saunders, 1983.

409. SHANMUHASUNTHARAM P *et al*. Transmigration of permanent mandibular canines. Aust Dent J 1991; 36: 209–13.

410. SHAPIRA J *et al*. Prevalence of tooth transposition, third molar agenesis, and maxillary canine impaction in individuals with Down syndrome. Angle Orthod 2000; 70: 290–6.

411. SHAPIRA Y. Transposition of canines. J Am Dent Assoc 1989; 100: 710–12.

412. SHAPIRA Y *et al*. Intrabony migration of impacted teeth. Angle Orthod 2003; 73: 738–43.

413. SHAPIRA Y *et al*. Early detection and prevention of mandibular tooth transposition. ASDC J Dent Child 2003; 70: 204–7.

414. SHAPIRA Y *et al*. An Unusual transposition of the maxillary central and lateral incisors. ASDC J Dent Child 1982; 49: 443–4.

415. SHAW L *et al*. Size and development of the dentition in endocrine deficiency. J Pedod 1989; 13: 155–60.

416. SHROFF B *et al*. Epidermal growth factor and epidermal growth factor–receptor expression in the mouse dental follicle during tooth eruption. Arch Oral Biol 1996; 41: 613–17.

417. SIAN JS. An impacted mandibular first permanent molar. ASDC J Dent Child 1982; 49: 39–40.

418. SIERRA AM. Assessment of dental and skeletal maturity. Angle Orthod 1987; 57: 194–208.

419. SILVESTRI AR. The unresolved problem of the third molar. J Am Dent Assoc 2003; 134: 450–5.

420. SMITH RA *et al*. Intranasal teeth. Oral Surg 1979; 47: 120–2.

421. STAAF V *et al*. Age estimation based on tooth development. Scand J Dent Res 1991; 99: 281–6.

422. STAFNE EC. Supernumerary upper central incisors. Dent Cosmos 1931; 73: 976–80.

423. STAHL F *et al*. Maxillary canine displacement and genetically determined predisposition to disturbed development of the dentition. J Orofac Orthop 2003; 64: 167–77.

424. STANLEY HR *et al*. Pathological sequelae of "neglected" impacted third molars. J Oral Pathol 1988; 17: 113–17.

425. STEEDLE JR *et al*. The pattern and control of eruptive tooth movements. Am J Orthod 1985; 87: 56–66.

426. STEIGMAN S *et al*. Submerged deciduous molars in preschool children: an epidemiologic study. J Dent Res 1973; 52: 322–6.

427. STEINER DR. Timing of extraction of ankylosed teeth to maximize ridge development. J Endod 1997; 23: 242–5.

428. STOELINGA PJW. De asymptomatische verstandskies. Ned Tandartsenbl 2000; 55 (11): 514–17.

429. SUNDE OE et al. Dental changes in a patient with hypoparathyreoidism. Br Dent J 1961; 111: 112–17.

430. SURI L et al. Delayed tooth eruption: pathogenesis, diagnosis, and treatment. Am J Orthod Dentofac Orthop 2004; 126: 432–45.

431. SUTTON PRN. Migrating nonerupted mandibular premolars. Oral Surg Oral Med Oral Pathol 1968; 25: 87–98.

432. SVENDSEN H et al. Third molar impaction – a consequence of late M3 mineralization and early physical maturity. Eur J Orthod 1988; 10: 1–12.

433. SVENDSEN H et al. Prediction of lower third molar impaction from the frontal cephalometric projection. Eur J Orthod 1985; 7: 1–16.

434. SYMONS AL et al. Disturbances of tooth form and eruption in the microphthalmic (mi) mouse. Arch Oral Biol 1989; 34: 71–6.

435. SZERLIP L. Displaced third molar with dentigerous cyst. J Oral Surg 1978; 36: 551–2.

436. TAGUCHI Y et al. Eruption disturbances of mandibular permanent canines in Japanese children. Int J Paediatr Dent 2001; 11: 98–102.

437. TAGUCHI Y et al. Retarded eruption of maxillary second premolars associated with late development of the germs. J Clin Pediatr Dent 2003; 27: 321–6.

438. TALBOT TQ et al. Transposed and impacted maxillary canine with ipsilateral congenitally missing lateral incisor. Am J Orthod Dentofac Orthop 2002; 121: 316–23.

439. TAN SPK et al. Ectopische eruptie van de eerste blijvende molaren in de bovenkaak. Ned Tijdschr Tandheelkd 2004; 111: 307–10.

440. TANGUAY R et al. Sexual dimorphism in the emergence of deciduous teeth: its relationship with growth components in height. Am J Phys Anthrop 1986; 69: 511–15.

441. TANGUAY R et al. Sexual dimorphism in the emergence of the deciduous teeth. J Dent Res 1984; 63: 65–8.

442. TAY F et al. Unerupted maxillary anterior supernumerary teeth: report of 204 cases. ASDC J Dent Child 1984; 51: 289–94.

443. TEAGUE AM et al. Management of the submerged deciduous tooth: I. Dent Update 1999; 26: 292–6.

444. TEAGUE AM et al. Management of the submerged deciduous tooth: 2. Dent Update 1999; 26: 350–2.

445. TEIVENS A et al. A modification of the Demirjian method for age estimation in children. J Forensic Odontostomatol 2001; 19 (2): 26–30.

446. TEIVENS A et al. A comparison between dental maturity rate in Swedish and Korean populations using a modified Demirjian method. J Forensic Odontostomatol 2001; 19 (2): 31–5.

447. THILANDER B et al. Local factors in impaction of maxillary canines. Acta Odontol Scand 1968; 26: 145–68.

448. THILANDER B, MYRBERG N. The prevalence of malocclusion in Swedish schoolchildren. Scand J Dent Res 1973; 81: 12–20.

449. TITLEY KC. A comparative investigation of permanent tooth emergence timing of Northern Ontaria Indians. J Can Dent Assoc 1984; 50: 775–8.

450. TONG DC et al. Atypical migration of an impacted lower third molar. N Z Dent J 1999; 95: 127–9.

451. TRACEY C et al. Root resorption: the aggressive, unerupted second premolar. Br J Orthod 1985; 12: 97–101.

452. TRACEY C et al. A radiographic study of dental development in the hypopituitary dwarf mouse. Arch Oral Biol 1985; 30: 805–11.

453. TSAI TP. Surgical repositioning of an impacted dilacerated incisor in mixed dentition. J Am Dent Assoc 2002; 133: 61–6.

454. TSUKAMOTO S et al. Unerupted second primary molar positioned inferior to the second premolar. ASDC J Dent Child 1986; 53: 67–9.

455. TUMER C et al. Ectopic impacted mandibular third molar in the subcondylar region associated with a dentigerous cyst. Quint Int 2002; 33: 231–3.

456. TURNBULL NR, LAI NN. Eruption of a permanent mandibular canine in a 5-year-old boy. Int J Paediatr Dent 2003; 13: 117–20.

457. UBIOS AM et al. Mandibular growth and tooth eruption after localized X-radiation. J Oral Maxillofac Surg 1992; 50: 153–6.

458. UEMATSU S et al. Orthodontic treatment of an impacted dilacerated maxillary central incisor combined with surgical exposure and apicoectomy. Angle Orthod 2004; 74: 132–6.

459. ULLBRO C et al. Cytokines, matrix metalloproteinases and tissue inhibitors of metalloproteinases-l in gingival crevicular fluid from patients with Papillon-Lefévre syndrome. Acta Odontol Scand 2004; 62: 70–4.

460. UMEDA S et al. Neonatal changes of osteoclasts in osteopetrosis (op/op) mice defective in production of functional macrophage colony-stimulating factor (M-CSF) protein and effects of M-CSF on osteoclasts development and differentiation. J Submicrosc Cytol Pathol 1996; 28: 13–26.

461. UNGER S et al. Severe cleidocranial dysplasia can mimic hypophosphatasia. Eur J Pediatr 2002; 161: 623–6.

462. UZAMIS M et al. Unusual impaction of inverted primary incisor. ASDC J Dent Child 2001; 68: 67–9, 32.

463. VANDANA KL et al. Prepubertal periodontitis. ASDC J Dent Child 2003; 70: 82–5.

464. VASKOVA J et al. Extreme Dystopie von Eckzähnen oder Prämolaren im Unterkiefer bedingt durch intraosseale Migration. Zahn Mund Kieferheilkd 1984; 72: 673–8.

465. VAN DER VELD RGM. Een gebitselement in de sinus maxillaris. Ned Tijdschr Tandheelkd 1966; 73: 175–82.

466. VAN DER WEIJDEN GA et al. Een geïmpacteerde melkmolaar. Tandartspraktijk 1997; 5: 4–5.

467. VASIR NS et al. The mandibular third molar and late crowding of the mandibular incisors. Br J Orthod 1991; 18: 59–66.

468. VENN RJ. Ectopic eruption of permanent first molars. J Pedod 1985; 10: 81–8.

469. VENTÄ I. Predictive model for impaction of lower third molars. Oral Surg Oral Med Oral Pathol 1993; 76: 699–703.

470. VENTÄ I et al. Clinical follow-up study of third molar eruption from ages 20 tot 26 years. Oral Surg Oral Med Oral Pathol 1991; 72: 150–3.

471. VENTÄ I *et al*. A device to predict lower third molar eruption. Oral Surg Oral Med Oral Pathol Oral Radiol Endod 1997; 84: 598–603.

472. VENTÄ I *et al*. Third molars as an acute problem in Finnish university students. Oral Surg Oral Med Oral Pathol 1993; 76: 135–40.

473. VENTÄ I *et al*. Clinical outcome of third molars in adults followed during 18 years. J Oral Maxillofac Surg 2004; 62: 182–5.

474. VIA FF. Submerged deciduous molars: familial tendencies. J Am Dent Assoc 1964; 69: 127–9.

475. VIRTANEN JI *et al*. Timing of eruption of permanent teeth: standard Finnish patient documents. Community Dent Oral Epidemiol 1994; 22: 286–8.

476. VISSER JB. Speciële pathologie van het menselijke gebit. Leiden: Stafleu & Tholen BV, 1974.

477. VORHIES JM *et al*. Ankylosed deciduous molars. J Am Dent Assoc 1952; 44: 68–72.

478. WEDL JS *et al*. Die durchbruchzeiten der bleibenden zähne bei jungen und mädchen in New York. Deutsch Zahnätrtzl Zeitschr 2004; 59: 288–91.

479. WERTZ RA. Treatment of transmigrated mandibular canines. Am J Orthod Dentofac Orthop 1994; 106: 419–27.

480. WES BJ *et al*. De geïmpacteerde cuspidaat in de bovenkaak. I. Ned Tijdschr Tandheelkd 1992; 99: 121–2.

481. WEYMAN J. The effect of irradiation on developing teeth. Oral Surg 1968; 25: 623–9.

482. WHITTAKER DK *et al*. Quantitative assessment of tooth wear, alveolar-crest height and continuing eruption in a Romano-British population. Arch Oral Biol 1985; 30: 493–501.

483. WHYMAN RA *et al*. An unusual case of hemifacial atrophy. Oral Surg Oral Med Oral Pathol 1992; 73: 564–9.

484. WILLIAMS SA *et al*. Failure of eruption associated with anomalies of the dentition in siblings. Pediatr Dent 1988; 10: 130–6.

485. WINTER GB *et al*. Severe infra-occlusion and failed eruption of deciduous molars associated with eruptive and developmental disturbances in the permanent dentition. Br J Orthod 1997; 24: 149–57.

486. WISE GE. The biology of tooth eruption. J Dent Res 1998; 77: 1576–9.

487. WISE GE *et al*. Ultrastructural features of the dental follicle associated with formation of the tooth eruption pathway in the dog. J Oral Pathol 1985; 14: 15–26.

488. WOOD GD *et al*. A dentonasal deformity. Oral Surg 1987; 63: 656–7.

489. WYSOLMERSKI JJ *et al*. Absence of functional type 1 parathyroidhormone (PTH)/PTH-related protein receptors in humans is associated with abnormal breast development and tooth impaction. J Clin Endocrinol Metab 2001; 86: 1788–94.

490. YAMAOKA M. Supernumerary impactions of the mandibular cuspids and bicuspids. Aust Dent J 1995; 40: 34–5.

491. YAMAOKA M *et al*. Completely impacted teeth in dentate en edentulous jaws. Aust Dent J 1996; 41: 169–72.

492. YAMAOKA M *et al*. Incidence of inflammation in completely impacted lower third molars. Aust Dent J 1997; 42: 153–5.

493. YEUNG KH *et al*. Compound odontoma associated with an unerupted and dilacerated maxillary central incisor in a young patient. Int J Paediatr Dent 2003; 13: 208–12.

494. YEUNG KH *et al*. Intranasal tooth in a patient with cleft lip and alveolus. Cleft Palate Craniofac J 1996; 33: 157–9.

495. YONEMOCHI H *et al*. Pericoronal hamartomatous lesions in the opercula of teeth delayed in eruption: an immunohistochemical study of the extracellular matrix. J Oral Pathol Med 1998; 27: 441–52.

496. YOUNAI F *et al*. Osteopetrosis. Oral Surg Oral Med Oral Pathol 1988; 65: 214–21.

497. YOUNG DH. Ectopic eruption of the first permanent molar. ASDC J Dent Child 1957; 24: 153–62.

498. YUEN SWH *et al*. Double primary teeth and their relationship with the permanent successors: a radiographic study of 376 cases. Pediatr Dent 1987; 9: 42–8.

499. ZEITLER DL. Management of impacted teeth other than third molars. Oral Maxillofac Surg Clin North Am 1993; 5: 95–103.

500. ZILBERMAN Y *et al*. Familial trends in palatal canines, anomalous lateral incisors and related phenomena. Eur J Orthod 1990; 12: 135–9.

501. HEINRICH J *et al*. CSF-1, RANKL and OPG regulate osteoclastogenesis during murine tooth eruption. Arch Oral Biol 2005; 50: 897–908.

502. QIN H, YANG FS. Calcitonin may be a useful therapeutic agent for osteoclastogenesis syndromes involving premature eruption of the tooth. Med Hypotheses 2008; 70: 1048–50.

503. SOLLECITO TP *et al*. Systemic conditions associated with periodontitis in childhood and adolescence. Med Oral Patol Oral Cir Bucal 2005; 10: 142–50.

504. GROLLMUS N *et al*. Periodontal disease associated to systemic genetic disorders. Med Oral Patol Oral Cir Bucal 2007; 12: E11–15.

505. LUZZI V *et al*. Malignant infantile osteopetrosis. Eur J Paediatr Dent 2006; 7: 39–44.

506. Change in third molar angulation and position in young adults and follow-up periodontal pathology. J Oral Maxillofac Surg 2006; 64: 424–8.

507. PHILLIPS C *et al*. Changes over time in position and periodontal probing status of retained third molars. J Oral Maxillofac Surg 2007; 65: 2011–17.

508. HILL CM *et al*. Conservative, non-surgical management of patients presenting with impacted lower tthird molars: A 5-year study. Br J Oral Maxillofac Surg 2006; 44: 347–50.

509. AHMAD S *et al*. The clinical features and aetiological basis of primary eruption failure. Eur J Orthod 2006; 28: 535–40.

510. FRAZIER-BOWES SA *et al*. Primary failure of eruption. Am J Orthod Dentofac Orthop 2007; 131: 578e1–578e11.

511. MOONEY GC *et al*. Ectopic eruption of first permanent molars. Eur Arch Paediatr Dent 2007; 8: 153–7.

512. BONDEMARK L *et al*. Prevalence of ectopic eruption, retention and agenesis of the permanent second molar. Angle Orthod 2007; 77: 773–8.

513. GRANT JER *et al*. Mandibular first and second molar transposition. Int J Paediatr Dent 2006; 16: 227–9.

514. CAMILLERI S. Double transmigration and hyperdontia. Angle Orthod 2007; 77: 742–4.

515. BUYUKKURT MC *et al.* Transmigrant mandibular canines. J Oral Maxillofac Surg 2007; 65: 2025–9.

516. GONZÁLEZ-SÁNCHEZ MA *et al.* Transmigrant impacted mandibular canines. J Am Dent Assoc 2007; 138: 1450–5.

517. CIARLANTI R *et al.* Maxillary tooth transposition: Correct or accept? Am J Orthod Dentofac Orthop 2007; 132: 385–94.

518. KARA MI *et al.* Analysis of different type of transmigrant mandibular teeth. Med Oral Patol Cir Bucal 2011; 16: e355–40.

Chapter 5: Caries

1. AALTONEN AS *et al.* Increased dental caries activity in pre-school children with low baseline levels of serum IgG antibodies against the bacterial species *Streptococcus mutans.* Arch Oral Biol 1987; 32: 55–60.

2. AAMDAL-SCHEIE A *et al.* Plaque pH and microflora on sound and carious root surfaces. J Dent Res 1994; 75: 1001–8.

3. AGUIRRE-ZERO O *et al.* Effect of chewing Xilitol chewing gum on salivary flowrate and the acidogenic potential of dental plaque. Caries Res 1993; 27: 55–9.

4. AHLUWALIA M *et al.* Dental caries, oral hygiene, and oral clearance in children with craniofacial disorders. J Dent Res 2004; 83: 175–9.

5. AINAMO J. Relative roles of toothbrushing, sucrose consumption and fluorides in the maintenance or oral health in children. Int Dent J 1980; 30: 54–60.

6. AINAMO J *et al.* Occurrence of plaque, gingivitis and caries as related to self reported frequency of toothbrushing in fluoride areas in Finland. Community Dent Oral Epidemiol 1979; 7: 142–6.

7. AKPATA ES *et al.* Cavitation at radiolucent areas on proximal surfaces of posterior teeth. Caries Res 1996; 30: 313–16.

8. ALANEN P *et al.* Sealants and xylitol chewing gum are equal in caries prevention. Acta Odontol Scand 2000; 58: 279–84.

9. ALANEN P *et al.* Effect of war-time dietary changes on dental health of Finns 40 years later. Community Dent Oral Epidemiol 1985; 13: 281–4.

10. ALBRECHT M *et al.* Dental and oral symptoms of diabetes mellitus. Community Dent Oral Epidemiol 1988; 16: 378–80.

11. AL-HIYASAT AS *et al.* Effects of resin based dental composites on fertility of male mice. Eur J Oral Sci 2002; 110: 44–7.

12. AL-KHATEEB S *et al.* Laser fluorescence quantification of remineralisation *in situ* of incipient enamel lesions: influence of fluoride supplements. Caries Res 1997; 31: 132–40.

13. AMMARI AB *et al.* Systematic review of studies comparing the anti-caries efficacy of children's toothpaste containing 600 ppm or less with high fluoride toothpastes of 1000 ppm or above. Caries Res 2003; 37: 85–92.

14. ANDERSON MH. Current concepts of dental caries and its prevention. Oper Dent 2001; suppl 6: 11–18.

15. ANDERSON M. Chlorhexidine and xylitol gum in caries prevention. Spec Care Dent 2003; 23: 173–6.

16. ANDERSON MH *et al.* A comparison of digital and optical criteria for detecting carious dentin. J Prosthet Dent 1985; 53: 643–6.

17. ANDERSON MH *et al.* Bacteriologic study of a basic fuchsin caries-disclosing dye. J Prosthet Dent 1985; 54: 51–5.

18. ANDO M *et al.* Relative ability of laser fluorescence techniques to quantitate early mineral loss *in vitro.* Caries Res 1997; 31: 125–31.

19. ANGERHOLM DM *et al.* Reasons given for extraction of permanent teeth by general dental practitioners in England and Wales. Br Dent J 1988; 164: 345–8.

20. ANGMAR-MÅNSSON BE *et al.* Caries diagnosis. J Dent Educ 1998; 62: 771–80.

21. ANKKURINIEMI O *et al.* Dental health and dental treatment needs among recruits of the Finnish defence forces, 1919–91. Acta Odontol Scand 1997; 55: 192–7.

22. ANTTONEN V *et al.* Clinical study of the use of the laser fluorescence device DIAGNOdent for detection of occlusal caries in children. Caries Res 2003; 37: 17–23.

23. ANTTONEN V *et al.* A follow-up study of the use of DIAGNOdent for monitoring fissue caries in children. Community Dent Oral Epidemiol 2004; 32: 312–18.

24. ANUSAVICE KJ. Efficacy of nonsurgical management of the initial carious lesion. J Dent Educ 1997; 61: 895–905.

25. ANUSAVICE KJ. Does art have a place in preservative dentistry? Community Dent Oral Epidemiol 1999; 27: 442–8.

26. ANUSAVICE KJ. Caries risk assessment. Oper Dent 2001; suppl 6: 19–26.

27. APEL C *et al.* Demineralization of ER:YAG and Er,Cr:YSGG laser-prepared enamel cavities in vitro. Caries Res 2003; 37: 34–7.

28. ARENDS J *et al.* SEM and microradiographic investigation of initial enamel caries. Scand J Dent Res 1987; 95: 193–201.

29. ARENDS J *et al.* Wirkung einer magnesiumhaltigen MFP-Zahnpaste auf die Zahnschmelz-Remineralisation *in situ.* Dtsch Zahnärztl Z 1998; 53: 26–31.

30. ARENDS J *et al.* Nature and role of loosely bound fluoride in dental caries. J Dent Res 1990; 69 (spec. issue): 601–5.

31. ARENDS J *et al.* Penetration of varnishes into demineralized root dentine *in vitro.* Caries Res 1997; 31: 201–5.

32. ARNEBERG P *et al.* Caries and defective restorations in elderly faculty patients. Gerodontics 1988; 4: 224–8.

33. ASHBY J *et al.* Lack of effects for low dose levels of bisphenol A and diethylbestrol on the prostate gland of CF1 mice exposed in utero. Regul Toxicol Pharmacol 1999; 30: 156–66.

34. ASHLEY PF *et al.* Occlusal caries diagnosis: an *in vitro* histological validation of the Eelectronic Caries Monitor (ECM) and other methods. J Dent 1998; 26: 83–8.

35. ASSEV S *et al.* Xylitol fermentation by human dental plaque. Eur J Oral Sci 1996; 104: 359–62.

36. ATASU M. Dermatoglyphic findings in dental caries: a preliminary report. J Clin Pediatr Dent 1998; 22: 147–9.

37. ASHLEY FP et al. The effect of a school-based plaque control programme on caries and gingivitis. Br Dent J 1981; 150: 41–5.

38. AUSCHILL TM et al. The effect of dental restorative materials on dental biofilm. Eur J Oral Sci 2002; 110: 48–53.

39. AWADIA AK et al. Caries experience and caries predictors – a study of Tanzanian children consuming drinking water with different fluoride concentration. Clin Oral Invest 2002; 6: 98–103.

40. BABAAHMADY KG et al. Ecological study of Streptococcus mutans, Streptococcus sobrinus and Lactobacillus spp. at sub-sites from approximal dental plaque in children. Caries Res 1998; 32: 51–8.

41. BACA P et al. Mutans streptococci and lactobacilli in saliva after the application of fissure sealants. Oper Dent 2002; 27: 107–11.

42. BACKER DIRKS O. Posteruptive changes in dental enamel. J Dent Res 1966; 45 (suppl 3): 503–11.

43. BACKER DIRKS O. The benefits of water fluoridation. Caries Res 1974; 8 (suppl 1): 2–15.

44. BACKER DIRKS O et al. Caries-preventive water fluoridation. Caries Res 1978; 12 (suppl 1): 7–14.

45. BADER JD et al. A systematic review of selected caries prevention and management methods. Community Dent Oral Epidemiol 2001; 29: 399–411.

46. BAECKE JAH et al. Gebitstoestand, behandelnoodzaak, mondhygiëne en jeugdtandzorg in "s-Hertogenbosch". Ned Tijdschr Tandheelkd 1985; 92: 464–8.

47. BANERJEE A et al. Autofluorescence and mineral content of carious dentine: scanning optical and backscattered electron microscopic studies. Caries Res 1998; 32: 219–26.

48. BANERJEE A et al. In vitro evaluation of five alternative methods of carious dentine excavation. Caries Res 2000; 34: 144–50.

49. BANERJEE A et al. Dentine caries excavation: a review of current clinical techniques. Br Dent J 2000: 188: 476–82.

50. BANZAHIM M et al. Secondary caries detection by DIAGNOdent and radiography. Acta Ondontol Scand 2004; 62: 61–4.

51. BARBER D et al. Permeability of active and arrested carious lesions to dyes and radioactive isotopes. J Dent Child 1964; 31: 26–33.

52. BARREGÅRD L et al. People with high mercury uptake from their own dental amalgam fillings. Occup Environ Med 1995; 52: 124–8.

53. BAYSAN A et al. Antimicrobial effect of a novel ozone-generating device on micro-organisms associated with primary root carious lesions in vitro. Caries Res 2000; 34: 498–501.

54. BAYSAN A et al. Effect of ozone on the oral microbiota and clinical severity of primary root caries. Am J Dent 2004; 17: 56–60.

55. BECK DJ. The epidemiology of dental caries. In: COHEN B et al. (ed.) Scientific foundations of dentistry. London: William Heinemann Medical Books, 1976.

56. BECK JD et al. Prevalence of root and coronal caries in a noninstitutionalized older population. J Am Dent Assoc 1985; 111: 964–7.

57. BECK JD et al. Identification of high caries risk adults: attitudes, social factors and diseases. Int Dent J 1988; 38: 231–8.

58. BECK JD et al. Root caries: physical, medical and psychosocial correlates in an elderly population. Gerodontics 1986; 3: 242–7.

59. BEDI R et al. Dental caries experience and prevalence of children afraid of dental treatment. Community Dent Oral Epidemiol 1992; 20: 368–71.

60. BEIGHTON D et al. Comparison of selected microflora of plaque and underlying carious dentine associated with primary root caries lesions. Caries Res 1995; 29: 154–8.

61. BELAZI MA et al. Salivary alterations in insulin-dependent diabetes mellitus. Int J Paediatr Dent 1998; 8: 29–33.

62. BELLINI HT et al. Oral hygiene and caries. A review. Acta Odontol Scand 1981; 39: 257–65.

63. BENCHABANE H et al. Inactivation of the Streoptococcus mutans fxpC gene confers resistance to xylitol, a caries preventive natural carbohydrate sweetener. J Dent Res 2002; 81: 380–6.

64. BERENIE J et al. The relationship of frequency of toothbrushing, oral hygiene, gingival health, and caries-experience in school children. J Public Health Dent 1973; 33 (3): 160–71.

65. BEVENIUS J. Caries risk in patients with Crohn's disease. Oral Surg Oral Med Oral Pathol 1988; 65: 304–7.

66. BIBBY BG. Dental caries. Caries Res 1978; 12 (suppl 1): 3–6.

67. BILLE J et al. Approximal caries progression in 13- to 15-year-old Danish children. Acta Odontol Scand 1989; 47: 347–54.

68. BILLINGS RJ et al. Contemporary treatment strategies for root surface dental caries. Gerodontics 1985; 1: 20–7.

69. BILLINGS RJ et al. Xerostomia and associated factors in a community–dwelling adult population. Community Dent Oral Epidemiol 1996; 24: 312–16.

70. BINDER K et al. Caries-preventive fluoride tablet programs. Caries Res 1978; 12 (suppl 1): 22–30.

71. BINUS W et al. Zur Rolle der Schmelzbüschel und Schmelzlamellen in Stadium der Initialkaries. Zahn Mund Kieferheilkd 1986; 74: 6–12.

72. BIRKELAND JM et al. Continual highly significant decrease in caries prevalence among 14-year-old Norwegians. Acta Odontol Scand 1987; 45: 135–40.

73. BIRKELAND JM et al. Caries–preventive fluoride mouthrinses. Caries Res 1978; 12 (suppl 1): 38–51.

74. BIRKHED D et al. Per capita consumption of sugar-containing products and dental caries in Sweden from 1960 to 1985. Community Dent Oral Epidemiol 1989; 17: 41–3.

75. BISSELING GH et al. Statistische gegevens omtrent den toestand van het gebit bij kinderen en volwassenen. Tijdschr Tandheelkd 1916; 23: 288–347.

76. BJØRNDAL L et al. A structural analysis of approximal enamel caries lesions and subjacent dentin reactions. Eur J Oral Sci 1995; 103: 25–31.

77. BJØRNDAL L et al. A quantitative light microscopic study of the odontoblastic reactions to active and arrested enamel lesions without cavitation. Caries Res 1998; 31: 59–69.

78. BJØRNDAL L et al. Changes in the cultivable flora in deep carious lesions following a stepwise excavation procedure. Caries Res 2000; 34: 502–8.

79. BJØRNDAL L, LARSEN T, THYLSTRUP A. A clinical and microbiological study of deep carious lesions during stepwise excavation using long treatment intervals. Caries Res 1997; 31: 411–17.

80. BJØRNDAL L et al. Pulp-dentin biology in restorative dentistry. Part 4: Dental caries – Characteristics of lesions and pulpal reactions. Quint Int 2001; 32: 717–36.

81. BJØRNDAL L et al. A practice-based study on stepwise excavation of deep carious lesions in permanent teeth. Community Dent Oral Epidemiol 1998; 26: 122–8.

82. BLACK GV. Operative dentistry. Chicago, IL: Medico-dental Publishing Company, 1908.

83. BLUME A et al. Untersuchungen zur Zahngesundheit asthmakranker Kinder und Jugendlichen. Deutsch Zahnärztl Zeitschr 2002; 57: 644–9.

84. BOKHOUT B et al. Prevalence of mutans streptococci and lactobacilli in 1.5-year-old children with cleft lip and/or palate. Cleft Palate Craniofac J 1996; 33: 424–8.

85. BOKHOUT B et al. Increased caries prevalence in 2.5-year-old children with cleft lip and/or palate. Eur J Oral Sci 1996; 104: 518–22.

86. BOSTON DW et al. Histobacteriological analysis of acid red dye-stainable dentin found beneath intact amalgam restorations. Oper Dent 1994; 19: 65–9.

87. BOUMA I et al. A. Het syndroom van Sjögren: een progressief ziektebeeld. Ned Tijdschr Tandheelkd 2003; 110: 316–20.

88. BOWDEN G et al. Oral ecology and dental caries. In: THYLSTRUP A et al. (eds) Textbook of clinical cariology. Copenhagen: Munksgaard, 1994.

89. BOWEN WH. Henry Klein – A forgotten icon? J Dent Res 2004; 83: 365–7.

90. BRADSHAW D et al. Effect of sugar alcohols on the composition and metabolism of a mixed culture of oral bacteria grown in a chemostat. Caries Res 1994; 28: 251–6.

91. BRAILSFORD SR et al. The isolation of Actinomyces naeslundii from sound root surfaces and root carious lesions. Caries Res 1998; 32: 100–6.

92. BRÄNNSTRÖM M et al. Experimental caries in young human permanent teeth implanted in removable dentures. Arch Oral Biol 1977; 22: 571–8.

93. BRATTHALL D et al. Diagnostic basis of causal treatment: tools and tests for evaluation of caries and periodontal disease. In: Professional prevention in dentistry. Baltimore, MD: Lippincott Williams & Wilkins, 1994.

94. BRECX M et al. Efficacy of Listerine®, Meridol®, and chlorhexidine mouthrinses as Supplement to regular tooth-cleaning measures. J Clin Periodontol 1992; 19: 202–7.

95. BRETZ WA et al. J Evidence of a heritable component to dental caries surface traits is obscured by the multifactorial etiology and mesurement of the phenotype. J Evid Base Dent Pract 2003; 3: 185–9.

96. BROWN JP. Indicators for caries management from the patient history. J Dent Educ 1997; 61: 855–60.

97. BROWN LR et al. Interrelations of oral microorganisms, immunoglobulins, and dental caries following radiotherapy. J Dent Res 1978; 57: 882–93.

98. BROWN WE. Physicochemical mechanisms of dental caries. J Dent Res 1974; 53 (suppl 2): 204–16.

99. BRUDEVOLD F et al. Caries-preventive fluoride treatment of the individual. Caries Res 1978; 12 (suppl 1): 52–64.

100. BRUHN G et al. Effect of a toothpaste containing triclosan on dental plaque, gingivitis and bleeding on probing. Clin Oral Invest 2002; 6: 124–7.

101. BÜYÜKYILMAZ T et al. The caries-preventive effect of titanium tetrafluoride on root surfaces in situ as evaluated by microradiography and confocal laser scanning microscopy. Adv Dent Res 1997; 11: 448–52.

102. CAHEN PM et al. Survey of the reasons for dental extractions in France. J Dent Res 1985; 64: 1087–93.

103. CAI F et al. Remineralization of enamel subsurface lesions in situ by sugar-free legenzes containing casein phosphopeptide-amorphous calcium phospahe. Aut Dent J 2003; 48: 240–3.

104. CAMLING E et al. The relationship between IgA antibodies to Streptococcus mutans antigens in human saliva and breast milk and the numbers of indigenous oral Streptococcus mutans. Arch Oral Biol 1987; 32: 21–5.

105. CARLSSON P. Distribution of mutans streptococci in populations with different levels of sugar consumption. Scand J Dent Res 1989; 97: 120–5.

106. CARVALHO JC et al. Results after 3 years of non-operative occlusal caries treatment of erupting permanent first molars. Community Dent Oral Epidemiol 1992; 20: 187–92.

107. CARLSSON P. Microbial aspects of frequent intake of products with high sugar concentrations. Scand J Dent Res 1989B; 97: 110–14.

108. CAUFIELD PW et al. Initial acquisition of mutans streptococci by infants. J Dent Res 1993; 72: 37–45.

109. CAYLEY AS et al. The influence of audit on the diagnosis of occlusal caries. Caries Res 1997; 31: 97–102.

110. CHADWICK C et al. Challenges with studies investigating longevity of dental restorations – a critique of a systematic review. J Dent 2001; 155–61.

111. CHAUNCEY HH et al. Dental caries. Principal cause of tooth extraction in a sample of US male adults. Caries Res 1989; 23: 200–5.

112. CHOSACK A. A dental caries severity index for primary teeth. Community Dent Oral Epidemiol 1986; 14: 86–9.

113. CHOW LC et al. Enhancing remineralisation. Oper Dent 2001: suppl 6: 27–38.

114. CLARK DC et al. The effectiveness of three different strengths of chlorhexidine mouthrinse. J Can Dent Assoc 1994; 60: 711–14.

115. CLARKSON BH et al. Effect of proteolytic enzymes on caries lesion formation in vitro. J Oral Pathol 1986; 15: 423–9.

116. CLARKSON BH et al. Rational use of fluorides in caries control. In: FEJERSKOV O et al. (eds) Fluoride in dentistry. Copenhagen: Munksgaard, 1996, 347–57.

117. CLASEN ABS et al. Caries development in fluoridated and non-fluoridated deciduous and permanent enamel in situ examined by microradiography and confocal laser scanning microscopy. Adv Dent Res 1997; 11: 442–7.

118. CLEARY MA et al. Oral health implications in children with inborn errors of intermediary metabolism: a review. Int J Paedatr Dent 1997; 7: 133–41.

119. COLLIN HL *et al.* Caries in patients with non-insulin-dependent diabeters mellitus. Oral Surg Oral Med Oral Pathol Oral Radiol Endod 1998; 85: 680–5.

120. COMMISSIE TANDHEELKUNDIGE MATERIALEN. Tandheelkundige restauratiematerialen. Rijswijk: Gezondheidsraad, 1998, Publication no. 1998/09.

121. COMMISSION OF THE EUROPEAN UNION, AD HOC WORKING GROUP. Dental amalgam. Brussels, 1997.

122. CONSEIL D'EVALUATION DEs TECHNOLOGIES DE LA SANTé DU QUEBEC. The safety of dental amalgam: a state of the art review. Montreal, 1997.

123. CÔRTEZ DF *et al.* Visual inspection, FOTI, combined FOTI/visual examination, DIAGNOdent and ECM for occlusal caries detection. Caries Res 2000; 34: 327.

124. CÔRTEZ DF *et al.* An in vitro comparison of a combined FOTI/visual examination of occlusal caries with other caries diagnostic methods and the effect of stain on their diagnostic performance. Caries Res 2003; 37: 8–16.

125. CURZON MEJ. The relation between caries prevalence and strontium concentrations in drinking water, plaque, and surface enamel. J Dent Res 1985; 64: 1386–8.

126. CURZON MEJ *et al.* Trace elements and dental disease. Boston: Wright, PSG, 1983.

127. CURZON MEJ *et al.* An association between strontium in drinking water Supplies and low caries prevalence in man. Arch Oral Biol 1978; 23: 317–21.

128. DAHLLÖF G *et al.* Caries, gingivitis, and dental abnormalities in preschool children with cleft lip and/or palate. Cleft Palate 1989; 26: 233–7.

129. DANIELS TE. Sjögren's syndrome: clinical spectrum and current diagnostic controversies. Adv Dent Res 1996; 10: 3–8.

130. DARLING MR *et al.* Review of the effects of cannabis smoking on oral health. Int Dent J 1992; 42: 19–22.

131. DAS S *et al.* Cariostatic effect of aspartame in rats. Caries Res 1997; 31: 78–83.

132. DASANAYAKE AP *et al.* Lack of effect of chlorhexidine varnish on Streptococcus mutans transmission and caries in mothers and children. Caries Res 2002; 36: 288–93.

133. DAWES C *et al.* Kinetics of fluoride in the oral fluids. J Dent Res 1990; 69 (spec. issue): 638–44.

134. DEN DEKKER J. Behandelingsplanning in de tandart-spraktijk. Amsterdam: Thesis, University of Amsterdam, 1990.

135. DE SOET JJ *et al.* Transmission of mutans streptococci between mother and children with cleft lip and/or palate. Clef Palate Craniofac 1998; 5: 460–4.

136. DE SOET JJ *et al.* Acidogenesis by oral streptococci at different pH values. Caries Res 1989; 23: 14–17.

137. DE SOET JJ *et al.* Differences in cariogenicity between fresh isolates of *Streptococcus sobrinus* and *Streptococcus mutans*. Caries Res 1991; 25: 116–22.

138. DE SOET JJ *et al.* A comparison of the microbial flora in carious dentine of clinically detectable and undetectable occlusal lesions. Caries Res 1995; 29: 46–9.

139. DE VRIES HCB *et al.* Röntgenologische versus klinische cariësdiagnostiek. Ned Tijdschr Tandheelkd 1987; 94: 331–4.

140. DINIS M *et al.* Therapeutic vaccine against streptococcus sobrinus-induced caries. J Dent Res 2004; 83: 354–8.

141. DISNEY JA *et al.* Comparative effects of a 4-year fluoride mouth-rinse program on high and low caries forming grade 1 children. Community Dent Oral Epidemiol 1989; 17: 139–43.

142. DOWNER MG *et al.* How long do routine dental restorations last? Br Dent J 1999; 187: 432–9.

143. DOWNER MC *et al.* Dental experience and defects of dental enamel among 12-year-old children in north London, Edinburgh, Glasgow and Dublin. Community Dent Oral Epidemiol 1994; 22: 283–5.

144. DUCHIN S *et al.* Relationship of *Streptococcus mutans* and Lactobacilli to incipient smooth surface dental caries in man. Arch Oral Biol 1978; 23: 779–86.

145. DUGGAL MS *et al.* A study of the relationship between trace elements in saliva and dental caries in children. Arch Oral Biol 1991; 36: 881–4.

146. DUGGAL MS *et al.* An evaluation of the cariogenic potential of baby and infant fruit drinks. Br Dent J 1989; 166: 327–30.

147. DUNG SZ *et al.* Effect of lactic acid and proteolytic enzymes on the release of organic matrix components from human root dentin. Caries Res 1995; 29: 483–9.

148. EDGAR WM. Prevention of caries: immunology and vaccination. In: MURRAY JJ (ed.) The prevention of dental disease. Oxford: Oxford University Press, 1983.

149. EDWARD S. Changes in caries diagnostic criteria over time related to the insertion of fillings. Acta Odontol Scand 1997; 55: 23–6.

150. EDWARDSSON S *et al.* Acid production from Lycasin, maltitol sorbitol and xylitol by oral streptococci and lactobacilli. Acta Odontol Scand 1977; 35: 257–63.

151. EIDELMAN E *et al.* Histopathology of the pulp in primary incisors with deep dentinal caries. Padiatr Dent 1992: 14: 1372–5.

152. EINWAG J *et al.* The relative caries-inhibiting efficacy of amine fluoride and sodium fluoride in compatible dentifrices. Quint Int 1995; 26: 707–13.

153. EKLUND SA *et al.* Time of development of occlusal and proximal lesions: implications for fissure sealants. J Public Health Dent 1986; 46 (2): 114–21.

154. EKSTRAND KR *et al.* Reproducibility and accuracy of three methods for assessment of demineralization depth on the occlusal surface: an *in vitro* examination. Caries Res 1997; 31: 224–31.

155. EKSTRAND KR *et al.* Do occlusal carious lesions spread laterally at the enamel–dentin junction? Clin Oral Invest 1998; 2: 15–20.

156. EKSTRAND KR *et al.* Detection, diagnosing, monitoring and logical treatment of occlusal caries in relation to lesion activity and severity: an in vivo examination with histological validation. Caries Res 1998; 32: 247–54.

157. ELIAS-BONETA AR *et al.* Dental caries prevalence of twelve year olds in Puerto Rico. Community Dent Health 2003; 20: 171–6.

158. ELIASSON S *et al.* Root caries. A consensus conference statement. Swed Dent J 1992; 16: 21–5.

159. EMILSON CG *et al.* Microbial flora associated with presence of root surface caries in periodontally treated patients. Scand J Dent Res 1988; 96: 40–9.

160. ERIKSEN HM *et al*. Concepts of health and disease and caries prediction. Scand J Dent Res 1991; 99: 476–83.

161. ESPELID I *et al*. Clinical and radiographic assessment of approximal carious lesions. Acta Odontol Scand 1986; 44: 31–7.

162. ESPELID I *et al*. Variations among dentists in radiographic detection of occlusal caries. Caries Res 1994; 28: 169–75.

163. FALLER RV *et al*. The comparative anticaries efficacy of Crest toothpaste relative to some marketed Chinese toothpastes. Int Dent J 1997; 47: 313–20.

164. FEJERSKOV O *et al*. Root caries in Scandinavia in the 1980's and future trends to be expected in dental caries experience in adults. Adv Dent Res 1993; 7: 4–14.

165. FEJERSKOV O *et al*. Fluoride in dentistry. Copenhagen: Munksgaard, 1996.

166. FEJERSKOV O *et al*. Dental caries. The disease and its clinical management. Oxford: Blackwell/Munksgaard, 1996.

167. FEJERSKOV O *et al*. Clinical and pathological features of dental caries. In: THYLSTRUP A *et al*. (eds) Textbook of clinical cariology. Copenhagen: Munksgaard, 1994.

168. FENNIS-IE YL *et al*. Effect of 6-monthly applications of chlorhexidine varnish on incidence of occlusal caries in permanent molars: a 3-year study. J Dent 1998; 3: 233–8.

169. FENNIS-IE YL *et al*. Performance of some diagnostic systems in the prediction of occlusal caries in permanent molars in 6- and 11-year-old children. J Dent 1998; 26: 403–8.

170. FESKANICH D *et al*. Vitamin A uptake and hip fractures among postmenal women. J Am Med Assoc 2002; 287: 102–4.

171. FINE DH *et al*. Efficacy of a triclosan/NaF dentifrice in the control of plaque and gingivitis and concurrent oral microflora monitoring. Am J Dent 1998; 11: 259–70.

172. FIRESTIONE AR *et al*. The effect of a knowledge-based, image analysis and clinical decision support system on observer performance in the diagnosis of approximal caries from radiographic images. Caries Res 1998; 32: 127–34.

173. FONTANA M *et al*. Inhibition of secondary caries lesion progression using fluoride varnish. Caries Res 2002; 36: 129–35.

174. FORSS H *et al*. Retention of a glass ionomer cement and a resin-based fissure sealant and effect on carious outcome after 7 years. Community Dent Oral Epidemiol 1998; 26: 21–5.

175. FORSS H *et al*. Reasons for restorative therapy and the longevity of restorations in adults. Acta Ondontol Scand 2004; 62: 82–6.

176. FRANK RM *et al*. Ultrastructure of the human odontoblast process and its mineralization during dental caries. Caries Res 1980; 14: 367–80.

177. FURE S. Five-year incidence of coronal and root caries in 60-, 70- and 80-year-old Swedish individuals. Caries Res 1997; 31: 249–58.

178. FURE S. Five-year incidence of caries, salivary and microbial conditions in 60-, 70- and 80-year-old Swedish individuals. Caries Res 1998; 32: 166–74.

179. FURE S *et al*. Evaluation of Carisolv™ for the chemomechanical removal of primary root caries in vivo. Caries Res 2000; 34: 275–80.

180. FURE S *et al*. Root surface caries and associated factors. Scand J Dent Res 1990; 98: 391–400.

181. FURE S *et al*. Prevalence of root surface caries in 55, 65 and 75-year-old Swedish individuals. Community Dent Oral Epidemiol 1990; 18: 100–5.

182. FUSAYAMA T. Two layers of carious dentin: diagnosis and treatment. Oper Dent 1979; 4: 63–70.

183. FUSAYAMA T. New concepts in operative dentistry. Chicago, IL: Quintessence Publishing, 1980.

184. FUSAYAMA T. Clinical guide to removing caries using a caries-detecting solution. Oper Dent 1988; 19: 397–401.

185. FUSAYAMA T *et al*. Structure and removal of carious dentin. Int Dent J 1972; 22: 401–11.

186. FUSAYAMA T *et al*. Relationship between hardness, discoloration, and mocrobial invasion in carious dentin. J Dent Res 1966; 45: 1033–46.

187. GAKENHEIMER DC. The efficacy of a computerized caries detector in intraoral digital radiography. J Am Dent Assoc 2002; 133: 883–90.

188. GALEA H *et al*. The dental caries and periodontal disease experience of patients with early onset insulin dependent diabetes. Int Dent J 1986; 36: 219–24.

189. GARG AK *et al*. Manifestations and treatment of xerostomia and associate oral defects secondary to head and neck radiotherapy. J Am Dent Assoc 1997; 128: 1128–33.

190. GEBEL T *et al*. Einfluss des Kaugummikonsums sowie einer dentalen Nachbarschaft von Amalgamfüllungen zu metallischen Restaurationen anderer Art auf dem Quecksilberuringehalt. Zbl Hyg 1996; 199: 69–75.

191. GEDALIA I *et al*. Dental caries protection with hard cheese consumption. Am J Dent 1994; 7: 331–2.

192. GEDDES DAM *et al*. Apples, salted peanuts and plaque pH. Br Dent J 1977; 142: 317–19.

193. GEIGER AM *et al*. Reducing white spot lesions in orthodontic populations with fluoride rinsing. Am J Orthod Dentofac Orthop 1992; 101: 403–7.

194. GEZONDHEIDSRAAD. Tandheelkundige restauratiematerialen. Rijswijk: Gezondheidsraad, 1998.

195. GHUA-CHOWDHURY N *et al*. Effect of low levels of fluorid on proton excretion and intracellular pH in glycolysing streptococcal cells under strictly anaerobic conditions. Caries Res 1997; 31: 373–8.

196. GIERTSEN E *et al*. Effects of chlorhexidine-fluoride mouthrinses on viability, acidogenic potential, and glycolytic profile of established dental plaque. Caries Res 1995; 29: 181–7.

197. GIERTSEN E *et al*. Plaque inhibition by hexetidine and zinc. Scand J Dent Res 1987; 95: 49–54.

198. GILLCRIST JA *et al*. Clinical sealant retention following two different tooth-cleaning techniques. J Public Health Dent 1998; 58: 254–6.

199. GILMOUR ASM *et al*. Prevalence and depth of artificial caries-like lesions adjacent to cavities prepared in roots and restored with a glass ionomer cement or a dentin-bonded composite material. J Dent Res 1997; 76: 1854–61.

200. GLASS BJ *et al*. Xerostomia: diagnosis and treatment planning considerations. Oral Surg 1984; 58: 428–52.

201. GLASS RL *et al*. Root caries prevalence in adults with and without fluorosis. Budapest: ORCA, 1987.

202. GORDON M, NEWBRUN E. Comparison of trends in the prevalence of caries and restorations in young adult populations of several countries. Community Dent Oral Epidemiol 1986; 14: 104–9.

203. GOTEINER D *et al*. Periodontal and caries experience in children with insulin-dependent diabetes mellitus. J Am Dent Assoc 1986; 113: 277–9.

204. GRAVES RC *et al*. University of North Carolina caries risk assessment study. III. J Public Health 1991; 51: 134–43.

205. GRAVES RC *et al*. Oral health status in the United States: prevalence of dental caries. J Dent Educ 1985; 49: 341–51.

206. GROBLER SR *et al*. The effect of a high consumption of apples or grapes on dental caries and periodontal disease in humans. Clin Prev Dent 1989; 11: 8–12.

207. GROENEVELD A *et al*. Caries experience of 15-year old children in Tiel and Culemborg after cessation of water-fluoridation. Budapest: ORCA, 1987.

208. GRÖNDAHL HJ. Radiologic diagnosis in caries management. In: THYLSTRUP A *et al*. (eds) Textbook of clinical cariology. Copenhagen: Munksgaard, 1994.

209. GRÖNDAHL HG *et al*. Approximal caries and frequency of bitewing examinations in Swedish children and adolescents. Community Dent Oral Epidemiol 1992; 20: 20–4.

210. GROOSMAN E *et al*. Chemische plaqueremmers. Ned Tijdschr Tandheelkd 1994; 101: 177–9.

211. GUGGENHEIM J *et al*. Xerostomia. Etiology, recognition and treatment. J Am Dent Assoc 2003; 134: 61–9.

212. GUO JH *et al*. Construction and immunogenic characterization of a fusion anti-caries DNA vaccine against Pac and glucosyltransferase I of Streptococcus mutans. J Dent Res 2004; 83: 266–70.

213. GUSTAFSSON A *et al*. Progression of approximal carious lesions in Swedish teenagers and the correlation between caries experience and radiographic behavior. Acta Odontol Scand 2000; 58: 195–200.

214. GUSTAVSEN F *et al*. Root caries prevalence in a Norwegian adult dental patient population. Gerodontics 1988; 4: 219–23.

215. HAGER TS *et al*. Complete prosthodontic rehabilitation of a patient with Graves' disease. Gen Dent 1997; 45: 482–4.

216. HAIKEL Y *et al*. Scanning electron microscopy of the human enamel surface layer of incipient carious lesions. Caries Res 1983; 17: 1–13.

217. HAKEBERG M *et al*. A radiographic study of dental health in adult patients with dental anxiety. Community Dent Oral Epidemiol 1993; 21: 27–30.

218. HALBACH S *et al*. Amalgam im spiegel kritscher auseinandersetzungen. Köln: Deutscher Ärzte-Verlag, 1999.

219. HALL AF *et al*. The effect of sucrose-containing chewing-gum use on *in situ* enamel lesion remineralization. Caries Res 1995; 29: 477–82.

220. HALL AF *et al*. *In vitro* studies of laser fluorescence for detection and quantitfication of mineral loss from dental caries. Adv Dent Res 1997; 11: 507–14.

221. HAND JS *et al*. Coronal and root caries in older Iowans: 36-month incidence. Gerodontics 1988; 4: 136–9.

222. HANDELMAN SL *et al*. Use of adhesive sealants over occlusal carious lesions: radiographic evaluation. Community Dent Oral Epidemiol 1981; 9: 256–9.

223. HANNIG M. Effect of Carisolv™ solution on sound, demineralized and denatured dentin – an ultrastructural ivestigation. Clin Oral Invest 1999; 3: 155–9.

224. HARRIS R *et al*. Risk factors for dental caries in young children. Community Dent Health 2004; 21 (suppl): 71–85.

225. HASHIZUME LN *et al*. Fluoride availability and stability of Japanese dentifrices. J Oral Sci 2003; 45: 193–9.

226. HATTA H *et al*. Passive immunization against dental plaque formation in humans: effect of a mouth rinse containing egg yolk antibodies (igY) specific to *Streptococcus mutans*. Caries Res 1997; 31: 268–74.

227. HATTAB FN *et al*. Caries risk in patients with thalassaemia major. Int Dent J 2000; 51: 35–8.

228. HAUGEJORDEN O *et al*. Direct evidence concerning the "major role" of fluoride dentifrices in the caries decline. Acta Odontol Scand 1997; 55: 173–80.

229. HAUKALI G, POULSEN S. Effect of varnish containing chlorhexidine and thymol (Cervitec®) on approximal caries in 13- to16-year-old schoolchildren in a low caries area. Caries Res 2003; 37: 185–9.

230. HAWLEY GM *et al*. A 30-moth study investigating the effect of adding triclosan/copolymer to a fluoride dentifrice. Caries Res 1995; 29: 163–7.

231. HAWTHORNE WS *et al*. Factors influencing long-term restoration survival in three private dental practices in Adelaide. Aust Dent J 1997; 42: 59–63.

232. HAYES C. Xylitol gum decreases the decayed, missing and filled surfaces (DMFS) score over a 3-year period by an average of 1.9. J Evid Base Dent Pract 2002; 2: 14–15.

233. HAYNES RB. Hoe moeten medische tijdschriften worden gelezen? II. Ned Tijdschr Geneesk 1983; 127: 2331–7.

234. HEIDMANN J *et al*. Comparative three-year caries protection from an aluminium-containing and a fluoride-containing toothpaste. Caries Res 1997; 31: 85–90.

235. HEIN JW. A study of the effect of frequency of tooth brushing on oral health. J Dent Res 1954; 33: 708, abstract.

236. HEINRICH R *et al*. Klinisch kontrollierte untersuchung zur caries-profunda-therapie am milchmolaren. Dtsch Zahnärztl Z 1991; 46: 581–4.

237. HELM S *et al*. Correlations between caries experience in primary and permanent dentition in birth-cohorts 1950–1970. Scand J Dent Res 1990; 98: 225–7.

238. HENNON DK *et al*. Prevalence and distribution of dental caries in preschool children. J Am Dent Assoc 1969; 79: 1405–14.

239. HENSTEN-PETTERSEN A *et al*. Skin and mucosal reactions associated with dental materials. Eur J Oral Sci 1998; 106: 707–12.

240. HEROD EL. The effect of cheese on dental caries: a review of the literature. Aust Dent J 1991; 36: 120–5.

241. HICKEL R *et al*. Clinical results and new developments of posterior restorations. Am J Dent 2000; 13: 14D–54D.

242. HICKS J *et al*. Biological factors in dental caries: role of remineralisation and fluoride in the dynamic process of demineralisation and remineralisation (part 3). J Clin Pediatr Dent 2004; 28: 203–14.

243. HIGHAM SM *et al.* Effects of Parafilm® and cheese chewing on human dental plaque and metabolism. Caries Res 1989; 23: 42–8.

244. HILDEBRANDT GH *et al.* Effect of slow-release chlorhexidine mouthguards on the levels of selected salivary bacteria. Caries Res 1992; 26: 268–74.

245. HILLMAN JD *et al.* Construction and characterization of an effector strain of *Streptococcus mutans* for replacement therapy for dental caries. Infect Immun 2000; 68: 543–9.

246. HILLMAN JD. Replacement therapy of dental caries. Oper Dent 2002; suppl 6: 39–49.

247. HINTZE H *et al.* Reliability of visual examination, fibre-optic transillumination, and bite-wing radiography, and reproducibility of direct visual examination following tooth separation for the identification of cavitated carious lesions in contacting approximal surfaces. Caries Res 1998; 32: 204–9.

248. HIROSE H *et al.* Close association between *Streptococcus sobrinus* in the saliva of young children and smooth-surface caries increment. Caries Res 1993; 27: 292–7.

249. HOLMEN L *et al.* Scanning electron microscopic study of progressive stages of enamel caries in vivo. Caries Res 1985; 19: 546–54.

250. HOLT RD *et al.* British Society of Paediatric Dentistry: a policy document on fluoride dietary Supplements and fluoride toothpastes for children. Int J Paediatr Dent 1996; 6: 139–42.

251. HÖLTTÄ P *et al.* Mutans streptococcal serotypes in children with gastroesophagal reflux disease. J Dent Child 1997; 64: 201–4.

252. HOMAN BT *et al.* The oral needs and demands of a geriatric population at Mt. Olivet, Brisbane, 1986. Aust Dent J 1988; 33: 424–32.

253. HONKALA E *et al.* Chewing of Xylitol gum – a well adopted practice among Finnish adolescents. Caries Res 1996; 30: 34–9.

254. HÖRSTED-BINDSLEV P *et al.* Dental amalgam – a health hazard. Copenhagen: Munksgaard, 1991.

255. HOSOYA Y *et al.* Influence of tooth-polishing pastes and sealants on DIAGNOdent values. Quint Int 2004; 35: 605–11.

256. HOUWINK B. Tandcariës bij ouderen; de histopathologie en dynamiek. Ned Tijdschr Tandheelkd 1982; 89: 513–17.

257. HOUWINK B *et al.* Tandbederf bij 5-jarige Amsterdammers in 1973 en 1981 en een onderzoek naar kennis, houding en gedrag met betrekking tot tandheelkunde bij hun begeleiders. Ned Tijdschr Tandheelkd 1983; 90: 78–86.

258. HOUWINK B *et al.* Een onderzoek naar mondgezondheid. Deel III. Ned Tijdschr Tandheelkd 1985; 92: 104–11.

259. HUNTER PB. Risk factors in dental caries. Int Dent J 1988; 38: 211–17.

260. HUYSMANS M-ChDNJM *et al.* Electrical methods in occlusal caries diagnosis: an in vitro comparison with visual inspection and bite-wing radiography. Caries Res 1998; 32: 324–9.

261. HUYSMANS M-ChDNJM *et al.* Surface-specific electrical occlusal caries diagnosis: reproducibility, correlation with histological lesion depth, and tooth type dependence. Caries Res 1998; 32: 330–6.

262. IE YL *et al.* Electrical conductance of fissure enamel in recently erupted molar teeth as related to caries status. Caries Res 1995; 29: 94–9.

263. IMFELD T *et al.* Effect of urea in sugar-free chewing gums on pH recovery in human dental plaque evaluated with three different methods. Caries Res 1995; 29: 172–80.

264. IMFELD TN *et al.* Prediction of future high caries increments for children in a school dental service and in private practice. J Dent Educ 1995; 59: 941–4.

265. INABA D *et al.* Effect of sodium hypochlorite treatment on remineralization of human root dentine *in vitro*. Caries Res 1996; 30: 218–24.

266. IRMISCH B. Röntgenologische Verlaufskontrollen approximaler Initialkaries Jugendlicher. Zahn- Mund-Kieferheilkd 1987; 75: 786–9.

267. ISMAIL AI. Food cariogenicity in Americans aged from 9 to 29 years assessed in a national cross-sectional survey, 1971–74. J Dent Res 1986; 65: 1435–40.

268. ISMAIL AI *et al.* Prevalence of dental caries and fluorosis in seven- to 12-year-old children in Northern Newfoundland and Forteau, Labrador. J Can Dent Assoc 1998; 64: 118–24.

269. ISOKANGAS P *et al.* Occurrence of dental decay in children after maternal consumption of Xylitol chewing gum, a follow-up from 0 to 5 years of age. J Dent Res 2000; 79: 1885–9.

270. IVANCAKOVA R *et al.* Effect of fluoridated milk on progression of root surface lesions in vireo under pH cycling conditions. Caries Res 2003; 37: 177–1.

271. IWAMI Y *et al.* Relationship between vacterial infection and evaluation using a laser fluorescence device, DIAGNOdent. Eur J Oral Sci 2004; 112: 419–23.

272. JACOBSEN P *et al.* The use of topical fluoride to prevent or reverse dental caries. Spec Care Dent 2003; 23: 177–9.

273. JANNESSON L *et al.* Effect of xylitol in an enzyme-containing dentifrice without sodium lauryl sulfate on mutans streptococci *in vivo*. Acta Odontol Scand 1997; 55: 212–16.

274. JANSMA J *et al.* Xerostomie-gerelateerde cariës. Ned Tijdschr Tandheelkd 1992; 99: 225–32.

275. JENKINS GN. The physiology and biochemistry of the mouth. Oxford: Blackwell, 1978.

276. JENKINS S *et al.* Studies on the effect of toothpaste rinses on plaque regrowth. J Clin Periodontol 1989; 16: 385–7.

277. JENKINS S *et al.* The effects of a chlorhexidine toothpaste on the development of plaque, gingivitis and tooth staining. J Clin Periodontol 1993; 20: 59–62.

278. JENSEN ME. Effects of chewing sorbitol gum and paraffin on human interproximal plaque. Caries Res 1986; 20: 503–9.

279. JENSEN OE *et al.* Effect of autopolymerizing sealant on viability of microflora occlusal dental caries. Scand J Dent Res 1980; 88: 382–8.

280. JENSEN ME *et al.* Plaque measurements by different methods on the buccal and proximal surfaces of human teeth after a sucrose rinse. J Dent Res 1983; 62: 1314–19.

281. JENTSCH H *et al.* Untersuchunen zur Konstanz der Ergebnisse bei Speicheltests zur Kariesdiagnostik. Dtsch Zahnärztl Z 1997; 52: 109–11.

282. JOHANSSON I *et al*. Salivary flow and dental caries in Indian children suffering from chronic malnutrition. Caries Res 1992; 26: 38–43.

283. JOHANSSON I *et al*. Saliva composition in Indian children with chronic protein-energy malnutrition. J Dent Res 1994; 73: 11–19.

284. JOHARJI RM *et al*. Prevention of pit and fissure caries using an antimicrobila varnish. J Dent 2001; 29: 247–54.

285. JOHNSON MF. Comparative efficacy of NaF and SMFP dentifrices in caries prevention. Caries Res 1993; 27: 328–36.

286. JONES LR *et al*. Effects of total body irradiation on salivary gland function and caries-associated oral microflora in bone marrow transplant patients. Oral Surg Oral Med Oral Pathol 1992; 73: 670–6.

287. JOYSTON-BECHAL S. The effect of X-radiation on the susceptibility of enamel to an artificial caries-like attack *in vitro*. J Dent 1985; 13: 41–4.

288. KAKUTA H *et al*. Xylitol inhibition of acid production and growth of mutans streptococci in the presence of various dietary sugars under strictly anaerobic conditions. Caries Res 2003; 37: 404–9.

289. KALSBEEK H. Het effect van T.G.V.O.-projecten bij de preventie van tandcariës. Ned Tijdschr Tandheelkd 1982; 89: 106–17.

290. KALSBEEK H *et al*. Landelijk epidemiologisch onderzoek tandheelkunde. Ned Tijdschr Tandheelkd 1989; 96: 223–5.

291. KALSBEEK H *et al*. Trends in caries prevalence in Dutch adults between 1983 and 1995. Caries Res 1998; 32: 160–5.

292. KALSBEEK H *et al*. Lange-termijneffecten van preventieve tandzorg bij kleuters. Ned Tijdschr Tandheelkd 1993; 100: 209–13.

293. KALSBEEK H *et al*. Changes in caries prevalence in children and young adults of Dutch and Turkish or Moroccan origin in the Netherlands between 1987 and 1993. Caries Res 1996; 30: 334–41.

294. KANAMOTO T *et al*. Genetic variation in experimental dental caries in four inbred strains of rats. Caries Res 1994; 28: 156–60.

295. KARJALAINEN KM *et al*. Relationship between caries and level of metabolic balance in children and adolescents with insulin-dependent diabetes mellitus. Caries Res 1997; 31: 13–18.

296. KASHANI H *et al*. Effect of NaF-, SnF_2- and chlorhexidine-impregnated birh toothpicks on mutans streptococci and pH in approximal dental plaque. Acta Odontol Scand 1998; 56: 197–201.

297. KATZ L *et al*. Nursing caries in Head Start children, St. Thomas U.S. Virgin Islands: assessed by examiners with different dental backgrounds. J Clin Pediatr Dent 1992; 16: 24–8.

298. KELLY M *et al*. The prevalence of baby bottle tooth decay among two native American populations. J Publich Health Dent 1987; 47 (2): 94–7.

299. KERR NW *et al*. Caries experience in the permanent dentition of late mediaeval Scots (1300–1600 AD). Arch Oral Biol 1988; 33: 143–8.

300. KETLEY CE *et al*. Visual and radiographic diagnosis of occlusal caries in first permanent molars and in second primary molars. Br Dent J 1993; 174: 364–70.

301. KHASKET S *et al*. Lack of correlation between food retention on the human dentition and consumer perception of food stickiness. J Dent Res 1991; 70: 1314–19.

302. KIDD EAM. The histopathology of enamel caries in young and old permanent teeth. Br Dent J 1983; 155: 196–8.

303. KIDD EAM *et al*. Update on fissure sealants. Dent Update 1994; 21: 323–6.

304. KIDD EAM *et al*. The use of a caries detector dye during cavity preparation: a microbiological assessment. Br Dent J 1993; 174: 245–8.

305. KIDD EAM *et al*. The use of a caries detector dye in cavity preparation. Br Dent J 1989; 167: 132–4.

306. KIDD EAM *et al*. Diagnosis of secondary caries: a laboratory study. Br Dent J 1994; 176: 135–9.

307. KIDD EAM *et al*. Secondary caries. Int Dent J 1992; 42: 127–38.

308. KIDD EAM *et al*. Criteria for caries removal at the enamel-dentine junction. Br Dent J 1996; 180: 287–91.

309. KIELBASSA AM *et al*. *In vivo* erzeugte Demineralisation bei tumortherapeutisch bestrahltem, menschlichem Zahnschmelz. Acta Med Dent Helv 1997; 2: 193–8.

310. KIELBASSA AM *et al*. Führt der Einsatz des Caries Detectors® bei der Exkavation zur Erntfernung von gesundem Dentin? Dtsch Zahnärztl Z 2000; 55: 109–13.

311. KILIAN M *et al*. Caries immunology. In: THYLSTRUP A *et al*. (eds) Textbook of cariology. Copenhagen: Munksgaard, 1994.

312. KINDELAN SA *et al*. A comparison of intraoral Candida carriage in Sjögren's syndrome patients with healthy xerostomic controls. Oral Surg Oral Med Oral Pathol Oral Radiol Endod 1998; 85: 162–7.

313. KLEBER CJ *et al*. Aluminum uptake and inhibition of enamel dissolution by sequential treatments with aluminum solutions. Caries Res 1994; 28: 401–5.

314. KLONT B. Organic matrix components in root caries. Thesis, University of Amsterdam, Amsterdam, 1990.

315. KLONT B *et al*. Degradation of bovine incisor root collagen in an *in vitro* caries model. Arch Oral Biol 1991; 36: 4: 299–304.

316. KNABBEN APS *et al*. De validiteit van een nieuwe cariësindicator bij het aantonen van carieus, geïnfecteerd dentine. Ned Tijdschr Tandheelkd 2001; 108: 273–6.

317. KNUUTTILA MLE *et al*. Effect of xylitol on the growth and metabolism of *Streptoccus mutans*. Caries Res 1975; 9: 177–89.

318. KOCH G *et al*. Oral hygiene and dental caries. In: THYLSTRUP A *et al*. (eds) Textbook of clinical cariology. Copenhagen: Munksgaard, 1994.

319. KÖHLER B *et al*. The effect of caries-preventive measures in mothers on dental caries and the oral presence of the bacteria *Streptococcus mutans* and lactobacilli in their children. Arch Oral Biol 1984; 29: 879–83.

320. KÖHLER B *et al*. A five-year clinical evaluation of class II composite resin restorations. J Dent 2000; 28: 111–16.

321. KOLAVIC SA *et al*. The level of cariogenic micro-organisms in patients with Sjögren's syndrome. Spec Care Dent 1997; 17: 65–9.

322. KÖNIG KG. Root lesions. Int Dent J 1990; 40: 283–8.

323. KÖNIG KG. Melk en zuivelproducten in relatie tot tand-gezondheid. Ned Tandartsenbl 1998; 53: 580–7.

324. KOONTONGKAEW S et al. Interaction of chlorhexidine with cytoplasmic membranes of Streptococcus mutans GS-5. Caries Res 1995; 29: 413–17.

325. KORPELA A et al. Lactoperoxidase inhibits glucosyltras-ferases from Streptococcus mutans in vitro. Caries Res 2002; 36: 116–21.

326. KOVARI H et al. Use of xylitol chewing gum in daycare centers: a follow-up study in Savonlinna, Finland. Acta Odontol Scand 2003; 61: 367–70.

327. KRASSE B et al. An anticaries vaccine: report on the status of research. Caries Res 1987; 21: 255–76.

328. KREULEN CM et al. Infant caries. Streptococcus mutans in children using nursing bottles. J Dent Child 1997; 64: 107–11.

329. KROBICKA A et al. The effects of cheese snacks on caries in desalivated rats. J Dent Res 1987; 66: 1116–19.

330. KRONMILLER JE et al. Evaluation of bitewing intervals in children. J Dent Child 1986; 53: 110–14.

331. KUBOKI Y et al. Mechanism of differential staining in carious dentin. J Dent Res 1983; 62: 713–14.

332. LAGERWEIJ MD et al. Demineralization of dentine grooves in vitro. Caries Res 1996; 30: 231–6.

333. LAGERWEIJ MD et al. Effect of fluoridated toothpaste on lesion development in plaque-filled dentine grooves: an intra-oral study. Caries Res 1997; 31: 141–7.

334. LAGERWEIJ MD et al. Remineralisation of enamel lesions with daily applications of a high-concentration fluoride gel and a fluoridated toothpaste: an in vitro study. Caries Res 2002; 36: 270–4.

335. LAKO CJ et al. De invloed van een aantal sociaal-culturele variabelen op de gebitstoestand van Rotterdamse kinderen. Ned Tijdschr Tandheelkd 1984; 91: 346–51.

336. LAMB WJ et al. In situ remineralization of subsurface enamel lesion after the use of a fluoride chewing gum. Caries Res 1993; 27: 111–16.

337. LANGELAND K. Tissue response to dental caries. Endod Dent Traumatol 1987; 3: 149–71.

338. LANGWORTH S et al. A case of high mercury exposure from dental amalgam. Eur J Oral Sci 1996; 104: 320–1.

339. LARSEN MJ et al. Chemical and structural challenges in remineralization of dental enamel lesions. Scand J Dent Res 1989; 97: 285–96.

340. LARSEN MJ et al. Solubility, unit cell dimensions and crystallinity of fluoridated human dental enamel. Arch Oral Biol 1989; 34; 12: 969–73.

341. LARSSON B et al. Prevalence of caries in adolescents in relation to diet. Community Dent Oral Epidemiol 1992; 20: 133–7.

342. LATINO C et al. Support of undermined occlusal enamel provided by restorative materials. Quint Int 2001; 32: 287–91.

343. LAWRENCE HP et al. Three-year root caries incidence and risk modelling in older adults in North Carolina. J Public Health Dent 1995; 55: 69–78.

344. LAWRENCE HP et al. Five-year incidence rates and intraoral distribution of root caries among community-dwelling older adults. Caries Res 1996; 30: 169–79.

345. LEACH SA et al. Remineralization of artificial caries-like lesions in human enamel in situ by chewing sorbitol gum. J Dent Res 1989; 68: 1064–8.

346. LEE SS et al. The antimicrobial potential of 14 natural herbal dentifrices. J Am Dent Assoc 2004; 135: 1133–41.

347. LEENSTRA TS et al. Radio- en/of chemotherapie in het hoofd-halsgebied. Ned Tijdschr Tandheelkd 1990; 97: 17–22.

348. LEGLER DW et al. Etiology, epidemiology and clinical implications. In: MEANAKER L (ed.) The biologic basis of dental caries. Hagerstown: Harper & Row Publishers, 1980.

349. LEGEROS RZ et al. Chemical stability of carbonate- and fluoride-containing apatites. Caries Res 1983; 17: 419–29.

350. LEKSELL E et al. Pulp exposure after stepwise versus direct complete excavation of deep carious lesions in young posterior permanent teeth. Endod Dent Traumatol 1996; 12: 192–6.

351. LEMKE CW et al. Controlled fluoridation: the dental effects of discontinuation in Antigo, Winsconsin. J Am Dent Assoc 1970; 80: 782–6.

352. LEVERETT DH et al. Randomized clinical trial of the effect of prenatal fluoride Supplements in preventing dental caries. Caries Res 1997; 31: 174–9.

353. LI Y et al. Caries experience in deciduous dentition of rural children 3–5 years old in relation to the presence or absence of enamel hypoplasia. Caries Res 1996; 30: 8–15.

354. LINDHE J. Parodontologie. Alphen aan den Rijn: Samson Stafleu, 1985.

355. LINDHE J et al. The effect of a triclosan containing dentifrice on established plaque and gingivitis. J Clin Periodontol 1993; 20: 327–34.

356. LINDQUIST B et al. Colonization of Streptococcus mutans and Streptococcus sobrinus genotypes and caries development in children to mothers harbouring both species. Caries Res 2004; 38: 95–103.

357. LILLY JP et al. Sjögren's syndrome: diagnosis and management of oral complications. Gen Dent 1996; 44: 404–8.

358. LITH A et al. Predicting development of approximal dentin lesions by means of past caries experience. Community Dent Oral Epidemiol 1992; 20: 25–9.

359. LIN BP et al. Dental caries in older adults with diabetes mellitus. Spec Care Dent 1999; 19: 8–14.

360. LIN YT et al. Caries prevalence and bottle-feeding practices in 2-year-old children with cleft lip, cleft palate, or both in Taiwan. Cleft Palate Craniofac J 1999; 36: 522–6.

361. LINGSTRÖM P et al. Dietary factors in the prevention of dental caries: a systematic review. Acta Odontol Scand 2003; 61: 331–40.

362. LO ECM et al. A community-based caries control program for pre-school children using topical fluorides. 18 months results. J Dent Res 2001; 80: 2071–4.

363. LOCKER D et al. Oral health-related quality of life of a population of medically compromised elderly people. Community Dent Health 2002; 19: 90–7.

364. LOCKER D et al. Prevalence of and factors associated with root decay in older adults in Canada. J Dent Res 1989; 68: 768–72.

365. LOESCHE WJ. Role of *Streptococcus mutans* in human dental decay. Microbiol Rev 1986; 50: 353–80.

366. LU KH *et al*. A three-year clinical comparison of a sodium monofluorophosphate dentifrice with a sodium fluoride dentifrice on dental caries. J Dent Child 1987; 54: 241–4.

367. LUNDER N *et al*. Approximal cavitation related to bitewing image and caries activity in adolescents. Caries Res 1996; 30: 143–7.

368. LUNDGREN M *et al*. Root caries and some related factors in 88-year-old carriers and non-carriers of *Streptococcus sobrinus* in saliva. Caries Res 1998; 32: 93–9.

369. LUSSI A. Impact of including or excluding cavitated lesions when evaluating methods for the diagnosis of occlusal caries. Caries Res 1996; 30: 389–93.

370. LUSSI A *et al*. *In vivo* diagnosis of fissure caries using a new electrical resistance monitor. Caries Res 1995; 29: 81–7.

371. LUSSI A *et al*. Performance of conventional and new methods for the detection of occlusal caries in deciduous teeth. Caries Res 2003; 37: 2–7.

372. LUSSI A *et al*. DIAGNOdent. J Dent Res 2004; 83 (spec. issue C): C80–3.

373. LYNCH E *et al*. A comparison of primary root caries lesions classified according to colour. Caries Res 1994; 28: 233–9.

374. MACEK MD *et al*. Is 75 percent of dental caries really found in 25 percent of the population? J Public Health Dent 2004; 64: 20–5.

375. MaCENTEE MI *et al*. Longitudinal study of caries and cariogenic bacteria in an elderly disabled population. Community Dent Oral Epidemiol 1990; 18: 149–52.

376. MACHIULSKIENE V *et al*. Caries preventive effect of sugar-substituted chewing gum. Community Dent Oral Epidemiol 2001; 29: 278–88.

377. MACKERT JR *et al*. Mercury exposure from dental amalgam fillings. Crit Rev Oral Biol Med 1997; 8: 410–36.

378. MAGNUSSON BO *et al*. Stepwise excavation of deep carious lesions in primary teeth. J Int Ass Dent Child 1977; 8: 34–40.

379. MAGRI F *et al*. Behandlungsstand und Kariesneubefall seit der Schulzeit im Vergleich mit Persönlichkeit und Lebensführung. Schweiz Monatschr Zahnmed 1986; 96: 844–60.

380. MAGUIRE A *et al*. Dental health of children taking antimicrobial and non-antimicrobial liquid oral medication long-term. Caries Res 1996; 30: 16–21.

381. MÄKINEN KK *et al*. Properties of whole saliva and dental plaque in relation to 40-month consumption of chewing gums containing xylitol, sorbitol or sucrose. Caries Res 1996; 30: 180–8.

382. MÄKINEN KK *et al*. Polyol chewing gums and caries rates in primary dentition. Caries Res 1996; 30: 408–17.

383. MÄKINEN KK *et al*. A descriptive report of the effects of a 16-month xylitol chewing-gum progamme subsequent to a 40-month sucrose gum programme. Caries Res 1998; 32: 107–12.

384. MALTZ M *et al*. A clinical, microbiologic, and radiographic study of deep caries lesions after incomplete caries removal. Quint Int 2002; 33: 151–9.

385. MANJI F *et al*. Pattern of dental caries in an adult rural population. Caries Res 1989; 23: 55–62.

386. MARINHO VC *et al*. Fluoride toothpastes for preventing dental caries in children and adolescents. Cochrane Database Syst Rev 2003; CD002278.

387. MARSH P. Oral Microbiology. Walton-on-Thames, Surrey: Thomas Nelson & Sons, 1980.

388. MARSH PD. Host defenses and microbial homeostasis: role of microbial interactions. J Dent Res 1989; 68 (spec. issue): 1567–75.

389. MARSH PD. Dentifrices containing new agents for the control of plaque and gingivitis: microbial aspects. J Clin Periodontol 1991; 18: 462–7.

390. MARSCH PD *et al*. Microbiological study of early caries of approximal surfaces in schoolchildren. J Dent Res 1989; 68: 1151–4.

391. MARTHALER TM. Heutiger Stand und Ausblicke in der Kariesprophylaxe. Dtsch Zahnärztl Z 1992; 47: 724–31.

392. MARTHALER TM *et al*. Caries-preventive salt fluoridation. Caries Res 1978; 12 (suppl 1): 15–21.

393. MARTHALER TM *et al*. The prevalence of dental caries in Europe 1990–1995. Caries Res 1996; 30: 237–55.

394. MASSSARA MLA *et al*. Atraumatic restorative treatment: clinical, ultrastructural and chemical analysis. Caries Res 2002; 36: 430–6.

395. MATEE MIN *et al*. Nursing caries, linear hypoplasia, and nursing and weaning habits in Tanzanian infants. Community Dent Oral Epidemiol 1994; 22: 289–93.

396. MATHIESEN AT *et al*. Oral hygiene as a variable in dental caries experience in 14-year-olds exposed to fluoride. Caries Res 1996; 30: 29–33.

397. MATSSON L *et al*. Caries frequency in children with controlled diabetes. Scand J Dent Res 1975; 83: 327–32.

398. MAUPOMÉ G *et al*. Patterns of dental caries following the cessation of water fluoridation. Community Dent Oral Epidemiol 2001; 29: 37–47.

399. McARTHUR CP *et al*. Dental professionals' role in diagnosing Sjögren's syndrome. Gen Dent 1997; 45: 62–5.

400. McCOMB D. Caries detector dyes – How accurate and useful are they? J Can Dent Assoc 2000; 66: 195–8.

401. McLEAN JW. New concepts in cosmetic dentistry using glass-ionomer cements and composites. J Cal Dent Ass 1986; 14: 20–7.

402. McLEAN JW *et al*. Fissure sealing and filling with an adhesive glass-ionomer cement. Br Dent J 1974; 136: 269–76.

403. MEEUWISSEN R *et al*. Twintig jaar tandheelkundige verzorging. II. Ned Tijdschr Tandheelkd 1984; 91: 111–14.

404. MEJÁRE I *et al*. Caries development from 11 to 22 years of age: a prospective radiographic study. Caries Res 1998; 32: 10–16.

405. MELLBERG JR *et al*. Fluoride in preventive dentistry. Chicago, IL: Quintessence Publishing, 1983.

406. MENAKER L. The biologic basis of dental caries. Hagerstown: Harper & Row Publishers, 1980.

407. MERTZ-FAIRHURST EJ *et al*. Ultraconservative and cariostatic sealed restorations: results at year 10. J Am Dent Assoc 1998; 129: 55–66.

408. MESSER LB et al. The retention of pit and fissure sealants placed in pimary school children by Dental Health Services, Victoria. Aust Dent J 1997; 42: 233–9.

409. MILEMAN PA et al. Decisions on restorative treatment and recall intervals based on bitewing radiographs. A comparison between national surveys of Dutch and Norwegian practitioners. Community Dent Health 1988; 5: 273–84.

410. MILEMAN PA et al. Factors influencing the likelihood of successful decisions to treat dentin caries from bitewing radiographs. Community Dent Oral Epidemiol 1992; 20: 175–80.

411. MILEMAN PA et al. Variation in radiographic caries diagnosis and treatment decisions among university teachers. Community Dent Oral Epidemiol 1982; 10: 327–43.

412. MILEMAN PA et al. Variation in radiographic caries diagnosis and degree of caries on treatment decisions by dental teachers using bitewing radiographs. Community Dent Oral Epidemiol 1983; 11: 536–62.

413. MILGROM P et al. Dental caries and its relationship to bacterial infection, hypoplasia, diet, and oral hygiene in 6- to 36-month-old children. Community Dent Oral Epidemiol 2000; 28: 295–306.

414. MILLER AJ et al. Oral health of United States adults. The national survey of oral health in U.S. employed adults and seniors: 1985–1986. Washington DC: U.S. Department of Health and Human Services, 1987.

415. MJÖR IA. Frequency of secondary caries at various anatomical locations. Oper Dent 1985; 10: 88–92.

416. MJÖR IA. The reasons for replacement and the age of failed restorations in general dental practice. Acta Odontol Scand 1997; 55: 58–63.

417. MJÖR IA et al. Age of restorations at replacement in permanent teeth in general dental practice. Acta Odontol Scand 2000; 58: 97–101.

418. MJÖR IA et al. Secondary caries. Quint Int 2000; 31: 165–79.

419. MJÖR IA et al. The relative cost of different restorations in the UK. Br Dent J 1997; 182: 286–9.

420. MOORER WR et al. Suikers, suikervervangers en zoetstoffen. In: VAN LOVEREN C et al. (eds) Preventieve tandheelkunde. Houten: Bohn Stafleu Van Loghum, 1996.

421. MULLER M. Nursing-bottle syndrome: risk factors. J Dent Child 1996; 63: 42–50.

422. MURRAH VA. Diabetes mellitus and associated oral manifestations: a review. J Oral Pathol 1985; 14: 271–81.

423. MURRAY JJ. The prevention of dental disease. Oxford: Oxford University Press, 1983.

424. MURRAY JJ. Appropriate use of fluorides for human health. Geneva: World Health Organization, 1986.

425. MURRAY JJ et al. Fluorides in caries prevention. Bristol: Wright, PSG, 1982.

426. NAGAMINE M et al. Effect of resin modified glass ionomer cements on secondary caries. Am J Dent 1997; 10: 173–8.

427. NAGEL SC et al. Relative binding activity-serum modified access (RBA-SMA) assay predicts the relative in vivo activity of xenoestrogens Bisphenol A and octylphenol. Environ Health Perspect 1997; 105: 70–6.

428. NAPHAUSEN MTP et al. Diagnostiek van occlusale cariëslesies met behulp van laserfluorescentiemetingen. Ned Tijdschr Tandheelkd 2002; 109: 3–7.

429. NARIYAMA M et al. Identification of chromosomes associated with dental caries susceptibility using quantitative trait locus analysis in mice. Caries Res 2004; 38: 79–84.

430. NATHAVITHARANA KA et al. Primary Sjögren's syndrome and rampant dental caries in a 5-year-old child. Int J Paediatr Dent 1995; 5: 173–6.

431. NEWBRUN E. Fluorides and dental caries. Springfield, IL: Charles C. Thomas, 1978.

432. NEWBRUN E. Cariology. Chicago, IL: Quintessence Publishing, 1989.

433. NEWBRUN E. Frequent sugar intake – then and now: interpretation of the main results. Scand J Dent Res 1989; 97: 103–9.

434. NIKAWA H et al. In vitro cariogenic potential of Candida albicans. Mycoses 2003; 46: 471–8.

435. NISHI M et al. Caries experience of some countries and areas expressed by the Significant Caries Index. Community Dent Oral epidemiol 2002; 30: 296–301.

436. NOWAK AJ et al. Summary of the conference on radiation exposure in pediatric dentistry. J Am Dent Assoc 1981; 103: 426–8.

437. NUNN J et al. The condition of the teeth in the UK in 1998 and implications for the future. Br Dent J 2000; 189: 639–44.

438. NYVAD B et al. Active root surface caries converted inactive caries as response to oral hygiene. Scand J Dent Res 1986; 94: 281–4.

439. NYVAD B et al. Reliability of a new caries diagnostic system differentiating between active and inactive lesions. Caries Res 1999; 33: 252–60.

440. NYVAD B et al. Construct and predictive validity of clinical caries diagnostic criteria assessing lesion activity. J Dent Res 2003; 82: 117–22.

441. OGAWA K et al. The ultrastructure and hardness of the transparent layer of human carious dentin. J Dent Res 1983; 62: 7–10.

442. OKAZAKI M et al. Unstable behavior of magnesium-containing hydroxyapatites. Caries Res 1986; 20: 324–31.

443. OLEA N. Olea's response (Letter). Environ Health Perspect 1999; 107: A290–2.

444. OLEA N et al. Estrogenicity of resin-based composites and sealants used in dentistry. Environ Health Perspect 1996; 104: 298–305.

445. OLLILA P et al. Prolonged pacifier-sucking and use of a nursing bottle at night: possible risk factors for dental caries in children. Acta Odontol Scand 1998; 56: 233–7.

446. O'MULLANE DM et al. A three-year clinical trial of a combination of trimetaphosphate and sodium fluoride in silica toothpastes. J Dent Res 1997; 76: 1776–81.

447. ÖRTENDAHL T et al. Mutans streptococci and incipient caries adjacent to glass ionomer cement or resin-base composite in orthodontics. Am J Orthod Dentofac Orthop 1997; 112: 271–4.

448. O'SULLIVAN EA et al. Prevalence and site characteristics of dental caries in primary molar teeth from prehistoric times to the 18th century in England. Caries Res 1993; 27: 147–53.

449. OZAKI K *et al.* A quantitative comparison of selected bacteria in human carious dentine by microscopic counts. Caries Res 1994; 28: 137–45.

450. ÖZOK AR *et al.* Effect of dentinal fluid composition on dentin demineralisation *in vitro.* Caries Res 2004; 83: 849–53.

451. PAMEYER CH *et al.* The disastrous effects of the "Total etch" technique in vital pulp capping in primates. Am J Dent 1998; 11: S45–54.

452. PARFITT GJ. The speed of development of the carious cavity. Br Dent J 1956; 100: 204–7.

453. PEERS A *et al.* Validity and reproducibility of clinical examination, fibre–optic transillumination, and bite-wing radiology for the diagnosis of small approximal carious lesions: an *in vitro* study. Caries Res 1993; 27: 307–11.

454. PENNING CH. Amalgaam. V. Een duurzaam restauratiemateriaal? Ned Tijdschr Tandheelkd 1993; 100: 225–8.

455. PENNING CH *et al.* Prepareren en restaureren met plastische materialen. Utrecht: Bohn, Scheltema & Holkema, 1984.

456. PENNING CH. Cariëslaesies: opsporen, behandelen. Amsterdam: ACTA, Afdeling Cariologie Endodontologie Pedodontologie, 1988.

457. PEREIRA AC *et al.* Dental caries and fluorosis prevalence study in a nonfluoridated Barzilian community: trend analysis and toothpaste association. ASDC J Dent Child 2000; 67: 132–5.

458. PETERSSON LG *et al.* Effect of semin-annual applications of a chlorhexidine/fluoride varnish mixture on approximal caries incidence in schoolchildren. Eur J Oral Sci 1998; 106: 623–7.

459. PIENIHÄKKINEN K *et al.* Comparison of the efficacy of 40% chlorhexidine varnish and 1% chlorhexidine-fluoride gel in decreasing the level of salivary mutans streptococci. Caries Res 1995; 29: 62–7.

460. PINDBORG JJ. Pathology of the dental hard tissues. Copenhagen: Munksgaard, 1970.

461. PINE CM *et al.* Dynamics of and diagnostic methods for detecting small carious lesions. Caries Res 1996; 30: 381–8.

462. PISCHINGER A. Das system der Grundregulation. Grundlagen für eine ganzheitsbiologische Theorie. Heidelberg: Haug, 1990.

463. PITTS NB. Regression of approximal carious lesions diagnosed from serial standardized bitewing radiographs. Caries Res 1986; 20: 85–90.

464. PITTS NB. Detection of approximal radiolucencies in enamel: a preliminary comparison between experienced clinicians and an image analysis method. J Am Dent Assoc 1987; 15: 191–7.

465. PITTS NB. Patient caries status in the context of practical, evidence-based management of the initial caries lesion. J Dent Educ 1997; 61: 861–5.

466. PITTS NB *et al.* Some of the factors to be considered in the prescription and timing of bitewing radiography in the diagnosis and management of dental caries. J Dent 1992; 20: 74–84.

467. PITTS NB *et al.* Reproducibility of computer-aided image-analysis-derived estaimates of the depths and area of radi-

468. POHJAMO L *et al.* Increment of caries in diabetic adults. A two-year longitudinal study. Community Dent Health 1991; 8: 343–8.

469. POLLARD MA. Potential cariogenicity of starches and fruits as assessed by the plaque-sampling method and intra-oral cariogenicity test. Caries Res 1995; 29: 68–74.

470. POORTERMAN JHG *et al.* Variatie onder tandartsen bij de beoordeling van cariës en restauraties. Ned Tijdschr Tandheelkd 1997; 104: 214–18.

471. POORTERMAN JHG *et al.* Radiographic dentinal caries and its progression in occlusal surfaces in Dutch 17-year-olds: a 6-year longitudinal study. Caries Res 2003; 37: 29–33.

472. POWELL LV. Caries prediction. Community Dent Oral Epidemiol 1998; 26: 361–71.

473. PRIOVOLOU CH *et al.* A comparative study of enamel defects and caries in children and adolescents with and without coeliac disease. Eur J Paediatr Dent 2004; 5: 102–6.

474. PULGAR R *et al.* Determination of Bisphenol A and related aromatic compounds released from Bis-GMA-based composites and sealants by high performance liquid Chromatography. Environ Health Perspect 2000; 108: 21–7.

475. QVIST V *et al.* Restorative treatment pattern and longevity of resin restorations in Denmark. Acta Odontol Scand 1986; 44: 351–6.

476. QVIST J *et al.* Placement and longevity of amalgam restorations in Denmark. Acta Odontol Scand 1990; 48: 297–303.

477. RAADAL M *et al.* Caries prevalence in primary teeth as a predictor of early fissure caries in permanent first molars. Community Dent Oral Epidemiol 1992; 20: 30–4.

478. RAVALD N *et al.* Caries and periodontal conditions in patients with primary Sjögren's syndrome. Swed Dent J 1998; 22: 97–103.

479. REEVES R *et al.* The relationship of bacterial penetration and pulpal pathosis in carious teeth. Oral Surg Oral Med Oral Pathol 1966; 22: 59–65.

480. REICH E *et al.* Mouthrinses and dental caries. Int Dent J 2002; 52: 337–45.

481. RENGGLI HH. Chemotherapie van de plaque. Ned Tijdschr Tandheelkd 1986; 93: 419–21.

482. RENSON CE *et al.* Changing patterns of oral health and implications for oral health manpower: part I. Int Dent J 1985; 35: 235–51.

483. REUTERVING CO *et al.* Root surface caries and periodontal disease in long-term alloxan diabetic rats. J Dent Res 1986, 65: 689–94.

484. RHODUS NL *et al.* A comparison of the three methods for detecting *Candida albicans* in patients with Sjögren's syndrome. Quint Int 1998; 29: 107–13.

485. RICHARDSON PS *et al.* Susceptibility of tooth surfaces to carious attack in young adults. Community Dent Health 1996; 13: 163–8.

486. RICKARD G *et al.* Ozone therapy for the treatment of dental caries. Cochran Database Syst Rev 2004; 3: CD004153.

487. RICKETTS DNJ *et al*. Histological validation of electrical resistance measurements in the diagnosis of occlusal caries. Caries Res 1996; 30: 148–55.

488. RICKETTS DNJ *et al*. Hidden caries: what is it? Does it exist? Does it matter? Int Dent J 1997; 47: 259–65.

489. RICKETTS DNJ *et al*. The effect of airflow on site-specific electrical conductance measurements used in the diagnosis of pit and fissure caries *in vitro*. Caries Res 1997; 31: 111–18.

490. RICKETTS DNJ *et al*. The electronic diagnosis of caries in pits and fissures: site-specific stable conductance readings or cumulative resistance readings? Caries Res 1997; 31: 119–24.

491. RIOS D *et al*. Wear and superficial roughness of glass ionomer cements used as sealants, after simulated tooth-brushing. Pesqui Odontol Bras 2002; 16: 343–8.

492. RIPA LW. Correlations between oral hygiene status, gingival health and dental caries in school children. J Prev Dent 1974; 1: 28–38.

493. RIPA LW. The current status of pit and fissure sealants. J Can Dent Ass 1985; 51: 367–80.

494. RIPA LW. Review of the anticaries effectiveness of professionally applied and self-applied topical fluoride gels. J Public Health Dent 1989; 49 (spec. issue): 297–309.

495. RIPA LW *et al*. Clinical study of the anticaries efficacy of three fluoride dentifrices containing anticalculus ingredients. J Clin Dent 1990; 2 (2): 29–33.

496. ROBERTS GJ *et al*. Patterns of breast and bottle feeding and their association with dental caries in 1-to 4-year-old South African children. 1. Dental caries prevalence and experience. Community Dent Health 1993; 10: 405–13.

497. ROCHA RO *et al*. In vivo effectiveness of laser fluorescence compared to visual inspection and radiography for the detection of occlusal caries in primary teeth. Caries Res 2003; 37: 437–41.

498. ROETERS FJM *et al*. Latobacilli, mutans streptococci and dental caries: a longitudinal study in 2-year-old children up to the age of 5 years. Caries Res 1995; 29: 272–9.

499. ROETERS FJM *et al*. Prediction of the need for bitewing radiography in detecting caries in the primary dentition. Community Dent Oral Epidemiol 1994; 22: 456–60.

500. RØLLA G. Why is sucrose so cariogenic? The role of glucosyltransferase and polysaccharides. Scand J Dent Res 1989; 97: 115–19.

501. RØLLA G *et al*. Critical evaluation of the composition and use of topical fluorides, with emphasis on the role of calcium fluoride in caries inhibition (review). J Dent Res 1990; 69 (spec. issue): 780–5; discussion 820–3.

502. ROSALEN PL *et al*. Effect of copper co-crystallized with sugar on caries development in desalivated rats. Caries Res 1996; 30: 367–72.

503. ROSEN S *et al*. Effect on caries of cross-breeding caries-resistant and caries-susceptible rats. J Dent Res 1962; 41: 1033–6.

504. ROTH KK-F *et al*. Die Anfärbung von Kariösem Dentin mit dem Kariesdetektor (Säurerot in Propylenglykol). Dtsch Zahnärztl Z 1989; 44: 460–2.

505. ROZIER RG. Effectiveness of methods used by dental professionals for the primary prevention of dental caries: a review of evidence. J Dent Educ 2001; 65: 1063–72.

506. RUDOLPHY MP *et al*. Grey discolouration for the diagnosis of secondary caries in teeth with Class II amalgam restorations: an *in vitro* study. Caries Res 1996; 30: 189–93.

507. RUGH JD *et al*. Psychophysiological changes and oral conditions. In: COHEN LK *et al*. (eds) Social sciences and dentistry. A critical bibliography. Volume 2. Kingston-upon-Thames: Quintessence Publishing, on behalf of the Fédération Dentaire Internationale, 1984.

508. RUIKEN HMHM. Tandcariës en gedrag bij kinderen. Thesis, University of Nijmegen, Nijmegen, 1983.

509. RUSSELL MW. Potential for vaccines in the prevention of caries lesions. Oper Dent 2001; suppl 6: 51–60.

510. SAKKI TK *et al*. Lifestyle, dental caries and number of teeth. Community Dent Oral Epidemiol 1994; 22: 298–302.

511. SALAKO NO *et al*. Oral findings in a child with Prader-Labhart-Willi syndrome. Quint Int 1995; 26: 339–41.

512. SÄLLSTEN G *et al*. Long-term use of nicotine chewing gum and mercury exposure from dental amalgam fillings. J Dent Res 1996; 75: 594–8.

513. SCHAEKEN MJM *et al*. Plax effectiever dan water? Ned Tijdschr Tandheelkd 1989; 97: 315–17.

514. SCHAEKEN MJM *et al*. Influence of contact time and concentration of chlorhexidine varnish on mutans streptococci in interproximal dental plaque. Caries Res 1991; 25: 292–5.

515. SCHAEKEN MJM *et al*. Effect of chlorhexidine varnish on streptococci in dental plaque from occlusal fissures. Caries Res 1994; 28: 262–6.

516. SCHAMSCHULA RG *et al*. Prevalence and interrelationships of surface root caries in Lufa, Papua New Guinea. Community Dent Oral Epidemiol 1974; 2: 295–304.

517. SCHEIE AAA. Modes of action of currently known chemical anti-plaque agents other than chlorhexidine. J Dent Res 1989; 68 (spec. issue): 1609–16.

518. SCHEIE AA *et al*. Xylitol in caries prevention: what is the evidence for clinical efficacy? Oral Dis 1998; 4: 268–78.

519. SCHEIE AA *et al*. The effects of xylitol-containing chewing gums on dental plaque and acidogenic potential. J Dent Res 1998; 77: 1547–52.

520. SCHEININ A *et al*. Turku sugar studies. XVII. Incidence of dental caries in relation to 1-year of xylitol chewing gum. Acta Odontol Scand 1975; 33: 269–78.

521. SCHEININ A *et al*. Multifactorial modeling for root caries prediction. Community Dent Oral Epidemiol 1992; 20: 35–7.

522. SCHMALZ G *et al*. Bisphenol-A content of resin monomers and related degradation products. Clin Oral Invest 1999; 3: 114–19.

523. SCHNEIDERMAN A *et al*. Assessment of dental caries with digital fiber–optic transillumination (DIFOTI™): *in vitro* study. Caries Res 1997; 31: 103–10.

524. SCHUKAR M *et al*. Proximo-cervical adaptation of Class II-composite restorations after thermocycling: a quantitative and qualitative study. J Oral Rehabil 1997; 24: 766–75.

525. SCHULLER AA *et al*. Effects of routine professional application of topical fluoride on caries and treatment experi-

ence in adolescents of low socio-economic status in the Netherlands. Caries Res 2003; 37: 172–7.

526. SCHULTZ J et al. Studien über die Ursache des Zahnverlustes. Stomatol DDR 1987; 37: 305–9.

527. SCHULZ SD et al. Härtegrad verschiedener kariöser Schichten an Zähnen mit chronischer Dentinkaries. Dtsch Zahnärzt Zeit 1991; 46: 420–2.

528. SCHÜPBACH P et al. Human root caries: histopathology of initial lesions in cementum and dentin. J Oral Pathol Med 1989; 18: 146–56.

529. SCHÜPBACH P et al. Human root caries: Microbotia in plaque covering sound, carious and arrested carious root surfaces. Caries Res 1995; 29: 382–95.

530. SCHÜPBACH P et al. Human root caries: microbiota of a limited number of root caries lesions. Caries Res 1996; 30: 52–64.

531. SCHUURS AHB et al. Amalgaam. De feiten. Nijmegen: STI, 1995.

532. SCHUURS AHB et al. Wanneer klasse I en II vullen met composiet? Ned Tandartsenbl 1998; 53: 884–90.

533. SCHUURS AHB. Reproductive toxicity of occupational mercury. A review of the literature. J Dent 1999; 27: 249–56.

534. SCHUURS AHB et al. Hormoonontregelaars. Pseudo-oestrogenen in tandheelkundige composieten en sealants. Ned Tijdschr Tandheelkd 2000; 107: 490–4.

535. SCHUURS AHB et al. Orale lichen planus, amalgaam en andere vulmaterialen. Ned Tijdschr Tandheelkd 2000; 107: 198–202.

536. SCHUURS AHB et al. Huid- en slijmvliesreacties door tandheelkundige materialen. Ned Tijdschr Tandheelkd 1999; 106: 334–9.

537. SCLAVOS S et al. Future caries development in children with nursing bottle caries. J Pedod 1988; 13: 1–10.

538. SCULLY C. Sjögren's syndrome: clinical and laboratory features, immunopathogenesis, and management. Oral Surg 1986; 62: 510–23.

539. SELA M et al. Enamel rehardening with cheese in irradiated patients. Am J Dent 1994; 7: 134–6.

540. SHELLIS RP. Effects of supersaturated pulpal fluid on the formation of caries-like lesions on the roots of human teeth. Caries Res 1994; 28: 14–20.

541. SHIP JA et al. An assessment of salivary function in healthy premenopausal and postmenopausal females. J Gerodont 1991; 46: M11–15.

542. SHULER CF. Inherited risks for susceptibility to dental caries. J Dent Educ 200; 65: 1038–45.

543. SHWARTZ M et al. A longitudinal analysis from bite-wing radiographs of the rate of progression of approximal carious lesions through human dental enamel. Arch Oral Biol 1984; 29: 529–36.

544. SHWARTZ M et al. The expected benefits from alternative frequencies of bitewing radiograms. Acta Odontol Scand 1986; 44: 11–16.

545. SHWARTZ M et al. The frequency of bitewing radiographs. Oral Surg 1986; 61: 300–5.

546. SIDI AD et al. A comparison of bitewing radiography and interdental transillumination as adjuncts to the clinical identification of approximal caries in posterior teeth. Br Dent J 1988; 164: 15–18.

547. SIGURJONS H et al. Cariogenic bacteria in a longitudinal study of approximal caries. Caries Res 1995; 29: 42–5.

548. SILVER DH. A longitudinal study of infant feeding practice, diet and caries, related to social class in children aged 3 and 8–10 years. Br Dent J 1987; 163: 296–300.

549. SILVERSTONE LM. The structure of carious lesions. In: COHEN B et al. (eds) Scientific foundations of dentistry. London: William Heinemann Medical Books, 1976.

550. SILVERSTONE LM. The current state of sealant research. CDA J 1985; 13: 10–15.

551. SILVERSTONE LM et al. The structure and ultrastructure of the carious lesion in human dentin. Gerodontics 1985; 1: 185–93.

552. SIMONS D et al. The effect of chlorhexidine/xylitol chewing-gum on cariogenic salivary microflora: a clinical trial in elderly patients. Caries Res 1997; 31: 91–6.

553. SIMONSEN RJ. Cost effectiveness of pit and fissure sealant at 10 years. Quint Int 1989; 20: 75–82.

554. SJÖGREN K et al. Effect of post-brushing water rinsing on caries-like lesions at approximal and buccal sites. Caries Res 1995; 29: 337–42.

555. SJÖGREN K et al. Effect of improved toothpaste usage on approximal caries in pre-school children. Caries Res 1995; 29: 435–41.

556. SJÖGREN K et al. Fluoride in the interdental area after two different post-brushing water rinsing procedures. Caries Res 1996; 30: 194–9.

557. SJÖGREN K et al. Effect of water rinsing after toothbrushing on fluoride ingestion and absorption. Caries Res 1994; 28: 455–9.

558. SKÖLD UM et al. Differences in caries recording with and without bitewing radiographs. Swed Dent J 1997; 21: 69–75.

559. SMITH AJ. Pulpal responses to caries and dental repair. Caries Res 2002; 36: 223–32.

560. SMITH DJ. Dental caries vaccines: prospects and concerns. Crit Rev Oral Biol Med 2002; 13: 335–49.

561. SÖDERHOLMK J et al. Bis-GMA-based resins in dentistry: are they safe? J Am Dent Assoc 1999; 130: 201–9.

562. SÖDERLING E et al. Influence of maternal xylitol consumption on mother–child transmission of mutans streptoccoci: 6-year follow-up. Caries Res 2001; 35: 173–7.

563. SÖDERLING E et al. Long-term xylitol consumption and mutans streptococci in plaque and saliva. Caries Res 1991; 25: 153–7.

564. SONGPAISAN Y et al. Mutans streptococci in a Thai population: relation to caries and changes in prevalence after application of fissure sealants. Caries Res 1994; 28: 161–8.

565. SPAK CJ et al. Caries incidence, salivary flow rate and efficacy of fluoride gel treatment in irradiated patients. Caries Res 1994; 28: 388–93.

566. SPIJKERVET FKL et al. Chlorhexidine inactivation by saliva. Oral Surg Oral Med Oral Pathol 1990; 69: 444–9.

567. SPLIETH C et al. Caries prevention with chlorhexidine-thymol varnish in high risk school children. Community Dent Oral Epidemiol 2000; 34: 419–23.

568. STECKSÉN-BLICKS C et al. Dental health, dental care, and dietary habits in children in different parts of Sweden. Acta Odontol Scand 1985; 43: 59–67.

569. STECKSÉN-BLICKS C *et al*. Impact of oral hygiene and use of fluorides on caries increment in children during one year. Community Dent Oral Epidemiol 1986; 14: 185–9.

570. STECKSÉN-BLICKS C *et al*. Diagnosis of approximal caries in pre-school children. Swed Dent J 1983; 7: 179–84.

571. STEIN M *et al*. Zur Problematik der Kariesdiagnostik-vergleichende Untersuchungen des Röntgenbildes mit dem Zahnschliff. Stomatol DDR 1986; 36: 702–4.

572. STEINBERG D *et al*. Formulation, development and characterization of sustained release varnishes containing amine and stannous fluorides. Caries Res 2002; 36: 411–16.

573. STEINER M *et al*. Dental predictors of high caries increment in children. J Dent Res 1992; 71: 1926–33.

574. STEINER M *et al*. Effect of 1000 ppm relative to 250 ppm fluoride toothpaste. A meta-analysis. Am J Dent 2004; 17: 85–8.

575. STEINMETZ R *et al*. The xenoestrogen bisphenol A induces growth, differentiation, and *c-fos* gene expression in the female reproductive tract. Endocrinology 1998; 139: 2741–7.

576. STENLUND H *et al*. Caries rates related to approximal caries at ages 11–13: a 10-year follow-up study in Sweden. J Dent Res 2002; 81: 455–8.

577. STEPHENS RG *et al*. Information yield from routine bitewing radiographs for young adults. J Can Dent Assoc 1981; 47: 247–52.

578. STOOKEY GK *et al*. A critical review of the relative anti-caries efficacy of sodium fluoride and sodium monofluorophosphate dentifrices. Caries Res 1993; 27: 337–60.

579. STÖRTEBECKER P. Mercury poisoning from dental amalgam – a hazard to human brain. Stockholm: Störtebecker Foundation for Research, 1985.

580. STRAETEMANS MME *et al*. De nieuwe strijd tegen mutans streptokokken. Ned Tijdschr Tandheelkd 1997; 104: 370–2.

581. STRAETEMANS MM *et al*. Colonization with mutans streptococci and lactobacilli and the caries experience of children after the age of five. J Dent Res 1998; 77: 1851–5.

582. SUDDICK RP *et al*. Caries activity estimates and implications: insights into risk versus activity. J Dent Educ 1997; 61: 876–84.

583. SULLIVAN RJ *et al*. In vivo detection of calcium from dicalcium phosphate dihydrate dentifrices in demineralised human enamel and plaque. Adv Dent Res 1997; 11: 380–7.

584. SUNDSTRÖM F *et al*. Laser-induced fluorescence from sound and carious tooth substance: spectroscopic studies. Swed Dent J 1985; 9: 71–80.

585. SUTCLIFFE P. A longitudinal clinical study of oral cleanliness and dental caries in school children. Arch Oral Biol 1973; 18: 765–70.

586. SUZUKI N *et al*. Dental caries susceptibility in mice is closely linked to the H-2 region on chromosome 17. Caries Res 1998; 32: 262–5.

587. SWANLJUNG O *et al*. Caries and saliva in 12–18-year-old diabetics and controls. Scand J Dent Res 1992; 100: 310–13.

588. SYRJÄLÄ A-M *et al*. Metabolic control as a modifier of the association between salivary factors and dental caries among diabetic patients. Caries Res 2003; 37: 142–7.

589. TAHMASSEBI JF *et al*. Comparison of the plaque pH response to an acidogenic challenge in children and adults. Caries Res 1996; 30: 342–6.

590. TAHMASSEBI J *et al*. Effect of a calcium carbonate-based toothpaste with 0.3% triclosan on pH changes in dental plaque *in vivo*. Caries Res 1994; 28: 272–6.

591. TAIFOUR D *et al*. Effects of glass ionomer sealants in newly erupted first molars after 5 years: a pilot study. Community Dent Oral Epidemiol 2003; 31: 314–19.

592. TAIYM S *et al*. A comparison of the hormone levels in patients with Sjögren's syndrome and healthy controls. Oral Surg Oral Med Oral Pathol Oral Radiol Endod 2004; 97: 579–83.

593. TAN HH. Het project Abcoude. Thesis, University of Amsterdam, Amsterdam, 1981.

594. TAN PLB *et al*. Caries bitewings, and treatment decisions. Aust Dent J 2002; 47: 138–41.

595. TANAKA M *et al*. Release of mineral ions in dental plaque following acid production. Arch Oral Biol 1999; 44: 253–8.

596. TANNER ACR *et al*. The microbiota of young children from tooth and tongue samples. J Dent Res 2000; 81: 53–7.

597. TANZER JM. On changing the cariogenic chemistry of coronal plaque. J Dent Res 1989; 68 (spec. issue): 1576–87.

598. TANZER JM. Salivary and plaque microbiological tests and the management of dental caries. J Dent Educ 1997; 61: 866–75.

599. TEE JH. Some characteristics of 5-year-old children with a dmf of six or more in Gloucestershire, England. Community Dent Health 1987; 4: 121–8.

600. TEN CATE JM *et al*. Alternating demineralization and remineralization of artificial enamel lesions. Caries Res 1982; 16: 201–9.

601. TEN CATE JM *et al*. The influence of fluoride in solution on tooth enamel demineralization. I. Chemical data. Caries Res 1983; 17: 193–6.

602. TEN CATE JM *et al*. Mechanistic aspects of the interactions between fluoride and dental enamel. Crit Rev Oral Biol Med 1991; 2: 283–96.

603. TEN CATE JM *et al*. Speeksel, cariës en diagnostiek. Ned Tijdschr Tandheelkd 1992; 99: 85–8.

604. TENOVUO J *et al*. Serum and salivary antibodies against streptococcus mutans in young children with and without detectable oral *S. mutans*. Caries Res 1987; 21: 289–96.

605. THEILADE E *et al*. Effect of fissure sealing on the microflora in occlusal fissures of human teeth. Arch Oral Biol 1977; 22: 251–9.

606. TREVONEN T *et al*. Constant proportions of decayed teeth in adults aged 25, 35, 50 and 65 years in a high-caries area. Caries Res 1988; 22: 45–9.

607. THEUNS HM. The influence of *in-vitro* and *in-vivo* demineralizing conditions on dental enamel. Thesis, University of Nijmegen, Nijmegen, 1987.

608. THIBODEAU EA et al. Salivary mutans streptococci and incidence of caries in preschool children. Caries Res 1995; 29: 148–53.

609. THOMSON ME et al. In vitro and intra-oral investigations into cariogenic potential of human milk. Caries Res 1996; 30: 434–8.

610. THORSTENSSON H et al. Some salivary factors in insulin-dependent diabetics. Acta Odontol Scand 1989; 47: 175–83.

611. THYLSTRUP A et al. (eds) Textbook of cariology. Copenhagen: Munksgaard, 1986.

612. THYLSTRUP A et al. (eds) Textbook of clinical cariology. Copenhagen: Munksgaard, 1994.

613. TOUYZ LZG et al. Anticariogenic effects of black tea (Camellia sinensis) in caries prone-rats. Quint Int 2001; 32: 647–50.

614. TRUIN GJ et al. Caries prevalence and gingivitis in 5-, 7-, and 10-year-old schoolchildren in The Hague between 1969–1984. Caries Res 1986; 20: 131–40.

615. TRUIN GJ et al. Caries prevalence amongst schoolchildren in the Hague between 1969 and 1993. Caries Res 1994; 28: 176–80.

616. TRUIN GJ et al. Cariësprevalentie bij de Haagse jeugd. Nemen de verschillen in gebitsgezondheid toe? Ned Tijdschr Tandheelkd 1999; 106: 362–9.

617. TRUIN GJ et al. Time trends in caries experience of 6- and 12-year-old children of different socioeconomic status in the Hague. Caries Res 1998; 32: 1–4.

618. TSENG CC et al. The periodontal status of patients with Sjögren's disease. J Clin Periodontol 1990; 17: 329–30.

619. TUCKER GJ et al. The relationship between oral hygiene and dental caries incidence in 11-year-old children. A 3-year study. Br Dent J 1976; 141: 75–9.

620. TUUTTI H et al. Comparison of dental caries experience of the parents of caries-free and caries-active children. J Paediatr Dent 1989; 5: 93–8.

621. TVEIT AB et al. Vertical angulation of the X-ray beam and radiographic diagnosis of secondary caries. Community Dent Oral Epidemiol 1991; 19: 333–5.

622. TWETMAN S et al. Effect of different chlorhexidine varnish regimens on mutans streptococci levels in interdental plaque en saliva. Caries Res 1997; 31: 189–93.

623. TWETMAN S et al. Efficacy of a chlorhexidine and a chlorhexidine-fluoride varnish mixture to decrease interdental levels of mutans streptococci. Caries Res 1997; 31: 361–5.

624. TWETMAN S et al. Comparison of the efficacy of three different chlorhexidine preparations in decreasing the levels of mutans streptococci in saliva and interdental plaque. Caries Res 1998; 32: 113–18.

625. TWETMAN S. Antimicrobials in future caries control. Caries Res 2004; 38: 223–9.

626. USDHHS, PHS. Dental amalgam: a scientific review and recommended public health service strategy for research, education and regulation. Washington, DC: USDHHS, PHS, 1993.

627. VAARKAMP J et al. Wavelength-dependent fibre-optic transillumination of small approximal caies lesions: the use of a dye, and a comparison to bitewing radiography. Caries Res 1997; 31: 232–7.

628. VACCA-SMITH AM et al. The effect of milk and kappa casein on streptococcal glucosyltransferase. Caries Res 1995; 29: 498–506.

629. VACHIRAROJPISAN T et al. Early childhood caries in children aged 6–19 months. Community Dent Oral Epidemiol 2004; 32: 133–42.

630. VALACHOVIC RW et al. Examiner reliability in dental radiography. J Dent Res 1986; 65: 432–6.

631. VAN AMERONGEN JP et al. Caries diagnosis in molars with discoloured fissuren by FOTI and visual inspection. Caries Res 1994; 28: 191–2.

632. VAN AMERONGEN JP et al. Validity of caries diagnosis in molars with discolored fissures by radiography. J Dent Res 1993; 72: 344.

633. VAN AMERONGEN JP et al. Accuracy of Erbium: Yag laser for the detection of occlusal caries. Caries Res 2000; 34: 327.

634. VAN AMERONGEN JP et al. Caries activity of radiopacities under amalgam restorations on bite-wing radiographs? Caries Res 1997; 31: 325.

635. VANDERAS AP et al. Urinary catecholamine levels in children with and without dental caries. J Dent Res 1995; 74: 1671–8.

636. VAN DER HOEVEN JS et al. De microbiologie van de mond. Zeist: NIB, 1986.

637. VAN DER HOEVEN JS et al. Streptococci and actinomyces inhibit regrowth of Streptococcus mutans on gnotobiotic rat molar teeth after chlorhexidine varnish treatment. Caries Res 1995; 29: 159–62.

638. VAN LOVEREN C. Evidence-based cariology. Ned Tijdschr Tandheelkd 2003; 110: 357.

639. VAN LOVEREN C. Sugar alcohols: what is the evidence for caries-preventive and caries-therapeutic effects? Caries Res 2004; 38: 286–93.

640. VAN LOVEREN C et al. Incidence of mutans streptococci and lactobacilli in oral cleft children wearing acrylic plates from shortly after birth. Oral Microbiol Immunol 1998; 13: 286–91.

641. VAN LOVEREN C et al. Plaque composition, fluoride tolerance and acid production of mutans streptococci before and after the suspension of the use of fluoride toothpastes. Caries Res 1995; 29: 442–8.

642. VAN LOVEREN C et al. Protection of bovine enamel and dentine by chlorhexidine and fluoride varnishes in a bacterial demineralization model. Caries Res 1996; 30: 45–51.

643. VAN LUIJK AM. Mondspoelmiddelen en tandpasta's. Ned Tijdschr Tandheelkd 1992; 99: 472–3.

644. VAN NIEUW AMERONGEN A et al. Salivary proteins: protective and diagnostic value in cariology. Caries Res 2004; 38: 247–53.

645. VAN PALENSTEIN HELDERMAN WH. Kwaliteitscontrole van tandpasta in Nederland. Ned Tandartsenbl 2004; 59 (4): 20–2.

646. VAN PALENSTEIN HELDERMAN WH et al. Cariogenicity depends more on diet than the prevailing mutans streptococcal species. J Dent Res 1996; 75: 535–45.

647. VAN PALENSTEIN HELDERMAN WH et al. Validation of a Swis method of caries prediction in Dutch children. Community Dent Oral Epidemiol 2001; 29: 341–5.

648. VAN RIJKOM HM *et al.* A meta-analysis of clinical studies on the caries–inhibiting effect of fluoride gel treatment. Caries Res 1998; 32: 83–92.

649. VAN STRIJP AJP. Bacterial colonization and degradation of dentine. Thesis, University of Amsterdam, Amsterdam, 1996.

650. VAN STRIJP AJP *et al.* Host-derived proteinases and degradation of dentine collagen in situ. Caries Res 2003; 37: 58–65.

651. VAN STRIJP AJP *et al.* The effects of chlorhexidine on the bacterial colonization and degradation of dentine and completely demineralised dentine in situ. Eur J Oral Sci 1997; 105: 27–36.

652. VARRELA TM *et al.*The prevalence and distribution of dental caries in a medieval Finnish population. Budapest: ORCA, 1987.

653. VEHKALAHTI M *et al.* Remaining teeth in Finnish adults related to the frequency of tooth-brushing. Acta Odontol Scand 1989; 47: 375–81.

654. VERDONSCHOT EH *et al.* The in vivo performance of laser fluorescence device compared to visual inspection in occlusal caries diagnosis. Caries Res 1999; 33: 151–8.

655. VERDONSCHOT EH *et al.* Performance of some diagnostic systems in examinations for small occlusal carious lesions. Caries Res 1992; 26: 59–64.

656. VILLA AE, GUERRERO S. Caries experience and fluorosis prevalence in Chilean children from different socioeconomic status. Community Dent Oral Epidemiol 1996; 24: 225–7.

657. VISSER JB. Tandheelkundige behandeling van alcoholisten. Enkele notities uit de literatuur. Ned Tijdschr Tandheelkd 1989; 96: 352–5.

658. VISSER RSH *et al.* Landelijk Epidemiologisch Onderzoek Tandheelkunde. Deel XIII. Voeding. Ned Tijdschr Tandheelkd 1989; 97: 350–3.

659. VISSINK A *et al.* De droge mond. De mogelijk oorzakelijke rol van geneesmiddelen. Ned Tijdschr Tandheelkd 1992; 99: 103–12.

660. VISSINK A *et al.* Het syndroom van Sjögren. Gevolgen voor de mondgezondheid. Ned Tijdschr Tandheelkd 1997; 104: 458–62.

661. VISSINK A *et al.* Oorzaak, gevolg en behandeling van hyposialie. Ned Tijdschr Tandheelkd 1992; 99: 92–6.

662. VON DER FEHR F. Epidemiology of dental caries. In: THYLSTRUP A *et al.* (eds) Textbook of cariology. Copenhagen: Munksgaard, 1986.

663. VON DER FEHR F *et al.* Caries-preventive fluoride dentifrices. Caries Res 1978; 12 (suppl 1): 31–7.

664. VOM SAAL FS *et al.* A physiologically based approach to the study of Bisphenol A and other estrogenic chemicals on the size of reproductive organs, daily sperm production and behaviour. Toxicol Ind Health 1998; 14: 239–60.

665. VOM SAAL FS *et al.* Prostate enlargement in mice due to fetal expsure to low doses of estradiol or diethylstillbestrol and opposite effects at high doses. Proc Natl Acad Sci 1997; 94: 2056–61.

666. VRBIC V. Retention of a fluoride-containing sealant on primary and permanent teeth 3 years after placement. Quint Int 1999; 30: 825–8.

667. VRBIC V *et al.* Trace element content of primary and permanent tooth enamel. Caries Res 1987; 21: 37–9.

668. WADA H *et al.* In vitro estrogenicity of resin composites. J Dent Res 2004; 83: 222–6.

669. WALKER BN *et al.* Enamel cracks. The role of enamel lammelae in caries initiation. Aust Dent J 1998; 43: 110–16.

670. WALKER JD *et al.* Phenylketonuria and dentistry. J Dent Child 1982; 49: 280–4.

671. WARREN DP *et al.* Topical fluorides: efficacy, administration, and safety. Gen Dent 1997; 45: 134–42.

672. WARREN JJ *et al.* Current and future role of fluoride in nutrition. Dent Clin North Am 2003; 47: 225–43.

673. WEERHEIJM KL. Cariësdiagnostiek en de beoordeling van het cariësrisico. Ned Tijdschr Tandheelkd 1995; 102: 392–4.

674. WEERHEIJM KL *et al.* Prevalence of hidden caries. J Dent Child 1992; 59: 408–12.

675. WEERHEIJM KL *et al.* The effect of fluoridation on the occurrence of hidden caries in clinically sound occlusal surfaces. Caries Res 1997; 31: 30–4.

676. WEERHEIJM KL *et al.* Prolonged demand breast-feeding and nursing caries. Caries Res 1998; 32: 46–50.

677. WEIGER R *et al.* Effect of chlorhexidine-containing varnish (Cervitec[R]) on microbial vitality and accumulation of supragingival dental plaque in humans. Caries Res 1994; 28: 267–71.

678. WEINTRAUB JA. Fluoride varnish for caries prevention: comparison with other preventive agents and recommendations for a community-based protocol. Spec Care Dent 2003; 23: 180–6.

679. WENNERHOLM K *et al.* Effects of sugar restriction on *Streptococcus mutans* and *Streptococcus sobrinus* in saliva and dental plaque. Caries Res 1995; 29: 54–61.

680. WENZEL A *et al.* Accuracy of visual inspection, fiber-optic transillumination and various radiographic image modalities for the detection of occlusal caries in extracted non-cavitated teeth. J Dent Res 1992; 71: 1934–7.

681. WENZEL A. Diagnosis of dental caries and treatment decision in children and adolescents. Ned Tijdschr Tandheelkd 2002; 109: 60.

682. WESTMAAS-JES MM *et al.* De gebitstoestand bij 6- en 12-jarige kinderen in noord-oost-Friesland. Ned Tijdschr Tandheelkd 1985; 92: 22–8.

683. WIKTORSSON AM *et al.* Caries prevalence among adults in communities with optimal and low fluoride concentrations. Community Dent Oral Epidemiol 1992; 20: 359–63.

684. WILSON NHF *et al.* Reasons for placement and replacement of restorations of direct restorative materials by a selected group of practitioners in the United Kingdom. Quint Int 1997; 28: 245–8.

685. WOODWARD SM *et al.* School milk as a vehicle for fluoride in the United Kingdom. An interim report. Community Dent Health 2001; 18: 150–6.

686. WORLD HEALTH ORGANIZATION. Fluoride and oral health. Technical report 846. Geneva: World Health Organization, 1994.

687. WORLD HEALTH ORGANIZATION. Environmental health criteria 118. Inorganic mercury. Geneva: World Health Organization, 1991.

688. WRIGHT WE *et al*. An oral disease prevention program for patients receiving radiation and chemotherapy. J Am Dent Assoc 1985; 110: 43–7.

689. WYNE A *et al*. The prevalence and pattern of nursing caries in Saudi preschool children. Int J Paediatr Dent 2001; 11: 361–4.

690. WYNN RL. Fluoride: after 50 years, a clearer picture of its mechanism. Gen Dent 2002; 50: 118–26.

691. YANAGIDA A *et al*. Inhibitory effects of apple polyphenols and related compounds on cariogenic factors of mutans streptococci. J Agric Food Chem 2000; 48: 5666–71.

692. YANOVER LR. Root surface caries. Epidemiology, etiology and control. J Can Dent Assoc 1987; 53: 839–42.

693. YEE R *et al*. Caries experience of 5–6-year-old and 12–13-year-old schoolchildren in central and western Nepal. Int Dent J 2002; 52: 453–60.

694. YIP HK *et al*. Glass ionomer cements used as fissure sealants with the atraumatic restorative (ART) approach: review of literature. Int Dent J 2002; 52: 67–70.

695. YIP HK *et al*. The specificity of caries detector dyes in cavity preparation. Br Dent J 1994; 176; 417–21.

696. ZACHARIA MA *et al*. Microbiological assessment of dentin stained with a caries detector dye. J Clin Pediatr Dent 1995; 19: 111–15.

697. ZACHARIASEN RD. Diabetes mellitus and xerostomia. Compend Contin Educ 1992; 13: 314–24.

698. ZAMIR T *et al*. A longitudinal radiographic study of the rate of spread of human approximal dental caries. Arch Oral Biol 1976; 21: 523–6.

699. ZAURA E. Plaque stagnation sites and dental caries. Thesis, University of Amsterdam, Amsterdam, 2002.

700. ZDANOWICZ JA *et al*. Inhibitory effect of barium on caries formation in rats. Caries Res 1989; 23: 65–9.

701. ZIFF S. Silver dental fillings. The toxic time bomb. New York: Aurora Press, 1984.

702. ZUCKERBRAUN HL *et al*. Triclosan: cytotoxicity, mode of action, and induction of apoptosis in human gingival cell *in vitro*. Eur J Oral Sci 1998; 106: 628–36.

703. CHAMBERS MS *et al*. Clinical evaluation of the intraoral fluoreide releasing system in radiation-induced xerostomic patients. Part 1: fluorides. Oral Oncol 2006; 42: 934–45.

704. WILLUMSEN T *et al*. Stannous fluoride in dentifrice: an effective anti-plaque agent in elderly? Geropdontology 2007; 24: 239–43.

705. HICKS J *et al*. Role of remineralizing fluid in in vitro enamel caries formation and progresion. Quint Int 2007; 38: 313–19.

706. CASALS E *et al*. Anticaries potential of commercial dentifrices as determined by fluoridation and remineralization efficiency. J Contemp Dent Pract 2007; 8 (7): 1–19.

707. ITTHAGARUN A *et al*. Effects of child formula dentifrices on artificial caries like lesions using in vitro pH cycling. Int Dent J 2007; 57: 307–13.

708. AMERICAN DENTAL ASSOCIATION COUNCIL ON SCIENTIFIC AFFAIRS. Professionally applied topical fluoride. J Dent Educ 2007; 71: 393–402.

709. WYATT CCL *et al*. Chlorhexidine and preservation of sound tooth structure in older adults. Caries Res 2007; 41: 93–101.

710. GERARDU VAM *et al*. The effect of a single application of 40% chlorhexidine varnish on the numbers of salivary mutans streptococci and acidogenicity of dental plaque. Caries Res 2003; 37: 369–73.

711. DU MQ *et al*. A two year randomized clinical trial of chlorhexidine varnish on dental caries in Chinese preschool children. J Dent Res 2006: 85: 557–9.

712. VAN STRYDONCK DA *et al*. Chlorhexidine mouthrinse in combination with an SLS-containing dentifrice and a dentifrice slurry. J Clin Periodontol 2006; 33: 340–4.

713. HOLGERSON PL *et al*. Dental plaque formation and salivary mutans streptococci in school children after use of xylitol-containg chewing gum. Int J Paediatr Dent 2007; 17: 79–85.

714. OSCARSON P *et al*. Influence of a low xylitol-dose on mutans streptococci colonisation and caries development in preschool children. Eur Arch Paediatr Dent 2006; 7: 142–7.

715. AHOVUO-SALORANTA A *et al*. Pit and fissure sealants for preventing dental decay in the permanent teeth of children and adolescents. Cochrane Database Syst Rev 2008; (4): CD001830.

716. GANESH M *et al*. Comparative evaluation of the marginal sealing ability of Fuji VII and Concise as pit and fissure sealants. J Contemp Dent Pract 2007; 8 (4): 10–18.

717. MULLER-BOLLA M. Rtention of resin-based oit and fissure selants. Community Dent Oral Epidemiol 2006; 34: 321–36.

718. DUKIC W. Clinical evaluation of three fissure sealants: 24 month follow-up. Eur Arch Paediatr Dent 2007; 8: 163–6.

719. DÄHNHARDT JE *et al*. Treating open carious lesions in anxious children with ozone. Am J Dent 2006; 19: 267–70.

720. LENNON AM *et al*. Quantity of remaining bacteria and cavity size after ecxcavation with face, caries detector and conventional excavation in vitro. Oper Dent 2007; 32: 236–41.

721. INGLEHART MR *et al*. Chemomechanical caries removal in children. J Am Dent Assoc 2007; 138: 47–55.

722. SASAKI N *et al*. Salivary bisphenol-A levels detected by ELISA after restoration with composite resin. Mat Med 2005; 16: 297–300.

723. AIDA J *et al*. Reasons for permanent tooth extractions in Japan. J Epidemiol 2006; 16: 214–19.

724. SCIENTIFIC COMMITTEE ON EEMERGING AND NEWLY IDENTIFIED HEALTH RISKS (SCENHIR). The safety of dental amalgam and alternativ dental restoration materials for patients and users. European Commission: Health & Consumer Protection, 2007.

725. GRUYTHUYSEN G. Niet-restauratieve caviteitsbehandeling. Ned Tijdschr Tandheelkd 2010; 117: 173–80.

726. SCHUURS AHB *et al*. Oplosmiddelen ter verwijdering van guttapercha uti wortelkanalen. 2. Nevenwerkingen van chloroform, halaothaan en xyleen. Ned Tijdschr Tandheelkd 2004; 111: 303–6.

Chapter 6: Erosion

1. ABRAMS RA *et al*. Oral signs and symptoms in the diagnosis of bulimia. J Am Dent Assoc 1986; 113: 761–4.

2. ABSI EG *et al*. Dentine hypersensitivity. A study of the patency of dentinal tubules in sensitive and non-sensitive cervical dentine. J Clin Periodontol 1987; 14: 280–4.

3. ADDY M *et al*. Can tooth brushing damage your health? Effects on oral and dental tissues. Int Dent J 2003; 53: 177–86.

4. AESCHBACHER M. Die Erweichung der Schmelzoberfläche durch Fruchtsäfte unter *in-vitro* Bedingungen. Schweiz Monatsschr Zahnheilkd 1967; 77: 58–62.

5. AL-DLAIGAN YH *et al*. Dental erosion in a group of British 14-year-old school children. Part 1. Br Dent J 2001; 190: 152–7.

6. AL-DLAIGAN YH *et al*. Dental erosion in a group of British 14-year-old school children. Part 2. Br Dent J 2001; 190: 258–61.

7. AL-DLAIGAN YH *et al*. Is there a relationship between asthma and dental erosion? Int J Paediatr Dent 2002; 12: 189–200.

8. ALLAN DN. Enamel erosion with lemon juice. Br Dent J 1967; 122: 300–2.

9. ALLAN DN. Dental erosion from vomiting. Br Dent J 1969; 126; 311–12.

10. AMAECHI BT *et al*. Thickness of acquired salivary pellicle as a determinant of the sites of dental erosion. J Dent Res 1999; 78: 1821–8.

11. AMIN WM *et al*. Oral health status of workers exposed to acid fumes in phosphate and battery industries in Jordan. Int Dent J 2001; 51: 169–74.

12. ANDREWS FFH. Dental erosion due to anorexia nervosa with bulimia. Br Dent J 1982; 152: 89–90.

13. ARAUJO MW *et al*. Oral and dental health among patients in treatment for alcohol use disorders. J Int Acad Periodontol 2004; 6: 125–30.

14. ASHER C *et al*. Early enamel erosion in children associated with the excessive consumption of citric acid. Br Dent J 1987; 162: 384–7.

15. ATTIN T *et al*. Beeinflussung des erosionsbedingten oberflächenhärteverlust von zahnschmelz durch fluorid. Dtsch Zahnärztl Z 1997; 52: 241–5.

16. ATTIN T *et al*. In vitro evaluation of different remineralisation periods in improving the resistance of previously eroded bovine dentine against tooth-brushing abrasion. Arch Oral Biol 2001; 46: 871–4.

17. ATTIN T *et al*. Effect of mineral supplements to citric acid on enamel erosion. Arch Oral Biol 2003; 48: 753–9.

18. ATTIN T *et al*. Brushing abrasion of eroded dentin after application of sodium fluoride solutions. Caries Res 1998; 32: 344–50.

19. AZZOPARDI A *et al*. The surface effects of erosion and abrasion on dentine with and without a protective layer. Br Dent J 2004; 196: 351–4.

20. BANFIELD N *et al*. Dentine hypersensitivity: development and evaluation of a model in situ to study tubule patency. J Clin Periodontol 2004; 31: 325–35.

21. BARBAKOW F *et al*. A critical comparison of dentifrice abrasion scores on dentine recorded by gravimetric and radiotracer methods. J Dent 1992; 20: 283–6

22. BARBOUR ME *et al*. Enamel dissolution in citric acid as a function of calcium and phosphate concentrations and degree of saturation with respect to hydroxyapatite. Eur J Oral Sci 2003; 111: 428–33.

23. BARBOUR ME *et al*. The laboratory assessment of enamel erosion. J Dent 2004; 32: 591–602.

24. BARTLETT DW *et al*. The prevalence of tooth wear in a cluster sample of adolescent schoolchildren and its relationship with potential explanatory factors. Br Dent J 1998; 184: 125–9.

25. BARTLETT DW *et al*. Oral regurgitation after reflux provoking meals: a possible cause of dental erosion? J Oral Rehabil 1997; 24: 102–8.

26. BARTLETT DW *et al*. A study of the association between gastro-oesophageal reflux and palatal dental erosion. Br Dent J 1996; 181: 125–32.

27. BASHIR E *et al*. Effect of citric acid clearance on the saturation with respect to hydroxyapatite in saliva. Caries Res 1996; 30: 213–17.

28. BERNAU R. Zur Erosion der Zahnhartsubstanzen. Schweiz Monatsschr Zahnmed 1970; 80: 906–13.

29. BEVENIUS J *et al*. Erosion: guidelines for the general practitioner. Aust Dent J 1988; 33: 407–11.

30. BHATTI SA *et al*. Ethanol and pH levels of proprietary mouthrinses. Community Dent Health 1994; 11: 71–4.

31. BICKEL M *et al*. The pH of human crevicular fluid measured by a new microanalytical technique. J Periodontol Res 1985; 20: 35–40.

32. BIRKHED D. Sugar content, acidity and effect of plaque pH of fruit juices, fruit drinks, carbonated beverages and sport drinks. Caries Res 1984; 18: 120–7.

33. BISHOP K *et al*. Dental erosion as a consequence of voluntary regurgitation in a jockey. Br Dent J 1996; 181: 343–5.

34. BLANKSMA CJ *et al*. Effecten van cocaïnegebruik op de mondgezondheid en de implicaties voor tandheelkundige behandelingen. Ned Tijdschr Tandheelkd 2004; 111: 486–9.

35. BLUME A *et al*. Untersuchungen zur Zahngesundheit asthmakranker Kinder und Jugendlichen. Deutsch Zahnärtzl Zeitschr 2002; 57: 644–9.

36. BÖHMER C. Gastro-oesopahgeal reflux disease in intellectually disabled individuals. Thesis, Vrije Universiteit, Amsterdam, 1996.

37. BRADY JM *et al*. Scanning microscopy of cervical erosion. J Am Dent Assoc 1977; 94: 726–9.

38. BRADY WF. The anorexia nervosa syndrome. Oral Surg 1980; 50: 509–16.

39. BRÄNNSTRÖM M. The elicitation of pain in human dentine and pulp by chemical stimuli. Arch Oral Biol 1962; 7: 59–62.

40. BRÄNSTRÖM M *et al*. A study on the mechanism of pain elicited from the dentin. J Dent Res 1964; 43: 619–25.

41. BRÄNSTRÖM M *et al*. Movements of the dentine and pulp liquids on application of thermal stimuli. Acta Odontol Scand 1970; 28: 59–70.

42. BRÄNSTRÖM M. Etiology of dentin hypersensitivity. Proc Finn Dent Soc 1992; 88 (suppl 1): 7–13.

43. BRODY AG *et al*. Erosionlike denture markings possibly related to hyperactivity of oral soft tissues. J Am Dent Assoc 1974; 88: 1012–17.

44. BRUGGEN TEN CATE HJ. Dental erosion in industry. Br J Ind Med 1968; 25: 249–66.
45. BÜHLMANN H. Anorexie and Bulimie. Schweiz Monatsschr Zahnheilkd 1993; 103: 1451–6.
46. BURKE FJT et al. Bulimia: implications for the practising dentist. Br Dent J 1996; 180: 421–6.
47. BURNETT GW. Dental caries. In: BURNETT GW et al. (eds) Oral microbiology and infection disease. Baltimore, MD: Lippincott Williams & Wilkins, 1976.
48. BYERS M et al. Sensory innervation of pulp and dentin in adult dog teeth as demonstrated by autoradiography. Anat Rec 1987; 218: 207–15.
49. CAIRNS AM et al. The pH and titratable acidity of a range of diluting drinks and their potential effect on dental erosion. J Dent 2002; 30: 313–17.
50. CALAMIA JR et al. Effect of amalgam bond on cervical sensitivity. Am J Dent 1996; 8: 283–4.
51. CAMPS J et al. In vivo sensitivity of human root dentin to air blast and scratching. J Periodontol 2003; 74: 1589–94.
52. CAMPS J et al. Effects of desensitizing agents on human dentin permeability. Am J Dent 1998; 11: 286–90.
53. CANADIAN ADVISORY BOARD ON DENTIN HYPERSENSITIVITY. Consensus-based recommendations for the diagnosis and management of dentin hypersensitivity. J Can Dent Assoc 2003; 69: 221–6.
54. CENTERWALL BS et al. Erosion of dental enamel among competitive swimmers at a gas-chlorinated swimming pool. Am J Epidemiol 1986; 123: 641–7.
55. CHABANSKI MB et al. Clinical evaluation of cervical dentine sensitivity in a population of patients referred to a specialist periodontology department. J Oral Rehabil 1997; 24: 666–72.
56. CHAUDRY SI et al. Dental erosion in a wine merchant: an occupational hazard? Br Dent J 1997; 182: 226–8.
57. CHERNG AM et al. Reduction in dentin permeability using mildly supersaturated calcium phosphate solutions. Arch Oral Biol 2004; 49: 91–8.
58. CIARAMICOLI MT et al. Treatment of cervical dentin hypersensitivity using neodymium: Yttrium-aliminum-garnet laser. Lasers Surg Med 2003; 33: 358–62.
59. CLARK CS et al. Gastroesophageal reflux induced by exercise in healthy volunteers. J Am Med Assoc 1989; 261: 3599–601.
60. CLARK DC. Oral complications of anorexia nervosa and/or bulimia: with a review of the literature. J Oral Med 1985; 40: 134–8.
61. COLEMAN TA et al. Cervical dentin hypersensitivity. Part III: resolution following occlusal equilibration. Quint Int 2003; 427–34.
62. COLLINGS KL et al. Esophageal reflux in conditioned runners, cyclists, and weightlifters. Med Sci Sport Exerc 2003; 35: 730–5.
63. DANNENBERG JL. Vitamin C enamel loss. J Am Dent Assoc 1982; 105: 172–4.
64. DAVIS WB et al. Dietary erosion of adult dentine and enamel. Br Dent J 1977; 143: 116–19.
65. DAVIS WB et al. The effect of abrasion on enamel and dentine after exposure to dietary acid. Br Dent J 1980; 148: 253–6.
66. DE LAS CASAS E et al. Abfraction and anisotropy – effects of prism orientation on stress distribution. Comput Methods Biomech Biomed Egin 2003; 6: 65–73.
67. DE MAGALHAES MF et al. A morphological study of the effects of Nd: YAG laser on irradiated dentin. Photomed Laser Surg 2004; 22: 527–32.
68. DONDI DALL'OROLOGIO G et al. Desensitizing effects of Gluma and Gluma 2000 on hypersensitive dentin. Am J Dent 1993; 6: 283–6.
69. DIJKMAN GEHM et al. Closing of dentinal tubules by glutaraldehyde treatment, a scanning electron microscopic study. Scand J Dent Res 1994; 102: 144–50.
70. DUGMORE CR et al. The prevalence of tooth erosion in 12-year-old children. Br Dent J 2004; 196: 279–82.
71. DURAN I et al. The long-term effectiveness of five current desensitizing products on cervical dentine hypersensitivity. J Oral Rehabil 2004; 31: 351–6.
72. DUXBURY AJ. Ectasty – Dental implications. Br Dent J 1993; 175: 38.
73. ECCLES JD. Dental erosion of nonindustrial origin. J Prosthet Dent 1979; 42: 649–53.
74. ECCLES JD. Erosion affecting the palatal surfaces of upper anterior teeth in young people. Br Dent J 1982; 152: 375–8.
75. ECCLES JD. Tooth surface loss from abrasion, attrition, and erosion. Dent Update 1982; 9: 373–81.
76. ECCLES JD et al. Dental erosion and diet. J Dent 1974; 2: 153–9.
77. EDWARDS M et al. A videofluoroscopic comparison of straw and cup drinking: the potential influence on dental erosion. Br Dent J 1998; 185: 244–9.
78. EDWARDS M et al. Buffering capacities of soft drinks: the potential influence on dental erosion. J Oral Rehabil 1999; 26: 923–7.
79. EISENBURGER M et al. Erosion and attrition of human enamel in vitro. Part I. J Dent 2002; 30: 349–52.
80. EISENBURGER M et al. The use of ultrasonication to study remineralisation of eroded enamel. Caries Res 2001; 35: 61–6.
81. EISENBURGER M et al. Comparative study of wear of enamel induced by alternating and simultaneous combinations of abrasion and erosion in vitro. Caries Res 2003; 37: 450–5.
82. ELLIS LN. Influence of dietary calcium upon composition of mineralized tissues and upon susceptibility of enamel to erosion in vivo. J Dent Res 1963; 42: 973–80.
83. ELSBURY WB. Hydrogen-ion concentration and acid erosion of the teeth. Br Dent J 1952; 92: 177–9.
84. ERICSSON Y. Investigations on the occurrence and significance of citric acid in the saliva. J Dent Res 1953; 32: 850–8.
85. ERICSSON SY. Chemical action of external fluids on enamel. J Dent Res 1960; 39: 1083–4.
86. FINCH LD. Erosion associated with diabetes insipidus. Br Dent J 1957; 103: 280–2.
87. FERRARI M et al. Clinical evaluation of a one-bottle bonding system for desensitizing exposed roots. Am J Dent 1999; 12: 243–9.

88. FISSCHER C *et al*. Prevalence and distribution of cervical hypersensitivity in a population in Rio de Janeiro. J Dent 1992; 20: 272–6.

89. FULLER JL *et al*. Citric acid consumption and the human dentition. J Am Dent Assoc 1977; 95: 80–4.

90. GABAI Y *et al*. Effect of pH levels in swimming pools on enamel of human teeth. Am J Dent 1988; 1: 241–3.

91. GAGARI E *et al*. Adverse effects of mouthwash use. A review. Oral Surg Oral Med Oral Pathol Radiol Endod 1995; 80: 432–9.

92. GALLO LG *et al*. Chronic vomiting and the effect on the primary dentition. ASDC J Dent Child 1981; 48: 382–3.

93. GANSS C *et al*. Effects of two fluoridation measures on erosion progression in human enamel and dentine in situ. Caries Res 2004; 38: 561–6.

94. GANSS C *et al*. Quantitative analysis of the impact of the organic matrix on the fluoride effect on erosion progression in human dentine using longitudinal microradiography. Arch Oral Biol 2004; 49: 931–5.

95. GANSS C *et al*. Characteristics of tooth wear in relation to different nutritional patterns including contemporary and medieval subjects. Eur J Oral Sci 2002; 110: 54–60.

96. GANSS C *et al*. Effectiveness of two fluoridation measures on erosion progression in human enamel and dentin in vitro. Caries Res 2001; 35: 325–30.

97. GEDALIA I *et al*. Tooth enamel softening with a cola type drink and rehardening with hard cheese or stimulated saliva *in situ*. J Oral Rehabil 1991; 18: 501–6.

98. GEDALIA I *et al*. Enamel softening with Coca-Cola and rehardening with milk or saliva. Am J Dent 1991; 4: 120–2.

99. GEDALIA I *et al*. Effect of hard cheese exposure, with and without fluoride prerinse, on the rehardening of softened human enamel. Caries Res 1992; 26: 290–2.

100. GEERLINGS G *et al*. Het dentine. Ned Tijdschr Tandheelkd 1987; 94: 13–18.

101. GEIGER S *et al*. The clinical effect of amorphous calcium phosphate (ACP) on root surface hypersensitivity. Oper Dent 2003; 28: 496–500.

102. GELSKEY SC *et al*. The effectiveness of the Nd: YAG laser in the treatment of dental hypersensitivity. J Can Dent Assoc 1993; 59: 377–86.

103. GILLAM DG *et al*. Dentifrice abrasivity and cervical dentinal hypersensitivity. results 12 weeks following cessation of 8 weeks' supervised use. J Periodontol 1992; 63: 7–12.

104. GILLAM DG *et al*. Perceptions of dentine hypersensitivity in a general practice population. J Oral Rehabil 1999; 26: 710–14.

105. GRACE EG *et al*. Tooth erosion caused by chewing aspirin. J Am Dent Assoc 2004; 135: 911–14.

106. GRAEHN G. Säureerosion der Zahnhartsubstanzen. 1. Dtsch Stomatol 1991; 41: 494–9.

107. GRAEHN G. Säureerosion der Zahnhartsubstanzen. 3. Dtsch Stomatol 1991; 41: 505–7.

108. GRAEHN G *et al*. Säureerosion der Zahnhartsubstanzen. 2. Dtsch Stomatol 1991; 41: 500–4.

109. GRANDO LJ *et al*. *In vitro* study of enamel erosion caused by soft drinks and lemon juice in deciduous teeth analysed by stereomicroscopy and scanning electron microscopy. Caries Res 1996; 30: 373–8.

110. GRAY A *et al*. Wine tasting and dental erosion. Aust Dent J 1998; 43: 32–4.

111. GREENHILL JD *et al*. The effects of desensitizing agents on the hydraulic conductance of human dentin in vitro. J Dent Res 1981; 60: 686–98.

112. GREGG T *et al*. A study in vitro on the abrasive effect of the tongue on enamel and dentine softened by acid erosion. Caries Res 2004; 38: 557–60.

113. GREGORY-HEAD BL *et al*. Evaluation of dental erosion in patients with gastroesophageal reflux disease. J Prosthet Dent 2000; 83: 675–80.

114. GRENBY TH. Methods of assessing erosion and erosive potential. Eur J Oral Sci 1996; 104: 207–14.

115. GRENBY TH. Lessening dental erosive potential by product modification. Eur J Oral Sci 1996; 104: 221–8.

116. GRIPPO JO *et al*. Dental "erosion" revisited. J Am Dent Assoc 1995; 126: 619–30.

117. GRIPPO JO *et al*. Attrition, abrasion, corrosion and abfraction revisited. J Am Dent Assoc 2004; 135: 1109–18.

118. GROBLER SR *et al*. The effects of the composition and method of drinking of soft drinks on plaque pH. Br Dent J 1985; 158: 293–6.

119. GROBLER SR *et al*. The degree of enamel erosion by five different kinds of fruit. Clin Prev Dent 1989; 11 (5): 23–8.

120. GUDMUNDSSON K *et al*. Tooth erosion, gastroesophageal reflux, and salivary buffer capacity. Oral Surg Oral Med Oral Pathol Oral Radiol Endod 1995; 79: 185–9.

121. GÜRGAN S *et al*. *In vitro* effects of alcohol-containing and alcohol-free mouthrinses on microhardness of some restorative materials. J Oral Rehabil 1997; 24: 244–6.

122. GWINNETT AJ. Histologic changes in human enamel following treatment with acidic adhesive conditioning agents. Arch Oral Biol 1971; 16: 731–8.

123. HALL AF *et al*. The effect of saliva on enamel and dentin erosion. J Dent 1999; 27: 333–9.

124. HAMMADEH MN *et al*. The erosive susceptibility of cervical versus occlusal enamel. Eur J Prosthodont Restor Dent 2001; 9: 13–17.

125. HANNIG M *et al*. Influence of in vivo formed salivary pellicle on enamel erosion. Caries Res 1999; 33: 372–9.

126. HANNING M *et al*. Die erosive Wirkung von Acetylsalicylsäure an Zahnschmelz und Dentin *in vitro*. Dtsch Zahnärztl Z 1993; 48: 298–302.

127. HARRISON JL *et al*. Dental erosion caused by cola beverages. Gen Dent 1991; 39: 23–4.

128. HARTLES RL *et al*. Erosive effect of drinking fluids on the molar teeth of the rat. Arch Oral Biol 1962; 7: 307–15.

129. HAYS GL *et al*. Salivary pH while dissolving vitamin C-containing tablets. Am J Dent 1992; 5: 269–71.

130. HAZEN SP *et al*. The problem of root caries. I. J Am Dent Assoc 1973; 86: 137–44.

131. HELLSTRÖM I. Anorexia nervosa – odontologiska problem. Swed Dent J 1974; 67: 253.

132. HELLSTRÖM I. Oral complications in anorexia nervosa. Scand J Dent Res 1977; 85: 71–86.

133. HERTER JM *et al.* Behandlung überempfindlicher Zahnhälse in den Jahren 1910 bis 1950. Dtsch Zahnärztl Z 2004; 59: 257–63.

134. HIGH AS. An unusual pattern of dental erosion. Br Dent J 1977; 143: 403–4.

135. HOLLOWAY PJ *et al.* Fruit drinks and tooth erosion. Br Dent J 1958; 104: 305–9.

136. HOOPER S *et al.* A comparison of enamel erosion by a new sports drink compared to two proprietary products: a controlled, crossover study in situ. J Dent 2004; 32: 541–5.

137. HOUWINK B. Tanderosie. In: VAN DER KWAST WAM *et al.* (eds) Tandheelkundig Jaar 1985. Utrecht: Bohn, Scheltema & Holkema, 1985.

138. HOWDEN GF. Erosion as the presenting symptom in hiatus hernia. Br Dent J 1971: 131: 455–6.

139. HUGHES JA *et al.* Development and evaluation of a low erosive blackcurrant juice drink in vitro and situ. I. J Dent 1999; 27: 285–9.

140. HUGHES JA *et al.* The protective effect of fluoride treatments against enamel erosion *in vitro.* J Oral Rehabil 2004; 31: 357–63.

141. IMFELD T. Dental erosion: definition, classification, and links. Eur J Oral Sci 1996; 104 (2 (Pt 2)): 151–5.

142. IMFELD T. Prevention of progression of dental erosion by professional and individual prophylactic measures. Eur J Oral Sci 1996; 104: 221–8.

143. IRELAND AT *et al.* An investigation into the ability of soft drinks to adhere to enamel. Caries Res 1995; 29: 470–6.

144. JAEGGI T *et al.* Toothbrush abrasion of erosively altered enamel after intraoral exposure to saliva. Caries Res 1999; 33: 455–61.

145. JAEGGI T *et al.* Erosionen und keilförmige Defekte bei Rekruten der Schweizer Armee. Schweiz Monatschr Zahnmed 1999; 109: 1171–8.

146. JAEGGI T *et al.* Erosionen bei Kindern im frühen Schulalter. Schweiz Monatschr Zahmed 2004; 114: 876–81.

147. JAMES PMC *et al.* Local effects of certain medicaments on the teeth. Br Med J 1953; 2: 1252–3.

148. JÄRVINEN V *et al.* Dental erosion and upper gastrointestinal disorders. Oral Surg Oral Med Oral Pathol 1988; 65: 298–303.

149. JÄRVINEN V *et al.* Risk factors in dental erosion. J Dent Res 1991; 70: 942–7.

150. JÄRVINEN V *et al.* Location of dental erosion in a referred population. Caries Res 1992; 26: 391–6.

151. JENSEN OE *et al.* Chemical and physical oral findings in a case of anorexia nervosa and bulimia. J Oral Pathol 1987; 16: 399–402.

152. JOHANSSON A *et al.* Analysis of possible factors influencing the occurrence of occlusal tooth wear in a young Saudi population. Acta Odontol Scand 1991; 49: 139–45.

153. JOHANSSON A-K *et al.* Dental erosion, soft-drink intake, and oral health in young Saudi men, and the development of a system for assessing erosive anterior tooth wear. Acta Odontol Scand 1996; 54: 369–78.

154. JOHANSSON A-K *et al.* Influence of drinking method on tooth-surface pH in relation to dental erosion. Eur J Oral Sci 2004; 112: 484–9.

155. JOHANSSON A-K *et al.* Comparison of factors potentially related to the occurrence of dental erosion in high- and low-erosion groups. Eur J Oral Sci 2002; 110: 204–11.

156. JONES L *et al.* Studies on dental erosion: an *in vivo-in vitro* model of endogenous dental erosion – its application to testing production by fluoride gel application. Aust Dent J 2002; 47: 304–8.

157. JONES RRH *et al.* Depth and area of dental erosions, and dental caries, in bulimic women. J Dent Res 1989; 68: 1275–8.

158. KAPILA YL *et al.* Cocaine-associated rapid gingival recession and dental erosion. J Periodontol 1997; 68: 485–8.

159. KAWASAKI A *et al.* Effects of plaque control on the patency and occlusion of dentine tubules in situ. J Oral Rehabil 2001; 28: 439–49.

160. KELLEHER M *et al.* Tooth surface loss.1 Br Dent J 1999; 186: 61–6.

161. KHAN F *et al.* Dental erosion and bruxism. A tooth wear analysis from South East Queensland. Aust Dent J 1998; 43: 117–27.

162. KLEIER DJ *et al.* Dental management of the chronic vomiting patient. J Am Dent Assoc 1984; 108: 618–21.

163. KNIGHT NN *et al.* Hypersensitive dentin: testing of procedures for mechanical and chemical obliteration of dentinal tubuli. J Periodontol 1993; 65: 287–8.

164. KRUTCHKOFF DJ *et al.* Cocaine-induced dental erosions. N Engl J Med 1990; 322: 408.

165. KUN L. Etude biophysique des modifications des tissus dentaires provoquées par l'application locale de strontium. Schweiz Monatsschr Zahnheilkd 1976; 86: 661–76.

166. LAMBRECHTS P *et al.* Restorative therapy for erosive lesions. Eur J Oral Sci 1996; 104: 229–40.

167. LAN WH *et al.* Morphologic study of Nd:YAG laser usage in treatment of dentinal hypersensitivity. J Endod 2004; 30: 131–4.

168. LARSEN MJ. Prevention by means of fluoride of enamel erosion as caused by soft drinks and orange juice. Caries Res 2001; 35: 229–34.

169. LARSEN MJ *et al.* Enamel erosion by some soft drinks and orange juices relative to their pH, buffering effect and contents of calcium phosphate. Caries Res 1999; 33: 81–7.

170. LARSEN MJ *et al.* Fluoride is unable to reduce dental erosion from soft drinks. Caries Res 2002; 36: 75–80.

171. LEE WC *et al.* Possible role of tensile stress in the etiology of cervical erosive lesions of teeth. J Prosthet Dent 1984; 52: 374–80.

172. LEVINE RS. Fruit juice erosion – an increasing danger? J Dent 1973; 2: 85–8.

173. LEVINSON N. Anorexia and bulimia: eating functions gone awry. Cal Dent Assoc J 1985; 13 (8): 18–22.

174. LEWIS KJ *et al.* The relationship of erosion and attrition in extensive tooth tissue loss. Br Dent J 1973; 135: 400–4.

175. LIER BB *et al.* Treatment of dentin hypersensitivity by Nd:YAG laser. J Clin Periodontol 2002; 29: 501–6.

176. LILJA J. Sensory differences between crown and root dentin in human teeth. Acta Odontol Scand 1980; 38: 285–91.

177. LILJA J *et al.* Dentinal innervation of impacted human third molars. Scand J Dent Res 1984; 92: 485–8.

178. LINKOSALO E *et al*. Dental erosions in relation to lac-tovegetarian diet. Scand J Dent Res 1985; 93: 436–41.

179. LINNETT V *et al*. Oral health of children with gastro-esophageal reflux disease. Aust Dent J 2002; 47: 156–62.

180. LITTLE JW. Eating disorders: dental implications. Oral Surg Oral Med Oral Pathol Oral Radiol Endod 2002; 93: 138–43.

181. LIU HC *et al*. Prevalence and distribution of cervical dentin hypersensitivity in a population in Tapein, Taiwan. J Endod 1998; 24: 45–7.

182. LOKIN PAM *et al*. Zwemmerserosie. Een Nederlands probleem? Ned Tijdschr Tandheelkd 2004; 111: 146.

183. LUSSI A. Dental erosion. Eur J Oral Sci 1996; 104: 191–8.

184. LUSSI A *et al*. Effect of Amine/Sodium fluoride rinsing on toothbrush abrasion of softened enamel in situ. Caries Res 2004; 38: 567–71.

185. LUSSI A *et al*. The role of diet in the aetiology of dental erosion. Caries Res 2004; 38 (suppl 1) 34–44.

186. LUSSI A *et al*. Prediction of the erosive potential of some beverages. Caries Res 1995; 29: 349–54.

187. LUSSI A *et al*. Progression of and risk factors for dental erosion and wedge-shaped defects over a 6-year period. Caries Res 2000; 34: 182–7.

188. LUSSI A *et al*. Erosion der Zahnhartsubstanz. Epidemiologie, klinisches Erscheinungsbild, Risikofaktoren und Verhaltensregeln. Schweiz Monatsschr Zahnmed 1992; 102: 321–7.

189. LUSSI A *et al*. Dental erosion in a population of Swiss adults. Community Dent Oral Epidemiol 1991; 19: 286–90.

190. MACKIE IC *et al*. Case reports – Dental erosion associated with unusual drinking habits in childhood. J Pediatr Dent 1986; 2: 89–94.

191. MAHONEY E *et al*. Preliminary in vitro assessment of erosive potential using the ultra-micro-indentation system. Caries Res 2003; 37: 218–24.

192. MAIR LH. Understanding wear in dentistry. Compend Contin Educ Dent 1999; 20: 19–30.

193. MALCOLM D *et al*. Erosion of the teeth due to sulphuric acid in the battery industry. Br J Ind Med 1961; 18: 63–9.

194. MANNERBERG F. Changes in the enamel surface in cases of erosion. Arch Oral Biol 1961; 4 (spec. suppl): 59–62.

195. MANNERBERG F. Effect of lemon juice on different types of tooth surface. Acta Odontol Scand 1962; 20: 153–64.

196. MANNERBERG F. Appearances of tooth surfaces as observed in shadowed replicas in various age groups, in long term studies, after toothbrushing, in cases of erosion and after exposure to citrus fruit juice. Odontol Revy 1960; 11 (suppl 6): 1–116.

197. MANNERBERG F. The reversible phenomenon of erosion. J Dent Res 1966; 45: 512–18.

198. MARKOWITZ K *et al*. Decreasing interdental nerve activity in the cat with potassium and divalent cations. Arch Oral Biol 1991; 36: 1–7.

199. MARON FS. Mucosal burn resulting from chewable aspirin. J Am Dent Assoc 1989; 119: 279–80.

200. MARON FS. Enamel erosion resulting from hydrochloric acid tablets. J Am Dent Assoc 1996; 127: 781–4.

201. MATHEW T *et al*. Relationship between sport drinks and dental erosion in 304 University athletes in Columbus, Ohio, USA. Caries Res 2002; 36: 281–7.

202. MAUPOMÉ G *et al*. *In vitro* quantitative assessment of enamel microhardness after exposure to eroding immersion in a cola drink. Caries Res 1998; 32: 148–53.

203. McDERRA EJC *et al*. The dental status of asthmatic British school children. Pediatr Dent 1998; 20: 281–7.

204. McDONALD JL Jr *et al*. Laboratory studies concerning the effect of acid–containing beverages on enamel dissolution and experimental dental caries. J Dent Res 1973; 52: 211–16.

205. McLURE FJ *et al*. The destructive effect of citrate vs. lactate ions on rats' molar tooth surfaces, in vivo. J Dent Res 1946; 25: 1–12.

206. McFALL WT Jr. A Review of the active agents available for treatment of dentinal hypersensitivity. Endod Dent Traumatol 1986; 2: 141–9.

207. McLACHLAN W. Tooth damage from use of citrus fruits. Br Dent J 1971; 131: 385.

208. MEURMAN JH *et al*. Experimental erosion of dentin. Scand J Dent Res 1991; 99: 457–62.

209. MEURMAN JH *et al*. Scanning electronic microscopic study of the effect of salivary pellicle on enamel erosion. Caries Res 1991; 25: 1–6.

210. MEURMAN JH *et al*. Experimental sport drinks with minimal dental erosion effect. Scand J Dent Res 1990; 98: 120–8.

211. MEURMAN JH *et al*. Buffering effects of antiacids in the mouth – a new treatment of dental erosion? Scand J Dent Res 1988; 96: 412–17.

212. MEURMAN JK *et al*. Hospital mouth-cleaning aids may cause dental erosion. Special Care Dent 1996; 16: 247–50.

213. MEURMAN JH *et al*. Pathogenesis and modifying factors of dental erosion. Eur J Oral Sci 1996; 104: 199–206.

214. MILES DA *et al*. Bulimic erosion. J Can Dent Assoc 1985; 51: 757–60.

215. MILLER WD. Experiments and observations of the wasting of tooth tissue variously designated as erosion, abrasion, chemical abrasion, denudation, etc. Dent Cosmos 1907; 49: 1–23.

216. MILWARD A *et al*. Continuous monitoring of salivary flow rate and pH at the surface of the dentition following consumption of acidic beverages. Caries Res 1997; 31: 44–9.

217. MILWARD A *et al*. The distribution and severity of tooth wear and the relationship between erosion and dietary constituents in a group of children. Int J Paediatr Dent 1994; 4: 151–7.

218. MILLWARD A *et al*. Dental erosion in four-year-old children from differing socio–economic backgrounds. ASDC J Dent Child 1994; 61: 263–6.

219. MILLWARD A *et al*. *In vitro* techniques for erosive lesion formation and examination in dental enamel. J Oral Rehabil 1995; 22: 37–42.

220. MILOSEVIC A. Eating disorders and the dentist. Br Dent J 1999; 186: 109–13.

221. MILOSEVIC A *et al*. Epidemiological studies of tooth wear and dental erosion in 14-year-old children in North West England. Part II. Br Dent J 2004; 197: 479–83.

222. MILOSEVIC A *et al*. Salivary factors in vomiting bulimics with and without pathological tooth wear. Caries Res 1996; 30: 361–6.

223. MILOSEVIC A *et al*. The orodental status of anorexics and bulimics. Br Dent J 1989; 167: 66–70.

224. MILOSEVIC A *et al*. Sports supplement drinks and dental health in competitive swimmers and cyclists. Br Dent J 1997; 182: 303–8.

225. MINKOFF S *et al*. Efficacy of strontium chloride in dental hypersensitivity. J Periodontol 1987; 58: 470–4.

226. MISTRY M *et al*. Erosion by soft drinks of rat molar teeth assessed by digital image analysis. Caries Res 1993; 27: 21–5.

227. MIYAWAKI S *et al*. Relationships among nocturnal jaw muscle activities, decreased esophageal pH, and sleep positions. Am J Orthod Dentofac Orthop 2004; 126: 615–19.

228. MOAZZEZ R *et al*. Dental erosion, gastro-oesophageal reflux diseases and saliva: how are they related? J Dent 2004; 32: 498–94.

229. MONTGOMERY MT *et al*. Eating disorders: phenomenology, identification, and dental intervention. Gen Dent 1988; 36: 485–8.

230. MORRIS MF *et al*. Clinical efficacy of two desensitizing agents. Am J Dent 1999; 12: 72–6.

231. MOSS SJ. Dental erosion. Int Dent J 1998; 48: 529–39.

232. MÜHLEMANN HR. Zur Erosion des Zahnschmelzes. Dtsch Zahnärztzebl 1962; 16: 328–33.

233. NATANSON D *et al*. Effect of fluoride pretreatment or rehardening with calcifying solutions on enamel softened by orange juice. J Dent Res 1973; 52: 625.

234. NUNN JH. Prevalence of dental erosion and the implications for oral health. Eur J Oral Sci 1996; 104: 156–61.

235. NUNN J *et al*. Tooth wear – dental erosion. Br Dent J 1996; 180: 349–52.

236. ORCHARDSON R *et al*. Clinical features of hypersensitive teeth. Br Dent J 1987; 162: 353–6.

237. ORCHARDSON R *et al*. The efficacy of potassium salts as agents for treating dentin hypersensitivity. J Orofac Pain 2000; 14: 9–19.

238. O'SULLIVAN EA *et al*. Salivary factors affecting dental erosion in children. Caries Res 2000; 34: 82–7.

239. O'SULLIVAN EA *et al*. A comparison of acidic dietary factors in children with and without dental erosion. ASDC J Dent Child 2000; 67: 186–92.

240. O'SULLIVAN EA *et al*. Gastroesophagal reflux in children and its relationship to erosion of primary and permanent teeth. Eur J Oral Sci 1998; 106: 765–9.

241. OWENS NM *et al*. Noncarious dental "abfraction" lesions in an aging population. Compend Contin Educ 1995; 16: 552–61.

242. PAES LEME AF *et al*. Occlusion of dentin tubules by desensitising agents. Am J Dent 2004; 17: 368–72

243. PALLAV P. Occlusal wear in dentistry. Thesis, Universiteit van Amsterdam, Amsterdam, 1996.

244. PANDURIĆ V *et al*. The efficiency of dentine adhesives in treating non-carious cervical lesions. J Oral Rehabil 2001; 28: 1168–74.

245. PARRY J *et al*. Investigation of mineral waters and soft drinks in relation to dental erosion. J Oral Rehabil 2001; 28: 766–72.

246. PASHLEY DH *et al*. Fluid shifts across human dentine *in vitro* in response to hydrodynamic stimuli. Arch Oral Biol 1996; 41: 1065–72.

247. PEARCE NX *et al*. Dentine hypersensitivity: a clinical trial to compare 2 strontium densensitizing toothpastes with a conventional fluoride toothpaste. J Periodontol 1994; 65: 113–19.

248. PETERSEN PE *et al*. Oral conditions among German battery factory workers. Community Dent Oral Epidemiol 1991; 19: 104–6.

249. PINDBORG JJ. Pathology of the dental hard tissues. Copenhagen: Munksgaard, 1970.

250. PLAGMANN H-C *et al*. A clinical study comparing two high-fluoride dentifrices for the treatment of dentinal hypersensitivity. Quint Int 1997; 28: 403–8.

251. POULSEN S *et al*. Potassium nitrate toothpaste for dentine hypersensitivity. Cochrane Database Syst Rev 2001; (2): CD001476.

252. REES JS *et al*. An in vitro assessment of the erosive potential of conventional and white ciders. Eur J Prosthdont Restor Dent 2002; 10: 167–71.

253. REES JS *et al*. The prevalence of dentine hypersensitivity in a hospital clinic population in Hong Kong. J Dent 2003; 31: 453–61.

254. REUTER JE. Unusual incisal dental erosion. Br Dent J 1978; 145: 274.

255. ROBB ND *et al*. Anorexia and bulimia nervosa (the eating disorders): conditions of interest to the dental practitioner. J Dent 1996; 24: 7–16.

256. ROBERTS MW *et al*. Oral findings in anorexia nervosa and bulimia nervosa. J Am Dent Assoc 1987; 115: 407–10.

257. ROOS EH *et al*. In vivo dental plaque pH variation with regular and diet soft drinks. Pediatr Dent 2002; 24: 350–3.

258. ROST T *et al*. Possible etiologic factors in dental erosion. J Dent Res 1961; 40: 385.

259. RUFF JC *et al*. Bulimia: dentomedical complications. Gen Dent 1992; 40: 22–5.

260. RYBERG M *et al*. Effect of B_2-adrenoceptor agonists on saliva proteins and dental caries in asthmatic children. J Dent Res 1987; 66: 1404–6.

261. RYTÖMAA I *et al*. *In vitro* erosion of bovine enamel caused by acidic drinks and other foodstuffs. Scand J Dent Res 1988; 96: 324–33.

262. SCHEUTZEL P. Zahnmedizinische Befunde bei psychogenen Essstörungen. Dtsch Zahärztl Z 1992; 47: 119–23.

263. SCHEUTZEL P. Etiology of dental erosions – intrinsic factors. Eur J Oral Sci 1996; 104: 178–90.

264. SCHEUTZEL P *et al*. Anorexie und Bulimie aus zahnärztlicher Sicht. München: Urban & Schwarzenberg, 1994.

265. SCHIFF T *et al*. Desensitizing efficacy of a new dentifrice containing 5.0% potassium nitrate and 0.454% stannous fluoride. Am J Dent 2000; 13: 111–15.

266. SCHIFFNER U *et al*. Erosionen und Keilförmige Zahnhalsdefekte bei deutschen Erwachsenen und Senioren. Dtsch Zahnärztl Zeitschr 2002; 57: 102–6.

267. SCHROEDER HE. Pathobiologie oraler Strukturen. Basel: Karger, 1983.

268. SCHULZE C. Developmental abnormalities of the teeth and jaws. In: GORLIN RJ, GOLDMAN HM (eds) Thoma's oral pathology. St Louis, MO: CV Mosby, 1970.

269. SCHUURS AHB et al. An unusual case of black teeth. Oral Surg 1987; 64: 427–31.

270. SCHUURS AHB et al. Dentists' views on cervical hypersensitivity and their knowledge of its treatment. Endod Dent Traumatol 1995; 11: 240–4.

271. SHABANIAN M et al. In vitro wear of materials under different loads and varying pH. J Prosthet Dent 2002; 87: 650–6.

272. SHAW L et al. Childhood asthma and dental erosion. ASDC J Dent Child 2000; 67: 102–6.

273. SHAW L et al. UK national clinical guidelines in paediatric dentistry. Int J Paediatr Dent 2000; 10: 356–65.

274. SHENKIN JD et al. Soft drink consumption and caries risk in children and adolescents. Gen Dent 2003; 51: 302–3.

275. SHULMAN EH et al. Salivary citrate content and erosion of the teeth. J Dent Res 1948; 27: 541–3.

276. SILVERMAN G. The sensitivity-reducing effect of brushing with a potassium nitrate-sodium monofluorophosphate dentifrice. Compendium Contin Educ 1985; 6: 131–6.

277. SIMMONS MS et al. Dental erosion secondary to ethanol-induced emesis. Oral Surg Oral Med Oral Pathol 1987; 64: 731–3.

278. SIVASITHAMPARAM K et al. Endodontic sequelae of dental erosion. Aust Dent J 2003; 48: 97–101.

279. SIVASITHAMPARAM K et al. Dental erosion in asthma. Aust Dent J 2002; 47: 298–303.

280. SKOGEDAL O et al. Pilot study on dental erosion in a Norwegian electrolytic zinc factory. Community Dent Oral Epidemiol 1977; 5: 248–51.

281. SMITH AJ et al. Baby fruit juices and tooth erosion. Br Dent J 1987; 162: 65–7.

282. SMITH BGN et al. The prevalence, etiology and management of tooth wear in the United Kingdom. J Prosthet Dent 1997; 78: 367–72.

283. SMITH BGN et al. A comparison of patterns of tooth wear with aetiological factors. Br Dent J 1984; 157: 16–19.

284. SMITH BGN et al. An index for measuring the wear of teeth. Br Dent J 1984; 156: 435–8.

285. SMITH BGN et al. Dental erosion in patients with chronic alcoholism. J Dent 1989; 17: 219–21.

286. SOGNNAES RF. Dental hard tissue destruction with special reference to idiopathic erosions. In: SOGNNAES RF (ed.) Mechanisms of hard tissue destruction. Washington: American Association for the advancement of Science, 1963.

287. SOGNNAES RF et al. Dental erosion. I. J Am Dent Assoc 1972; 84: 571–6.

288. SORVARI R et al. Erosive effect of a sport drink mixture with and without addition of fluoride and magnesium on the molar teeth of rats. Scand J Dent Res 1988; 96: 226–31.

289. SORVARI R et al. Effect of fluoride varnish and solution on enamel erosion in vitro. Caries Res 1994; 28: 227–32.

290. SORVARI R et al. Surface ultrastructure of rat molar teeth after experimentally induced erosion and attrition. Caries Res 1996; 30: 163–8.

291. SPIGSET O. Oral symptoms in bulimia nervosa. Acta Odontol Scand 1991; 49: 335–9.

292. STABHOLZ A et al. Tooth enamel dissolution from erosion or etching and subsequent caries development. J Pedodont 1983; 7: 100–8.

293. STAFNE EC et al. Dissolution of tooth substance by lemon juice, acid beverages and acids from some other sources. J Am Dent Assoc 1947; 34: 586–92.

294. STEINMAN RR. Is caries susceptibility an internal problem of the tooth? Quint Int 1978; 9 (10): 95–9.

295. STEINMAN RR et al. Effect of infusing selected chemical compounds on dentinal fluid movement in the rat. J Dent Res 1975; 54: 567–9.

296. STEPHENS P et al. An investigation of the interaction between alcohol and fibroblasts in wound healing. Int J Oral Maxillofac Surg 1996; 25: 161–4.

297. SUGE T et al. Calcium phosphate precipitation method for the treatment of dentin hypersensitivity. Am J Dent 2002; 15: 220–6.

298. SULLIVAN RE et al. Iatrogenic erosion of teeth. ASDC J Dent Child 1983; 50: 192–6.

299. SWIFT EJ Jr et al. Clinical evaluation of prime & Bond 2.1 for treating dentin hypersensitivity. Am J Dent 2001; 14: 13–16.

300. TAANI Q et al. Clinical evaluation of cervical dentin sensitivity (CDS) in patients attending general dental clinics (GDC) and periodontal speciality clinics (PSC). J Clin Periodontol 2002; 29: 118–22.

301. TARBET WJ et al. Clinical evaluation of a new treatment for dentinal hypersensitivity. J Periodontol 1980; 51: 535–40.

302. TAVVS EA et al. The scientific rationale and development of an optimised dentifrice for the treatment of dentin hypersensitivity. Am J Dent 2004; 17: 61–70.

303. TEN CATE JM et al. Dental erosion, summary. Eur J Oral Sci 1996; 104: 241–4.

304. THEUNS HM. The influence of in-vitro and in-vivo demineralizing conditions on dental enamel. Thesis, University of Nijmegen, Nijmegen, 1987.

305. TOUYZ LZG et al. Anticariogenic effects of black tea (Camellia sinensis) in caries prone-rats. Quint Int 2001; 32: 647–50.

306. TOUYZ LZG. The acidity (pH) and buffering capacity of Canadian fruit juice and dental implications. J Can Dent Assoc 1994; 60: 454–8.

307. TOUYZ LZG et al. Citrus, acid and teeth. Dent Health 1982; 21 (2): 10.

308. TOUYZ LZ et al. Increased acidity in frozen fruit juices and dental implications. ASDC J Dent Child 1993; 60: 223–5.

309. TUOMINEN ML et al. Tooth surface loss and associated factors among factory workers in Finland and Tanzania. Community Dent Health 1992; 9: 143–50.

310. TUOMINEN ML et al. Tooth surface loss and exposure to organic and inorganic acid fumes in workplace air. Community Dent Oral Epidemiol 1991; 19: 217–20.

311. TURSSI CP et al. An in situ investigation into the abrasion of eroded dental hard tissues by a whitening dentifrice. Caries Res 2004; 38: 473–7.

312. UCHIDA A *et al*. Controlled clinical evaluation of a 10% strontium chloride dentifrice in treatment of dentin hypersensitivity following periodontal surgery. J Periodontol 1980; 51: 578–81.

313. VAN DER SLUIS LW *et al*. Cervical dentine hypersensitivity. Ned Tijdschr Tandheelkd 2001; 108: 492–5.

314. VAN LOVEREN C *et al*. Voeding en gebitsziekten. In: VAN LOVEREN C *et al*. (eds) Preventieve tandheelkunde. Houten: Bohn Stafleu Van Loghum, 1996, pp. 109–11.

315. VAN NIEUW AMERONGEN A. Speeksel en gebitselementen. Ned Tandarstenbl 1995; 50: 104–5.

316. VAN NIEUW AMERONGEN A. Tanderosie en abrasie. Ned Tijdschr Tandheelkd 1997; 52: 166–9.

317. VAN NIEUW AMERONGEN A *et al*. De invloed van "vruchten"– en ijsthee op de pH en de buffercapaciteit van speeksel. Ned Tijdschr Tandheelkd 2004; 111: 804.

318. VAN NIEUW AMERONGEN A *et al*. Speeksel en gebitselementen. Bussum: Coutinho, 1999.

319. VAN MEERBEEK B *et al*. A randomised, controlled trial evaluating the three-year clinical effectiveness of two etch & rinse adhesives in cervical lesions. Oper Dent 2004; 29: 376–85.

320. VAN RIJKOM HM *et al*. Prevalence, distribution and background variables of smooth-bordered tooth wear in teenagers in The Hague, The Netherlands. Caries Res 2002; 36: 147–54.

321. VANUSPRONG W *et al*. Cervical tooth wear and sensitivity: erosion, softening and rehardening of dentine; effects of pH, time and ultrasonication. J Clin Periodontol 2002; 29: 351–7.

322. VASSILAKOS N *et al*. Oral electrochemical action after soft drink rinsing and consumption of sweets. J Dent Res 1990; 98: 336–40.

323. VERRET TRG. Analyzing the etiology of an extremely worn dentition. J Prosthodont 2001; 10: 224–33.

324. VISSER JB. Speciële pathologie van het menselijke gebit. Leiden: Stafleu & Tholen BV, 1974.

325. VISSINK A *et al*. Oorzaak, gevolg en behandeling van hyposialie. Ned Tijdschr Tandheelkd 1992; 99: 92–6.

326. VON FRAUNHOFER JA *et al*. Dissolution of dental enamel in soft drinks. Gen Dent 2004; 52: 308–12.

327. WALDMAN HB. Is your next young patient pre-anorexic or pre-bulemic? ASDC J Dent Child 1998; 65: 52–6.

328. WARREN JJ *et al*. Tooth wear patterns in the deciduous dentition. Am J Orthod Dentofac Orthop 2002; 122: 614–18.

329. WEST NX *et al*. Dentine hypersensitivity and the placebo response. A comparison of the effect of strontium acetate, potassium nitrate and fluoride toothpastes. J Clin Periodontol 1997; 24: 209–15.

330. WEST NX *et al*. The effect of pH on the erosion of dentine and enamel by dietary acids *in vitro*. J Oral Rehabil 2001; 28: 860–4.

331. WEST NX *et al*. Dentine hypersensitivity: the effect of brushing toothpaste on etched and unetched dentine in vitro. J Oral Rehabil 2002; 29: 167–74.

332. WEST NX *et al*. Development and evaluation of a low erosive blackcurrant juice drink. 2. J Dent 1999; 27: 341–4.

333. WEST NX *et al*. Modification of soft drinks with xanthan gum to minimise erosion: a study *in situ*. Br Dent J 2004; 196: 478–81.

334. WIEGAND A *et al*. Influence of buffering effects of dentifrices and fluoride gels on abrasion on eroded dentine. Arch Oral Biol 2004; 49: 259–65.

335. WHITE DK *et al*. Loss of tooth structure associated with chronic regurgitation and vomiting. J Am Dent Assoc 1978; 97: 833–5.

336. WIKTORSSON A-M *et al*. Erosive tooth wear: prevalence and severity in Swedish winetasters. Eur J oral Sci 1997; 105: 544–50.

337. WILLERSHAUSEN B *et al*. In vitro study on dental erosion provoked by various beverages using electron probe microanalysis. Eur J Med Res 2004; 29: 432–8.

338. WILLIAMS D *et al*. The prevalence of dental erosion in the maxillary incisors of 14-year-old school-children in Tower Hamlets and Hackney, London, Uk. Int Dent J 1999; 49: 211–16.

339. WÖLTGENS JHM *et al*. Enamel erosion and saliva. Clin Prev Dent 1985; 7 (3): 8–10.

340. WÖLTGENS JHM *et al*. Speekseltesten en erosie van glazuur. Ned Tijdschr Tandheelkd 1986; 93: 237–9.

341. WYNN W *et al*. The erosive action of various fruit juices on the lower molar teeth of the albino rat. J Nutr 1948; 35: 489–97.

342. XHONGA FA *et al*. The influence of hyperthyroidism on dental erosions. Oral Surg 1973; 36: 349–57.

343. XHONGA FA *et al*. Dental erosion: progress of erosion measured clinically after various fluoride applications. J Am Dent Assoc 1973; 87: 1223–8.

344. XHONGA FA *et al*. Geographic comparisons of the incidence of dental erosion. J Oral Rehabil 1983; 10: 269–77.

345. XHONGA-OJA FA *et al*. Factor analysis of dental erosion occurrence. J Oral Rehabil 1986; 13: 247–56.

346. XHONGA FA *et al*. Dental erosions. II. J Am Dent Assoc 1972; 84: 577–82.

347. YIP H-K *et al*. Fluoride release, weight loss and erosive wear of modern aesthetic restoratives. Br Dent J 1999; 187: 265–70.

348. YIP H–K *et al*. Management of tooth tissue loss from erosion. Quint Int 2002; 33: 516–20.

349. ZERO DT. Etiology of dental erosion – extrinsic factors. Eur J Oral Sci 1996; 104: 162–77.

350. ZIMMER S *et al*. Untersuchung einer neue Zahnpasta zur Therapie überempfindlicher Zahnhälse. Deutsch Zahnärztl Z 1998; 53: 517–21.

351. ZIPKIN I *et al*. Salivary citrate and dental erosion. Procedure for determining citric acid in saliva – dental erosion and citric acid in saliva. J Dent Res 1949; 28: 613–26.

352. NEKRASHEVYCH Y *et al*. Protective influence of experimentally formed salivary pellicle on enamel erosion. Caries Res 2003; 37: 225–31.

353. JENSDOTTIR T *et al*. Immediate erosive potential of Coal drinks and orange juices. J Dent Res 2006; 85: 226–30.

354. HEMMINGWAY CA. Erosion of enamel by non–carbonated soft drinks with and without toothbrushing abrasion. Br Dent J 2006; 201: 447–50.

355. ESCARTIN JL *et al*. A study of dental staining among competitive swimmers. Community Dent Oral Epidemiol 2000; 28: 10–17.

356. ROSE KJ *et al*. Intensive swimming: can it affect your patients' smile? J Am Dent Assoc 1995; 126: 1402–6.

357. LEADER DM. Scleroderma and dentistry. J Mass Dent Soc 2007; 56: 16–19.

358. MILLER AJ *et al*. Oral health of United States adults. The national survey of oral health in U.S. employed adults and seniors: 1985–1986. Washington, DC: U.S. Department of Health and Human Services, 1987.

359. LUSSI A *et al*. Erosive tooth wear: diagnosis, risks factors and prevention. Am J Dent 2006; 19: 319–25.

360. WIEGAND A *et al*. Influence of rotating-oscillating, sonic and ultrasonic action of power toothbrushes on abrasion of sound and eroded dentine. J Periodont Res 2006; 41: 221–7.

361. GANSS C *et al*. Efficacy of waiting periods and topical fluoride treatment on toothbrush abrasion of eroded enamel. Caries Res 2007; 41: 146–51.

362. SCHLUETER N *et al*. Effect of pepsin on erosive tissue loss and the efficacy of fluoridation in dentine in vitro. Acta Odontol Scand 2007; 65: 298–305.

363. HOOPER SM *et al*. The protective effects of toothpaste against erosion by orange juice. J Dent 2007; 35: 476–81.

364. HOVE L *et al*. The protective effect of TiF4, SnF2 and NaF on erosion of enamel by hydrochloric acid in vitro measured by white light interferometry. Caries Res 2006; 40: 440–3.

Chapter 7: Tooth Resorption

1. ABBOTT PV *et al*. Antibiotics and endodontics. Aust Dent J 1990; 35: 50–60.

2. ABRAHAM-INPIJN L *et al*. Lack of evidence for link between intradental lesions and chronic renal failure. Oral Surg Oral Med Oral Pathol 1990; 70: 734–7.

3. ALATLI I *et al*. Orthodontically induced root resorption in rat molars after 1-hydroxyethylidene-1,1-biphosphanate injection. Acta Odontol Scand 1996; 54: 102–8.

4. ALATLI-KUT I *et al*. Disturbances of cementum formation induced by a single dose of 1-hydroxyethyledene-1,1-biphosphanate (HEBP) in rats. Scand J Dent Res 1994; 102: 260–8.

5. ALBAIR WB *et al*. Connective tissue attachment to periodontally diseased roots after citric acid demineralization. J Peridontol 1982; 53: 515–26.

6. AL-BADRI S *et al*. Factors affecting resorption in traumatically intruded permanent incisors in children. Dent Traumatol 2002; 18: 73–6.

7. ALEXANDER SA. Levels of root resorption associated with continuous arch and sectional arch mechanics. Am J Orthod Dentofac Orthop 1996; 10: 321–4.

8. ALEXANDER SA *et al*. Identification and localization of a mucopolysaccharidase in human deciduous teeth. J Dent Res 1980; 59: 594–601.

9. AL-NAZAH S. External root resorption after bleaching. Oral Surg Oral Med Oral Pathol 1991; 72: 607–9.

10. ANDERSEN E *et al*. Effects of cooling and heating of the tooth on pulpal blood flow in man. Endod Dent Traumatol 1994; 10: 256–9.

11. ANDERSSON L *et al*. Avulsed human teeth replanted within 15 minutes. Endod Dent Traumatol 1990; 6: 37–42.

12. ANDERSSON L *et al*. Progression of root resorption following replantation of human teeth after extended extraoral storage. Endod Dent Traumatol 1989; 5: 38–47.

13. ANDERSSON L *et al*. Tooth ankylosis. Int J Oral Surg 1984; 13: 423–31.

14. ANDREASEN FM. Transient apical breakdown and its relation to color and sensibility changes after luxation injuries to the teeth. Endod Dent Traumatol 1986; 2: 9–19.

15. ANDREASEN FM *et al*. Diagnosis of luxation injuries: the importance of standardized clinical, radiographic and photographic techniques in clinical investigations. Endod Dent Traumatol 1985; 1: 160–9.

16. ANDREASEN JO. Luxation of permanent teeth due to trauma. Scand J Dent Res 1970; 78: 273–86.

17. ANDREASEN JO. The effect of splinting upon periodontal healing after replantation of permanent incisors in monkeys. Acta Odontol Scand 1975; 33: 313–23.

18. ANDREASEN JO *et al*. Traumatic injuries to the teeth. Copenhagen: Munksgaard, 1981.

19. ANDREASEN JO. Relationship between cell damage in the periodontal ligament after replantation and subsequent development of root resorption. Acta Odontol Scand 1981; 39: 15–25.

20. ANDREASEN JO. Relationship between surface and inflammatory resorption and changes in the pulp after replantation of permanent incisors in monkeys. J Endod 1981; 7: 294–301.

21. ANDREASEN JO. Effect of extra-alveolar period and storage media upon periodontal and pulpal healing after replantation of mature permanent incisors in monkeys. Int J Oral Surg 1981; 10: 43–53.

22. ANDREASEN JO *et al*. Textbook and color atlas of traumatic injuries to the teeth, 3rd edn. Copenhagen: Munksgaard, 1994.

23. ANDREASEN JO. Challenges in clinical dental traumatology. Endod Dent Traumatol 1985; 1: 45–55.

24. ANDREASEN JO. The effect of pulp extirpation or root canal treatment on periodontal healing after replantation of permanent incisors in monkeys. J Endod 1981; 7: 245–52.

25. ANDREASEN JO *et al*. Replantation of 400 avulsed permanent incisors. 2. Endod Dent Traumatol 1995; 11: 59–68.

26. ANDREASEN JO *et al*. Replantation of 400 avulsed permanent incisors. 4. Endod Dent Traumatol 1995; 11: 76–89.

27. ANDREASEN JO *et al*. Replantation of teeth. I. Acta Odontol Scand 1966; 24: 263–86.

28. ANDREASEN JO *et al*. Replantation of teeth. II. Acta Odont Scand 1966; 24: 287–306.

29. ANDREASEN JO *et al*. Intraalveolar root fractures. J Oral Surg 1967 25: 414–26.

30. ANDREASEN JO *et al.* The effect of limited drying or removal of the periodontal ligament. Acta Odontol Scand 1981; 39: 1–13.

31. ANDREASEN JO *et al.* Damage of the Hertwig's epithelial root sheath: effect upon root growth after autotransplantation of teeth in monkeys. Endod Dent Traumatol 1988; 4: 145–51.

32. ANDREASEN JO *et al.* A long-term study of 370 autotransplanted premolars. Part III. Eur J Orthod 1990; 12: 14–24.

33. ANIL N *et al.* Temperature change in the pulp chamber during application of heat to composite and amalgam cores and its returning time to oral heat. Int Dent J 1996; 46: 362–6.

34. ANNEROTH G *et al.* Periodontal ligament injection. Int J Oral Surg 1985; 14: 538–43.

35. ARMSTRONG C *et al.* Histopathology of the teeth in segmental odontomaxillary dysplasia: new findings. J Oral Pathol Med 2004; 33: 246–8.

36. ATRIZADEH F *et al.* Ankylosis of teeth following thermal injury. J Periodontol Res 1971; 6: 159–67.

37. AUKHIL I *et al.* Root resorption potentials of granulation tissue from bone and flap connective tissue. J Periodontol Res 1986; 21: 531–42.

38. AUKHIL I *et al.* An experimental study of new attachment procedure in beagle dogs. J Periodontol Res 1983; 18: 643–54.

39. AZAZ B *et al.* Resorption of the crown in impacted maxillary canine. Int J Oral Surg 1978; 7: 167–71.

40. BALDISSARA P *et al.* Clinical and histological evaluation of thermal injury thresholds in human teeth. J Oral Rehabil 1997; 24: 791–801.

41. BARBAKOW FH *et al.* Experimental replantation of root-canal-filled and untreated teeth in the velvet monkey. J Endod 1977 3: 89–93.

42. BARBAKOW FH *et al.* Histologic response of replanted teeth pretreated with acidulated sodium fluoride. Oral Surg 1978; 45: 621–8.

43. BARNETT F *et al.* Paget's disease of the mandible. Endod Dent Traumatol 1985; 1: 39–42.

44. BARRETT EJ *et al.* Avulsed permanent teeth. Endod Dent Traumatol 1997; 13: 153–63.

45. BARRETT EJ *et al.* Survival of avulsed permanent maxillary incisors in children following delayed replantation. Endod Dent Traumatol 1997; 13: 269–75.

46. BARTHEL CR *et al.* Resorptionen. Erscheinungsbild und Therapie. Endodontie 1996; 2: 143–56.

47. BAUMRIND S *et al.* Apical root resorption in orthodontically treated adults. Am J Orthod Dentofac Orthop 1996; 110: 311–20.

48. BEATTY RG *et al.* Thermomechanical compaction of gutta-percha. Int Endod J 1988; 21: 367–75.

49. BEAVERS RA *et al.* Periodontal wound healing following intentional root perforations in permanent teeth of Macaca mulatta. Int Endod J 1986; 19: 36–44.

50. BECK BW *et al.* Apical root resorption in orthodontically treated subjects: analysis of edgewise and light wire mechanics. Am J Orthod Dentofac Orthop 1994; 105: 350–61.

51. BECKS H. Histologic study of tooth structure in osteogenesis imperfecta. Dent Cosmos 1931; 73: 437–54.

52. BECKTOR KB *et al.* Segmental odontomaxillary dysplasia. Oral Dis 2002; 8: 106–10.

53. BEERTSEN W *et al.* Continuous growth of acellular extrinsic fiber cementum. Acta Med Dent Helv 1997; 2: 103–15.

54. BELANGER GK *et al.* Idiopathic external root resorption of the entire permanent dentition. ASDC J Dent Child 1985; 52: 359–63.

55. BENENATI FW. Root resorption: types and treatment. Gen Dent 1997; 45: 42–5.

56. BERGLUNDH T *et al.* Tissue characteristics of root resorption areas in transplanted maxillary canines. Acta Odontol Scand 1997; 55: 206–11.

57. BJORVATN K *et al.* Effect of fluorides on root resorption in replanted rat molars. Acta Odontol Scand 1971; 28: 17–29.

58. BJORVATN K *et al.* Effect of tetracycline and SnF_2 on root resorption in replanted incisors in dogs. Scand J Dent Res 1989; 97: 477–82.

59. BLAIR HC *et al.* Macrophage-mediated bone resorption occurs in an acidic environment. Calcif Tissue Int 1985; 37: 547–50.

60. BLOMLÖF L *et al.* Periodontal healing of exarticulated monkey teeth stored in milk or saliva. Scand J Dent Res 1981; 89: 251–9.

61. BLOMLÖF L *et al.* Periodontal healing of replanted monkey teeth prevented from drying. Acta Odontol Scand 1983; 41: 117–23.

62. BLOMLÖF L *et al.* Cervical root resorption associated with guided tissue regeneration. J Periodontol 1998; 69: 392–5.

63. BLOMLÖF L *et al.* Storage of experimentally avulsed teeth in milk prior to replantation. J Dent Res 1983; 62: 912–16.

64. BLOMLÖF L *et al.* Viability of human periodontal ligament cells after storage in milk or saliva. Scand J Dent Res 1980; 88: 436–40.

65. BOEKENOOGEN DI *et al.* The effects of exogenous prostaglandin E_2 on root resorption in rats. Am J Orthod Dentofac Orthop 1996; 109: 277–86.

66. BORAZ RA. Hypophosphatasia. J Pedod 1988 13: 44–52.

67. BOUYSSOU M *et al.* Les critéres radiologiques pour le diagnostic différentiel des processus de résorption intradentaires progressifs. Schweiz Monatschr Zahnheilkd 1957; 67: 319–41.

68. BOYD DH *et al.* A prospective study of factors affecting survival of replanted permanent incisors in children. Int J Paediatr Dent 2000; 10: 200–5.

69. BOYDE A *et al.* Resorption of dentine by isolated osteoclasts *in vitro.* Br Dent J 1984; 156: 216–20.

70. BOYDE A *et al.* Electron microscopy of resorbing surfaces of dental hard tissues. Zeitschr Zellforschung 1967; 83: 538–48.

71. BRADY J *et al.* Internal resorption complicating orthodontic tooth movement. Br J Orthod 1984; 11: 155–7.

72. BRAMANTE CM *et al.* Root perforations dressed with calcium hydroxide or zinc oxide and eugenol. J Endod 1987; 13: 392–5.

73. BRÄNNSTRÖM M *et al.* Periodontal tissue changes after intraligamentary anesthesia. ASDC J Dent Child 1982; 49: 417–23.

74. BREIVIK M *et al.* Histometric study of root resorption on human premolars following experimental replantation. Scand J Dent Res 1987; 95: 273–80.

75. BREZNIAK N *et al.* Root resorption after orthodontic treatment: part 1. Am J Orthod Dentofac Orthop 1993; 103: 62–6.

76. BREZNIAK N *et al.* Root resorption after orthodontic treatment: part 2. Am J Orthod Dentofac Orthop 1993; 103: 138–46.

77. BRISENO B *et al.* Rise in pulp temperature during finishing and polishing of resin composite restorations. Quint Int 1995 26: 361–5.

78. BROOKS JK. An unusual case of idiopathic internal root resorption beginning in an unerupted permanent tooth. J Endod 1986; 12: 309–10.

79. BRÖSJÖ M *et al.* An experimental model for cervical resorption in monkeys. Endod Dent Traumatol 1990; 6: 118–20.

80. BRUDVIK P *et al.* The repair of orthodontic root resorption: an ultrastructural study. Eur J Orthod 1995; 17: 189–98.

81. BRYSON EC *et al.* Effect of *immediate* intracanal placement of Ledermix Paste® on healing of replanted dog teeth after extended dry times. Dent Traumatol 2002; 18: 316–21.

82. BRYSON EC *et al.* Effect of minocycline on healing of replanted dog teeth after extended dry times. Dent Traumatol 2003; 19: 90–5.

83. BURGER EH *et al. In vitro* formation of osteoclasts from long-term cultures of bone marrow momonuclear phagocytes. J Exp Med 1982; 156: 1604–14.

84. BURGER EH *et al.* Cellular origin and theories of osteoclast differentiation. In: HALL BK. Bone. Volume 2. Boca Raton: CRC Press, 1991.

85. ÇALISKAN MK *et al.* Prognosis of permanent teeth with internal resorption: a clinical review. Endod Dent Traumatol 1997; 13: 75–81.

86. CAMERON JA. The endodontic management of a replanted avulsed tooth with severe root resorption. Int Endod J 1984; 17: 76–9.

87. CARTER L. Paget's disease: important features for the general practitioner. Compend Cointin Educ Dent 1990; 11: 662–9.

88. CARTER LC. Resorption of tooth substance: diagnosis and management. Compend Contin Educ Dent 1992; 13: 1008–15.

89. CASA MA *et al.* Root resorptions in upper first premolars after application of continuous torque moment. J Orofac Orthop 2001; 62: 285–95.

90. CHRISTIANSEN RL. Commentary: thyroxine administration and its effects on root resorption. Angle Orthod 1994 64: 399–400.

91. CLARK DB. Dental findings in patients with chronic renal failure. J Can Dent Assoc 1987; 53: 781–5.

92. CONKLIN WW. Long-term follow-up and evaluation of transplantation of fully developed teeth. Oral Surg 1978; 46: 477–85.

93. COPELAND S *et al.* Root resorption in maxillary central incisors following active orthodontic treatment. Am J Orthod 1986; 89: 51–5.

94. CORNELIUS CP *et al.* Replantationsergebnisse nach traumatischer Zahneluxation. Dtsch Zahnärtzl Z 1987; 42: 211–15.

95. COSTOPOULOS G *et al.* An evaluation of root resorption incident to orthodontic intrusion. Am J Orthod Dentofac Orthop 1996; 109: 543–8.

96. CRIGGER M *et al.* The effect of topical citric acid application on the healing of experimental furcation defects in dogs. J Periodontol Res 1978; 13: 538–49.

97. CVEK M *et al.* Pulp revascularization in reimplanted immature monkey incisors. Endod Dent Traumatol 1990; 6: 157–69.

98. CVEK M *et al.* External root resorption following bleaching of pulpless teeth with oxygen peroxide. Endod Dent Traumatol 1985; 1: 56–60.

99. CZOCHROWSKA EM *et al.* Outcome of tooth transplantation. Am J Orthod Dentofac Orthop 2002; 121: 110–19.

100. DAHLSTROM SW *et al.* Hydroxyl radical activity in thermo-catalytically bleached root-filled teeth. Endod Dent Traumatol 1997; 13: 119–25.

101. DARBAR UR *et al.* Multiple external root resorption. Aus Dent J 1993; 38: 433–5.

102. DÉRAND T. Mercury vapor from dental amalgams. Swed Dent J 1989; 13: 169–75.

103. DERMAUT LR *et al.* Apical root resorption of upper incisors caused by intrusive tooth movement. Am J Orthod Dentofac Orthop 1986; 90: 321–6.

104. DESHIELDS RW. A study of root resorption in treated Class II, division 1 malocclusions. Angle Orthod 1969; 39: 231–45.

105. DOMON T *et al.* Mononuclear odontoclast participation in tooth resorption. Anatom Record 1997; 249: 449–57.

106. DONALDSON M *et al.* Factors affecting the time of onset of resorption in avulsed and replanted incisor teeth in children. Dent Traumatol 2001; 17: 205–9.

107. DOYLE DL *et al.* Effect of soaking in Hank's balanced salt solution or milk on PDL cell viability of dry stored human teeth. Endod Dent Traumatol 1998; 14: 221–4.

108. DIJKMAM GEHM *et al.* Orthodontische behandeling en wortelresorptie. Ned Tijdschr Tandheelkd 1996; 103: 301–3.

109. DRAGOO MR *et al.* A clinical and histological evaluation of autogenous iliac bone grafts in humans. Part II. J Periodontol 1973; 44: 614–25.

110. DREYER WP *et al.* Hypothermic insult to the periodontium: a model for the study of aseptic tooth resorption. Endod Dent Traumatol 2000; 16: 9–15.

111. DREYER WP *et al.* The effect of citric acid on the healing of periodontal ligament–free, healthy roots, horizontally implanted against bone and gingival connective tissue. J Periodontol Res 1986; 21: 210–20.

112. DURR DP *et al.* Pulpal responses after the avulsion and replantation of permanent teeth. J Pedod 1987; 11: 301–10.

113. DUMSHA T *et al.* Evaluation of long-term calcium hydroxide treatment in avulsed teeth. Int Endod J 1995; 28: 7–11.

114. EBELESEDER KA *et al*. A study of replanted permanent teeth in different age groups. Endod Dent Traumatol 1998; 14: 274–8.

115. EBELESEDER KA *et al*. Externe Wurzelresorptionen nach Zahnluxation und Draht-Komposit-Schienung. Dtsch Zahnärztl Z 1997; 52: 22–7.

116. EBENSBERGER U *et al*. PCNA-expression of cementoblasts and fibroblasts on the root surface after extraoral rinsing for decontamination. Dent Traumatol 2002: 18: 262–6.

117. EL-BIALY T *et al*. Repair of orthodontically induced root resorption by ultrasound in humans. Am J Orthod Dentofac Orthop 2004; 126: 186–93.

118. ELIASSON S *et al*. Pathological changes related to long-term impaction of third molars. Int J Oral Maxillofac Surg 1989; 18: 210–12.

119. ELIASSON S *et al*. Autotransplanted teeth with early-stage endodontic treatment. Oral Surg Oral Med Oral Pathol 1988; 65: 598–603.

120. ENGSTROM C. Root resorptions during orthodontic tooth movement and bone remodeling dynamics during hypocalcaemia and treatment with bisphosphonate. In: DAVIDOVITCH Z (ed.) Biological mechanisms of tooth eruption and root resorption. Birmingham: EBSCO Media, 1988.

121. EPSTEIN JB *et al*. Maxillofacial manifestations of multiple myeloma. Oral Surg 1984; 57: 267–71.

122. ERAUSQUIN J *et al*. Alveolodental ankylosis induced by root canal treatment in rat molars. Oral Surg 1970; 30: 105–16.

123. ERICSON S *et al*. Radiographic examination of ectopically erupting maxillary canines. Am J Orthod Dentofac Orthop 1987; 91: 483–92.

124. ERICSON S *et al*. Incisor resorption caused by maxillary cuspids. Angle Orthod 1987; 57: 332–45.

125. FAYAD S *et al*. Root resorptions in a patient with hemifacial atrophy. J Endod 1994; 6: 299–303.

126. FIGDOR D *et al*. Heat generation in the McSpadden compaction technique. J Dent Res 1983; 62: 405.

127. FILIPPI A. Resorptionen der Zahnhartsubstanzen durch retinierte und verlagerte dritte Molaren. Quintessenz 1994; 45: 779–87.

128. FILIPPI A *et al*. Replantation of avulsed primary anterior teeth: treatment and limitations. ASDC J Dent Child 1997; 64: 272–5

129. FILIPPI A *et al*. Treatment of replacement resorption with Emdogain®. Dent Traumatol 2002; 18: 138–43.

130. FOLLIN ME *et al*. Occurrence and distribution of root resorption in orthodontically moved premolars in dogs. Angle Orthod 1986; 56: 164–75.

131. FORD GS *et al*. A case report of severe external resorption. J Can Dent Assoc 1994; 60: 503–10.

132. FORS U *et al*. Measurement of the root surface temperature during thermo-mechanical root canal filling *in vitro*. Int Endod J 1985; 18: 199–202.

133. FRANK AL. Inflammatory resorption caused by an adjacent necrotic tooth. J Endod 1990; 16: 339–41.

134. FRANK AL. Extracanal invasive resorption. Compend Contin Educ 1995; 16: 250–62.

135. FRANK AL *et al*. Nonsurgical therapy for the perforative defect of internal resorption. J Am Dent Assoc 1973; 87: 863–8.

136. FEINMAN RA *et al*. Bleaching teeth. Chicago, IL: Quintessence Publishing, 1987.

137. FRIEDMAN S. Internal bleaching. J Am Dent Assoc 1997; 128: 51S–8S.

138. FRIEDMAN S *et al*. Incidence of external root resorption and esthetic results in 58 bleached pulpless teeth. Endod Dent Traumatol 1988; 4: 23–6.

139. FUJIYAMA K *et al*. Denervation resulting in dento-alveolar ankylosis associated with decreased Malassez epithelium. J Dent Res 2004; 83: 625–9.

140. FUKS AB *et al*. Assessment of a 2% buffered glutaraldehyde solution in pulpotomized primary teeth of school children: a preliminary report. J Pedod 1986; 10: 323–30.

141. FUSS Z *et al*. Root resorption – diagnosis, classification and treatment choices based on stimulation factors. Dent Traumatol 2003; 19: 175–82.

142. GALILI D *et al*. Intraligamentary anesthesia. Int J Oral Surg 1984; 13: 511–16.

143. GARCIA RI *et al*. Internal resorption of an unerupted third molar. Spec Care Dent 1986; 6: 205–7.

144. GARTNER AH *et al*. Differential diagnosis of internal and external root resorption. J Endod 1976; 2: 329–34.

145. GASKELL PHF. A case of gross internal root resorption. Br Dent J 1979; 147: 126.

146. GEORGE DI *et al*. Idiopathic resorption of teeth. Am J Orthod 1986; 89: 13–20.

147. GERNER NW *et al*. External root resorption in patients with secondary bone-grafting of alveolar clefts. Endod Dent Traumatol 1986; 2: 263–6.

148. GIUNTA D *et al*. Influence of imdomethacin on bone turnover related to orthodontic tooth movement in miniature pigs. Am J Orthod Dentofac Orthop 1995; 108: 361–6.

149. GHOLSTON LR *et al*. An endodontic-orthodontic technique for esthetic stabilization of externally resorbed teeth. Am J Orthod 1983; 83: 435–40.

150. GLASS RT. Oral manifestations in primary hyperoxaluria and oxalosis. Oral Surg 1973; 35: 502–9.

151. GOLDIE RS *et al*. Root resorption and tooth movement in orthodontically treated, calcium-deficient, and lactating rats. Am J Orthod 1984; 85: 424–30.

152. GOLDMAN HM. Spontaneous intermittent resorption of teeth. J Am Dent Assoc 1954; 49: 522–32.

153. GOON WWY *et al*. External cervical root resorption following bleaching. J Endod 1986; 12: 414–18.

154. GOTTLOW J *et al*. Healing following citric acid conditioning of roots implanted into bone and gingival connective tissue. J Periodont Res 1984; 19: 214–220.

155. GOULTSCHIN J *et al*. Root resorption. Oral Surg 1982; 54: 586–90.

156. GRUNDY GE *et al*. Intra-coronal resorption of unerupted molars. Aust Dent J 1984; 29: 175–9.

157. GUPTA S *et al*. Suture splint: an alternative for luxation injuries of teeth in pediatric patients. J Clin Pediatr Dent 1997; 22: 19–21.

158. GUTMAN JL *et al*. Evaluation of heat transfer during root canal obturation with thermoplasticized gutta-percha. Part II. J Endod 1987; 13: 441–8.

159. HALL EH *et al.* Early, aggressive cemento-ossifying fibroma. Oral Surg 1987; 36: 132–6.

160. HAMMARSTRÖM LE *et al.* Effect of calcium hydroxide treatment on periodontal repair and root resorption. Endod Dent Traumatol 1986; 2: 184–9.

161. HAMMARSTRÖM L *et al.* Replantation of teeth and antibiotic treatment. Endod Dent Traumatol 1986; 2: 51–7.

162. HAMMARSTRÖM L *et al.* General morphological aspects of resorption of teeth and alveolar bone. Int Endod J 1985; 18: 93–108.

163. HAMMARSTRÖM L *et al.* Tooth avulsion and replantation. Endod Dent Traumatol 1986; 2: 1–8.

164. HANDELMAN CS. The anterior alveolus: its importance in limiting orthodontic treatment and its influence on the occurrence of iatrogenic sequelae. Angle Orthod 1996; 66: 95–110.

165. HARDIE EM. Heat transmission to the outer surface of the tooth during the thermo-mechanical compaction technique of root canal obturation. Int Endod J 1986; 19: 73–7.

166. HARDIE EM. Further studies on heat generation during obturation techniques involving thermally softened gutta-percha. Int Endod J 1987; 20: 122–7.

167. HARRINGTON GW *et al.* External resorption associated with bleaching of pulpless teeth. J Endod 1979; 5: 344–8.

168. HARRIS EF *et al.* Patterns of incisor root resorption before and after orthodontic correction in cases with anterior open bites. Am J Orthod Dentofac Orthop 1992; 101: 112–19.

169. HARRIS EF *et al.* An analysis of causes of apical root resorption in patients not treated orthodontically. Quint Int 1993; 24: 417–28.

170. HARRIS EF *et al.* A heritable component for external apical resorption in patients treated orthodontically. Am J Orthod Dentofac Orthop 1997; 111: 301–9.

171. HARRY MR *et al.* Root resorption in bicuspid intrusion. Angle Orthod 1982; 52: 235–58.

172. HARVEY BLC *et al.* Root surface resorption of periodontally diseased teeth. Oral Surg 1959; 12: 1439–43.

173. HEDEMARK A *et al.* Dental and jaw changes in primary hyperoxaluria. J Oral Pathol Med 1989; 18: 586–9.

174. HEIMDAHL A *et al.* Replantation of avulsed teeth after long extra-alveolar periods. Int J Oral Surg 1983; 12: 413–17.

175. HEITHERSAY GS. Replantation of avulsed teeth. Aust Dent J 1975; 20: 63–72.

176. HEITHERSAY GS *et al.* Tissue responses in the rat to tricholacetic acid – an agent used in the treatment of invasive cervical resorption. Aust Dent J 1988; 33: 451–61.

177. HEITHERSAY GS. Clinical, radiologic, and histopathologic features of invasive cervical resorption. Quint Int 1999; 30: 27–37.

178. HEITHERSAY GS. Invasive cervical resorption: an analysis of potential predisposing factors. Quint Int 1999; 30: 83–95.

179. HEITHERSAY GS. Treatment of invasive cervical resorption: an analysis of results using topical application of tricholoacetic acid, curettage, and restoration. Quint Int 1999; 30: 96–110.

180. HELLER D *et al.* Effect of intracoronal bleaching on external cervical root resorption. J Endod 1992; 18: 145–8.

181. HENDRIX I *et al.* A radiographic study of posterior apical root resorption in orthodontic patients. Am J Orthod Dentofac Orthop 1994; 105: 345–9.

182. HENEFER EP. Root resorption by an impacted tooth. Oral Surg 1968; 26: 658.

183. HENRY JL *et al.* The pattern of resorption and repair of human cementum. J Am Dent Assoc 1951; 42: 270–90.

184. HERR P *et al.* Mantle dentine in man. J Biol Buccale 1986; 14: 139–46.

185. HICKS MJ *et al.* Formocresol pulpotomies in primary molars: a radiographic study in a pediatric dentistry practice. J Pedod 1986; 10: 331–9.

186. HICKS MJ *et al.* External root resorption of a primary molar. Oral Surg Oral Med Oral Pathol Oral Radiol Endod 2001; 92: 4–8.

187. HILL FJ. Iatrogenic root resorption of upper first permanent molars associated with orthodontic treatment. Br J Orthod 1987; 14: 109–13.

188. HOKETT SD *et al.* Inflammatory cervical root resorption following segmental orthognathic surgery. J Periodontol 1998; 69: 219–26.

189. HOLAN G. Idiopathic internal resorption followed by calcification deposits in primary molars. Int J Paediatr Dent 1998; 8: 213–17.

190. HOLAN G *et al.* Pre-eruptive coronal resorption of permanent teeth. Pediatr Dent 1994; 16(5): 373–7.

191. HOLCOMB JB *et al.* Endodontic treatment modalities for external root resorption associated with impacted mandibular third molars. J Endod 1983; 9: 335–7.

192. HOLMSTRUP G *et al.* Bleaching of discoloured root-filled teeth. Endod Dent Traumatol 1988; 4: 197–201.

193. HOPKINS R *et al.* Multiple idiopathic resorption of the teeth. Br Dent J 1979; 146: 309–12.

194. HOSSEINI AA. A clinical evaluation of root resorption by formocresol treatment in 120 cases of pulpotomy in permanent molars. J Clin Pediatr Dent 1992; 17: 11–13.

195. HOUSTON F *et al.* Healing after root reimplantation in the monkey. J Clin Periodontol 1985; 12: 716–27.

196. HOVINGA J. Autotransplantatie van kiemen van derde molaren. Resultaten van voortgezette observatie. Ned Tijdschr Tandheelkd 1986; 93: 235–7.

197. HUPP JG *et al.* Periodontal ligament vitality and histologic healing of teeth stored for extended periods before transplantation. Endod Dent Traumatol 1998; 14: 79–83.

198. HUSSEY DL *et al.* Thermographic measurement of temperature change during resin composite polymerization *in vivo.* J Dent 1995; 23: 267–71.

199. HUSSEY DL *et al.* Thermographic assessment of heat generated on the root surface during post space preparation. Int Endod J 1997; 30: 187–90.

200. HUTTON CE. Intradental lesions and their reversal in a patient being treated for end–stage renal disease. Oral Surg 1985; 60: 258–61.

201. IBBOTT CG. Root resorption associated with placement of a ceramic implant. J Periodontol 1985; 56: 419–21.

202. IGNELZI MA *et al.* Intracoronal radiolucencies within unerupted teeth. Oral Surg Oral Med Oral Pathol 1990; 70: 214–20.

203. IGARASHI K *et al*. Inhibitory effect of topical administration of bisphosphonate (risedronate) on root resorption incident to orthodontic tooth movement in rats. J Dent Res 1994; 75: 1644–9.

204. ITO K *et al*. Root resorption associated with hydroxyapatite particles. Quint Int 1995; 26: 377–83.

205. JIMÉNEZ-RUBIO A *et al*. The effect of the bleaching agent sodium perborate on macrophage adhesion *in vitro*: implications in external cervical root resorption. J Endod 1998; 24: 229–32.

206. JIMENEZ-PELLEGRIN C *et al*. Root resorption in human mandibular first premolars after rotation as detected by scanning electron microscopy. Am J Orthod Dentofac Orthop 2004; 126: 178–85.

207. JOHNSON WT *et al*. Replantation of avulsed teeth with immature root development. Oral Surg 1985; 60: 420–7.

208. JONES ML *et al*. Tooth resorption in the two-stage transplantation technique. Br J Orthod 1983; 10: 157–8.

209. JONES SJ *et al*. The resorption of dentine and cementum *in vivo* and *in vitro*. In: DAVIDOVITCH Z (ed.) Biological mechanisms of tooth eruption and root resorption. Birmingham: EBSCO Media, 1988.

210. JONSSON T *et al*. Autotransplantation of premolar to premolar sites. A long-term follow-up study of 40 consecutive patients. Am J Orthod Dentofac Orthop 2004; 125: 668–75.

211. KAFFE I *et al*. A radiographic survey of apical root resorption in pulpless permanent teeth. Oral Surg 1984; 58: 109–12.

212. KAHNBERG K-E. Autotransplantation of teeth. (I). Int J Oral Maxillofac Surg 1987; 16: 577–85.

213. KALEY J *et al*. Factors related to root resorption in edgewise practice. Angle Orthod 1991; 61: 125–32.

214. KALKWARF KL *et al*. Effect of apical root resorption on periodontal support. J Prosthet Dent 1986; 56: 317–19.

215. KARRING T *et al*. Potentials for root resorption during periodontal wound healing. J Clin Periodontol 1984; 11: 41–52.

216. KARSTEN J *et al*. Effect of phenytoin on periodontal tissues exposed to orthodontic force. Br J Orthod 1997; 24: 209–15.

217. KEHOE JC. pH reversal following *in vitro* bleaching of pulpless teeth. J Endod 1987; 13: 6–9.

218. KEIL A, SPETH-ESCHENBRENNER J. Über Zahnanomalien bei 3400 Patienten nach Röntgenstaten. Dtsch Zahn Mund Kieferheilkd 1963; 40: 360–76.

219. KEMP WB *et al*. Evaluation of 71 replanted teeth. J Endod 1977; 3: 30–5.

220. KENNY DJ *et al*. Avulsions and intrusions: the controversial displacement injuries. J Can Dent Assoc 2003; 69: 308–13.

221. KENWOOD M *et al*. Sequelae of trauma to the primary dentition. J Pedod 1989; 13: 230–8.

222. KERR DA *et al*. Multiple idiopathic root resorption. Oral Surg 1970; 29: 552–65.

223. KIM PH *et al*. Multiple idiopathic resorption in the primary dentition. Oral Surg Oral Med Oral Pathol Oral Radiol Endod 1999; 88: 501–5.

224. KINERET SE. Heritability of external apical root resorption in orthodontically treated siblings. Am J Orthod Dentofac Orthop 1996; 109: 106.

225. KING GJ *et al*. The effect of force magnitude on extractable bone resorptive activity and cemental cratering in orthodontic tooth movement. J Dent Res 1982; 61: 775–9.

226. KINIRONS MJ *et al*. Inflammatory and replacement resorption in reimplanted permanent incisor teeth. Endod Dent Traumatol 1999; 15: 269–72.

227. KINIRONS MJ *et al*. Variations in the presenting and treatment features in reimplanted permanent incisors in children and their effect on the prevalence of root resorption. Br Dent J 2000; 189: 263–6.

228. KINOMOTO Y *et al*. Internal root resorption associated with inadequate caries removal and orthodontic therapy. J Endod 2002; 28: 405–7.

229. KLING M *et al*. Rate and predictability of pulp revascularization in therapeutically reimplanted permanent incisors. Endod Dent Traumatol 1986; 2: 83–9.

230. KNIGHT H. Tooth resorption associated with the eruption of maxillary canines. Br J Orthod 1987; 14: 21–31.

231. KOCH H *et al*. Indications for surgical removal of supernumerary teeth in the premaxilla. Int J Oral Maxillofac Surg 1986; 15: 273–81.

232. KOGON SL *et al*. Hemifacial hypertrophy affecting the maxillary dentition. Oral Surg 1984; 58: 549–53.

233. KOJIMA R *et al*. External root resorption of the maxillary permanent incisors cause by ectopically erupting canines. J Clin Pediatr Dent 2002; 26: 193–7.

234. KOULAOUZIDOU E *et al*. Role of cementoenamel junction on the radicular penetration of 30% hydrogen peroxide during intracoronal bleaching *in vitro*. Endod Dent Traumatol 1996; 12: 146–50.

235. KRISTERSON L. Autotransplantation of human premolars. A clinical and radiographic study of 100 teeth. Int J ORal Surg 1985; 14: 200–13.

236. KRISTERSON L *et al*. Influence of root development on periodontal and pulpal healing after replantation of incisors in monkeys. Int J Oral Surg 1984; 13: 313–23.

237. KUROL J *et al*. Hyalinization and root resorption during early othodontic tooth movement in adolescents. Angle Orthod 1998; 68: 161–5.

238. KUROL J *et al*. Resorption of maxillary second primary molars caused by ectopic eruption of the maxillary first permanent molar. ASDC J Dent Child 1982; 49: 273–9.

239. KUROL J *et al*. Time-related root resorption after application of a controlled continuous orthodontic force. Am J Orthod Dentofac Orthop 1996; 110: 303–10.

240. L'ABEE EM *et al*. Apical root resorption during Begg treatment. J Clin Orthod 1985; 19: 60–1.

241. LADO EA *et al*. Cervical resorption in bleached teeth. Oral Surg 1983; 55: 78–80.

242. LADO EA. Bleaching of endodontically treated teeth: an update on cervical resorption. Gen Dent 1988; 36: 500–1.

243. LAMBRECHT JT. Antibiotische Prophylaxe unde Therapie. Schweiz Monatschr Zahnmed 2004; 114: 601–7.

244. LANGELAND K. The histopathologic basis in endodontic treatment. Dent Clin North Am 1967; 11: 515.

245. LANGFORD SR. Root resorption extremes resulting from clinical RME. Am J Orthod 1982; 81: 371–7.

246. LANGORD SR et al. Root surface resorption, repair, and periodontal attachment following rapid maxillary expansion in man. Am J Orthod 1982; 81: 108–15.

247. LANTZ B et al. Periodontal tissue reactions after surgical treatment of root perforations in dogs' teeth. Odont Revy 1970; 21: 51–62.

248. LAPOINTE HJ et al. Oral manifestations of oxalosis secondary to ileojejunal intestinal bypass. Oral Surg Oral Med Oral Pathol 1988; 65: 76–80.

249. LATCHAM NL. Postbleaching cervical resorption. J Endod 1986; 12: 262–4.

250. LATCHAM NL. Management of a patient with severe postbleaching cervical resorption. A clinical report. J Prosthet Dent 1991; 65: 603–5.

251. LEE A et al. Root resorption: the possible role of extracellular matrix proteins. Am J Orthod Dentofac Orthop 2004; 126: 173–7.

252. LEKIC PC et al. The influence of storage conditions on the clonogenic capacity of periodontal ligament cells. Int Endod J 1998; 31: 137–40.

253. LESAR CG et al. Tooth transplantation with the periodontium intact: a histometric analysis. Am J Orthod 1984; 85: 260–6.

254. LEVANDER E et al. Early radiographic diagnosis of apical root resorption during orthodontic treatment. Eur J Orthod 1998; 20: 57–63.

255. LEVANDER E et al. Evaluation of the risk of root resorption during orthodontic treatment. Eur J Orthod 1988; 10: 30–8.

256. LEVANDER et al. Evaluation of root resorption in relation to two orthodontic treatment regimes. Eur J Orthod 1994; 16: 223–8.

257. LINDHE J. Textbook of clinical periodontology. Copenhagen: Munksgaard, 1989.

258. LINDSKOG S et al. Evidence in favour of an anti-invasion factor in cementum or periodontal membrane of human teeth. Scand J Dent Res 1980; 88: 161–3.

259. LINDSKOG S et al. Repair of periodontal tissues in vivo and in vitro. J Clin Periodontol 1983; 10: 188–205.

260. LINDSKOG S et al. Cellular colonization of denuded root surfaces in vivo: cell morphology in dentin resorption and cementum repair. J Clin Periodontol 1987; 14: 390–5.

261. LINDSKOG S et al. Comparative effects of parathyroid hormone on osteoblasts and cementoblasts. J Clin Periodontol 1987; 14: 386–9.

262. LINDSKOG S et al. Influence of osmolality and composition of some storage media on human periodontal ligament cells. Acta Odontol Scand 1982; 40: 435–41.

263. LINDSKOG S et al. Chlorhexidine as a root canal medicament for treating inflammatory lesions in the periodontal space. Endod Dent Traumatol 1998; 14: 186–90.

264. LINGE L et al. Patient characteristics and treatment variables associated with apical root resorption during orthodontic treatment. Am J Orthod Dentofac Orthop 1991; 99: 35–43.

265. LIPSKI M. Root surface temperature rises in vitro during root canal obturation with thermoplasticized gutta-percha on a carrier or by injection. J Endod 2004; 30: 441–3.

266. LOBERG EL et al. Thyroid administration to reduce root resorption. Angle Orthod 1994; 64: 395–9.

267. LOË H et al. Experimental replantation of teeth in dogs and monkeys. Arch Oral Biol 1961; 3: 176–228.

268. LU LH et al. Histological and histochemical quantification of root resorption incident to the application of intrusive force to rat molars. Eur J Orthod 1999; 21: 57–63.

269. LUPI JE et al. Prevalence and severity of apical root resorption and alveolar bone loss in orthodontically treated adults. Am J Orthod Dentofac Orthop 1996; 109: 28–37.

270. LYDIATT DD et al. Multiple idiopathic root resorption. Oral Surg Oral Med Oral Pathol 1989; 67: 208–10.

271. LYROUDIA KM et al. Internal root resorption studied by radiography, microscope and computerized 3D reconstructive method. Dent Traumatol 2002; 18: 148–52.

272. MACKIE IC et al. An investigation of replantation of traumatically avulsed permanent incisor teeth. Br Dent J 1992; 172: 17–20.

273. MACKIE IC et al. Investigation of the children referred to a dental hospital with avulsed permanent incisor teeth. Endod Dent Traumatol 1993; 9: 106–10.

274. MADISON S et al. Cervical root resorption following bleaching of endodontically treated teeth. J Endod 1990; 16: 570–4.

275. MAGNUSSON B. Therapeutic pulpotomy in primary molars. I. Calcium hydroxide paste as wound dressing. Odontol Revy 1970; 21: 415–31.

276. MAGNUSSON B. Therapeutic pulpotomy in primary molars II. Zinc Oxide-eugenol as wound dressing. Odontol Revy 1971; 22: 45–54.

277. MAGNUSSON I et al. Root resorption following periodontal flap procedures in monkeys. J Periodontol Res 1985; 20: 79–85.

278. MAKKES PCH. Wortelresorptie aan de tweede molaren onder invloed van opdringende derde molaren. Ned Tijdschr Tandheelkd 1973; 80: 163–7.

279. MAKKES PC et al. Cervicale externe wortelsresorptie. Ned Tijdschr Tandheelkd 1977; 84: 158–62.

280. MALMGREN B et al. Surgical treatment of ankylosed and infrapositioned reimplanted incisors in adolescents. Scand J Dent Res 1984; 92: 391–9.

281. MALMGREN O et al. Root resorption after orthodontic treatment of traumatized teeth. Am J Orthod 1982; 82: 487–91.

282. MALTHA JC et al. Incidence and severity of root resorption in orthodontically moved premolars in dogs. Orthod Craniofac Res 2004; 7: 115–21.

283. MARCUSSON KAM et al. Autotransplantation of premolars and molars in patients with tooth aplasia. J Dent 1996; 24: 355–8.

284. MARKS SC Jr. The origin of osteoclasts: evidence, clinical implications and investigative challenges of an extraskeletal source. J Pathol 1983; 12: 226–56.

285. MARTIN DM. The management of root resorption in replanted and transplanted teeth. Int Endod J 1983; 16: 156–66.

286. MARTINS WD et al. Tooth replantation after traumatic avulsion. Dent Traumatol 2004; 20: 101–5.

287. MATUSOW RJ. Clinical observations regarding the treatment of traumatically avulsed mature teeth. Oral Surg 1985; 60: 94–9 and 428–35.

288. MASSLER M et al. Root resorption in human permanent teeth. Am J Orthod 1954; 40: 619–33.

289. MASSLER M et al. Root resorption in the permanent teeth of young adults. ASDC J Dent Child 1954; 21: 158–64.

290. McCORMICK JE et al. Tissue pH of developing periapical lesions in dogs. J Endodont 1983; 9: 47–52.

291. McCULLAGH JJP et al. Thermographic assessment of root canal obturation using thermomechanical compaction. Int Endod J 1997; 30: 191–5.

292. McFADDEN WM et al. A study of the relationship between incisor intrusion and root shortening. Am J Orthod Dentofac Orthop 1989; 96: 390–6.

293. McNABB S et al. External apical root resorption of posterior teeth in asthmatics after orthodontic treatment. Am J Orthod Dentofac Orthop 1999; 116: 545–51.

294. MEISTER F Jr et al. Treatment of external resorption by a combined endodontic-periodontic procedure. J Endod 1986; 12: 542–5.

295. MELCHER AH. Repair of wounds in the periodontium. Arch Oral Biol 1970; 15: 1183–206.

296. MICHAILESCO PM et al. An in vivo recording of variations in oral temperature during meals: a pilot study. J Prosthet Dent 1995; 73: 214–18.

297. MIDDLETON CT et al. Histologic evaluation of cementogenesis on periodontitis-affected roots in humans. Int J Periodont Rest Dent 1990; 10: 429–35.

298. MIRABELLA AD et al. Risk factors for apical root resorption of maxillary anterior teeth in adult orthodontic patients. Am J Orthod Dentofac Orthop 1995; 108: 48–55.

299. MIRABELLA AD et al. Prevalence and severity of apical root resorption of maxillary anterior teeth in adult orthodontic patients. Eur J Orthod 1995; 17: 93–9.

300. MOCK ES et al. Rapidly progressing extracanal invasive resorption. Gen Dent 1997; 45: 66–7.

301. MONSOUR FNT. Pulpal changes following the reimplantation of teeth in dogs: a histological study. Aust Dent J 1971; 16: 227–31.

302. MONSOUR FNT et al. Responses of periodontal tissues and cementum following transplantation of teeth. J Oral Maxillofac Surg 1984; 42: 441–6.

303. MONTGOMERY S. External cervical resorption after bleaching a pulpless tooth. Oral Surg 1984; 57: 203–6.

304. MOODY AB. Multiple idiopathic external resorption of teeth. Int J Oral Maxillofac Surg 1990; 19: 200–2.

305. MOODY GH et al. Multiple idiopathic root resorption. J Clin Periodontol 1991; 18: 577–80.

306. MORLEY BS et al. Analysis of functional splinting upon autologously reimplanted teeth. J Dent Res 1978; 57 (spec. issue A): 223.

307. MOSKOW BS. Periodontal manifestations of hyperoxaluria and oxalosis. J Periodontol 1989; 60: 271–8.

308. MOULE AJ et al. Cervical external root resorption following trauma. Int Endod J 1985; 18: 277–81.

309. MOUNT GJ. Idiopathic internal resorption. Oral Surg 1972; 33: 801–9.

310. MUMMERY JH. Some further cases of chronic perforating hyperplasia of the pulp (the so-called "pink spot"). Br Dent J 1926; 47: 801–11.

311. MURPHY J et al. Atypical central neurilemmoma of the mandible. Oral Surg 1984; 59: 275–8.

312. MYRLUND S et al. Root length in transplanted premolars. Acta Odontol Scand 2004; 62: 132–6.

313. NAIR PNR. Pathogenesis of apical periodontitis and the causes of endodontic failures. Crit Rev Oral Biol Med 2004; 15: 348–81.

314. NAKAMURA I et al. Chemical and physical properties of the extracellular matrix are required for the active ring formation in osteoclasts. J Bone Miner Res 1996; 11: 1873–9.

315. NAKANE S et al. Root resorption caused by mechanical injury of the periodontal soft tissues in rats. J Periodontol Res 1987; 22: 390–5.

316. NALBANDIAN J et al. Direct histological comparison of periodontal wound healing in the beagle dog with and without citric acid conditioning. J Periodontol Res 1982; 17: 552–62.

317. NASJLETI CE et al. The effects of different splinting times on replantation of teeth in monkeys. Oral Surg 1982; 53: 557–66.

318. NATIELLA JR et al. The replantation and transportation of teeth. Oral Surg 1970; 29: 397–419.

319. NEDIR R et al. Recurrent peripheral giant cell granuloma associated with cervical resorption. J Periodontol 1997; 68: 381–4.

320. NEMCOVSKY CE et al. Effect of non-erupted third molars on roots of approximal teeth. J Oral Pathol Med 1997; 26: 464–9.

321. NETHANDER G et al. Autogenous free tooth transplantation in man by a 2-stage operation technique. A longitudinal intra-individual radiographic assessment. Int J Oral Maxillofac Surg 1988; 17: 330–6.

322. NEVINS AJ et al. Replantation of enzymatically treated teeth in monkeys. Part I. Oral Surg 1980; 50: 277–81.

323. NICKEL AA et al. Internal resorption of four bony impacted third molars. Oral Surg 1980; 49: 187.

324. NISHIOKA M et al. Tooth replantation in germ-free and conventional rats. Endod Dent Traumatol 1998; 14: 163–73.

325. NITZAN D et al. Does an impacted tooth cause root resorption of the adjacent one? Oral Surg 1981; 51: 221–4.

326. ODENRICK L et al. Nailbiting: frequency and association with root resorption during orthodontic treatment. Br J Orthod 1985; 12: 78–81.

327. OGUCHI H. In vitro studies of bone resorption by the root resorbing tissue from the bovine deciduous tooth. Bull Tokyo Med Dent Univ 1975; 22: 175–83.

328. OIKARINEN K. Replacing resorbed maxillary central incisors with mandibular premolars. Endod Dent Dent Traumatol 1990; 6: 43–6.

329. ORBAN B. The epithelial network in the periodontal membrane. J Am Dent Assoc 1952; 44: 632–5.

330. OSHIRO T et al. Immunolocalization of vacuolar-type H^+-ATPase. Cathepsin K, matrix metalloproteinase-9, and receptor activator of Nfkappa ligand in odontoclasts

during physiological root resorption of human deciduous teeth. Anat Rec 2001; 264: 305–11.

331. OSWALD RJ *et al*. A postreplantation evaluation of air-dried and saliva-stored avulsed teeth. J Endod 1980; 6: 546–51.

332. OTTL P *et al*. Temperature response in the pulpal chamber during ultrahigh-speed tooth preparation with diamond burs of different grit. J Prosthet Dent 1998; 80: 12–19.

333. OWMAN-MOLL P *et al*. Continuous versus interrupted continuous orthodontic force related to early tooth movement and root resorption. Angle Orthod 1995A; 65: 395–402.

334. OWMAN-MOLL P *et al*. Repair of orthodontically induced root resorption in adolescents. Angle Orthod 1995; 65: 403–8.

335. OWMAN-MOLL P *et al*. Effects of a doubled orthodontic force magnitude on tooth movement and root resorptions. Eur J Orthod 1996; 18: 141–50.

336. OWMAN-MOLL P *et al*. The effects of a four-fold increased orthodontic force magnitude on tooth movement and root resorptions. Eur J Orthod 1996; 18: 287–94.

337. PACKOTA GV *et al*. Radiographic features of segmental odontomaxillary dysplasia: study of 12 cases. Oral Surg Oral Med Oral Pathol Oral Radiol Endod 1996; 82: 577–84.

338. PANKHURST CL *et al*. Multiple idiopathic external root resorption. Oral Surg Oral Med Oral Pathol 1988; 65: 754–6.

339. PARKER WS. Root resorption – long term outcome. Am J Orthod Dentofac Orthop 1997; 112: 119–23.

340. PERETZ B *et al*. Early root resorption of maxillary primary first molars in a child with severe congenital heart disease. J Clin Pediatr Dent 1997; 21: 163–6.

341. PERTOT W-J *et al*. Bone and root resorption. Effects of the force developed during periodontal ligament injections in dogs. Oral Surg Oral Med Oral Pathol 1992; 74: 357–65.

342. PETERS LB. Endodontic infections and apical periodontitis. Thesis, University of Amsterdam, Amsterdam, 2002.

343. PETERSON JE *et al*. Cementum and epithelial attachment response to the sulcular and periodontal ligament injection techniques. Pediatr Dent 1983; 5: 257–60.

344. PETTIETE M *et al*. Periodontal healing of extracted dog's teeth air-dried for extended periods and soaked in various media. Endod Dent Traumatol 1997; 13: 113–18.

345. PHILLIPS JR. Apical root resorption under orthodontic therapy. Angle Orthod 1955; 25: 1–22.

346. PINDBORG JJ. Pathology of the dental hard tissues. Copenhagen: Munksgaard, 1970.

347. POHL Y *et al*. Nachuntersuchung zur intentionalen auto-alloplastischen Reimplantation pulpatoter wurzelunreifer Frontzähne. Dtsch Zahnärztl Z 1997; 52: 180–5.

348. POSTLETHWAITE KR *et al*. Multiple idiopathic external root resorption. Oral Surg Oral Med Oral Pathol 1989; 68: 640–3.

349. POUMPROS E *et al*. Thyroid function and root resorption. Angle Orthod 1994; 64; 389–93.

350. POVOLNY B. Commentary: thyroid function and root resorption. Angle Orthod 1994; 64: 394.

351. PROYE MP *et al*. Effect of root surface alterations on periodontal healing. I. Surgical denudation. J Clin Periodontol 1982; 9: 428–40.

352. PRUSACK N *et al*. Segmental odontomaxillary dysplasia. A case report and review of the literature. Oral Surg Oral Med Oral Pathol Oral Radiol Endod 2000; 90: 483–8.

353. RABINOWITCH BZ. Internal resorption. Oral Surg 1972; 33: 263–82.

354. RAHIMA MM *et al*. Primary hyperoxaluria in a pediatric dental patient. Pediatr Dent 1992; 14: 260–2.

355. RANKOW H *et al*. Preeruptive idiopathic coronal resorption of permanent teeth in children. J Endod 1986; 12: 36–9.

356. REICHART PA. ^{224}Ra-induced dental resorptions. Oral Surg 1982; 54: 281–4.

357. REMINGTON DN *et al*. Long-term evaluation of root resorption occurring during orthodontic treatment. Am J Orthod Dentofac Orthop 1989; 96: 43–6.

358. REUKERS EAJ *et al*. Radiographic evaluation of apical root resorption with 2 different types of edgewise appliances. Results of a randomized clinical trial. J Orthofac Orthop 1998; 59: 100–9.

359. RINDERER LA. Zur unterminierenden Resorption der zweiten Milchmolaren beim Durchbruch der 6-Jahr-Molaren. Schweiz Monatschr Zahnmed 1984; 94: 471–97.

360. ROBERTS MW. Multiple familial dental anomalies. ASDC J Dent Child 1973; 40: 482–3.

361. RODRIGUEZ-PATO RB. Root resorption in chronic periodontitis: a morphometrical study. J Periodontol 2004; 75: 1027–32.

362. ROMERO CJ. Root resorption of second molar related to impacted third molar. Oral Surg 1971; 32: 502.

363. ROSENBERG EH *et al*. Hyperparathyroidism. A review of 220 proved cases with special emphasis on findings in the jaws. Oral Surg 1962; 15: 84–94.

364. ROTSTEIN I *et al*. Effect of cementum defects on radicular penetration of 30% H_2O_2 during intracoronal bleaching. J Endod 1991; 17: 230–3.

365. ROTSTEIN I *et al*. Effect of bleaching agents on inorganic components of human dentin and cementum. J Endod 1992; 18: 290–3.

366. RUBEL I. Atypical root resorption of maxillary primary central incisors due to digital sucking: a report of 82 cases. ASDC J Dent Child 1986; 53: 201–4.

367. RUBIN PL *et al*. Experimental tooth ankylosis in the monkey. Angle Orthod 1984; 54: 67–72.

368. RUNE B *et al*. Root resorption and submergence in retained deciduous second molars. Europ J Orthod 1984; 6: 123–31.

369. RYGH P. Orthodontic root resorption studied by electron microscopy. Angle Orthod 1977; 47: 1–16.

370. SAE-LIM V *et al*. Local dexamethasone improves periodontal healing of replanted dogs' teeth. Endod Dent Traumatol 1998; 14: 232–6.

371. SAGNE S *et al*. Transalveolar transplantation of maxillary canines. A follow-up study. Eur J Orthod 1990; 12: 140–7.

372. SALAMA F *et al*. Successive internal resorption. J Pedod 1990; 14: 165–8.

373. SAMESHIMA GT *et al*. Predicting and preventing root resorption: Part I. Diagnostic features. Am J Orthod Dentofac Orthop 2001; 119: 505–10.

374. SAMESHIMA GT *et al*. Predicting and preventing root resorption: Part II. Am J Orthod Dentofac Orthop 2001; 119: 511–15.

375. SAROFF SA *et al*. External tooth resorption following periodontal ligament injection. J Oral Med 1986; 41: 201–3.

376. SASAKI T. Differentiation and functions of osteoclasts and odontoclasts in mineralized tissue resorption. Microsc Res Tech 2003; 61: 483–95.

377. SASAKI T *et al*. Possible role of cementoblasts in resorbant organ of human deciduous teeth during root resorption. J Periodontol Res 1990; 25: 143–51.

378. SASSAKURA H *et al*. Root resorption of upper permanent incisor caused by impacted canine. Int J Oral Surg 1984; 13: 299–306.

379. SAUNDERS ME. *In vivo* findings associated with heat generation during thermo-mechanical compaction of gutta percha. Part II. Histological response to temperature elevation on the external surface of the root. Int Endod J 1990; 23: 268–74.

380. SAVAGE NW *et al*. Preeurptive intracoronal radiolucencies. ASDC J Dent Child 1998; 65: 36–40.

381. SCHATZ JP *et al*. A retrospective clinical and radiographic study of teeth re-implanted following traumatic avulsion. Endod Dent Traumatol 1995; 11: 235–9.

382. SCHROEDER HE. Pathobiologie oraler Strukturen. Basel: Karger, 1983.

383. SCHROEDER HE *et al*. Focal root resorption lacunae causing retention of subgingival plaque in periodontal pockets. Acta Parodontol 1983; 12: 1033–41.

384. SCHRÖDER U. Effect of an extra-pulpal blood clot on healing following experimental pulpotomy and capping with calcium hydroxide. Odontol Revy 1973; 24: 257–68.

385. SCHRÖDER U. A 2-year follow-up of primary molars, pulpotomized with a gentle technique and capped with calcium hydroxide. Scand J Dent Res 1978; 86: 273–8.

386. SCHRÖDER U *et al*. A one-year follow-up of partial pulpotomy and calcium hydroxide capping in primary molars. Endod Dent Traumatol 1987; 3: 304–6.

387. SCHWARTZ O *et al*. Cryopreservation of mature teeth before replantation in monkeys. Int J Oral Surg 1983; 12: 425–36.

388. SEDDON RP *et al*. Early arrested development and coronal resorption of an impacted maxillary canine. ASDC J Dent Child 1996; 63: 208–12.

389. SEALE NS *et al*. Pulpal response to bleaching of teeth in dogs. Pediatr Dent 1985; 7: 209–14.

390. SEOW WK. Diagnosis and management of unusual dental abscesses in children. Aust Dent J 2003; 48: 156–68.

391. SHAFER WG *et al*. A textbook of oral pathology. Philadelphia, PA: WB Saunders, 1983.

392. SHARPE MS. Internal resorption in a deciduous incisor. J Am Dent Assoc 1970; 81: 947–8.

393. SHAW L *et al*. Size and development of the dentition in endocrine deficiency. J Pedod 1989; 13: 155–60.

394. SILVERMAN S *et al*. The dental structures in primary hyperparathyroidism. Oral Surg 1962; 15: 426–35.

395. SIMON BI *et al*. The destructive potential of electrosurgery on the periodontium. J Periodontol 1976; 47: 342–7.

396. SINGER S *et al*. Idiopathic coronal radiolucencies in unerupted permanent teeth. Aust Dent J 1991; 36: 32–7.

397. SISMANIDOU C *et al*. Healing of the root surface-associated periodontium: an immunohistochemical study of orthodontic root resorption in man. Eur J Orthod 1996; 18: 435–44.

398. SKAFF DM *et al*. Lesions resembling caries in unerupted teeth. Oral Surg 1978; 45: 643–6.

399. SKOGLUND A *et al*. A microangiographic study of vascular changes in replanted and autotransplanted immature teeth of dogs. Oral Surg 1978; 45: 17–28.

400. SLAGSVOLD O *et al*. Indications for autotransplantation in cases of missing premolars. Am J Orthod 1978; 74: 241–57.

401. SMITH NHH. Monostotic Paget's disease of the mandible presenting with progressive resorption of the teeth. Oral Surg 1978; 46: 246–53.

402. SÖDER P-Ö *et al*. Effect of drying on viability of periodontal membrane. Scand J Dent Res 1977; 85: 164–8.

403. SOLOMON CS *et al*. Herpes zoster revisited: implicated in root resorption. J Endod 1986; 12: 210–13.

404. SPERLING I *et al*. A new treatment of heterotransplanted teeth to prevent progression of root resorption. Endod Dent Traumatol 1986; 2: 117–20.

405. SPURRIER SW *et al*. A comparison of apical root resorption during orthodontic treatment in endodontically treated and vital teeth. Am J Orthod Dentofac Orthop 1990; 97: 130–4.

406. STAFNE EC *et al*. Resorption of embedded teeth. J Am Dent Assoc 1945; 32: 1003–9.

407. STANLEY HR *et al*. Pathological sequelae of "neglected" impacted third molars. J Oral Pathol 1988; 17: 113–17.

408. STANLEY HR *et al*. The detection and prevalence of reactive physiologic sclerotic, reparative dentin and dead tracts beneath various types of dental lesions according to tooth surface and age. J Pathol 1983; 12: 257–89.

409. STOCK CJR. Calcium hydroxide: root resorption and perio-endo lesions. Br Dent J 1985; 158: 325–34.

410. STRUTHERS P *et al*. Root resorption by ameloblastomas and cysts of the jaws. Int J Oral Surg 1976; 5: 128–32.

411. SYMONS AL. Root resorption: a complication following traumatic avulsion. ASDC J Dent Child 1986; 53: 271–4.

412. TAITHONGCHAI R *et al*. Facial and dentoalveolar structure and the prediction of apical root shortening. Am J Orthod DentofacOrthop 1996; 110: 296–302.

413. TAYLOR MH *et al*. Effect of digit-sucking habits on root morphology in primary incisors. Pediatr Dent 1983; 5: 61–3.

414. TAYLOR NG *et al*. Resorption of the crown of an unerupted permanent molar. Int J Paediatr Dent 1991; 2: 89–92.

415. THODEN VAN VELZEN SK *et al*. Endodontologie. Alphen aan den Rijn: Stafleu & Tholen BV, 1995.

416. TRACEY C *et al*. Root resorption: the aggressive, unerupted second premolar. Br J Orthod 1985; 12: 97–101.

417. TRONSTAD L. Pulp reactions in traumatized teeth. In: GUTMAN JL et al. (eds) Proceedings of the international conference on oral trauma. Chicago, IL: American Association of Endodontists Endowment & Memorial Foundation, 1986.

418. TRONSTAD L. Root resorption. Endod Dent Traumatol 1988; 4: 241–52.

419. TRONSTAD L et al. pH changes in dental tissues after root canal filling with calcium hydroxide. J Endod 1981; 7: 17–21.

420. TROPE M. Cervical root resorption. J Am Dent Assoc 1997; 128: 56S–9S.

421. TROPE M. Luxation injuries and external root resorption. CDA J 2000; 28: 860–6.

422. TROPE M. Root resorption due to dental trauma. Endodont Topics 2002; 1: 79–100.

423. TROPE M. Clinical management of the avulsed tooth: present strategies and future directions. Dent Traumatol 2002; 18: 1–11.

424. TROPE M et al. The role of the socket in the periodontal healing of replanted dog's teeth stored in Viaspan for extended periods. Endod Dent Traumatol 1997; 13: 171–5.

425. TROPE M et al. Periodontal healing of replanted dog teeth stored in Viaspan, milk and Hank's balanced salt solution. Endod Dent Traumatol 1992; 8: 183–8.

426. TSUKIBOSHI M. Autotransplantation of teeth: requirements for predictable results. Dent Traumatol 2002; 18: 157–80.

427. VANDERAS AP. Effects of intracanal medicaments on inflammatory resorption or occurrence of ankylosis in mature traumatized teeth: a review. Endod Dent Traumatol 1993; 9: 175–84.

428. VAN DER WAAL I. Een geresorbeerde verstandskies: wat te doen? Ned Tijdschr Tandheelkd 1995; 102: 357.

429. VINCENTELLI R et al. Les <<taches rosées de la couronne>> (<<pink spots>>). Schweiz Monatschr Zahnheilkd 1973; 83: 1132–50.

430. WALLS AWG. Amelogenesis imperfecta with progressive root resorption. Br Dent J 1987; 162: 466–7.

431. WALTON JL. Dentin radiolucencies in unerupted teeth. ASDC J Dent Child 1980; 47: 183–6.

432. WALTON RE et al. The periodontal ligament injection: histologic effects on the periodontium in monkeys. J Endod 1982; 8: 22–6.

433. WATERHOUSE PJ et al. Crown and root resorption of a maxillary permanent first molar by an impacted second premolar. Int J Paediatr Dent 1995; 5: 259–62.

434. WEDENBERG C. Evidence for a dentin-derived inhibitor of macrophage spreading. Scand J Dent Res 1987; 95: 381–8.

435. WEDENBERG C et al. Experimental internal resorption in monkey teeth. Endod Dent Traumatol 1985; 1: 221–7.

436. WEDENBERG C et al. Evidence for an inhibitor of osteoclast attachment in dentinal matrix. Endod Dent Traumatol 1990; 6: 255–9.

437. WEDENBERG C et al. Internal resorption in human teeth – a histological, scanning electron microscopic, and enzyme histochemical study. J Endod 1987; 13: 255–9.

438. WEIGER R et al. Radicular penetration of hydrogen peroxide during intra-coronal bleaching with various forms of sodium perborate. Int Endod J 1994; 27: 313–17.

439. WEINSTEIN FM et al. The effect on periodontal and pulpal tissues of various cleansing procedures prior to replantation of extracted teeth. Acta Odontol Scand 1981: 39: 251–5.

440. WESSELINK PR et al. Resorption of the mouse incisor after the application of cold to the periodontal attachment apparatus. Calcif Tissue Int 1986; 39: 11–21.

441. WESSELINK PR et al. Initiating factors in dental root resorption. In: DAVIDOVITCH Z (ed.) Biological mechanisms of tooth eruption and root resorption. Birmingham: EBSCO Media, 1988.

442. WHITE C. Repair of a root resorption lesion. J Periodontol 1998; 69: 596–600.

443. WILLIAMS CG et al. Suspected idiopathic external root resorption of a mandibular molar. Br Dent J 1983; 155: 193–5.

444. WINTER GB. 3. Local pathological conditions influencing the development of the upper labial segment. Dent Pract 1966; 17: 153–9.

445. WONG KS et al. The effect of intracanal Lexdermix on root resorption of delayed-replanted monkey teeth. Dent Traumatol 2002; 18: 309–15.

446. WYSOCKI GP et al. Oral findings in primary hyperoxaluria and oxalosis. Oral Surg 1982; 53: 267–72.

447. YAACOUB HB. The resistant dentine shell of teeth suffering from idiopathic external resorption. Aust Dent J 1980; 25: 73–5.

448. YANPISET K et al. Pulp revascularisation of replanted immature dog teeth after different treatment methods. Endod Dent Traumatol 2000; 16: 211–17.

449. YUSOF WZ et al. Multiple external root resorption. J Am Dent Assoc 1989; 118: 453–5.

450. ZACH L et al. Pulp response to externally applied heat. Oral Surg Oral Med Oral Pathol 1965; 19: 515–30.

451. ZERVAS P et al. The effect of citric acid treatment on periodontal haling after replantation of permanent teeth. Int Endod J 1991; 24: 317–25.

452. HOHMANN A. Periodontal ligament hydrostatic pressure with areas of root resorption after application of continuous torque movement. Angle Orthod 2007; 77: 653–9.

453. CHAN E et al. Physical properties of root cementum: Part 7. Am J Orthod Dentofac Orthop 2006; 129: 504–10.

454. ESTEVEZ T et al. Orthodontic root resorption of endodontically treated teeth. J Endod 2007; 33: 119–22.

455. VARGAS KG et al. Preliminary evaluation of sodium hypochlorite for pulpotomies in primary molars. Pediatr Dent 2006; 28: 511–17.

456. EL-MELIGI OA et al. Comparison of mineral trioxide and calcium hydroxide as pulpotomy agents in young peremanent teeth (apexogenesis). Pediatr Dent 2006; 28: 399–404.

457. PENG L et al. Evaluation of formocresol versus ferric sulphate primary molar pulpotomy. Int Endod J 2007; 40: 751–7.

458. IZUMI N et al. Periodontal regeneration of transplanted rat teeth subcutaneously after cryptopreservation. Int J Oral Maxillofac Surg 2007; 36: 838–44.

459. KLAMBANI M *et al*. Radiolucent lesion of an unerupted mandibular molar. Am J Orthod Dentofac Orthop 2005; 127: 67–71.

460. PANZARINI SR *et al*. Minreal trioxide aggregate as a root canal filling material in reimplanted teeth. Dent Traumatol 2007; 23: 265–72.

461. MORI GG *et al*. Morphometric and microscopic evaluation of the effect of a solution of alendronate as intracanal therapeutic agent in rat teeth submitted to late reimplantation. Dent Traumatol 2007; 23: 218–21.

462. POI WR *et al*. Influence of enamel matrix derivate (Emdogain) and sodium fluoride on the healing process in delayed tooth replantation. Dent Traumatol 2007; 23: 35–41.

463. FILIPPI A *et al*. Treatment of replacement resorption by intentional replantation, resection of the ankylosed sites, and Emdogain®. Dent Traumatol 2006; 22: 307–11.

464. FLORES MT *et al*. Guidelines for the management of traumatic dental injuries. II. Dent Traumatol 2007; 23: 130–6.

Chapter 8: Tooth Wear and Other Signs of Ageing

1. ABRAHAM-INPIJN L. Ziekte van Paget. Tandartspraktijk 2003; May: 21–2.

2. ADDY M *et al*. The distribution of plaque and gingivitis and the influence of toothbrushing hand in a group of South-Wales 11–12 year-old children. J Clin Periodontol 1987; 14: 564–72.

3. ADDY M *et al*. Development of a method in situ to study toothpaste abrasion of dentin. Comparison of two products. J Clin Periodont 2002; 29: 896–900.

4. AHLBERG J *et al*. Reported bruxism and stress experience. Community Dent Oral Epidemiol 2002; 30: 405–8.

5. AHLBERG J *et al*. Reported bruxism and biopsychological symptoms: a longitudinal study. Community Dent Oral Epidemiol 2004; 32: 307–11.

6. AHMAD R. Bruxism in children. J Pedodont 1986; 10: 105–26.

7. AL-HIYASAT AS *et al*. Investigation of human enamel wear against four dental ceramics and gold. J Dent 1998; 26: 487–95.

8. AL-OITABI M. The miswak (chewing stick) and oral health. Studies on oral hygiene practices of urban Saudi Arabians. Swed Dent J 2004; 167 (suppl): 2–75.

9. ALPOZ AR *et al*. Bruxism in Rett syndrome. J Clin Pediatr Dent 1999; 23: 161–3.

10. American dental association health foundation research. Clinical methods for determining dentifrice-cleaning ability. J Am Dent Assoc 1984; 109: 759–62.

11. ANSELM WISKOTT HW *et al*. In vivo wear of three types of veneering materials using implant–supported restorations: a method evaluation. Eur J Oral Sci 2002; 110: 61–7.

12. ARNOLD LV. Problemen verbonden aan de preventie van parodontale aandoeningen door overbelasting. Ned Tijdschr Tandheelkd 1954; 61: 790–9.

13. ASHMORE H. Dental enamel abrasion. An in vitro method using interference microscopy. Br Dent J 1966; 120: 309–14.

14. AYANOGLOU CM *et al*. New cementum formation induced by cyclosporine A: a histological, ultrastructural and histomorphometric study in the rat. J Periodont Res 1997; 32: 543–55.

15. AYER WA *et al*. Extinction of bruxism by massed practice therapy. J Can Dent Assoc 1969; 35: 492–4.

16. AZAZ B *et al*. Correlation between age and thickness of cementum in impacted teeth. Oral Surg 1974; 38: 6914.

17. BADER JD *et al*. How dentists classified and treated non-carious lesions. J Am Dent Assoc 1993; 124: 46–54.

18. BADER JD *et al*. Case-control study of non-carious cervical lesions. Community Dent Oral Epidemiol 1996; 24: 286–91.

19. BADR SE *et al*. Reconstruction of a severely abraded dentition using an overdenture. Quint Int 1986; 17: 293–7.

20. BAILEY JO *et al*. Effect of occlusal adjustment on bruxism as monitored by nocturnal EMG recordings. J Dent Res 1980; 59: 317.

21. BAKKE M *et al*. Distortion of maximal elevator activity by unilateral tooth contact. Scand J Dent Res 1980; 80: 67–75.

22. BAGHDADY VS *et al*. Prevalence of pulp stones in a teenage Iraqi group. J Endod 1988; 14: 309–11.

23. BANG G *et al*. Determination of age in humans from root dentin transparency. Acta Odontol Scand 1970; 28: 3–35.

24. BARBAKOW F *et al*. A review of methods to determine the relative abrasion of dentifrices and prophylaxis pastes. Quint Int 1987; 18: 17–22 and 23–8.

25. BARBAKOW F *et al*. A critical comparison of dentifrice abrasion scores on dentine recorded by gravimetric and radiotracer methods. J Dent 1992; 20: 283–6.

26. BARGHI N *et al*. Experimentally induced occlusal disharmonies, nocturnal bruxism and MPD. J Dent Res 1979; 58: 317.

27. BAUER W *et al*. Wear in upper and lower incisors in relation to incisal and condylar guidance. J Orofac Orthop 1997; 58: 306–19.

28. BAXTER PM *et al*. Toothpaste abrasive requirements to control naturally stained pellicle. J Oral Rehabil 1981; 8: 19–26.

29. BECKER JL. Een geval van ziekte van Paget van de mandibula gecompliceerd door een fractuur als gevolg van een extractie. Ned Tijdschr Tandheelkd 1958; 65: 3558.

30. BECKETT H *et al*. Occupational tooth abrasion in a dental technician: loss of tooth surface resulting from exposure to porcelain powder. Quint Int 1995; 26: 217–20.

31. BEGG PR. Stone age man's dentition. Am J Orthod 1954; 40: 298–312, 373–83, 462–75 and 517–31.

32. BERGSTRÖM J *et al*. Cervical abrasion in relation to toothbrushing and periodontal health. Scand J Dent Res 1988; 96: 405–11.

33. BERGSTRÖM J *et al*. An epidemiologic approach to toothbrushing and dental abrasion, Community Dent Oral Epidemiol 1979; 7: 57–64.

34. BERNARDON JK *et al*. Diagnosis and management of maxillary incisors affected by incisal wear. J Esthet Restor Dent 2002; 14: 331–9.

35. BERRY DC *et al*. Attrition: possible mechanisms of compensation. J Oral Rehabil 1976; 3: 201–6.

36. BEVENIUS J *et al*. Conservative management of erosion-abrasion: a system for the general practitioner. Aust Dent J 1994; 39: 4–10.

37. BEYRON H. Occlusal relations and mastication in Australian aborigines. Acta Odontol Scand 1964; 22: 597–678.

38. BILLER HR *et al*. Enamel loss during a prophylaxis polish in vitro. J Int Assoc Dent Child 1980; 11: 7–12.

39. BISHOP K *et al*. Wear now? An update on the etiology of tooth wear. Quint Int 1997; 28: 305–13.

40. BJÖRN H *et al*. On the mechanics of toothbrushing. Odont Revy 1966; 17: 9–16 and 17–27.

41. BJÖRN H *et al*. The abrasion of dentine by commercial dentifrices. Odont Revy 1966; 17: 109–20.

42. BORCIC J *et al*. The prevalence of non-carious cervical lesions. J Oral Rehabil 2004; 117–23.

43. BOWLES WH *et al*. Abrasive particles in tobacco products: a possible factor in dental attrition. J Am Dent Assoc 1995; 126: 327–31.

44. BOYENS PJ. Value of autosuggestion in the therapy of "bruxism" and other biting habits. J Am Dent Assoc 1940; 27: 1773–7.

45. BRADY JM *et al*. Scanning microscopy of cervical erosion. J Am Dent Assoc 1977; 94: 726–9.

46. BRASHER WJ *et al*. Sequestration of root cementum in an endodonticperiodontally involved tooth. J Endod 1982; 8: 4136.

47. BUCCINO MA *et al*. Rett syndrome – a rare and often misdiagnosed syndrome. Pediatr Dent 1989; 11: 151–7.

48. BUDTZ-JØRGENSEN E. A 3-month study in monkeys of occlusal dysfunction and stress. Scand J Dent Res 1980; 88: 171–80.

49. BUDTZ-JØRGENSEN E. Bruxism and trauma from occlusion: an experimental model in Macaca monkeys. J Clin Periodontol 1980; 7: 149–62.

50. BUDTZ-JØRGENSEN E. Occlusal dysfunction and stress. J Oral Rehabil 1981; 8: 1–9.

51. BULL WH *et al*. The abrasion and cleaning properties of dentifrices. Br Dent J 1968; 125: 331–7.

52. CAMARDA AJ *et al*. The use of nuclear medicine in the diagnosis of Paget's disease of the mandible. J Can Dent Assoc 1989; 55: 49–53.

53. CAMARGO IM *et al*. Abrasiveness evaluation of silica and calcium carbonate used in the production of dentifrices. J Cosmet Sci 2001; 52: 163–7.

54. CARLSSON GE *et al*. Dental abrasion and alveolar bone loss in the white rat. I. Effect of ligation of the major salivary gland ducts. Odont Revy 1965; 16: 308–16.

55. CARLSSON GE *et al*. Occlusal wear. A follow-up study of 18 subjects with extensively worn dentitions. Acta Odontol Scand 1985; 43: 83–90.

56. CARTER LC. Paget's disease: important features for the general practitioner. Compend Contin Educ Dent 1990; 9: 662–9.

57. CHAPMAN RJ *et al*. Excessive wear of natural tooth structure by opposing composite restorations. J Am Dent Assoc 1983; 106: 51–3.

58. CLARK GT *et al*. Nocturnal electromyographic evaluation of myofacial pain dysfunction in patients undergoing occlusal splint therapy. J Am Dent Assoc 1979; 99: 607–11.

59. CLARKE NG *et al*. Distribution of nocturnal bruxing patterns in man. J Oral Rehabil 1984; 11: 529–34.

60. CLARKE NG *et al*. Bruxing patterns in man during sleep. J Oral Rehabil 1984; 11: 123–7.

61. COHEN RB *et al*. A case of acromegaly identified after patient complaint of apertognathia. Oral Surg Oral Med Oral Pathol 1993; 75: 583–6.

62. COLBY RA *et al*. Color atlas of oral pathology. Philadelphia, PA: JB Lippincott Company, 1961, p. 56.

63. COLQUITT T. The sleep-wear syndrome. J Prosthet Dent 1987; 57: 33–41.

64. COPPES L. Occlusie en parodontologie. In: VAN DER KWAST WAM *et al*. (eds) Tandheelkundig Jaar 1980. Utrecht: Bohn, Scheltema & Holkema, 1980.

65. CORRUCINI RS. Australian aboriginal tooth succession, interproximal attrition, and Begg's theory. Am J Orthod Dentofac Orthop 1990; 97: 349–57.

66. COUNCIL ON DENTAL THERAPEUTICS. Abrasivity of current dentifrices. J Am Dent Assoc 1970; 81: 1177–8.

67. COWAN A. Leontiasis ossea. Oral Surg 1959; 12: 98395.

68. COX CF *et al*. Reparative dentin: factors affecting its deposition. Quint Int 1992; 23: 257–70.

69. CROTHERS A *et al*. Vertical height differences in subjects with severe dental wear. Eur J Orthod 1993; 15: 519–25.

70. DAHL BL *et al*. Pathologic attrition and maximal bite force. J Oral Rehabil 1985; 12: 337–42.

71. DAVIES GN. Social customs and habits and their effect on oral disease. J Dent Res 1963; 42 (suppl 1): 209–32.

72. DAVIES TGH *et al*. The degree of attrition of the deciduous teeth and first permanent molars of primitive and urbanised Greenland natives. Br Dent J 1955; 99: 35–43.

73. DAVIS WB. Cleaning and polishing of teeth by brushing. Community Dent Oral Epidemiol 1980; 8: 237–43.

74. DAVIS WB *et al*. Measurement in vitro of enamel abrasion by dentifrice. J Dent Res 1976; 55: 970–5.

75. DAWID E *et al*. Keilförmige Defekte als mögliche Folge von Stress? Dtsch Zahnärztl Z 1994; 49: 522–4.

76. DE BOER JG. Hypercementose. Ned Tijdschr Tandheelkd 1976; 83: 3489.

77. DE BOER P *et al*. Influence of tooth paste particle size and tooth brush stiffness on dentine abrasion in vitro. Caries Res 1985; 19: 232–9.

78. DE GEE AJ *et al*. Abrasion of dentin and enamel by 32 different dentifrices. J Dent Res 1997; 76: 50.

79. DE LAAT DE *et al*. Bruxisme: alom gekend maar moeilijk te vatten. Ned Tijdschr Tandheelkd 2000; 107: 271–4.

80. DELONG R *et al*. The wear of enamel when opposed by ceramic systems. Dent Mater 1989; 5: 266–71.

81. DE QUINCEY GN *et al*. Zijn de dagen van elektrisch danwel handmatig poetsen geteld? Ned Tandartsenbl 1992; 47: 103–4.

82. DERKSEN HB *et al*. Herstel van tandslijtage. Restauratief-prosthetische aspecten. Ned Tijdschr Tandheelkd 2000; 107: 301–7.

83. DONACHIE MA *et al*. Assessment of tooth wear in an ageing population. J Dent 1995; 23: 157–64.

84. DUINKERKE ASH *et al*. Aandacht voor psychosociale factoren bij de behandeling van pijn en dysfunctie van het kauwstelsel. Ned Tijdschr Tandheelkd 1986; 93: 127–32.

85. DUKE SA *et al*. The conditions occurring in vivo when brushing with toothpastes. Br Dent J 1982; 152: 52–4.

86. DULIO P *et al*. Dentifrices en parodontie: revue de la littérature – II. Abrasion, sensibilité dentinaire, effets secondaires. Schweiz Monatschr Zahnheilkd 1983; 93: 572–80.

87. DYER D *et al*. Studies in vitro of abrasion by different manual toothbrush heads and a standard toothpaste. J Clin Periodontol 2000; 27: 99–103.

88. DYER D *et al*. Abrasion and stain removal by different manual toothbrushes and brush actions: studies in vitro. J Clin Periodontol 2001; 28: 121–7.

89. EATON SB *et al*. Paleolithic nutrition. A consideration of its nature and current implications. N Engl J Med 1985; 312: 283–9.

90. EGERMARK-ERIKSSON I *et al*. A long-term epidemiologic study of the relationship between occlusal factors and mandibular dysfunction in children and adolescents. J Dent Res 1987; 66: 67–71.

91. EKFELDT A *et al*. An individual tooth wear index and an analysis of factors correlated to incisal and occlusal wear in an adult Swedish population. Acta Odontol Scand 1990; 48: 343–9.

92. ELMER E *et al*. Reflectometry and micromorphology of polished, etched and repolished teeth. Helv Odont Acta 1975; 19: 40–7.

93. EL-MOWAFY OM. Characteristic abrasion of permanent incisors in Jordanians caused by a bad eating habit. Quint Int 1988; 19: 739–44.

94. ELVERY MW *et al*. Radiographic study of the broadbeach aboriginal dentition. Am J Phys Anthropol 1998; 107: 211–19.

95. ENBOM L *et al*. Occlusal wear in miners. Swed Dent J 1986; 10: 165–70.

96. ESTAFAN D *et al*. Clinical efficacy of an herbal toothpaste. J Clin Dent 1998; 9: 31–3.

97. EVERSOLE LR *et al*. Dental occlusal wear and degenerative disease of the temporomandibular joint: a correlational study utilizing skeletal material from a contemporary population. J Oral Rehabil 1985; 12: 401–6.

98. FAULKNER KDB. Bruxism: a review of the literature. Part I. Aust Dent J 1990; 35: 266–76.

99. FAULKNER KDB. Bruxism: a review of the literature. Part I. Aust Dent J 1990; 35: 355–61.

100. FEELDERS RA *et al*. Acromegalie. Behandeling van de oorzaak en de oral gevolgen. Ned Tijdschr Tandheelkd 2004; 111: 20–2.

101. FORWARD GC. Role of toothpastes in the cleaning of the teeth. Int Dent J 1991; 41: 164–70.

102. FRISCH J *et al*. A study on the relationship between bruxism and aggression. J Periodontol 1960; 31: 409–12.

103. FUNCH DP *et al*. Factors associated with nocturnal bruxism and its treatment. J Behav Med 1980; 3: 385–97.

104. GANSS C *et al*. Characteristics of tooth wear in relation to different nutritional patterns including contemporary and medieval subjects. Eur J Oral Sci 2002; 110: 54–60.

105. GARDNER BS *et al*. The significance of hypercementosis. Dent Cosmos 1931; 73: 10659.

106. GERLACH RW *et al*. Extrinsic stain prevention with a combination dentifrice containing calcium phosphate surface active builders compared to two marketed controls. J Clin Dent 2002; 13: 15–18.

107. GERLACH RW *et al*. Extrinsic stain removal with a sodium hexamethaphosphate–containing dentifrice: comparisons to marketed controls. J Clin Dent 2002; 13: 10–14.

108. GIBBS CH *et al*. Limits of human bite strength. J Prosthet Dent 1986; 56: 226–9.

109. GLAROS AG *et al*. Bruxism: a critical review. Psychol Bull 1977; 84: 767–81.

110. GLICKMAN I. Inflammation and trauma from occlusion, co-destructive factors in chronic periodontal disease. J Periodontol 1963; 34: 5–10.

111. GLICKMAN I. Role of occlusion in the etiology and treatment of periodontal disease. J Dent Res 1971; 50 (suppl 2): 199–204.

112. GLICKMAN I *et al*. Role of trauma from occlusion in initiation of periodontal pocket formation in experimental animals. J Periodontol 1955; 26: 14–20.

113. GOURDON AM *et al*. Development of an abrasion index. J Prosthet Dent 1987; 57: 358–61.

114. GRABER G. Psychische Einflüsse auf die Funktion des Kausystems. Dtsch Zahnärztl Z 1992; 47: 155–6.

115. GREENE CS *et al*. Epidemiologic studies of mandibular dysfunction: a critical review. J Prosthet Dent 1982; 48: 184–90.

116. GRIPPO JO *et al*. Dental "erosion" revisited. J Am Dent Assoc 1995; 126: 619–30.

117. GRIPPO JO *et al*. Attrition, abrasion, corrosion and abfraction revisited. J Am Dent Assoc 2004; 135: 1109–18.

118. GROSFELD O *et al*. Musculo-articular disorders of the stomatognathic system in school children examined according to clinical criteria. J Oral Rehabil 1977; 4: 117–20.

119. GROSSMAN E *et al*. A comparative clinical study of extrinsic tooth stain removal with two electric toothbrushes [Braun D7 and D9] and a manual brush. Am J Dent 1996; 9: S25–9.

120. GUSTAFSON G. Age determinations on teeth. J Am Dent Assoc 1950; 41: 45–54.

121. HACHMANN A *et al*. Efficacy of the nocturnal bite plate in control of bruxism for 3 to 5 year old children. J Clin Pediatr Dent 1999; 24: 9–15.

122. HAND JS *et al*. The prevalence and treatment implications of cervical abrasion in the elderly. Gerodontics 1986; 2: 167–70.

123. HARGREAVES AS *et al*. Acromegaly: an unusual presentation and unexpected sequelae to treatment. Br Dent J 1987; 163: 196–7.

124. HARRINGTON E *et al*. Toothbrush-dentifrice abrasion. A suggested standard method. Br Dent J 1982; 153: 135–8.

125. HARRINGTON JH *et al*. Automatic and hand toothbrushing abrasion studies. J Am Dent Assoc 1964; 68: 343–50.

126. HEANUE M *et al.* Manual versus powered toothbrushing for oral health. Cochrane Database Syst Rev 2005; 2: CD002281.

127. HEATH JR *et al.* Abrasion of restorative materials by toothpaste. J Oral Rehabil 1976; 3: 121–38.

128. HEBEL KS *et al.* Abrasion of enamel and composite resin by removable partial denture clasps. J Prosthet Dent 1984; 52: 389–97.

129. HEFFERREN JJ. A laboratory method for assessment of dentifrice abrasivity. J Dent Res 1976; 55: 563–73.

130. HEITHERSAY GS. Attritional values for Australian aborigines, Haast's Bluff. Aust Dent J 1960; 5: 84–8.

131. HELLER RF *et al.* An evaluation of bruxism control: massed negative practice and automated relaxation training. J Dent Res 1975; 54: 1120–3.

132. HILL TJ. Pathology of the dental pulp. J Am Dent Assoc 1934; 21: 820–44.

133. HINTON RJ. Changes in articular eminence morphology with dental function. Am J Phys Anthropol 1981; 54: 439–55.

134. HINTON RJ. Form and patterning of anterior tooth wear among aboriginal human groups. Am J Phys Anthropol 1981; 54: 555–64.

135. HINTON RJ. Differences in interproximal and occlusal tooth wear among prehistoric Tennessee Indians: implications for masticatory function. Am J Phys Anthropol 1982; 57: 103–15.

136. HLUSKO LJ. The oldest hominid habit? Experimental evidence for toothpicking with grass stalks. Curr Anthropol 2003; 44: 738–41.

137. HOLMGREN K *et al.* Effect of a full-arch maxillary occlusal splint on parafunctional activity during sleep in patients with nocturnal bruxism and signs and symptoms of craniomandibular disorders. J Prosthet Dent 1993; 69: 293–7.

138. HOUWINK B. Elektrische tandenborstels; gebruik blijven ontraden. Ned Tandartsenbl 1992; 47: 7.

139. HUDSON JD *et al.* Enamel wear caused by three different restorative methods. J Prosthet Dent 1995; 74: 647–54.

140. HUGOSON A *et al.* Incisal and occlusal tooth wear in children and adolescents in a Swedish population. Acta Odontol Scand 1996; 54: 263–70.

141. HUNTER ML *et al.* The role of toothpastes and toothbrushes in the aetiology of toothwear. Int Dent J 2002; 52 (suppl 2): 399–405.

142. IKEDA T *et al.* The effect of light premature occlusal contact on tooth pain threshold in humans. J Oral Rehabil 1998; 25: 589–95.

143. IMFELD T. Dental erosion. Definition, classification and links. Eur J Oral Sci 1996; 104: 151–5.

144. IDE M *et al.* A case report of severe attrition of primary dentition. Pediatr Dent J 1992; 2: 115–20.

145. INGERSLEV H. Functional disturbances of the masticatory system in school children. ASDC J Dent Child 1983; 50: 445–50.

146. IVANOVIC V *et al.* Rate of formation of tertiary dentin in dogs' teeth in response to lining materials. Oral Surg Oral Med Oral Pathol 1989; 67: 684–8.

147. HILLMANN G *et al.* Dentikel und diffuse Verkalkungen in unterschiedlich alten Zahnpulpen. Dtsch Zahnärztl Z 1996; 51: 456–61.

148. HUMSI ANK *et al.* The immediate effects of a stabilization splint on the muscular symmetry in the masseter and anterior temporal muscles of patients with a craniomandibular disorder. J Prosthet Dent 1989; 62: 339–43.

149. JAGGER DC *et al.* An in vitro investigation into the wear effects of unglazed, glazed, and polished porcelain on human enamel. J Prosthet Dent 1994; 72: 320–3.

150. JOHANSSON A *et al.* Analysis of possible factors influencing the occurrence of occlusal tooth wear in a young Saudi population. Acta Odontol Scand 1991; 49: 139–45.

151. JOHANSSON A *et al.* An investigation of some factors associated with occlusal tooth wear in a selected high-wear sample. Scand J Dent Res 1993; 101: 407–15.

152. JOHANSSON A *et al.* Covariation of some factors associated with occlusal tooth wear in a selected high-wear sample. Scand J Dent Res 1993; 101: 398–406.

153. JOST-BRINKMAN P-G. The influence of air-polishers on tooth enamel. An in vitro study. J Orofac Orthop 1998; 59: 1–13.

154. KALNINS V. Origin of enamel drops and cementicles in the teeth of rodents. J Dent Res 1952; 31: 58290.

155. KAMPE T *et al.* Personality traits in a group of subjects with long-standing bruxing behaviour. J Oral Rehabil 1997; 24: 588–93.

156. KAMPE T *et al.* Dental filling therapy as a possible etiological factor regarding mandibular dysfunction. Acta Odontol Scand 1983; 41: 1–9.

157. KAMPE T *et al.* Reported symptoms and clinical findings in a group of subjects with longstanding bruxism behavior. J Oral Rehabil 1997; 24: 581–7.

158. KANTOR M *et al.* Alveolar bone regeneration after removal of inflammatory and traumatic factors. J Periodontol 1976; 47: 687–95.

159. KARDACHI BJR, BAILEY JO, ASH MM. A comparison of biofeedback and occlusal adjustment on bruxism. J Periodontol 1978; 49: 367–72.

160. KATO T *et al.* Evidence that experimentally induced sleep bruxism is a consequence of transient arousal. J Dent Res 2003; 82: 284–8.

161. KEIL A, SPETH-ESCHENBRENNER J. Über Zahnanomalien bei 3400 Patienten nach Röntgenstaten. Dtsch Zahn Mund Kieferheilkd 1963; 40: 360–76.

162. KEYES G *et al.* Successful surgical endodontics for benign cementoblastoma. J Endod 1987;13: 566–9.

163. KHOORY T. The use of chewing sticks in preventive oral hygiene. Clin Prev Dent 1983; 5 (4): 11–14.

164. KIESER JA *et al.* Patterns of dental wear in the Lengua Indians of Paraguay. Am J Phys Anthropol 1985; 66: 21–9.

165. KILIARIDIS S *et al.* Craniofacial morphology, occlusal traits, and bite force in persons with advanced occlusal tooth wear. Am J Orthod Dentofac Orthop 1995; 107: 286–92.

166. KITCHIN PC *et al.* The abrasiveness of dentifrices as measured on the cervical areas of extracted teeth. J Dent Res 1948; 27: 195–200.

167. KLETT R. Zur Biomechanik des Kiefergelenkknackens. Dtsch Zahnärztl Z 1985; 40: 206–10.

168. KLIMM W *et al.* Klinische Variationen des sogenannten keilförmigen Defektes. Zahn Mund Kieferheilkd 1990; 78: 713–16.

169. KNIGHT DJ *et al*. A longitudinal study of tooth wear in orthodontically treated patients. Am J Orthod Dentofac Orthop 1997; 112: 194–202.

170. KÖNÖNEN M *et al*. Prevalence of nocturnal and diurnal bruxisme in patients with psoriasis. J Prosthet Dent 1988; 60: 238–41.

171. KREISBURG MK. Alternative view of the bruxism phenomenon. DMJ 1982; 30: 121–3.

172. KREYNS JM. Post mortem. Tanden na de dood. Tandartspraktijk 2003; November: 11–13.

173. KROGSTAD O *et al*. Dento-facial morphology in patients with advanced attrition. Europ J Orthod 1985; 7: 57–62.

174. KUCH EV *et al*. Bruxing and non-bruxing children: a comparison of their personality traits. Pediatr Dent 1979; 1: 182–7.

175. KUMAR S *et al*. Pulp calcifications in primary teeth. J Endod 1990; 16: 218–20.

176. KVAAL S *et al*. Fluorescence from dentin and cementum in human mandibular second premolars and its relation to age. Scand J Dent Res 1989; 97: 131–8.

177. LAMBRECHTS P *et al*. Quantitative in vivo wear of human enamel. J Dent Res 1989; 68: 1752–4.

178. LAVIGNE GL *et al*. Cigarette smoking as a risk factor or an exacerbating factor for restless legs syndrome and sleep bruxism. Sleep 1997; 20: 290–3.

179. LAVIGNE GJ *et al*. Sleep bruxism: validity of clinical research criteria in a controlled polysomnographic study. J Dent Res 1996; 75: 546–52.

180. LEE WC *et al*. Possible role of tensile stress in the etiology of cervical erosive lesions of teeth. J Prosthet Dent 1984; 52: 374–80.

181. LEEK FF. Teeth and bread in ancient Egypt. J Egypt Archeol 1972; 58: 126–32.

182. LEHNE RK *et al*. Abrasivity of sodium bicarbonate. Clin Prev Dent 1983; 5: 17–18.

183. LEIDER AS *et al*. Generalized hypercementosis. Oral Surg 1987; 63: 37580.

184. LEIGH RW. Notes on the somatology and pathology of ancient Egypt. J Am Dent Assoc 1935; 22: 199–222.

185. LEOF M. Clamping and grinding habits: their relation to periodontal disease. J Am Dent Assoc 1944; 31: 184–94.

186. LEWIS KJ *et al*. The relationship of erosion and attrition in extensive tooth tissue loss. Br Dent J 1973; 135: 400–4.

187. LIETHA-ELMER E *et al*. Polishing effect and abrasion of five tooth pastes on dental enamel. Schweiz Monatschr Zahnheilkd 1979; 89: 987–95.

188. LINDHE J *et al*. Influence of trauma from occlusion on progression of experimental periodontitis in the beagle dog. J Clin Periodontol 1974; 1: 3–14.

189. LINDHE J. Parodontologie. Alphen aan den Rijn: Samson Stafleu, 1985.

190. LINDQVIST B. Bruxism and emotional disturbance. Odont Revy 1972; 23: 231–42.

191. LINDQVIST B. Occlusal interferences in children with bruxism. Odont Revy 1973; 24: 141–8.

192. LOBBEZOO F *et al*. Veroorzaakt bruxisme klachten van TMD? Ned Tijdschr Tanadheelkd 1997; 104: 24.

193. LOBBEZOO F *et al*. Morfologische, parofysiologische en psychologische factoren. Ned Tijdschr Tandheelkd 2000; 107: 275–80.

194. LOBBEZOO F *et al*. Bruxism is mainly related centrally, not peripherally. J Oral Rehabil 2001; 28: 1085–91.

195. LUKE DA *et al*. The significance of cusps. J Oral Rehabil 1983; 10: 197–206.

196. LUSSI AR *et al*. Epidemiology and risk factors of wedge-shaped defects in a Swiss population. Schweiz Monatschr Zahnmed 1993; 103: 276–80.

197. LUTZ F *et al*. Elimination of polymerization stresses at the margins of posterior composite resin restorations: a new restorative technique. Quint Int 1986; 17: 777–84.

198. LUTZ F *et al*. Self-adjusting abrasiveness: a new technology for prophylaxis pastes. Quint Int 1993; 24: 63–63.

199. LUTZ F *et al*. Comparison of the efficacy of prophylaxis pastes with conventional abrasives or a new self-adjusting abrasive. Quint Int 1993; 24: 193–201.

200. LYONS MF *et al*. A preliminary electromyographic study of bite force and jaw-closing muscle fatigue in human subjects with advanced tooth wear. J Oral Rehabil 1990; 17: 311–18.

201. MACALUSO GM *et al*. Sleep bruxism is a disorder related to periodic arousals during sleep. J Dent Res 1998; 77: 565–73.

202. MACDONALD JWC *et al*. Relationship between occlusal contacts and jaw–closing muscle activity during tooth clenching: Part I. J Prosthet Dent 1984; 52: 718–29.

203. MADRID G *et al*. Cigarette smoking and bruxism. Percept Mot Skills 1998; 87 (3 Pt 1): 898.

204. MAHALICK JA *et al*. Occlusal wear in prosthodontics. J Am Dent Assoc 1971; 82: 154–9.

205. MAIR LH. Understanding wear in dentistry. Compend Cont Educ 1999; 20: 19–30.

206. MANDEL ID. The new toothpastes. J Can Dent Assoc 1998; 26: 186–90.

207. MANLY RS *et al*. Relative abrasiveness of natural and synthetic toothbrush bristles on cementum and dentin. J Am Dent Assoc 1957; 55: 779–80.

208. MANLY RS *et al*. Influence of method of testing on dentifrice abrasiveness. J Dent Res 1974; 53: 835–9.

209. MARIE *et al*. Bruxomania (gritting of the teeth). Dent Cosmos 1907; 49: 525.

210. MARKITZIU A *et al*. Tooth wear, solubility and fluoride concentration of molar–tooth surfaces in rats maintained on simultaneous or separate intake of food and fluoridated drinking water. Arch Oral Biol 1985; 30: 167–9.

211. MEHTA JD *et al*. A study of attrition of teeth in the Arkansas Indian skulls. Angle Orthod 1966; 36: 248–57.

212. MEISTER F *et al*. Endodontic involvement resulting from dental abrasion or erosion. J Am Dent Assoc 1980; 101: 651–3.

213. MELLBERG JR. The relative abrasivity of dental prophylactic pastes and abrasives on enamel and dentin. Clin Prev Dent 1979; 1: 13–18.

214. MENDIS BRRM *et al*. Distribution with age and attrition of peritubular dentine in the crowns of human teeth. Arch Oral Biol 1979; 24: 131–9.

215. MIERAU H-D *et al*. Zur Epidemiologie der Gingivarezessionen und möglicher klinischer Begleiterscheinungen. Dtsch Zahnärztl Z 1987; 42: 512–20.

216. MIKAMI DB. A review of psychogenic aspects and treatment of bruxism. J Prosthet Dent 1977; 37: 411–18.

217. MILES JRE. In: COHEN B *et al.* (eds) Scientific foundations of dentistry. London: Williman Heinemann Medical Books, 1976.

218. MILES AEW. In: COHEN B *et al.* (eds) Scientific foundations of dentistry. London: Williman Heinemann Medical Books, 1976.

219. MILLER WD. Experiments and observations on the wasting of tooth tissue variously designated as erosion, abrasion, chemical abrasion, denudation, etc. Dent Cosmos 1907; 49: 1–23.

220. MILOSEVIC A *et al.* Sports supplement drinks and dental health in competitive swimmers and cyclists. Br Dent J 1997; 182: 303–8.

221. MILOSEVIC A *et al.* Risk factors associated with tooth wear in teenagers. Community Dent Health 1997; 14: 143–7.

222. MILOSEVIC A *et al.* The prevalence of tooth wear in 14-year-old school children in Liverpool. Community Dent Health 1994; 11: 83–6.

223. MIYAWAKI S *et al.* Relationships among nocturnal jaw muscle activities, decreased esophageal pH, and sleep positions. Am J Orthod Dentofac Orthop 2004; 126: 615–19.

224. MOLIN C. From bite to mind TMD. Int J Prosthodont 1999; 12: 297–88.

225. MOLIN C *et al.* A psycho-odontologic investigation of patients with bruxism. Acta Odontol Scand 1966; 24: 373–91.

226. MOLINA OF *et al.* Prevalence of headaches and bruxism among patients with craniomandibular disorder. J Craniomandib Pract 1997; 15: 314–25.

227. MOLNAR S. Human tooth wear, tooth function and cultural variability. Am J Phys Anthropol 1971; 34: 175–90.

228. MOLNAR S *et al.* Measurement of tooth wear among Australian aborigines: I. Serial loss of the enamel crown. Am J Phys Anthropol 1983; 61: 51–65.

229. MOLNAR S *et al.* Tooth wear rates among contemporary Australian aborigines. J Dent Res 1983; 62: 562–5.

230. MOMOI Y *et al.* In vitro toothbrush-dentifrice abrasion of resin-modified glass ionomers. Dent Mater 1997; 13: 82–8.

231. MONSOUR FNT *et al.* Responses of periodontal tissues and cementum following transplantation of teeth. J Oral Maxillofac Surg 1984; 42: 4416.

232. MONSOUR FNT *et al.* Histological changes following transplantation of developing teeth to more advanced functional positions. Aust Dent J 1987; 32: 1049.

233. MORSE DR *et al.* A cross-sectional radiographic study of aging changes of teeth and supporting structures. Compend Contin Educ Dent 1993; 14: 241–7.

234. MUHLE G. Akromegalie. Quintessenz 1988; 9: 1563–7.

235. NADLER SC. Bruxism, a classification: critical review. J Am Dent Assoc 1957; 54: 615–22.

236. NANNINGA C *et al.* Abrasivität von Zahnpasten. Phillip J 1993; 10: 279–84.

237. NANNINGA C *et al.* Abrasivität von Zahnbürsten. Phillip J 1996; 13: 289–94.

238. NEWESELY H. Bewertung der Abrasivität von Zahnpflegemitteln und ihrer Auswirkung auf die beteiligten Gewebe. Dtsch Zahnärztl Z 1985; 40: 767–70.

239. NEWBRUN E. Cariology. Williams and Wilkins, Baltimore, 1983.

240. NEWBRUN E. The use of sodium bicarbonate in oral hygiene products and practice. Compend Contin Educ Dent Suppl 1997; 18: S2–7.

241. NEWMAN HN. Attrition, eruption, and the periodontium. J Dent Res 1999; 78: 730–4.

242. NEWMAN HN *et al.* Tooth eruption and function in an early Anglo-Saxon population. J R Soc Med 1979; 72: 341–50.

243. NIEMI M-L. Gingival abrasion and plaque removal after toothbrushing with an electric and a manual toothbrush. Acta Odontol Sacnd 1987; 45: 367–70.

244. NIEMI M-L *et al.* The effect of toothbrush grip on gingival abrasion and plaque removal during toothbrushing. J Clin Periodontol 1987; 14: 19–21.

245. NILNER M. Relationships between oral parafunctions and functional disturbances and diseases of the stomatognathic system among children aged 7–14 years. Acta Odontol Scand 1983; 41: 167–72.

246. NILNER M *et al.* Prevalence of functional disturbances and diseases of the stomatognathic system in 7–14 year olds. Swed Dent J 1981; 5: 173–87.

247. NITZAN DW *et al.* The effect of aging on tooth morphology: a study on impacted teeth. Oral Surg 1986; 61: 54–60.

248. NORDBO H *et al.* The rate of cervical abrasion in dental students. Acta Odontol Scand 1982; 40: 45–7.

249. NOORDMANS J *et al.* A new profilometric method for determination of enamel and dentinal abrasion in vivo using computer comparisons: a pilot study. Quint Int 1991; 22: 653–7.

250. NUNN J *et al.* The condition of the teeth in the UK in 1998 and implications for the future. Br Dent J 2000; 189: 639–44.

251. NYSTRÖM M *et al.* Development of horizontal tooth wear in maxillary anterior teeth from five to 18 years of age. J Dent Res 1990; 69: 1765–70.

252. OGINNI AO *et al.* Non-carious cervical lesions in a Nigerian population: abrasion or abfraction? Int Dent J 2003; 53: 275–9.

253. ØILO G *et al.* An index for evaluating wear of teeth. Acta Ondontol Scand 1987; 45: 361–5.

254. OKESON JP. The effects of hard and soft occlusal splints on nocturnal bruxism. J Am Dent Assoc 1987; 114: 788–91.

255. OTIS LL *et al.* Paget's disease of bone. J Oral Med 1986; 41: 214–20.

256. OTT K *et al.* A. Rasterelektronenmikroskopische Untersuchungen an Abrasionsfacetten im Schmelz und im Dentin. Dtsch Zahnärztl Z 1981; 36: 51–4.

257. OTT RW *et al.* Einflüsse der Zahnputztechnik auf die Entstehung keilförmiger Defekte. Dtsch Stomatol 1991; 41: 463–5.

258. OWENS NM *et al.* Noncarious dental "abfraction" lesions in an aging population. Compend Contin Educ 1995; 16: 552–61.

259. PADBURY AD *et al.* Abrasion caused by three methods of toothbrushing. J Periodontol 1974; 45: 434–8.

260. PALLAV P. Occlusal wear in dentistry. Thesis, Universiteit van Amsterdam, Amsterdam, 1996.

261. PAMEIJER JHN. Occlusiestoornissen, gewrichtsklachten en inslijpen. In: VAN DER KWAST WAM *et al.* (eds) Tandheelkundig Jaar 1980. Utrecht: Bohn, Scheltema & Holkema, 1980.

262. PAVONE BW. Bruxism and its effect on the natural teeth. J Prosthet Dent 1985; 53: 692–6.

263. PEAK J *et al.* Oral manifestations of Rett's syndrome. Br Dent J 1992; 172: 248–9.

264. PERLSTEIN MA *et al.* Nature and recognition of cerebral palsy in infancy. J Am Med Assoc 19 1952; 148: 1389–97.

265. PFARRER AM *et al.* Anticaries and hard tissue abrasion effects of a "dual-action" whitening, sodium hexametaphosphate tartar control dentifrice. J Clin Dent 2002; 13: 50–4.

266. PHANEUF EA *et al.* Automatic toothbrush: a new reciprocating action. J Am Dent Assoc 1962; 65: 26–39.

267. PHILIPPAS G. Effects of function on healthy teeth: the evidence of ancient Athenian remains. J Am Dent Assoc 1952; 45: 443–52.

268. PHILIPPAS GG. Influence of occlusal wear and age on formation of dentin and size of pulp chamber. J Dent Res 1961; 40: 1186–98.

269. PHILIPPAS GG *et al.* Age change in the permanent canine teeth. J Dent Res 1968; 47: 411–17.

270. PINDBORG JJ *et al.* Pilot survey of oral mucosa in areca (betel) nut chewers on Hainan Island of the people's Republic of China. Community Dent Oral Epidemiol 1984; 12: 195–6.

271. PIERCE CJ *et al.* Stress, anticipatory stress, and psychologic measures related to sleep bruxism. J Orofac Pain 1995; 9: 21–44.

272. PINDBORG JJ. Pathology of the dental hard tissues. Copenhagen: Munksgaard, 1970.

273. PINGITORE G *et al.* The social and psychologic factors of bruxism. J Prosthet Dent 1991; 65: 443–6.

274. PINTADO MR *et al.* Variation in tooth wear in young adults over a two year period. J Prosthet Dent 1997; 77: 313–20.

275. PLATA M *et al.* Clinical evaluation of induced occlusal disharmonies. J Dent Res 1982; 62: 204.

276. POLSON AM. Trauma and progression of marginal periodontitis in squirrel monkeys. II. Co-destructive factors of periodontitis and mechanically-produced injury. J Periodontol Res 1974; 9: 108–13.

277. POPOVICIU AM. Verstümmelung der Frontzähne durch Sonnenblumenkern knacken. Dtsch Zahnärztl Z 1961; 16: 1018–22.

278. POULSEN S *et al.* Potassium nitrate toothpaste for dentine hypersensitivity. Cochrane Database Syst Rev 2001; 2: CD001476.

279. POWELL RN. Tooth contact during sleep: association with other events. J Dent Res 1965; 44: 959–67.

280. PUTT MS *et al.* Enamel polish and abrasion by prophylaxis pastes. Dent Hyg 1982; 56: 38–43.

281. RATCLIF PA *et al.* The effect of dihydrotachysterol and ferric dextran on the teeth and periodontium. J Periodontol 1964; 35: 320–5.

282. RADENTZ WH *et al.* A survey of factors possibly associated with cervical abrasion of tooth surfaces. J Periodontol 1976; 47: 148–54.

283. RAJAN BP. Attrition pattern in first permanent molar – a marker in diabetes mellitus? J Indian Dent Assoc 1982; 54: 403–7.

284. RAMFJORD SP. Bruxism, a clinical and electromyographic study. J Am Dent Assoc 1961; 62: 21–44.

285. RAMP MH *et al.* Evaluation of wear: enamel opposing three ceramic materials and a gold alloy. J Prosthet Dent 1997; 77: 523–30.

286. RANDOW K *et al.* The effect of an occlusal interference on the masticatory system. An experimental investigation. Odontol Revy 1976; 27: 245–56.

287. RAO SM *et al.* Electromyographic correlates of experimentally induced stress in diurnal bruxists and normals. J Dent Res 1979; 58: 1872–8.

288. RAO SR *et al.* Pulpal dysplasia. Oral Surg 1970; 30: 682–9.

289. REDING GR *et al.* Incidence of bruxism. J Dent Res 1966; 45: 1198–204.

290. REDING GR *et al.* Nocturnal teeth-grinding: all-night psychophysiologic studies. J Dent Res 1968; 47: 786–97.

291. REDMALM G. Dentifrice abrasivity. The use of laser light for determination of the abrasive properties of different silicas. An in vitro study. Swed Dent J 1986; 10: 243–50.

292. REDMALM G *et al.* Dentifrice abrasivity. The use of laser beams for comparative studies in vitro of surface changes. Swed Dent J 1979; 3: 91–100.

293. REDMALM G *et al.* Dentifrice abrasivity. The use of laser light and supplemental techniques for characterizing toothpastes containing different abrasives. An in vitro study. Swed Dent J 1984; 8: 57–66.

294. REICHART PA. Oral cancer and precancer related to betel and miang chewing in Thailand: a review. J Oral Pathol Med 1995; 24: 241–3.

295. REINHARDT GA. Attrition and the edge-to-edge bite. An anthropological study. Angle Orthod 1983; 53: 157–64.

296. REINHARDT GA. Relationships between attrition and lingual tilting in human teeth. Am J Phys Anthropol 1983; 61: 227–37.

297. RICHARDS LC *et al.* Dental attrition and degenerative arthritis of the temporomandibular joint. J Oral Rehabil 1981; 8: 293–307.

298. ROBB ND *et al.* Anorexia and bulimia nervosa (the eating disorders): conditions of interest to the dental practitioner. J Dent 1996; 24: 7–16.

299. ROBERTS CA *et al.* Comparison of internal derangements of the TMJ with occlusal findings. Oral Surg 1987; 63: 645–50.

300. ROBERTSON A *et al.* Incidence of pulp necrosis subsequent to pulp canal obliteration from trauma of permanent incisors. J Endod 1996; 22: 557–60.

301. ROBINSON JE *et al.* Nocturnal teeth-grinding: a reassessment for dentistry. J Am Dent Assoc 1969; 78: 1308–11.

302. ROELOFS SA *et al.* Behandeling van locale slijtage in het front. Deel I: klinische evolatie van het Dahl-platvorm. Tandartspraktijk 2002; 23 (7): 2–8.

303. ROSENZWEIG KA. Dentition of Bedouins in Israel: I. Epidemiology. J Dent Res 1968; 47: 407–10.

304. RUGH JD *et al.* Experimental occlusal discrepancies and nocturnal bruxism. J Prosthet Dent 1984; 51: 548–33.

305. RUGH JD *et al.* Psychophysiological changes and oral conditions. In: COHEN LK *et al.* (eds) Social sciences and dentistry. A critical bibliography. Volume 2. Kingston-upon-Thames: Quintessence Publishing, on behalf of the Fédération Dentaire Internationale, 1984.

306. RUGH JD *et al.* Orale Gewohnheiten. In: INGERSOLL B. Psychologische Aspekte der Zahnheilkunde. Berlin: Quintessenz Verlags-GmbH, 1987.

307. RUGH JD *et al.* Electromyographic studies of bruxist behavior before and during treatment. J Calif Dent Assoc 1975; 3: 56–9.

308. SAHIMA M *et al.* Age-related changes of the cementogenesis in the senescence-accelerated mouse (SAM). J Periodont Res 1996; 31: 470–6.

309. SANGNES G. Traumatization of teeth and gingiva related to habitual tooth cleaning procedures. J Clin Periodontol 1976; 3: 94–103.

310. SANGNES G *et al.* Prevalence of oral soft and hard tissue lesions related to mechanical toothcleansing procedures. Community Dent Oral Epidemiol 1976; 4: 77–83.

311. SAWYER DR *et al.* The effect of attrition on the pre-Columbian Indian arch length. J Dent 1983; 11: 154–8.

312. SAXTON CA *et al.* Clinical investigation of the effects of dentifrices on dentin wear at the cementoenamel junction. J Am Dent Assoc 1981; 102: 38–43.

313. SAXTON CA *et al.* Clinical investigation of the effect of dentifrices on dentin wear at the cementoenamel junction. J Am Dent Assoc 1981; 102: 38–43.

314. SCHAERER P *et al.* Occlusal interferences and mastication: an electromyographic study. J Prosthet Dent 1967; 17: 438–49.

315. SCHEMEHORN BR *et al.* The dentin abrasivity potential of a new electric toothbrush. Am J Dent 1996; 9: S19–20.

316. SCHIFFNER U. Keilförmige Zahnhalsdefekte bei regelmässiger Bürstapplikation eines Aminfluorid-haltigen Gelees. Schweiz Monatschr Zahnmed 1995; 105: 760–4.

317. SCHROEDER HE. Pathobiologie oraler Strukturen. Basel: Karger, 1983.

318. SCHROEDER HE. Altersveränderung der Pulpakammer und ihre Wandung in menschlichen Eckzähnen. Schweiz Monatschr Zahnmed 1993; 103: 141–9.

319. SCHULZ PD. Task activity and anterior tooth grooving in prehistoric California Indians. Am J Phys Anthropol 1970; 46: 87–92.

320. SCHULZE C. Developmental abnormalities of the teeth and jaws. In: GORLIN RJ, GOLDMAN HM (eds) Thoma's oral pathology. St Louis, MO: CV Mosby, 1970.

321. SCHWARZ WD. Erosion affecting the palatal surfaces of upper anterior teeth in young people. Br Dent J 1982; 153: 49.

322. SEDANO HO *et al.* Autosomal dominant cemental dysplasia. Oral Surg 1982; 54: 6426.

323. SEICHTER U. REM-Untersuchungen über den zervikalen Randspalt bei Komposit-Restaurationen mit Haftvermittlern. Dtsch Zahnärztl Z 1986; 41: 739–42.

324. SEGHI RR *et al.* Abrasion of human enamel by different dental ceramics in vitro. J Dent Res 1991; 70: 221–5.

325. SELIGMAN DA *et al.* The degree to which dental attrition in modern society is a function of age and of canine contact. J Orofacial Pain 1995; 9: 266–75.

326. SELIGMAN DA *et al.* The prevalence of dental attrition and its association with factors of age, gender, occlusion, and TMJ symptomatology. J Dent Res 1988; 67: 1323–33.

327. SENGUPTA A *et al.* Difficulties in estimating age using root dentine translucency in human teeth of varying antiquity. Arch Oral Biol 1999; 44: 889–99.

328. SENGUPTA A *et al.* The effects of dental wear on third molar eruption and on the curve of Spee in human archaeological dentitions. Arch Oral Biol 1999; 44: 925–34.

329. SHAFER WG *et al.* A textbook of oral pathology. Philadelphia, PA: WB Saunders, 1983.

330. SHATZ A *et al.* Monostotic Paget's disease of the mandible. J Oral Med 1986; 41: 1646.

331. SICHER H. The biology of attrition. Oral Surg 1953; 6: 406–12.

332. SILNESS J *et al.* Prevalence, pattern, and severity of incisal wear in dental students. Acta Odontol Scand 1994; 52: 178–81.

333. SILNESS J *et al.* Longitudinal study of incisal tooth wear in children and adolescents. Eur J Oral Sci 1995; 103: 90–4.

334. SILNESS J *et al.* Relationship between incisal tooth wear and the increasing number of permanent teeth in children and adolescents. J Oral Rehabil 1997; 24: 410–13.

335. SISKOS GJ *et al.* Unusual case of general pulp calcification (pulp stones) in a young Greek girl. Endod Dent Traumatol 1990; 6: 282–4.

336. SJÖHOLM TT *et al.* Sleep movements in teethgrinders. J Craniomandib Disord Facial Oral Pain 1992; 6: 184–91.

337. SLOP D *et al.* Abrasion of enamel. I. An in vitro investigation. Caries Res 1983; 17: 242–8.

338. SMITH BGN *et al.* An index for measuring the wear of the teeth. Br Dent J 1984; 156: 435–8.

339. SMITH BGN *et al.* The prevalence of toothwear in 1007 dental patients. J Oral Rehabil 1996; 23: 232–9.

340. SMITH BJ *et al.* Paget's disease of bone with particular reference to dentistry. J Oral Pathol 1981; 10: 233–47.

341. SÖDERLING E *et al.* Betadine-containing toothpaste relieves subjective symptoms of dry mouth. Acta Odontol Scand 1998; 56: 65–9.

342. SOGNNAES RF. Dental hard tissue destruction with special reference to idiopathic erosions. In: SOGNNAES RF (ed.) Mechanisms of hard tissue destruction. Washington, DC: American Association for the advancement of Science, 1963.

343. SOGNNAES RF *et al.* Dental erosion. I. J Am Dent Assoc 1972; 84: 571–6.

344. SOLHEIM T. Dental attrition as an indicator of age. Gerodontics 1988; 4: 299–304.

345. SOLLBERG WK *et al.* Temperomandibular joint pain and dysfunction: a clinical study of emotional and occlusal components. J Prosthet Dent 1972; 28: 412–22.

346. SPONHOLZ H *et al.* Anatomischhistologische Untersuchungen zur Zementapposition unter besonderer Berücksichtigung funktioneller Reize. Zahn Mund Kieferheilkd 1986; 74: 5636.

347. STANLEY HR et al. The detection and prevalence of reactive physiologic sclerotic, reparative dentin and dead tracts

beneath various types of dental lesions according to tooth surface and age. J Pathol 1983; 12: 257–89.

348. STEENKS MH. Occlusie en temperomandibulaire dysfunctie. Ned Tijdschr Tandheelkd 1996; 103: 279–83.

349. STEGENGA B et al. Bruxisme en temperomandibulaire stoornissen. Ned Tijdschr Tandheelkd 2000; 107: 285–8.

350. STEIN TJ et al. Anatomy of the root apex and its histologic changes with age. Oral Surg Oral Med Oral Pathol 1990; 69: 238–42.

351. STEIN TJ et al. Pararadicular cementum deposition as a criterion for age estimation in human beings. Oral Surg Oral Med Oral Pathol 1994; 77: 266–70.

352. STOCK P et al. Monitoring bruxism. Med Biol Eng Comput 1983; 21: 295–300.

353. STOOKEY GK. In vitro estimates of enamel and dentin abrasion associated with prophylaxis. J Dent Res 1978; 57: 36.

354. STOOKEY GK, MUHLER JC. Laboratory studies concerning the enamel and dentin abrasion properties of common dentifrice polishing agents. J Dent Res 1968; 47: 524–32.

355. STOTT GG et al. Cemental annulations as an age criterion in forensic dentistry. J Dent Res 1982; 61: 814–17.

356. SUZUKI JB. Etiology of parafunction: a brief review of psychological and occlusal genesis. J West Soc Periodontol Periodontal Abstr 1979; 27: 48–52.

357. SUZUKI S et al. Evaluating the antagonistic wear of restorative materials. J Am Dent Assoc 1996; 127: 74–80.

358. SVINNSETH PN et al. Abrasivity of toothpastes. An in vitro study of toothpastes marketed in Norway. Acta Odontol Scand 1987; 45: 195–202.

359. TALLGREN A et al. Correlations between EMG jaw muscle activity and facial morphology in complete denture wearers. J Oral Rehabil 1983; 10: 105–20.

360. TAMSE A et al. Statistical evaluation of radiologic survey of pulp stones. J Endod 1982; 8: 455–8.

361. TISHLER B. Occlusal habit neuroses. Dent Cosmos 1928; 70: 690–4.

362. THODEN VAN VELZEN SK et al. Endodontologie. Alphen aan den Rijn: Stafleu & Tholen BV, 1995.

363. THOMA KH et al. The pathology of dental cementum. J Am Dent Assoc 1939; 26: 1943–53.

364. TINANOFF N et al. Effect of a pumice prophylaxis on fluoride uptake in tooth enamel. J Am Dent Assoc 1974; 88: 384–9.

365. TOLLENS HL. Een merkwaardig pygmeeëngebit. Ned Tijdschr Tandheelkd 1960; 67: 193–9.

366. UNGAR PS et al. A review of interproximal wear grooves on fossil hominin teeth with new evidence from Olduvai Gorge. Arch Oral Biol 2001; 46: 285–92.

367. VANDENBERGHE JM et al. Pulp stones throughout the dentition of monozygotic twins. Oral Surg Oral Med Oral Pathol Oral Radiol Endod 1999; 87: 49–51.

368. VAN DER MEULEN MJ et al. De rol van de psycholoog bij de behandeling van bruxisme. Ned Tijdschr Tandheelkd 2000; 107: 297–300.

369. VAN DER WAALI et al. Pathologie van de mondholte. Houten: Bohn Stafleu Van Loghum, 1996.

370. VANDEWALLE KS. Guidelines for the restoration of Class V lesions. Gen Dent 1997; 45: 254–60.

371. VAN DER WEIJDEN GA et al. Moeten we nog wel poetsen? Ned Tandartsenbl 1992; 47: 102–3.

372. VAN NIEUW AMERONGEN A et al. Salivary proteins: protective and diagnostic value in cariology. Caries Res 2004 38: 247–53.

373. VAN DER ZAAG J et al. Tandheelkundige en farmacologische behandelingsstrategieën voor bruxisme. Ned Tijdschr Tandheelkd 2000; 107: 289–92.

374. VAN NIEUW AMERONGEN A et al. Werking van het speeksel tijdens het kauwproces. Ned Tijdschr Tandheelkd 1995; 102: 443–5.

375. VAN PALENSTEIN HELDERMAN et al. Mondhygiëne. In: VAN LOVEREN C et al. Preventieve tandheelkunde. Houten: Bohn Stafleu Van Loghum, 1996, pp. 174–7.

376. VELLY MIGUEL AM et al. Bruxism and other orofacial movements during sleep. J Craniomandib Disord Facial Oral Pain 1992; 6: 71–81.

377. VESTERGAARD CHRISTENSEN L. Facial pain and internal pressure of masseter muscle in experimental bruxism in man. Arch Oral Biol 1971; 16: 1021–31.

378. VILLAROSA GA et al. Oral behavioral patterns as factors contributing to the development of head and facial pain. J Prosthet Dent 1985; 54: 427–30.

379. VISSCHER CM, LOBBEZOO F, NAIJE M. Behandeling van bruxisme: de fysiotherapeutische benadering. Ned Tijdschr Tandheelkd 2000; 107: 293–6.

380. VISSER JB. Speciële pathologie van het menselijke gebit. Leiden: Stafleu & Tholen BV, 1974.

381. VISSINK A et al. Veranderingen in de secretie en samenstelling van speeksel met het ouder worden. Ned Tijdschr Tandheelkd 1997; 104: 186–9.

382. VISSINK A et al. Zwelling van de lippen als eerste uiting van acromegalie. Ned Tijdschr Tandheelkd 2004; 111: 17–19.

383. VÖLK W et al. Beitrag zur Ätiologie der keilförmigen Defekte. Dtsch Zahnärztl Z 1987; 42: 499–504.

384. VOLPE AR et al. A long term clinical study evaluating the effect of two dentifrices on oral tissues. J Periodontol 1975; 46: 113–18.

385. WALKER PL. A quantitative analysis of dental attrition rates in the Santa Barbara Channel area. Am J Phys Anthropol 1978; 48: 101–6.

386. WALTIMO A et al. Bite force and dentofacial morphology in men with severe dental attrition. Scand J Dent Res 1994; 102: 92–6.

387. WARREN JJ et al. Tooth wear patterns in the deciduous dentition. Am J Orthod Dentofac Orthop 2002; 122: 614–18.

388. WASSELL RW. Do occlusal factors play a part in temporomandibular dysfunction? J Dent 1989; 17: 101–10.

389. WATAHA JC et al. Effect of toothbrushing on the toxicity of casting alloys. J Prosthet Dent 2002; 87: 94–8.

390. WEDEL A et al. Tooth wear and temporomandibular joint morphology in a skull material from the 17th century. Swed Dent J 1998; 22: 85–95.

391. WEINBERGER A. The clinical significance of hypercementosis. Oral Surg 1954; 7: 79–87.

392. WENNEBERG B et al. Subjective symptoms from the stomatognathic system in ankylosing spondylitis. Acta Odont Scand 1982; 40: 215–22.

393. WHITE DJ. A new and improved "dual action" whitening dentifrice technology – sodium hexametaphosphate. J Clin Dent 2002; 13: 1–5.

394. WHITTAKER DK *et al*. Racial variations in the extent of tooth root translucency in ageing individuals. Arch Oral Biol 1996; 41: 15–19.

395. WHITTAKER DK *et al*. Tooth loss, attrition and temporomandibular joint changes in a Romano-British population. J Oral Rehabil 1985; 12: 407–19.

396. WHITTAKER DK *et al*. Quantitative assessment of tooth wear, alveolar–crest height and continuing eruption in a Romano-British population. Arch Oral Biol 1985; 30: 493–501.

397. WHITTAKER DK *et al*. Continuing tooth eruption and alveolar crest height in an eighteenth-century population from Spitalfields, East London. Arch Oral Biol 1990; 35: 81–5.

398. WICTORIN L. Effect of toothbrushing on acrylic resin veneering material. II. Abrasive effect of selected dentifrices and toothbrushes. Acta Odontol Scand 1972; 30: 383–95.

399. WIEDERKEHR M *et al*. Zahnärztliche untersuchung mittelalterlicher Schädel aus drei Regionen des Kantons Bern. Schweiz Monatschr Zahnheilkd 1982; 92: 127–36.

400. WILLIAMS DR. A rationale for the management of advanced tooth wear (ATW). J Oral Rehabil 1987; 14: 77–89.

401. WRUBBLE MK *et al*. Sleep-related bruxism and sleep variables: a critical review. J Craniomandib Disord Fac Oral Pain 1989; 3: 152–8.

402. WÜLKNITZ P. Cleaning power and abrasivity of European toothpastes. Adv Dent Res 1997; 11: 576–9.

403. XHONGA FA. Bruxism and its effect on the teeth. J Oral Rehabil 1977; 4: 65–76.

404. YANG MS *et al*. Prevalence and related risk factors of betel quid chewing by adolescent students in southern Taiwan. J Oral Pathol Med 1996; 25: 69–71.

405. YOUNG W *et al*. Syndromes with salivary dysfunction predispose to tooth wear. Oral Surg Oral Med Oral Pathol Oral Radiol Endod 2001; 92: 38–48.

406. ZANDER HA *et al*. Continuous cementum apposition. J Dent Res 1958; 37: 1035–44.

407. ELMARIA A *et al*. An evaluation of wear when enamel is opposed by various ceramic materials and gold. J Prosthet Dent 2006; 96: 345–53.

Chapter 9: Tooth Fractures and Traumatic Dentoalveolar Injuries

1. ABBOTT PV *et al*. Complicated crown fracture of an unerupted permanent tooth. Endod Dent Traumatol 1998; 14: 48–56.

2. ABOU-RASS M. Crack lines: the precursors of tooth fractures. Quint Int 1983; 14: 437–47.

3. AGAR JR *et al*. Occlusal adjustment for initial treatment and prevention of the cracked tooth syndrome. J Prosthet Dent 1988; 60: 145–7.

4. AL-BADRI S *et al*. Factors affecting resorption in traumatically intruded permanent incisors in children. Dent Traumatol 2002; 18: 73–6.

5. ALEXANDER RE. The appropriate use of antibiotics in dentistry. Quint Int 1997; 12: 815–23.

6. AL-JUNDI SH. Type of treatment, prognosis, and estimation of time spent to manage dental trauma in later presentation cases at a dental teaching hospital. Dent Traumatol 2004; 20: 1–5.

7. ALLANDER L *et al*. Reasons for replacement of class II amalgam restorations in private practice. Swed Dent J 1990; 14: 179–84.

8. ALLARD RHB *et al*. Diagnostiek en beleid bij (verdenking op) kindermishandeling. Ned Tijdschr Tandheelkd 2002; 109: 91–4.

9. AL-MAJED I *et al*. Prevalence of dental trauma in 5–6- and 12–14-year-old boys in Riyadh, Saudi Arabia. Dent Traumatol 2001; 17: 153–8.

10. ANDREASEN FM. Transient apical breakdown and its relation to color and sensibility changes after luxation injuries to the teeth. Endod Dent Traumatol 1986; 2: 9–19.

11. ANDREASEN F. Complications after traumatic dental injuries – stationary and transistory changes. In: GUTMANN JL *et al*. (eds) Proceedings of the international conference on oral trauma. Chicago, IL: American Association of Endodontists Endownment & Memorial Foundation, 1986.

12. ANDREASEN FM. Pulpal healing after luxation injuries and root fracture in the permanent dentition. Endod Dent Traumatol 1989; 5: 111–31.

13. ANDREASEN FM *et al*. Diagnosis of luxation injuries: the importance of standardized clinical, radiographic and photographic techniques in clinical investigations. Endod Dent Traumatol 1985; 1: 160–9.

14. ANDREASEN FM *et al*. Resorption and mineralization processes following root fracture of permanent incisors. Endod Dent Traumatol 1988; 4: 202–14.

15. ANDREASEN FM *et al*. Prognosis of root-fractured permanent incisors. Endod Dent Traumatol 1989; 5: 11–22.

16. ANDREASEN FM *et al*. Bonding of enamel-dentin crown fractures with glumar and resin. Endod Dent Traumatol 1986; 2: 277–80.

17. ANDREASEN FM *et al*. Prognosis of luxated permanent teeth. Endod Dent Traumatol 1985; 1: 207–20.

18. ANDREASEN FM *et al*. Occurrence of pulp canal obliteration after luxation injuries in permanent teeth. Endod Dent Traumatol 1987; 3: 103–15.

19. ANDREASEN FM *et al*. Relationship between pulp dimensions and development of pulp necrosis after luxation injuries in the permanent dentition. Endod Dent Traumatol 1986; 2: 90–8.

20. ANDREASEN JO. Luxation of permanent teeth due to trauma. A clinical and radiographic follow-up study of 189 injured teeth. Scand J Dent Res 1970; 78: 273–86.

21. ANDREASEN JO. The effect of splinting upon periodontal healing after replantation of permanent incisors in monkeys. Acta Odontol Scand 1975; 33: 313–23.

22. ANDREASEN JO *et al*. Traumatic injuries to the teeth. Copenhagen, Munksgaard, 1981.

23. ANDREASEN JO. Challenges in clinical dental traumatology. Endod Dent Traumatol 1985; 1: 45–55.

24. ANDREASEN JO et al. Textbook and color atlas of traumatic injuries to the teeth. Copenhagen: Munksgaard, 1994.

25. ANDREASEN JO et al. Healing of 400 intra-alveolar root fractures. 1. Effect of pre–injury and injury factors such as sex, age, stage of root development, fracture type and severity of dislocation. Dent Traumatol 2004; 20: 192–202.

26. ANDREASEN JO et al. Healing of 400 intra-alveolar root fractures. 2. Effect of treatment factors such as treatment delay, repositioning, splinting type and period and antibiotics. Dent Traumatol 2004; 20: 203–11.

27. ANDREASEN JO et al. Effect of treatment delay upon pulp and periodontal healing of traumatic injuries. Endod Dent Traumatol 2002; 18: 116–28.

28. ANDREASEN JO et al. Replantation of 400 avulsed permanent incisors. 3. Factors related to root growth. Endod Dent Traumatol 1995; 11: 69–75.

29. ANDREASEN JO et al. Long-term calcium hydroxide as a root canal dressing may increase risk of root fracture. Dent Traumatol 2002; 18: 134–7.

30. ANDREASEN JO et al. Intraalveolar root fractures: radiographic and histologic study of 50 cases. J Oral Surg 1967; 25: 414–26.

31. ANDREASEN JO et al. Damage of the Hertwig's epithelial root sheath: effect upon root growth after autotransplantation of teeth in monkeys. Endod Dent Traumatol 1988; 4: 145–51.

32. ANDREASEN JO et al. Epidemiology of traumatic dental injuries to primary and permanent teeth in a Danish population sample. Int J Oral Surg 1972; 1: 235–9.

33. ANDREASEN JO et al. The effect of traumatic injuries to primary teeth on their permanent successors. I. Scand J Dent Res 1971; 79: 219–83.

34. ANGMAR-MÅNSSON B et al. Root fractures due to corrosion. I. Metallurgical aspects. Odontol Revy 1969; 20: 245–64.

35. ANTRIM D et al. A functional splint for traumatized teeth. J Endod 1982; 8: 328–31.

36. APICELLA MJ et al. A comparison of root fracture resistance using two canal sealers. Int Endod J 1999; 32: 376–80.

37. ARIËNS EJ et al. Het geneesmiddel in de tandheelkunde. Alphen aan den Rijn: Samsom Stafleu, 1984.

38. ARMSTRONG SR et al. Mode of failure in the dentin-adhesive resin-resin composite bonded joint as determined by strength-based (μTBS) and fracture-based (CNSB) mechanical testing. Dent Mater 2001; 17: 201–10.

39. AROLA D et al. A comparison of the mechanical behavior of posterior teeth with amalgam and composite MOD restorations. J Dent 2001; 29: 63–7.

40. AUSIELLO P et al. Fracture resistance of endodontically treated premolars adhesively restored. Am J Dent 1997; 10: 237–41.

41. AUSIELLO P et al. Debonding of adhesively restored deep Class II restorations after functional loading. Am J Dent 1999; 12: 84–8.

42. BADER JD et al. Preliminary estimates of the incidence and consequences of tooth fracture. J Am Dent Assoc 1995; 126: 1650–4.

43. BADER JD et al. Incidence rates for complete cusp fracture. Community Dent Oral Epidemiol 2001; 29: 346–53.

44. BADER JD et al. Risk indicators for posterior tooth fracture. J Am Dent Assoc 2004B; 135: 883–92.

45. BADER JD et al. Consequences of posterior cusps fracture. Gen Dent 2004; 52: 128–31.

46. BADER JD et al. Case-control study of non-carious cervical lesions. Community Dent Oral Epidemiol 1996; 24: 286–91.

47. BARBAKOW FH et al. Experimental replantation of root-canal-filled and untreated teeth in the velvet monkey. J Endod 1977 3: 89–93.

48. BARRETT EJ et al. Survival of avulsed permanent maxillary incisors in children following delayed replantation. Endod Dent Traumatol 1997; 13: 269–75.

49. BAUSS O et al. Prevalence of traumatic injuries to the permanent incisors in candidates for orthodontic treatment. Dent Traumatol 2004; 20: 61–6.

50. BAXTER PW. Management of vertical incomplete fractures of posterior teeth with composite resin. Br Dent J 1987; 162: 219–20.

51. BEAN TA et al. Effect of esterase on methacrylates and methacrylate polymers in an enzyme simulator for biodurability and biocompatibility testing. J Biomed Mater Res 1994; 28: 59–63.

52. BEAN TA et al. Acetylcholinesterase degradation of a series of methacrylate monomers. J Dent Res 1995; 74: 186.

53. BENDER IB et al. Adult root fracture. J Am Dent Assoc 1983; 107: 413–19.

54. BENSON P. An unusual vertical root fracture. Br Dent J 1991; 170: 147–8.

55. BERNAU R et al. Spätergebnisse nach traumatischem Frontzahnverlust und nachfolgendem Lückenschluss. Stomatol DDR 1983; 33: 846–52.

56. BHASKAR SN et al. Dental vitality tests and pulp status. J Am Dent Assoc 1973; 86: 409–11.

57. BIJELLA MFTB et al. Occurrence of primary incisor traumatism in Brazilian children: a house-by-house survey. ASDC J Dent Child 1990; 87: 424–7.

58. BIRCH R et al. The incidence of complications following root fracture in permanent anterior teeth. Br Dent J 1986; 160: 119–22.

59. BONILLA E et al. Fatigue of resin-bonded amalgam restorations. Oper Dent 1996; 21: 122–6.

60. BORUM MK et al. Sequelae of trauma to primary maxillary incisors. I. Complications in the primary dentition. Endod Dent Traumatol 1998; 14: 31–44.

61. BORSSÉN E et al. Traumatic dental injuries in a cohort of 16-year-olds in northern Sweden. Endod Dent Traumatol 1997; 13: 276–80.

62. BOWDEN DEJ et al. Autotransplantation of premolar teeth to replace missing maxillary central incisors. Br J Orthod 1990; 17: 21–8.

63. BRALY BV et al. Potential for tooth fracture in restorative dentistry. J Prosthet Dent 1981; 45: 411–14.

64. BRAEM M *et al*. Stress-induced cervical lesions. J Prosthet Dent 1992; 67: 718–22.

65. BREMER BD *et al*. Molar fracture resistance after adhesive restoration with ceramic inlays or resin-based composites. Am J Dent 2001; 14: 216–20.

66. BROWN WS *et al*. Thermal fatigue in teeth. J Dent Res 1972; 51: 461–7.

67. BRUNTHALER A *et al*. Longevity of direct resin composite restorations in posterior teeth. Clin Oral Invest 2003; 7: 63–70.

68. BRUNTON PA *et al*. Fracture resistance of teeth restored with onlays of three contemporary tooth-colored resin-bonded restorative materials. J Prosthet Dent 1999; 82: 167–71.

69. BRUSZT P. Secondary eruption of teeth intruded into the maxilla by a blow. Oral Surg 1958; 11: 146–9.

70. BÜHLER H. Extrusion und apikale Verlängerung tief frakturierter Zähne. Quintessenz 1992; 43: 967–77.

71. BURTON J *et al*. Traumatized anterior teeth amongst high school students in northern Sydney. Aust Dent J 1985; 30: 346–8.

72. BRYNJULFSEN A *et al*. Incompletely fractured teeth associated with diffuse longstanding orofacial pain. Int Endod J 2001; 35: 461–6.

73. ÇALIŞKAN MK. Surgical extrusion of crown-root-fractured teeth. Int Endod J 1999; 32: 146–51.

74. ÇALIŞKAN MK *et al*. Prognosis of root-fractures permanent incisors. Endod Dent Traumatol 1996; 11: 129–36.

75. CAMERON CE. Cracked-tooth syndrome. J Am Dent Assoc 1964; 68: 405–11.

76. CAMERON CE. The cracked tooth syndrome. J Am Dent Assoc 1976; 93: 971–5.

77. CAMP JH. Recommended guidelines for treatment of the avulsed tooth. J Endod 1983; 9: 571.

78. CARON GA *et al*. Resistance to fracture of teeth with various preparations for amalgam. J Dent 1996; 24: 407–10.

79. CARVALHO JC *et al*. Malocclusion, dental injuries and dental anomalies in the primary dentition of Belgian children. Int J Paediatr Dent 1998; 8: 137–41.

80. ÇASKAN MK *et al*. Prognosis of root-fractured permanent incisors. Endod Dent Traumatol 1996; 12: 129–36.

81. CASTERLINE AC. Replantation of avulsed central incisor with advanced periodontal disease. Endod Dent Traumatol 1999; 15: 135–7.

82. CAVEL WT *et al*. An in vivo study of cuspal fracture. J Prosthet Dent 1985; 53: 38–42.

83. CHAPMAN PJ *et al*. Prevalence of orofacial injuries and use of mouthguards in high school Rugby Union. Aust Dent J 1996; 41: 252–5.

84. CHAWLA HS. Apical closure in a nonvital permanent tooth using one Ca(OH)2 dressing. ASDC J Dent Child 1986; 53: 44–7.

85. CHEUNG GSP *et al*. Long-term survival of primary root canal treatment carried out in a dental teaching hospital. Int Endod J 2003; 36: 117–28.

86. CLARK LL *et al*. Restorative treatment for the cracked tooth. Oper Dent 1984; 9: 136–42.

87. COTERT HS *et al*. In vitro comparison of cuspal fracture resistances of posterior teeth restored with various adhesive restorations. Int J Prothod 2001; 14: 374–8.

88. CRONA-LARSSON G *et al*. Effect of luxation injuries on permanent teeth. Endod Dent Traumatol 1991; 7: 199–206.

89. CRONA-LARSSON G *et al*. Luxation injuries to permanent teeth. Endod Dent Traumatol 1989; 5: 176–9.

90. CVEK M. Treatment of non-vital permanent incisors with calcium hydroxide. Part IV. Odontol Revy 1974; 25: 239–46.

91. CVEK M *et al*. Healing of 208 intraalveolar root fractures in patients aged 7–17 years. Dent Traumatol 2001; 17: 53–62.

92. CVEK M *et al*. Pulp reactions to exposure after experimental crown fractures or grinding in adult monkeys. J Endod 1982; 8: 391–7.

93. CVEK M *et al*. Healing and prognosis of teeth with intra-alveolar fractures involving the cervical part of the root. Dent Traumatol 2002; 18: 57–65.

94. DARENDELILER KABA *et al*. A fourteen-year follow-up study of traumatic injuries to the permanent dentition. ASDC J Dent Child 1989; 56: 417–25.

95. DAVIS GT *et al*. Dental trauma in Australia. Aust Dent J 1984; 29: 217–21.

96. DAWID E *et al*. Keilförmige Defekte als mögliche Folge von Stress? Dtsch Zahnärztl Z 1994; 49: 522–4.

97. DE CLEEN M. Apexifikation – Eine Literaturübersicht und klinische Emphelungen. Endodontie 1994; 1: 39–50.

98. DE BLANCO LP. Treatment of crown fractures with pulp exposure. Oral Surg Oral Med Oral Pathol Oral Radiol Endod 1996; 82: 564–8.

99. DE FREITAS CRB *et al*. Resistance to maxillary premolar fractures after restoration of class II preparations with resin composite ceromer. Quint Int 2002; 23: 589–94.

100. DE LAS CASAS EB *et al*. Abfraction and anisotropy. Comput Methods Biomech Biomed Engin 2003; 6: 65–73.

101. DEMARCO FF *et al*. Fracture resistance of re-attached coronal fragments. Dent Traumatol 2004; 20: 157–63.

102. DE MUNCK J *et al*. Four-year water degradation of total etch adhesives bonded to dentin. J Dent Res 2003; 82: 136–40.

103. DENNISON JB *et al*. Effect of variable light intensity on composite shrinkage. J Prosthet Dent 2000; 84: 499–505.

104. DESPAIN RR *et al*. Scanning electron microscope investigation of cracks in teeth through replication. J Am Dent Assoc 1974; 88: 580–4.

105. DEUTSCH AS *et al*. Root fracture and the design of prefabricated posts. J Prosthet Dent 1985; 53: 637–40.

106. DEUTSCH AS *et al*. Root fracture during insertion of prefabricated posts related to root size. J Prosthet Dent 1985; 53: 786–9.

107. DEWBERRY JJ. Vertical fractures of posterior teeth. In: WEINE FS (ed.) Endodontic therapy. St Louis, MO: CV Mosby, 1996.

108. DIAS DE SOUZA GM *et al*. Fracture resistance of premolars with bonded Class II amalgams. Oper Dent 2002; 27: 349–53.

109. DRÜKE B *et al*. Versprengte Zahnfragmente im Weichgewebe nach Frontzahntrauma. Quintessenz 1995; 46: 173–82.

110. DUMSHA T *et al*. Pulp prognosis following extrusive luxation injuries in permanent teeth with closed apexes. J Endod 1982; 8: 410–12.

111. DURHAM TM *et al*. Rapid forced eruption. Gen Dent 2004; 52: 167–75.

112. EAKLE WS. Reinforcement of fractured posterior teeth with bonded composite restorations. Quint Int 1985; 16: 481–2.

113. EAKLE WS. Effect of thermal cycling on fracture strength and microleakage in teeth restored with a bonded composite resin. Dent Mater 1986; 2: 114–17.

114. EAKLE WS *et al*. Fractures of posterior teeth in adults. J Am Dent Assoc 1986; 112: 215–18.

115. EBELESEDER KA *et al*. An analysis of 58 traumatically intruded and surgically extruded permanent teeth. Endod Dent Traumatol 2000; 16: 34–9.

116. EBELESEDER KA *et al*. A study of replanted permanent teeth in different age groups. Endod Dent Traumatol 1998; 14: 274–8.

117. EHRMANN EH *et al*. Cracked tooth syndrome: diagnosis, treatment and correlation between symptoms and post-extraction findings. Aust Dent J 1990; 35: 105–12.

118. ELLIS SG. Incomplete tooth fracture – proposal for a new definition. Br Dent J 2001; 190: 424–8.

119. ELLIS SG *et al*. Influence of patient age on the nature of tooth fracture. J Prosthet Dent 1999; 82: 226–30.

120. ERVERDI N *et al*. Complete intrusion of maxillary permanent central incisors. J Clin Pediatr Dent 2002; 27: 9–11.

121. FA-LIAN H *et al*. Clinical classification and therapeutic design of dental cervical abrasion. Gerodontics 1988; 4: 101–3.

122. FALOMO B. Fractured permanent incisors among Nigerian school children. ASDC J Dent Child 1986; 53: 119–21.

123. FARIK B *et al*. Adhesive bonding of fragmented anterior teeth. Endod Dent Traumatol 1998; 14: 119–23.

124. FARIK B *et al*. Drying and rewetting anterior crown fragments prior to bonding. Endod Dent Traumatol 1999; 15: 113–16.

125. FEIGLIN B. Clinical management of transverse root fractures. Dent Clin North Am 1995; 39 (1): 53–78.

126. FEILZER AJ *et al*. Curing contraction of composites and glass-ionomer cements. J Prosthet Dent 1988; 59: 297–300.

127. FEILZER AJ *et al*. Influence of light intensity on polymerization shrinkage and integrity of restoration – cavity interface. Eur J Oral Sci 1995; 103: 322–6.

128. FENNIS WMM *et al*. A survey of cusp fractures in a population of general dental practices. Int J Prosthodont 2002; 15: 559–63.

129. FERGUSON FS *et al*. Prevalence and type of traumatic injuries to the anterior teeth of preschool children. J Pedod 1979; 3: 3–8.

130. FILIPPI A *et al*. Replantation of avulsed primary anterior teeth: treatment and limitations. ASDC J Dent Child 1997; 64: 272–5.

131. FERRARI M *et al*. Technique sensitivity in bonding to vital, acid-etched dentin. Oper Dent 2003; 28: 3–8.

132. FISSORE B *et al*. Load fatigue of teeth restored by a dentin bonding agent and a posterior composite. J Prosthet Dent 1991; 65: 80–5.

133. FLANDERS R *et al*. The incidence of orofacial injuries in sports: a pilot study in Illinois. J Am Dent Assoc 1995; 126: 491–6.

134. FLORES MT. Traumatic injuries in the primary dentition. Dent Traumatol 2002; 18: 287–98.

135. FORSBERG C-M *et al*. Traumatic injuries to teeth in Swedish children living in an urban area. Swed Dent J 1990; 14: 115–22.

136. FORSBERG C-M *et al*. Etiological and predisposing factors related to traumatic injuries to permanent teeth. Swed Dent J 1993; 17: 183–90.

137. FRIED I *et al*. Subluxation injuries of maxillary primary anterior teeth: epidemiology and prognosis of 207 traumatized teeth. Pediatr Dent 1996; 18: 145–51.

138. FUKS AB *et al*. Long-term follow-up of traumatized incisors treated by partial pulpotomy. Pediatr Dent 1993; 15: 334–6.

139. FULLING HJ *et al*. Influence of maturation status and tooth type of permanent teeth upon electrometic and thermal pulp-testing. Scand J Dent Res 1976; 84: 286–90.

140. FUSS Z *et al*. Prevalence of vertical root fractures ion extracted endodontically treated teeth. Int Endod J 1999; 32: 283–6.

141. GALEA H. An investigation of dental injuries treated in an acute care general hospital. J Am Dent Assoc 1984; 109: 434–8.

142. GARCIA-GODOY F. A classification for traumatic injuries to primary and permanent teeth. J Pedod 1981; 5: 295–7.

143. GARCIA-GODOY FM. Prevalence and distribution of traumatic injuries to the permanent teeth of Dominican children from private schools. Community Dent Oral Epidemiol 1984; 12: 136–9.

144. GARCIA-GODOY F *et al*. Primary teeth traumatic injuries at a private pediatric dental center. Endod Dent Traumatol 1987; 3: 126–9.

145. GARCIA-GODOY F *et al*. Traumatic dental injuries in schoolchildren from Santo Domingo. Community Dent Oral Epidemiol 1985; 13: 177–9.

146. GARFIELD RE. Esthetic correction of incisal fractures without using restorative materials. Oper Dent 1987; 12: 24–6.

147. GARON MW *et al*. Mouth protectors and oral trauma: a study of adolescent football players. J Am Dent Assoc 1986; 112: 663–5.

148. GARRETT GB. Forced eruption in the treatment of transverse root fracture. J Am Dent Assoc 1985; 111: 270–2.

149. GASSNER R *et al*. Prevalence of dental trauma in 6000 patients with facial injuries. Implications for prevention. Oral Surg Oral Med Oral Pathol Oral Radiol Endod 1999; 87: 27–33.

150. GASSNER R *et al*. Traumatic dental injuries and Alpine skiing. Endod Dent Traumatol 2000; 16: 122–7.

151. GAUBERT SA *et al*. Periodontal mechano-sensory responses following traumata to permanent incisor teeth in children. Dent Traumatol 2003; 19: 145–53.

152. GAZELIUS B *et al*. Restored vitality in luxated teeth assessed by laser Doppler flowmeter. Endod Dent Traumatol 1988; 4: 265–8.

153. GELBIER MJ *et al*. Traumatised incisors treated by vital pulpotomy. Br Dent J 1988; 164: 319–23.

154. GENET JM *et al*. Klinische Instructie Endodontologie. Amsterdam: Universiteit van Amsterdam, 1984.

155. GERAMY A *et al*. Abfraction: 3 D analysis by means of the finite element method. Quint Int 2003; 34: 526–33.

156. GEURTSEN W *et al*. Bonded restorations for the prevention and treatment of the cracked tooth syndrome. Am J Dent 1999; 12: 266–70.

157. GEURTSEN W *et al*. Diagnosis, therapy, and prevention of the cracked tooth syndrome. Quint Int 2003; 34: 409–17.

158. GHER ME *et al*. Clinical survey of fractured teeth. J Am Dent Assoc 1987; 114: 174–7.

159. GIANGREGO E. Child abuse: recognition and reporting. Spec Care Dent 1986; 20: 62–7.

160. GÖRÜCÜ J *et al*. Fracture resistance of teeth with Class II bonded amalgam and new tooth-colored restorations. Oper Dent 2003; 28: 501–7.

161. GOEL VK *et al*. Stresses at the dentinal junction of human teeth – a finite element investigation. J Prosthet Dent 1991; 66: 451–9.

162. GRAEHN G *et al*. Zur Epidemiologie keilförmiger Defekte. Dtsch Stomatol 1991; 41: 210–13.

163. GREER JM *et al*. Resumed tooth development following avulsion of a permanent central incisor. Int Endod J 1996; 29: 266–70.

164. GRIPPO JO. Abfractions: a new classification of hard tissue lesions of teeth. J Esthet Dent 1991; 3: 14–19.

165. GRIPPO JO *et al*. Role of biodental engineering factors in the etiology of root caries. J Ethet Dent 1991; 3: 71–6.

166. GRIPPO JO *et al*. Dental "erosion" revisited. J Am Dent Assoc 1995; 126: 619–30.

167. GUPTA S *et al*. Suture splint: an alternative for luxation injuries of teeth in pediatric patients. J Clin Pediatr Dent 1997; 22: 19–21.

168. GUTHRIE FC *et al*. Treating the cracked tooth with a full crown. J Am Dent Assoc 1991; 122: 71–3.

169. GWINNETT AJ *et al*. Effect of long-term water storage on dentin bonding. Am J Dent 1995; 8: 109–11.

170. HAMDAN MA *et al*. A study comparing the prevalence and distribution of traumatic dental injuries among 10–12-year-old children in an urban and a rural area of Jordan. Int J Paediatr Dent 1995; 5: 237–41.

171. HAMILTON FA *et al*. An investigation of dento-alveolar trauma and its treatment in an adolescent population. Part 1. Br Dent J 1997; 182: 91–5.

172. HAMMARSTRÖM L *et al*. Tooth avulsion and replantation. Endod Dent Traumatol 1986; 2: 1–8.

173. HANDTMANN S *et al*. Korrosionserscheinungen an Silberstiften im Wurzelkanal (I). Dtsch Zahnärztl Z 1987; 42: 362–7.

174. HANSEN EK. In vivo cusp fracture of endodontically treated premolars restored with MOD amalgam or MOD resin fillings. Dent Mater 1988; 4: 169–73.

175. HANSEN EK *et al*. In vivo fractures of endodontically treated posterior teeth restored with enamel bonded resin. Endod Dent Traumatol 1990; 6: 218–25.

176. HANSEN EK *et al*. In vivo fractures of endodontically treated posterior teeth restored with amalgam. Endod Dent Traumatol 1990; 6: 49–55.

177. HANSEN EK *et al*. In vivo fractures of endodontically treated posterior teeth restored with enamel-bonded resin. Endod Dent Traumatol 1990; 6: 218–25.

178. HANSEN EK *et al*. Cusp fracture of endodontically treated posterior teeth restored with amalgam. Teeth restored in Denmark before 1975 versus after 1979. Acta Ododontol Scand 1993; 51: 73–7.

179. HARGREAVES JA *et al*. Trauma to primary teeth of South African pre-school children. Endod Dent Traumatol 1999; 15: 73–6.

180. HARRISON JW *et al*. The beginning of the end of the antibiotic era? Part I. Quint Int 1998; 29: 151–62.

181. HASHIMOTO M *et al*. Resin-tooth adhesive interfaces after long-term function. Am J Dent 2001; 14: 211–15.

182. HASHIMOTO M *et al*. Micromorphological changes in resin-dentin bonds after 1 year water storage. J Biomed Mater Res 2002; 63: 306–11.

183. HASHIMOTO M *et al*. In vitro degradation of resin-dentin bonds analyzed by microtensile bond test, scanning and transmission electron microscopy. Biomater 2003; 24: 3795–803.

184. HASHIMOTO M *et al*. Degradation patterns of different adhesives and bonding procedures. J Biomed Mater Res Part B: Appl Biomater 2003; 66: 324–30.

185. HEDEGÅRD B *et al*. A study of traumatized permanent teeth in children aged 7–15 years. Part I. Swed Dent J 1973; 66: 431–50.

186. HEITHERSAY GS. Combined endodontic-orthodontic treatment of transverse root fractures in the region of the alveolar crest. Oral Surg 1973; 36: 404–15.

187. HEITHERSAY GS. Replantation of avulsed teeth. A review. Aust Dent J 1975; 20: 63–72.

188. HELFER AR *et al*. Determination of the moisture content of vital and pulpless teeth. Oral Surg 1972; 34: 661–70.

189. HELING I. Intrusive luxation of an immature incisor. J Endod 1984; 10: 387–90.

190. HELING I *et al*. Bone-like tissue growth in the root canal of immature permanent teeth after traumatic injuries. Endod Dent Traumatol 2000; 16: 298–303.

191. HENRY RJ *et al*. Rationale and treatment of an avulsed permanent tooth. Compend Contin Educ 1991; 11: 346–53.

192. HEYDECKE G *et al*. Fracture strength after dynamic loading of endodontically treated teeth restored with different post-and-core systems. J Prosthet Dent 2002; 87: 438–45.

193. HEYDECKE G *et al*. The restoration of endodontically treated, single-rooted teeth with cast or direct posts and cores: a systematic review. J Prosthet Dent 2002; 87: 380–6.

194. HEYMANN HO *et al*. Examining tooth flexure effects. J Am Dent Assoc 1991; 122: 41–7.

195. HIATT WH. Incomplete crown-root fracture in pulpal-periodontal disease. J Periodontol 1973; 44: 369–79.

196. HILL CM *et al*. Dental and facial injuries following sports accidents. Br J Oral Maxillofac Surg 1985; 23: 268–74.

197. HOFFMANN J *et al*. Experimental comparative study of various mouthguards. Endod Dent Traumatol 1999; 15: 157–63.

198. HOLAN G *et al*. The diagnostic value of coronal dark-gray discoloration in primary teeth following traumatic injuries. Pediatr Dent 1996; 21: 224–7.

199. HOMEWOOD CI. Cracked tooth syndrome. Aust Dent J 1998; 43: 217–22.

200. HOOD JAA. Biomechanics of the intact, prepared and restored tooth. Int Dent J 1991; 41: 25–32.

201. HOTZ PR. Zahunfälle. Schweiz Monatschr Zahnmed 1990; 100: 849–58.

202. HUANG TJ *et al*. Effects of moisture content and endodontic treatment on some mechanical properties of human dentin. J Endod 1991; 18: 209–15.

203. HUANG MS *et al*. The effect of thermocycling and dentine pre-treatment on the durability of the bond between composite resin and dentine. J Oral Rehabil 2004; 31: 492–9.

204. HUF G. Diagnostik und Therapie des Crack-syndroms. Quintessenz 1988; 5: 1319–22.

205. HUMPHREY JM *et al*. Clinical outcomes for permanent incisor luxations in a pediatric population. I. Intrusions. Dent Traumatol 2003; 19: 266–73.

206. HUNTER ML *et al*. Traumatic injury to maxillary incisor teeth in a group of South Wales school children. Endod Dent Traumatol 1990; 6: 260–4.

207. HÜRMÜZLÜ F *et al*. In vitro fracture resistance of root-filled teeth using new-generation dentine bonding adhesives. Int Endod J 2003; 36: 770–3.

208. INGBER JS. Forced eruption: Part II. J Periodontol 1976; 47: 203–16.

209. JACOBSEN I. Clinical follow-up study of permanent incisors with intrusive luxation after acute trauma. J Dent Res 1983; 62: 486.

210. JACOBSEN I *et al*. Diagnosis and treatment of pulp necrosis in permanent anterior teeth with root fracture. Scand J Dent Res 1980; 88: 370–6.

211. JACOBSEN I *et al*. Traumatized primary anterior teeth. Prognosis related to calcific reactions in the pulp cavity. Acta Odontol Scand 1978; 36: 199–204.

212. JACOBSEN I *et al*. Repair characteristics of root fractures in permanent anterior teeth. Scand J Dent Res 1975; 83: 355–64.

213. JÄRVINEN S. Incisal overjet and traumatic injuries to upper permanent incisors. Acta Odontol Sacnd 1978; 36: 359–62.

214. JÄRVINEN S. Fractured and avulsed permanent incisors in Finnish children. Acta Odontol Scand 1979; 37: 47–50.

215. JÄRVINEN S. Traumatic injuries to upper permanent incisors related to age and incisal overjet. Acta Ondontol Scand 1979; 37: 335–8.

216. JESSEE SA. Detecting and reporting child maltreatment. Gen Dent 1994; 42: 218–21.

217. JOHNSON GK *et al*. Forced eruption in crown-lengthening procedures. J Prosthet Dent 1986; 56: 424–7.

218. JOHNSON R. Traumatic injuries to the teeth and supporting tissues. In: STEWART RE *et al*. (eds) Pediatric dentistry. St Louis, MO: CV Mosby, 1982.

219. KAHABUKA FK *et al*. Initial treatment of traumatic dental injuries by dental practitioners. Endod Dent Traumatol 1998; 14: 206–9.

220. KANIA MJ *et al*. Risk factors associated with incisor injury in elementary school children. Angle Orthod 1996; 66: 423–31.

221. KARGUL B *et al*. Dental trauma in Turkish children, Istanbul. Dent Trauamatol 2003; 19: 72–5.

222. KASSEBAUM DK *et al*. Recognition and reporting of child abuse: a survey of dentists. Gen Dent 1991; 39: 159–62.

223. KAWANAMI M *et al*. Infraposition of ankylosed permanent maxillary incisors after replantation related to age and sex. Endod Dent Traumatol 1999; 15: 50–6.

224. KENNY DJ *et al*. Avulsions and intrusions: the controversial displacement injuries. J Can Dent Assoc 2003; 69: 308–13.

225. KFIR A *et al*. Vertikale Wurzelfrakturen bei wurzelkanalbehandelten Zähnen. Endodontie 2002; 11: 115–21.

226. KHAN F *et al*. Dental cervical lesions associated with occlusal erosion and attrition. Aust Dent J 1999; 44: 176–86.

227. KINIRONS MJ *et al*. Inflammatory and replacement resorption in reimplanted permanent incisor teeth: a study of the characteristics of 84 teeth. Endod Dent Traumatol 1999; 15: 269–72.

228. KINIRONS MJ *et al*. Variations in the presenting and treatment features in reimplanted permanent incisors in children and their effect on the prevalence of root resorption. Br Dent J 2000; 189: 263–6.

229. KINIRONS MJ *et al*. Traumatically intruded permanent incisors: a study of treatment and outcome. Br Dent J 1991; 170: 1446.

230. KINOSHITA S *et al*. Prognosis of replanted primary incisors after injuries. Endod Dent Traumatol 2000; 16: 175–83.

231. KISHEN A *et al*. Stress-strain response in human dentine: rethinking fracture predilection in postcore restored teeth. Dent Traumatol 2004; 20: 90–100.

232. KITTLE PE *et al*. Examining for child abuse and child neglect. Pediatr Dent 1986; 8 (spec. issue 1): 80–2.

233. KLING M *et al*. Rate and predictability of pulp revascularization in therapeutically reimplanted permanent incisors. Endod Dent Traumatol 1986; 2: 83–9.

234. KOPEL HM *et al*. Examination and neurologic assessment of children with oro-facial trauma. Endod Dent Traumatol 1985; 1: 155–9.

235. KOSHIRO K *et al*. In vivo degradation of resin-dentin bonds produced by a self-etch vs. a total-etch adhesive system. Eur J Oral Sci 2004; 112: 368–75.

236. KREJCI I *et al*. Marginal adaptation, retention and fracture resistance of adhesive composite restorations on devital teeth with and without posts. Oper Dent 2003; 28: 127–35.

237. KRENKEL C *et al.* Behandlung total luxierter jugendlicher Frontzähne bei zertrümmerter Alveole. Quint 1986; 37: 2011–20.

238. KREYNS JM. Oud zeer (14). Tand om tand. Tandartspraktijk 2003; 24 (11): 42–3.

239. KUROE T *et al.* Potential for load-induced cervical stress concentration as a function of periodontal support. J Esthet Dent 1999; 11: 215–22.

240. LAMBRECHT JT. Antibiotische Prophylaxe unde Therapie. Schweiz Monatschr Zahnmed 2004; 114: 601–7.

241. LAVOUGARDOS P *et al.* Coronal fractures in posterior teeth. Oper Dent 1989; 14: 28–32.

242. LEE R *et al.* Clinical outcomes for permanent incisor luxations in a pediatric population. II. Extrusions. Dent Traumatol 2003; 19: 274–9.

243. LEE WC *et al.* Possible role of tensile stress in the etiology of cervical erosive lesions of teeth. J Prosthet Dent 1984; 52: 374–80.

244. LEE WC *et al.* Stress-induced cervical lesions. J Prosthet Dent 1996; 75: 487–94.

245. LEONARDO MR *et al.* Effect of intracanal dressings on repair and apical bridging of teeth with incomplete root formation. Endod Dent Traumatol 1993; 9: 25–30.

246. LETCHIRAKARN V *et al.* Effects of root canal sealer on vertical root fracture resistance of endodontically treated teeth. J Endod 2002; 28: 217–19.

247. LETZEL H *et al.* A controlled clinical study of amalgam restorations. Dent Mater 1989; 5: 115–21.

248. LEVIN L *et al.* Dental and oral trauma and mouthguard use during sport activities in Israel. Dent Traumatol 2003; 19: 237–42.

249. LEVITCH LC *et al.* Non-carious cervical lesions. J Dent 1994; 22: 195–207.

250. LI HP *et al.* The effect of long-term storage on nanoleakage. Oper Dent 2001; 26: 609–16.

251. LIEW VP *et al.* Anterior dental trauma treated after-hours in Newcastle, Australia. Community Dent Oral Epidemiol 1986; 14: 362–6.

252. LIM BS *et al.* Reduction of polymerization contraction stress for dental composites by two-step light-activation. Dent Mater 2002; 18: 436–44.

253. LINDEMANN W *et al.* Korrosions-erscheinungen an Silberstiften im Wurzelkanal (II). Dtsch Zahnärztl Z 1987; 42: 639–46.

254. LINDAUER PA *et al.* Vertical root fractures in curved roots under simulated clinical conditions. J Endod 1989; 15: 345–9.

255. LITONJUA LA *et al.* Noncarious cervical lesions and abfractions: a re-evaluation. J Am Dent Assoc 2003; 34: 2845–50.

256. LIU HH *et al.* Cracked teeth. Quint Int 1995; 26: 485–92.

257. LÖST C *et al.* Zahninfraktion. Die unvollständige Zahnfraktur. Schweiz Monatschr Zahnmed 1989; 99: 1033–7.

258. LOUVARDOS P *et al.* Coronal fractures in posterior teeth. Oper Dent 1989; 14: 28–32.

259. LUSTIG JP *et al.* Pattern of bone resorption in vertically fractured, endodontically treated teeth. Oral Surg Oral Med Oral Pathol Oral Radiol Endod 2000; 90: 224–7.

260. LUTZ F *et al.* Enamel cracks caused by vitality tests with carbon dioxide snow. Schweiz Monatschr Zahnmed 1974; 84: 709–25.

261. LYNCH CD *et al.* The cracked tooth syndrome. J Can Dent Assoc 2002; 68: 470–5.

262. LYONS K. Aetiology of abfraction lesions. N Z Dent J 2001; 97: 93–8.

263. MACKENZIE DF. The reinforcing effect of mesio-occlusodistal acid-etch composite restorations on weakened posterior teeth. Br Dent J 1986; 161: 410–14.

264. MACKO DJ *et al.* A study of fractured anterior teeth in a school population. ASDC J Dent Child 1979; 46: 130–3.

265. MAHLER DB *et al.* Clinical evaluation of amalgam bonding in Class I and Class II restorations. J Am Dent Assoc 2000; 131: 43–9.

266. MARCENES W *et al.* Epidemiology of traumatic injuries to the permanent incisores of 9–12-year-old schoolchildren in Damascus, Syria. Endod Dent Traumatol 1999; 15: 117–23.

267. MARCENES W *et al.* Social deprivation and traumatic dental injuries among 14-year-old schoolchildren in Newham, London. Dent Traumatol 2001; 17: 17–21.

268. MATA E *et al.* Divergent types of repair associated with root fractures in maxillary incisors. Endod Dent Traumatol 1985; 1: 150–3.

269. McCOMB D *et al.* Shear bond strength of resin-mediated amalgam-dentin attachment after cyclic loading. Oper Dent 1995; 20: 236–40.

270. McDOWELL JD *et al.* Recognizing and reporting victims of domestic violence. J Am Dent Assoc 1992; 123: 44–50.

271. McCOY G. The etiology of gingival erosion. J Oral Implantol 1982; 10: 361–2.

272. MEADOW D *et al.* Oral trauma in children. Pediatr Dent 1984; 6: 248–51.

273. MEHLMAN ES. Traumatic injuries of the teeth: current treatment modalities. Dent Today 2003; 22: 98–101.

274. MEIER B *et al.* Infraktionen. Quintessenz 1997; 48: 1621–38.

275. MEREDITH N *et al.* In vitro measurement of cuspal strain and displacement in composite restored teeth. J Dent 1997; 25: 331–7.

276. MEYER G *et al.* Zur Pathomorphologie keilförmiger Defekte. Dtsch Zahnärztl Z 1991; 46: 629–32.

277. MILLER N *et al.* Analysis of etiologic factors and periodontal conditions involved with 309 abfractions. J Clin Periodontol 2003; 30: 828–32.

278. MJÖR IA *et al.* Placement and replacement of amalgam restorations in Italy. Oper Dent 1992; 17: 70–3.

279. MORGANTINI J *et al.* Traumatism dentaires chez l'enfant en âge préscolaire et répercussions sur les dents permanentes. Rev Mens Suisse Odonto Stomatol 1986; 96: 37–40.

280. MIYASHIN M *et al.* Tissue reactions after experimental luxation injuries in immature rat teeth. Endod Dent Traumatol 1991; 7: 26–35.

281. MONDELLI J *et al.* Fracture strength of human teeth with cavity preparations. J Prosthet Dent 1980; 43: 419–22.

282. MORFIS AS. Enamel hypoplasia of a maxillary central incisor. Endod Dent Traumatol 1989; 5: 204–6.

283. MORIN DL *et al.* Biophysical stress analysis of restored teeth: experimental strain measurement. Dent Mater 1988; 4: 41–8.

284. MOTSCH A. Pulpitische Symptome als Problem in der Praxis. Deutsch Zahärtzl Zeit 1992; 47: 73–83.

285. MOULE AJ *et al.* Diagnosis and management of teeth with vertical root fractures. Aust Dent J 1999; 44: 75–87.

286. MURGEL CAF *et al.* Vertical root fracture and dentin deformation in curved roots: the influence of spreader design. Endod Dent Traumatol 1990; 6: 273–8.

287. NAMMOUR S *et al.* Use of the laser for welding cracks on the dental enamel. J Biol Buccale 1987; 15: 37–43.

288. NASJLETI CE *et al.* The effects of different splinting times on replantation of teeth in monkeys. Oral Surg 1982; 53: 557–66.

289. NEEDLEMAN HL. Orofacial trauma in child abuse. Pediatr Dent 1986; 8 (spec. issue 1): 71–80.

290. NEWMAN MP *et al.* Fracture resistance of endodontically treated teeth restored with composite posts. J Prosthet Dent 2003; 89: 360–7.

291. NGUYEN QV *et al.* A systematic review of the relationship between overjet size and traumatic dental injuries. Eur J Orthod 1999; 21: 503–15.

292. NIK-HUSSEIN NN. Traumatic injuries to anterior teeth among schoolchildren in Malaysia. Dent Treaumatol 2002; 17: 149–52.

293. NIKOUI M *et al.* Clinical outcomes for permanent incisor luxations in a pediatric population. III. Dent Traumatol 2003; 19: 280–5.

294. NORTHWAY W. Autogenic dental transplants. Am J Orthod Dentofac Orthop 2002; 121: 592–3.

295. OGINNI AO *et al.* Non-carious cervical lesions in a Nigerian population: abrasion or abfraction? Int Dent J 2003; 53: 275–9.

296. OIKARINEN K. Pathogenesis and mechanism of traumatic injuries to teeth. Endod Dent Traumatol 1987; 3: 220–3.

297. OIKARINEN K. Comparison of the flexibility of various splinting methods for tooth fixation. Int J Oral Maxillofac Surg 1988; 17: 125–7.

298. OIKARINEN K *et al.* Rigidity of various fixation methods used as splints. Endod Dent Traumatol 1992; 8: 113–19.

299. OIKARINEN K *et al.* Causes and types of traumatic tooth injuries treated in a public dental health clinic. Endod Dent Traumatol 1987; 3: 172–7.

300. OIKARINEN KS *et al.* Introduction to four custom-made mouth protectors constructed of single and double layers for activists in contact sports. Endod Dent Traumatol 1993; 9: 19–24.

301. OLGART L *et al.* Invasion of bacteria into dentinal tubules. Experiments in vivo and in vitro. Acta Odontol Scand 1974; 32: 61–70.

302. OLGART L *et al.* Laser Doppler flowmetry in assessing vitality in luxated permanent teeth. Int Endod J 1988; 21: 300–6.

303. OLUWOLE TO *et al.* Clinical and epidemiological survey of adolescents with crown fractures of permanent anterior teeth. Pediatr Dent 1986; 8: 221–5.

304. O'MULLANE DM. Some factors predisposing to injuries of permanent incisors in school children. Br Dent J 1973; 134: 328–32.

305. O'NEIL DW *et al.* Oral trauma in children: a hospital survey. Oral Surg Oral Med Oral Pathol 1989; 68: 691–6.

306. O'REILLY PM. Management of a vertically fractured endodontically treated tooth. Oral Surg 1985; 60: 208–11.

307. OSBORNE-SMITH KL *et al.* The aetiology of the non-carious cervical lesion. Int Dent J 1999; 49: 139–43.

308. OTT RW, PRÖSCHEL P. Zur Ätiologie des keilformigen Defektes. Dtsch Zahnärztl Z 1985; 40: 1223–7.

309. OTT RW *et al.* Einflüsse der Zahnputztechnik auf die Entstehung keilförmiger Defekte. Dtsch Stomatol 1991; 41: 463–5.

310. OTUYEMI OD. Traumatic anterior dental injuries related to incisor overjet and lip competence in 12-year-old Nigerian children. Int J Paediatr Dent 1994; 4: 81–5.

311. OULIS CJ *et al.* Dental injuries of permanent teeth treated in private practices in Athens. Endod Dent Traumatol 1996; 11: 60–5.

312. OULIS C *et al.* Management of intrusive luxation injuries. Endod Dent Traumatol 1996; 12: 113–19.

313. OWENS NM *et al.* Noncarious dental "abfraction" lesions in an aging population. Compend Contin Educ 1995; 16: 552–61.

314. PADILLA R *et al.* Prevention of oral injuries. J Cal Dent Assoc 1996; 24 (3): 30–6.

315. PALAMARA D *et al.* Strain patterns in cervical enamel of teeth subjected to occlusal loading. Dent Mater 2000; 16: 412–19.

316. PANITVISAI P *et al.* Cuspal deflection in molars in relation to endodontic and restorative procedures. J Endod 1995; 21: 57–61.

317. PAPA J *et al.* Moisture content of vital vs endodontically treated teeth. Endod Dent Traumatol 1994; 10: 91–3.

318. PASHLEY DH *et al.* Collagen degradation by host-derived enzymes during aging. J Dent Res 2004; 83: 216–21.

319. PAUL SJ *et al.* Nanonleakage at the dentin adhesive interface vs microtensile bond strength. Oper Dent 1999; 24: 181–8.

320. PEARSON GJ *et al.* Cusp movement in molar teeth using dentine adhesives and composite filling materials. Biomat 1987; 8: 473–6.

321. PERES R *et al.* Dental trauma in children. Endod Dent Traumatol 1991; 7: 212–13.

322. PIEPER K *et al.* Zur Prävalenz von Zahninfraktionen. Dtsch Zahnärztl Z 1994; 49: 822–4.

323. PILO R *et al.* Cusp reinforcement by bonding of amalgam restorations. J Dent 1998; 26: 467–72.

324. PILO R *et al.* Effect of core stiffness of the in vitro fracture of crowned, endodontically treated teeth. J Prosthet Dent 2002; 88: 302–6.

325. PINTADO MR *et al.* Correlation of noncarious cervical lesion size and occlusal wear in a single adult over a 14-year time span. J Prosthet Dent 2000; 84: 436–43.

326. PUGLIESI DMC *et al.* Influence of the type of dental trauma on the pulp vitality and the time elapsed until treatment. Dent Traumatol 2004; 20: 139–42.

327. QUALTROUGH AJ *et al.* Influence of different transitional restorations on the fracture resistance of premolar teeth. Oper Dent 2001; 26: 267–72.

328. RAKOCZ M *et al.* Traumatic impaction of a maxillary primary incisor into the nasal cavity. J Pedod 1985; 4: 338–43.

329. RANDOW K *et al.* On cantilever loading of vital and nonvital teeth. Acta Odontol Scand 1986; 44: 271–7.

330. RATCLIFF S *et al.* Type and incidence of cracks in posterior teeth. J Prosthet Dent 2001; 86: 168–72.

331. RAVN JJ. Dental injuries in Copenhagen schoolchildren. Community Dent Oral Epidemiol 1974; 2: 231–45.

332. RAVN JJ. Follow-up study of permanent incisors with enamel cracks as a result of an acute trauma. Scand J Dent Res 1981; 89: 117–23.

333. RAVN JJ. Follow-up study of permanent incisors with enamel fractures as a result of an acute trauma. Scand J Dent Res 1981; 89: 213–17.

334. RAVN JJ. Follow-up study of permanent incisors with enamel-dentin fractures after acute trauma. Scand J Dent Res 1981; 89: 355–65.

335. RAVN JJ. Follow-up study of permanent incisors with complicated crown fractures after acute trauma. Scand J Dent Res 1982; 90: 363–72.

336. REES JS. A review of the biomechanics of abfraction. Eur J Prosthodont Rest Dent 2000; 8: 139–44.

337. REES JS. The effect of variation in occlusal loading on the development of abfraction lesions: a finite element study. J Oral Rehabil 2002; 29: 188–93.

338. REES JS, *et al.* Abfraction lesion formation in maxillary incisors, canines and premolars: a finite element study. Eur J Oral Sci 2003; 111: 149–54.

339. REES JS *et al.* Undermining of enamel as a mechanism of abfraction lesion formation: a finite element study. Eur J Oral Sci 2004; 112: 347–52.

340. REIS A *et al.* Re-attachment of anterior fractured teeth: fracture strength using different techniques. Oper Dent 2001; 26: 287–94.

341. REIJNTJES RJ *et al.* Het extruderen van radices van eenwortelige gebitselementen. Ned Tijdschr Tandheelkd 1986; 93: 295–7.

342. RITTER AL *et al.* Pulp revascularization of replanted immature dog teeth after treatment with minocycline and doxycycline assess by laser Doppler flowmetry, radiography, and histology. Dent Traumatol 2004; 20: 75–84.

343. ROBERTSON A. A retrospective evaluation of patients with uncomplicated crown fractures and luxation injuries. Endod Dent Traumatol 1998; 14: 245–56.

344. ROBERTSON A *et al.* Incidence of pulp necrosis subsequent to pulp canal obliteration from trauma of permanent teeth. J Endod 1996; 22: 557–60.

345. ROBERTSON A *et al.* Long-term prognosis of crown-fractured permanent incisors. The effect of stage of root development and associated luxation injury. Int J Paediatr Dent 2000; 10: 191–9.

346. ROBERTSON A *et al.* Pulp calcifications in traumatized primary incisors. A morphological and inductive analysis study. Eur J Oral Sci 1997; 105: 196–206.

347. ROCK WP *et al.* The effect of luxation and subluxation upon the prognosis of traumatized incisor teeth. J Dent 1981; 9: 224–30.

348. RODD HD *et al.* Sports-related oral injury and mouthguard use among Sheffield school children. Community Dent Health 1997; 14: 25–30.

349. ROETERS JJM *et al.* Problems after trauma of maxillary central permanent incisors. Quint Int 1985; 22: 639–47.

350. ROSEN H. Cracked tooth syndrome. J Prosthet Dent 1982; 47: 36–43.

351. ROTHMAN DL. Pediatric orofacial injuries. J Cal Dent Assoc 1996; 24 (3): 37–42.

352. RUSMAH M. Traumatized anterior teeth in children. A 24-month follow-up study. Aust Dent J 1990; 35: 430–3.

353. SAE-LIM V *et al.* The effect of systemic tetracycline on resorption of dried replanted dogs' teeth. Endod Dent Traumatol 1998; 14: 127–32.

354. SAE-LIM V *et al.* Effect of systemic tetracycline and amoxicillin on inflammatory root resorption of replanted dogs' teeth. Endod Dent Traumatol 1998; 14: 216–20.

355. SALIS SG *et al.* Patterns of indirect fracture in intact and restored human premolar teeth. Endod Dent Traumatol 1987; 3: 10–14.

356. SANCHEZ AV *et al.* Traumatic dental injuries in 3- to 13-year-old boys in Monterrrey, Mexico. Endod Dent Traumatol 1990; 6: 63–5.

357. SANE J *et al.* Dental trauma in contact team sports. Endod Dent Traumatol 1988; 4: 164–9.

358. SAXE MD *et al.* Child abuse: a survey of ASDC members and a diagnostic-data-assessment for dentists. ASDC J Dent Child 1991; 58: 361–6.

359. SCHATZ JP *et al.* A retrospective clinical and radiographic study of teeth re-implanted following traumatic avulsion. Endod Dent Traumatol 1995; 11: 235–9.

360. SCHMITT BD. Types of child abuse and neglect: an overview for dentists. Pediatr Dent 1986; 8 (spec. issue 1): 67–71.

361. SCHNEIDER PE. Dental trauma and central nervous system injury. Quint Int 1986; 17: 749–53.

362. SCHRÖDER UE *et al.* Traumatized primary incisors – Follow-up program based on frequency of periapical osteitis related to tooth color. Swed Dent J 1977; 1: 95–8.

363. SCHWARTZ RS *et al.* Post placement and restoration of endodontically treated teeth. J Endod 2004; 30: 289–301.

364. SCOTT J *et al.* A review of dental injuries and the use of mouthguards in contact team sports. Br Dent J 1994; 176: 310–14.

365. SEDGLEY CM *et al.* Are endodontically treated teeth more brittle? J Endod 1992; 18: 332–5.

366. SELTZER S *et al.* Hypersensitivity and pain induced by operative procedures and the "cracked tooth" syndrome. Gen Dent 1997; 45: 148–59.

367. SHAPIRA J *et al.* Re-eruption of completely intruded immature permanent incisors. Endod Dent Traumatol 1986; 2: 113–16.

368. SHEROAN MM *et al.* Management of a complex dentoalveolar trauma with multiple avulsions. Dent Traumatol 2004; 20: 222–5.

369. SHETH JJ *et al.* Cuspal deformation and fracture resistance of teeth with dentin adhesives and composites. J Prosthet Dent 1988; 60: 560–9.

370. SHETTY V *et al.* Teeth in the line of fracture: a review. J Oral Maxillofac Surg 1989; 47: 1303–6.

371. SHIBUE T *et al.* Pulp and root development after partial extrusion in immature rat molars. Endod Dent Traumatol 1998; 14: 174–81.

372. SHINOGAYA T *et al.* Bite force and occlusal load distribution in normal complete dentitions of young adults. Eur J Prosthodontol Rest Dent 1999; 7: 65–70.

373. SHOCKLEDGE RR *et al.* Oral soft tissue trauma: gingival degloving. Endod Dent Traumatol 1996; 11: 109–11.

374. SHULLMAN JD *et al.* The association between incisor trauma and occlusal characteristics in individuals 8–50 years of age. Dent Traumatol 2004; 20: 67–74.

375. SILVESTRI AR *et al.* Treatment rationale of fractured posterior teeth. J Am Dent Assoc 1978; 97: 806–10.

376. SIMONSEN RJ. Restoration of a fractured central incisor using original tooth fragment. J Am Dent Assoc 1982; 105: 646–8.

377. SKAARE AB *et al.* Etiological factors related to dental injuries in Norwegians aged 7–18 years. Dent Traumatol 2003; 19: 304–8.

378. SKEIE A *et al.* Traumatic injuries of the teeth in connection with general anaesthesia and the effect of use of mouthguards. Endod Dent Traumatol 1999; 15: 33–6.

379. SNYDER DE. The cracked-tooth syndrome and fractures posterior cusp. Oral Surg 1976; 41: 698–704.

380. SONIS AL. Longitudinal study of discolored primary teeth and effect on succedaneous teeth. J Pedod 1987; 11: 247–51.

381. SOPOROWSKI NJ *et al.* Luxation injuries of primary anterior teeth. Pediatr Dent 1994; 16: 96–101.

382. SORENSEN JA *et al.* Intracoronal reinforcement and coronal coverage. J Prosthet Dent 1984; 51: 780–4.

383. SPAHR A *et al.* Expression of amelin and trauma-induced dentin formation. Clin Oral Invest 2002; 6: 51–7.

384. SPINAS E. A biological conservative approach to complex traumatic dento-alveolar lesions. J Clin Pediatr Dent 2003; 28: 1–10.

385. STAMPALIA LL *et al.* Fracture resistance of teeth with resin-bonded restorations. J Prosthet Dent 1986; 55: 694–8.

386. STÅLHANE I *et al.* Traumatized permanent teeth in children aged 7–15 years. Svensk Tandläk T 1975; 68: 157–69.

387. STANDLEE JP *et al.* The retentive and stress-distributing properties of a threaded endodontic dowel. J Prosthet Dent 1980; 44: 398–404.

388. STAPLEFORD RG. The management of dento-alveolar trauma. J Can Dent Assoc 1990; 56: 39–41.

389. STEELMAN R *et al.* Traumatic avulsion of the mandibular right primary lateral incisor and cuspid. J Clin Pediatr Dent 1991; 15: 249–50.

390. SPRANGER H. Investigation into the genesis of angular lesions at the cervical region of teeth. Quint Int 1995; 26: 149–54.

391. STEELE A *et al.* In vitro fracture strength of endodontically treated premolars. J Endod 1999; 25: 6–8.

392. STEWART GG. The detection and treatment of vertical root fractures. J Endod 1988; 14: 47–53.

393. STOCKWELL AJ. Incidence of dental trauma in the Western Australian school dental service. Community Dent Oral Epidemiol 1988; 16: 294–8.

394. STOKES AN *et al.* Diminutive lateral incisor as replacement for an avulsed permanent central incisor. Endod Dent Traumatol 1987; 3: 141–3.

395. STROBL H *et al.* Evaluation of pulpal blood flow after tooth splinting of luxated permanent maxillary incisors. Dent Traumatol 2004; 20: 36–41.

396. SWEPSTON JH *et al.* The incompletely fractured tooth. J Prosthet Dent 1986; 55: 413–16.

397. SYMONS AL *et al.* Dental aspects of child abuse. Aust Dent J 1987; 32: 42–7.

398. TAKEDA T *et al.* The influence of impact object characteristics on impact force and force absorption by mouthguard material. Dent Traumatol 2004; 20: 12–20.

399. TAKUSHIGE T *et al.* Endodontic treatment of primary teeth using a combination of antibacterial drugs. Int Endod J 2004; 37: 132–8.

400. TALIM ST *et al.* Management of coronal fractures of permanent posterior teeth. J Prosthet Dent 1974; 31: 172–8.

401. TAMSE A. Iatrogenic vertical root fractures in endodontically treated teeth. Endod Dent Traumatol 1988; 4: 190–6.

402. TANIGUCHI K *et al.* The effect of mechanical trauma on the tooth germ of rat molars at various developmental stages: a histopathological study. Endod Dent Traumatol 1999; 15: 17–25.

403. TANTBIROJN D *et al.* Tooth deformation patterns in molars after composite restoration. Dent Mater 2004; 20: 535–42.

404. TAPIAS MA *et al.* Prevalence of traumatic crown fractures to permanent incisors in a childhood population. Dent Traumatol 2003; 19: 119–23.

405. TER HORST G *et al.* Kindermishandeling en tandartsen. Ned Tijdschr Tandheelkd 1993; 100: 333–5.

406. THODEN VAN VELZEN SK *et al.* Endodontologie. Houten: Bohn Stafleu Van Loghum, 1995.

407. THYLSTRUP A *et al.* The influence of traumatic intrusion of primary teeth on their permanent successors in monkeys. A macroscopic, polarized light and scanning electron microscopic study. J Oral Pathol 1977; 6: 296–306.

408. TROPE M. Protocol for treating the avulsed tooth. J Cal Dent Assoc 1996; 24 (3): 43–9.

409. TROPE M. Clinical management of the avulsed tooth: present strategies and future directions. Dent Traumatol 2002; 18: 1–11.

410. TROPE M *et al.* Resistance to fracture of restored endodontically treated premolars. Endod Dent Traumatol 1986; 2: 35–8.

411. TRUSHKOWSKY RD. Esthetic, biologic and restorative considerations in coronal segment reattachment for a fractured tooth. J Prosthet Dent 1998; 79: 115–19.

412. TÜRP JC, GOBETTI JP. The cracked tooth syndrome. J Am Dent Assoc 1996; 127: 1502–7.

413. VELTMAAT A *et al.* In-vivo-Studie zur Epidemiologie der Kroneninfraktionen bei gefüllten Seitenzähnen. Dtsch Zahnärztl Z 1997; 52: 137–40.

414. VOLKERS AM.Preventieve en curatieve orthodontie in verband met fronttandtraumata. In: VAN DER KWAST WAM *et al*. (eds) Het tandheelkundig jaar 1982. Utrecht: Bohn, Scheltema & Holkema BV, 1982.

415. VON ARX T. Developmental disturbances of permanent teeth following trauma to the primary dentition. Aust Dent J 1993; 38: 1–10.

416. VON ARX T. Milchzahnintrusionen und odontogenese der bleibenden Zähne. Schweiz Monatschr Zahnmed 1995; 105: 11–17.

417. VON ARX T. Milchzahnintrusionen und Odontogenese der bleibende Zähne. Schweiz Monatschr Zahnmed 1995; 105: 11–17.

418. VON ARX T. Developmental disturbances of permanent teeth following trauma to the primary dentition. Aust Dent J 1993; 38: 1–10.

419. WAHL MJ *et al*. Prevalence of cusp fractures in teeth restored with amalgam and with resin-based composite. J Am Dent Assoc 2004; 135: 1127–32.

420. WARBURTON AL *et al*. Alcohol-related violence and the role of oral and maxillofacial surgeons in multi-agency prevention. Int J Oral Maxillofac Surg 2002; 31: 657–63.

421. WEIGER R *et al*. Management of an avulsed primary incisor. Endod Dent Traumatol 1999; 15: 138–43.

422. WIENS JP. Acquired maxillofacial defects from motor vehicle accidents: statistics and prosthodontic considerations. J Prosthet Dent 1990; 63: 172–81.

423. WU M-K *et al*. Comparison of mandibular premolars and canines with respect to their resistance to vertical root fracture. J Dent 2004; 32: 265–8.

424. YAGOT KH *et al*. Traumatic dental injuries in nursery schoolchildren from Baghdad, Iraq. Community Dent Oral Epidemiol 1988; 16: 292–3.

425. YAMADA Y *et al*. Effect of restoration method on fracture resistance of endodontically treated maxillary premolars. Int J Prosthodont 2004; 17: 94–8.

426. YANPISET K *et al*. Pulp revascularisation of replanted immature dog teeth after different treatment methods. Endod Dent Traumatol 2000; 16: 211–17.

427. YATES JA. Barrier formation time in non-vital teeth with open apices. Int Endod J 1988; 21: 313–19.

428. YATES JA. Root fractures in permanent teeth: a clinical review. Int Endod J 1992; 25: 150–7.

429. ZACHRISSON BU *et al*. Long-term prognosis of 66 permanent anterior teeth with root fracture. Swed Dent J Res 1975; 83: 345–54.

430. ZADIK D *et al*. A survey of traumatized incisors in Jerusalem school children. ASDC J Dent Child 1972; 39: 185–8.

431. ZADIK D *et al*. The prognosis of traumatized permanent anterior teeth with fracture of the enamel and dentin. Oral Surg 1979; 47: 173–5.

432. ZADIK D *et al*. Traumatized teeth: two-year results. J Pedod 1980; 4: 116–23.

433. ZAMON EL *et al*. Replantation of avulsed primary incisors: a risk-benefit assessment. J Can Dent Assoc 2001; 67: 386.

434. ZERMAN N *et al*. Traumatic injuries to permanent incisors. Endod Dent Traumatol 1993; 9: 61–4.

435. ZIDAN O *et al*. The effect of amalgam bonding on the stiffness of teeth weakened by cavity preparation. Dent Mater 2003; 19: 680–5.

436. ROG BD *et al*. Analysis of 154 cases of teeth with cracks. Dent Traumatol 2006; 22: 118–23.

437. BONFANTE G *et al*. Fracture strength of teeth with flared root canals restored with glas fibre posts. Int Dent J 2007, 57: 153–60.

438. SIGNORE A *et al*. A 4–6-year retrospective clinical study of cracked teeth restored with bonded indirect resin composite onlys. Int J Prosthodont 2007; 20: 609–16.

439. SAGSEN B *et al*. Effect of bonded restorations on the fracture resistance of root filled teeth. Int Endod J 2006; 39: 900–4.

440. HABEKOST LDV *et al*. Fracture resistance of thermal cycled and endodontically treated premolars with adhesive restorations. J Prosthet Dent 2007; 98 : 186–92.

441. BARTLETT DW *et al*. A critical review of non-carious cervical (wear) lesions and the role of abfraction, erosion, and abrasion. J Dent Res 2006; 85: 306–12.

442. FLORES MT *et al*. Guidelines for the management of traumatic dental injuries, I, II and III. Dent Traumatol 2007; 23: 66–71 and 130–6 and 196–202.

443. ANDREASEN JO *et al*. Traumatic intrusion of permanent teeth. Part 3. Dent Traumatol 2006; 22: 99–111.

444. GOPISRISHNA V *et al*. Comparison of electrical, thermal, and pulse oximetry methods for assessing pulp vitality in recently traumatized teeth. J Endod 2007; 33: 531–5.

445. HOLAN GL. Long-term effect of different treatment modalities for traumatized primary incisors presenting dark coronal discoloration with no other signs of injury. Dent Traumatol 2006; 22: 14–17.

446. RAFTER M. Apexification. Dent Traumatol 2005; 21: 1–8.

447. ROSENBERG B *et al*. The effect of calcium hydroxide root filling on dentin fracture strength. Dent Traumatol 2007; 23: 26–9.

448. TAMSE A *et al*. Radiographic features of vertically fractured endodontically treated mesial roots of mandibular molars. Oral Surg Oral Med Oral Pathol Oral Radiol Endod 2006; 101: 792–802.

449. MORA MA *et al*. Effect of number of basis images on the detection of longitudinal tooth fractures using local computed tomography. Dentomaxillofac Radiol 2007; 36: 382–6.

450. CVEK M *et al*. Conservative endodontic treatment of teeth fractured in the middle or apical part of the root. Dent Traumatol 2004; 20: 261–9.

451. CAMPBELL KM *et al*. Diagnosis of ankylosis in permanent incisors by expert ratings, Periotest® and digital sound wave analysis. Dent Traumatol 2005; 21: 206–12.

452. CAMPBELL KM *et al*. Development of ankylosis in permanent incisors following delayed replantation and svere intrusion. Dent Traumatol 2007; 23: 162–6.

453. TORRIANI DD *et al*. Histological evaluation of dog permanent teeth after traumatic intrusion of their primary predecessors. Dent Traumatol 2006; 22: 198–204.

454. DÍAZ JA *et al*. Conservative treatment of an ankylosed tooth after delayed replantation. Dent Traumatol 2007; 23: 313–17.

455. POI WR *et al*. Influence of enamel matrix derivate (Emdogain) and sodium fluoride on the healing process in delayed tooth replantation. Dent Traumatol 2007; 23: 35–41.
456. KNAPIK JJ *et al*. Mouthguards in sport activities. Sports Med 2007; 37: 117–44.
457. KAHLER B *et al*. An evidence-based appraisal of splinting luxated, avulsed and root-fractured teeth. Dent Traumatol 2008; 24: 2–10.
458. DIKBAS I *et al*. Evaluation of the effect of different ferrule designs on the fracture resistance of endodontically treated maxillary central incisors incorporating fiber posts, composite cores and crown restorations. J Contemp Dent Pract 2007; 8 (7): 1–10.

Chapter 10: Discoloration of Teeth

1. Abbott P *et al*. Internal bleaching of teeth: an analysis of 255 teeth. Aust Dent J 2009; 54: 326–33.
2. ABOU-RAS M. The elimination of tetracycline discoloration by intentional endodontics and internal bleaching. J Endod 1982; 8: 101–6.
3. ABOU-RAS M. Long-term prognosis of intentional endodontics and internal bleaching of tetracycline stained teeth. Compend Contin Educ Dent 1998; 19: 1034–40.
4. ADDY M *et al*. The effects of a 0.2% chlorhexidine gluconate mouth rinse on plaque, toothstaining and candida in aphthous ulcer patients. J Clin Periodontol 1987; 14: 267–73.
5. ADDY M *et al*. Extrinsic tooth discoloration by metals and chlorhexidine. II. Br Dent J 1985; 159: 331–4.
6. ADDY M *et al*. Extrinsic tooth discoloration by metals and chlorhexidine. I. Br Dent J 1985; 159: 281–5.
7. AFSETH J *et al*. Factors affecting retention of Cu in the human oral cavity after mouth rinses. Scand J Dent Res 1986; 94: 141–5.
8. ALDECOA EA *et al*. Modified internal bleaching of severe tetracycline discoloration: a 6-year clinical evaluation. Quint Int 1992; 23: 83–9.
9. ALLEN DR *et al*. A clinical study to compare the anticalculus efficacy of three dentifrice formulations. J Clin Dent 2002; 13: 69–72.
10. ALKHATIB NN *et al*. Prevalence of self-assessed tooth discolouration in the United Kingdom. J Dent 2004; 32: 561–6.
11. ANDREASEN FM *et al*. Bonding of enamel-dentin crown fractures with glumar and resin. Endod Dent Traumatol 1986; 2: 277–80.
12. ANDREASEN FM. Transient apical breakdown and its relation to color and sensibility changes after luxation injuries to the teeth. Endod Dent Traumatol 1986; 2: 9–19.
13. ANITUA E *et al*. Internal bleaching of severe tetracycline discolorations: four-year clinical evaluation. Quint Int 1990; 21: 783–8.
14. ASFORA KK *et al*. Evaluation of biocompatibility of sodium perborate and 30% hydrogen peroxide using analysis of the adherence capacity and morphology of macrophages. J Dent 2005; 33: 155–62.
15. ASHKENAZI M *et al*. Microabrasion of teeth with discoloration resembling hypomaturation defects: four-year follow up. J Clin Pediatr Dent 2000; 25: 29–34.
16. ATTIN T *et al*. Review of current status of tooth whitening with the walking bleach technique. Int Endod J 2003; 36: 313–29.
17. ATTIN T *et al*. Influence of different bleaching systems on fracture toughness and hardness of enamel. Oper Dent 2004; 29: 188–95.
18. ATTIN T *et al*. Subsurface microhardness of enamel and dentin after external bleaching procedures. Am J Dent 2005; 18: 8–12.
19. ATTIN T *et al*. Potential of fluoridated carbamide peroxide gels to support post-bleaching enamel re-hardening. J Dent 2007; 35: 755–9.
20. AUSCHILL TM *et al*. Efficacy, side-effects and patients' acceptance of different bleaching techniques. Oper Dent 2005; 30: 156–63.
21. AYAD F *et al*. Clinical efficacy of a new tooth whitening dentifrice. J Clin Dent 2002; 13: 82–5.
22. BACHMANN L *et al*. Dental discolouration after thermal treatment. Arch Oral Biol 2004; 49: 233–8.
23. BADER H *et al*. Clinical and laboratory evaluation of powered electric toothbrushes: comparative efficacy of two powered brushing instruments in furcations and interproximal areas. J Clin Dent 1997; 8: 91–4.
24. BAIG AA *et al*. Laboratory studies on the chemical whitening effects of a sodium hexametaphosphate dentifrice. J Clin Dent 2002; 13: 19–24.
25. BAIK JW *et al*. Effect of light-enhanced bleaching on in vitro surface and intrapulpal temperature rise. J Esthet Restor Dent 2001; 13: 370–8.
26. BALDISSARA P *et al*. Clinical and histological evaluation of thermal injury thresholds in human teeth. J Oral Rehabil 1997; 24: 791–801.
27. BARBOSA CM *et al*. Influence of time on bond strength after bleaching with 35% hydrogen peroxide. J Contemp Dent Pract 2008; 9: 81–8.
28. BARKHORDAR RA *et al*. Effect of nonvital tooth bleaching on microleakage of resin composite restorations. Quint Int 1997; 28: 341–4.
29. BARNES CM *et al*. A comparison of the Braun Oral-B Plaque Remover (D5) Electric and a manual toothbrush in affecting gingivitis. J Clin Dent 1993; 4: 48–51.
30. BARTA JE *et al*. ABO blood group incompatibility and primary tooth discoloration. Pediatr Dent 1989; 11: 316–18.
31. BASTING RT *et al*. The effect of 10% carbamide peroxide bleaching material on microhardness of sound and demineralized enamel and dentin in situ. Oper Dent 2001; 26: 531–9.
32. BASTING RT *et al*. The effect of 10% carbamide peroxide, carbopol and or glycerine on enamel and dentin microhardness. Oper Dent 2005; 30: 608–16.
33. BEN-AMAR A *et al*. Effect of mouthguard bleaching on enamel surface. Am J Dent 1995; 8: 29–32.
34. BIESBROCK AR *et al*. A chewing gum containing 7.5% sodium hexametaphosphate inhibits stain deposition compared with a placebo chewing gum. Compend Contin Educ Dent 2004; 25: 253–67.

35. BISTEY T *et al*. In vitro FT-IR study of the effects of hydrogen peroxide on superficial enamel. J Dent 2007; 35: 325–30.

36. BITTER NC *et al*. The effect of four bleaching agents on the enamel surface: a scanning electron microscopic study. Quint Int 1993; 24: 817–24.

37. BILLER IR *et al*. Enamel loss during a prophylaxis polish *in vitro*. J Int Assoc Den Child 1980; 11: 7–12.

38. BJORVATN K. Antibiotic compounds and enamel demineralization. Acta Odontol Scand 1982; 40: 341–52.

39. BLAKENAU R *et al*. The current status of vital tooth whitening techniques. Compend Contin Educ Dent 1999; 20: 781–94.

40. BOERE G. Elektrochemische activiteit in de mond. In: SCHUURS AHB *et al*. (eds) Amalgaam, de feiten. Nijmegen: STI, 1995.

41. BORUM MK *et al*. Sequelae of trauma to primary maxillary incisors. I. Complications in the primary dentition. Endod Dent Traumatol 1998; 14: 31–44.

42. BOWLES WH *et al*. Vital bleaching: the effects of heat and hydrogen peroxide on pulpal enzymes. J Endod 1986; 12: 108–12.

43. BOWLES WH *et al*. Pulp chamber penetration by hydrogen peroxide following vital bleaching procedures. J Endod 1987; 13: 375–7.

44. BOWLES WH. Protection against minocycline pigment formation by ascorbic acid (vitamin C). J Esthet Dent 1998; 10: 182–6.

45. BOWLES WH *et al*. Staining of adult teeth by minocycline: binding of minocycline by specific proteins. J Esthet Dent 1997; 9: 30–4.

46. BRIN I *et al*. Trauma to the primary incisors and its effect on the permanent successors. Pediatr Dent 1984; 6: 78–82.

47. ONDUM N *et al*. Postmortem red coloration of teeth. Am J Forensic Med Pathol 1987; 8: 127–30.

48. BROWN RS *et al*. The management of a dental abscess in a patient with acute intermittent porphyria. Oral Surg Oral Med Oral Pathol 1992; 73: 575–8.

49. BROWNING WD *et al*. Safety and efficacy of a nightguard bleaching agent containing sodium fluoride and potassium nitrate. Quint Int 2004; 35: 693–8.

50. BROWNING WD *et al*. Duration and timing of sensitivity related to bleaching. J Esthet Restor Dent 2007; 19: 256–64.

51. BROWNING WD *et al*. Comparison of traditional and low sensitivity whiteners. Oper Dent 2008; 33: 379–85.

52. BUCCI F *et al*. Oral lesions in lepromatous leprosy. J Oral Med 1987; 42: 4–6.

53. BURKINSHAW SM. Colour in relation to dentistry. Fundamentals of colour science. Br Dent J 2004; 196: 33–41.

54. CADENARO M *et al*. Effect of two in-office whitening agents on the enamel surface in vivo. Oper Dent 2008; 33: 127–34.

55. CALE AE *et al*. Pigmentation of the jawbones and teeth secondary to minocycline hydrochloride therapy. J Periodontol 1988; 59: 112–14.

56. CAMPS J *et al*. Time-course diffusion of hydrogen peroxide through human dentine: clinical significance for young tooth internal bleaching. J Endod 2007; 33: 455–9.

57. CAMPOS I *et al*. Effects of bleaching with carbamide peroxide gels on microhardness of restoration materials. J Esthet Restor Dent 2003; 15: 175–83.

58. CASEY LJ *et al*. The use of dentinal etching with endodontic bleaching procedures. J Endod 1989; 15: 535–8.

59. CESAR ICR *et al*. Analyses by photoreflectance spectroscopy of Vickers hardness of conventional and laser-assisted tooth bleaching. Am J Dent 2005; 18: 219–22.

60. CHERRY DV *et al*. Acute toxicological effects of ingested tooth whiteners in female rats. J Dent Res 1993; 72: 1298–303.

61. CHNG HK *et al*. Effects of traditional and alternative intracoronal bleaching agents on microhardness of human dentine. J Oral Rehabil 2004; 31: 811–16.

62. CIMILLI H *et al*. Effect of carbamide peroxide bleaching agents on the physical properties and chemical composition of enamel. Am J Dent 2001; 14: 63–6.

63. CHEEK CC *et al*. Dental and oral discolorations associated with minocycline and other tetracycline analogs. J Esthet Dent 1999; 11: 43–8.

64. CHEN JW *et al*. A study on betel quid chewing behavior among Kaohsiung residents aged 15 years and above. J Oral Pathol Med 1996; 25: 140–3.

65. CHIAPINELLI JA *et al*. Tooth discoloration resulting from long-term tetracycline therapy. Quint Int 1992; 23: 539–41.

66. CHIESARA E *et al*. The safety of tooth whitening. Munksgaard: Blackwell, 2002.

67. CLAYDON NCA *et al*. Clinical study to compare the effectiveness of a test whitening toothpaste with a commercial whitening toothpaste at inhibiting dental stain. J Clin Periodontol 2004; 31: 1088–91.

68. CLINICAL RESEARCH ASSOCIATES NEWSLETTER. Tooth bleaching, state-of-art. 1997; April: 1–3.

69. COBANKARA FK *et al*. Effect of home bleaching agents on the roughness and surface morphology of human enamel and dentine. Int Dent J 2004; 54: 211–16.

70. COCKINGS JM *et al*. Minocycline and oral pigmentation. Aust Dent J 1998; 43: 14–16.

71. COHENCA N *et al*. Transient apical breakdown following tooth luxation. Dent Traumatol 2003; 19: 289–91.

72. COLLYS K *et al*. Tandsteenremmende tandpasta's. Een nieuw tijdperk in de preventieve tandheelkunde? Ned Tijdschr Tandheelkd 1989; 96: 554–8.

73. COOPER JS *et al*. Penetration of the pulp chamber by carbamide peroxide bleaching agents. J Endod 1992; 18: 315–17.

74. COVINGTON J *et al*. Carbamide peroxide bleaching: effects on enamel composition and topography. J Dent Res 1990; 69: Abstract 530.

75. CRIM GA. Prerestorative bleaching: effect on microleakage of Class V cavities. Quint Int 1992; 23: 823–5.

76. CROLL TP. Das bleichen von Zähnen bei Kindern und Jugendlichen –Vorgehensweise und Beispiele. Quintessenz 1995; 46: 213–24.

77. CROLL TP *et al*. Tooth color improvement for children and teens: enamel microabrasion and dental bleaching. ASDC J Dent Child 1996; 63: 17–22.

78. CROLL TP. Enamel microabrasion: observations after 10 years. J Am Dent Assoc 1997; 128: 45S–50S.

79 CROLL TP. Esthetic correction for teeth with fluorosis and fluorosis-like enamel dysmineralization. J Esthet Dent 1998; 10: 21–9.

80. CROLL TP et al. Enamel color modification by controlled hydrochloric acid-pumice abrasion. I. Technique and examples. Quint Int 1986A; 17: 81–7.

81. Croll TP et al. Enamel color modification by controlled hydrochloric acid-pumice abrasion. II. Further examples. Quint Int 1986B; 17: 157–64.

82. Croll TP et al. Carbamide peroxide bleaching of teeth with dentinogenesis imperfecta discoloration. Qunit Int 1995; 26: 683–6.

83. CRONIN MJ et al. Comparison of two over-the-counter tooth whitening products using a novel system. Compen Contin Educ Dent 2005; 26: 140–8.

84. CULLEN DR et al. Peroxide bleaches: effect on tensile strength of composite resins. J Prosthet Dent 1993; 69: 247–9.

85. CVITKO E et al. Improved esthetics with a combined bleaching technique. Quint Int 1992; 23: 91–3.

86. DAHL JE et al. Acute toxicity of carbamide peroxide and a commercially available tooth-bleaching agent in rats. J Dent Res 1995; 74: 710–14.

87. DAHLSTROM SW et al. Hydroxyl radical activity in thermo-catalytically bleached root-filled teeth. Endod Dent Traumatol 1997; 13: 119–25.

88. DAVIES AK et al. Photo-oxidation of tetracycline adsorbed on hydroxyapatite in relation to the light-induced staining of teeth. J Dent Res 1985; 64: 936–9.

89. DAYAN D et al. Tooth discoloration. Quint Int 1983; 14: 195–9.

90. DA SILVA AP et al. Effect of peroxide-based bleaching agents on enamel ultimate tensile strength. Oper Dent 2005; 30: 318–24.

91. DELIPERI S et al. Two-year clinical evaluation of nonvital tooth whitening and resin composite restorations. J Esthet Dent Res 2005; 17: 369–79.

92. DE SILVA GOTARDI M et al. Number of in-office light activated bleaching treatments to achieve patient satisfaction. Quint Int 2006; 37: 115–20.

93. DE WIT MEC et al. Meldingen van tandverkleuringen door geneesmiddelen. Ned Tijdschr Tandheelkd 1996; 103: 3–4.

94. Đozić A. Capturing tooth color. Thesis, Academisch Centrum voor Tandheelkunde Amsterdam (ACTA), 2005.

95. DUSCHNER H et al. Effects of hydrogen peroxide gels on dental restoration in vitro. J Dent Res 2003; 82 (spec. issue C): C–529, #398.

96. DUYVENSZ F. Porfyrie en de betrekking tot het gebit. Ned Tijdschr Tandheelkd 1963; 70: 159–70.

97. EFEOGLU N et al. Microcomputerized tomography evaluation of 10% carbamide peroxide applied to enamel. J Dent 2005; 33: 561–7.

98. EISENBERG E et al. Anomalies of the teeth with stains and discolorations. J Prev Dent 1975; 2: 7–20.

99. ELLINGSEN JE et al. Extrinsic dental stain caused by stannous fluoride. Scand J Dent Res 1982; 90: 9–13.

100. ELLINGSEN JE et al. Extrinsic dental stain caused by chlorhexidine and other denaturing agents. J Clin Periodontol 1982; 9: 317–22.

101. ERIKSEN HM et al. Evaluation of extrinsic tooth discoloration. Acta Ondotol Scand 1979; 37: 371–5.

102. ERIKSEN HM et al. Characterization of saliva proteins from "stainers" and "non-stainers" adsorbed to hydroxyapatite. Acta Odontol Scand 1985; 43: 115–20.

103. ERIKSEN HM et al. Extrinsic discoloration of teeth. J Clin Periodontol 1978: 5: 229–36.

104. ERIKSEN HM et al. Chemical plaque control and extrinsic tooth discoloration. J Clin Periodontol 1985; 12: 345–50.

105. ERIKSEN HM et al. Chemical plaque control and prevention of extrinsic tooth discoloration in vivo. Acta Odontol Scand 1983; 41: 87–91.

106. ERNST C-P et al. Effects of hydrogen peroxide-containing bleaching agents on the morphology of human enamel. Quint Int 1996; 27: 53–6.

107. ESBERARD R et al. Effect of bleaching on the cemento-enamel junction. Am J Dent 2007; 20: 245–9.

108. FARAONI-ROMANO JJ et al. Bleaching agents with varying concentrations of carbamide peroxide and/or hydrogen peroxide: effect on dental microhardness and roughness. J Esthet Restor Dent 2008; 20: 403–4.

109. FARDAL O et al. A review of the literature on use of chlorhexidine in dentistry. J Am Dent Assoc 1986; 112: 863–9.

110. FASARANO TS. Bleaching teeth. J Esthet Dent 1992; 4: 71–8.

111. FAUNCE F. Management of discolored teeth. Dent Clin North Am 1983; 27: 657–70.

112. FAYLE SA et al. Congenital erythropoietic porphyria. Quint Int 1994; 25: 551–4.

113. FEIGLIN B. A 6-year recall study of clinically chemically bleached teeth. Oral Surg 1987;63: 610–13.

114. FEINMAN RA. Bleaching. A combination therapy. Cal Dent Assoc J 1987; April: 10–13.

115. FEINMAN RA et al. Bleaching teeth. Chicago, IL: Quintessence Publishing, 1987.

116. FELDER RS et al. Oral manifestations of drugs therapy. Spec Care Dent 1988; 8: 119–24.

117. FLAITZ CM et al. Effects of carbamide peroxide whitening agents on enamel surfaces and caries-like lesion formation: a SEM and polarized light microscopic in vitro study. ASDC J Dent Child 1996; 63: 249–56.

118. FLOYD RA. The effect of peroxides and free radicals on body tissues. J Am Dent Assoc 1997; 128: 37S–340S.

119. FRECCIA WF et al. An in vitro comparison of nonvital bleaching techniques in the discolored tooth. J Endod 1982; 8: 70–8.

120. FREDMOND AF et al. Acute illness and recovery in adult female rats following ingestion of a tooth whitener containing 6% hydrogen peroxide. Am J Dent 1997; 10: 268–71.

121. FRIEDMAN S et al. Incidence of external root resorption and esthetic results in 58 bleached pulpless teeth. Endod Dent Traumatol 1988; 4: 23–6.

122. FUSAYAMA T et al. Relationship between hardness, discoloration, and mocrobial invasion in carious dentin. J Dent Res 1966; 45: 1033–46.

123. GAGE JP. Dentinogenesis imperfecta. Aust Dent J 1985; 30: 285–90.

124. GALLAGHER A *et al*. Clinical study to compare two in-office (chairside) whitening systems. J Clin Dent 2000; 13: 219–24.

125. GALLO JR *et al*. Evaluation of 30% carbamide peroxide at-home bleaching gels with and without potassium nitrate. Quint Int 2009; 40: e1–6.

126. GAMBARINI G *et al*. Clinical evaluation of a novel liquid whitening gel. Am J Dent 2003; 16: 147–51.

127. GARCIA-GODOY F *et al*. Composite resin bonding strength after enamel bleaching. Oper Dent 1993; 18: 144–7.

128 128GEGAUFF AG *et al*. Evaluating tooth color change from carbamide peroxide gel. J Am Dent Assoc 1993; 124: 65–72.

129. GERLACH RW *et al*. Clinical trial comparing whitening strips and a paint-on tooth whitener. Presented at the annual meeting of the AADR, 12–15 March 2003.

130. GERLACH RW *et al*. Objective and subjective whitening response of two self-directed bleaching systems. Am J Dent 2002; 15 (spec. issue): 7A–12A.

131. GERLACH RW *et al*. Extrinsic stain removal with a sodium hexametaphosphate-containing dentifrice. J Clin Dent 2002; 12: 10–14.

132. GERLACH RW *et al*. Removal of extrinsic stain using a tartar control whitening dentifrice: a randomized clinical trial. J Clin Dent 2001; 12: 42–6.

133. GERLACH RW *et al*. Vital bleaching with whitening strips: summary of clinical research on effectiveness and tolerability. J Contemp Dent Pract 2001; 2(3): 1–15.

134. GERLACH RW. Whitening paradigms 1 year later: introduction of a novel professional tooth-bleaching system. Compend Contin Educ Dent 2002: 23 (spec. issue 1A): 4–8.

135. GERLACH RW *et al*. Clinical response of three direct-to-consumer whitening products. Compend Contin Educ Dent 2003; 24: 461–4.

136. GIUNTA JL *et al*. Stains and discolorations of teeth. J Pedod 1978; winter: 175–82.

137. GLASS RT. Oral manifestations in primary hyperoxaluria and oxalosis. Oral Surg 1973; 35: 502–9.

138. GLOCKNER K *et al*. Das Bleichen von verfärbten Frontzähnen. Schweiz Monatschr Zahnmed 1997; 107: 413–20.

139. GLOCKNER K *et al*. Five-year follow-up of internal bleaching Braz Dent J 1999; 10: 105–110

140. GODDER B *et al*. Evaluation of two at-home bleaching systems. J Clin Dent 1994; 5: 86–8.

141. GÖKAY O *et al*. *In vitro* peroxide penetration into the pulp chamber from newer bleaching products. Int Endod J 2005; 38: 516–20.

142. GOLDSTEIN RE. In-office bleaching: where we came from, where we are today. J Am Dent Assoc 1997; 128: 11S–15S.

143. GOLDSTEIN RE *et al*. Complete dental bleaching. Chicago, IL: Quintessence Publishing, 1995.

144. GROSSMAN E *et al*. A comparative clinical study of extrinsic tooth stain removal with two electric tooth-brushes [Braun D7 and D9] and a manual brush. Am J Dent 1996; 9: S25–9.

145. GRÜNDEMANN LJMM *et al*. Stain, plaque and gingivitis reduction by combining chlorhexidine and peroxxyborate. J Clin Periodontol 2000; 27: 9–15.

146. GOLDSTEIN GR *et al*. Bleaching: is it safe and effective? J Prosthet Dent 1993; 69: 325–8.

147. GOLDSTEIN RE. In-office bleaching: where we came from, where we are today. J Am Dent Assoc 1997; 128: 11S–15S.

148. GOON WWY *et al*. External cervical root resorption following bleaching. J Endod 1986; 12: 414–18.

149. GÜNAY H *et al*. Zahnverfärbungen bei Kindern und Jugendlichen mit Leberererkrankungen. Dtsch Zahnärztl Z 1994; 49: 461–3.

150. GURGAN S. Different light-activated in-office bleaching systems. Laser Med Sci 2010; 25: 817–22.

151. HANKS CT *et al*. Cytotoxicity and dentin permeability of carbamide peroxide and hydrogen peroxide vital bleaching materials *in vitro*. J Dent Res 1993; 72: 931–8.

152. HARA AT *et al*. Nonvital tooth bleaching. Quint Int 1999; 30: 748–54.

153. HARGREAVES I *et al*. Acromegaly: an unusual presentation and unexpected sequelae to treatment. Br Dent J 1987; 163: 196–7.

154. HALS E *et al*. Electron probe microanalysis of secondary carious lesions associated with silver amalgam fillings. Acta Odontol Scand 1975; 33: 149–60.

155. HANNING C *et al*. Efficacy and tolerability of two home bleaching systems having different peroxide delivery. Clin Oral Investig 2007; 11: 321–9.

156. HARRINGTON GW *et al*. External resorption associated with bleaching of pulpless teeth. J Endod 1979; 5: 344–8.

157. HATTAB FN *et al*. Dental discoloration: an overview. J Esthet Dent 1999; 11: 291–310.

158. HATTAB FN *et al*. Fluoride content in khat (Catha edulis) chewing leaves. Arch Oral Biol 2000; 45: 253–5.

159. HATTON PV *et al*. Treatment of dental amalgam with carbamide peroxide. J Dent Res 2003; 82 (spec. issue C): C–578, #709.

160. HAYES PA *et al*. The etiology and treatment of intrinsic discolourations. J Can Dent Assoc 1986; 52: 217–20.

161. HAYWOOD VB *et al*. Nightguard vital bleaching. Quint Int 1989; 20: 173–6.

162. HAYWOOD VB *et al*. Nightguard vital bleaching: effects on enamel surface texture and diffusion. Quint Int 1990; 21: 801–4.

163. HAYWOOD VB *et al*. Effectiveness, side effects and long term status of nightguard vital bleaching. J Am Dent Assoc 1994; 125: 1219–26.

164. HAYWOOD VB *et al*. History, safety, and effectiveness of current bleaching techniques and applications of the night-guard vital bleaching technique. Quint Int 1992; 23: 471–88.

165. HAYWOOD VB *et al*. Efficacy of six months of nightguard vital bleaching of tetracycline-stained teeth. J Esthet Dent 1997; 9: 13–19.

166. HAYWOOD VB. Nightguard vital bleaching: current concepts and research. J Am Dent Assoc 1997; 128: 19S–25S.

167. HAYWOOD VB. Greening of the tooth-amalgam interface during extended 10% carbamide peroxide bleaching of tetracycline-stained teeth: a case report. J Esthet Restor Dent 2002; 14: 12–17.

168. HAYWOOD VB. Tooth whitening. Chicago, IL: Quintessence Publishing, 2007.

169. HEITHERSAY GS. Invasive cervical resorption. Quint Int 1999; 30: 83–95.

170. HELLER D et al. Effect of intracoronal bleaching on external cervical root resorption. J Endod 1992; 18: 145–8.

171. HERBERT FL et al. Unusual case of green teeth resulting from neonatal hyperbilirubinemia. ASDC J Dent Child 1987; 54: 54–6.

172. HIGASHI C. One-year follow-up of non-vital discoloured teeth after bleaching with an association of techniques. Gen Dent 2007; 55 (spec. issue): 676–82.

173. HOLAN G. Development of clinical and radiographic signs associated with dark discolored primary incisors following traumatic injuries. Dent Traumatol 2004; 20: 276–87.

174. HOLMSTRUP G et al. Bleaching of discoloured root-filled teeth. Endod Dent Traumatol 1988; 4: 197–201.

175. HOOD ML, HUSSEY DL. Minocycline: stain devil? Br J Dermatol 2003; 149: 237–9.

176. HORN DJ et al. Effect of smear layer removal on bleaching of human teeth in vitro. J Endod 1998; 24: 791–5.

177. HOWELL RA. The prognosis of bleached root-filled teeth. Int Endod J 1981; 14: 22–6.

178. HURSEY RJ et al. Dentinogenesis imperfecta in a racial isolate with multiple hereditary effects. Oral Surg 1956; 9: 641–58.

179. JAHANGIRI L et al. Relationship between tooth shade value and skin color. J Prosthet Dent 2002; 87: 149–52.

180. JENKINS S et al. The effects of a chlorhexidine toothpaste on the development of plaque, gingivitis and tooth staining. J Clin Periodontol 1993; 20: 59–62.

181. JOHANSSON BI. An in vitro study of galvanic currents between amalgam and gold alloy electrodes in saliva and in saline solutions. Scand J Dent Res 1986; 94: 562–8.

182. JOHO J-P et al. Trauma in the primary dentition. ASDC J Dent Child 1980; 47: 167–74.

183. JOINER A. Tooth colour. J Dent 2004; 32 (suppl 1): 3–12.

184. JOINER A et al. In vitro evaluation of a novel 6% hydrogen peroxide tooth whitening product. J Dent 2004 (suppl 1); 32: 19–25.

185. JOINER A et al. Whitening toothpastes: effects on tooth stain and enamel. Int Dent J 2002; 52: 424–30.

186. JOINER A et al. The measurement of enamel wear of two toothpastes. Oral Health Prev Dent 2004; 2: 383–8.

187. JOINER A et al. Review of the effects of peroxide on enamel and dentine properties. J Dent 2007; 35: 889–96.

188. JONGENELIS APJM et al. A comparison of plaque removal effectiveness of an electric versus a manual toothbrush in children. ASDC J Dent Child 1997; 64: 176–82.

189. JOSEY AL et al. The effect of a vital bleaching technique on enamel surface morphology and the bonding of composite resin to enamel. J Oral Rehabil 1996; 23: 244–50.

190. JUSTINO LM et al. In situ and in vitro effects of bleaching with carbamide peroxide on human enamel. Oper Dent 2004; 29: 219–25.

191. KAYSER F. Verkleurde tanden. Ned Tijdschr Tandheelkd 1975; 82: 450–3.

192. KELLEHER MGD et al. The safety-in-use of 10% carbamide peroxide (Opalescence) for bleaching teeth under the supervision of a dentist. Br Dent J 1999; 187: 190–4.

193. KIDD EA et al. Staining of residual caries under freshly-packed amalgam restorations exposed to tea/chlorhexidine in vitro. Int Dent J 1990; 40: 219–24.

194. KILLIAN CM. Conservative color improvement for teeth with fluorosis-type stain. J Am Dent Assoc 1993; 124: 72–4.

195. KINIRONS MJ et al. The relationship between black extrinsic staining of teeth and the pH and buffering capacity of saliva in cystic-fibrosis patients. J Paediatr Dent 1990; 6: 27–37.

196. KLEBER CJ et al. Laboratory assessment of tooth whitening by sodium bicarbonate dentifrices. J Clin Dent 1998; 9: 72–5.

197. KLETER GA et al. Modification of amino acids residues in carious dentin matrix. J Dent Res 1998; 77: 488–95.

198. KOCH MJ et al. Prävalenz schwarzer Zahnbeläge bei Schulkindern. Dtsch Zahnärztl Z 1996; 51: 664–5.

199. KOERTGE TE et al. Comparison of two dentifrices in the control of chlorhexidine-induced stain. J Clin Dent 1993; 4: 1–5.

200. KOULAOUZIDOU E et al. In vitro evaluation of the cytotoxicity of a bleaching agent. Endod Dent Traumatol 1998; 14: 21–5.

201. KRAUSE F et al. Subjective intensities of pain and contentment with treatment outcomes during tray bleaching of vital teeth employing different carbamide peroxide concentrations. Quint Int 2008; 39: 202–9.

202. KUGEL G et al. Tooth whitening efficacy and safety: a randomized and controlled clinical trial. Compend Contin Educ Dent Dent 2003; 21 (suppl 29): 22–8.

203. KUGEL G et al. Daily use of whitening strips on tetracycline-stained teeth: comparative results after two months. Compend Contin Educ Dent 2000; 23 (spec. issue 1A): S29–S53.

204. KUROSAKI N et al. Penetration of elements from amalgam into dentin. J Dent Res 1973; 52: 309–17.

205. LADO EA et al. Cervical resorption in bleached teeth. Oral Surg 1983; 55: 78–80.

206. LATCHAM NL. Postbleaching cervical resorption. J Endod 1986; 12: 262–4.

207. LANGSTEN RE et al. Higher-concentration carbamide peroxide effects on surfaces of composites. J Esthet Restor Dent 2004; 14: 92–6.

208. LEE JH et al. Effect of bleaching agents on the fluoride release and microhardness of dental materials. J Biomed Mater Res 2002; 63: 535–41.

209. LEONARD RH et al. Risk factors for developing tooth sensitivity and gingival irritation associated with nightguard vital bleaching. Quint Int 1997; 28: 527–34.

210. LEONARD RH et al. Nightguard vital bleaching of tetracycline-stained teeth 54 months post treatment. J Esthet Dent 1999B; 11: 265–77.

211. LEONARD RH Jr. Nightguard vital bleaching: dark stains and long-term results. Compend Contin Educ Dent Suppl 2000; S18–S27.

212. LEONARD RH et al. Nightguard vital bleaching: a long-term study on efficacy, shade retention, side effects, and patients' perception. J Esthet Restor Dent 2001;13: 357–69.

213. LEONARD RH et al. Nightguard vital bleaching and its effects on enamel surface morphology. J Esthet Res 2001A; 13: 132–9.

214. LEONARD RH et al. Nightguard vital bleaching of tetracycline-stained teeth: 90 months post treatment. J Esthet Restor Dent 2003; 15: 142–53.

215. LEONARD RH et al. effect on enamel microhardness of two consumer-available bleaching solutions with a dentist-prescribed home-applied bleaching solution and a control. J Esthet Dent Res 2005; 17: 343–50.

216. LEUNG SW. Naturally occurring stains on the teeth of children. J Am Dent Assoc 1950; 41: 191–7.

217. LEWINSTEIN I et al. Effect of different peroxide bleaching regimens and subsequent fluoridation on the hardness of human enamel and dentin. J Prosthet Dent 2004; 92: 337–42.

218. LI Y et al. Safety evaluation of Opalescence sustained release whitening gel. J Dent Res 1996; 75: Abstrat 3304.

219. LI Y. Toxicological considerations of tooth bleaching using peroxide-containing agents. J Am Dent Assoc 1997; 128: 31S–36S.

220. LI Y, LEE SS et al. Comparison of clinical efficacy and safety of three professional at-home tooth whitening systems. Compend Contin Educ Dent 2003; 24: 357–76.

221. LIEBENBERG WH. Intracoronal lightening of discolored pulpless teeth: a modified walking bleach technique. Quint Int 1997; 28: 771–7.

222. LO ECM et al. A community-based caries control program for pre-school children using topical fluorides. 18 months results. J Dent Res 2001; 80: 2071–4.

223. LOPES GC et al. Effect of bleaching agents on the hardness and morphology of enamel. J Esthet Restor Dent 2002; 14: 24–30.

224. LOOS BG. Tandsteen: prevalentie, pathofysiologie en preventie. Ned Tijdschr Tandheelkd 1996; 103: 142–5.

225. LUFFINGHAM JK et al. Dentinal dysplasia. Br Dent J 1986; 160: 281–3.

226. LUK K et al. Effect of light energy on peroxide tooth bleaching. J Am Dent Assoc 2004; 135: 194–201.

227. MAACKE C. Die Histologie der Porphyriezähne. Vierteljahrschr Zahnheilkd 1931; 47: 191–202.

228. MADISON S et al. Cervical root resorption following bleaching of endodontically bleached teeth. J Endod 1990; 16: 570–4.

229. MAGGIO B et al. Whitening gel designed to accelerate whitening. Compend Contin Educ Dent 2003; 24: 519–32.

230. MAIA E et al. The influence of two home-applied bleaching agents on enamel microhardness. J Dent 2008; 36: 2–7.

231. MAIR L et al. The measurement and degradation and wear of three glass ionomers following peroxide bleaching. J Dent 2004; 32: 41–5.

232. MAJEWSKI RF et al. Dental findings in a patient with biliary atresia. J Clin Pediatr Dent 1993; 18: 33–7.

233. MARIN PD et al. Tooth discoloration by blood: an in vitro histochemical study. Endod Dent Traumatol 1997; 13: 132–8.

234. MARIN PD et al. A quantitative comparison of traditional and non-peroxide bleaching agents. Dental Traumatol 1998; 14: 64–7.

235. MARKOWITZ K. Pretty painful: why does bleaching hurt? Med Hypotheses 2010; 74: 835–40.

236. MASSLER M et al. Action of amalgam on dentin. J Am Dent Assoc 1953; 47: 415–22.

237. MATHESON JR et al. Effect of toothpaste with natural calcium carbonate/perlite on extrinsic tooth stain. Int Dent J 2004; 54 (suppl 1): 321–5.

238. MATIS BA et al. The efficacy and safety of a 10% carbamide peroxide. Quint Int 1998; 29: 555–63.

239. MATIS BA et al. In vivo degradation of bleaching gel used in whitening teeth. J Am Dent Assoc 1999; 130: 227–35.

240. MATIS BA et al. Extended at-home bleaching of tetracycline-stained teeth with different concentrations of carbamide peroxide. Quint Int 2002; 33: 645–55.

241. MATIS BA et al. A clinical evaluation of bleaching using whitening wraps and strips. Oper Dent 2005; 30: 588–92.

242. McCRACKEN et al. Effects of 10% carbamide peroxide on the subsurface hardness of enamel. Quint Int 1995; 26: 21–4.

243. McCRACKEN et al. Demineralization effects of 10% carbamide peroxide. J Dent 1996; 26: 395–8.

244. McEVOY SA. Removing intrinsic stains from vital teeth by microabrasion and bleaching. J Esthet Dent 1995;7: 104–9.

245. McCORMICK JE et al. Tissue pH of developing periapical lesions in dogs. J Endod 1983; 9: 47–52.

246. MEIRELES SS et al. Efficacy and safety of 10% and 16% carbamide peroxide tooth-whitening gels. Oper Dent 2008; 33: 606–12.

247. MERCK INDEX. Rahway, NJ: Merck & Co., 1976, pp. 1172–3.

248. METZ MJ et al. Clinical evaluation of 15% carbamide peroxide on the surface microhardness and shear bond strength of human enamel. Oper Dent 2007; 32: 427–36.

249. MILES AEW. Age changes in dental tissues. In: COHEN B et al. (eds) Scientific foundations of dentistry. London: William Heinemann Medical Books, 1976.

250. MONTALVAN E et al. The shear bond strength of acetone and ethanol-based bonding agents to bleached teeth. Pediatr Dent 2006; 28: 531–6.

251. MONTGOMERY S. External cervical resorption after bleaching a pulpless tooth. Oral Surg 1984; 57: 203–6.

252. MORAES RR et al. Carbamide peroxide bleaching agents: effects on roughness of enamel, composite and porcelain. Clin Oral Investig 2005; 10: 23–8.

253. MORAN J et al. A clinical study to assess the ability of a powered toothbrush to remove chlorhexidine/tea dental stain. J Clin Periodontol 2004; 31: 95–8.

254. MOSKOW BS. Periodontal manifestations of hyperoxaluria and oxalosis. J Periodontol 1989; 60: 271–8.

255. NATHOO SA. The chemistry and mechanisms of extrinsic and intrinsic discoloration. J Am Dent Assoc 1997; 128: 6S–10S.

256. NATHOO S *et al*. Comparative 3-week clinical tooth-shade evaluation of a novel liquid whitening gel containing 18% carbamide peroxide and a commercial available whitening dentifrice. Compend Contin Educ Dent 2002; 23 (suppl 1): 12–17.

257. MÜLLER ARCANI G *et al*. Influence of the duration of treatment using 19% carbamide peroxide gel on dentin surface microhardness. Quint Int 2005; 36: 15–24.

258. MURCHISON DF *et al*. Carbamide peroxide leaching: effects on enamel surface hardness and bonding. Oper Dent 1992; 17: 181–5.

259. NATHANSON D. Vital tooth bleaching: sensitivity and pulpal considerations. J Am Dent Assoc 1997; 128: 41S–44S.

260. NEWBRUN E. Fluorides and dental caries. Springfield, IL: Charles C. Thomas, 1978.

261. NIEDERMAN R *et al*. Effectiveness of dentist-prescribed, home-applied tooth whitening: a meta-analysis. J Contemp Dent Pract 2000; 1 (4 Fall Issue): 1–6.

262. NORDBÖ H *et al*. Iron staining of the acquired enamel pellicle after exposure to tannic acid or chlorhexidine: preliminary report. Scand J Dent Res 1982; 90: 117–23.

263. ONTIVEROS J *et al*. Color change of vital teeth exposed to bleaching performed with and without supplementary light. J Dent 2009; 37: 840–7.

264. PATEL K *et al*. Oral and systemic effects of prolonged minocycline therapy. Br Dent J 1998; 185: 560–2.

265. PARK H-J *et al*. Changes in bovine enamel after treatment with 30% hydrogen peroxide bleaching agent. Dent Mater 2004; 23: 517–21.

266. PARKINS FM *et al*. Minocycline use discolors teeth. J Am Dent Assoc 1992; 123: 87–9.

267. PARSONS JR *et al*. In vitro longitudinal assessment of coronal discoloration from endodontic sealers. J Endod 2001; 27: 699–702.

268. PERDIGÃO J *et al*. Ultra-morphological study of the interaction of dental adhesives with carbamide-peroxide bleached enamel. Am J Dent 1998; 11: 291–301.

269. PFARRER AM *et al*. Anticaries and hard tissue abrasion effects of a "dual-action" whitening, sodium hexametaphosphate tartar control dentifrice. J Clin Dent 2002; 13: 50–4.

270. PINDBORG JJ. Pathology of the dental hard tissues. Copenhagen: Munksgaard, 1970.

271. PINDBORG JJ. Aetiology of developmental enamel defects not related to fluorosis. Int Dent J 1982; 32: 123–34.

272. POHJOLA R *et al*. Sensitivity and tooth whitening agents. J Esthet Restor Dent 2002; 14: 85–91.

273. POLYDOROU O *et al*. Effect of in-office bleaching on the microhardness of six dental esthetic restorative materials. Dent Mater 2007; 23: 153–8.

274. PONTEFRACT H *et al*. Development of methods to enhance extrinsic tooth discoloration for comparison of toothpastes. 2. J Clin Periodontol 2004; 31: 7–11.

275. POTOČNIK I *et al*. Effect of 10% carbamide peroxide bleaching gel on enamel microhardness, microstructure, and mineral content. J Endod 2000; 26: 203–6.

276. POWELL KR *et al*. A simple technique for the aesthetic improvement of fluorotic-like lesions. ASDC J Dent Child 1982; 49: 112–17.

277. POWELL LV *et al*. Tooth bleaching: its effect on oral tissues. J Am Dent Assoc 1991; 122: 50–4.

278. PUGH G *et al*. High levels of hydrogen peroxide in overnight tooth-whitening formulas: effects on enamel and pulp. J Esthet Restor Dent 2005; 17: 40–7.

279. RAHIMA MM *et al*. Primary hyperoxaluria in a pediatric dental patient. Pediatr Dent 1992; 14: 260–2.

280. RAO SR *et al*. Pulpal dysplasia. Oral Surg 1970; 30: 682–9.

281. RAPLEY JW *et al*. Subgingival and interproximal plaque removal using a counter-rotational electric toothbrush and a manual toothbrush. Quint Int 1994; 25: 39–42.

282. RAVNHOLT G. Accelerated corrosion analysis of dental amalgams. Scand J Dent Res 1986; 94: 553–61.

283. REED AJ *et al*. The dark primary incisor. Dent Survey 1978; July: 16–19.

284. REICHART PA. Oral cancer and precancer related to betel and miang chewing in Thailand: a review. J Oral Pathol Med 1995; 24: 241–3.

285. REICHART PA *et al*. The black layer on the teeth of betel chewers. J Oral Pathol 1985; 14: 466–75.

286. REID JS *et al*. Investigations into black extrinsic tooth stain. J Dent Res 1977; 56: 895–9.

287. REINHARDT JW *et al*. A clinical study of nightguard vital bleaching. Quint Int 1993; 24: 379–84.

288. RENDALL JR *et al*. Reddening of the upper central incisors associated with periapical granuloma in lepromatous leprosy. Br J Oral Surg 1976; 13: 271–7.

289. ROBERTELLO FJ *et al*. Effect of home bleaching products on mercury release from an admixed amalgam. Am J Dent 1999; 12: 227–30.

290. ROBINSON PJ *et al*. Clinical comparison of two electric toothbrushes on periodontitis patients. J Clin Dent 1997; 8: 4–9.

291. RODRÍGUES JA *et al*. Effects of 10% carbamide peroxide bleaching materials on enamel microhardness. Am J Dent 2001; 14: 67–71.

292. RODRÍGUES JA *et al*. Microhardness evaluation of in situ vital bleaching on human dental enamel using a novel study design. Dent Mater 2005; 21: 1059–67.

293. ROTSTEIN I *et al*. Effect of bleaching agents on inorganic components of human dentin and cementum. J Endod 1992; 18: 290–3.

294. ROTSTEIN L *et al*. Histochemical analysis of dental hard tissues following bleaching. J Endod 1996; 22: 23–6.

295. ROTSTEIN L *et al*. Changes in surface levels of mercury, silver, tin and copper of dental amalgam treated with carbamide peroxide and hydrogen peroxide in vitro. Oral Surg Oral Med Oral Pathol Radiol Endod 1997; 83: 506–9.

296. ROTSTEIN L *et al*. Bleaching discoloured teeth. In: WALTON R *et al*. Principles and practices of endodontics Philadelphia: WB Saunders, 2002, pp. 405–423.

297. ROTSTEIN I *et al*. Factors affecting mercury release from dental amalgam exposed to carbamide peroxide bleaching agent. Am J Dent 2004; 17: 347–50.

298. ROSENSTIEL SF *et al.* Duration of tooth color change after bleaching. J Am Dent Assoc 1991; 123: 54–9.

299. ROSENSTRITT M *et al.* Discoloration of restorative materials after bleaching application. Quint Int 2005; 36: 33–9.

300. RUDOLPHY MP *et al.* Radiopacities in dentine under amalgam restorations. Caries Res 1994; 28: 240–5.

301. SANTINI A *et al.* The effect of 10% carbamide peroxide bleaching agent on phosphate concentration of tooth enamel assessed by Raman spectroscopy. Dent Traumatol 2008; 24: 220–3.

302. SANZ M *et al.* The effect of a dentifrice containing chlorhexidine and zinc on plaque, gingivitis, calculus and tooth staining. J Clin Periodontol 1994; 21: 431–7.

303. SARKER S *et al.* Clinical and laboratory evaluation of powered electric toothbrushes: laboratory determination of relative interproximal cleaning efficiency of four powered toothbrushes. J Clin Dent 1997; 8: 81–5.

304. SAWYER DR *et al.* Facial and oral manifestations of leprosy. J Oral Med 1987; 42: 143–9.

305. SCHEMEHORN B *et al.* A SEM evaluation of a 6% hydrogen peroxide tooth whitening gel on dental materials *in vitro*. J Dent 2004; 32 (suppl 1): 35–9.

306. SCHEMEHORN BR *et al.* Stain removal with power toothbrushes at optimal tension on tooth. J Dent Res 1996; 75: 46.

307. SCHEMEHORN BR *et al.* A laboratory investigation of stain removal from enamel surface: comparative efficacy of three electric toothbrushes. Am J Dent 1996; 9: S21–24.

308. SCHOONOVER IC *et al.* Corrosion of dental alloys. J Am Dent Assoc 1941; 28: 1278–91.

309. SCHROEDER HE. Pathobiologie oraler Strukturen. Basel: Karger, 1983.

310. SCHUURS AHB *et al.* An unusual case of black teeth. Oral Surg 1987; 64: 427–31.

311. SCHUURS AHB *et al.* Tanden bleken [Bleaching teeth], 2nd edn. Houten: Bohn Stafleu van Loghum, 2008.

312. SCHWARTZ S *et al.* Oral findings in osteogenesis imperfecta. Oral Surg 1984; 57: 161–7.

313. SEEDAT HA *et al.* The oral features of betel nut chewers without submucous fibrosis. J Biol Buccale 1988; 16: 123–8.

314. SEDANO HO *et al.* Clinical orodental abnormalities in Mexican children. Oral Surg Oral Med Oral Pathol 1989; 68: 300–11.

315. SELTZER S *et al.* Histologic changes in dental pulps of dogs and monkeys following application of pressure, drugs, and microorganisms on prepared cavities. Oral Surg 1961; 14: 327–46.

316. SEOW WK *et al.* Oral changes associated with end-stage liver disease and liver transplantation: implications for dental management. ASDC J Dent Child 1991; 58: 474–80.

317. SHARIF N *et al.* The chemical stain removal properties of "whitening" toothpaste products: studies in vitro. Br Dent J 2000; 188: 620–4.

318. SHAY DE *et al.* An inorganic qualitative and quantitative analysis of green stain. J Am Dent Assoc 1955; 50: 156–60.

319. SHIELDS ED *et al.* A proposed classification for heritable human dentine defects with a description of a new entity. Arch Oral Biol 1973; 18: 543–53.

320. SHINOHARA MS *et al.* The effect of nonvital bleaching on the shear bond strength of composite resin using three adhesive systems. J Adhes Dent 2004; 6: 205–9.

321. SIELSKI C *et al.* A study to assess the tooth whitening efficacy of a new dentifrice formulation variant containing a special grade of silica. J Clin Dent 2002; 13: 77–81.

322. SLEZAK B *et al.* Safety profile of a new liquid whitening gel. Compend Cont Educ Dent 2002; 23 (suppl 1): 4–11.

323. SLOTS J. The microflora of black stain on human primary anterior teeth. Scand J Dent Res 1974; 82: 484–90.

324. SMALL BW. Bleaching with 10 percent carbamide peroxide: an 18-month study. Gen Dent 1994; 42: 142–6.

325. SPYRIDES GM *et al.* Effect of whitening agents on dentin bonding. J Esthet Dent 2000; 12: 264–70.

326. SOLHEIM H *et al.* Oral retention and discoloration tendency from a chlorhexidine mouth rinse. Acta Odontol Scand 1983; 41: 193–6.

327. SOLHEIM T. Dental color as an indicator of age. Gerodontics 1988; 4: 114–18.

328. SONIS AL. Longitudinal study of discolored primary teeth and effect on succedaneous teeth. J Pedod 1987; 11: 247–51.

329. SOPARKAR P *et al.* A clinical investigation to evaluate reduction in dental stain provided by the once-daily use of a breath mint or chewing gum. Compen Contin Educ Dent 2001; 22 (7A): 33–5.

330. SÖREMARK R *et al.* Penetration of metallic ions from restorations into teeth. J Prosthet Dent 1968; 20: 531–40.

331. SOXMAN JA *et al.* Pulpal pathology in relation to discoloration of primary teeth. ASDC J Dent Child 1984; 51: 282–4.

332. STANGEL I *et al.* Absorption of iron by dentin: its role in discoloration. J Biomed Mater Res 1996; 31: 287–92.

333. STANLEY HR. The effect of systemic diseases on the human pulp. Oral Surg 1972; 33: 606–48.

334. STEIDLER NE *et al.* Dentinal dysplasia. Br J Oral Maxillofac Surg 1984; 22: 274–86.

335. STEINBERG D *et al.* Formation of Streptococcus mutans biofilm following toothbrushing with regular and whitening toothpastes. Am J Dent 2003; 16: 58–60.

336. SULIEMAN M *et al.* Comparison of three in-office bleaching systems based upon 35% hydrogen peroxide with different light activators. Am J Dent 2000; 18: 194–6.

337. SUTCLIFFE P. Extrinsic tooth stains in children. Dent Pract 1967; 17: 175–9.

338. SWIFT EJ. Restorative considerations with vital tooth bleaching. J Am Dent Assoc 1997; 128: 60S–64S.

339. TAHER NM. The effect of bleaching agents on the surface hardness of tooth colored restorative materials. J Contemp Techniques Dent Pract 2005; 15: 18–26.

340. TAM L. The safety of home bleaching analysis. Quint Int 1998; 29: 28–37.

341. TANTBIROJN D *et al.* Stain removal efficacy: an in vitro evaluation using quantitative image analysis. Quint Int 1998; 29: 28–37.

342. TEIXEIRA ECN *et al*. Use of 37% carbamide peroxide in the walking bleach technique. Quint Int 2003; 35: 97–102.

343. TEREZHALMY GT *et al*. Clinical evaluation of the effect of an ultrasonic toothbrush on plaque, gingivitis, and gingival bleeding: a six-month study. J Prosthet Dent 1995; 73: 97–103.

344. THEILADE J *et al*. The ultrastructure of black stain on human primary teeth. Scand J Dent Res 1973; 81: 528–32.

345. THITINANTHAPAN W *et al*. In vitro penetration of the pulp chamber by three brands of carbamide peroxide. J Esthet Dent 1999; 11: 259–64.

346. THODEN VAN VELZEN SK *et al*. Endodontologie. Alphen aan den Rijn: Stafleu & Tholen BV, 1995.

347. TIMPAWAT S *et al*. Effect of bleaching agents on bonding to pulp chamber dentine. Int Endod J 2005; 38: 211–17.

348. TITLEY KC *et al*. Scanning electron microscopy observations on the penetration and structure of the resin tags in bleached and unbleached bovine enamel. J Endod 1991; 17: 72–5.

349. TITLEY KC *et al*. The effect of carbamide-peroxide gel on the shear bond strength of a microfil resin to bovine enamel. J Dent Res 1992; 71: 20–4.

350. TITLEY KC *et al*. Adhesion of a resin composite to bleached and unbleached human enamel. J Endod 1993; 19: 112–25.

351. TREDWIN CJ *et al*. Drug-induced disorders of teeth. J Dent Res 2005; 84: 596–602.

352. TREDWIN CJ *et al*. Hydrogen peroxide tooth-whitening (bleaching) products: review of adverse effects and safety issues. Br Dent J 2006 200: 371–6.

353. TRONSTAD L. Pulp reactions in traumatized teeth. In: GUTMAN JL *et al*. (eds) Proceedings of the international conference on oral trauma. Chicago, IL: American Association of Endodontists Endowment & Memorial Foundation, 1986.

354. TREISTER NS *et al*. Oral mucosal pigmentation secondary to minocycline therapy. Oral Surg Oral Med Oral Pathol Oral Radiol Endod 2004; 97: 18–25.

355. TSE CS *et al*. Is home tooth bleaching gel cytotoxic? J Esthet Dent 1991; 3: 162–8.

356. TÜRKER SB *et al*. Effect of three bleaching agents on the surface properties of three different aesthetic restorative materials. J Prosthet Dent 2003; 89: 466–73.

357. TURSSI CP *et al*. An in situ investigation into the abrasion of eroded dental hard tissues by a whitening dentifrice. Caries Res 2004; 38: 473–7.

358. UNLU N *et al*. Effect of elapsed time following bleaching on the shear bond strength of composite resin to enamel. J Biomed Mater Res Part B: Applied Biomater 2008; 84B: 363–8.

359. VAN DER BURGT TP *et al*. Tandverkleuring door endodontische materialen. Ned Tijdschr Tandheelkd 1986; 93: 117–20.

360. VAN DER BURGT TP *et al*. Tooth discoloration induced by dental materials. Oral Surg 1985; 60: 666–9.

361. VAN DER BURGT TP *et al*. Tooth discoloration induced by endodontic sealers. Oral Surg 1986; 61: 84–9.

362. VAN DER LINDEN LWJ *et al*. The origin of localized increased radiopacity in the dentin. Oral Surg Oral Med Oral Pathol 1973; 35: 862–71.

363. VAN DIS ML *et al*. The thalassemias: oral manifestations and complications. Oral Surg 1986; 62: 229–33.

364. VAN DER WEIJDEN GA *et al*. A comparative study of electric toothbrushes for the effectiveness of plaque removal in relation to toothbrushing duration. J Clin Periodontol 1993; 20: 476–81.

365. VAN DER WEIJDEN GA *et al*. The long-term effect of an oscillating/rotating electric toothbrush on gingivitis. J Clin Periodontol 1994; 21: 139–45.

366. VAN DER WEIJDEN GA *et al*. Comparison of 2 electric toothbrushes in plaque-removing ability; professional and supervised brushing. J Clin Periodontol 1995; 22: 648–52.

367. VISSER JB. Speciële pathologie van het menselijke gebit. Leiden: Stafleu & Tholen BV, 1974.

368. VOGEL RI. Intrinsic and extrinsic discoloration of the dentition. J Oral Med 1975; 30: 99–104.

369. VOGEL RI *et al*. Tetracycline-induced extrinsic discoloration of the dentition. Oral Surg 1977; 44: 50–3.

370. WAERHAUG M *et al*. Comparison of the effect of chlorhexidine and CUSO$_4$ on plaque formation and development of gingivitis. J Clin Periodontol 1984; 11: 176–80.

371. WANDERA A *et al*. Home-use tooth bleaching agents; an in vitro study on quantitative effects on enamel, dentin, and cementum. Quint Int 1994; 25: 541–6.

372. WARNER RR *et al*. Analytical electron microscopy of chlorhexidine-induced tooth stain in humans: direct evidence for metal-induced stain. J Periodontol Res 1993; 28: 255–65.

373. WARREN DP *et al*. Topical fluorides: efficacy, administration, and safety. Gen Dent 1997; 45: 134–42.

374. WATANABE K *et al*. Bilirubin pigmentation of human teeth caused by hyperbulinrubinaemia. J Oral Pathol Med 1999; 28: 128–30.

375. WATERHOUSE PJ *et al*. Intracoronal bleaching of nonvital teeth in children and adolescents: interim results. Quint Int 1996; 27: 447–53.

376. WATTS A *et al*. Tooth discolouration and staining. Br Dent J 2001; 190: 309–16.

377. WEI SHY *et al*. Analyses of the amalgam-tooth interface using the electron microprobe. J Dent Res 1969; 48: 317–20.

378. WELLOCK WD *et al*. Caries increments, tooth discoloration, and state of oral hygiene in children given single annual applications of acid phosphate-fluoride and stannous fluoride. Arch Oral Biol 1965; 10: 453–60.

379. WESTBURY LW *et al*. Minocycline-induced intraoral pharmacogenic pigmentation. J Periodontol 1997; 68: 84–91.

380. WHITE DJ *et al*. Anticalculus effects of a novel, dual-phase polypyrophosphate dentifrice: chemical basis, mechanism, and clinical response. J Contemp Dent Pract 2000; 15: 1–19.

381. WIEGAND A *et al*. Efficacy of different whitening modalities on bovine enamel and dentin. Clin Oral Investig 2005; 9: 91–7.

382. WIEGAND A *et al*. 12-month color stability of enamel dentine and enamel dentine samples after bleaching. Clin Oral Investig 2008; 12: 303–10.

383. WOOLVERTON CJ *et al*. Toxicity of two carbamide peroxide products used in nightguard vital bleaching. Am H Dent 1993; 6: 310–14.

384. WYSOCKI GP *et al*. Oral findings in primary hyperoxaluria and oxalosis. Oral Surg 1982; 53: 267–72.

385. YANG MS *et al*. Prevalence and related risk factors of betel quid chewing by adolescent students in southern Taiwan. J Oral Pathol Med 1996; 25: 69–71.

386. YANKELL SL *et al*. Efficacy of chewing gum in preventing extrinsic tooth staining. J Clin Dent 1997; 8: 169–72.

387. YAP AUJ *et al*. Effects of in-office tooth whiteners on hardness of tooth-colored restoratives. Oper Dent 2002; 27: 137–41.

388. YEH S-T *et al*. Surface changes and acid dissolution of enamel after carbamide peroxide bleach treatment. Oper Dent 2005; 30: 507–15.

389. ZAIA AA *et al*. Oral changes associated with biliary atresia and liver transplantation. J Clin Pediatr Dent 1993; 18: 39–42.

390. ZACH L *et al*. Pulp response to externally applied heat. Oral Surg Oral Med Oral Pathol 1965; 19: 515–30.

391. ZALKIND M *et al*. Surface morphology changes in human enamel dentin and cementum following bleaching. Endod Dent Traumatol 1996; 12: 82–8.

392. ZEKONIS R *et al*. Clinical evaluation of in-office and at-home bleaching treatments. Oper Dent 2003; 28: 114–21.

Chapter 11: Congenital Syndromes with Dental Anomalies

1. AHN BD *et al*. Hallermann-Streiff syndrome: those are not supernumerary teeth. J Pediatr 2006; 148: 415.

2. ALBUM MM. Ectodermal dysplasia – a crown and bridge approach in treatment technique. J Int Assoc Dent Child 1980; 11: 53–61.

3. ALPÖZ AR *et al*. Taurodontism in children associated with trisomy 21. J Clin Pediatr Dent 1997; 22: 37–9.

4. ALVESALO L *et al*. 47,XXY males: sex chromosomes and tooth size. Am J Hum Genet 1980; 32: 955–9.

5. AMARATUNGA NA DE S. The prevalence of dental abnormalities in children with cleft lip and palate. J Paediatr Dent 1987; 3: 69–73.

6. AMARATUNGA NA DE S. A comparative clinical study of Pierre Robin syndrome and isolated cleft. Br J Oral Maxillofac Surg 1989; 27: 451–8.

7. ANDERSON PJ *et al*. The feet in Crouzon syndrome. J Craniofac Genet Dev Biol 1997; 17: 43–7.

8. ARCHER WH *et al*. Cleidocranial dysostosis. Oral Surg 1951; 4: 1201–13.

9. ARVYSTAS MG. Familial generalized delayed eruption of the dentition with short stature. Oral Surg 1976; 41: 235–43.

10. ARWILL T *et al*. Epidermolysis bullosa hereditaria. Oral Surg 1965; 19: 723–44.

11. ATASU M, AKYUZ S. Congenital hypodontia: a pedigree and dermatoglyphic study. J Clin Pediatr Dent 1995; 19: 215–24.

12. ATASU M *et al*. Multiple supernumerary teeth in association with cleidocranial dysplasia. J Clin Pediatr Dent 1996; 21: 87–93.

13. ATASU M *et al*. Local, hypoplastic type of amelogenesis imperfecta: a clinical, genetic, radiological and dermatoglyphic study. J Clin Pediatr Dent 1996; 20: 337–42.

14. BAKRI H *et al*. Clinical management of ectodermal dysplasia. J Clin Pediatr Dent 1995; 19: 167–72.

15. BANKS PA *et al*. Prader-Willi syndrome. Br J Orthod 1996; 23: 299–304.

16. BARABAS GM. The Ehlers–Danlos syndrome. Abnormalities of the enamel, dentine, cementum and the dental pulp. Br Dent J 1969; 509–15.

17. BARKER D *et al*. Dental findings in Morquio syndrome (Mucopolysaccharidoses Type IVA). ASDC J Dent Child 2000; 67: 431–3.

18. BARNETT ML *et al*. The prevalence of periodontitis and dental caries in a Down's syndrome population. J Periodontol 1986; 57: 288–93.

19. BARTLETT RC *et al*. Autosomal recessive hypohidrotic ectodermal dysplasia: dental manifestations. Oral Surg 1972; 33: 736–42.

20. BATHI RJ, MASUR VN. Pyknodysostosis. Int J Oral Maxillofac Surg 2000; 29: 439–42.

21. BAUSS O *et al*. Temporomandibular joint dysfunction in Marfan syndrome. Oral Surg Oral Med Oral Pathol Oral Radiol Endod 2004; 97: 592–8.

22. BAXTER AM *et al*. Dental and oral lesions in two patients with focal dermal hypoplasia (Goltz syndrome). Br Dent J 2000; 189: 550–3.

23. BAZOPOULOU-KYRKANIDOU E *et al*. Prader–Willi syndrome. J Clin Pediatr Dent 1992; 17: 37–40.

24. BECKER A *et al*. Cleidocranial dysplasia: part 2 – treatment protocol for the orthodontic and surgical modality. Am J Orthod Dentofac Orthop 1997; 111: 173–83.

25. BEDI R *et al*. Goldenhar's syndrome – interdisciplinary approach to management. ASDC J Dent Child 1984; 51: 215–17.

26. BEEMER FA. Het velo-cardio-faciaal (VCF/Shprintzen) syndroom. Ned tijdschr Tandheelkd 1998; 105: 287–88.

27. BELL EJ *et al*. Tooth wear in children with Down syndrome. Aust Dent J 2002; 47: 30–5.

28. BERGENDAL B. Children with ectodermal dysplasia need early treatment. Spec Care Dent 2002; 22: 212–13.

29. BOHATY B *et al*. Epidermolysis bullosa. J Clin Pediatr Dent 1998; 22: 243–5.

30. BOJ JR *et al*. Dentures for a 3-yr-old child with ectodermal dysplasia. Am J Dent 1993; 6: 165–7.

31. BOKHOUT B *et al*. Incidence of dental caries in the primary dentition in children with a cleft lip and/or palate. Caries Res 1997; 31: 8–12.

32. BORAZ RA. Cockayne's syndrome. Pediatr Dent 1991; 13: 227–30.

33. BOREA G *et al*. The oral cavity in Down syndrome. J Pedod 1990; 14: 139–40.

34. BORSTLAP WA *et al*. Schedeldakreconstructies bij kinderen. Ned Tijdschr Tandheelkd 1996; 103: 9–13.

35. BOTTOMLEY WK *et al*. Dental anomalies in the Roth-mund-Thomson syndrome. Oral Surg 1976; 41: 321–6.

36. BOYADJIEV SA *et al*. Physical map of the chromosome 6q22 region containing the ocuslodentodigital dysplasia locus: analysis of thirteen candidate genes and identification of novel SSTs and DNA polymorphisms. Cyogenet Genome Res 2000; 98: 29–37.

37. BRAIN EB *et al*. Developing teeth in epidermolysis bullosa hereditaria letalis. Br Dent J 1968; 124: 255–60.

38. BROOK AH *et al*. Dental anomalies in association with achondroplasia. Br Dent J 1970; 129: 519–20.

39. BRITTAIN JM *et al*. Odontohypophosphatasia. ASDC J Dent Child 1976; 43: 106–11.

40. BRUCKNER RJ *et al*. Hypophosphatasia with premature shedding of the teeth and aplasia of cementum. Oral Surg 1962; 15: 1351–9.

41. BUCCI E *et al*. Oral and dental anomalies in Goltz syndrome. J Pedod 1989; 13: 161–8.

42. BURDICK AB. Genetic epidemiology and control of genetic expression in van der Woude syndrome. J Craniofac Genet Dev Biol 1986; suppl 2: 99–105.

43. CARL W *et al*. Dental abnormalities and bone lesions associated with familial adenomatous polyposis. J Am Dent Assoc 1989; 119: 137–9.

44. CARRETERO QUEZADA MG *et al*. Dental anomalies in patients with familial and sporadic cleft lip and palate. J Biol Buccale 1988; 16: 185–90.

45. CHEN HJ *et al*. "Otodental" dysplasia. Oral Surg Oral Med Oral Pathol 1988; 66: 353–8.

46. CHEUNG WS. A mild form of hypophosphatasia as a cause of premature exfoliation of primary teeth. Pediatr Dent 1987; 9: 49–52.

47. CHIPPS JE. Multiple supernumerary teeth in cleidocranial dysostosis. Oral Surg 1951; 4: 25–8.

48. CHOW KMC *et al*. Concomitant occurrence of hypodontia and supernumerary teeth in a patient with Down syndrome. Spec Care Dent 1997; 17: 54–7.

49. CICHON P *et al*. Early-onset periodontitis associated with Down's syndrome. Ann Periodontol 1998; 3: 370–80.

50. CICHON JC, PACK RS. Taurodontism. J Am Dent Assoc 1985; 111: 453–5.

51. COHEN MM. Syndromology: an updated conceptual overview. I. Syndrome concepts, designations, and population characteristics. Int J Oral Maxillofac Surg 1989; 18: 216–22.

52. COHEN MM. Syndromology: an updated conceptual overview. IV. Perspectives on malformation syndromes. Int J Oral Maxillofac Surg 1989; 18: 286–90.

53. COHEN MM. Syndromology: an updated conceptual overview. II. Syndrome classifications. Int J Oral Maxillofac Surg 1989; 18: 223–8.

54. COHEN MM. Syndromology: an updated conceptual overview. IX. Facial dysmorphology. Int J Oral Maxillofac Surg 1989; 19: 81–8.

55. COHEN MM *et al*. Perspectives on craniofacial syndromes. Acta Odontol Scand 1998; 56: 315–20.

56. COHEN SR *et al*. Intracranial pressure in single-suture craniosynsostosis. Cleft Palate Craniofac J 1998; 35: 194–6.

57. COOK PA. Pyknodysostosis. J Paediatr Dent 1987; 3: 81–3.

58. COYLE JT *et al*. Down syndrome, Alzheimer's disease and the trisomy 16 mouse. Trends Neurosci 1988; 11: 390–4.

59. CUTANDO A *et al*. Oral health management implications in patients with tuberous sclerosis. Oral Surg Oral Med Oral Pathol Oral Radiol Endod 2000; 89: 430–5.

60. CUTANDO-SORIANO A *et al*. Free inteleukin-2 receptors in children with trisomy 21 (Down's syndrome) and different levels of periodontal disease. Int J Paediatr Dent 1998; 8: 177–80.

61. DA FONSECA MA *et al*. Hallerman–Streiff syndrome. ASDC J Dent Child 1994; 61: 334–7.

62. DALY CG. Blood blisters on the soft palate in Angina bullosa haemorrhagica. Vase reports. Aust Dent J 1988; 33: 400–3.

63. DAHLLÖF G *et al*. Caries, gingivitis, and dental abnormalities in preschool children with cleft lip and/or palate. Cleft Palate J 1989; 26: 233–7.

64. DAMM DD *et al*. Intraosseous fibrous lesions of the jaws. A manifestation of tuberous sclerosis. Oral Surg Oral Med Oral Pathol Oral Radiol Endod 1999; 87: 334–40.

65. DAVIES TM *et al*. The surgical and orthodontic management of unerupted teeth in cleidocranial dysostosis. Br J Orthod 1987; 14: 43–7.

66. DAVIS RK *et al*. Tuberous sclerosis with oral manifestations. Oral Surg 1964; 17: 395–400.

67. DAYAL PK *et al*. Aarskog syndrome. Oral Surg Oral Med Oral Pathol 1990; 69: 403–5.

68. DEAN JA *et al*. Dental management of oculodentodigital dysplasia. ASDC J Dent Child 1986; 53: 131–4.

69. DE COSTER PJ. Harde tandweefsels en bindweefselstoornissen. In: De BAAT C *et al*. (eds) Het tandheelkundig jaar 2005. Houten: Bohn Stafleu van Loghum, 2004.

70. DE COSTER PJ *et al*. Unusual findings in dermatosparaxis (Ehlers–Danlos syndrome type VIIC). J Oral Pathol Med 2003; 32: 568–70.

71. DEFRAIA E *et al*. Case report: orofacial characteristics of Hallermann–Streiff syndrome. Eur J Paediatr Dent 2003; 4: 155–8.

72. DE HAAS JM. Syndroom van Cornelia de Lange. Ned Tijdschr Tandheelkd 1972; 79: 246–7.

73. DE JONGE TE *et al*. Het syndroom van Gardner. Ned Tijdschr Tandheelkd 1990; 97: 252–4.

74. DESAI SS. Down syndrome. Oral Surg Oral Med Oral Pathol Radiol Endod 1996; 84: 279–85.

75. DOMINGUEZ REYES A *et al*. General and dental characteristics of Bloch-Sulzberger syndrome. Medicina Oral 2002; 7: 296–7.

76. DUNLAP C *et al*. The Noonan syndrome/cherubism association. Oral Surg Oral Med Oral Pathol 1989; 67: 698–705.

77. EHMER U. Humangenetische Studien an Patienten mit trisomie 21 unter besonderer Wertung von Morphologie und Pathogenese im orofazialen Bereich. Zahn Mund Kieferheilkd 1977; 65: 399–405.

78. EIDELMAN E *et al*. Orodigitofacial dysostosis and oculodentodigital dysplasia. Oral Surg 1967; 23: 311–19.

79. ENDRUSCHAT AJ *et al.* Anesthetic and dental management of a child with epidermolysis bullosa dystrophica. Oral Surg 1973; 36: 667–71.

80. FADER M *et al.* Gardner's syndrome (intestinal polyposis, osteomas, sebaceous cysts) and a new dental discovery. Oral Surg 1962; 15: 153–72.

81. FADHIL M *et al.* Odontoonychodermal dysplasia. A previously apparently undescribed ectodermal dysplasia. Am J Med Genet 1983; 14: 335–46.

82. FARIAS M, VARGERIK K. Dental development in hemifacial microsomia I. Eruption and agenesis. Pediatr Dent 1988; 10: 140–3.

83. FEICHTINGER C *et al.* Taurodontism in human sex chromosome aneuploidy. Arch Oral Biol 1977; 22: 327–9.

84. FELIX-SCHOLLAART B. Solitary, non-syndromic cleft lip and/or palate. Thesis, Vrije Universiteit te Amsterdam, 1989.

85. FISCHER-BRANDIES H *et al.* Craniofacial development in patients with Down's syndrome from birth to 14 years of age. Eur J Orthod 1986; 8: 35–42.

86. FLANAGAN N *et al.* Developmental enamel defects in tuberous sclerosis; a clinical genetic marker? J Med Genet 1997; 34: 637–9.

87. FLEISCHER-PETERS A *et al.* Zahnbefunde bei Incontinentia pigmenti (Bloch-Sulzberger-Syndrom). Dtsch Zahnärztl Z 1982; 37: 841–9.

88. FRAME K *et al.* Progressive development of supernumerary teeth in cleidocranial dysplasia. Br J Orthod 1989; 16: 103–6.

89. FREIHOFER HPM. Dysostosis cleidocranialis. Ned Tijdschr Tandheelkd 1998; 105: 204–5.

90. FREIHOFER HPM. Morbus Crouzon. Ned Tijdschr Tsandheelkd 1998; 105: 451–2.

91. FREIHOFER HPM. Syndroom van Treacher Collins. Ned Tijdschr Tandheelkd 1999; 106: 226–8.

92. FRIDRICH KL. Management of impacted teeth in patients with congenital clefts. Oral Maxillofac Surg Clin North Am 1993; 5: 105–10.

93. FRIDRICH KL *et al.* Dental implications in Ehlers–Danlos syndrome. Oral Surg Oral Med Oral Pathol 1990; 69: 431–5.

94. FUNG DE. Hypophosphatasia. Br Dent J 1983; 154: 49–50.

95. GARDNER DG. The oral manifestations of Hurler's syndrome. Oral Surg 1971; 32: 46–57.

96. GARDNER DG *et al.* The disturbances in odontogenesis in epidermolysis bullosa hereditaria letalis. Oral Surg 1975; 40: 483–93.

97. GIANSANTI JS *et al.* The "tooth and nail" type of autosomal dominant ectodermal dysplasia. Oral Surg 1974; 37: 576–82.

98. GOEPFERD SJ *et al.* Hypohidrotic ectodermal dysplasia. J Am Dent Assoc 1981; 102: 867–9.

99. GOLAN I *et al.* Zur Variabilität der CBFA1/RUNX2-Genexpression bei dysostosis cleidocranialis. Fortschr Kieferprthop 2002; 63: 190–8.

100. GOLDSTEIN E *et al.* Mohr syndrome or oral-facial-digital II. J Am Dent Assoc 1974; 89: 377–82.

101. GOODMAN RM, GORLIN RJ. Atlas of the face in genetic disorders. St Louis, MO: CV Mosby, 1977.

102. GORLIN RJ. Chromosomal abnormalities and oral anomalies. J Dent Res 1963; 42 (suppl 6): 1297–306.

103. GORLIN RJ. Epidermolysis bullosa. Oral Surg 1971; 32: 760–6.

104. GORLIN R. Syndromes, syndromes, and more syndromes. J Dent Res 1996; 75: 732–5.

105. GORLIN RJ *et al.* Oral manifestations of the Fitzgerald–Gardner, Pringle–Bourneville, Robin, Androgenital, and Hurler–Pfaundler syndromes. Oral Surg 1960; 13: 1233–44.

106. GORLIN RJ *et al.* Syndromes of head and neck. New York, NY: Oxford University Press, 2001.

107. GRAU H *et al.* Verlaufsformen und therapiemassnahmen beim cherubismus. Schweiz Monatschr Zahnheilkd 1986; 96: 835–43.

108. GRIFFIN GJ. Case report: a possible variant of otodental syndrome. J Pediatr Dent 1985; 1: 27–9.

109. GRUBE M *et al.* Zur Häufigkeit von Initialkaries und Strukturanomalien des Zahnschmelzes bei Patienten mit Lippen-Kiefer-Gaumensplaten. Zahn- Mund- Kieferheilkd 1987; 75: 816–20.

110. GUCKES AD *et al.* Prospective clinical trial in persons with ectodermal dysplasia. J Prosthet Dent 2002; 88: 21–5.

111. GUNBAY S *et al.* Orofaciodigital syndrome I. J Clin Pediatr Dent 1996; 20: 329–32.

112. HALL RK. Congenitally missing teeth – a diagnostic feature in many syndromes of the head and neck. J Int Assoc Dent Child 1983; 14: 69–75.

113. HALL RK. Care of adolescents with cleft lip and palate. Int Dent J 1986; 36: 120–30.

114. HAMEL BCJ. Syndromen 8. De diagnostiek van aangeboren afwijkingen en syndromen. Ned Tijdschr Tandheelkd 1999; 106: 51–3.

115. HARRIS RJ *et al.* Mandibular prognathism and apertognathia associated with cleidocranial dysostosis in a father and son. Oral Surg 1977; 44: 830–6.

116. HARRIS EF *et al.* Delayed dental development in children with isolated cleft lip and palate. Arch Oral Biol 1990; 35: 469–73.

117. HATA S *et al.* The dentofacial manifestations of XXXXY syndrome. Int J Paediatr Dent 2001; 11: 138–42.

118. HATTAB FN *et al.* Oligodontia of the permanent dentition in two sisters with polycystic ovarian syndrome. Oral Surg Oral Med Oral Pathol Oral Radiol Endod 1997; 84: 368–71.

119. HATTAB FN *et al.* Oral manifestations of Ellis-van Creveld syndrome: report of two siblings with unusual dental anomalies. J Clin Pediatr Dent 1998; 22: 159–65.

120. HELIOVAARA A *et al.* Dental abnormalities in permanent dentition in children with submucous cleft palate. Acta Ondontol Scand 2004; 62: 129–31.

121. HIBBERT SA *et al.* Molecular basis of familial cleft lip and palate. Oral Dis 1996; 2: 238–41.

122. HITCHIN AD. The defects of cementum in epidermolysis bullosa dystrophica. Br Dent J 1973; 135: 437–42.

123. HOCHBER MS *et al.* Epidermolysis bullosa. Oral Surg Oral Med Oral Pathol 1993; 75: 54–7.

124. HOFF M *et al.* Het Williams-Beuren-syndroom. Ned Tijdschr Tandheelkd 1999; 105: 368–9.

125. HOFF M *et al*. Het tubereuze sclerose-complex. Ned Tijd-schr Tandheelkd 2000; 107: 203–5.

126. HOFF M. Dental manifestations in Ehlers-Danlos syndrome. Oral Surg 1977; 44: 864–71.

127. HOFF M *et al*. Enamel defects associated with tuberous sclerosis. Oral Surg 1975; 40: 261–9.

128. HORGAN JE *et al*. Analysis of extracraniofacial anomalies in hemifacial microsomia. Cleft Palate Craniofac J 1995; 32: 405–12.

129. HU JC-C *et al*. Characterization of a family with dominant hypophosphatasia. Eur J Oral Sci 2000; 108: 189–94.

130. HUANG MHS *et al*. The differential diagnosis of abnormal head shapes: separating craniosynostosis from positional deformities and normal variants. Cleft Palate Craniofac J 1998; 35: 204–11.

131. HUDSON CD *et al*. Autosomal dominant hypodontia with nail dysgenesis. Oral Surg 1975; 39: 409–23.

132. HUNT NP *et al*. The dental, craniofacial, and biochemical features of pyknodysostosis. J Oral Maxillofac Surg 1998; 56: 497–504.

133. IWASAKI H *et al*. Dental findings in a case of Bloch–Sulzberger syndrome (incontinentia pigmenti). Pediatr Dent J 2001; 11: 89–96.

134. ITTHAGARUN A *et al*. Ectodermal dysplasia. Quint Int 1997; 28: 595–601.

135. JASPERS MT. Taurodontism in the down syndrome. Oral Surg 1981; 51: 632–6.

136. JENSEN BL. Craniofacial morphology in Turner syndrome. J Craniofac Genet Dev Biol 1985; 5: 327–40.

137. JENSEN BL *et al*. Dental treatment strategies in cleidocranial dysplasia. Br Dent J 1992; 172: 243–7.

138. JENSEN BL *et al*. Cleft lip and palate in Denmark, 1976–1981: epidemiology, variability, and early somatic development. Cleft Palate J 1988; 25: 258–69.

139. JOHNSON T JR *et al*. Chondrodysplasia punctata. Pediatr Dent 1986; 8: 171–4.

140. JONES CM *et al*. Pycnodysostosis. Br Dent J 1988; 164: 218–20.

141. JONES MC. Etiology of facial clefts. Cleft Palate J 1988; 25: 16–20.

142. JONES ML. Orthodontic treatment in Ehlers-Danlos syndrome. Br J Orthod 1984; 11: 158–62.

143. KÄLLÉN B *et al*. The epidemiology of orofacial clefts. 2. J Craniofac Genet Dev Biol 1996; 16: 242–8.

144. KALLIALA E *et al*. Cleidocranial dysostosis. Oral Surg 1962; 15: 808–22.

145. KEELER C. Taurodont molars and shovel incisors in Klinefelter's syndrome. J Heredity 1973; 64: 234–7.

146. KEITH O *et al*. Orofacial features of Scheie (Hurler-Scheie) syndrome (α-L-iduronidase deficiency). Oral Surg Oral Med Oral Pathol 1990; 70: 70–4.

147. KING NM *et al*. An intranasal tooth in a patient with a cleft lip and palate. J Am Dent Assoc 1987; 114: 475–8.

148. KING NM *et al*. Oral-facial-digital syndrome, Type I. J Clin Pediatr Dent 2002; 26: 211–15.

149. KINIRONS MJ *et al*. Dental findings in mucopolysaccharidosis type IV A (Morquio's disease type A). Oral Surg Oral Med Oral Pathol 1990; 70: 176–9.

150. KIRVESKARI P *et al*. Dental morphology in Turner's syndrome (45,X females). In: KURTÉN B (ed.) Teeth. New York, NY: Columbia University Press, 1982.

151. KLINGBERG G *et al*. Oral manifestations in 22q11 deletion syndrome. Int J Paediatr Dent 2002; 12: 14–23.

152. KOCABALKAN O *et al*. Repeated mandibular lengthening in Treacher Collins syndrome. Int J Oral Maxillofac Surg 1995; 24: 406–8.

153. KOLAR JC *et al*. Patterns of dysmorphology in Crouzon syndrome. Cleft Palate J 1988; 25: 235–44.

154. KRAUS BS *et al*. The dentition in Rothmund's syndrome. J Am Dent Assoc 1970; 81: 894–915.

155. KRAUS BS *et al*. Dental abnormalities in the deciduous and permanent dentitions of individuals with cleft lip and palate. J Dent Res 1966; 45: 1736–46.

156. KREIBORG S *et al*. Cephalometric study of the Apert syndrome in adolescence and adulthood. J Craniofac Genet Dev Biol 1999; 19: 1–11.

157. KREIBORG S *et al*. Anomalies of craniofacial skeleton and teeth in cleidocranial dysplasia. J Craniofac Genet Dev Biol 1999; 19: 75–9.

158. KREIBORG S *et al*. Is craniofacial morphology in Apert and Crouzon syndromes the same? Acta Odontol Scand 1998; 56: 339–41.

159. LANDAU H *et al*. Zahnärztlich-kieferorthopädische Befunde bei Patienten mit Mukopolysaccharidosen. Fortschr Kieferorthop 1988; 49: 132–43.

160. LAINE T *et al*. A study in 47,XYY men of the expression of sex-chromosme anomalies in dental occlusion. Arch Oral Biol 1992; 37: 923–8.

161. LAITINEN SH *et al*. Craniofacial morphology in young adults with the Pierre Robin sequence and isolated cleft palate. Acta Odontol Scand 1997; 55: 223–8.

162. LANIER PA *et al*. Epidermolysis bullosa – dental management and anesthetic considerations. Pediatr Dent 1990; 12: 246–9.

163. LAPEER GL *et al*. Hypodontia, impacted permanent teeth, spinal defects, and cardiomegaly in a previously diagnosed case of the Yunis–Varon syndrome. Oral Surg Oral Med Oral Pathol 1992; 73: 456–60.

164. LEE CS *et al*. Ectodermal dysplasia: Christ–Siemens–Touraine syndrome in a female patient. Gen Dent 1990; 38: 292–5.

165. LIDRAL AC *et al*. Studies of the candidate genes TGFB2, MSX1, TGFA, and TGFB3 in the etiology of cleft lip and palate in the Philippines. Cleft Palate Craniofac J 1997; 34: 1–6.

166. LIU H-H *et al*. Epidermolysis bullosa simplex. ASDC J Dent Child 1998; 65: 349–53.

167. LUKINMAA P-L *et al*. Dental findings in osteogenesis imperfecta: II. J Craniofac Genet Dev Biol 1987; 7: 127–35.

168. LUKINMAA P-L *et al*. Microanatomy of the dental enamel in autoimmune polyendocrinopathy-candidiasis-ectodermal dystrophy (APECED). J Craniofac Genet Dev Biol 1996; 16: 174–81.

169. LYGIDAKIS NA *et al*. Oral fibromatosis in tuberous sclerosis. Oral Surg Oral Med Oral Pathol 1989; 68: 725–8.

170. MACCAULEY FJ. Incontinentia pigmenti (Bloch–Sulzberger syndrome). Br Dent J 1968; 125: 169–72.

171. MACEY LV *et al.* Inontinentia pigmentii. Int J Paediatr Dent 1999; 9: 193–7.

172. MaCFARLANE JD *et al.* Dental aspects of hypophosphatasia. Oral Surg Oral Med Oral Pathol 1989; 67: 521–6.

173. MACKLER SB *et al.* Tuberous sclerosis with gingival lesions. Oral Surg 1972; 34: 619–24.

174. MALERMAN AJ *et al.* Hallermann–Streiff syndrome. ASDC J Dent Child 1986; 53: 287–92.

175. MARKOVIC M. The role of the orthodontist in the treatment of adolescents with orofacial clefts. Int Dent J 1986; 36: 131–9.

176. MASSLER M, SAVARA BS. Natal and neonatal teeth. A review of twenty–four cases reported in the literature. J Pediatr 1950; 36: 349–59.

177. MAYHALL JT *et al.* Dental morphology of 45,X0 human females: molar cusp area, volume, shape and linear measurements. Arch Oral Biol 1992; 37: 1039–43.

178. McCORMICK J *et al.* Hypophosphatasia. J Am Dent Assoc 1968; 77: 618–25.

179. McFARLAND PH *et al.* Gardner's syndrome. J Oral Surg 1968; 26: 632–8.

180. McLAUGHLIN WS. Congenital absence of all primary and permanent lateral incisors in a carrier of X-linked hypohidrotic ectodermal dysplasia. Int J Paediatr Dent 1991; 2: 99–103.

181. McNAMARA CM *et al.* Cleidocranial dysplasia: radiological appearances on dental panoramic radiography. Dentomaxillofac Radiol 1999; 28: 89–97.

182. McNAMARA T *et al.* Focal dermal hypoplasia (Goltz-Gorlin) syndrome with taurodontism. Spec Care Dent 1996; 16: 26–8.

183. MÉGARBANÉ H *et al.* Further delineation of the odonto-onycho-dermal dysplasia syndrome. Am J Med Genet 2004; 129: 193–7.

184. MEIJNDERT L *et al.* Epidermolysis bullosa.Ned Tijdschr Tandheelkd 1999; 106: 302–5.

185. MELAMED Y *et al.* Multiple supernumerary teeth (MSNT) and Ehlers–Danlos syndrome (EDS). J Oral Pathol Med 1994; 23: 88–91.

186. MERKX MAW *et al.* Ectodermale dysplasie: een heterogene afwijking. Ned Tijdschr Tandheelkd 1995; 102: 334–6.

187. MESAROS AJJ *et al.* Otodental syndrome. Gen Dent 1996; 44: 427–9.

188. MIDTBØ M *et al.* Skeletal maturity, dental maturity, and eruption in young patients with Turner syndrome. Acta Odontol Scand 1992; 50: 303–12.

189. MIDTBØ M *et al.* Tooth crown size and morphology in Turner syndrome. Acta Odontol Scand 1994; 52: 7–19.

190. MILLER VJ *et al.* Ehlers-Danlos, fibromyalgia and temporomandibular disorder. J Craniomand Pract 1997; 15: 267–9.

191. MODÉER T *et al.* Periodontal disease in children with Down's syndrome. Scand J Dent Res 1990; 98: 228–34.

192. MOLLER KT *et al.* Oligodontia, taurodontia and sparse hair growth – a syndrome. J Speech Hear Dis 1973; 38: 268–271.

193. MONREAL AW *et al.* Mutations in the human homologue of mouse *dl* cause autosomal recessive and dominant hypohidrotic ectodermal dysplasia. Nat Genet 1999; 22: 366–9.

194. MOORE RS *et al.* A classification of medically handicapping conditions and the health risks they present in the dental care of children. Part II – neoplastic, renal, endocrine, metabolic, hepatic, musculo-skeletal, central-nervous-system and skin disorders. J Paediatr Dent 1990; 6: 1–14.

195. MORISAKI I *et al.* Localized dentin dysplasia of primary teeth in children with Williams syndrome. Pediatr Dent J 1997; 7: 55–9.

196. MORTIER K *et al.* Ectodermale dysplasie syndromen. Ned Tijdschr Tandheelkd 2003; 110: 190–2.

197. MOTOYAMA LCJ *et al.* Natal teeth in cleft lip and palate patients. Braz Dent J 1996; 7: 115–19.

198. MUELLER-LESSMANN V *et al.* Orofacial findings in the Klippel–Trènaunay syndrome. Int J Paediatr Dent 2001; 11: 225–9.

199. MÜSSIG D *et al.* Milchzahndurchbruch bei unterschiedlichen Formen des Down-Syndroms und kongenitalen Herzfehlern. Dtsch Zahnärztl Z 1990; 45: 157–9.

200. MUTO T *et al.* Pycnodysostosis. Oral Surg Oral Med Oral Pathol 1991; 72: 449–55.

201. MYLLÄRNIEMI S *et al.* Oral findings in the autoimmune polyendocrinopathhy-candidosis syndrome (APECS) and other forms of hypoparathyroidism. Oral Surg 1978; 45: 721–9.

202. MYLNARCZYK G. Enamel pitting: a common symptom of tuberous sclerosis. Oral Surg Oral Med Oral Pathol 1991; 71: 63–7.

203. NICCOLI-FILHO DA *et al.* Incontinentia pigmenti (Bloch-Sulzberger syndrome). J Clin Pediatr Dent 1993; 17: 251–3.

204. NORTON LA. Orthodontic tooth movement response in Ehlers–Danlos syndrome. J Am Dent Assoc 1984; 109: 259–62.

205. NYSTRÖM M *et al.* Dental age and asymmetry in the formation of mandibular teeth in twins concordant or discordant for oral clefts. Scand J Dent Res 1988; 96: 393–8.

206. O'DONNELL D. Dental management problems related to self-image in Crouzon's syndrome. Aust Dent J 1985; 30: 355–7.

207. O'DONNELL D *et al.* Bilateral, asymmetrical, complete oro-ocular facial clefts and supernumerary teeth in a young Chinese female. ASDC J Dent Child 1985; 52: 191–4.

208. O'DONNELL D *et al.* Management problems associated with Cornelia de Lange syndrome. Spec Care Dent 1985; 5: 160–3.

209. OHISHI M *et al.* Hallermann–Streiff syndrome and its oral implications. ASDC J Dent Child 1986; 53: 32–7.

210. OLSEN CB *et al.* Recessive dystrophic epidermolysis bullosa. Aust Dent J 1997; 42: 1–7.

211. ONLINE MENDELIAN INHERITANCE IN MAN (OMIM™). McKusick-Nathans Institute for Genetic Medicine, John Hopkins University (Baltimore, MD) and National Center for Biotechnology Information, National Library of Medicine (Bethesda, MD), 2000. Available at: www.ncbi.nlm.nih.gov/omim/.

212. ORELAND A *et al.* Malocclusions in physically and/or mentally handicapped children. Swed Dent J 1987; 11: 103–19.

213. ORNER G. Posteruptive tooth age in children with Down's syndrome and their sibs. J Dent Res 1975; 54:581–7.

214. OUELLET B *et al.* La dysplasie ectodermique: expressions multiples d'une maladie héréditaire. J Can Dent Assoc 1997; 63: 377–81.

215. PETERKA M *et al.* Tooth size in children with cleft lip and palate. Cleft Palate J 1983; 20: 307–13.

216. PINHEIRO M *et al.* Ectodermal dysplasias: a clinical classification and a causal review. Am J Med Genet 1994; 53: 153–62.

217. PINHEIRO M *et al.* A previously undescribed condition: tricho-odonto-onycho-dermal syndrome. A review of the tricho-odonto-onychial subgroup of ectodermal dysplasias. Br J Dermatol 1981; 105: 371–82.

218. PIRTTINIEMI P *et al.* Asymmetry in the occlusal morphology of first permanent molars in 45,X/46,XX mosaics. Arch Oral Biol 1998; 43: 25–32.

219. POLAND C III *et al.* Histochemical observations of hypophosphatasia. J Dent Res 1972; 51 (suppl 2): 333–8.

220. POYTON HG *et al.* Thalassemia. Changes visible in radiographs used in dentistry. Oral Surg 1968; 25: 564–76.

221. PRABHU NT *et al.* Branchio-oto-renal syndrome with generalized microdontia. Oral Surg Oral Med Oral Pathol Oral Radiol Endod 1999; 87: 180–3.

222. PRAHL-ANDERSEN B *et al.* Characteristics of permanent teeth in persons with Trisomy G. J Dent Res 1976; 55: 633–8.

223. RAJIC Z *et al.* Taurodontism in Down's syndrome. Coll Antropol 1998; 22 (suppl): 63–7.

224. RANTA R. Comparison of tooth formation in noncleft and cleft-affected children with and without hypodontia. ASDC J Dent Child 1982; 49: 197–9.

225. RANTA R. Incomplete median cleft of lower lip associated with cleft palate, the Pierre Robin anomaly or hypodontia. Int J Oral Surg 1984; 13: 555–8.

226. RANTA R. Associations of some variables to tooth formation in children with isolated cleft palate. Scand J Dent Res 1984; 92: 496–502.

227. RANTA R. Hereditary agenesis of ten maxillary posterior teeth: a family history. ASDC J Dent Child 1985; 52: 125–7.

228. RANTA R. A review of tooth formation in children with cleft lip/palate. Am J Orthod Dentofac Orthop 1986; 90: 11–18.

229. RANTA R. Numeric anomalies of teeth in concomitant hypodontia and hyperodontia. J Craniofac Genet 1988; 8: 245–51.

230. RANTA R, TULENSALO T. Symmetry and combinations of hypodontia in non-cleft and cleft palate children. Scand J Dent Res 1988; 96: 1–8.

231. RANTA R *et al.* Tooth anomalies associated with congenital sinuses of the lower lip and cleft lip/palate. Angle Orthod 1982; 52: 212–21.

232. RATEITSCHAK KH *et al.* Parodontologie (1). Langdon Down-Syndrom: Mongolismus – Trisomie 21. Schweiz Monatsschr Zahnmed 1987; 97: 1145–8.

233. REISNER RM *et al.* Oral changes in incontinentia pigmenti. J Am Dent Assoc 1968; 76: 795–7.

234. REULAND BOSMA W. Parodontale aandoeningen bij het syndroom van Down. Ned Tijdschr Tandheelkd 1990; 97: 468–71.

235. RICHTSMEIER JT *et al.* Analysis of craniofacial growth in Crouzon syndrome using landmark data. J Craniofac Genet Dev Biol 1990; 10: 39–62.

236. RITSERT EF *et al.* Supernumerary teeth associated with cleft lip. J Am Dent Assoc 1959; 59: 552–3.

237. ROBERT E *et al.* The epidemiology of orofacial clefts. 1. J Craniofac Genet Dev Biol 1996; 16: 234–41.

238. RØLLING I *et al.* Dental findings in three siblings with Morquio's syndrome. Int J Paediatr Dent 1999; 9: 219–24.

239. RUBIN MM *et al.* Tuberous sclerosis complex and a calcifying epithelial odontogenic tumor of the mandible. Oral Surg Oral Med Oral Pathol 1987; 64: 207–11.

240. RUPRECHT A *et al.* Incidence of oligodontia (hypodontia). J Oral Med 1986; 41: 43–6.

241. RUPRECHT A *et al.* Ectodermal dysplasia associated with cleft palate and lobster claw deformity of hands and feet. J Can Dent Assoc 1986; 52: 147–50.

242. RUSSELL DL *et al.* Incontinentia pigmenti (Bloch–Sulzberger syndrome). ASDC J Dent Child 1967; 34: 494–500.

243. SALAKO NO *et al.* Oral findings in a child with Prader–Labhart–Willi syndrome. Quint Int 1995; 26: 339–41.

244. SALINAS CF. Orodental findings and genetic disorders. Birth Defects Orid Artic Ser 1982; 18: 79–120.

245. SALINAS CF. In: SALINAS CF *et al.* (eds) Dentistry in the interdisciplinary treatment of genetic diseases. New York, NY: AR Liss, 1980.

246. SARVAN I *et al.* Hypohidrotic ectodermal dysplasia. SADJ 2000; 55: 34–7.

247. SAUK JJ *et al.* An electron optic analysis and explanation for the etiology of dentinal dysplasia. Oral Surg 1972; 33: 763–71.

248. SCHNEIDER PE. Dental findings in a child with Cockayne's syndrome. ASDC J Dent Child 1983; 50: 58–64.

249. SCHUDY FF. Treatment of Crouson's and Apert's syndromes. J Clin Orthod 1986; 20: 114–17.

250. SCHULLER MG *et al.* Oculodentodigital dysplasia. Oral Surg 1986; 61: 418–21.

251. SCULLY C. Down's syndrome. J Dent 1976; 4: 167–74.

252. SEDANO HO *et al.* Epidermolysis bullosa. Oral Surg Oral Med Oral Pathol 1989; 67: 555–63.

253. SEDANO HO *et al.* Otodental syndrome. Oral Surg Oral Med Oeal Pathol Oral Radiol Endod 2001; 92: 312–17.

254. SEDANO HO *et al.* Oral manifestations of inherited disorders. Woburn: Butterworth (Publishers) Inc., 1977.

255. SEOW WK *et al.* Morphometric analysis of the primary and permanent dentitions in hemifacial microsomia: a controlled study. J Dent Res 1998; 77: 27–38.

256. SHAIKH R *et al.* Delayed dental maturation in cleidocranial dysplasia. ASDC J Dent Child 1998; 65: 325–9.

257. SHAPIRA J *et al.* Prevalence of tooth transposition, third molar agenesis, and maxillary canine impaction in individuals with Down syndrome. Angle Orthod 2000; 70: 290–6.

258. SHAPIRA Y *et al.* Congenitally missing second premolars in cleft lip and palate children. Am J Orthod Dentofac Orthop 1999; 115: 396–400.

259. SHAW M *et al.* Oral facial digital syndrome. Br J Oral Surg 1981; 19: 142–7.

260. SHAW RM. Prosthetic management of hypohidrotic ectodermal dysplasia with anodontia. Aust Dent J 1990; 35: 113–16.

261. SILVA LCP *et al.* Clinical evaluation of patients with epidermolysis bullosa. Spec Care Dent 2004; 24: 22–7.

262. SINGER SL *et al.* Dentofacial features of a family with Crouzon syndrome. Aust Dent J 1997; 42: 11–17.

263. SIQUEIRA WL *et al.* Electrolyte concentrations in saliva of children ages 6–10 years with Down syndrome. Oral Surg Oral Med Oral Pathol Oral Radiol Endod 2004; 98: 76–9.

264. SLAVKIN HC. Entering the era of molecular dentistry. J Am Dent Assoc 1999; 130: 413–17.

265. SLOOTWEG PJ *et al.* Dento-alveolar abnormalities in oculomandibulodyscephaly (Hallermann–Streiff syndrome). J Oral Pathol 1984; 13: 147–54.

266. SMITH KS *et al.* Mucopolysaccharidosis: MPS VI and associated delayed tooth eruption. Int J Oral Maxillofac Surg 1995; 24: 176–80.

267. SMITH NHH. A histologic study of cementum in a case of cleidocranial dysostosis. Oral Surg 1968; 25: 470–8.

268. SOFAER JA. Single genetic disorders. In: JONES JH *et al.* (eds) Oral manifestations of inherited disorders. London: WB Saunders, 1980.

269. SØNDERGAARD JO *et al.* Dental anomalies in familial adenomatous polyposis coli. Acta Odontol Scand 1987; 45: 61–3.

270. SOUREN JPHJA *et al.* Gebitsontwikkeling bij kinderen met schisis. Ned Tijdschr Tandheelkd 1994; 101: 104–6.

271. SPITZER R. Observations on congenital dentofacial disorders in Mongolism and microcephaly. Oral Surg 1967; 24: 325–32.

272. STELLZIG A *et al.* Non-surgical treatment of upper airway obstructions in oculoauriculovertebral dysplasia. Eur J Orthod 1998; 20: 111–14.

273. STENVIK A *et al.* Taurodontism and concomitant hypodontia in siblings. Oral Surg 1972; 33: 841–5.

274. STEWART RE. Taurodontism in X_chromosome aneuploid syndromes. Clin Genet 1974; 6: 341–4.

275. STEWART RE. Craniofacial anomalies. In: STEWART RE *et al.* (eds) Pediatric dentistry. St. Louis, MO: CV Mosby, 1982.

276. STEWART RE. In: SALINAS CF *et al.* (eds) Dentistry in the interdisciplinary treatment of genetic diseases. New York, NY: AR Liss, 1980.

277. STEWART RE *et al.* Unusual dental findings in a patient with a rare bone dysplasia (dyschondrosteosis) and a chromosomal anomaly. Oral Surg 1971; 32: 596–604.

278. SURI L *et al.* Delayed tooth eruption: pathogenesis, diagnosis, and treatment. Am J Orthod Dentofac Orthop 2004; 126: 432–45.

279. TAN H *et al.* Het hypohydrotische type van de ectodermale dysplasie. Ned Tijdschr Tandheelkd 1976; 83: 213–16.

280. TEREZHALMY GT *et al.* Ectodermal dysplasia. Quint Int 2003; 34: 482–3.

281. THOMAS S *et al.* Hurler syndrome. J Clin Pediatr Dent 2000; 24: 335–8.

282. TILLMAN HH *et al.* Tuberous sclerosis. Oral Surg Oral Med Oral Pathol 1991; 71: 301–2.

283. TOWNSEND GC. Fluctuating dental asymmetry in Down's syndrome. Aust Dent J 1983; 28: 39–44.

284. TOWNSEND GC. Tooth size in children and young adults with trisomy 21 (Down) syndrome. Arch Oral Biol 1983; 28: 159–66.

285. TOWNSEND G *et al.* Tooth size in 47,XYY males: evidence for a direct effect of the Y chromosome on growth. Aust Dent J 1985; 30: 268–72.

286. TOWNSEND G *et al.* Reduced tooth size in 45,X (Turner syndrome) females. Am J Phys Athropol 1984; 65: 367–71.

287. TSUTSUMI T *et al.* Labial talon cusp in a child with incontinentia pigmenti achromians. Pediatr Dent 1991; 13: 236–7.

288. ULUSU T *et al.* The relation of ectodermal dysplasia and hypodontia. J Clin Pediatr Dent 1990; 15: 46–50.

289. URELES SD *et al.* Focal dermal hypoplasia syndrome (Goltz syndrome). Pediatr Dent 1986; 8: 239–44.

290. VAN DEN AKKER AMEA *et al.* Schisis in Nederland. Ned Tijdschr Tandheelkd 1987; 94: 520–5.

291. VAN DE ENDE JJ *et al.* Schisis: denk aan bijkomende afwijkingen. Ned Tijdschr Tandheelkd 1997; 104: 81–2.

292. VAN DER WAL KGH. Gnathoschisis en de laterale incisief. Ned Tijdschr Tandheelkd 1993; 100: 442–4.

293. VAN DOORNE L *et al.* Otodental syndrome. Int J Oral Maxillofac Surg 1998; 27: 121–4.

294. VAN MERKESTEYN JPR *et al.* Osteomyelitis of the jaws in pycnodysostosis. Int J Oral Maxillofac Surg 1987; 16: 615–19.

295. VARRELA J *et al.* Taurodontism in 47,XXY males. J Dent Res 1988; 67: 501–2.

296. VICHI M *et al.* Abnormalities of the maxillary incisors in children with cleft lip and palate. ASDC J Dent Child 1995; 62: 412–17.

297. VIEIRA AR *et al.* Maternal age and oral clefts. Oral Surg Oral Med Oral Pathol Oral Radiol Endod 2002; 94: 530–5.

298. VISSER A *et al.* Het Sanfilipo-syndroom. Ned Tijdschr Tandheelkd 1998; 105: 324–5.

299. VISSINK A *et al.* Het foetaal alcoholsyndroom. Ned Tijdschr Tandheelkd 2000; 107: 97–9.

300. VOGT J *et al.* Incontinentia pigmenti (Bloch-Sulzberger syndrome). Oral Surg Oral Med Oral Pathol 1991; 71: 454–6.

301. VON WOWERN N. Cherubism. Oral Surg Oral Med Oral Pathol Oral Radiol Endod 2000; 90: 765–72.

302. WALLERSTEIN R *et al.* Partial trisomy 11q in a female infant with Robin sequence and congenital heart disease. Cleft Palate Craniofac J 1992; 29: 77–8.

303. WALLS AWG *et al.* Dental manifestations of autoimmune hypoparathyroidism. Oral Surg Oral Med Oral Pathol 1993; 75: 452–4.

304. WANG RR *et al.* Hemifacial microsomia and treatment options for auricular replacement. J Prosthet Dent 1999; 82: 197–204.

305. WELBURY RR *et al.* Goldenhar's syndrome and hypodontia. ASDC J Dent Child 1987; 54: 62–4.

306. WESTLING L *et al.* Craniofacial manifestations in the Marfan syndrome. J Craniofac Genet Dev Biol 1998; 18: 211–18.

307. WICOMB GM *et al.* Dental implications of tooth-nail dysplasia (Witkop syndrome). J Clin Pediatr Dent 2004; 28: 107–12.

308. WINTER GB. Hereditary and idiopathic anomalies of tooth number, structure and form. Dent Clin North Am 1969; 13 (2): 355–73.

309. WINTER GB *et al.* Enamel hypoplasia and anomalies of the enamel. Dent Clin North Am 1975; 19 (1): 3–24.

310. WINTER GB. The association of ocular defects with the otodental syndrome. J Int Assoc Dent Child 1983; 14: 83–7.

311. WINTHER JE *et al.* Cleidocranial dysostosis. Dent Pract 1972; 22: 215–19.

312. WITKOP CJ *et al.* Hypoplastic enamel, onycholysis, and hypohidrosis inherited as an autosomal dominant trait. Oral Surg 1975; 39: 71–86.

313. WRIGHT JT *et al.* Epidermolysis bullosa. Associated with enamel hypoplasia and taurodontism. J Oral Pathol 1983; 12: 73–83.

314. WRIGHT JT *et al.* Developmental defects of enamel in humans with hereditary epidermolysis bullosa. Arch Oral Biol 1993; 38: 945–55.

315. YOKOZEKI M *et al.* A case of Japanese cleidocranial dysplasia with a CBFA1 frameshift mutation. J Craniofac Genet Dev Biol 2000; 20: 121–6.

316. ZACH GA. Oculodento-osseous dysplasia syndrome. Oral Surg 1975; 40: 122–5.

317. ZACHARIADES N. Gardner's syndrome. J Oral Maxillofac Surg 1987; 45: 438–40.

318. ZACHARIADES N *et al.* Cherubism. Int J Oral Surg 1985; 14: 138–45.

319. ZILBERMAN U *et al.* The effects of hereditary disorders on tooth components: a radiographic morphometric study of two syndromes. Arch Oral Biol 2004; 49: 621–9.

320. ZLOTOGORA J *et al.* Microtia in infantys with chromosomal trisomy. J Craniofac Genet Dev Biol 1988; 8: 205–6.

321. ZSCHIESCHE S *et al.* Möglichkeiten der interdisziplinären Versorgung von Kindern mit Ektodermaldysplasie. Fortschr Kieferorthop 1989; 50: 207–12.

322. LETRA A *et al.* Intraoral features of Apert's syndrome. Oral Syrg Oral Med Oral Pathol Oral Radiol Endod 2007; 103: e38–41.

323. HOHOFF A *et al.* The spectrum of Apert syndrome: phenotype, particularities in orthodontic treatment, and characteristics of orthognathic surgery. Head Face Med 2007; 3: 10–34.

324. TANAKA JLO *et al.* Cleidocranial dysplasia: importance of radiographic images in diagnosis of the condition. J Oral Sci 2006; 48: 161–6.

325. SUDA N *et al.* Diversity of supernumerary tooth formation in siblings with cleidocranial dysplasia having identical mutation in RUNX2: possible involvement of non-genetic or epigenetic regulation. Orthod Craniofac Res 2007; 10: 222–5.

326. CARBÓ G *et al.* Cornelia de Lange syndrome. Med Oral Patol Oral Cir Bucal 2007; 12: E445–8.

327. PRÄGER TM *et al.* Dental findings in patients with ectodermal dysplasia. J Orofac Orthop 2006; 67: 347–55.

328. GREGORIOU S *et al.* Should we consider hypohidrotic ectodermal dysplasia as a possible risk factor for malignant melanoma? J Cutan Med Surg 2007; 11: 188–90.

329. BARBERÍA E *et al.* Multiple agenesis and anhydrotic ectodermal dysplasia. Eur J Paediatr Dent 2006; 7: 113–21.

330. BADAUY CM *et al.* Ehlers–Danlos syndrome (EDS) type IV. Clin Oral Investig 2007; (online): 1–10.

331. DE COSTER PJ *et al.* Abnormal dentine structure in two novel gene mutations [COL1A1, Arg134Cys] and [ADAMTS2, Trp795-to-ter] causing rare type I collagen disorders. Arch Oral Biol 2007; 52: 101–9.

332. KLEINE-HAKAL M *et al.* Effect of mandibular distraction osteogenesis on developing molars. Orthod Craniofac Res 2007: 10; 196–202.

333. SHIGA M *et al.* Characteristic phenotype of immortalized periodontal cells isolated from Marfan type I patient. Cell Tissue Res 2008; 331: 461–72.

334. GARCIA DE PAULA E SILVA FW. Solitary median maxillary central incisor in association with Goldenhar's syndrome. Spec Care Dent 2007; 27: 105–7.

335. MADANI M *et al.* Gardner's syndrome presenting with dental complaints. Arch Iran Med 2007; 10: 535–9.

336. SCARDINA GA *et al.* Oral diseases in a patient affected with Prader–Willi syndrome. Eur J Paediatr Dent 2007; 8: 96–9.

337. DEVADAS S *et al.* Witkop tooth and nail syndrome. Int J Paediatr Dent 2005; 15: 364–9.

338. AKYUZ S *et al.* Tooth and nail syndrome: genetic, clinical and dermatoglyphic findings. J Clin Pediatr Dent 1993; 17: 105–8.

339. DE LA LUZ ARENAS SORDO M *et al.* Cockayne's syndrome. Med Oral Patol Cir Bucal 2006; 11: E236–8.

340. KURIAN K *et al.* Chondroectodermal dysplasia (Ellis van Creveld syndrome). Indian J Dent Res 2007; 18: 31–4.

341. BAUJAT G *et al.* Ellis-Van Creveld sundrome. Orphanet J Rare Dis 2007; 2: 27–14.

342. MORNET E. Hypophosphatasia. Orpahnet J Rare Dis (online) 2007; 2: 40–51.

343. GUVEN G *et al.* Mucopolysaccharidosis type I (Hurker syndrome). Oral Surg Oral Med Oral Pathol Oral Radiol Endod 2008; 105: 72–8.

344. FREITAS DQ *et al.* Bilateral dentigerous cysts. Dentomaxillofac Radiol 2006; 35: 464–8.

345. ALPÖZ AR *et al.* The oral manifestations of Maroteaux-Lamy syndrome (mucopolysacchariddosis VI). Oral Surg Oral Med Oral Pathol Oral Radiol Endod 2006; 101: 632–7.

346. ÖNCAG G *et al.* Multidisciplinary treatment approach of Morquio syndrome (mucopolysaccharidosis type IVA). Angle Orthod 2006; 76: 335–40.

347. SA RORIS FONTELES C *et al.* Cephalometric characteristics and dentofacial abnormalities of pycnodysostosis. Oral Surg Oral Med Oral Pathol Oral Radiol Endod 2007; 104: e83–0.

348. FLEMING KW *et al.* Dental and facial bone abnormalities in pyknodysostosis. Am J Neuroradiol 2007; 28: 132–4.

349. EHRENREICH M *et al*. Incontinentia pigmenti (Bloch–Sulzerbeerger syndrome): systemic disorder. Cutis 2007; 79: 355–62.

350. ARDELEAN D *et al*. Incontinentia pigmenti in boys. Pediatr Dermatol 2006; 23: 523–7.

351. WU HP *et al*. Dental anomalies in two patients with incontinentia pigmenti. J Formos Med Assoc 2005; 104: 427.

352. MORAES ME *et al*. Dental anomalies in patients with Down syndrome. Braz Dent J 2007; 18: 346–50.

353. ZIGMOND M *et al*. The outcome of a preventive dental care programme on the prevalence of localized aggressive periodontitis in Down's syndrome individuals. J Intellect Disabil Res 2006; 50: 492–500.

354. FAGGELLA A *et al*. Dental features in patients with Turner syndrome. Eur J Paediatr Dent 2006; 7: 165–8.

355. DE LANGE J *et al*. Central giant cell granuloma of the jaw. Oral Surg Oral Med Oral Pathol Oral Radiol Endod 2007; 104: 603–15.

356. LEXNER MO *et al*. Anomalies of tooth formation in hypohidrotic ectodermal dysplasia. Int J Paediatr Dent 2007; 17: 10–18.

357. BLOCH-ZUPAN A *et al*. Otodental syndrome. Orphanet J Rare Dis 2006; 1: 5–10.

358. FONSECA LC *et al*. Radiographic assessment of Gardner's syndrome. Dentomaxillofac Radiol 2007; 36: 121–4.

359. BAILLEUL-FORESTIER I *et al*. The oro-dental phenotype in Prader–Willi syndrome. Int J Paediatr Dent 2008; 18: 40–7.

360. YAKUT T *et al*. PISH investigation of 22q11.2 deletion in patients with immunodeficiency and/or cardiac abnormalities. Pediatr Surg Int 2006; 22: 380–3.

361. ARENAS-SORDO Mde L *et al*. Cockayne's syndrome. Med Oral Patol Oral Cir Bucal 2006; 11: E236–8.

362. KUSIAK A *et al*. Root morphology of mandibular premolars in 40 patients with Turner syndrome. Int Endod J 2005; 38: 822–6.

363. YAVUZ I *et al*. Ectodermal dysplasia. Arch Med Res 2006; 37: 403–9.

364. LÄHDESMÄKI R *et al*. Root lengths in the permanent teeth of Klinefelter (47,XXY) men. Arch Oral Biol 2007; 52: 822–7.

Appendix
Chronology of Dental Development

The age at which the calcification of the teeth starts and at which the calcification of the crowns are completed as given in Table A.1 are based upon the work of Logan & Kronfeld (1893). The data are meant as a general guide.

The reader should note that the association between skeletal and dental age is low (Chapter 4) and there are considerable group differences in eruption times.

Table A.1 Chronology of dental development

Tooth	Initiation of the tooth germ	Calcification of the crown		Root completed
		Start of calcification	Enamel formation complete	
Deciduous maxillary teeth				
Central incisor	7 weeks *in utero*	3–4 months *in utero*	1–4 months	1.5–2 years
Lateral incisor	7 weeks *in utero*	4.5 months *in utero*	2–5 months	1.5–2 years
Canine	7.5 weeks *in utero*	5.5 months *in utero*	9 months	2.5–3.3 years
First molar	8 weeks *in utero*	5 months *in utero*	6 months	2–2.5 years
Second molar	10 weeks *in utero*	6 months *in utero*	10–12 months	3 years
Deciduous mandibular teeth				
Central incisor	7 weeks *in utero*	4.5 months *in utero*	4 months	1.5–2 years
Lateral incisor	7 weeks *in utero*	4.5 months *in utero*	4.5 months	1.5–2 years
Canine	7.5 weeks *in utero*	5 months *in utero*	9 months	2.5–3.3 years
First molar	8 weeks *in utero*	5 months *in utero*	6 months	2–2.5 years
Second molar	10 weeks *in utero*	6 months *in utero*	10–12 months	3 years
Permanent maxillary teeth				
Central incisor	5–51/4 months *in utero*	3–4 months after birth	4–5 years	10 years
Lateral incisor	5–5.3 months *in utero*	10 months after birth	4–5 years	11 years
Canine	5.5–6 months *in utero*	4–5 months after birth	6–7 years	13–15 years
First premolar	Birth	1.5 years	5–6 years	12–13 years
Second premolar	7.5–8 months	2 years	6–7 years	12–14 years
First molar	3.5–4 months *in utero*	0 years	2–3 years	9–10 years
Second molar	8.5–9 months	2.5 years	7–8 years	14–16 years
Third molar	3.5–4 years	7–9 years	12–16 years	18–25 years
Permanent mandibular teeth				
Central incisor	5–5.3 months *in utero*	3–4 months after birth	4–5 years	9 years
Lateral incisor	5–5.3 months *in utero*	3–4 months after birth	4–5 years	10 years
Canine	5.5–6 months *in utero*	4–5 months after birth	6–7 years	12–14 years
First premolar	Birth	1–2 years	5–6 years	12–13 years
Second premolar	7.5–8 months	2–2.5 years	6–7 years	13–14 years
First molar	3.5–4 months *in utero*	0 years	2.5–3 years	9–10 years
Second molar	8.5–9 months	2–3 years	7–8 years	14–15 years
Third molar	3.5–4 years	8–10 years	12–16 years	18–25 years

Pathology of the Hard Dental Tissues, First Edition. Albert Schuurs.
© 2013 Albert Schuurs. Published 2013 by Blackwell Publishing Ltd.

Index

Note: page numbers in *italic* refer to tables and figures.

Aarskog(–Scott) syndrome 290
abfraction 194
  cervical 215–16
ABO incompatibility, maternal–fetal 57,
  238
abrasion
  defined 194
  discoloured teeth *see* micro-
    abrasive(-erosive) technique
abrasives
  prophylactic pastes *208*, 208–9
  in toothpastes 205–7
abscesses
  dentine dysplasia 88
  dentinogenesis imperfecta 93
  Turner teeth after 78
  vitamin D-resistant rickets 65
abuse, physical 210–11
accessory roots 47
achondroplasia 271
acid erosion 157–60, 164
acids
  bacterial production 126, 127
  caries formation 127–8, 129
  dietary 158
  erosive effects 156, 157–64
  titrability 159
acidulated phosphorous fluoride (APF)
  168
acrocephalosyndactyly type I 271
acrofacial dysostosis 280–2, *282*
acromegaly 193
Actinomyces sp. 124, *125*, 125–6, 246
additional roots 46, 46–7
adrenal gland disorders 67
age
  chronological, estimation 101–2, 192
  dental 101–2
  replanted/transplanted teeth 184–5
  skeletal 101–2

tooth development stages by *431*
tooth wear and 196–7
ageing 191–4, 242
  see also elderly people
agenesis, dental 3–11
  definitions 3
  hyperdontia with 11–12
  isolated 3–9
    aetiology 5–7
    consequences 8
    epidemiology 3–5
    prevention and treatment 8–9
AIH1 gene mutations 81
Albright's disease 67
alcohol abuse 162, 269
allele ix
aluminium oxide 206, *208*
amalgam restorations
  cracks/fractures in teeth with 212,
    215
  discolouring surrounding tooth 243,
    248
  effects of bleaching 263
  erosion 166
  longevity 154
  side effects 154
ameloblastic fibro-dentinoma 11
ameloblastic fibroma 11
ameloblastic fibro-odontoma 11, 106
ameloblastin gene 81
ameloblasts 50, *51*
  fluoride sensitivity 73
amelogenesis imperfecta, hereditary 52,
  79–86
  anterior open bite and deep overbite
    85, *85*
  classification *80*, 80–1
  dentinogenesis imperfecta with 89
  eruption delays 107
  genetics 81

hypocalcified (type III) 80, 84, 85
hypomaturative (type II) 80, 83–4, *84*,
  85
hypomaturative-hypoplastic with
  taurodontism (type IV) 80, 84–5
hypoplastic (type I) 80, 82, 82–3, *83*,
  85
microdontia 37
pathogenesis 85
prevalence 81, *81*
tooth discoloration 236, *237*
tooth wear 197
treatment 85–6, *86*
amelogenins 50, 53, 81
AMELX gene mutations 81
angiomas, macrodontia with 36
angio-osteo-hypertrophy (Klippel-
  Trénaunay) syndrome 103, 280
ankyloglossia, cleft palate with 273
ankylosis
  deciduous molars 79
  delayed eruption 106
  external replacement resorption 180,
    182
  infra-occlusion 111–12
  replanted teeth 184, 189, 230–1
anodontia 3, 10–11
anorexia nervosa 162, 162–3, 164–5
antacids 168
anterior open bite, amelogenesis
  imperfecta 85, *85*
anterior teeth
  crown-root fractures 220–1
  talon *42*, 42–3
  see also canines; incisors
antibiotics
  tooth discoloration 244
  transplantation/replantation 184, 231
  see also tetracyclines
antihypertensive medicines 160